ALLERGY, ASTHMA, AND IMMUNOLOGY FROM INFANCY TO ADULTHOOD

THIRD EDITION

ALLERGY, ASTHMA, AND IMMUNOLOGY FROM INFANCY TO ADULTHOOD

C. WARREN BIERMAN, M.D.
Seattle, Washington

DAVID S. PEARLMAN, M.D.
Denver, Colorado

GAIL G. SHAPIRO, M.D.
Seattle, Washington

WILLIAM W. BUSSE, M.D.
Madison, Wisconsin

W.B. SAUNDERS COMPANY
A Division of Harcourt Brace & Company
Philadelphia • London • Toronto • Montreal • Sydney • Tokyo

W.B. SAUNDERS COMPANY
A Division of
Harcourt Brace & Company

The Curtis Center
Independence Square West
Philadelphia, Pennsylvania 19106

Library of Congress Cataloging-in-Publication Data

Allergy, Asthma, and Immunology from Infancy to Adulthood / [edited by]
C. Warren Bierman . . . [et al.].—3rd ed.

    p.   cm.

Rev. ed. of: Allergic diseases from infancy to adulthood / [edited by] C. Warren Bierman, David S. Pearlman. 2nd ed. 1988.

Includes bibliographical references and index.

ISBN 0-7216-5587-4

1. Allergy.   I. Bierman, C. Warren (Charles Warren).   II. Allergic diseases from infancy to adulthood.
[DNLM: 1. Hypersensitivity.   2. Asthma.   3. Immune System—physiology. WD 300 A4336 1996]
RC584.A343 1996
616.97—dc20
DNLM/DLC
                                                                                                                               94-37063

ALLERGY, ASTHMA, AND IMMUNOLOGY FROM INFANCY   ISBN 0-7216-5587-4
TO ADULTHOOD

Copyright © 1996, 1988, 1980 by W.B. Saunders Company.

All rights reserved. No part of this publication may be reproduced or transmitted in any form or by any means, electronic or mechanical, including photocopy, recording, or any information storage and retrieval system, without permission in writing from the publisher.

Printed in the United States of America.

Last digit is the print number: 9   8   7   6   5   4   3

*To our families and to our patients,
who made this book possible*

CONTRIBUTORS

ALLEN D. ADINOFF, M.D.
Associate Clinical Professor, Departments of Pediatrics and Medicine, University of Colorado Health Sciences Center, Denver; Colorado Allergy and Asthma Clinic, Aurora, Colorado
Atopic Dermatitis

JOHN L. AELING, M.D.
Professor of Dermatology, University of Colorado Health Sciences Center, Denver, Colorado
Contact Dermatitis

LEONARD C. ALTMAN, M.D.
Clinical Professor of Medicine, Environmental Health and Oral Biology, University of Washington; Chief of Allergy, Harborview Medical Center, Seattle, Washington
Industrial Hygiene Aspects of Preventing Occupational Asthma

JOHN A. ANDERSON, M.D.
Professor of Pediatrics, Case Western Reserve University School of Medicine, Cleveland, Ohio; Head, Division of Allergy and Immunology, Department of Pediatrics, Henry Ford Health System, Detroit, Michigan
Food-Induced Systemic Reactions and Anaphylaxis

JAMES L. BALDWIN, M.D.
Lecturer, Division of Allergy, Department of Internal Medicine, University of Michigan Medical Center, Ann Arbor, Michigan
Drug-Induced Asthma

DAVID I. BERNSTEIN, M.D.
Associate Professor of Medicine, Division of Immunology, University of Cincinnati College of Medicine, Cincinnati, Ohio
Occupational Asthma

I. LEONARD BERNSTEIN, M.D.
Clinical Professor of Medicine, Co-Director, Allergy Research Laboratory, University of Cincinnati College of Medicine; Attending Physician, University Hospital, Deaconess Hospital, and Jewish Hospital, Cincinnati, Ohio
Occupational Asthma

JONATHAN A. BERNSTEIN, M.D.
Assistant Professor of Medicine, University of Cincinnati College of Medicine; Attending Physician, University Hospital, Deaconess Hospital, Jewish Hospital, Cincinnati, Ohio
Occupational Asthma

C. WARREN BIERMAN, M.D.
Clinical Professor of Pediatrics, University of Washington School of Medicine, Division of Allergy, Seattle; Attending Physician, Children's Hospital and Medical Center, Seattle, Washington
Evaluation and Treatment of the Patient with Asthma—Pediatric Asthma

ROBERT K. BUSH, M.D.
Professor of Medicine (CHS), Allergy and Immunology Section, University of Wisconsin; Chief of Allergy Section, William S. Middleton Veterans Administration Hospital, Madison, Wisconsin
Evaluation and Treatment of the Patient with Asthma—Adult Asthma

WILLIAM W. BUSSE, M.D.
Professor of Medicine, Head, Allergy and Immunology, University of Wisconsin Medical School, Madison, Wisconsin
Evaluation and Treatment of the Patient with Asthma—Adult Asthma

DEBORAH ORTEGA CARR, M.D.
Staff Physician, Midwest Allergy, Asthma, and Immunology; Riverside Methodist Hospital, Columbus, Ohio
Evaluation and Treatment of the Patient with Asthma—Adult Asthma

MARGARETHA L. CASSELBRANT, M.D., PH.D.
Associate Professor of Otolaryngology, University of Pittsburgh School of Medicine; Director of Clinical Research and Education, Department of Pediatric Otolaryngology, Children's Hospital of Pittsburgh, Pittsburgh, Pennsylvania
Diseases of the Ear

RICHARD A. F. CLARK, M.D.
Professor and Chairman, SUNY Stony Brook Department of Dermatology, Health Sciences Center, Stony Brook, New York
Atopic Dermatitis

DENISE M. COLEMAN, M.D.
Pediatric Pulmonary Fellow, Department of Pediatrics, University of New Mexico School of Medicine, Albuquerque, New Mexico
Bronchopulmonary Dysplasia

JONATHAN CORREN, M.D.
Assistant Clinical Professor of Medicine, Assistant Director, Allergy Fellowship Program, University of California Los Angeles; Director, Allergy Research Foundation, Los Angeles, California
Sinusitis

WILLIAM K. DOLEN, M.D.
Associate Professor of Pediatrics and Medicine, Medical College of Georgia, Augusta, Georgia
Common Allergenic Pollen and Fungi; Other Allergenic Plants and Animals

PEYTON A. EGGLESTON, M.D.
Professor of Pediatrics, Johns Hopkins University, Baltimore, Maryland
Exercise-Induced Asthma

RICHARD EVANS III, M.D., M.P.H.
Professor of Pediatrics and Medicine, Northwestern University Medical School; Head, Division of Allergy, Children's Memorial Hospital, Chicago, Illinois
Epidemiology of Allergy and Asthma

JORDAN N. FINK, M.D.
Professor of Medicine, Chief, Allergy/Immunology Division, Medical College of Wisconsin; Associate Staff, John L. Doyne Hospital, Children's Hospital of Wisconsin, and Froedtert Lutheran Memorial Hospital, Milwaukee, Wisconsin
Hypersensitivity Pneumonitis

EDWIN B. FISHER, JR., PH.D.
Professor of Psychology and Medicine, Director, Center for Health Behavior Research, Washington University, St. Louis, Missouri
Identification and Management of Psychosocial Factors

DAVID J. FRAENKEL, B.M., B.S., FRACP
Respiratory Physician, Intensive Care Unit, Flinders Medical Centre, Bedford Park, South Australia
Etiology of Asthma: Pathology and Mediators

MITCHELL H. FRIEDLAENDER, M.D.
Division of Ophthalmology, Scripps Clinic and Research Foundation, La Jolla, California
Allergic Disorders of the Eye

NOAH J. FRIEDMAN, M.D.
Assistant Clinical Professor of Pediatrics, University of California, San Diego, La Jolla; Staff Allergist, Kaiser Permanente Medical Center, San Diego, California
Risk Factors and Prevention of Allergy

VINCENT A. FULGINITI, M.D.
Chancellor and Professor of Pediatrics, University of Colorado Health Sciences Center; Chairman, Board of Directors, University Hospital Authority, University Hospital, Denver, Colorado
Adverse Reactions to Vaccines: The Complexity of Vaccine Safety

CLIFTON T. FURUKAWA, M.D.
Clinical Professor of Pediatrics, Chief, Division of Allergy, University of Washington School of Medicine, Seattle, Washington
Allergies in the School

STEPHEN J. GAIONI, PH.D.
Research Assistant Professor of Psychology in Internal Medicine, Center for Health Behavior Research, Washington University School of Medicine, St. Louis, Missouri
Identification and Management of Psychosocial Factors

PETER J. GERGEN, M.D., M.P.H.
Director, Office of Epidemiology and Clinical Trials, Division of Allergy, Immunology, and Trans-

plantation, National Institute of Allergy and Infectious Diseases, National Institutes of Health, Bethesda, Maryland
Epidemiology of Allergy and Asthma

DAVID B. K. GOLDEN, M.D.
Assistant Professor of Medicine, Johns Hopkins University, Baltimore, Maryland
Allergic Reactions to Insect Stings

LESLIE C. GRAMMER, M.D.
Professor of Medicine, Northwestern University School of Medicine; Attending Physician, Northwestern Memorial Hospital, Chicago, Illinois
Surgery in Allergic and Asthmatic Patients

FRANK M. GRAZIANO, M.D., PH.D.
Professor of Medicine, University of Wisconsin Medical School; Chief, Section of Rheumatology, University of Wisconsin Hospital and Clinics, Madison, Wisconsin
Autoimmune Diseases

PAUL A. GREENBERGER, M.D.
Professor of Medicine, Division of Allergy and Immunology, Northwestern University Medical School; Attending Staff, Northwestern Memorial Hospital, Chicago, Illinois
Allergic Bronchopulomonary Aspergillosis

TERRY O. HARVILLE, M.D., PH.D.
Assistant Professor of Pediatrics, Division of Allergy and Immunology, Duke University Medical Center, Durham, North Carolina
Primary and Secondary Immunodeficiency Diseases

KATHRYN F. HOBBS, M.D.
Research Fellow, National Jewish Center for Immunology and Respiratory Medicine, Denver, Colorado
Urticaria and Angioedema

KRISTINA M. HOFFMAN, M.D.
Staff, Allergy and Immunology, David Grant USAF Medical Center, 60th Medical Group, Travis Air Force Base, Fairfield, California
Evaluation and Management of Patients with Adverse Food Reactions

STEPHEN T. HOLGATE, M.D., D.SC., FRCP
MRC Clinical Professor of Immunopharmacology, University of Southampton, Southampton General Hospital, Southampton, United Kingdom
Etiology of Asthma: Pathology and Mediators

RICHARD F. HORAN, M.D.
Assisatnt Clinical Professor of Dermatology, Harvard Medical School; Physician and Consultant in Allergy, Brigham and Women's Hospital; Physician, Section on Allergy, New England Deaconess Hospital, Boston, Massachusetts
Exercise-Induced Anaphylaxis

RICHARD S. IRWIN, M.D.
Professor of Medicine, University of Massachusetts Medical School; Director, Division of Pulmonary, Allergy, and Critical Care Medicine, University of Massachusetts Medical Center, Worcester, Massachusetts
Chronic Cough

CYNTHIA STEICHEN KABALIN, M.D.
Fellow, Northwestern University Medical School, Division of Allergy and Immunology, Chicago, Illinois
Allergic Bronchopulmonary Aspergillosis

ROGER M. KATZ, M.D.
Clinical Professor of Pediatrics, University of California Los Angeles School of Medicine, Los Angeles, California
Headaches

ERIC C. KLEERUP, M.D.
Clinical Instructor, Division of Pulmonary and Critical Care Medicine, Department of Medicine, University of California Los Angeles School of Medicine; Co-Director, Asthma and Cough Center, University of California Los Angeles, Center for the Health Sciences, Los Angeles, California
Chronic Obstructive Pulmonary Diseases in Adults

JANE Q. KOENIG, PH.D.
Professor, Department of Environmental Health, School of Public Health and Community Medicine, University of Washington, Seattle, Washington
Nonallergenic Environmental Factors

JOANNE KRIEGE, M.D.
Fellow, Section of Rheumatology, University of Wisconsin Hospital and Clinics, Madison, Wisonsin
Autoimmune Diseases

GARY L. LARSEN, M.D.
Professor of Pediatrics, Head, Section of Pediatric Pulmonary Medicine, University of Colorado School of Medicine; Senior Faculty Member, Head, Division of Pediatric Pulmonary Medicine, National Jewish Center for Immunology and Respiratory Medicine, Denver, Colorado
Assessment of Lung Function: Pulmonary Function Testing

JOHN LATALL, M.D.
Fellow, Division of Allergy/Immunology, Northwestern University Medical School, Chicago, Illinois
Surgery in Allergic and Asthmatic Patients

DENNIS K. LEDFORD, M.D.
Associate Professor of Medicine, Division of Allergy and Immunology and Division of Rheumatology; Director, Clinical and Laboratory Immunology Training Program, University of South Florida College of Medicine; Staff Physician, James A. Haley Veterans Hospital, Tampa, Florida
Immunotherapy for Allergic Disease

ROBERT F. LEMANSKE, JR., M.D.
Professor of Medicine and Pediatrics, University of Wisconsin Medical School; Head, Division of Pediatric Allergy, University of Wisconsin Hospitals, Madison, Wisconsin
Asthma (Bronchial Asthma): Principles of Diagnosis and Treatment

DONALD Y. M. LEUNG, M.D., PH.D.
Professor of Pediatrics, University of Colorado Health Sciences Center; Head, Division of Pediatric Allergy and Immunology, National Jewish Center for Immunology and Respiratory Medicine, Denver, Colorado
Allergic Immune Response

DOUGLAS S. LEVINE, M.D.
Associate Professor of Medicine, University of Washington School of Medicine; Attending Staff Physician, University of Washington Medical Center and Affiliated Teaching Hospitals, Seattle, Washington
Inflammatory Bowel Diseases

PHILLIP L. LIEBERMAN, M.D.
Clinical Professor of Medicine and Pediatrics, Departments of Medicine and Pediatrics, University of Tennessee College of Medicine, Memphis, Tennessee
Specific and Idiopathic Anaphylaxis: Pathophysiology and Treatment

RICHARD F. LOCKEY, M.D.
Professor of Medicine, Pediatrics, and Public Health; Director, Division of Allergy and Immunology, University of South Florida College of Medicine; Chief, Allergy and Immunology, James A. Haley Veterans Hospital, Tampa, Florida
Immunotherapy for Allergic Disease

MICHAEL S. MORGAN, Sc.D.
Associate Professor of Environmental Health, University of Washington, Seattle, Washington
Industrial Hygiene Aspects of Preventing Occupational Asthma

SHIRLEY J. MURPHY, M.D.
Professor and Chairman, Department of Pediatrics, University of New Mexico School of Medicine, Albuquerque, New Mexico
Bronchopulmonary Dysplasia

ROBERT M. NACLERIO, M.D.
Professor and Chief of Otolaryngology, University of Chicago School of Medicine, Chicago, Illinois
Physiology and Diseases of the Nose

DENNIS R. OWNBY, M.D.
Director, Allergy Research, Henry Ford Health System, Detroit, Michigan
Tests for IgE Antibody

DAVID S. PEARLMAN, M.D.
Clinical Professor of Pediatrics, University of Colorado School of Medicine; Physician, Colorado Allergy and Asthma Clinic, Denver, Colorado
Asthma (Bronchial Asthma): Principles of Diagnosis and Treatment

GEORGE PHILIP, M.D.
Associate Director of Medical Affairs, Immunologic Pharmaceutical Corporation, Waltham, Massachusetts
Physiology and Diseases of the Nose

THOMAS A. PLATTS-MILLS, M.D., PH.D.
Professor of Medicine, Head, Asthma and Allergic Disease Center, University of Virginia, Charlottesville, Virginia
Principles of Avoidance

DON WARREN PRINTZ, M.D.
Staff Physician, DeKalp Medical Center, Decatur, Georgia
Other Skin Disorders

GARY S. RACHELEFSKY, M.D.
Clinical Professor of Pediatrics; Assistant Director, Allergy Fellowship Program, University of California Los Angeles; Director, Allergy Research Foundation, Los Angeles, California
Patient Education: Creating a Partnership for Effective Asthma Care; Sinusitis

GARY P. RAKES, M.D.
Fellow, Department of Pediatrics, Division of Allergy and Immunology, University of Virginia Health Sciences Center, Charlottesville, Virginia
Principles of Avoidance

ELIZABETH ROSE, M.D.
Fellow, Pediatric Otolaryngology, University of Pittsburgh; Children's Hospital of Pittsburgh, Pittsburgh, Pennsylvania
Obstructive Diseases of the Larynx and Trachea

JOHN E. SALVAGGIO, M.D.
Henderson Professor and Vice-Chancellor, Tulane University Medical Center; Medical Staff, Tulane University Hospital and Charity Hospital, New Orleans, Louisiana
Controversial Concepts in Allergy and Clinical Immunology

HUGH A. SAMPSON, M.D.
Professor of Pediatrics, Division of Allergy and Immunology, Johns Hopkins University School of Medicine; Director, Pediatric Clinical Research Center, Johns Hopkins Hospital, Baltimore, Maryland
Evaluation and Management of Patients with Adverse Food Reactions

ERIC T. SANDBERG, M.D.
Assistant Professor of Pediatrics, Baylor College of Medicine, Houston, Texas
Normal Immune Responses

MICHAEL SCHATZ, M.D.
Clinical Professor, Department of Medicine, University of California San Diego, School of Medicine; Staff Allergist, Department of Allergy, Kaiser Permanente Medical Center, San Diego, California
Asthma and Allergy During Pregnancy

RICHARD I. SCHIFF, M.D., Ph.D.
Associate Professor of Pediatrics, Division of Allergy and Immunology, Duke University Medical Center, Durham, North Carolina
Primary and Secondary Immunodeficiency Diseases

ALAN SCHOCKET, M.D.
Associate Clinical Professor, University of Colorado School of Medicine; Staff Physician, National Jewish Hospital; Medical Director, Qual Med, Denver, Colorado
Urticaria and Angioedema

ROBERT H. SCHWARTZ, M.D.
Clinical Professor of Pediatrics, University of Rochester School of Medicine and Dentistry; Director, Pediatric Allergy, University of Rochester Medical Center and Strong Memorial Hospital, Rochester, New York
Chronic Pulmonary Disease in Children: Including Cystic Fibrosis and Primary Ciliary Dyskinesia

GAIL G. SHAPIRO, M.D.
Clinical Professor of Pediatrics, University of Washington School of Medicine, Seattle; Attending Physician, Children's Hospital, Seattle, Washington
Inhalation Bronchoprovocation; Sinusitis; Evaluation and Treatment of the Patient with Asthma—Pediatric Asthma

WILLIAM T. SHEARER, M.D., Ph.D.
Professor, Department of Pediatrics and Microbiology/Immunology, Baylor College of Medicine; Chief, Allergy and Immunology Service, Texas Children's Hospital, Houston, Texas
Normal Immune Responses

ALBERT L. SHEFFER, M.D.
Clinical Professor of Medicine, Harvard Medical School; Director, Allergy Clinic, Brigham and Women's Hospital; Chief, Section on Allergy, New England Deaconess Hospital, Boston, Massachusetts
Exercise-Induced Anaphylaxis

SHELDON C. SIEGEL, M.D.
Clinical Professor in Pediatrics; Co-Director of Pediatric Allergy-Immunology Training Program, University of California Los Angeles, School of Medicine, Los Angeles, California
Headaches

RONALD A. SIMON, M.D.
Head, Division of Allergy and Immunology, Scripps Clinic and Research Foundation, La Jolla, California
Diagnostic Challenges; Drug-Induced Asthma

F. ESTELLE R. SIMONS, M.D.
Professor and Deputy Chairman, Department of Pediatrics and Child Health, University of Manitoba; Head, Section of Allergy and Clinical Immunology, Children's Hospital, Winnipeg, Manitoba, Canada
Pharmacology and Therapeutics

DAVID P. SKONER, M.D.
Associate Professor of Pediatrics, University of Pittsburgh School of Medicine; Chief, Laboratory

Research, Division of Allergy/Immunology/Rheumatology, Children's Hospital of Pittsburgh, Pittsburgh, Pennsylvania
Diseases of the Ear

RAYMOND G. SLAVIN, M.D.
Professor of Medicine; Director, Division of Allergy and Immunology, St. Louis University School of Medicine, St. Louis, Missouri
Sinusitis

WILLIAM R. SOLOMON, M.D.
Professor of Internal Medicine and Chief, Division of Allergy, University of Michigan Medical School; Attending Physician, University Hospital, Ann Arbor; Consultant, University of Michigan Student Health Service; Consultant, United States Veterans Administration Hospital, Ann Arbor, Michigan
Common Allergenic Pollen and Fungi

SHELDON L. SPECTOR, M.D.
Clinical Professor, Department of Medicine, University of California Los Angeles, School of Medicine, Los Angeles, California
Inhalation Bronchoprovocation

SYLVAN E. STOOL, M.D.
Professor of Otolaryngology and Pediatrics, Department of Otolaryngology/Head and Neck Surgery, University of Pittsburgh School of Medicine; Director of Otolaryngology Education, Department of Pediatric Otolaryngology, Children's Hospital of Pittsburgh, Pittsburgh, Pennsylvania
Obstructive Diseases of the Larynx and Trachea

ROBERT C. STRUNK, M.D.
Professor of Pediatrics, Washington University School of Medicine, St. Louis, Missouri
Identification and Management of Psychosocial Factors

VIRGINIA SILVER TAGGART, M.P.H.
National Heart, Lung, and Blood Institute, Division of Lung Diseases, Bethesda, Maryland
Patient Education: Creating a Partnership for Effective Asthma Care

DONALD P. TASHKIN, M.D.
Professor of Medicine, Division of Pulmonary and Critical Care Medicine, Department of Medicine, University of California Los Angeles, School of Medicine; Co-Director, Asthma and Cough Center; Director, Pulmonary Function Laboratory, University of California Los Angeles Center for the Health Sciences, Los Angeles, California
Chronic Obstructive Pulmonary Diseases in Adults

ABBA I. TERR, M.D.
Clinical Professor of Medicine, Stanford University Medical School; Director, Allergy Clinic, Stanford University Medical Center, Stanford, California
Controversial Concepts in Allergy and Clinical Immunology

DAVID G. TINKELMAN, M.D.
Clinical Professor of Pediatrics, Division Allergy and Immunology, Medical College of Georgia, Augusta, Georgia
Evaluation of the Patient with Chronic Respiratory Symptoms

PAUL P. VanARSDEL, Jr., M.D.†
Professor Medicine and Head, Section of Allergy, University of Washington School of Medicine; Chief, Allergy Section, University Hospital; Associate Attending Physician, Harborview Medical Center; Consultant, Children's Hospital and Medical Center, Seattle, Washington
Drug Hypersensitivity
†Deceased 1994

FRANK S. VIRANT, M.D.
Clinical Associate Professor of Pediatrics, University of Washington School of Medicine; Attending Physician, Children's Hospital and Medical Center, Seattle, Washington
Radiocontrast, Local Anesthetic, and Latex Reactions

RICHARD W. WEBER, M.D.
Associate Professor of Medicine, University of Colorado Health Sciences Center; Staff Physician, Allergy/Immunology, National Jewish Center for Immunology and Respiratory Medicine, Denver, Colorado
Common Allergenic Pollen and Fungi; Other Allergenic Plants and Animals

SCOTT T. WEISS, M.D., M.S.
Associate Professor of Medicine, Harvard Medical School; Attending Physician, Brigham and Women's Hospital and Beth Israel Hospital, Boston, Massachusetts
Asthma Epidemiology; Risk Factors and Natural History

SALLY E. WENZEL, M.D.
Assistant Professor, University of Colorado Health Sciences Center; Staff Physician, National Jewish Center for Immunology and Respiratory Medicine, Denver, Colorado
Assessment of Lung Function: Pulmonary Function Testing

PAUL V. WILLIAMS, M.D.

Clinical Professor of Pediatrics and Environmental Health, University of Washington School of Medicine; Allergist, Northwest Asthma and Allergy Center, Seattle, Washington

Nonallergenic Environmental Factors; Inhalation Bronchoprovocation

JOHN W. YUNGINGER, M.D.

Professor of Pediatrics, Mayo Medical School; Consultant in Pediatric and Adolescent Medicine, Mayo Medical Center, Rochester, Minnesota

Biology of Allergens

MICHAEL C. ZACHARISEN, M.D.

Clinical Professor, University of Nevada; Associate Staff, Sunrise Hospital and Children's Hospital, Las Vegas, Nevada

Hypersensitivity Pneumonitis

ROBERT S. ZEIGER, M.D., Ph.D.

Clinical Professor of Pediatrics, University of California San Diego, La Jolla; Chief of Allergy, Kaiser Permanente Medical Center, San Diego, California

Risk Factors and Prevention of Allergy; Asthma and Allergy During Pregnancy

FOREWORD

Eight years have elapsed since the second edition of the book now titled *Allergy, Asthma, and Immunology from Infancy to Adulthood,* years that have established the worth of this volume to the practicing physician. Careful blending of the clinical and immunologic background needed for the care of the allergic patient and the clarity of presentation have made the text an invaluable source of information.

The recent explosion of knowledge in the fields of immunobiologic and immunochemical reactions, the recognition of new immunogenic agents, the increased importance of immunodeficiency states and autoimmune diseases, the increased knowledge of respiratory pathophysiology, and an increased understanding of chemical mediators have had a tremendous impact on the diagnosis and treatment of allergic diseases. Integrating this new information with present knowledge is essential.

No text can hope to be as current as today's journals, but the third edition of this text succeeds admirably in meeting current needs. It emphasizes the clinical aspects of allergy and immunology, with sufficient inclusion of the fundamentals to ensure understanding of basic mechanisms. The text is well-organized, is eminently readable, and will continue to be the definitive reference in the field for those physicians caring for patients with allergy, clinical immunologic problems, and/or asthma.

WILLIAM A. HOWARD, M.D.

NOTICE

Medicine is an ever-changing field. Standard safety precautions must be followed, but as new research and clinical experience broaden our knowledge, changes in treatment and drug therapy become necessary or appropriate. The editors of this work have carefully checked the generic and trade drug names and verified drug dosages to ensure that the dosage information in this work is accurate and in accordance with the standards accepted at the time of publication. Readers are advised, however, to check the product information currently provided by the manufacturer of each drug to be administered to be certain that changes have not been made in the recommended dose or in the contraindications for administration. This is of particular importance in regard to new or infrequently used drugs. It is the responsibility of the treating physician, relying on experience and knowledge of the patient, to determine dosages and the best treatment for the patient. The editors cannot be responsible for misuse or misapplication of the material in this work.

THE PUBLISHER

PREFACE

Allergy, asthma, and other immune diseases are among the most common chronic health disorders in children and adults. They are responsible for a significant proportion of emergency room visits and hospitalizations and for high health system costs related in large part to poor disease recognition and management. Furthermore, these diseases cause substantial absenteeism from school and work and pose a wide range of problems for both patients and family, including physical disability, abnormal psychosocial development or relationships, and potential limitations to normal lifestyle. They often impose an enormous economic burden on patients or families as well. Unfortunately, many physicians are inadequately prepared to manage these problems. This is particularly disheartening since, for the most part, these are highly treatable disorders with much better outcomes than is currently achieved. This book is written for all health care providers who deal in any way with allergy, asthma, and immune diseases, with the hope of increasing understanding that is necessary for proper diagnosis and management of these disorders.

The term "allergy" suffers from diverse and often vague usage. We define "allergy" as an adverse manifestation of an immune event not totally limited to situations involving IgE antibody. Atopic disorders are considered to represent a subgroup of allergic disorders, including perennial and seasonal allergic rhinitis, atopic dermatitis, and asthma. Allergic factors can play an important role in causing these disorders in the first place, as well as precipitating their manifestations. In fact, exposure to increased concentrations of house dust mite and other allergens may be largely responsible for the increased prevalence and severity of asthma recorded in recent years. These disorders also are often multifactorial. For example, although allergic factors induce pulmonary inflammation and increase disease severity in asthma, asthma also may be associated with viral respiratory infections, bacterial sinusitis, drugs such as nonsteroidal anti-inflammatory drugs (NSAIDs), air pollutants, and occupational exposures.

An early breakthrough in the understanding of clinical immunology occurred a generation ago with the discovery of X-linked agammaglobulinemia by Bruton. Subsequently, a variety of congenital and acquired immunologic syndromes in children and adults involving both B and T cells were discovered. The past two decades have seen the rapid accumulation of knowledge relating to the complexity and importance of the immune system in regard to many diseases, including allergic disorders. In part, this advance has been stimulated more recently by the worldwide epidemic of acquired immunodeficiency syndrome (AIDS) and the transplantation of human organs. Similarly, clinical immunology has become important in the diagnosis and management of collagen-vascular syndromes and autoimmune diseases.

This book is written as a guide for physicians and other health care providers who care for patients with these diseases. Although ultimate orientation is toward patient management, the book also considers mechanisms, manifestations, differential diagnoses, as well as methods of disease management. We hope that the information presented will foster a more informed understanding of diagnosis and management of allergic, asthmatic, and other immune diseases and, in so doing, will help to minimize the physical, psychosocial, and economic issues associated with these disorders.

The editors are grateful to the authors of the individual chapters; to Grace Strodtbeck, Executive Assistant of A.S.T.H.M.A., Inc., for her outstanding work in keeping this book on track; and to the editorial and production staffs of the W.B. Saunders Company for their help in its preparation.

C. WARREN BIERMAN, M.D.
DAVID S. PEARLMAN, M.D.
GAIL G. SHAPIRO, M.D.
WILLIAM W. BUSSE, M.D.

CONTENTS

Section One
THE IMMUNE SYSTEM: PHYSIOLOGY AND CLINICAL CONSIDERATIONS

Chapter 1
Normal Immune Responses 1
Eric T. Sandberg, M.D., and William T. Shearer, M.D., Ph.D.

Chapter 2
Primary and Secondary Immunodeficiency Diseases 20
Richard I. Schiff, M.D, Ph.D., and Terry O. Harville, M.D., Ph.D.

Chapter 3
Autoimmune Diseases 55
JoAnne Kriege, M.D., and Frank M. Graziano, M.D., Ph.D.

Chapter 4
Allergic Immune Response 68
Donald Y. M. Leung, M.D., Ph.D.

Section Two
ETIOLOGY AND PATHOGENETIC FACTORS IN ALLERGY AND ASTHMA

Chapter 5
Epidemiology of Allergy and Asthma 79
Richard Evans III, M.D., M.P.H., and Peter J. Gergen, M.D., M.P.H.

Chapter 6
Biology of Allergens 89
John W. Yunginger, M.D.

Chapter 7
Common Allergenic Pollen and Fungi 93
William R. Solomon, M.D., Richard W. Weber, M.D., and William K. Dolen, M.D.

Chapter 8
Other Allergenic Plants and Animals 115
Richard W. Weber, M.D., and William K. Dolen, M.D.

Chapter 9
Nonallergenic Environmental Factors 124
  Jane Q. Koenig, Ph.D., and Paul V. Williams, M.D.

Section Three
PRINCIPLES OF DIAGNOSIS AND MANAGEMENT

Chapter 10
Evaluation of the Patient with Chronic Respiratory Symptoms 135
  David G. Tinkleman, M.D.

Chapter 11
Tests for IgE Antibody 144
  Dennis R. Ownby, M.D.

Chapter 12
Assessment of Lung Function: Pulmonary Function Testing 157
  Sally E. Wenzel, M.D., and Gary L. Larsen, M.D.

Chapter 13
Inhalation Bronchoprovocation 173
  Gail G. Shapiro, M.D., Paul V. Williams, M.D., and Sheldon L. Spector, M.D.

Chapter 14
Diagnostic Challenges 187
  Ronald A. Simon, M.D.

Chapter 15
Principles of Avoidance 195
  Gary P. Rakes, M.D., and Thomas A. Platts-Mills, M.D., Ph.D.

Chapter 16
Pharmacology and Therapeutics 208
  F. Estelle R. Simons, M.D.

Chapter 17
Immunotherapy for Allergic Disease 237
  Dennis K. Ledford, M.D., and Richard F. Lockey, M.D.

Chapter 18
Identification and Management of Psychosocial Factors 256
  Stephen J. Gaioni, Ph.D., Edwin B. Fisher, Jr., Ph.D., and Robert C. Strunk, M.D.

Chapter 19
Patient Education: Creating a Partnership for Effective Asthma Care ... 268
  Virginia Silver Taggart, M.P.H., and Gary S. Rachelefsky, M.D.

Chapter 20
Risk Factors and Prevention of Allergy 282
  Noah J. Friedman, M.D., and Robert S. Zeiger, M.D., Ph.D.

Section Four
SYSTEMIC REACTIONS AND ANAPHYLAXIS

Chapter 21
Specific and Idiopathic Anaphylaxis: Pathophysiology and Treatment 297
  Phillip L. Lieberman, M.D.

Chapter 22
Drug Hypersensitivity 320
  Paul P. VanArsdel, Jr., M.D.

Chapter 23
Allergic Reactions to Insect Stings 348
  David B. K. Golden, M.D.

Chapter 24
Radiocontrast, Local Anesthetic, and Latex Reactions 355
  Frank S. Virant, M.D.

Chapter 25
Food-Induced Systemic Reactions and Anaphylaxis 366
  John A. Anderson, M.D.

Chapter 26
Exercise-Induced Anaphylaxis 376
  Richard F. Horan, M.D., and Albert L. Sheffer, M.D.

Chapter 27
Adverse Reactions to Vaccines: The Complexity of Vaccine Safety 384
  Vincent A. Fulginiti, M.D.

Section Five
UPPER RESPIRATORY TRACT DISEASES

Chapter 28
Physiology and Diseases of the Nose 393
  George Philip, M.D., and Robert M. Naclerio, M.D.

Chapter 29
Diseases of the Ear 411
  David P. Skoner, M.D., and Margaretha L. Casselbrant, M.D., Ph.D.

Chapter 30
Sinusitis 428
  Jonathan Corren, M.D., Gary S. Rachelefsky, M.D., Gail G. Shapiro, M.D., and Raymond G. Slavin, M.D.

Chapter 31
Obstructive Diseases of the Larynx and Trachea 436
  Elizabeth Rose, M.D., and Sylvan E. Stool, M.D.

Section Six
ASTHMA

Chapter 32
Etiology of Asthma: Pathology and Mediators 443
   David J. Fraenkel, B.M., B.S., FRACP, and Stephen T. Holgate, M.D., D.Sc., FRCP

Chapter 33
Asthma Epidemiology: Risk Factors and Natural History 472
   Scott T. Weiss, M.D., M.S.

Chapter 34
Asthma (Bronchial Asthma): Principles of Diagnosis and Treatment 484
   David S. Pearlman, M.D., and Robert F. Lemanske, Jr., M.D.

Chapter 35
Evaluation and Treatment of the Patient with Asthma 498
   PEDIATRIC ASTHMA
   C. Warren Bierman, M.D., and Gail G. Shapiro, M.D.

   ADULT ASTHMA
   Deborah Ortega Carr, M.D., Robert K. Bush, M.D., and William W. Busse, M.D.

Chapter 36
Exercise-Induced Asthma 520
   Peyton A. Eggleston, M.D.

Chapter 37
Occupational Asthma 529
   Jonathan A. Bernstein, M.D., David I. Bernstein, M.D., and
   I. Leonard Bernstein, M.D.

Chapter 38
Drug-Induced Asthma 549
   Ronald A. Simon, M.D., and James L. Baldwin, M.D.

Section Seven
IMMUNE AND NONIMMUNE CHRONIC PULMONARY DISEASE

Chapter 39
Hypersensitivity Pneumonitis 559
   Michael C. Zacharisen, M.D., and Jordan N. Fink, M.D.

Chapter 40
Allergic Bronchopulmonary Aspergillosis 566
   Cynthia Steichen Kabalin, M.D., and Paul A. Greenberger, M.D.

Chapter 41
Chronic Pulmonary Disease in Children: Including Cystic Fibrosis and Primary Ciliary Dyskinesia 572
   Robert H. Schwartz, M.D.

Chapter 42
Bronchopulmonary Dysplasia 592
   Denise M. Coleman, M.D., and Shirley J. Murphy, M.D.

Chapter 43
Chronic Obstructive Pulmonary Diseases in Adults 600
 Eric C. Kleerup, M.D., and Donald P. Tashkin, M.D.

Section Eight
MANAGEMENT OF SKIN DISEASE

Chapter 44
Atopic Dermatitis 613
 Allen D. Adinoff, M.D., and Richard A. F. Clark, M.D.

Chapter 45
Contact Dermatitis 633
 John L. Aeling, M.D.

Chapter 46
Urticaria and Angioedema 643
 Kathryn F. Hobbs, M.D., and Alan Schocket, M.D.

Chapter 47
Other Skin Disorders 653
 Don Warren Printz, M.D.

Section Nine
ADVERSE REACTIONS TO FOOD

Chapter 48
Evaluation and Management of Patients with Adverse Food Reactions 665
 Kristina M. Hoffman, M.D., and Hugh A. Sampson, M.D.

Chapter 49
Inflammatory Bowel Diseases 687
 Douglas S. Levine, M.D.

Section Ten
SPECIAL ISSUES

Chapter 50
Allergic Disorders of the Eye 703
 Mitchell H. Friedlaender, M.D.

Chapter 51
Chronic Cough 713
 Richard S. Irwin, M.D.

Chapter 52
Headaches 719
 Roger M. Katz, M.D., and Sheldon C. Siegel, M.D.

Chapter 53
Asthma and Allergy During Pregnancy 729
 Michael Schatz, M.D., and Robert S. Zeiger, M.D., Ph.D.

Chapter 54
Surgery in Allergic and Asthmatic Patients 743
  John Latall, M.D., and Leslie C. Grammer, M.D.

Chapter 55
Controversial Concepts in Allergy and Clinical Immunology 749
  Abba I. Terr, M.D., and John E. Salvaggio, M.D.

Chapter 56
Allergies in the School 761
  Clifton T. Furukawa, M.D.

Chapter 57
Industrial Hygiene Aspects of Preventing Occupational Asthma 769
  Michael S. Morgan, Sc.D., and Leonard C. Altman, M.D.

Index 779

Section One

THE IMMUNE SYSTEM: PHYSIOLOGY AND CLINICAL CONSIDERATIONS

Chapter 1

Normal Immune Responses

Eric T. Sandberg, M.D., and William T. Shearer, M.D., Ph.D.

Innate to the beliefs of mankind is the trust that natural factors exist that can protect humans from infection by microorganisms and the development of malignancy. Students of the discipline of immunology have been carefully delineating these factors for centuries, but in the past two decades spectacular advances have been made in the understanding of the power and complexities of the immune system. A particularly illuminating area has been the discovery of how the apparent excesses of the immune response create clinical problems in humans with allergic disease and asthma. This textbook is devoted to the study of treatments for aberrations in the human immune response: both those that result from insufficient immune responses and, equally important, those that emanate from unrestrained immune responses. The chapters that follow will detail these abnormal conditions and their treatments. It is the purpose of this chapter to describe the essential components of immunity and how they produce normal immune responses. An initial consideration of the normal immune response will facilitate the understanding of abnormal immune responses seen in the immunodeficiency diseases, autoimmune diseases, allergic disorders, and asthmatic conditions to be described in this textbook.

LYMPHOCYTES

The bone marrow is the site of production and initial maturation for cells of the immune system. The pluripotent bone marrow stem cell receives signaling cues from the microenvironment to produce both lymphoid and myeloid cell lines. The lymphoid stem cell gives rise to T lymphocytes, B lymphocytes, and non-T, non-B large granular lymphocytes. Final differentiation of lymphocytes occurs in the periphery, most prominently in the thymus, spleen, and lymph nodes. The maturation of these cells depends on a complex array of cytokine and cell-cell interactions. Description of the maturation process involves a large number of surface membrane molecules, many of which have been assigned an arbitrary number in the cluster of differentiation (CD) nomenclature. Recent research has led toward a greater understanding of the signaling pathways and molecular events that direct the maturational changes of cell surface markers.

T Lymphocytes

The functions of T lymphocytes include orchestration of B lymphocyte and macrophage responses, antigen-specific cell killing, and elaboration of cytokines. The principal stimulus of T cells by antigen occurs through interaction of antigen with the T cell receptor (TCR). Expression of the TCR is dependent on genomic rearrangement that permits expression of either an α/β heterodimer or a γ/δ heterodimer. Only 10 percent of mature T cells express the γ/δ TCR. Most of these cells are $CD4^-CD8^-$, and their physiologic function is not yet well defined. The remaining 90 percent of mature T lymphocytes express the α/β TCR. The TCR α/β^+ cells fall into two mutually exclusive groups defined by expression of CD4 or CD8. The $CD4^+$ cells, often referred to as helper T cells, have recently been appreciated for their ability to recognize antigens within the context of class II major histocompatibility complex (MHC) molecules. $CD8^+$ lymphocytes, also referred to as cytotoxic/suppressor T cells, recognize antigens within the context of class I MHC molecules.

The pathway from lymphoid stem cell to mature T cell in the periphery is complex and remains only partially delineated (Fig. 1–1). Stem cells destined to become T cells are delivered to the thymus as early as the eighth week of gestation. On arrival in the thymus, these immature thymocytes lack CD4 and CD8 and are designated double negative cells ($CD4^-CD8^-$). An early step in the "education" of these progenitor T cells results in expression of CD2, which was first identified by its unusual property of binding sheep erythrocytes. Although the biologic function of CD2 is unknown, cross-linking of CD2 with monoclonal antibody leads to T cell activation and thereby suggests a role in T cell development or function. Increasing thymocyte maturity is marked by the appearance of CD1. Final events in the developmental process are marked by the loss of CD1 and the expression of the TCR complex, composed of the hetero-

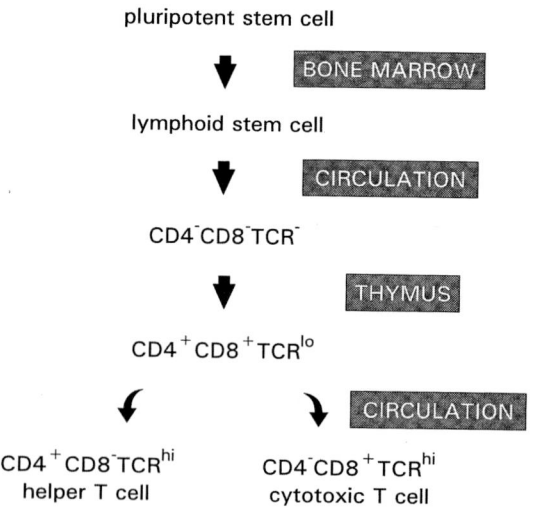

FIGURE 1–1. T lymphocyte development. Cells initially mature in the bone marrow before homing to the thymus where the T cell receptor is first expressed at low concentration (TCR^{lo}). TCR interactions with thymic cell MHC expression allow efficient selection of the mature single positive T cells, $CD4^+$ or $CD8^+$, which express TCR at high concentration (TCR^{hi}). These mature T cells exit the thymus to reenter the circulation.

dimeric TCR and the CD3 polypeptide. (See section on Lymphocyte Function for a discussion of CD3.) Low-level expression of the TCR coincides with dual expression of CD4 and CD8, resulting in "double positive" cells (CD4$^+$CD8$^+$TCR^{lo}). Presence of the α/β TCR permits thymocyte differentiation to progress to the single positive CD4 or CD8 stage. A major goal of thymocyte education is the selection of cells that have the capability to protect the host from foreign insult. In addition, cells that might react against host antigens must be eliminated. As described below, two distinct forms of selection accomplish these objectives (Blackman et al, 1990).

The presence of the TCR complex permits the thymus to select in a positive manner those developing lymphocytes that will be capable of recognizing antigen within the context of the host's MHC molecules. Recent evidence points to a proposed stochastic mechanism for positive selection (Chan et al, 1993; Davis et al, 1993). The TCR of double positive cells engages MHC and is followed by random down-regulation of CD4 or CD8 leading to a cell line of intermediate maturity. Full maturity is not achieved until a second engagement of the same MHC occurs, this time within the context of either CD4 or CD8. CD4$^+$ cells with a TCR compatible with MHC class II molecules or CD8$^+$ cells with a TCR compatible with MHC class I molecules escape programmed cell death to reach full maturity. Thus, positive selection involves three molecules: TCR, MHC, and CD4 or CD8. The end result is a peripheral T cell repertoire dramatically skewed toward recognition of antigen within the context of the host's MHC.

The same triad of molecules operates in negative selection. Maturing thymocytes are deleted when their TCR engages self antigen within the context of MHC. A second possible mechanism in negative selection involves clonal anergy. Thymocytes carrying self-reactive TCR can be made permanently unresponsive. Both mechanisms potentially act to negatively select potentially harmful clones of T cells. Because both positive and negative selection involve the same set of surface markers, future research will strive to address the different underlying mechanisms.

B Lymphocytes

The primordial bone marrow lymphoid stem cell also gives rise to B lymphocytes responsible for antibody production. B cells interact with antigen through cell surface immunoglobulin (Ig). A fundamental distinction between T cells and B cells is the latter's capability to engage native antigen directly as opposed to the T cell's requirement of MHC presentation of antigen. Early maturation of the B cell occurs in the bone marrow or in the fetal liver and is independent of antigen. Further differentiation occurs after migration to the spleen and lymph nodes, where B cells respond to specific antigen. Activated B cells can develop into plasma cells capable of Ig secretion. A small number of activated B cells develop into memory cells that are responsible for the secondary immune response that takes place with re-exposure to antigen.

Molecular analysis has facilitated the understanding of B cell differentiation, which was first described in terms of the cellular localization of Ig. Cytoplasmic μ chains mark the pre-B cell, the first stage of maturation. These cytoplasmic chains are produced from a genetically rearranged Ig heavy chain. Further maturity is denoted by expression of IgM on the cell surface followed by expression of membrane-bound IgD. The molecular correlate of surface Ig expression is genetic rearrangement of the Ig light chain. B cells expressing IgM and IgD are released from the bone marrow into the periphery. Subsequent isotype switching, the association of the original variable region to different heavy chain components, is facilitated by T cell interactions. Final differentiation requires exposure to antigen. After antigen activation, surface Ig is lost, and the B cell is converted into a plasma cell capable of secreting large amounts of specific immunoglobulin directed against the inciting antigen. The signaling pathways that allow B cell differentiation to occur have begun to be unraveled. Recent studies in children with X-linked agammaglobulinemia have suggested strongly that the cascade of B cell expansion is dependent on a cytoplasmic tyrosine kinase (Tsukada et al, 1993). Lack of this kinase activity prevents B cell maturation and production of Ig without effect on T cell development.

Large Granular Lymphocytes

A third lineage of lymphocytes, large granular lymphocytes (LGLs), derives from the lymphoid stem cell and lacks cell surface markers CD3, TCR, and Ig, which define T cells and B cells. These lymphocytes, which comprise 5 percent of peripheral blood lymphocytes, contain characteristic cytoplasmic granules and stain positive for CD16 and CD56. LGLs are nonphagocytic, nonadherent cells with spontaneous cytotoxicity against various target cells including tumors, a function that defines natural killer activity. Additionally, LGLs express cell surface receptors for the Fc portion of immunoglobulin, which allow binding to antibody coated target cells and mediate antibody-dependent cellular cytotoxicity (ADCC). This class of lymphocytes also has been noted to participate in B cell differentiation and the release of cytolysins. The beta chain of the interleukin-2 (IL-2) receptor (CD25) is expressed on the LGL cell surface, resulting in functional and therapeutic implications. Clinical trials have shown that LGLs obtained from patients can be directly activated by IL-2 in vitro to proliferate into lymphokine-activated killer (LAK) cells that can be returned to the patient to slow tumor spread and development (Gray and Horwitz, 1988).

MYELOID STEM CELL LINEAGE

The myeloid stem cell gives rise to mononuclear phagocytes and granulocytes. The mononuclear cells reach full maturity in the soft tissues of the body. Granulocytes mature predominately in the blood stream and are classified according to their defining cytoplasmic granules. Four granulocytic forms will be discussed below: polymorphonuclear neutrophils, eosinophils, basophils, and mast cells. The development of these myeloid cells occurs under the influence of the bone marrow microenvironment, which includes cell-cell interactions as well as cytokine effects. In simple terms, the function of these cells is to provide a controlled nonspecific inflammatory response to insult. In contrast to lymphocytes, these cells are not genetically determined for a specific immune response and are not capable of immune memory.

Mononuclear Phagocytes

Various forms of mononuclear phagocytes exist in different locations of the body. After initial maturation in the bone marrow, cells emerge into the blood stream as monocytes. Circulating monocytes can traverse the endothelial lining of the blood stream into the soft tissue compartment where they are referred to as macrophages. Within the central nervous system, macrophages are designated microglia, and within the liver, Kupffer's cells. Their primary function in promoting general inflammatory responses is production of cytokines and phagocytosis. Importantly, they also participate in specific responses in concert with lymphocytes by processing antigen. Monocytes and macrophages can express both class I and class II MHC molecules, which are capable of presenting antigen to either $CD4^+$ or $CD8^+$ T cells. Specific immune responses are enhanced by macrophage-produced cytokines acting on T lymphocytes.

Polymorphonuclear Neutrophils

Neutrophils are the most numerous of the peripheral leukocytes, and they function as the major cell in the acute inflammatory response. Surface receptors for complement and the Fc portions of immunoglobulin confer the ability to phagocytose opsonized particles. Mature forms are marked by their multilobed nuclei and characteristic azurophilic granules, which contain acid hydrolases, myeloperoxidase, and lysozyme. Secondary neutrophil granules contain lactoferrin in addition to lysozyme. Granules that provide primarily for intracellular killing also can be released extracellularly when neutrophils are activated by immune complexes.

Eosinophils

Eosinophils exhibit brightly staining granules that contain basic proteins toxic to many helminthic parasites. Although eosinophils express the low-affinity Fc receptor for IgE, which facilitates phagocytosis of IgE-targeted fragments, their primary function is mediated through extracellular release of granule contents. This defensive strategy is utilized against large targets such as parasites, which cannot be easily phagocytosed. Interleukin-5 (IL-5) is the principal eosinophilic activating factor. The strong link between eosinophils and IgE is suggested by evidence that T cells producing IL-5 may have functional overlap with those lymphocytes producing IL-4, the IgE switching factor.

Basophils and Mast Cells

Basophils are inflammatory granulocytes that can be recruited from the circulation to sites of local inflammation. They express Fc receptors for IgE, but in contrast to eosinophils, these receptors are of high affinity. Basophilic granules exhibit a deep violet color with Wright's stain. Basophils also differ from eosinophils in that they utilize interleukin-3 (IL-3) as a primary differentiation factor.

Several characteristics exemplify the overlap between basophils and a fourth group of granulocytes, mast cells. Both express the high-affinity Fc receptor for IgE, and both cell types proliferate in the presence of IL-3. Secretory granules of both cell types contain histamine complexed with proteoglycans. For both cell types, activation occurs by cross-linking IgE on the cell surface by an allergen. Activation results in the intracytoplasmic fusion of granules and subsequent degranulation. Extracellular release of histamine from granules mediates many allergic symptoms. Despite these structural and functional similarities, the relationship of the mast cell and the basophil is not completely defined. In addition to the common heparin proteoglycans, the granules in basophils and mast cells vary qualitatively in their enzyme content. Granular peroxidases are characteristic of basophils, whereas acid and alkaline phosphatases are detected in mast cells. Another significant point of difference is the mast cell's localization in tissues rather than in the blood stream.

LYMPHOCYTE FUNCTION

The adaptive immune response depends strongly on proper activation of naive or resting lymphocytes to mature effector T cells and to memory B cells. Lymphocyte activation is central to the development of protective immunity as well as a contributing factor to human disease such as allergy and autoimmunity. As noted previously, T cell activation is initiated by the engagement of membrane-bound TCR to antigen that has been properly processed. Recent studies have greatly clarified the mechanisms of antigen processing, also known as antigen presentation.

Antigen Presentation

Before T cells can be activated, antigen must be processed and presented by an accessory or antigen-presenting cell (APC). As depicted in Figure 1–2, fragments of peptide antigens are displayed on the APC surface in a form that can be recognized by the TCR. The conversion of native antigenic protein to peptide fragments on the cell surface is called antigen processing. $CD8^+$ T cells recognize antigen within the context of MHC class I cells. The prototypic example of antigen presentation to $CD8^+$ T cells occurs in the course of a viral infection. The virus enters the cell and directs assembly of viral proteins. These cytosolic proteins can be processed within the Golgi apparatus and brought to the cell surface in conjunction with MHC class I complex (Yewdell and Bennink, 1992). The degraded protein is represented by an 8–12 amino acid peptide. The cell presenting the viral protein represents a potential target for $CD8^+$ cell killing.

$CD4^+$ T cells are restricted to interact with APC expressing the MHC class II phenotype. Such APCs include macrophages, B cells, and dendritic cells. The APC internalizes exogenous protein antigen and subsequently degrades the antigen within lysosomal vesicles. Macrophages acting as APC have a variety of mechanisms at their disposal for uptake of antigen. Opsonized protein can enter the macrophage through the Ig Fc receptor as well as the C3 receptor. Glycoproteins can attach to the surface of the macrophage through carbohydrate receptors. Proteins that have been internalized by the macrophage are processed within the acidic environment of the intracellular vesicle. This biochemical processing results in degradation of the native protein into a 14–18 amino acid peptide that associates with the MHC class II molecule and subsequently is expressed on the cell surface. The entire process of attachment of protein to the APC followed by degradation and cell surface expression with MHC often is accomplished within 60 minutes.

Antigen presentation can result in an amplification cascade of lymphocyte activation. T lymphocytes activated by antigen presentation are stimulated to secrete various cytokines. Secretion of interferon gamma can induce MHC class II expression of nearby phagocytes and thus increase the pool of potential APC. Increasing numbers of APC also secrete interleukin-1 (IL-1), which further promotes T cell activation.

T Cell Activation

T cell activation requires two stimulatory steps. The first step is recognition of antigen

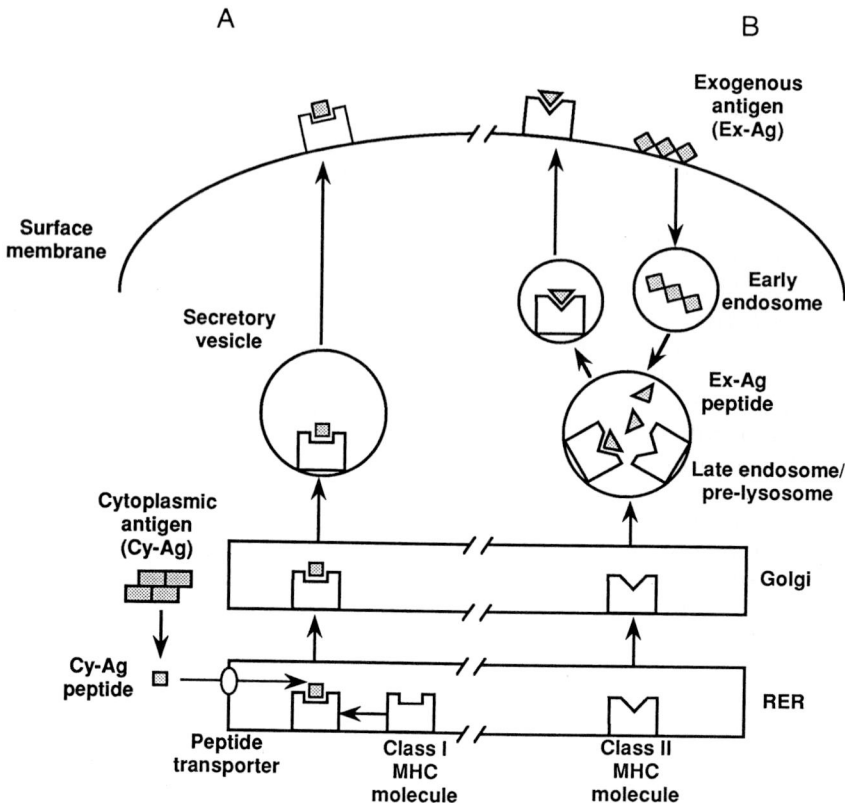

FIGURE 1–2. Pathways of antigen presentation. *A,* Cytoplasmic antigens (Cy-Ag) are degraded in the cytoplasm through the action of proteosomes, then enter the rough endoplasmic reticulum (RER) through a peptide transporter. In the RER, Cy-Ag derived peptides are loaded into class I MHC molecules that move through the Golgi apparatus into secretory vesicles and are then expressed on the cell surface, where they may be recognized by TCR expressed by $CD8^+$ T cells. *B,* Exogenous antigens (Ex-Ag) enter the cell through endocytosis and are transported from early endosomes to late endosomes or pre-lysosomes, where they are fragmented and where peptide resulting from Ex-Ag is loaded into class II MHC molecules. The latter have been transported from the RER through the Golgi apparatus to the peptide-containing vesicles. Class II MHC molecules with antigen peptides are then transported to the cell surface, where they may be recognized by TCR expressed on $CD4^+$ T cells. (Modified from Paul WE. Development and function of lymphocytes. In Gallin JI, Goldstein IM, Snyderman R (eds). Inflammation: Basic Principles and Clinical Correlates. 2nd ed. New York, Raven Press Ltd, 1992.)

by the TCR. More recently described, the second stimulatory step is that of CD28 on the T cell surface adhering to its ligand, B7, on the surface of an antigen-presenting cell (Linsley et al, 1990). Understanding the stimulus provided by the interaction of antigen with the TCR requires some appreciation of the co-expressed CD3 molecule. CD3 consists of five polypeptides composed of five distinct species (γ, δ, ε, ζ, η). (The nomenclature of the γ and δ species of the CD3 molecule should not be confused with the γ/δ TCR with which they can reside.) An individual CD3 molecule consists of a single chain each of γ, δ, and ε together with either a ζ-ζ or ζ-η dimer. The CD3 molecule functions to transduce signals that originate with engagement of the TCR. Cytokine production and cell proliferation are two readily defined end points of T cell activation. The intermediate steps between antigen engagement and mature activation include plasma membrane hydrolysis and resulting increased levels of diacylglycerol and inositol triphosphate (IP_3). Calcium mobilized by IP_3 leads to activation of various tyrosine kinases. The resulting phosphorylation events favor increased transcription of cellular proto-oncogenes, cytokine genes, and cytokine receptor genes.

A fundamental tenet of T cell activation

involves cell-cell contact and adhesion that differs from the classic activation pathways triggered by the interaction of a soluble hormone and its receptor. The primary interaction is direct contact between the TCR and the MHC of the antigen-presenting cell. This cell-cell contact is facilitated and strengthened by accessory molecules. As mentioned above, co-stimulation is achieved by an interaction of B7 and CD28. Additional adhesion molecules such as LFA-1 (lymphocyte function–associated antigen) and LFA-2 (CD2) can stabilize the binding of T cells through their ligands. LFA-1 binds to three species of intercellular adhesion molecule (ICAM-1, ICAM-2, and ICAM-3). LFA-2 promotes cell-cell adhesion through binding with LFA-3 (CD58).

In summary, recognition of antigen by T lymphocytes involves a complex array of cell surface molecules. Antigen must first be processed and presented in the context of the MHC. Recognition of the processed antigenic peptide is the responsibility of the TCR. This recognition is restricted by CD4 and CD8 molecules. Accessory molecules provide important interactions between the antigen-presenting cell and the T cell. Subsequent signal events are mediated by CD3 through kinase-dependent pathways to the cell interior to influence gene transcription.

B Cell Activation

The initial signal of B cell activation is cross-linking of surface Ig by antigen or bivalent anti-Ig antibody. Membrane-bound Ig lacks the cytoplasmic structure to propagate signal transduction to the cytoplasm directly. A peptide complex that acts as a cytoplasmic intermediary for signal transduction has been described (Campbell and Cambier, 1990; Wienands et al, 1990). Conceptually, this complex promotes signal propagation in an analogous function to the ζ chain of the CD3 molecule. As is the case with T cells, B cells utilize second messengers such as increased cytoplasmic calcium to begin the cascade of gene transcription and cell proliferation. For B cell maturation to occur, an important result of this cascade is the switch from IgM production to different isotypes with specialized function.

IMMUNOGLOBULIN STRUCTURE AND FUNCTION

Immunoglobulin (Ig) proteins are designed not to perform a single well-defined task, as are most proteins, but to respond to the myriad possible microbes that currently exist or may evolve in the future. Secreted or membrane-bound forms of immunoglobulin exert their biologic effect by binding antigen. Immunoglobulin capable of binding antigen is often referred to as antibody, though many use the terms interchangeably. The ability to mount a specific response to a variety of antigens implies that immunoglobulin diversity is paramount to evolutionary success. Many structural features of immunoglobulin contribute to this diversity.

The core design of immunoglobulin includes one pair of identical light chains that complex with another pair of identical heavy chains (Fig. 1–3). Each chain of the complex shows striking variability at the amino terminus and an invariant region at the carboxyl end. Simple functional correlates exist for these different structures: the variable end of

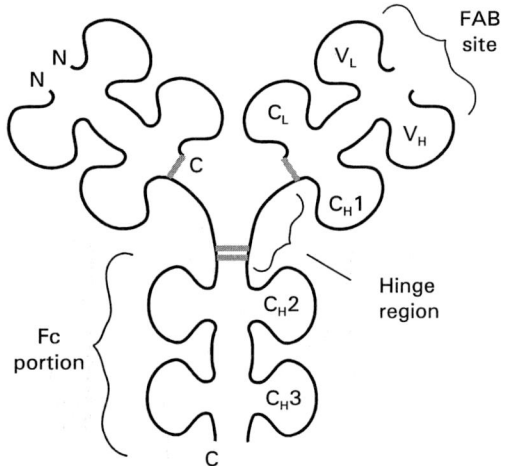

FIGURE 1–3. Schematic structure of IgG. Immunoglobulin glycoproteins consist of two identical heavy chains and two identical light chains. Interchain disulfide bonds (depicted by gray lines) provide linkage between the chains. The amino-terminal ends (N) are characterized by significant sequence variability most marked in the complementarity determining regions (see text). The variable portions of the heavy and light chains are referred to as V_H and V_L, respectively. This region of the molecule is capable of binding antigen and is termed the fragment antigen binding (FAB) site. The remaining portion of the molecule, including the carboxy terminus (C), has a relatively constant structure. The constant portion of the light chain is designated C_L and the constant regions of the heavy chain are called C_H1, C_H2, and C_H3. The hinge region is a site of protein flexibility located between the C_H1 and C_H2 domains. The Fc (fragment crystallizable) region represents the portions of the heavy chain that are below the hinge region.

the molecule presents a binding region for the wide variety of possible antigens and the constant region performs a more limited array of functions, which include binding to cell surface receptors and fixing complement. Within each variable region of both the heavy (V_H) and light (V_L) chains there exists a conserved framework region and three hypervariable regions. Most of the amino acid sequence diversity is confined to the hypervariable regions. These hypervariable regions contribute to the antigen binding by forming a surface complementary to the antigen, leading to the term "complementarity determining region" (CDR).

Immunoglobulin Classes

Five immunoglobulin classes or isotypes have been described on the basis of different component heavy chains (Table 1-1). The heavy chains γ, α, μ, δ, and ϵ define the Ig classes IgG, IgA, IgM, IgD, and IgE, respectively. The same light chain can associate with multiple heavy chains. Light chains exist as two variants: κ and λ. The κ chains account for 60 percent of light chains in human immunoglobulins. However, it is the heavy chain that endows the different Ig classes with their variant conformational and functional characteristics. The various Ig classes are associated with differing clinical and biologic characteristics.

IgG is the predominant species of immunoglobulin in the serum, constituting 75 percent of the total pool. It bears primary responsibility for the humoral response to microbes and toxins. Four different subclasses—IgG1, IgG2, IgG3, and IgG4—are defined by small variations of the Fc portion of the heavy chain. The average half-life of IgG is about three weeks, although IgG3 is notable for a half-life of only one week. IgG1 and IgG3 are produced most efficiently within the context of T cell help. IgG4 has been implicated in the protective response elicited by immunotherapy. The unique capacity of IgG to cross the placenta gives it a critical role in the immunity of infants during the first six months of life. Transport of IgG to the fetus involves the Fc portion of the molecule. Not all subclasses cross the placenta at equal rates, with IgG2 being the most slowly transported. A critical feature of IgG function is the ability to activate complement. The subclasses vary in their efficiency, as follows: IgG3 > IgG1 > IgG2 >> IgG4. The first protein of the classical complement pathway, C1q, binds to the C_H2 portion of the IgG molecule. IgG also plays a role in phagocytosis by granulocytes and mononuclear cells. The Fc portion of the IgG molecule interacts with a variety of Fc receptors (FcR). When antigenic peptides are coated with IgG, subsequent phagocytosis is enhanced by interaction of the FcR on the phagocyte and the Fc portion of immunoglobulin.

IgA is found in secretions of mucous membranes and functions as an early-acting defense mechanism. The respiratory, gastrointestinal, and genitourinary tracts all secrete a specialized form of dimeric IgA that is resistant to proteolytic cleavage. This resistance is attributable to an additional protein in dimeric IgA, called the secretory piece, which is synthesized by epithelial cells. An additional component of IgA is the J (joining) chain, a low-molecular-weight glycopeptide that appears to facilitate polymerization of IgA and the pentameric form of IgM. Smaller proportions of IgA circulate as a monomer without a J chain. Infant immunity is enhanced by secreted IgA passed from mother to child in breast milk.

IgM (macroglobulin) circulates in a large pentameric form that is unable to cross the placenta. The presence of cytoplasmic IgM and surface IgM marks important steps in B

TABLE 1-1. CHARACTERISTICS OF IMMUNOGLOBULIN CLASSES

Ig Class	Secretory Form Structure	Heavy Chain Domains	Half-life (days)	Complement Fixation	Placental Transfer	Mucosal Transfer
IgG	Monomer	4	23	+	+	−
IgA	Monomer or dimer	4	6	−	−	+
IgM	Pentamer	5	10	+	−	+
IgD	Monomer	4	3	−	−	−
IgE	Monomer	5	2	−	−	−

cell maturation. IgM is the earliest antibody formed as a result of primary infection. It plays a critical role in the immune response to gram-negative organisms. Specialized antibodies such as isohemagglutinins, cold agglutinins, and heterophile antibodies fall in this class. Similar to IgG, it is an efficient activator of complement through the classical pathway.

The function of IgD remains to be elucidated. Similar to IgG, it is formed by two identical light chains and two identical heavy chains. It is expressed on the surface of maturing B cells and circulates at low concentration in the blood.

The IgE class of antibodies participates in immediate hypersensitivity and is of critical importance to the allergist. The biologic properties of IgE depend on interaction between its Fc portion and specialized FcR on eosinophils, basophils, and mast cells. Triggering of these cells releases a wide variety of mediators, which manifest as the wheal and flare response seen in skin tests of atopic individuals. In the general population, serum concentrations of IgE correlate with clinical manifestations of atopy. However, the strength of this association is inadequate for generalized application to individual patients. The serum concentration of IgE is orders of magnitude less than other Ig species. Despite a low serum concentration, high avidity interaction with its receptor results in potent biologic effects. Further aspects of IgE biology are discussed at length in a later chapter of the book.

Regulation of IgE Production by T Cells

T lymphocyte control of B cell IgE production deserves special consideration. This immune regulation is well illustrated by cases of childhood T cell deficiency in which patients present with extremely high levels of IgE that return to normal after curative bone marrow transplantation. Recent evidence suggests that $CD4^+$ T cell subsets may play a crucial role in IgE regulation (Del Prete et al, 1991). In mouse and human systems, these subsets of $CD4^+$ cells are designated T_{H1} and T_{H2}. T_{H1} cells secrete IL-2, interferon-γ (IFN-γ), and tumor necrosis factor-β, and turn off IgE synthesis. T_{H2} cells secrete IL-4, IL-5, IL-6, and IL-10—resulting in increased IgE production. The regulation of T_{H1} and T_{H2} responses is partially attributable to reciprocal inhibition by cytokines. The IFN-γ of T_{H1} cells inhibits proliferation of T_{H2} cells. Analogously, IL-10 is produced by T_{H2} cells and inhibits T_{H1} cytokine production. High levels of T_{H2} cells and low levels of T_{H1} cells have been identified in dust mite allergy and atopic dermatitis (Wieranga et al, 1990a and 1990b).

Immunotherapy of allergic disease induces antigen-specific suppressor T cells that down-regulate IgE responses to allergen. The demonstration that IL-4 directs B cell switching to IgE synthesis suggests possible therapeutic avenues. Modification of interactions between IL-4 and its receptor may be accomplished through antibody interactions or blocking peptides. Down-regulating IL-4 synthesis presents another therapeutic option. Research in allergy promises continued contributions in defining the pathways of IgE regulation as well as testing new concepts in clinical practice.

IMMUNOGENETICS

Immunogenetics is the study of polymorphic genetic systems that influence the immune response. The most thoroughly studied of these systems include immunoglobulin, T cell receptors, and major histocompatibility (MHC) antigens. All are members of the immunoglobulin supergene family. This common structural motif suggests a common evolutionary ancestor. Immunogenetic studies have had implications for basic science research, as noted in the analysis of the mechanism of V(D)J recombination of immunoglobulin (see below), which permits study of DNA double-strand break repair and chromatin structure (Lieber, 1992). Immunogenetics also has come to play an increasingly important role in clinical medicine as many diseases become associated with specific determinants of the immune response. Diabetes and hyperthyroidism have long been recognized to often occur in the context of specific MHC antigens. Many other autoimmune diseases, ranging from organ-specific entities (e.g., Hashimoto's thyroiditis) to systemic diseases such as systemic lupus erythematosus, have been associated with certain MHC antigens (Table 1–2). One possible explanation of some of these associations is immunologic cross-tolerance. For example, in ankylosing spondylitis, it is proposed that infection by *Klebsiella* may induce autoantibodies responsible for the subsequent pathology. Specific

TABLE 1–2. HLA AND DISEASE ASSOCIATION

	HLA ASSOCIATIONS*	RACE†	APPROXIMATE RELATIVE RISK
Acute anterior uveitis	B27	C	14
Ankylosing spondylitis	B27	A, B, C	156
Behçet's disease	B5	A, C	7
Celiac disease	DR3, B8, DR7, A1	C	3–12
Dermatitis herpetiformis	DR3	C	28
Goodpasture's syndrome	DR2	C	14
Graves' disease	Bw35, DR3	A, C	4–5
IgA deficiency	B8	C	4
Insulin-dependent diabetes mellitus	DR3, DR4	A, B, C	4–5
Multiple sclerosis	Dw2, DR2, DR6	A, C	4–6
Myasthenia gravis	B8	C	3
Narcolepsy	DR2	A, C	227
Pemphigus vulgaris	DR4	C	12
Psoriasis vulgaris	Cw6, B17, B37, B13	A, C	5–9
Reactive arthritis	B27	C	13–54
Reiter's disease	B27	C	53
Rheumatoid arthritis	DR4, Dw4	A, B, C	5–6
Juvenile rheumatoid arthritis	B27, DR5, DR8	C	3–5
Sjögren's syndrome	Dw3, B8	C	4–9
Systemic lupus erythematosus	B8, DR3	C	3

*In relative order of strength.
†A = Asian; B = Black; C = Caucasian.
Data from Baines M, Ebringer A: HLA and disease. Molec Aspects Med 13:263–378, 1992.

amino acid polymorphisms of MHC have been shown to strongly influence disease susceptibility. One example is the resistance to insulin-dependent diabetes mellitus conferred by having aspartate encoded at position 57 of a DQ β chain (Todd et al, 1987). Interestingly, this observation originally made in a Caucasian population does not extend completely to Asian diabetics (Awata et al., 1990).

HLA Complex

A major task of the immune system is discrimination between "self" and "nonself." Failure to accomplish such discrimination may result in unchecked invasion of foreign microbes or immune-mediated self destruction. This important distinction is mediated by molecules of the major histocompatibility complex, which in humans is referred to as the human leukocyte antigen (HLA) complex. Three different classes of HLA molecules are recognized within a 3 megabase region of the short arm of chromosome 6 (Fig. 1–4). Class I and class II molecules are highly polymorphic membrane-bound proteins that serve a critical role in T cell recognition of foreign antigen. Class III HLA genes, located between class I and class II genes, code for soluble factors such as C2, C4, and factor B of the complement system as well as tumor necrosis factor, which will be discussed later in the chapter.

The HLA class I region, located at the telomeric aspect of the gene complex, codes for three polymorphic heavy chains designated A, B, and C. Nearly every nucleated cell of the body expresses class I HLA molecules. Each heavy chain associates with the non-polymorphic β_2-microglobulin (β_2m), coded on chromosome 15, to form the class I molecule (Fig. 1–5A). The heavy chain contains three distinct extracellular domains, α_1, α_2, and α_3, as well as a transmembrane region and a cytoplasmic tail. The single domain of β_2m and the α_3 domain of the heavy chain are homologous to the structure of immunoglobulin. The α_1 and α_2 domains form a groove with helices at the lateral aspects and a β-pleated sheet at the base. This groove, or cleft, acts as the protein-binding site that presents antigenic peptides to CD8$^+$ lymphocytes.

The structure and genetics of HLA class II molecules are more complicated than for class I. The HLA class II region is divided into three subregions: DP, DQ, and DR. Each subregion expresses at least one α chain and one β chain. HLA class II molecules differ substantially from class I molecules in their tissue

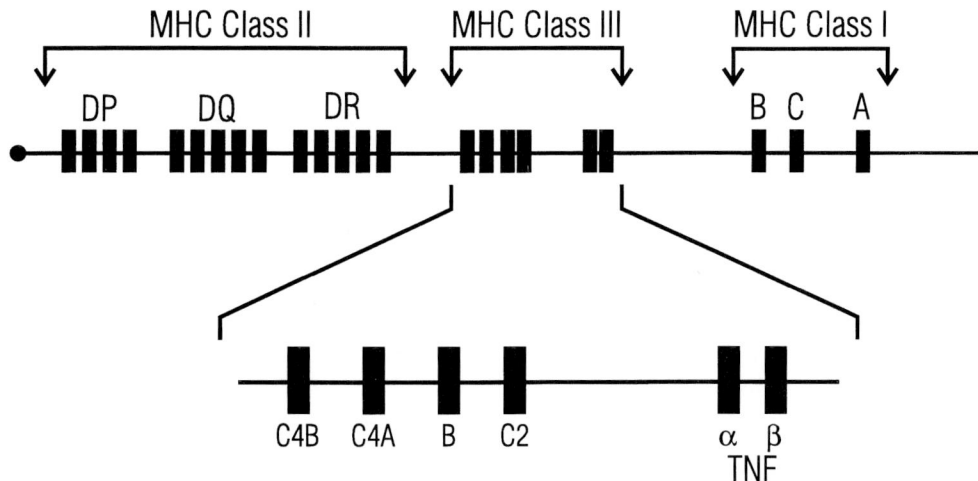

FIGURE 1–4. Molecular map of the human MHC chromosomal region. MHC genes lie on the short arm of chromosome 6 encompassing 3.5 megabases of DNA. In this depiction (not drawn to exact scale) the centromere is to the left. The class II region contains the subregions DP, DQ, and DR. The DP subregion contains four genes, two of which are expressed. The DQ and DR subregions each contain 5 genes, of which two are expressed in every haplotype. Depending on the haplotype, two additional genes in the DR subregion can code for expressed protein. The class III region contains the complement genes C2, C4, and factor B. Two genes encode functionally indistinguishable C4 proteins, C4A and C4B. The genes for the cytokines TNF-α and TNF-β also are found in this region. The class I genes include A, B, and C, which code for highly polymorphic proteins that associate with the $β_2$ macroglobulin, which is encoded on chromosome 15.

distribution. Class II markers are found on B cells, monocytes, and dendritic cells, as well as on activated T cells. Other cells such as endothelial cells can be induced to express class II molecules by interferon-γ. Class II molecules are composed of two subunits, α and β, which are both polymorphic and encoded at the MHC chromosomal region. As with class I molecules, there are four external domains in class II complexes. Two domains, $α_2$ and $β_2$, show homology to the Ig superfamily (Fig. 1–5B). Analogous to class I molecules, a primary function of class II cells is presentation of antigen to a specific group of lymphocytes, in this case $CD4^+$ T cells.

A patient's extended HLA haplotype describes the combination of alleles occurring within the entire HLA gene locus. Since these genes are in relatively close proximity to each other, they tend to be inherited as a block, with children receiving one extended haplotype from one parent and a different haplotype from the other parent. For bone marrow transplantation, this implies that siblings have a 25 percent chance of sharing identical MHC haplotypes. A second clinical implication is the association of rare extended haplotypes with disease. For example, common variable immunodeficiency has been associated with specific extended haplotypes (Volanakis et al, 1992). Whether these haplotypes predispose to disease in a manner analogous to classic HLA associations or whether they contain a disease-specific gene within the haplotype is unknown.

Immunoglobulin and T Cell Receptor Gene Rearrangement

The question of how immunoglobulin genes can code for the great diversity that they exhibit has been of tremendous interest over the past 30 years. The novel consideration that two genes could code for a single peptide has matured into theories concerning the mechanism of gain and loss of individual nucleotides at sites of greatest diversity. As discussed earlier, immunoglobulin consists of a heavy chain and a light chain. Both utilize somatic recombination of separated gene segments to generate biologic diversity. Although Ig heavy chain rearrangement takes place prior to light chain rearrangement during B cell maturation, light chain mechanisms will be discussed first because of their relative simplicity.

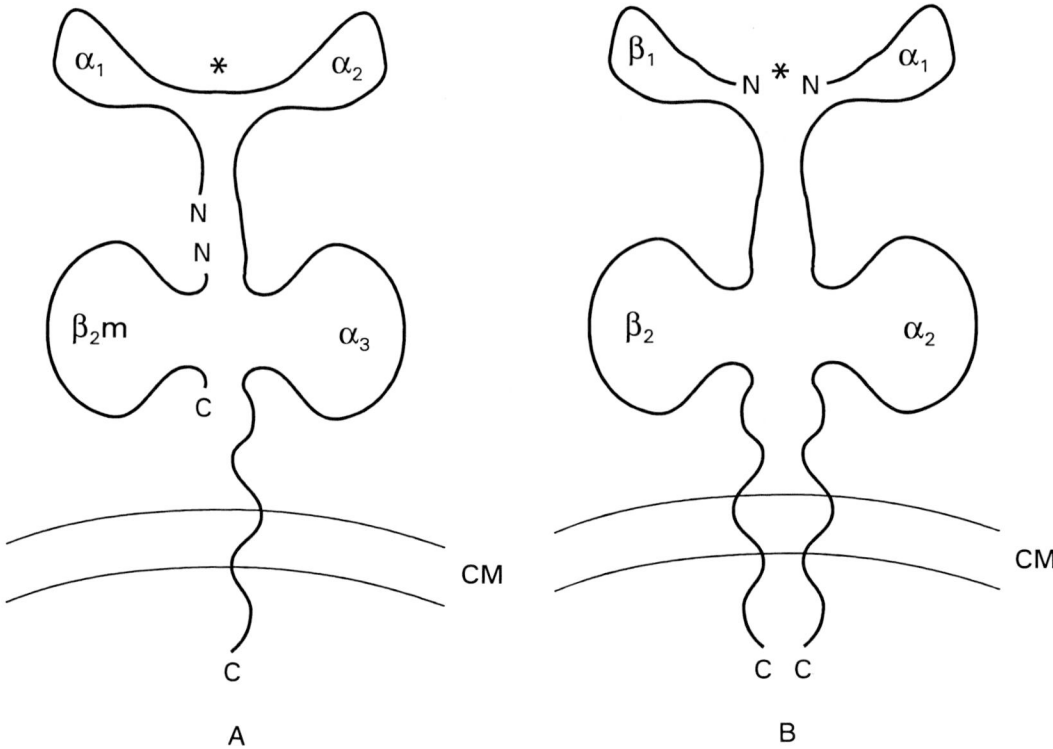

FIGURE 1–5. Schematic drawings of HLA class I and class II molecules. The carboxy (C) terminus of the heavy chain traverses the cell membrane (CM) and the amino (N) terminal portion forms the hypothetical antigen binding site (*). *A,* The polymorphic heavy chain of the class I molecule is represented by the three α domains, the transmembrane domain, and the cytoplasmic carboxy-terminal domain. The β_2-microglobulin (β_2-m) is positioned opposite the α_3 domain, both of which belong to the immunoglobulin supergene family. *B,* In the class II molecule, the α_1 and β_1 domains of the two non-covalently associated chains represent the polymorphic regions. The α_2 and β_2 domains belong to the immunoglobulin supergene family.

Recombination of the κ light chain is exemplified in Figure 1–6. Germline DNA contains a single constant (C) region with multiple alternative variable (V) and joining (J) regions. These regions are separated by long stretches of noncoding DNA (introns) which play a crucial role in recombination. Early in B cell development a variable region is brought together with a joining (J) region so that the intervening germline DNA, which can include coding regions as well as introns, is excised. The rearranged allele with the adjacent VJ segment is transcribed into RNA. Remaining introns are removed by splicing mechanisms, and the mature message contains the VJ segment flanked on one side by the constant (C) region of the light chain and on the other side by a leader (L) peptide, which permits transmembrane passage of the molecule. Only a single type of light chain can be produced by an individual B cell, a phenomenon known as isotope exclusion. Each cell contains two κ and two λ light chain genes. Rearrangement first occurs on a κ gene, and if successful, other rearrangements are blocked. If the first rearrangement is unproductive, another rearrangement takes place at another gene. Since κ genes are rearranged before λ genes, a κ-producing B cell has unarranged λ genes and a λ-producing B cell has deleted or unsuccessfully rearranged κ genes.

The genetic shuffle of immunoglobulin heavy chains functions at a higher level of complexity compared to light chain recombination. An additional family of genes, the diversity (D) segments, is located between the variable and joining region. Initial gene rearrangement results in adjacent VDJ segments followed by a constant region for each of the heavy chain classes and subclasses. Transcription at this stage is amenable to al-

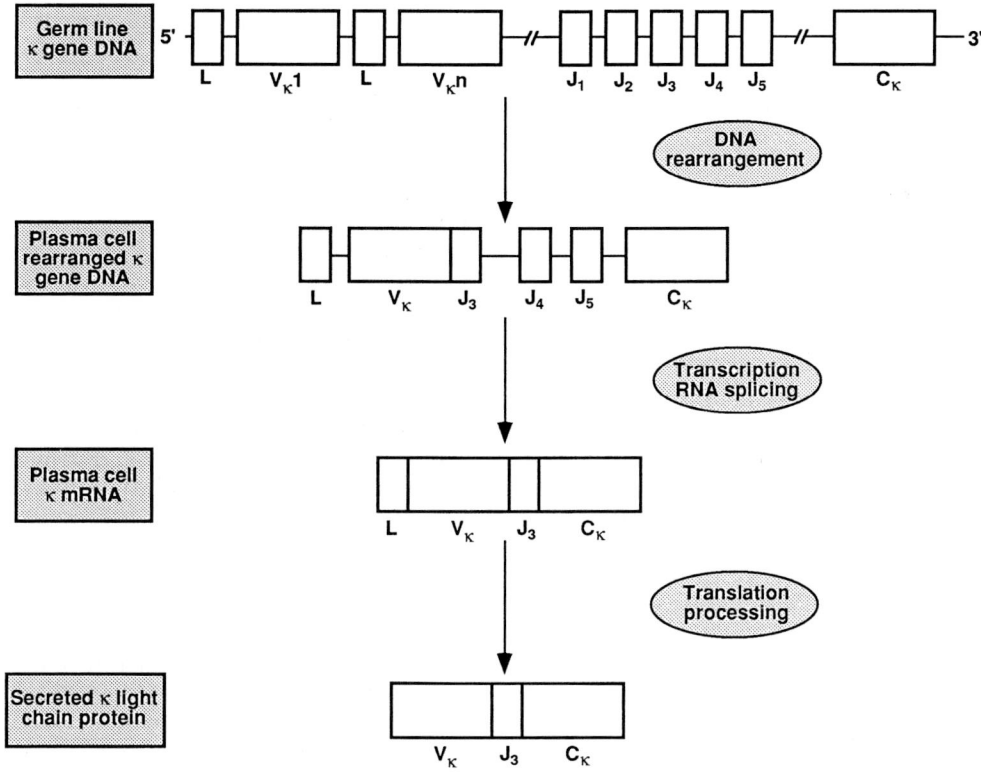

FIGURE 1–6. Immunoglobulin κ light chain recombination. Genomic DNA for the κ light chain contains multiple exons (boxes) with intervening sequences. Of the many potential variable (V) regions, one is brought into juxtaposition with one of the five joining (J) segments during gene rearrangement. Messenger RNA is subsequently transcribed and spliced to bring the VJ segment together with the single constant (C) region. The leader (L) segment is cleaved prior to secretion of the light chain. (Modified from Korsmeyer SJ. Immunoglobulin: proteins and genes. In Schwartz BD (ed). Immunology. Kalamazoo, The Upjohn Company, 1991.)

ternative splicing of messenger RNA to produce the IgM and IgD of the maturing B cell. The IgM and IgD have the same light chain and same VDJ segment of the heavy chain. They differ at the heavy chain constant region, C_μ for IgM and C_δ for IgD. Later in maturation, a second rearrangement of heavy chain DNA leads to deletion of segments coding for the C_μ and C_δ, and this results in positioning of the previously rearranged VDJ segments closer to alternative heavy chain constant regions. This second rearrangement, referred to as heavy chain class switch, is important for generating the appropriate antibody response to a variety of microbes that are susceptible to different effector mechanisms. Molecular studies have revealed that the CD40 molecule of B cells interacts with its ligand on T cells to enable this switch. An inability to make this switch is seen in children with X-linked hyper-IgM syndrome (Allen et al, 1993; Aruffo et al, 1993). Patients who lack the T cell ligand for CD40 are unable to complete B cell development and thus lack sufficient production of IgG and IgA, despite having elevated IgM levels.

The genetic rearrangements of TCR polymorphism employ many of the same principles as those discussed for Ig production. The TCR consists of two nonidentical chains, each containing Ig gene superfamily domains. Most T cells express α/β TCR and a smaller number express γ/δ TCR. As with immunoglobulin, each chain is derived from a selection of multiple genetic segments representing variable, diversity, and joining regions. Somatic gene rearrangements bring these VDJ segments into close proximity to the constant regions. Each TCR chain is encoded by a separate chromosomal locus. The β and λ genes are located on different arms of chromosome 7. Interestingly, the δ locus is located within the α gene on chromosome 14.

Diversity of Immune Response

Multiple mechanisms have been described that contribute to the vast diversity of immunoglobulin and TCR expression. At a first level, one chain of the heterodimeric molecule can pair with another member from the opposite family. For example, every Ig light chain could theoretically pair with any Ig heavy chain. Further diversity is provided by the multiple V, D, and J segments that exist for both Ig and TCR. This multiplicity allows for combinatorial associations that generate enormous variety. Immunoglobulin genes contain more V and D segments and fewer J segments than TCR genes. Both chains of the TCR and the immunoglobulin heavy chain exhibit variation in the genomic sequence at the VD, DJ, and VJ junctions. This sequence diversity arises as the result of random deletion and insertion of single nucleotides. The insertion of a few nucleotides without need for a template is catalyzed by terminal deoxynucleotidyl transferase (TdT).

A critical difference between immunoglobulin and TCR diversity is the existence of somatic mutation within the immunoglobulin genes. Frequent point mutations are noted in the assembled variable regions but not in the constant regions of immunoglobulin. It is hypothesized that somatic mutation is avoided in T cell diversity because such mutations would be potentially reactive against self antigens, leading to autoimmunity. Since B cells are under the control of T cells, somatic mutations of B cell genes may pose less threat of untoward self-destructive events. A second difference between Ig and TCR diversity involves the presence of isotope switching noted in Ig heavy chains. Such switching allows multiple secretory forms of Ig to exist. Lack of a switching mechanism in the TCR correlates with the absence of a secretory form.

CYTOKINES

Cytokines represent a diverse group of soluble proteins that play an important role in mediation and regulation of the immune response. Both general and specific inflammatory responses are influenced by cytokines. Additionally, cytokines act as growth factors for developing cells of the immune system. A key aspect of cytokine biology is that a single cytokine can be produced by multiple cell types and subsequently act on many different types of cells. In addition to this pleiotropism, cytokines can influence the synthesis of other cytokines. An overview of cytokines and their function is presented in Table 1–3. To simplify the presentation of these complex functions and interactions, three groups of cytokines will be discussed in the context of their primary effect: mediators of nonspecific inflammation, activators of lymphocytes, and hematopoietic growth factors.

Nonspecific Inflammatory Mediators

Three different classes of interferons (IFN-α, IFN-β, and IFN-γ) have been described, all of which inhibit cell growth in general and impair viral replication as a result. These interferons increase MHC class I expression and thereby enhance CD8$^+$ cytotoxic killing of virally infected cells. Interferons also activate natural killer cell activity. IFN-γ differs from the other interferons in its ability to induce MHC class II expression on a wide variety of cells. In contrast, IFN-α and IFN-β both inhibit MHC class II expression. A second distinguishing function of IFN-γ is the activation of macrophages, evidenced by increased gene transcription. The combined effect of IFN-γ on macrophages, increased MHC class II expression and activation, promotes the activity of CD4$^+$ helper cells.

Additional cytokines that mediate nonspecific immune response are tumor necrosis factor-α (TNF-α) and interleukin-1 (IL-1). The activated mononuclear phagocyte is the primary source for both cytokines. Both act as endogenous pyrogens in the face of infection and are key mediators of septic shock. Lipopolysaccharide (LPS) from gram-negative bacteria induces the secretion of both TNF-α and IL-1, with TNF-α playing a greater role through activation of phagocytes and B cells. TNF-α also is considered to be the principal mediator of the Schwartzman reaction, which describes the coagulation pathology associated with serial administration of LPS.

Another cytokine that mediates nonspecific

TABLE 1–3. IMMUNOLOGIC PROPERTIES OF CYTOKINES

Cytokine	Principle Cell Sources	Primary Type of Activity	Predominant Effects
IL-1	Macrophages and others	Immunoaugmentation	Inflammatory and hematopoietic; promotes B cell activation
IL-2	T lymphocytes	B and T cell growth factor	Activates T and NK cells; promotes B cell growth and Ig production
IL-3	T lymphocytes	Hematopoietic growth factor	Promotes growth of early myeloid progenitor cells, eosinophils, mast cells, and basophils
IL-4	T lymphocytes	B and T cell growth factor; promotes IgE switch; mast cell growth cofactor*	Promotes B cell activation and IgE switch; promotes T cell growth; synergizes with IL-3 for mast cell growth*
IL-5	T lymphocytes	Eosinophil growth factor; B and T cell growth factor*	Promotes eosinophil growth, terminal differentiation factor for B cell Ig production*; co-stimulant of T cell proliferation*
IL-6	Fibroblasts and others	Hybridoma growth factor; augments inflammation	Terminal differentiation factor for B cells and polyclonal Ig production; enhances IL-4 induced IgE production
IL-7	Stromal cells	Lymphopoietin	Promotes growth of pre-B and pre-T cells
IL-8	Macrophages and others	Chemoattractant for neutrophils and T lymphocytes	Regulates lymphocyte homing and neutrophil infiltration
IL-9	T lymphocytes	Erythroid precursor; T cell tumor; macrophage and mast cell growth factor	Maturation of erythroid progenitors; T cell tumor growth; synergizes with IL-3 for mast cell growth
IL-10	B lymphocytes T lymphocytes	Thymocyte proliferation; cytokine synthesis inhibitory factor	Synergizes with IL-2 and IL-4 for thymocyte growth; inhibits TH_1 function; inhibits macrophage function
IL-11	Stromal cells	Megakaryocyte and plasma cell growth factor	Enhances IL-3 effect for megakaryocytes; mitogenic for plasma cells
IL-12	B lymphocytes	Cytotoxic lymphocyte maturation factor	Synergizes with IL-2 for generation of CTL and LAK
IL-13	T lymphocytes	Monocyte activation; B cell proliferation	Directs B cell switching to IgE and IgG4; synergizes with IL-2 to regulate IFN-γ in LGL
IL-14	T lymphocytes	IL-4–like effects	Promotes B cell activation
IL-15	Not yet described	T cell proliferation	Promotes T cell activation
G-CSF	Monocytes and others	Neutrophil growth factor	Neutrophil proliferation
M-CSF	Monocytes and others	Monocyte growth factor	Macrophage proliferation
GM-CSF	T lymphocytes and others	Monomyelocytic growth factor	Myelopoiesis
IFN-α	Leukocytes	Antiviral; antiproliferative; immunomodulating	Inhibits viral replication; stimulates macrophages and NK cells
IFN-β	Fibroblasts	Antiviral; antiproliferative; immunomodulating	Inhibits viral replication; stimulates macrophages and NK cells
IFN-γ	T lymphocytes and LGL	Immunomodulating; antiproliferative; antiviral	Induces cell membrane antigens (e.g., MHC, FcR); enhances IL-2 effects; antagonizes IL-4 effects; enhances macrophage, CTL, and LGL effector function
TNF-α	Macrophages and others	Inflammatory; immunoenhancing and tumoricidal	Vascular thromboses and tumor necrosis
TNF-β	T lymphocytes	Inflammatory, immunoenhancing and tumoricidal	Vascular thromboses and tumor necrosis
TGF-β	T and B lymphocytes	Fibroplasma and immunosuppression	Wound healing and remodeling; broadly immunosuppressive but increases IgA production

Key: CTL = cytotoxic lymphocyte; FcR = receptor for crystallizing fragment of immunoglobulin; G-CSF = granulocyte colony-stimulating factor; GM-CSF = granulocyte-macrophage colony-stimulating factor; IFN = interferon; IL = interleukin; LAK = lymphokine-activated killer cells; LGL = large granular lymphocytes; M-CSF = monocyte colony-stimulating factor; MHC = major histocompatibility complex; TGF = transforming growth factor; TNF = tumor necrosis factor.
*Not shown for human cells.
Modified from Shearer WT, Huston DP. The immune system: An overview. *In* Middleton E, et al (eds). Allergy Principles and Practice. 4th ed. St. Louis, Missouri, Mosby-Year Book, Inc., 1993, pp 3–21.

inflammatory responses is TNF-β (sometimes referred to as lymphotoxin). Similarities to TNF-α include a 30 percent genetic homology and gene localization in the MHC on chromosome 6 in tandem with TNF-α. Although the biologic effects of TNF-α and TNF-β are similar, two important differences exist. TNF-β is produced exclusively by T cells, whereas only a minor fraction of TNF-α derives from T cells. A second difference is that TNF-β is a secretory protein without a transmembrane domain. TNF-α is synthesized as a transmembrane protein that can be cleaved at the cell surface and form a homotrimer in the circulation.

In response to IL-1 and TNF-α, mononuclear phagocytes and endothelial cells can produce interleukin-6 (IL-6). IL-6 is the principal mediator of the acute phase response, a rapid change in plasma protein levels coordinated by hepatocytes. For example, C-reactive protein levels rise while albumin protein decreases in concentration. Additionally, IL-6 functions as a primary stimulus for terminal differentiation of B cells. As does IL-6, interleukin-5 (IL-5) also mediates general inflammatory responses and promotes B cell growth and differentiation. However, the most critical function of IL-5 is the activation of eosinophils and the resulting increased killing of helminths.

Lymphocyte Activators

Interleukin-2 (IL-2), initially called T cell growth factor, is a major regulator of T cell growth. It is produced by T cells, a greater quantity being derived from $CD4^+$ cells than from $CD8^+$ cells. IL-2 acts both in an autocrine fashion, stimulating the same cell that produced it, and in a paracrine manner, stimulating nearby T cells. IL-2 is also a potent stimulator for large granular lymphocytes and B cells. The central importance of IL-2 is underscored by recent studies of children with severe combined immunodeficiency characterized by a profound lack of T cells. A small subset of these patients have been identified to have defective IL-2 production (Pahwa et al, 1989). Other patients have been shown to have a mutation in the IL-2 receptor (Noguchi et al, 1993). These studies strongly suggest that the IL-2/IL-2 receptor system is critical for thymocyte maturation. Another critical cytokine produced by $CD4^+$ lymphocytes is interleukin-4 (IL-4), which acts as an important growth factor for B cells. Other important functions of IL-4 include mast cell stimulation (along with IL-3) and macrophage activation. Recent studies have implicated IL-13 as a significant B cell activator (Minty et al, 1993; Punnonen et al, 1993). Its role in promoting B cell switching to IgG4 and IgE production should prove to be of great interest to the field of allergy.

The role of cytokines in immune regulation is well exemplified by transforming growth factor-β (TGF-β). This cytokine was originally described by tumor biologists, and its name reflects their early studies more than it describes its immunologic significance. TGF-β acts primarily to antagonize lymphocyte response and thus serves as a negative regulator. Mice with a mutation that inactivates the TGF-β gene are unable to produce TGF-β and die in the first weeks of life with a generalized chronic inflammatory response (Shull et al, 1992).

Hematopoietic Growth Factors

As stated earlier, immune cells originate in the bone marrow. Cytokines that influence the early development of these immune cells are of obvious importance. In analogous fashion, interleukin-3 (IL-3) and interleukin-7 (IL-7) promote the growth of early myeloid and lymphoid stem cells, respectively. Acting further downstream in the maturation process is granulocyte-macrophage colony-stimulating factor (GM-CSF). Myeloid cells already committed to the leukocyte lineage are stimulated by GM-CSF to differentiate into granulocytes and mononuclear phagocytes. Further development is promoted by monocyte colony-stimulating factor (M-CSF) and granulocyte colony-stimulating factor (G-CSF).

COMPLEMENT

Serum complement was first described in the nineteenth century as the fraction of serum that could be inactivated by heat. Nearly one hundred years later and after the description of more than 25 component proteins, the complexity of nomenclature often obscures the vital role complement plays in natural immunity. The primary source of complement is the liver, with smaller contributions made by monocytes and fibroblasts. From a simplistic viewpoint, complement is an independent humoral immune system that protects the host from infection. Often it acts in concert with the other humoral system, antibody, to promote both physical clearance of pathogens and nonspecific inflammation. Clearance is achieved by direct lysis and by opsonization. Opsonization refers to the process of coating a foreign membrane with complement proteins that allow other cellular components to easily ingest the pathogen. Anaphylatoxins and chemotactic factors derived from complement proteins mediate nonspecific inflammation. Anaphylatoxins can trigger the release of histamine from eosinophils and mast cells, promoting easy entry of inflammatory cells from the blood stream to the tissue compartment. Chemotactic factors attract nonspecific inflammatory cells to sites of complement activation.

Two distinct avenues have been described for initiating complement activity. The classical pathway requires existing antibody capable of activating complement, notably IgM and most subclasses of IgG. The so-called alternative pathway directs complement function in the absence of existing antibody, thus providing early immune protection for the naive host. Although these pathways differ in their utilization of C3 and production of C5 convertase, a convergence occurs at the level of generation of opsonins and chemotactic factors as well as formation of the membrane attack complex (MAC) (Fig. 1-7).

Classical Pathway

The link between the humoral immune system and complement is provided by the Fc portion of the antigen-bound immunoglobulin molecule. The C1 complex is activated when one of its components, C1q, binds to antibody. Activated C1 permits sequential activation of C4 and C2 to produce the enzyme complex C4b2a on the antigen surface. C4b2a acts as C3 convertase. Splitting of C3 results in C3a, a potent anaphylatoxin, and C3b, an important opsonin. Opsonic C3b permits the involvement of phagocytes in the killing process. A secondary function of C3b is an interaction with C4b2a to form a C5 convertase that can produce C5a and C5b. As is C3a, C5a is released into the fluid phase to act as an anaphylatoxin and chemotactic factor. C5b remains on the membrane surface where it can recruit C6, C7, C8, and C9 in forming the MAC, which has lytic capability. From a quantitative standpoint, it is important to note that C3b is generated in much greater quantity than the other complement products.

Alternative Pathway

Complement component C3 also plays a critical role in the alternative pathway. C3 is joined by factor B, factor D, and properdin. In the absence of specific antibodies, foreign membranes are coated with C3b. The source of the initial C3b is unclear, perhaps being generated at a continuous low level. Serum factors B and D join C3b on the surface membrane and are stabilized by properdin. The resulting C3bBb acts as C3 convertase in a manner similar to that of C4b2a in the classical pathway. Production of opsonins, anaphylatoxins, and chemotactic factors including C3b, C3a, and C5a, as well as generation of the lytic MAC, can all result from activation of the alternative pathway.

SUMMARY

Reviewing the multiple, complex components of the normal human immune response inevitably leads to the conclusion that the system is designed for host survival through several interlocking mechanisms of distinguishing self from nonself. Although immune reactions against nonself antigens are the basis of protective responses, a too vigorous response may result in clinical symptoms of allergy. Analogously, reactions against self antigens are seen in the clinical arena as autoimmune reactions. T lymphocytes developing in the thymus are selected for survival based on their ability to distinguish self antigens from nonself antigens. Cells that are not reactive to self antigens may progress to become mature T lymphocytes, which can exert a lifelong protective effect. Cells that react to self antigens fail to mature and possibly undergo apoptosis, a mechanism of controlled cell death. In addition to independent functions, T cells strongly influence the antibody component of the immune system. B lymphocyte production of efficient antibodies requires T cell assistance, and T cell dysfunction can precede B cell production of autoantibodies. Another limb of the immune response, the complement cascade, acts in concert with

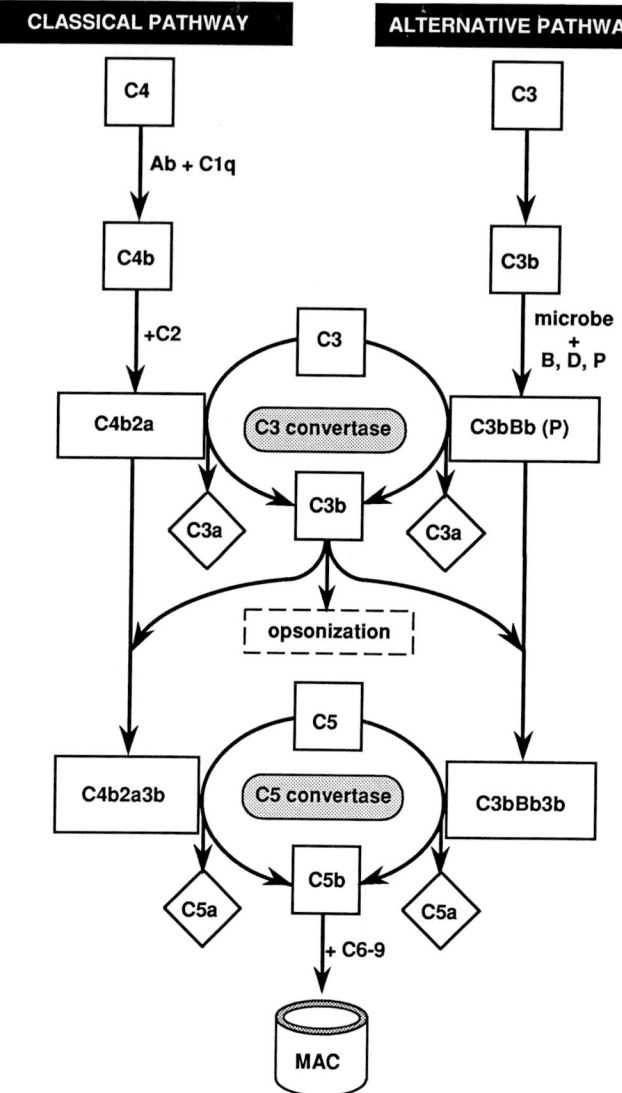

FIGURE 1–7. Comparison of classical and alternative pathways of complement. A major function of both pathways is generation of C3b, an important opsonin, and production of the membrane attack complex (MAC). These common goals are achieved by different routes of initiation and differing mechanisms for conversion of C3 and C5. The alternative pathway is initiated by any mechanism that increases the rate of C3b production or reduces the rate of C3b breakdown, such as the presence of microorganisms. The classical pathway initiates with the interaction of preexisting antibody (Ab) and C1q to facilitate the subsequent cleavage of C4. The alternative pathway C3 convertase forms through the interaction of C3b, factor B (B), and factor D (D). The resulting C3bBb, stabilized by properdin (P), converts C3 to C3b, which can act as an opsonin or contribute to the C5 convertase (C3bBb3b). The classical pathway utilizes C4b2a to convert C3 to C3b, which subsequently participates in the C5 convertase (C4b2a3b). Production of C5b by either C5 convertase allows progression to the lytic pathway where C6, C7, C8, and C9 participate in the generation of the MAC. In the course of both pathways, cleavage of C3 and C5 generates C3a and C5a (◊) which possess anaphylatoxin activity.

antibodies to facilitate their protective response. Complement is also capable of reacting directly to nonself antigens, such as the polysaccharide wall of microorganisms, through activation of the alternative pathway. Added to these well-known themes of host protection and the ability to discriminate between self and nonself antigens is new knowledge of intra- and intercellular signal molecules, cytokines, interleukins, and cellular growth factors. An understanding of the fields of signal transduction and the molecular biology of the cells of the immune system will lead to a much better comprehension of precisely how these protective arms of immunity function. A careful study of the normal immune response can lead to a greater appreciation of the extraordinary diversity of this system, which enables us to survive in a hostile environment.

REFERENCES

Allen RC, Armitage RJ, Conley ME, Rosenblatt HM, Jenkins NA, Copeland NG, Bedell MA, Edelhoff S, Disteche CM, Simoneaux DK, et al. CD40 ligand gene defects responsible for X-linked hyper-IgM syndrome. Science 259:990–993, 1993.

Aruffo A, Farrington M, Hollenbaugh D, Li X, Milatovich A, Nonoyama S, Bajorath J, Grosmaire LS, Stenkamp R, Neubauer M, et al. The CD40 ligand, gp39, is defective in activated T cells from patients with X-linked hyper-IgM syndrome. Cell 72:291–300, 1993.

Awata T, Kuzuya T, Matsuda A, Iwamoto Y, Kanazawa Y, Okuyama M, Juji T. High frequency of aspartic acid at position 57 of HLA-DQ beta-chain in Japanese IDDM patients and nondiabetic subjects. Diabetes 39:266–269, 1990.

Blackman M, Kappler J, Marrack P. The role of the T cell receptor in positive and negative selection of developing T cells. Science 248:1335–1341, 1990.

Campbell KS, Cambier JC. B lymphocyte antigen receptors (mIg) are non-covalently associated with a disulfide linked, inducibly phosphorylated glycoprotein complex. EMBO J 9:441–448, 1990.

Chan SH, Cosgrove D, Waltzinger C, Benoist C, Mathis D. Another view of the selective model of thymocyte selection. Cell 73:225–236, 1993.

Davis CB, Killeen N, Crooks ME, Raulet D, Littman DR. Evidence for a stochastic mechanism in the differentiation of mature subsets of T lymphocytes. Cell 73:237–247, 1993.

Del Prete GF, De Carli M, Mastromauro C, Biagiotti R, Macchia D, Falagiani P, Ricci M, Romagnani S. Purified protein derivative of *Mycobacterium tuberculosis* and excretory-secretory antigen(s) of *Toxocara canis* expand in vitro human T cells with stable and opposite (type 1 T helper or type 2 T helper) profile of cytokine production. J Clin Invest 88:346–350, 1991.

Gray JD, Horwitz DA. Lymphocytes expressing type 3 complement receptors proliferate in response to interleukin 2 and are the precursors of lymphokine-activated killer cells. J Clin Invest 81:1247–1254, 1988.

Lieber MR. The mechanism of V(D)J recombination: a balance of diversity, specificity, and stability. Cell 70:873–876, 1992.

Linsley PS, Clark EA, Ledbetter JA. T-cell antigen CD28 mediates adhesion with B cells by interacting with activation antigen B7/BB-1. Proc Natl Acad Sci USA 87:5031–5035, 1990.

Minty A, Chalon P, Derocq JM, Dumont X, Guillemot JC, Kaghad M, Labit C, Leplatois P, Liauzun P, Miloux B, et al. Interleukin-13 is a new human lymphokine regulating inflammatory and immune responses. Nature 362:248–250, 1993.

Noguchi M, Yi H, Rosenblatt HM, Filipovich AH, Adelstein S, Modi WS, McBride OW, Leonard WJ. Interleukin-2 receptor gamma chain mutation results in X-linked severe combined immunodeficiency in humans. Cell 73:147–157, 1993.

Pahwa R, Chatila T, Pahwa S, Paradise C, Day NK, Geha R, Schwartz SA, Slade H, Oyaizu N, Good RA. Recombinant interleukin-2 therapy in severe combined immunodeficiency disease. Proc Natl Acad Sci USA 86:5069–5073, 1989.

Punnonen J, Aversa G, Cocks BG, McKenzie AN, Menon S, Zurawski G, de Waal Malefyt R, de Vries JE. Interleukin-13 induces interleukin-4-independent IgG4 and IgE synthesis and CD23 expression by human B cells. Proc Natl Acad Sci USA 90:3730–3734, 1993.

Shull MM, Ormsby I, Kier AB, Pawlowski S, Diebold RJ, Yin M, Allen R, Sidman C, Proetzel G, Calvin D, et al. Targeted disruption of the mouse transforming growth factor-beta 1 gene results in multifocal inflammatory disease. Nature 359:693–699, 1992.

Todd JA, Bell JI, McDevitt HO. HLA-DQ beta gene contributes to susceptibility and resistance to insulin-dependent diabetes mellitus. Nature 329:599–604, 1987.

Tsukada S, Saffran DC, Rawlings DJ, Parolini O, Allen RC, Klisak I, Sparkes RS, Kubagawa H, Mohandas T, Quan S, et al. Deficient expression of a B cell cytoplasmic tyrosine kinase in human X-linked agammaglobulinemia. Cell 72:279–290, 1993.

Volanakis JE, Zhu ZB, Schaffer FM, Macon KJ, Palermos J, Barger BO, Go R, Campbell RD, Schroeder HW, Jr., Cooper MD. Major histocompatibility complex class III genes and susceptibility to immunoglobulin A deficiency and common variable immunodeficiency. J Clin Invest 89:1914–1922, 1992.

Wienands J, Hombach J, Radbruch A, Riesterer C, Reth M. Molecular components of the B cell antigen receptor complex of class IgD differ partly from those of IgM. EMBO J 9:449–455, 1990.

Wierenga EA, Snoek M, Bos JD, Jansen HM, Kapsenberg ML. Comparison of diversity and function of house dust mite-specific T lymphocyte clones from atopic and non-atopic donors. Eur J Immunol 20:1519–1526, 1990a.

Wierenga EA, Snoek M, deGroot C, Chrétien I, Bos JD, Jansen HM, Kapsenberg ML. Evidence for compartmentalization of functional subsets of $CD2^+$ T lymphocytes in atopic patients. J Immunol 144:4651–4656, 1990b.

Yewdell JW, Bennink JR. Cell biology of antigen processing and presentation to major histocompatibility complex class I molecule-restricted T lymphocytes. Adv Immunol 52:1–123, 1992.

Chapter 2

Primary and Secondary Immunodeficiency Diseases

Richard I. Schiff, M.D., Ph.D., and Terry O. Harville, M.D., Ph.D.

Patients with immunodeficiency diseases may present with recurrent or persistent infections, especially with opportunistic organisms, or with a bewildering variety of autoimmune and inflammatory conditions. Although the final classification of the particular immunodeficiency disease usually requires referral to a specialist in such disorders, it is the physician in primary care who must recognize the signs and symptoms of immune dysregulation and identify the patient who needs further evaluation. Many of these diseases can be effectively treated, and others may be cured by bone marrow transplantation, but a successful outcome requires early recognition and treatment before permanent tissue damage or severe, untreatable infections occur.

CONGENITAL IMMUNODEFICIENCY DISEASES

The first human immunodeficiency disease was reported nearly 40 years ago by Colonel Ogden Bruton, who recognized that a child with recurrent infections lacked the recently identified gamma globulin fraction in his serum. Since then, a wide variety of congenital immunodeficiency diseases have been described; however, we understand the underlying biologic defect at the molecular level for only two defects of the purine salvage pathway. Nonetheless, evaluation of these experiments of nature has provided us with invaluable information to help us understand the normal function of the immune system.

Genetically determined immunodeficiency diseases are rare. It has been estimated that hypogammaglobulinemia occurs with a frequency of 1:50,000 and severe combined immunodeficiency (SCID) with a frequency of 1:500,000 live births. The most common immune deficiency, selective IgA deficiency, has a reported incidence of 1:300 to 1:3000, depending on the population studied. The incidence of many of these diseases may be much higher; many of the children die of infections before immune deficiency is suspected. Early recognition is vital, for many of these diseases can be treated by replacement immunoglobulin or cytokines, or they may be cured by bone marrow transplantation.

Classification of Primary Immunodeficiency Diseases

The most recent classification of the primary immunodeficiency diseases was proposed by a Committee of the World Health Organization in 1989 (WHO Scientific Group, 1992). The classification (Table 2–1) is based on the clinical and immunologic evaluation of patients and undoubtedly will change as the genetic abnormality for each is identified. Our concept of the organization of the lymphocyte-mediated immune system was developed from studies in animals. The loss of delayed hypersensitivity reactions and other so-called cellular immune functions with the

TABLE 2-1. DISORDERS OF HUMORAL AND CELLULAR IMMUNITY

Disorder	Functional Deficiency	Cellular or Genetic Defect
Predominantly Antibody Defects		
X-linked agammaglobulinemia	Absent antibody	Bruton tyrosine kinase deficiency
X-linked agammaglobulinemia with hyper-IgM	Antibody deficiency Low IgA and IgG	Defect in CD40 ligand on T cells (majority of patients)
Common variable immunodeficiency	Poor antibody formation Autoimmunity	Unknown; variable defects in B cells, T helper, or excessive T suppressor cells
Antibody deficiency with normal immunoglobulins		
IgG subclass deficiency	May be associated with antibody deficiency	Unknown; may be a defect in antigen processing, switch T cells, or switch region in heavy chain
Poor response to polysaccharide antigens	Antibody deficiency	Unknown; possibly defect in antigen processing
Selective IgA deficiency	IgA antibody deficiency Allergy, autoimmunity	Possible switch defect, possible abnormal switch T cells
Transient hypogammaglobulinemia of infancy	Prolonged physiologic trough; usually no antibody deficiency	Unknown; slow maturation of B and T lymphocytes
X-linked lymphoproliferative syndrome	Abnormal response to Epstein-Barr virus, immune deficiency, malignancy	Unknown; abnormal regulation of B cell activation
Immunodeficiency with thymoma	Antibody deficiency	Unknown; possible excessive T cell suppression
Primary Defect in Cellular Immunity–Combined Immunodeficiency		
Thymic hypoplasia (DiGeorge anomaly)	Variable T and (secondary) B cell defects	Developmental field defect Often associated with deletion on chromosome 22q11
Severe combined immune deficiency		
X-linked	Severe B and T cell defects	Defect in γ-chain of the IL-2 receptor
Autosomal recessive	Severe B and T cell defects	Unknown, variable(?)
Adenosine deaminase deficiency	Severe B and T cell defects	Deletions or base substitutions in ADA gene
Defective expression of HLA antigens	Severe B and T cell defects	Absent expression of class I or II antigens; genetic defect unknown
Deficiency of T cell receptors	Variable B and T cell defects	Defective expression of CD3ε
Cellular immunodeficiency with immunoglobulins (Nezelof syndrome)	Severe T cell, variable B cell defects; autoimmune disease	Unknown; variable
PNP deficiency	Severe T cell, variable B cell defects; autoimmune disease	Defect in gene for purine nucleoside phosphorylase
Omenn syndrome	Variable T cell and antibody defects; "GVH-like" syndrome	Unknown; possible T regulatory defects
Immune Deficiency Associated with Other Defects		
Wiskott-Aldrich syndrome	Variable T cell defect; poor antibody response to antigens, thrombocytopenia, malignancy	Defect in CD43 expression Gene identified on X-chromosome but not yet characterized
Chronic mucocutaneous candidiasis	Specific defect in T cell function, possible defect in antigen processing	Unknown; possible defect in processing of mannan
Hyper-IgE syndrome	Excessive IgE; poor specific antibody responses	Unknown; possible defect in T cell regulation; possible overexpression of IL-4
Ataxia-telangiectasia	Variable T and B cell defect; malignancy	Unknown; defect in DNA repair involving many cells
Cartilage-hair hypoplasia	Moderate to severe T and B cell defect	Unknown; defect in G1 cycle of many cells, including lymphoid

removal of the thymus in mice led to the identification of the thymus-derived or T lymphocyte. Similarly, studies in chickens indicated that removal of the bursa of Fabricius led to a selective defect in antibody formation due to loss of bursal or B lymphocytes. Although this concept has been immensely useful, there are few examples of a pure defect in human disease. The pattern of human disease does differ, however, depending on whether the primary defect affects the T cells, B cells, phagocytic cells, or complement system.

Infections in Patients with Immunodeficiency Diseases

For the most part, susceptibility to infections in patients with immunodeficiency diseases has a specific cause depending on the nature of the immune deficiency; however, important exceptions exist. Patients with antibody deficiency most commonly suffer from purulent bacterial infections, including pneumonia, meningitis, arthritis, sinusitis, otitis, conjunctivitis, and gastroenteritis. These infections are most frequently caused by encapsulated organisms such as *Haemophilus influenzae* and *Streptococcus pneumoniae*, but other organisms, including *Staphylococcus aureus, Meningococcus, Pseudomonas, Campylobacter, Ureaplasma,* and *Mycoplasma*, are commonly isolated. Most viral infections are adequately controlled, but several viruses can result in devastating consequences. Poliomyelitis, often secondary to live virus vaccine, results in several cases of paralytic disease each year. Viral hepatitis, particularly with hepatitis C, is particularly severe in patients with agammaglobulinemia. Another important exception is chronic meningoencephalitis caused by ECHO and Coxsackie enteroviruses, which occurs primarily in patients with X-linked agammaglobulinemia but has also occurred in a few patients with other forms of agammaglobulinemia. Some protozoal infections, notably *Giardia lamblia*, cause significant difficulty for patients with humoral immunodeficiency, and *Pneumocystis carinii* occasionally occurs despite apparently normal T cell function.

Patients with T cell immunodeficiency are susceptible to a variety of opportunistic organisms. Growth failure and early death are more common than in patients with humoral immunodeficiency. Oral and cutaneous candidiasis is common, and disseminated infections with *Candida* species, *Cryptococcus, Histoplasma,* and *Nocardia* occur frequently. Protozoal infections, particularly with *P. carinii*, are a frequent cause of death unless recognized and rapidly treated. *Toxoplasma* can cause chronic infections leading to blindness, and *Cryptosporidium* is a common cause of chronic diarrhea. T cell immunity is particularly important for defense against a variety of viral infections, especially the herpesviruses, cytomegalovirus (CMV), herpes simplex, and varicella-zoster. The respiratory viruses—adenovirus, parainfluenza, and respiratory syncytial virus—often cause a fulminant pneumonia and may disseminate throughout the body. Bacterial infections with both pathogenic and nonpathogenic organisms are also a significant problem, probably because nearly all patients have associated deficiency in antibody formation; however, atypical organisms such as *Mycobacterium tuberculosis* and *intracellulare,* and *Listeria monocytogenes* cause infections primarily in those patients with cellular immunodeficiencies.

Defects in the phagocytic system or complement result in increased susceptibility to bacterial and fungal infections. Decreased cell number results in sepsis or disseminated infections with a variety of gram-negative and gram-positive bacteria and fungi such as *Candida albicans* and *Aspergillus*. Defective function, as in chronic granulomatous disease, can result in granulomatous lesions or abscesses. Absence of the early complement components results in susceptibility to gram-positive bacteria, whereas the lack of the late components leads to a high incidence of neisserial infections.

Immunodeficiency Diseases with Primary Defect in Humoral Immunity

Defects in this category include a primary defect in the ability to make immunoglobulins or to make specific antibodies, but some are associated with T cell defects as well. The genetic defect has been identified for X-linked agammaglobulinemia and X-linked hyperimmunoglobulinemia-M (hyper-IgM) syndrome and may eventually lead to correction by gene therapy.

X-linked Agammaglobulinemia (XAG)

Boys afflicted with this disorder usually present after the sixth month of life, after the transplacentally derived IgG has been catabolized. They acquire pyogenic infections with high-grade bacteria such as pneumococci, *Haemophilus,* and streptococci. Unusual organisms may be seen as well, such as *Ureaplasma urealyticum,* which causes an erosive septic arthritis. Infections of the sinopulmonary tract predominate, including sinusitis, pharyngitis, otitis, bronchitis, and pneumonia, but others such as furunculosis, arthritis, and meningitis frequently occur. Growth failure is not a common problem unless chronic diarrhea is present, often as a result of infection with *G. lamblia*. Most viral infections are handled as well as in normal hosts, but a few can lead to devastating illness. Poliovirus, either live or vaccine strain, can cause paralytic disease; nearly all cases of vaccine-related paralytic poliomyolitis occur in patients with immunodeficiency. Children excrete the virus in the stool for weeks to months after immunization, which increases the opportunity for the virus to mutate to a more neurotropic form. The hepatitis viruses can lead to severe, even fatal, chronic active hepatitis. Enteroviruses of the ECHO and Coxsackie families can cause a chronic meningoencephalitis (McKinney et al, 1987). The CNS disease is chronic and often leads to progressive neurologic deterioration despite high doses of intravenous gamma globulin. Some patients have improved when gamma globulin has been infused directly into the cerebral ventricles, but the disease can never be totally cured. Patients may also develop a dermatomyositis-like illness and progress to sclerodermatous changes with atrophic skin and joint contractures. The disease is almost exclusively confined to patients with XAG, although a few females lacking B lymphocytes and others with forms of common variable immunodeficiency have also contracted this illness.

Patients with XAG have a nearly complete absence of immunoglobulins of all isotypes, although small amounts of IgM may be present. Isohemagglutinins are absent, and there is no response to immunizations with a wide variety of antigens, including tetanus and diphtheria, *H. influenzae, S. pneumoniae*, poliomyelitis, measles, or bacteriophage ΦX-174. A few exceptional families have been described who have immunoglobulins and even some specific antibody early in life, but progress to typical XAG within a few years. The mechanism of this "late onset" illness is not known, but provides a cautionary note when evaluating young infants; longitudinal follow-up is crucial for all infants suspected of having immunodeficiency.

The most characteristic immunologic finding is the nearly complete absence of B lymphocytes as detected by surface immunoglobulins or surface receptors CD21 (EBV receptor), CD19, or CD20. No germinal centers can be identified upon histologic examination of lymph nodes or tonsils, which accounts for the absence of these structures on physical examination. T cell percentages are increased as a result of the loss of B cells; T cell activity is usually normal and thymic architecture is intact.

X-linked Immunodeficiency with Hyper-IgM

Patients with hyper-IgM have a clinical presentation similar to those with X-linked agammaglobulinemia. They present within the first few months of life with pyogenic infections including pneumonia, otitis, sinusitis, and pharyngitis. *P. carinii* pneumonia has also been reported. In fact, distinguishing the two diseases may be difficult, particularly in the young child, since the IgM concentrations may initially be normal or even low. However, unlike XAG, patients with hyper-IgM often have lymphoid hypertrophy. Autoimmune hematologic diseases including hemolytic anemia, thrombocytopenia, and cyclic or persistent neutropenia are frequent. Although an X-linked mode of inheritance can be identified in most patients, a few females have been reported with a similar clinical picture.

IgG and IgA concentrations in serum are usually extremely low, and antibody responses are absent. IgM concentrations can be normal to markedly elevated, usually with a polyclonal pattern. T lymphocyte numbers and function seem to be normal and B cell numbers may be normal or slightly reduced. Patients' B cells stimulated with polyclonal activators such as EBV synthesize only IgM, which is similar to the immature B cell of the neonate. Recently, an abnormality was identified in the ligand for CD40 (gp 39), normally found on T cells, that interact with CD40 on B cells. If B cells from those patients are stimulated with anti-CD40 they produce immunoglobulins normally. Not every patient has had an abnormal CD40 ligand and the presence of females with the hyper-IgM phenotype indicates that there is more than one genetic cause.

Common Variable Immune Deficiency (CVID)

CVID represents a variety of immune defects that undoubtedly have different genetic origins (Cunningham-Rundles, 1989). The onset can be early in infancy, like that of XAG, or the disease may present later in life. In a few patients the evolution of the immunodeficiency has been documented, often first with a decrease in the ability to form specific antibodies and later a decline in immunoglobulin concentrations. The spectrum and severity of infections is similar to that of patients with XAG except that ECHO virus meningoencephalitis is uncommon. On physical examination lymphoid tissue is present and may be increased, with lymphadenopathy, enlarged tonsils, nodular lymphoid hyperplasia of the intestine, and splenomegaly. Some patients have had an intersitital pneumonitis due to B cell hyperplasia. This nonmalignant condition resolves once gamma globulin therapy is initiated.

CVID is more complex than XAG, with a high incidence of autoimmune disorders that may dominate the clinical picture. Nearly every organ system can be involved. Hematologic disorders include hemolytic anemia, thrombocytopenia, and neutropenia. Alopecia areata and vitiligo are not uncommon, and the incidence of other skin diseases such as warts is increased. Autoimmune endocrine disorders and collagen vascular disease, with rheumatoid arthritis, sicca syndrome, and systemic lupus erythematosus are all seen with increased incidences. Gastrointestinal disorders are common, including a sprue-like syndrome, with or without lymphoid hyperplasia, atrophic gastritis, achlorhydria, and pernicious anemia. Bowel infections with unusual organisms such as *Giardia* and *Helicobacter pylori* and *jejuni* are frequent and resistant to therapy. Malignancy is also common, with non-Hodgkin's lymphoma, gastric carcinoma, and a variety of carcinomas of the skin and genital tract predominating. In a series of 103 adult and pediatric patients observed for 1 to 13 years by Charlotte Cunningham-Rundles, 22 percent developed chronic lung disease, 22 percent autoimmune disease, 15 percent cancer, 13 percent hepatitis, and 9 percent malabsorption.

The immune defect varies in its severity, but all patients have a marked reduction in serum immunoglobulin concentrations and poor responses to specific antigens. B lymphocytes can be present in the peripheral blood in normal numbers. B cells taken from some patients are capable of proliferating and secreting IgM when stimulated with the polyclonal activator pokeweed mitogen or EBV. T cell activity, including T cell help, is normal in most patients with CVID. However, a subset have a significant defect in cellular immunity, suggestive of Nezelof's syndrome (discussed below), although immunoglobulin concentrations are low rather than elevated. In some patients, mostly adults, a very potent T suppressor cell has been identified. However, most patients have an intrinsic B cell disorder.

Antibody Deficiency with Normal Immunoglobulin Concentrations

Patients have been described who have normal serum immunoglobulin concentrations but poor specific antibody titers to a variety of antigens, including tetanus and diphtheria, blood group substances, and pneumococcal polysaccharide. Primary responses to bacteriophage ΦX-174 are also far below normal. In some patients abnormalities of IgG subclasses are present, but the critical abnormality is the inability to respond to antigen challenge. Despite the normal immunoglobulin concentrations, these patients should be treated with intravenous gamma globulin if they cannot produce functional antibody.

IgG Subclass Deficiency

Selective deficiency of IgG subclasses in patients with normal total IgG concentrations was described in 1968. Within a few years there were numerous reports of an association of frequent infections, primarily of the sinopulmonary tract, with a deficiency of one or more IgG subclasses (Aucouturier et al, 1989; Preud'Homme and Hanson, 1990). Nearly every combination of subclass deficiency has been described, but some appear to be more relevant than others. Deficiency of IgG2 with or without concurrent IgA deficiency seems to have the greatest association with recurrent infections. Heiner described several patients with complete absence of IgG4 who developed recurrent sinusitis and pneumonia that often progressed to bronchiectasis. Deficiency of IgG1 was associated with pyogenic infections of the lung, and IgG3 deficiency with recurrent respiratory infections and viral infections of the urinary tract. Other disorders have been associated with a variety of subclass deficiencies. Juvenile diabetes is associated with IgG2,3 deficiency, idiopathic thrombocytopenic purpura and systemic lupus with decreased IgG2 and absent IgG4, childhood epilepsy with IgG2 deficiency, and mothers of infants with group B streptococcal sepsis with deficiency of IgG1,2,3. Despite these clinical associations, it is still not clear if the absent subclass is of clinical significance or if subclass deficiency is merely an indicator of immune dysregulation. Individuals have been identified with absent IgG1,2,4 due to gene deletions who were completely healthy. This suggests that it is not the lack of a subclass per se that is relevant to the increased incidence of infection. Responses to certain antigens are made preferentially in a particular subclass. For example, responses to polysaccharide antigens such as *H. influenzae* are preferentially made of the IgG2 subclass; however, IgG2-deficient patients make perfectly functional antipolysaccharide antibody of the IgG1 subclass. There are biologic differences between the subclasses, but no subclass has a biologic activity that is so unique that other subclasses cannot assume its function. There is a higher incidence of poor antibody responses, particularly to polysaccharide antigens, in patients with subclass deficiencies, but when groups of patients were studied, the increased incidence of infection was related to poor antibody responses regardless of IgG subclass concentrations.

Polysaccharide Antibody Deficiency

Ambrosino and her colleagues (1988) reported a 30-year-old man with a life-long history of pneumonia, particularly with *Pneumococcus*. His serum immunoglobulins and IgG subclasses were normal. He made antibodies normally to tetanus and diphtheria, but had no response at all to pneumococcal polysaccharide, *H. influenzae*, or *Neisseria meningitidis*. Since this report there has been a great deal of attention on the ability to respond to polysaccharide antigens. As discussed in the preceding section, there is an association between IgG2 subclass deficiency and poor responses to polysaccharides. Infants all fail to respond to polysaccharides, and a normal response is not achieved until at least 3 years of age (Sell et al, 1981). A number of children between the ages of 2 and 5 years have been identified who have poor responses to polysaccharide antigens such as *H. influenzae* (unconjugated) vaccine; most of these children eventually become normal, so that this may represent a delay in maturation rather than a true immunodeficiency. These patients are different from the children with transient hypogammaglobulinemia (THI) (discussed in the next section) in that these children have normal immunoglobulin concentrations but fail to respond appropriately to antigens, whereas those with THI have low immunoglobulins but normal antibody responses. Patients who fail to respond to polysaccharides may suffer from recurrent and severe infections and, if they fail to improve with antibiotics and reduced exposure in day care, may benefit from therapy with intravenous gamma globulin.

Selective IgA Deficiency

Isolated deficiency of IgA is the most common of the primary immunodeficiency diseases, with an incidence recorded as high as 1:333 blood bank donors. Most investigators do not consider a patient to be deficient unless the concentration is less than 0.1 or 0.15 gm/L. Many patients with IgA deficiency are clinically normal, but there are higher incidences of infectious, allergic, collagen-vascular, and gastrointestinal disorders in patients with reduced IgA concentrations. There is also an increased incidence of malignancy, particularly of the gastrointestinal tract, in IgA-deficient patients. The increased incidence of infections of the respiratory and genitourinary tracts is to be expected since IgA is primarily an immunoglobulin found in the external secretions. Bacterial infections predominate with a spectrum of organisms that is similar to that of other humoral immunodeficiency diseases. Antibodies to food antigens, especially cow's milk and ruminant serum proteins, are common and may be related to the high incidence of malabsorption and a sprue-like condition. Autoantibodies are also frequent and are often related to clinically relevant autoimmune disease.

The etiology of this defect, as with most of the other primary immunodeficiency diseases, is unknown. There is a high degree of association with selective subclass deficiency, and some patients have been noted to have impaired responses to polysaccharide antigens. T cell numbers and subsets and B cell numbers are normal. IgA is near the end of the immunoglobulin heavy-chain gene region, so that errors in switching are likely to be more common. Recent studies indicate that T cells are involved in immunoglobulin isotype switching, so that the primary defect may be in the regulatory T cell rather than the B cell. The concurrence of other forms of immune dysregulation such as autoimmune disease lends support to this hypothesis.

Transient Hypogammaglobulinemia of Infancy (THI)

If compared to normal adults, all children are immunodeficient at birth and require several years for immunoglobulins and antibody responses to become "normal." A small number of children with recurrent infections have been identified who have depressed immunoglobulin concentrations that eventually normalize. This disorder appears to be fairly rare, with only 11 patients reported by Tiller and Buckley (1978) over a 13-year period and five patients described by Dressler and his colleagues in an 11-year period and with 8000 sera tested. By definition, all of these patients recover, usually by age 2 to 4 years. These patients can be distinguished from those with more serious immunodeficiency in that their ability to form specific antibody to immunization is intact despite the low immunoglobulin levels. Unfortunately, it is not possible to make a definitive diagnosis without a prolonged period of reevaluation.

A subset of patients with low immunoglobulins has been described who do not show complete recovery. Some developed selective IgA deficiency. Others have had depressed responses to antigens, especially the carbohydrate antigens from *H. influenzae* and *S. pneumoniae*. There is some disagreement as to whether these children should be considered to have THI or if they have a separate syndrome. It is likely that they represent one end of the spectrum of immunologic maturation, and although most will eventually recover, they are at increased risk of infection as long as antibody production is abnormal. The decision to treat such patients should be based on the incidence of infection and severity of the antibody deficiency, not immunoglobulin concentrations alone.

X-linked Lymphoproliferative Syndrome (XLP)

The X-linked lymphoproliferative syndrome is characterized by selective inability to respond to infection with Epstein-Barr virus (EBV), which results in severe or fatal infectious mononucleosis and acquired immunodeficiency (Sullivan, 1989). The disease was originally reported by Purtillo in the male children in three families of the Duncan kindred. Since then more than 25 kindred with more than 160 affected children have been described world-wide. The most common presentation, which occurs in approximately 75 percent of patients, is fatal mononucleosis with hepatic necrosis and bone marrow aplasia. If they survive the initial infection, many patients have severe defects in humoral immunity and 20 to 25 percent develop lymphomas.

Patients have a marked impairment in the ability to make specific antibodies to EBV nuclear antigen, EBNA, whereas anti-capsid antibody is normal or elevated. T cell immunity is only mildly impaired, with inverted CD4:CD8 ratios and decreased proliferative responses to mitogens. However, some patients had decreased cytotoxic responses to EBV-infected cells. Natural killer (NK) cell activity was significantly depressed in many of the patients studied.

There is no effective therapy for XLP. Acyclovir and ganciclovir have not been particularly effective, probably because it has been shown that the EBV is no longer in the replication phase. There have been several reports of a beneficial response to γ-interferon, but too few patients have been treated to reach any conclusions. Prophylactic use of gamma globulin with high titers of antibody to EBV is being used in an attempt to prevent the initial infection. Trials have been proposed using cytotoxic agents to eliminate the activated CD8 cytotoxic cells, but no data are yet available. Patients that survive the initial infection and do not develop lymphomas are likely to develop agammaglobulinemia and recurrent infections. These symptoms improve markedly after they begin treatment with intravenous gamma globulin.

Immunodeficiency with Thymoma

Immunodeficiency associated with thymoma is a disease predominantly of adults in the fourth decade or older in association with benign thymoma of the spindle cell variety. They may develop eosinophilia or eosinopenia, hemolytic or agenerative anemia, agranulocytosis, thrombocytopenia, or pancytopenia. Recurrent infections occur and are associated with panhypogammaglobulinemia and poor antibody responses. The percentage of B cells is low or even absent. T cell numbers and function appear to be normal, although excessive suppressor activity has been reported in some patients.

Immunodeficiency Diseases with Primary Defect in Cellular Immunity

Thymic Hypoplasia (DiGeorge Anomaly)

DiGeorge anomaly (DGA) was initially considered to be an example of pure T cell deficiency, but the severity and nature of the immunologic defect is highly variable. It is what the embryologists term a developmental field defect, or a defect in induction during organogenesis, primarily involving the third and fourth branchial arches, which leads to thymic, parathyroid, and conotruncal cardiac defects. However, all of the branchial arches may be involved, as evidenced by abnormal development of the ears, maxilla, and mandible. Other more remote organs such as the kidney and gastrointestinal tract may also be abnormal, and mild-to-moderate mental retardation has been common. There are occasional reports of autosomal dominant transmission, but most cases are sporadic. DGA has been related to chromosomal abnormalities, such as hemizygous 22q11 and 10p13, single gene defects, of teratogenic exposures to agents such as ethanol and isotretinoin. The degree and severity of each of the defects is variable, and patients who have less severe manifestations are considered to have "partial DGA." Infants with interrupted aortic arch type B, right-side aortic arch, or truncus arteriosus, especially if associated with hypocalcemia, are at increased risk of having DGA. It is important to consider the diagnosis in such infants so that appropriate treatment, especially ensuring that all blood products are irradiated prior to transfusions, can be initiated.

The immunologic defect in DGA is variable and is not confined to cellular immune function (Bastian et al, 1989). In a review of 18 patients, only four had a severe, permanent T cell defect, even though no thymus could be identified at surgery in 11 of 14 patients; the histology of the thymus in the other three was normal. Several patients had low T cell numbers or function, which improved over the first few months of life. Immunoglobulin levels were often normal, but no specific antibody was formed after appropriate immunization in the four children with severe T cell dysfunction. The overall experience with DGA suggests that many of the children will improve over time and that only a small subset have sufficient abnormality of T cell function to put them at risk of serious infections.

The variability in the expression of the immunologic defect has made evaluation of therapy difficult. Many patients were treated with thymic implants, thymic epithelium, or thymic hormones such as thymosin. Although some of them demonstrated improvement in immunologic function, it was not possible to prove that it was due to the therapy. Patients with severe immunologic defects do require reconstitution, but the best form of therapy is still a controversial issue.

Severe Combined Immunodeficiency Disease (SCID)

Severe combined immunodeficiency disease actually represents a large number of heterogeneous syndromes characterized by severe deficiency of both B and T cell function. T lymphocytes are severely reduced in nearly all patients, but B cell and NK numbers are variable. B cell function is probably normal in all but the X-linked patients, as indicated by the ability of patients' B cells to cooperate with normal donor T cells in post-transplant bone marrow chimeras; however, B cell function is reduced prior to transplant because of the lack of T cell help (Buckley et al, 1993). These are the most severe of the immunologic disorders; onset is early in life, and nearly all patients will die of opportunistic infection or malignancy before their first birthday unless kept in isolation and reconstituted with normal bone marrow.

Autosomal Recessive and X-linked SCID

Patients with SCID usually present within the first few months of life with mucocutaneous candidiasis, recurrent sepsis, pneumonia, otitis, and diarrhea. Early growth is normal, but once infections start the children exhibit extreme wasting. Opportunistic infections intervene, especially *P. carinii* pneumonia, *C. albicans,* and overwhelming infections with vaccinia, varicella, measles, and bacille Calmette-Guerin (BCG) occur and provide the strongest clue to the diagnosis. These infants are susceptible to graft-versus-host disease (GVHD) if given histoincompatible immunocompetent lymphocytes, and they may die of overwhelming GVHD if transfused with non-irradiated blood products.

Nearly all patients are severely lymphopenic, but only if one uses age-related normal values rather than the 1000 lymphocytes/mm^3 that is considered to be the lower limits of normal for adults. Some patients have normal lymphocyte counts, however, and that may delay diagnosis if a high index of suspicion is not maintained. In most cases the lymphocytes are either B cells or NK cells; T cell numbers are almost always low. An exception is the infant in whom maternal T cells have crossed the placenta and engrafted in the infant. Responses to mitogens and antigens in vitro are uniformly very low or absent and are the most reliable means of making the diagnosis of SCID. Serum immunoglobulin levels are severely depressed and there is no response to specific antigens.

In addition to the lymphopenia, there is cutaneous anergy and inability to reject skin grafts. On examination lymphoid tissue is absent, and no thymus is detectable by x-ray examination; at surgery or autopsy a very tiny thymus may be found, usually in the neck, that histologically lacks corticomedullary distinction and Hassall's corpuscles.

The etiologies of two forms of SCID are known: adenosine deaminase deficiency (described below) and X-linked SCID, which is due to a defect in the γ chain of the IL-2 receptor. Because this chain is also shared by other cytokine receptors, including IL-4, IL-7, and IL-13, functions of B and NK cells are also abnormal, which is in contrast to autosomal forms of SCID. A few patients have been described who have a block at the level of production of IL-2, and some of these patients improve with injections of recombinant IL-2, although there is never complete restoration of function. Regardless of the phenotype, bone marrow transplantation is the most effective means of therapy. It is clear that the chances of success are dependent on making an early diagnosis and on transplanting before serious infections occur.

Adenosine Deaminase (ADA) Deficiency

Approximately 15 percent of patients with SCID have been found to lack this enzyme in the purine salvage pathway (Hirshhorn, 1990). ADA deficiency leads to a build-up of high levels of 2'-adenosine, which leads to expansion of intracellular pools of deoxyadenosine triphosphate (dATP) and S-adenosylhomocysteine. The dATP is toxic to many cells, but T cells are particularly sensitive. ADA-deficient patients usually present early in life, but a few have been reported in whom serious infections did not begin for several years. Even in this disease, in which the genetic defect has been identified, there is heterogeneity. Patients with major deletions in the ADA gene have a more severe form than those with a point mutation, which may be "leaky" and allow some active enzyme to be produced. This is an autosomal recessive condition, and parents have half the normal level of enzyme in their cells, which permits carrier detection. Only a small percentage of enzyme is necessary to prevent the build-up of toxic metabolites and prevent immunodeficiency.

The majority of ADA-deficient patients are similar to other patients with SCID. Some patients differ, however, in that they have skeletal abnormalities, which include rib cage abnormalities similar to a rachitic rosary and chondro-osseous dysplasia of long bones throughout the body. Unlike patients treated with the ADA inhibitor deoxycoformycin, other tissues of the body are relatively healthy and only the T cells are severely affected.

The treatment of choice in this form of SCID is also bone marrow transplant, although there is a higher incidence of graft failure in ADA-deficient patients unless some form of cytoreduction is done before the transplant. Patients can also be treated with enzyme replacement. Initially, infusions of normal red blood cells were used, but the levels of ADA that were achieved were not adequate to reduce the adenosine to acceptable levels, and patients suffered from iron overload from the many transfusions. Patients are now treated with bovine ADA linked to polyethylene glycol (PEG-ADA), which prolongs its half-life (Hershfield et al, 1987). Patients treated with PEG-ADA achieve good levels of ADA, and the adenosine levels fall to normal. There is clinical and immunologic improvement, although the level of reconstitution is not as good as that achieved by bone marrow transplant. PEG-ADA is a valuable form of therapy for these children but should be reserved for those in whom bone marrow transplant is contraindicated or has failed.

Defective Expression of Major Histocompatibility Antigens

The lack of either class I (the bare lymphocyte syndrome) or class I plus class II histocompatibility antigens prevents cooperation between cells of the immune system and results in a syndrome similar to the other forms of SCID. Patients present with *Pneumocystis carinii* pneumonia, oral candidiasis, recurrent bacterial pneumonia and septicemia, increased susceptibility to viral infections, especially the herpesviruses and enteroviruses, and chronic diarrhea and malabsorption. Survival is unlikely unless the patient can be successfully reconstituted with bone marrow.

B and T cell numbers are usually normal or slightly reduced, but germinal follicles are absent, immunoglobulin concentrations are reduced, and antibody formation is poor. Lymphoid organs, including the thymus, are severely hypoplastic. T cell and NK function is markedly reduced *in vitro*, but usually is not absent as in other forms of SCID. The disorder is autosomal recessive and thought to be due to regulatory gene defects, as it is possible to induce some antigen expression by stimulation *in vitro*.

Deficiency of T Cell Receptors

Several patients have been identified with a clinical syndrome of SCID who were found to lack the TCR/CD3 complex. Lymphocytes from these patients failed to proliferate in response to mitogens or antigens, but did respond to TCR-independent signals such as anti-CD2, phorbol esters, or IL-2. The TCR/CD3 complex consists of at least seven chains; two chains form the clonotypic heterodimer, which determines antigen specificity. The other chains comprise the CD3 complex, which is believed to be important for signal transduction. In one family the biochemical defect was found to be localized to expression of the CD3ε chain, but undoubtedly other defects will be identified as molecular biology techniques are applied more widely.

Cellular Immunodeficiency with Immunoglobulins (Nezelof's Syndrome)

Severe but incomplete T cell dysfunction results in a clinical syndrome characterized by failure to thrive, chronic mucocutaneous candidiasis, diarrhea, susceptibility to viral infections, especially the herpesviruses varicella and herpes simplex, chronic progressive pulmonary infections, gram-negative sepsis, and urinary tract infections. Autoimmune disorders, especially hemolytic anemia and thrombocytopenia, are common, and there is an increased incidence of lymphoreticular malignancies.

Most patients are profoundly lymphopenic with proportional reduction in CD4 and CD8 T cells. T cell function *in vivo* and *in vitro* to mitogens and antigens is markedly reduced but is not absent as in the classic SCID. Serum immunoglobulins are normal or elevated, but specific antibody formation is absent. This variant of SCID can be treated by bone marrow transplantation, but it is always necessary to use myeloablative therapy to eliminate the residual T cell function so that the transplant will not be rejected.

This syndrome is distinguished from other forms of SCID by the presence of immunoglobulins and lymphoid tissue. The histologic structure of the thymus and lymph nodes is abnormal, with poor corticomedullary distinction and reduced or absent Hassall's corpuscles in the thymus and poor follicle formation in peripheral lymphoid organs. Some patients present with lymphadenopathy and hepatosplenomegaly. This description is obviously suggestive of AIDS, but this is a genetic disorder that can be distinguished by several features. Total T cells are reduced, but there usually is a normal CD4:CD8 ratio. T cell function is usually relatively normal early in HIV infection but is low at all times in the genetic disorder. The architecture of the thymus is different, but this is not usually known antemortem. Since antibody formation is poor, antibodies to HIV-1 are unreliable in the patient, but can be evaluated in the mother since vertical transmission would be the most likely mode of infection. Cultures for HIV-1 are the most reliable means of distinguishing between these two diseases.

Purine Nucleoside Phosphorylase (PNP) Deficiency

A few patients with severe cellular immunodeficiency with immunoglobulins have been identified who lack the enzyme of the purine salvage pathway purine nucleoside phosphorylase (PNP) (Markert, 1991). This disorder is similar to other forms of Nezelof's syndrome but differs from ADA deficiency in that immunoglobulin levels are usually normal, uric acid is low or absent, and there are no associated skeletal abnormalities. Immunologically, T cell numbers are severely reduced, but NK cell numbers and activity are normal or increased. Thymic architecture is usually abnormal, but Hassall's corpuscles are present. B and T cell function are markedly reduced, as in other forms of Nezelof's syndrome. Thus far enzyme replacement therapy has not been as successful as it has been in ADA deficiency. Bone marrow transplantation is still the treatment of choice, but the success rate is very low due to failure of engraftment and the occurrence of overwhelming infections.

Omenn Syndrome

In 1965 Gilbert Omenn reported 12 patients in 6 sibships who had developed a fatal illness characterized by a generalized erythematous scaling skin eruption, hepatosplenomegaly, generalized lymphadenopathy, eosinophilia, and fever. Death was usually secondary to overwhelming infection with *S. aureus, C. albicans, P. carinii,* pneumonia, and a variety of other organisms. Subsequent immunologic studies revealed B lymphopenia with reduced serum concentrations of IgG, IgA, and IgM, increased levels of IgE, and a marked depression of T cell activation not restored by the addition of exogenous IL-2 (Businco et al, 1987). IL-2 and γ-interferon production were depressed. Lymphocyte counts were normal or elevated in many patients, with normal percentages of T cells and variable CD4:CD8 ratios. Biopsy of lymph nodes showed effacement of the normal architecture with a proliferation of histiocytes that were positive for the surface antigens S-100, T6, and Ia, which are characteristic of Langerhans' or interdigitating reticulum cells.

The pathologic findings are similar to those of acute graft-versus-host disease, and some studies have suggested that this is the etiology of Omenn's syndrome. Indeed, these patients clinically resemble patients with severe combined immunodeficiency and maternal engraftment. However, the familial association with an autosomal recessive mode of inheritance and the inability to detect maternal cells in the majority of patients who have been studied support this as a distinct disease entity. It is reminiscent of those patients with a Letterer-Siwe syndrome and SCID. In both cases there appears to be excessive proliferation of reticuloendothelial cells. Several patients have been cured by bone marrow transplant, although the mortality rate remains high.

Reticular Dysgenesis

This extremely rare disorder is the most severe form of SCID. Patients have severe lymphopenia and depressed B and T cell function, but also lack granulocytes. Red cells and platelets are usually normal. Some patients have had small numbers of granulocytes or T cells, arguing against a stem cell defect. Seven of the eight patients reported thus far have died of overwhelming infections within the first 3 months of life; only the one patient that was reconstituted with a bone marrow transplant has survived.

Combined Immunodeficiency Diseases

Wiskott-Aldrich Syndrome (WAS)

The combination of eczema, thrombocytopenia, and recurrent pyogenic infections is an X-linked disorder first reported in 1954. Clinically, children with WAS present with bloody diarrhea and petechiae early in infancy. Platelet numbers are reduced and individual platelets are small. Platelets from patients with WAS have abnormal survival times, whereas normal platelets infused into patients with WAS have normal survival times. Eczema also develops early in life and may be related to specific allergy, although often no allergen can be identified. The most striking abnormality is the high incidence of bacterial infections especially otitis, sinusitis, pneumonia, and meningitis, often caused by encapsulated organisms such as *S. pneumoniae* and *H. influenzae.* There is often increased susceptibility to viruses such as varicella and to *P. carinii;* however, mucocutaneous candidiasis and other opportunistic infections are uncommon. There is an extremely high incidence of malignancy, nearly 15 percent in the immunodeficiency registry (Kersey et al, 1988). Nearly all of the tumors have been lymphomas, including those in the CNS that were initially thought to be brain tumors but were actually lymphomas metastatic from the abdomen.

The most consistent immunologic abnormality is an impaired humoral response to polysaccharide antigens, with diminished or absent isohemagglutinins, low concentrations of natural antibodies to *Escherichia coli,* and poor antibody response following immunization with carbohydrate antigens such as *H. influenzae,* and pneumococcal polysaccharide. The response to other antigens, including polio, diphtheria, and tetanus, is also reduced, but not as severely as that to carbohydrate antigens. Serum IgG concentrations are usually normal, IgM slightly low, and IgA and IgE are often elevated. All immunoglobulins are catabolized at a markedly increased rate; IgG at three times and IgA and IgM at twice the usual rate. Thus, the synthetic rates are increased in proportion to maintain the serum concentrations. The concentrations of IgG2 have been found to be normal, despite the poor response to polysaccharide antigens and the apparent linkage of IgG2 to responses to those antigens.

Patients with WAS frequently have cutaneous anergy by delayed-hypersensitivity skin testing. Proliferative responses to the usual mitogens and antigens are moderately decreased. In contrast, cells from these patients do not proliferate in response to periodate, which oxidizes carbohydrate residues on glycoproteins. The numbers and proportions of T lymphocytes in peripheral blood are modestly decreased with normal CD4:CD8 ratios. The numbers of B lymphocytes as indicated by CD20 are normal, although a high proportion of these are negative for CD21, the complement and EBV receptor, which is a pattern seen on immature B cells. B cell lines derived from patients with WAS respond normally to IL-4, IL-6, and low-molecular-weight B cell growth factor.

Lymphocytes and platelets from patients with WAS have been reported to lack a surface sialoglycoprotein of MW 115,000 known as gpL115 or sialophorin and now designated CD43 (Remold-O'Donnell and Rosen, 1990). The gene for sialophorin is located in the p11.2 band of chromosome 16. Most WAS patients, however, have CD43 on their lymphocytes. Since WAS is an X-linked disease, the abnormal gene must code for a surface anchoring protein or an enzyme necessary for modifying the protein. The gene on the X chromosome has been isolated and the actual biochemical abnormality should be elucidated in the near future.

Chronic Mucocutaneous Candidiasis (CMC)

CMC is a group of syndromes that are characterized by persistent infections of the skin, nails, and mucous membranes with *Candida* species and occasionally other fungal organisms (Kirkpatrick, 1988). Although many other defects of cellular immunity are associated with an increased susceptibility to fungal infection, only in CMC do patients develop disfiguring hyperkeratotic lesions. Despite the extensive superficial infection, disseminated infection leading to pneumonia, sepsis, or parenchymal organs is unusual. Five subgroups were identified by Kirkpatrick based on associated abnormalities and the pattern of the candidiasis: (1) chronic oral candidiasis, (2) chronic candidiasis with endocrinopathy, (3) *Candida* granuloma, (4) chronic diffuse candidiasis, and (5) chronic candidiasis associated with thymoma. Endocrine abnormalities are common, especially in the second group, and include hypoparathyroidism, hypothyroidism, hypoadrenalism, gonadal dysfunction, as well as polyendocrinopathy syndromes. Autoimmune disease is also a common feature and may involve the endocrine organs with antibodies to thyroid, adrenal, and islet cells. Anti–parietal cell antibody can lead to pernicious anemia, and autoimmune disease in the skin can result in alopecia totalis, vitiligo, and chronic keratitis. Gastrointestinal disorders also occur with chronic malabsorption that may be related to gluten sensitivity, chronic active hepatitis, and dental enamel dysplasia.

Despite the initial impression that infection in CMC patients was confined to *Candida* species, the majority of patients suffer from multiple infections including pyogenic infections of the skin, sinopulmonary tract, and urinary tract (Herrod, 1990). Recurrent pneumonia with bronchiectasis has been a significant cause of morbidity and mortality. Isolated cases of bacterial sepsis and meningitis have been reported. A few patients have had severe infections with varicella, herpes simplex, measles, and respiratory syncytial virus, suggesting a defect in cell-mediated immunity. Superficial but persistent infections with dermatophytes are relatively common. Although disseminated infections with fungi are uncommon, at least five children are known to have had life-threatening disseminated infections with *Histoplasma capsulatum.*

The underlying immunologic defect is as

yet uncharacterized. The majority of patients are anergic to *Candida in vivo*, but many will demonstrate positive responses, especially if tested while the disease is under good control. Similar results are observed when their lymphocytes are stimulated with *Candida* antigen *in vitro*. Although some are completely anergic, the majority can respond to other recall antigens such as tetanus or streptokinase. Responses to mitogens are almost always normal. Serum immunoglobulins and antibody responses are normal in the majority of patients. B and T cell numbers and subsets have also been within normal limits, but transient abnormalities have been observed in patients tested during the acute phase of their illness. The studies of Durandy and his colleagues found that *in vitro* production of antibody to mannan isolated from the cell wall of *C. albicans* was absent during the active phase of the disease. T lymphocytes from patients with CMC were not able to proliferate in response to mannan or provide helper activity for B cell antibody activity. This was associated with the presence of mannan-specific T suppressor cells. They hypothesized that defective processing of mannan by monocytes could lead to the accumulation of mannan and the induction of suppressor T lymphocytes.

Hyperimmunoglobulinemia E Syndrome

Patients with this disorder suffer from recurrent severe staphylococcal abscesses of the skin and lung and an eczematous skin rash (Buckley and Sampson, 1981). They were noted to have extremely high serum concentrations of IgE, usually several thousand units per milliliter. Recurrent infections occur in skin, lungs (which often lead to pneumatocele formation), joints, and other sites. Most infections are caused by *S. aureus*, but a variety of other bacteria and fungi, especially *C. albicans* and *Aspergillus*, have been isolated. Some patients develop skin infections with *Candida* that are similar to those of patients with chronic mucocutaneous candidiasis. Both males and females are affected, as are members of successive generations, suggesting an autosomal dominant form of inheritance with incomplete penetrance.

The underlying immunologic defect has not been identified. Disorders of phagocytosis and chemotaxis have been reported and are discussed in the section on the Phagocytic Disorders. Serum immunoglobulin concentrations are usually normal, except for the elevated IgE; specific antibody responses are variable but impaired to a wide variety of protein and carbohydrate antigens. Some patients failed to switch from IgM to IgG when immunized with bacteriophage ΦX-174, and others showed a rapid decline in antibody titers. Most patients have normal numbers of circulating B and T lymphocytes and subsets, and responses to mitogens are usually normal. The ability of T cells from these patients to produce γ-interferon is a point of controversy, with some studies indicating impaired responses and others showing good production. Mononuclear cells from patients produce IgE *in vitro* but do not increase production when stimulated with IL-4, suggesting that they are already maximally stimulated. The importance of these abnormalities and of the elevated IgE and its relationship to the high incidence of infections is still unclear.

Ataxia-Telangiectasia (AT)

Ataxia-telangiectasia is a complex multisystem disease in which the immune system is variably involved (Swift, 1990). The predominant abnormality is progressive cerebellar ataxia, which is manifest about the time the child starts to walk and in severe cases progresses until he or she is confined to a wheelchair, usually by 10 or 12 years of age. Oculomotor abnormalities are prominent and may precede truncal ataxia. Oculocutaneous telangiectasia develops between the ages of 3 and 6 years and helps to distinguish this form from other forms of ataxia. Immunologic abnormalities manifest as recurrent sinopulmonary infections, and chronic pneumonia and bronchiectasis are a frequent cause of death. Although these are the cardinal manifestations of the disease, all organ systems are involved. The skin and hair show progeric changes with graying of the hair and loss of elastic tissue. The skin may become atrophic, even resembling mild scleroderma. Nearly all of the patients develop seborrheic dermatitis and common warts. One of the most dramatic and devastating aspects of AT is the remarkable incidence of malignancy. Nearly 15 percent of patients will develop malignancy, often of the lymphoreticular system; T cell malignancies have been especially common (Kersey et al, 1988). Cutaneous, hepatic, and renal tumors have been frequent, especially in patients over 15 years of age. While treating these malignancies it was noted that chemotherapy and irradiation led to severe, ultimately fatal, reactions and are therefore contraindicated in these patients.

The immunologic abnormalities are available. Sinopulmonary infections are most common. There is not a high incidence of infections with opportunistic organisms and the response to most viral infections is normal, although one patient died from disseminated varicella. The most frequent humoral abnormality is absent IgA, found in 50 to 80 percent of patients. IgE is also often low, and IgM levels, while normal, may be monomeric. IgG concentrations are usually normal, but subclass deficiency, especially of IgG2, is frequent. Specific antibody titers may be reduced but seldom absent. T cell immunity is mildly decreased *in vivo*, as evidenced by cutaneous anergy and prolonged allograft survival. Percentages of T cells in the peripheral blood are only mildly reduced although there may be a selective decrease in CD4 lymphocytes. Proliferative responses to mitogens and antigens *in vitro* are also low, but never absent. Production of γ-interferon and IL-2 are also reduced. Thymic histology is abnormal, with poor corticomedullary distinction and absence of Hassall's corpuscles. Serum alpha-fetoprotein levels are elevated.

Cartilage-Hair Hypoplasia (CHH)

Immune deficiency has been associated with short-limbed dwarfism, especially those with CHH. The biochemical defect is not known. Patients have short and pudgy hands, hyperextensible joints of the hands and feet, sparse light hair, and redundant skin. Some have had megacolon or other gastrointestinal disorders. Radiologically, the bones show sclerotic or cystic changes in the metaphysis and flaring of the costochondral junctions. Severe, often fatal infections with varicella, vaccinia, and poliovirus have been reported, and opportunistic infections such as oral candidiasis can occur. There appears to be a defect in cellular proliferation that affects all cells of the body, including those of the immune system.

The immunologic defect is highly variable, ranging from nearly normal to that resembling SCID. In one series, 11 of 77 patients died before the age of 20 years. Some patients have only defective humoral immunity, which nonetheless may be severe enough to require replacement with gamma globulin. A subset of patients have severe T cell defects with decreased T cell numbers and impaired proliferation to mitogens due to an arrest in the G_1 phase of the cell cycle. NK activity is normal or increased, which may account for the lack of an increased incidence of malignancy in this disorder.

Phagocytic Disorders

The macrophage/phagocytic system plays a major role in the host defense against microorganisms (Roberts and Gallin, 1983). Macrophages are also critical for antigen presentation to B and T lymphocytes and provide cytokines that activate lymphocytes and endothelial cells. Most investigations have concentrated on the circulating phagocytes because of availability, and the more numerous neutrophils or polymorphonuclear leukocytes (PMNs) have been the most extensively studied. Despite major advances in our knowledge over the past 15 years, especially in the realm of molecular biology, the phagocyte remains one of the least understood of the cells of the immune system. Only three disorders—deficiency of a surface glycoprotein necessary for intracellular adhesion (leukocyte function antigen-1 or LFA-1), myeloperoxidase deficiency, and chronic granulomatous disease—have been well characterized at the molecular level. Many of the assays of phagocytic function are difficult to standardize, and since a great number of diseases can cause transient depression of phagocytic function, the diagnosis of a primary disorder is difficult. Despite these difficulties, knowledge of phagocytic function is critical to an understanding of host defense.

Abnormalities in the phagocytic system can result from defects in cell number or from abnormal function of morphologically normal cells (Table 2–2). Neutropenia can be caused by deficient production or excessive consumption. The most common acquired causes of neutropenia are infection, chemotherapeutic agents, and autoimmune disease. This section will focus primarily on the intrinsic disorders of leukocyte function.

Disorders of Production

There are several congenital forms of neutropenia, some of which are severe, even fatal. Kostmann's syndrome is severe, with

TABLE 2–2. DISORDERS OF PHAGOCYTIC FUNCTION

Disorders of production and consumption
  Abnormal production
    Kostmann's syndrome
    Schwachman's syndrome
    Cyclic neutropenia
    Primary B and T lymphocyte disorders
      X-linked hyper-IgM
      X-linked agammaglobulinemia
      Ataxia-telangiectasia
      Cartilage-hair hypoplasia
      IgA deficiency
  Abnormal consumption
    Maternal autoimmune neutropenia
    Felty's syndrome
    Immunodeficiency associated with thymoma
Disorders of migration and chemotaxis
  General defects in leukocyte mobility
    Abnormal adhesion
    Abnormal locomotion
    Abnormal chemotactic responses
  Kartagener's syndrome
  Lazy leukocyte syndrome
  Hyper-IgE syndrome
  Chediak-Higashi syndrome
Disorders of intracellular killing
  Chronic granulomatous disease
  Myeloperoxidase deficiency
  Glutathione reductase and peroxidase deficiency
  Glucose-6-phosphate dehydrogenase deficiency
Deficiency of leukocyte function antigen 1 (LFA-1)

neutrophil counts <100/mm^3, but there are other less severe idiopathic forms of neutropenia. Neutropenia is also found associated with pancreatic insufficiency (Shwachman syndrome) and in several primary immunologic disorders including X-linked agammaglobulinemia, X-linked hyper-IgM syndrome, ataxia-telangiectasia, and IgA deficiency. Neutropenia has been observed in cartilage-hair hypoplasia, which also is associated with severe B and T cell immunologic defects. Cyclic neutropenia is an autosomal dominant disorder, which usually presents in infancy and occurs as an isolated abnormality or may be associated with other immunologic disorders such as X-linked hyper-IgM syndrome. The etiology of the neutropenia is not known for any of these defects, but the association with other immunologic disorders suggests that at least some defects may be due to abnormal cytokine production. Others may be secondary to intrinsic defects in neutrophil development.

Neutropenia may be secondary to autoimmune reactions. Some congenital neutropenias are due to the transplacental passage of maternal IgG directed against fetal white blood cells. High levels of antineutrophil antibodies have been observed in the neutropenia associated with splenomegaly and rheumatoid arthritis (Felty's syndrome). Neutropenia has also been associated with thymoma and abnormal suppressor T cell activity.

Disorders of Migration and Chemotaxis

Abnormal movement of neutrophils and macrophages may be due to intrinsic abnormalities in the cells or to abnormal mediators or accessory substances (Yang and Hill, 1991). Little is known of these accessory substances. Lactoferrin and fibronectin are both thought to be important for adhesiveness, but specific disorders due to their absence have not been described. Leukocytes from patients with severe genetic defects of the complement system display abnormal chemotactic responses, presumably secondary to inability of their serum to generate chemoattractive factors.

Abnormalities of neutrophil mobility may involve several different functions, including adherence, deformability, nondirected locomotion, and chemotaxis, but none are well characterized. Neutrophils from neonates are less adherent and more rigid than those from adults, and as a result show impaired diapedesis and chemotaxis. A number of abnormalities have been described in individual patients, including defects in actin polymerization, ability to respond to f-met-leu-phe, and a defect in specific granules. The biochemical bases for these defects have not been elucidated.

Kartagener's Syndrome

In its complete form this autosomal recessive syndrome is characterized by recurrent sinopulmonary infections and situs inversus; however, variations without situs inversus are common. The underlying defect is abnormal formation of the microstructure of the cilia. Since the cilia are intimately related to the microtubular system, there undoubtedly is a more generalized defect, which affects the motion of a variety of cells including white blood cells and spermatozoa. Abnormal locomotion and chemotaxis have been observed in the leukocytes from patients with Kartagener's syndrome and, along with abnormal clearance due to immotility of the cilia, are responsible for the high incidence of infections of the respiratory tract.

Hyper-IgE Syndrome

The hyper-IgE syndrome involves defects in B and T cell function and was previously discussed in the section on combined immunodeficiency. A number of investigators have reported a chemotactic defect in the PMNs from these patients. However, the defect is not present in all patients and in some patients the defect is present only intermittently. Serum inhibitors of chemotaxis have been reported but could not be found by all investigators. Although IgE anti-staphylococcal antibodies and immune complexes have been identified, they are probably not responsible for the immunologic defect since the same abnormalities have been observed in patients with severe atopic dermatitis. Phagocytosis and killing are consistently normal. Defective production of γ-interferon has been reported in some studies, but this abnormality could not be confirmed by others. In another report, neutrophil chemotaxis was markedly reduced but became normal after incubation *in vitro* with γ-interferon. The importance of the dramatically elevated IgE is not known, but since γ-interferon can down-regulate IgE synthesis *in vivo* and *in vitro*, its role in this disease is worthy of further investigation.

Chediak-Higashi Syndrome

This rare disease is characterized by recurrent pyogenic infections, predominantly of the respiratory tract, and partial oculocutaneous albinism (Stoltz et al, 1989). Approximately 85 percent of the patients develop an accelerated phase of the disease with fever, jaundice, hepatosplenomegaly, lymphadenopathy, pancytopenia, bleeding diathesis, and neurologic changes. Once the accelerated phase occurs, the disease is almost always fatal within 29 months unless treated with chemotherapeutic agents to deplete cellular immunity followed by bone marrow transplantation.

The hallmark of the disease is the presence of giant lysosomal granules not only in PMNs, but also in most of the other cells of the body, including renal tubular cells, gastric mucosa, pneumocytes, hepatocytes, Langerhans' cells of the skin, and adrenal and neural cells. The granules in neutrophils are positive for peroxidase, acid phosphatase, and esterase. They are believed to be abnormal lysosomes that undergo abnormal fusion with phagosomes so that ingested bacteria cannot be properly lysed.

Of the several immunologic abnormalities that have been reported in Chediak-Higashi syndrome, the most dramatic is a nearly complete absence of natural killer cell activity, which is most likely a result of the abnormal function of the lysosomal granules. Abnormal chemotaxis has been reported, and there is evidence of a profound alteration of the cytoskeleton of the cells. Leukocyte degranulation, capping of concanavalin A receptors, and migration in a chemotactic gradient are all the same as in cells treated with colchicine, which disrupts microtubule formation. The genetic defect in this autosomal recessive disorder is not known, but it is probably due to abnormal microtubule function, which causes disordered fusion of cell membranes.

Disorders of Intracellular Killing

Chronic Granulomatous Disease (CGD)

CGD is the best described and best understood disorder of the phagocyte (Lomax et al, 1989; Malech and Gallin, 1987; Segal, 1989). Patients have an increased incidence of infections with catalase-positive organisms, such as *S. aureus, E. coli, Serratia marcescens, Salmonella, Chromobacterium, C. albicans*, and *Aspergillus*, but not with catalase-negative organisms such as *Streptococcus pneumoniae* (Mouy et al, 1989). Most patients develop extensive inflammatory lesions that are poorly responsive to antibiotics and form granulomatous lesions, especially in the gastrointestinal and urinary tracts. Draining lesions of the lymph nodes in the neck and axilla often develop, and abscesses of the lung and liver may require surgical drainage. Osteomyelitis with bacteria and fungi, especially *Aspergillus*, is a frequent complication. In one study, 50 percent of the patients died before 10 years of age; the prognosis is better for patients diagnosed after 1978, presumably because of advances in diagnosis and therapy. Studies of the defect in CGD have resulted in major advances in the comprehension of host defense. Chemotaxis and phagocytosis are normal, and the phagocytes are filled with viable microorganisms. Thus, the defect is in the ability of the phagocyte to kill the ingested organism.

When appropriately stimulated, phagocytes activate a NADPH oxidase-dependent respiratory burst resulting in the univalent reduction of molecular oxygen to superoxide, which then dismutates further to hydrogen peroxide. Hydrogen peroxide is directly toxic to microorganisms or interacts with chloride ion to produce hypochlorite. A 66 kD flavoprotein appears to be the receptor for NADPH in the membrane, and links it with a cytochrome. The cytochrome, b-558, has the capability of directly reducing oxygen to superoxide, and thus is the terminal component of the electron transport chain.

Patients with X-linked CGD lack the cytochrome b-558 in the cell membrane. Approximately 65 percent of patients with CGD follow an X-linked mode of inheritance, and the remainder are autosomal recessive (AR-CGD). In the majority of patients with autosomal recessive CGD the cytochrome is present but nonfunctional. Evaluation of cytochrome-positive AR-CGD patients led to the identification of cytosolic proteins. The majority lack a 47 kD phosphoprotein, but in a few patients a 65 kD protein is missing or defective.

The diagnosis of CGD is made by demonstrating the inability of the activated phagocytes from the patient to undergo a respiratory burst to generate superoxide ions. The generation of superoxide ions can be demonstrated by measuring chemiluminescence or by the ability to reduce a dye such as nitrotetrazolium blue (NBT). In addition, the cells can phagocytose but not kill bacteria such as *Staphylococcus aureus*. The diagnosis can be confirmed by molecular biology techniques to determine the absence of the specific components of the NADPH oxidase system.

When CGD was first diagnosed it was considered to be a fatal granulomatous disease of childhood. Patients diagnosed today have a better prognosis, but morbidity and mortality are still significant (Mouy et al, 1989). Aggressive treatment with antibiotics, especially those such as sulfonamides, chloramphenicol, and rifampin, that can penetrate into, and even concentrate in, neutrophils has reduced the severity of bacterial infections. Prophylaxis with trimethoprim-sulfamethoxazole has been helpful to reduce the incidence of infection. Fungal infections, especially with *Aspergillus*, have assumed greater prominence. Ketoconazole has decreased the incidence of infection with *C. albicans* but not *Aspergillus*.

Itraconazole holds greater promise, but the majority of patients require at least initial therapy with amphotericin B. The use of white blood cell transfusions is controversial, but in several studies patients with *Aspergillus* osteomyelitis have improved following granulocyte transfusions after they failed treatment with amphotericin B alone. A large double-blind placebo-controlled study of 128 patients conducted by the National Institutes of Health reported a significant reduction in the number of infections and days of hospitalization in patients treated subcutaneously three times a week with γ-interferon (International CGD Cooperative Study Group, 1991). *In vitro* studies have shown that γ-interferon can up-regulate expression of cytochrome b-558, but interestingly, both X-linked and AR-CGD patients responded to interferon therapy, even though the cytochrome is abnormal only in the patients with X-linked inheritance. It was not possible to demonstrate an increase in the ability of neutrophils from the treated patients to kill microorganisms. Thus, γ-interferon may stimulate other aspects of host defense in addition to increasing the cytochrome. Although the mechanism is not fully elucidated, the data were convincing enough for the FDA to approve γ-interferon for the treatment of CGD. Further studies will be needed to determine optimal dose and dosing schedule. Not even γ-interferon provides optimal restoration of cell function, however. A few patients have been successfully treated with bone marrow transplantation, but patients must be transplanted early, before severe infections are present, and only those with HLA-matched donors are suitable candidates with current methods for marrow ablation and treatment of graft-versus-host disease. Further advances in the understanding of the molecular basis of CGD may permit correction of the defect using gene therapy, with the appropriate gene being inserted into hematopoietic stem cells.

Myeloperoxidase Deficiency

Free oxygen radicals and hydrogen peroxide generated by the cytochrome system can be directly toxic to microorganisms, but in the presence of chloride ions, H_2O_2 and myeloperoxidase (MPO) generate hypochlorous acid, a potent agent with 50 times the microbicidal activity of H_2O_2 alone. MPO is a heme-containing protein present in the azurophilic granules of monocytes and neutrophils. It comprises 7 percent of the dry weight of neutrophils and is responsible for the green color of pus. The MPO-H_2O_2-Cl system is not only capable of killing bacteria and fungi, but also can destroy tumor cells, natural killer cells, and round worms.

The first reports of MPO deficiency were of patients with recurrent infections of the skin (Nauseef, 1990). However, with the introduction of automated systems for performing differential blood counts, which use MPO as a marker for neutrophils, it has become apparent that MPO deficiency is common, occurring in as many as 1 in 2000 apparently healthy individuals. It is inherited in an autosomal recessive pattern and has been mapped to chromosome 17 at q21-q23 or q22-q24. MPO deficiency can also occur as an acquired condition, usually as a result of a myelodysplastic condition, such as acute myelogenous leukemia, myelodysplastic syndrome, aplastic anemia, or megaloblastic anemia. Several patients have had severe visceral or disseminated candidiasis, but most of them have had concomitant diabetes mellitus. In one report, seven of 12 patients with complete MPO deficiency and two of 48 patients with partial MPO deficiency had associated tumors. The fact that the majority of patients with MPO deficiency are healthy suggests that other mechanisms of killing may be able to compensate; however, differences in clinical expression may also be due to different genetic defects in the MPO molecule.

Glutathione Reductase and Peroxidase

Hydrogen peroxide molecules generated by the cytochrome system can diffuse into the cytosol or cell organelles and damage the phagocyte. Peroxide in the organelles is destroyed by catalase. In the cytosol, peroxide is destroyed by the glutathione cycle. Glutathione (GSH) is oxidized to two molecules of glutathione linked by disulfide bonds (GSSG) by glutathione oxidase, with the reduction of H_2O_2 to water. The GSSG is reduced back to two molecules of GSH by glutathione reductase. A defect in glutathione oxidase can lead to a condition resembling CGD and initially was thought to be the only cause of CGD in females. Defects in glutathione reductase do not seem to result in clinically apparent disease.

Glucose-6-Phosphate Dehydrogenase Deficiency

G-6-PD is critical in the hexose monophosphate shunt to generate NADPH. Complete deficiency in leukocytes has been associated with defects in intracellular killing leading to mild clinical disease, similar in severity to myeloperoxidase deficiency. These patients also have hemolytic anemia due to deficiency of the enzyme in red blood cells. Microbicidal activity is normal if the level of G-6-PD in PMNs at least 20 percent of normal levels.

Leukocyte Adhesion Molecule Defects

In the early 1980s Springer and his colleagues reported a clinical syndrome characterized by delayed separation of the umbilical cord, marked leukocytosis with neutrophil counts of 20,000 to 100,000, and recurrent necrotic infections of skin, mucous membranes, and gastrointestinal tract (Kishimoto and Springer, 1989; Fischer et al, 1990). Despite the leukocytosis, few leukocytes were found in the large ulcerative lesions. The defect in these patients is the absence of an adhesion molecule, which they named leukocyte function antigen-l (LFA-1). LFA-1 is one of the integrin family of adhesion molecules, which includes Mac-1 or complement receptor 3 (CR3) and p150,95 or complement receptor 4 (CR4). These molecules are $\alpha\beta$ heterodimers; the α units of LFA-1, Mac-1, and p150,95 are distinct proteins now designated CD11a, b, and c, respectively. The 95,000 dalton β subunit, designated CD18 and located on chromosome 21, is common to all three, and all patients with LFA-1 deficiency have lacked this protein. Expression is linked, so that a defect in β chain expression results in a lack of all three adhesion molecules. The CD11a/CD18 complex, or LFA-1, is found on nearly all immune cells and mediates both antigen-specific and antigen-independent interactions, including lymphocyte adhesion, natural killing, T cell cytotoxicity, and T cell helper activity. The CD11b/CD18 complex is found on monocytes, granulocytes, macrophages, and natural killer cells. It is a receptor for C3bi and mediates phagocyte adhesion and antibody-dependent cellular cytotoxicity.

The CD11c/Cd18 complex or CR4 is found on monocytes and neutrophils and is similar in function to CR3. The ligand for these molecules is intracellular adhesion molecule-1 (ICAM-1), which is widely distributed on lymphocytes and macrophages but also is prominent on endothelial cells, especially after activation by a variety of cytokines, particularly interleukin-1 (IL-1), tumor necrosis factor, and γ-interferon. In addition to binding ICAM-1, Mac-1 can also bind to the C3bi fragment of complement to promote phagocytosis and opsonized particle-induced respiratory burst activity.

The adhesion molecules mediate mobilization of leukocytes through binding to endothelial cells. Natural killer cell activity is also absent since these molecules are critical for effector-to-target binding. Similarly, cell-mediated lympholysis is deficient. Killing of microorganisms is intact, but since the cells cannot be mobilized to the point of inflammation and complement-mediated phagocytosis is impaired, the result is a lack of an inflammatory response. Patients with <0.5 percent activity die of overwhelming microbial infections within the first few years of life, whereas those with 3 to 10 percent activity have recurrent ulcers of the mucous membranes, severe periodontal disease, and recurrent abscesses of the skin, but have a much better prognosis for survival. In several children, severe defects have been successfully corrected with an allogeneic bone marrow transplant with marrow from HLA-identical sibling donor or a haploidentical T-depleted transplant from a parent. In the future it will be possible to correct the defect by inserting the gene for the β chain into hematopoietic stem cells.

Disorders of Complement

Complement deficiency is one of the rarest of the immunologic disorders. The complement system comprises more than 25 plasma and membrane-bound glycoproteins, and defects have been described for most of these components (Frank, 1987; Ross and Densen, 1984). In general, absence of one of the early components of the classic pathway results in autoimmune disease such as systemic lupus erythematosus (SLE) or increased susceptibility to infection with gram-positive bacteria, whereas defects in the later components of the classic pathway or in the alternative pathway result in an increased incidence of neisserial infections. A defect in one of the inhibitory proteins can result in secondary defects in one of the other components due to uncontrolled utilization.

DEFECTS RESULTING IN AUTOIMMUNE DISEASE. The most common manifestation of C1q deficiency is SLE, often with renal involvement. Absence of C1r or C1s, C4 or C2 also may result in a SLE-like syndrome. Patients with C2 deficiency, which is the most common complement deficiency, also have an increased incidence of rheumatoid arthritis. Absence of C3 is extremely rare, with only 16 patients reported, five of whom had glomerulonephritis or an SLE-like syndrome. The reason these defects lead to autoimmune disease is unknown, but is thought to be due to inability to clear immune complexes via C1q or C3 receptors on phagocytic cells. Absence of C1 inhibitor results in uncontrolled activation of C1, C2, and C4 and results in hereditary angioedema, characterized by recurrent episodes of nonpruritic, nonurticarial swelling of the face, extremities, upper airways, and abdominal viscera. Patients may present with upper airway obstruction, occasionally leading to death. Episodes involving abdominal viscera may result in symptoms suggestive of an acute abdomen and have led to needless surgery when the true cause of the pain was overlooked.

DEFECTS RESULTING IN RECURRENT INFECTIONS. A defect in one of the early components of the classic pathway, C1, C2, C4, or C3, may result in an increased incidence of pyogenic infections with the gram-positive bacteria *Streptococcus* and *Staphylococcus*. This suggests that phagocytosis and intracellular killing are critical for host defense against these organisms. Patients with the most common defect, C2 deficiency, may present with sepsis, pneumonia, meningitis, or pyogenic arthritis with *S. pneumoniae*. Several of these patients who have been evaluated have been unable to make specific antibodies to the pneumococcal polysaccharide antigens when immunized with the pneumococcal vaccine, suggesting that development of immune complexes with complement is critical for antigen processing that leads to antibody formation against these antigens.

Defects in C3, the alternative pathway components, or any of the terminal components of the classic pathway result in an increased incidence of neisserial infections, including meningitis, sepsis, and pyogenic arthritis. Infections with other organisms, such as brucellosis and toxoplasmosis, have been reported. Defects in the C3 factors, factor I and factor H, result in decreased levels of C3 and a similar clinical presentation. Since the terminal complement components are necessary for the development of the membrane attack complex, susceptibility to *Neisseria* suggests that extracellular lysis by complement is important for defense against these organisms. However, some patients with deficiency of complement are healthy, and the rarity of these defects makes it difficult to understand the mechanisms that lead to increased susceptibility.

DEFICIENCY IN CELL-SURFACE COMPLEMENT RECEPTORS. Membrane receptors for activated complement components mediate many of the biologic activities of the system, such as chemotaxis, phagocytosis, and leukocyte activation. CR1 is a receptor for C3b and serves as an adhesion receptor to enhance phagocytosis by macrophages. However, the bulk of CR1 is on erythrocytes, where its primary purpose appears to be transporting and clearing immune complexes from the circulation. CR3 and CR4 are receptors for iC3b and belong to the integrin family of adhesion molecules. Defects in these proteins are associated with lack of the CD18 molecule, known as LFA-1 deficiency, and lead to the disease leukocyte adhesion defect (LAD), discussed earlier. Since isolated defects of CR3 and CR4 have not been described, the relative importance of defective complement binding compared to intracellular adhesion is not known.

DEFECTS IN CELL-SURFACE COMPLEMENT COMPONENTS. Several complement components are found on the surface of cells and mainly serve to regulate complement and protect cells from the consequences of complement activation. Some, such as decay-accelerating factor, C8bp, and CD59, serve to limit complement damage to homologous cells. Defects in these proteins lead to paroxysmal nocturnal hemoglobinuria, a clonal bone marrow disorder characterized by chronic intravascular hemolysis and thrombosis. The underlying defect is an abnormality in the synthesis of the glycolipid anchors, which attach proteins to the cell membrane. These molecules are found on leukocytes and platelets as well as red blood cells, which may explain the thrombocytopenia, leukopenia, and thrombosis seen in this disease.

Immunodeficiency Associated with Other Disorders

Chromosomal Abnormalities

Immunologic defects have been identified in association with a variety of chromosomal disorders, but none has been well characterized. Patients with Down syndrome have an increased incidence of respiratory infections, hepatitis, and leukemia. IgG subclass deficiencies, impaired antibody responses, deficient T cell function, especially decreased interferon production, and abnormal phagocytic function have all been reported, but no consistent abnormality has been identified. Patients with Bloom syndrome, xeroderma pigmentosum, and Fanconi's anemia all have chromosomal repair abnormalities and increased incidence of malignancies reminiscent of ataxia-telangiectasia. They also have increased incidences of sinopulmonary infections. Patients with Bloom syndrome may have decreased concentrations of one or more immunoglobulin isotypes and impaired antibody responses. Some have had decreased *in vitro* cellular immune responses. Similar abnormalities have been observed in Fanconi's anemia, but few patients have been studied in any detail.

Nutritional Disorders

Severe protein-calorie malnutrition can result in profound B and T cell defects, but this problem is beyond the scope of this chapter. Of the inherited defects, an inability to absorb zinc is an autosomal recessive disease that leads to a clinical syndrome known as acrodermatitis enteropathica. The disease is characterized by eczema, especially around the mouth and rectum, chronic diarrhea and malabsorption, and recurrent sinopulmonary infections. Patients may have hypogammaglobulinemia, but it may be secondary to enteric losses. There also may be an associated T lymphocyte defect. Therapy with parenteral zinc or high doses of oral zinc results in clearing of the diarrhea, skin rash, and immunologic defect.

Metabolic Diseases

Several hereditary metabolic disorders have associated immunologic defects. Few patients have been studied, and the relationship of the metabolic defect to the immune dysfunction is not clear. Biotin-dependent carboxylase deficiency results in convulsions, ataxia, alopecia, and keratoconjunctivitis. Patients may have *Candida* dermatitis, isolated IgA deficiency, and a reduced number of T cells in the peripheral blood. Biotin corrects both the biochemical and clinical abnormalities. Patients with type I hereditary orotic aciduria have growth failure, recurrent diarrhea, megaloblastic anemia, and an increased incidence of infections including meningitis and severe varicella. They are lymphopenic, with decreased numbers of T cells and impaired T cell function.

HUMAN IMMUNODEFICIENCY VIRUS-ASSOCIATED ACQUIRED IMMUNODEFICIENCY SYNDROME (AIDS)

During the past decade, human immunodeficiency virus (HIV)-associated acquired immunodeficiency has come to the forefront as the major cause of acquired immunodeficiency syndrome (AIDS) (Pizzo and Wilfert, 1991). Initially believed to be a disease process limited to homosexual men, it was soon realized to have no race, life style, or social status boundaries. In the early 1980s, absence of "safer sex" practices and transmission through blood and blood products led to identification of the affected population as the so-called "four-Hs": homosexuals, hemophiliacs, Haitians, and other "high-risk" individuals (which included intravenous-drug users, bisexual persons, and individuals having sex with those exhibiting AIDS or at risk for HIV infection). All too soon, infants and children were also showing signs of AIDS. In contrast to the fact that the initial population affected consisted of males in California, infants exhibiting symptoms of AIDS were mainly on the east coast in New York, New Jersey, and Florida. These infants were born to mothers who were, in general, infected with HIV through heterosexual contact, although drug abuse was a contributing factor in many cases. While being an urban disease in the Northeast and West, it spread as a more rural disease in Florida. Indeed, many of the young mothers infected in North Florida (a rural setting) were not displaying behavior outside of their social group norm when they would become infected. In many cases, the woman's first awareness of her HIV infection was when her infant would be hospitalized for severe pneumonia, and both the infant and its young mother would test positive for HIV.

The overall HIV antibody seroprevalence rate within the continental United States is estimated to be ~0.5 percent. In urban areas, an estimated 2.5 percent of the population are positive for HIV, and in certain locations within large cities, such as New York City, the seroprevalence rate has been documented to be as high as 10 percent of the population. A disproportionately large number of minorities are seropositive for HIV, but in actuality, the incidence correlates better with socioeconomic status. In 1988, anonymous testing of sera collected from 50,000 women of childbearing age visiting an outpatient obstetrics clinic revealed a seroprevalence rate of 2.5 percent. This places a large number of infants and children at risk for infection with HIV. Despite apparent disparity of seropositivity based on socioeconomic or racial backgrounds, HIV infection and AIDS should always be on the differential diagnosis for a patient of any age presenting with an unusual disease or infection.

Biology of the Human Immunodeficiency Viruses

HIV-1 (the major virus that causes AIDS) and HIV-2 are members of the *Lentivirinae* subfamily of retroviruses. These are enveloped viruses, and one of the major coat proteins, gp120, targets the virus to bind to cells that express CD4 (helper/inducer subset of T lymphocytes, macrophages/monocytes, Langerhans' dendritic cells, microglia, some renal tubular epithelia, some intestinal cells, and possibly others). Once bound by a target cell, the viral envelope allows the virus to fuse with the cell membrane and release into the cell's cytoplasm the inner nucleoprotein structure, which includes two genomic strands of RNA and reverse transcriptase (RT) bound to each. There the RT generates cDNA copies of the HIV genomic RNA. The cDNA translocates to the cell's nucleus, where a viral genome-encoded integrase protein (IN) incorporates HIV cDNA strands into the nuclear DNA. From this point forward, the infected cell contains HIV genome within its own genome, and therefore when it replicates, HIV genome is passed into each of the daughter cells. Most other retroviruses "transform" a cell after the integration of their genome, which then results in malignancy. In contrast, HIV contains proteins (TAT, REV, and NEF) that appear to be present to attenuate its control of the host cell and therefore down-regulate its replication of new viral particles. In this manner, the infection is more indolent, allowing infected cells to be reservoirs of virus rather than causing lytic death or loss of regulatory control via transformation resulting in early lymphoma.

Immunodeficiency viruses are not unique to humans. Similar viruses—SIV, FIV, and MIV—have been found to cause AIDS-like disorders in various African monkeys (macaques, mangabeys, mandrills, and African green monkeys), cats, and mice, respectively. These viruses are different from the previously discovered feline and murine leukemia viruses, FeLV and MuLV, respectively.

Unfortunately for attempts at devising therapy for HIV infection, there is the propensity of the virus to undergo mutations. An individual might be infected with a predominant virus among a population of viruses in the inoculum or possibly by multiple equally prevalent viruses, each with slightly different cellular tropism and virulence. After infection, the predominant viral population may change via mutation and subsequently alter the disease manifestations. Host factors, including HLA-type and immune system responsiveness, apply selective pressure (in a Darwinian sense) to the viral populations, allowing the selection of viruses that can survive the host immune system attack. An example of this occurs in HIV-infected women who give birth to several HIV-infected infants. Each of a mother's children will have different HIV genomic consensus sequences, but each consensus sequence can be found as a predominant form within blood taken from their mother during that infant's gestation or perinatal period. In addition, greater severity of illness in an infant correlates with poorer health status in the mother. This is taken to indicate that a more virulent form of HIV has evolved within the mother, adversely affecting her health while causing a more rapid progression to AIDS with more severe symptoms in the infant.

Transmission of HIV

Acquisition of HIV does not result from casual contact but requires contact with infected blood, tissue, or body fluid from an HIV-infected individual so that the infected material enters the circulation (Jones et al, 1989). This can occur during unprotected sex, when a needle or sharp object penetrates deep into tissue or muscle, or when receiving infected blood products. Blood-bank testing has virtually eliminated the latter circumstance, but the others require careful thought. Individuals participating in sex outside of long-term monogamous relationships place themselves at risk unless practicing safer sex. In general safer sex practice means to always use a condom that contains a detergent spermicide. This is critical for women who are at some 29 times greater risk of becoming infected during unprotected sex with infected men than men having unprotected sex with HIV-infected women. Universal precautions are important in types of medical practice in which sharp instruments are used and blood is exposed. All people should be treated as being potentially infected with HIV, to avoid the appearance of discrimination against anyone and to maintain a proper guard against transmission of the disease. Planning ahead is the best way to reduce risks (Table 2–3).

According to epidemiologic studies of health-care workers who have been injured via infected needles or sharp objects, the transmission rate is less than 0.1 percent. Any health-care worker that receives a puncture injury should report it to the local infection control agency (hospital infection control or

TABLE 2–3. PREVENTION OF HIV TRANSMISSION IN THE CLINICAL SETTING

Procedures must be planned ahead and be organized (e.g., starting IV, blood draw, arterial blood gas, lumbar puncture)
One person, generally the physician in charge, should be designated as the leader
The leader assigns each person's task (e.g., who will and how to restrain an infant or child)
One person is placed in charge of the "sharps" and maintains control of any "sharps" for the entire procedure, discarding them into puncture-resistant containers at the end of the procedure (generally the physician in charge)
Wear gloves
Never recap a used needle
Never use needles to transfer blood into various vacutainers (pop the top and use the needleless syringe to transfer blood into the open tube; alternatively use appropriately designed devices that shield the needle from accidental puncture)

health department) or contact the CDC in Atlanta and should consider a course of prophylactic zidovudine (AZT).

Transmission of HIV to infants is thought to occur during gestation, with free viral particles or infected leukocytes passing through the placenta, but it might also result from the mixing of blood during delivery or occur in the perinatal period from breast milk. Sexual abuse is another potential source of infection (Gutman et al, 1993). Currently, ~20 to 30 percent of infants born to HIV-infected mothers are actually infected. Almost all infants born to infected mothers will test positive via the ELISA test during the first 18 (and possibly as long as 24) months of life, owing to the transplacental acquisition of maternal antibody against HIV viral proteins. Therefore, it can be difficult to accurately diagnose infants that are truly infected early in their infancy.

Casual contact does not spread HIV. Touching, as during a routine physical examination, will not spread HIV. Holding an infant or child will not spread HIV. Instances of changing diapers, using the same food utensils, drinking from the same glass, using the same toothbrush, sleeping in the same bed, and even using the same razor for shaving have been monitored in families with an HIV-infected child or adult with no evidence of disease spread. However, such practices, which could allow infected body fluids to enter into one's blood, as through an open sore or abrasions, should be avoided.

HIV Disease Progression and Development of AIDS

Manifestations of congenital or perinatal infection of infants and of disease progression differ from those of adults or older children who become infected. Hallmarks of infant HIV infection and AIDS that differentiate the disease from that of adults include a shorter latency of infection to diagnosis of AIDS, greater degree of earlier immune system dysfunction, increased incidence of encapsulated bacterial infections with organisms that commonly cause childhood sepsis, lymphoid interstitial pneumonitis (LIP), increased incidence of CNS disease (exhibited as poor attainment or loss of developmental milestones), failure to thrive, multiple opportunistic infections, absence of Kaposi's sarcoma, lower incidence of lymphoma, and greater degree of hypergammaglobulinemia (Table 2–4). The majority of infants infected with HIV exhibit signs of AIDS by 9 to 12 months of age (MaWhinney et al, 1993). It is now clear that some do not develop problems until they are much older, having more of an "adult-like" disease that does not lead to symptoms until 7 to 13 years of age.

Adult infections are believed to be more stereotypical than those in infants. After inoculation, there is a 2- to 8-week period during which HIV infects its CD4+ target cells and the individual exhibits a flu-like illness. During this time, the viral p24 antigen can usually be detected in the blood by an antigen capture assay, and initially no antibodies against viral proteins are detected. Generally, specific antibodies against viral proteins are detected by the second month of infection, although it might take several months to generate a titer. This immune response against the virus helps to promote latency, which is also helped by the viral control proteins—TAT, NEF, and REV—which further reduce viral expansion. With the immune responsiveness, p24 antigen becomes difficult to detect. After recovery from the flu-like phase, there may be no outward sign of disease or any other indication of HIV infection. During a period that can be longer than 10 to 12

TABLE 2–4. COMPARISON OF INFANTILE AND ADULT AIDS

INFANTILE AIDS	ADULT AIDS
Shorter incubation and latency (<12 months)	Longer latency (>10 years)
Greater immune dysfunction earlier	Immune function declines slowly
Greater number of encapsulated bacterial infections (usual childhood pathogens)	Encapsulated bacterial infections less common
Unusual opportunistic infections early	Later opportunistic infections
Lymphoid interstitial pneumonitis (LIP)	LIP not present
Loss or lack of gain of developmental milestones	Dementia
Failure to thrive and wasting	Wasting
Rare occurrence of lymphoma	Kaposi's sarcoma, CNS lymphoma
Hypergammaglobulinemia and parotitis	Less hypergammaglobulinemia
Viral reservoir in macrophages, Langerhans' dendritic cells, and microglia	Langerhans' dendritic cells and microglia felt to be less important as viral reservoirs

years, there is attrition of CD4+ T lymphocytes with decreasing immune function. The onset of opportunistic infections or other AIDS-defining illnesses, such as Kaposi's sarcoma, or other malignancy such as cervical carcinoma in women, along with the fall in CD4+ T lymphocytes to less than 400/µL, signal the point at which AIDS can be diagnosed.

Some children appear to follow the adult-type AIDS onset, in that despite congenital infection, there is a prolonged latency before AIDS can be diagnosed. The majority of HIV-infected infants present during the first year of life. Typically, these infants may appear relatively normal at birth and begin having definite signs of disease by 3 months of age. Careful follow-up of growth parameters reveals that infected infants lag both in weight and in height, the latter being more important, especially in comparison to non-HIV-associated FTT. Demonstration of reduced height on growth charts can be an early indicator of AIDS. In addition to the small size of infected infants, lymphadenopathy and hepatosplenomegaly are generally present and, in some cases, were present at birth. It is interesting to note that rarely do HIV-infected infants present with opportunistic infections or sepsis before the age of 3 months. This probably corresponds to the loss of protective maternal antibody, both to the encapsulated organisms that cause sepsis and against HIV proteins that might in some way help retard HIV infection or delay its immunodeficiency effects. If the latter is true, loss of maternal antibody might allow a rapid onset of AIDS in the infant whose immune system has been more severely damaged by the *in utero* presence of HIV. *P. carinii* pneumonia (PCP) is the most common early opportunistic infection that allows AIDS to be diagnosed. Many of these infants will have had thrush, diarrhea, or fevers that herald the PCP. Unfortunately, these symptoms are many times overlooked because the infant might not appear to be ill or there are alternative explanations for the symptoms.

HIV infection and AIDS in infants and children can be divided into two major categories based on clinical presentation: (1) lymphoid interstitial pneumonitis-prone, or (2) *P. carinii* pneumonia-prone. These categories further divide infected infants into two somewhat different prognostic categories. The LIP-prone infant has greater hepatosplenomegaly, lymphadenopathy, hypergammaglobulinemia, parotitis, and typically milder disease with somewhat longer life expectancy. The PCP-prone infant generally presents with a more severe disease and PCP in infancy, has greater wasting and FTT, smaller liver and spleen, less lymphadenopathy, immunoglobulin levels slightly elevated, normal, or decreased, and a somewhat shorter life expectancy.

Older children might present with wheezing that is mistakenly diagnosed as asthma. Indeed, several children have gone for weeks with "walking PCP" that was being partially treated with bronchodilators and prednisone. Recurrent or exceptionally severe cases of zoster have also been the presenting symptoms of older children. Immunologic evaluation reveals these children to have low CD4 counts and they tend to be developing signs of wasting. The progress of their disease is similar to that of adult cases of AIDS.

Diagnosis of HIV Infection and AIDS

Adults and Children Older Than 18 to 24 Months

As with any disease, presenting signs and symptoms must arouse a suspicion in the examiner. Diagnosis of HIV infection in the adult or older child is relatively straightforward and can be applied to most children past 18 to 24 months of age. A screen for the presence of antibodies against HIV is performed by ELISA, which is performed in most clinical laboratories. However, many individuals might prefer anonymous testing through their community health department. All positive screens are confirmed via Western Blot testing, which is also commonly performed in most clinical laboratories. This tests for the presence of antibodies against specific HIV proteins. Rare false-positive tests occur, mainly in the ELISA assay, whereby individuals with other disorders that cause polyclonal B lymphocyte activation, such as SLE or after certain viral infections (especially with EBV), have nonspecific antibody production. Under these circumstances, the Western Blot analysis generally fails to demonstrate specific anti-HIV antibodies. Again, in rare circumstances, an "indeterminate" result is detected via the Western Blot. This is the apparent detection of specific anti-HIV antibody, but fewer or unusual protein bands are detected. Tests with such indeterminate results bear repeating every 3 to 6 months to ascertain whether the individual will truly exhibit evidence of an HIV infection or whether the nonspecific antibody titers will decline.

False-negative ELISA tests are extremely rare and can occur in at least two circumstances. A recently infected individual might not have generated antibodies against HIV at the time of testing but would be expected to test positive in the future. Individuals with antibody deficiency syndromes, X-linked agammaglobulinemia or common variable immunodeficiency, have an inability to produce specific antibodies and will continually test negative. In these latter subjects, alternative testing is required.

Antigen capture for detection of HIV p24 protein is a highly specific test, since it directly detects the presence of HIV protein. Unfortunately, at any one time only ~25 percent of truly infected individuals will test positive. Since one of the reasons for low sensitivity might be the inaccessibility of p24 antigen that is complexed with anti-p24, this test has greater potential sensitivity in individuals with hypogammaglobulinemic disorders. The p24 antigen capture tests are generally available through clinical laboratories.

The gold standard for HIV testing would be culture of the virus. This test is laborious, expensive, and not readily available, so that its utility is limited. If a physician is located near a research facility that performs HIV culture, a culture can be ordered, especially for diagnosis in infants and patients with hypogammaglobulinemia.

Polymerase chain reaction (PCR) amplification of HIV genome is an extremely sensitive method for the detection of HIV. This test should be performed only in reputable laboratories where quality control dictates the use of multiple negative control specimens so that false-positive amplifications can be detected. New specimens should be obtained to confirm the positive result and to verify that it was not positive due to contamination. PCR is useful for determining HIV infection status in infants and patients with hypogammaglobulinemia.

Infants Younger Than 18 Months

HIV diagnosis in newborns and infants less than 18 months of age can be challenging. Almost all infants born to HIV-infected mothers will test positive to HIV via the ELISA test during early infancy as a result of passively acquired maternal antibody. Generally, those not infected will demonstrate a loss of titer in the ELISA assay during the first 6 to 9 months of life. However, some will continue to have positive titers until almost 2 years of age. A reduction in specific titer is probably a good indicator for ruling out HIV infection, whereas an initial fall with a subsequent rise in titer indicates the presence of HIV infection. All positive ELISA tests need Western Blot analysis confirmation. In children who have reached 2 years of age, the standard ELISA and Western Blot assays can identify those truly infected with HIV, but earlier diagnosis is imperative so that appropriate therapy can be instituted early. An earlier diagnosis allows an avoidance of morbidity or death.

Useful tests in newborns and infants include (1) p24 antigen capture, (2) HIV culture, and (3) PCR for HIV genome. As with older individuals, the p24 antigen capture is highly specific, but its sensitivity may allow detection of only ~25 percent of those truly HIV-infected at any one time. Except at certain research institutions, culture for HIV is impractical. On the other hand, PCR for HIV genome is sensitive and can be readily obtained. As discussed above, quality control is important to prevent false-positive results. It is usually wise to confirm a positive PCR test with a second independently obtained specimen.

Quantitative immunoglobulin levels can be useful in making the diagnosis of HIV in an infant. Elevated levels of IgG, IgA, and IgM are distinctly unusual for a newborn or young infant and should raise suspicion of HIV infection. Many laboratories can determine immunoglobulin levels and return the results within a day or so, whereas other tests discussed may take longer to have results returned.

The guidelines shown in Tables 2–5 and 2–6 have been used successfully for the diagnosis and management of newborns and infants. Early diagnosis allows the institution of prophylactic and anticipatory therapy.

Pre- and Post-Test Counseling

Testing for HIV carries responsibility for both the patient being tested and the physician performing the tests. Before a sample is obtained for testing, each patient (including

TABLE 2–5. DETERMINATION OF MATERNAL RISK FOR HIV INFECTION

Mother or expectant mother in high-risk category
  Partner HIV+
  IV drug abuser
  Crack cocaine abuser/prostitute
  Inner city resident (especially underprivileged socioeconomic groups)
  From high seroprevalence region (urban or rural)
  Evidence or history of multiple STDs
  No prenatal care
Offer testing for HIV to all regardless of apparent risk (ELISA screen and Western Blot confirmation)
  Provide pre- and post-test counseling
Negative for HIV
  Further counsel patient for reduction in risks
  Get patient enrolled in community programs that provide support to reduce risks
  Offer further testing for HIV at routine intervals of 3–6 months
Positive for HIV
  Further counsel patient for reduction in risks of transmission of HIV to others
  If seropositivity determined during pregnancy, patient should be enrolled in AZT trial for the prevention of fetal acquisition of HIV
  If already delivered, counsel against breast-feeding of infants
  Evaluate newborn for the possibility of HIV infection (see Table 2–6)
  Establish immune status of patient (CD4 count) for initiating trimethoprim/sulfa PCP prophylaxis and consideration of anti-retroviral therapy

---

the parents of infants and young children) requires individual counseling. The test must be clearly described with emphasis on interpretation of the results. This becomes even more important for those whose test results might be equivocal or indeterminate due to another underlying disorder. Post-test counseling is equally important. Test results require timely and accurate presentation to the patient. A plan for future testing in those who test negative should be outlined, and in particular, a plan for therapy should be outlined in those who test positive. Pre- and post-test counseling should be performed face to face in a nonthreatening location where the patient will not be distracted. Most important for counseling is reassurance of strict confidentiality of the results.

Management of Patients with HIV Infection and AIDS

Adults and children are at risk for PCP when their absolute CD4+ T lymphocyte count falls below 400 to 500/μl and should be placed on trimethoprim/sulfamethoxazole (10 mg/kg/day based on trimethoprim) prophylaxis. Rashes occur in 50 percent or more of HIV-infected infants and children on trimethoprim/sulfamethoxazole. Discontinuance for one week generally allows resolution of the rash, and restarting the medication does not lead to recurrence of rash in the majority of patients. In those that have recurrence, dapsone (0.5 mg/kg/day up to 25 mg) alone is given for one week, after which trimethoprim (10 mg/kg/day) is added. An alternate but less efficacious treatment consists of monthly inhalations of pentamidine.

Intravenous gamma globulin therapy (400 mg/kg/month) may reduce the number of hospitalizations of children with HIV, but will not alter their long-term outcome. A decision to initiate IVIG therapy should be based on clinical data (recurrent infections with encapsulated organisms, such as *Pneumococcus*) and laboratory data (failure to respond to challenge with tetanus toxoid, diphtheria toxoid, and Pneumovax). Children with demonstrable humoral dysfunction will probably derive benefit from IVIG therapy; those without should not be treated unnecessarily.

Fever should be judiciously evaluated in infants and children, considering their susceptibility to pyogenic infections.

Diarrhea often can be attributed to *Giardia*, but other intestinal parasites such as *Cryptosporidium* and *Isospora belli* also have been incriminated. Flagyl treatment can be useful; Furoxone typically is not.

CMV infection is serious in HIV-infected infants and children and should be aggressively treated with ganciclovir or foscarnet if a resistant strain is suspected. Presenting signs typically include fever, leukopenia, anemia, and thrombocytopenia. Pneumonia and colitis are common. Flashing lights or descriptions of "fireworks" going off in the eyes can indicate CMV retinitis with retinal detachment and subsequent blindness. This is an ophthalmologic emergency to salvage sight and requires aggressive anti-CMV therapy.

Infection of the gastrointestinal tract with *M. avium-intracellulare* complex commonly occurs, leading to diarrhea and eventually to wasting. Treatment with some of the newer macrolide antibiotics (clarithromycin and azithromycin) offers some benefit.

Treatment of the primary HIV infection has become more controversial (Goodwin and Shipp, 1992). There was initial promise that

TABLE 2-6. EVALUATION OF NEWBORN AND INFANTS AT RISK FOR HIV INFECTION (MOTHER AT RISK OR POSITIVE FOR HIV INFECTION)

Clinical examination
   Growth retardation or inappropriate size for gestational age?
   Hepatosplenomegaly?
   Lymphadenopathy?
   Evidence of TORCH infections?
   Evidence of withdrawal symptoms from maternal drug abuse?
Laboratory examination for HIV
   ELISA and Western Blot analyses of newborn's serum paired with simultaneous analyses of maternal serum (higher titers or stronger bands from the newborn's serum in contrast to the maternal serum could indicate a response by the infant and therefore HIV infection in the infant)
   p24 antigen capture (high specificity, low sensitivity)
   PCR for HIV genome (high sensitivity, but false-positives occur so that quality control is critical)
   Positive PCR tests should be repeated for confirmation on a separately obtained specimen
   HIV culture (not readily available everywhere)
Further laboratory examination
   Quantitative immunoglobulin levels (elevated IgA and IgM indicate existence of prenatal infection, HIV, or other, such as TORCH)
   Consider additional risks, such as maternal STDs or possibility of TORCH infections and test appropriately
   Drug screen?
   Enumeration of T lymphocyte subsets (not predictive, except if abnormal; generally not performed unless other tests indicate newborn is truly HIV infected)
Negative for HIV
   Counsel parents for reducing risks of HIV exposure and spread
   Future evaluation for HIV to be based on future clinical status
   Routine follow-up evaluation for HIV probably not required
Positive for HIV: ELISA and Western Blot only (no clinical evidence of HIV, absence of hepatosplenomegaly and lymphadenopathy)
   Follow-up at 2 weeks of age
     Repeat clinical examination
     If no suspicious findings, follow-up at 1 month of age
     If hepatosplenomegaly, lymphadenopathy, FTT, or other suspicious findings are present, initiate further testing or repeat testing for the presence of HIV
   Follow-up at 1 month of age
     Repeat clinical examination as above
     Base repeat testing on clinical suspicion
     Consider initiating trimethoprim/sulfa PCP prophylaxis
   Follow-up at 6 weeks of age
     Optional reevaluation, follow up on FTT, suspected developmental delay, or other problems that have arisen
   Follow-up at 2 months of age
     Repeat routine evaluation and clinical examination, carefully checking growth parameters
     Repeat laboratory examinations based on clinical suspicion, FTT, and decreased rate of height growth, hepatosplenomegaly, lymphadenopathy, thrush, diarrhea, rashes, or other
     Substitute IPV for OPV (oral polio vaccine should not be given to an infant suspected of having an HIV infection or if someone in the family has an HIV infection)
     If not done earlier, consider initiating trimethoprim/sulfa PCP prophylaxis
   Follow-up at 10 weeks of age
     Optional reevaluation, based on clinical need
   Follow-up at 3 months of age
     Repeat routine evaluation and clinical examination as above, checking growth parameters and other clinical parameters that would indicate HIV infection
     Repeat ELISA and Western Blot analyses
     Pair the infant's 3-month serum with that obtained from same as a newborn and with maternal serum (fall in titer and loss of specific bands, respectively, in comparison with the newborn and maternal sera, make HIV infection less likely)
   Continue monthly clinical evaluations for evidence of possible HIV infection, especially if growth or other clinical parameters are not normal. Repeat paired ELISA and Western Blot studies every 2 to 4 months until the infant has persistently negative titers. Repeat ELISA and Western Blot studies at 2 years of age and then every 6 months to 1 year subsequently.
   If laboratory tests indicate and/or clinical condition warrants, initiate zidovudine therapy. T lymphocyte subsets should be enumerated. Trimethoprim/sulfa prophylaxis of PCP should definitely be initiated in any infant or child with a CD4+ T lymphocyte count of <500/μl.

early treatment with zidovudine in the HIV-infected individual led to a longer period before the onset of AIDS. Owing to the rapid mutability of HIV, resistance to zidovudine can readily occur so that its effectiveness might be lost. Because of continuing change as new data are collected, it is advisable to check with the CDC and in recent issues of the MMWR for current zidovudine therapy guidelines. For those that have failed zidovudine, dideoxyinosine and dideoxycytidine are two available alternatives. Neurotoxicity and pancreatitis are possible side effects of these latter two agents.

Treatment of primary HIV infection in infants and children, although somewhat controversial, demands careful thought. As discussed above, HIV-infected infants and children have a more rapid course to full-blown AIDS and exhibit more serious disease features, including infections related to the immunodeficiency and developmental delay problems related to CNS involvement. Therefore, one has less leeway in waiting to initiate therapy with one of the chain-terminator nucleoside analogs. As a result of delayed therapy, these children will have greater morbidity and poorer function in daily living. It is recommended that zidovudine therapy be instituted earlier in symptomatic infants and probably also in those truly infected to prevent HIV-associated morbidity. Again it is advisable to consult the CDC and MMWR for the most current guidelines for therapy.

Summary

HIV-associated immunodeficiency has become the most significant cause of acquired immunodeficiencies in both adults and children. Early diagnosis affords prophylaxis against PCP and allows the institution of therapy as warranted for the primary HIV infection or against opportunistic infections. Infants and young children with congenital HIV infections differ from adults with HIV infection in the latency before the onset of AIDS and the propensity to have recurrent infection with encapsulated bacteria. HIV infections involve the entire family, and all must receive appropriate therapy.

EVALUATION OF THE PATIENT FOR IMMUNODEFICIENCY

The most difficult decision is to determine which patient requires an immunologic evaluation. Otherwise healthy adults and children can have six or more respiratory infections per year, each of which can last for 1 to 2 weeks. Children in day care or adults who are exposed to large numbers of people are more likely to become infected. Nearly all of the congenital immunodeficiency diseases present in early childhood, although exceptions exist. Common variable immune deficiency or selective IgA deficiency may present in adulthood, and adults have been identified who are unable to make specific antibodies to polysaccharide antigens. Patients with immune deficiency may present with signs and symptoms suggestive of autoimmune disease, and the underlying immunodeficiency may be missed if the physician does not consider an underlying immune defect. A careful history and physical examination, combined with a few screening laboratory studies, can usually rule out a significant immune deficiency (Table 2–7). Other, more common, causes of recurrent infections, including allergy, asthma, cystic fibrosis, gastroesophageal reflux, and anatomic abnormalities of the nasopharynx should be ruled out.

Abnormalities detected by the screening studies are indications for a more detailed evaluation. The interpretation of many of the specific tests of immunity is difficult and as much an art as a science. Patients who require such studies should be referred to an immunologist, who can request the appropriate tests and aid in their interpretation.

History and Physical Examination

The history is the most important step in evaluating the patient suspected of having an immunodeficiency. Details of infections are particularly important, including age of onset, incidence and type of infection, severity, associated complications, response to therapy, and documentation of the type of organism. The history should include details of exposure in day care or the workplace, foreign travel, and risk factors for HIV infection. Seasonal variation may be helpful in distinguishing infections from allergic disease. One should inquire about immunization history and any adverse reactions to vaccines. A family history should be obtained with emphasis on a history of recurrent infections, early childhood deaths, allergy, autoimmune disease, lymphoreticular malignancy, or HIV infection. Details of growth and development, especially

TABLE 2-7. LABORATORY EVALUATION OF THE PATIENT WITH SUSPECTED IMMUNODEFICIENCY

	SCREENING TESTS	ADVANCED TESTS	CONFIRMATORY/RESEARCH TESTS
General	CBC and differential Sedimentation rate Chest film Sinus film/lateral neck	Sweat test Hemoglobulin electrophoresis Sinus CT scan Skin/lymph node biopsy	

Humoral immunity	Immunoglobulins	Specific antibodies
		  Tetanus
		  Diphtheria
		  H. influenzae
		  Pneumococci
		  Isohemagglutinins
			In vitro immunoglobulin synthesis
			Assays for T suppressor cells
			Enumeration of surface Ig-bearing cells

Complement/phagocytic	CH50/CH100	NBT Chemiluminescence Levels of C3, C4 C1-esterase inhibitor	Leukocyte adhesion markers Phagocytosis/chemotaxis Bactericidal assays Myeloperoxidase/G-6-PD levels

Cellular immunity	HIV antibody/antigen
	DH skin tests
	  Tetanus
	  Candida albicans
		Lymphocyte enumeration
		NK activity
			T and B subsets/activation markers
			Mitogen/antigen proliferation
			Cytokine production
			Cell-mediated lympholysis

lack of weight gain, are important indicators for children, whereas appetite and history of weight loss are more useful indicators for adults. Associated problems may suggest a specific immunodeficiency, such as hypocalcemia in a newborn with congenital heart disease that may indicate DiGeorge anomaly, or eczema and thrombocytopenia that could lead to a diagnosis of Wiskott-Aldrich syndrome. Other important historical points include intolerance to medications, particularly antibiotics, food allergy, diarrhea, and history of surgical procedures such as tonsillectomy, adenoidectomy, or splenectomy.

The physical examination is equally important, with emphasis on general health and growth, the presence of tonsillar tissue, lymph nodes, or hepatosplenomegaly, and, for children, the presence of congenital anomalies such as low-set ears, abnormal facies, or heart murmur. The skin may provide a variety of clues, such as petechiae indicating thrombocytopenia, a seborrheic or desquamating rash characteristic of Omenn syndrome or SCID with maternal GVHD, telangiectasia suggesting ataxia-telangiectasia, eczema suggesting either the hyper-IgE syndrome or Wiskott-Aldrich syndrome, or vitiligo, which could be a manifestation of CVID.

Initial Laboratory Evaluation

The initial laboratory studies should include an automated blood count and differential, sedimentation rate, and chest and sinus roentgenograms when clinically indicated (see Table 2-7). Immunoglobulin profile—IgG, IgA, IgM, and IgE—can be obtained through most hospital or commercial laboratories and can rule out severe defects in humoral immunity such as X-linked agammaglobulinemia or CVID, selective IgA deficiency, or hyper-IgE syndrome. Either the CH50 or CH100 is an adequate screening test for any of the congenital defects of complement. A test for HIV should be considered for any patient with unusual infections, failure to thrive, or history or physical examination suggestive of HIV. Adults can be screened by evaluating antibody to gp120, but young children or patients in whom a humoral immune defect is suspected should be evaluated by testing for p24 core antigen by antigen capture, pro-viral DNA in cells by PCR, or by culture. Cellular immunity can be readily assessed by delayed hypersensitivity skin testing using a 1:10 dilution of tetanus toxoid and a 1:1000 dilution of C. albicans for adults or 1:100 for children. More extensive DH skin test panels may be employed, including mumps, *Trichophyton*, streptokinase, histoplasmin, and coccidioidin, but they do not add significant information if either tetanus or Candida is positive.

Advanced Laboratory Studies

The selection of specific tests of immunity should be based on the clinical presentation.

Patients with several serious pyogenic infections should have an evaluation of humoral immunity. Sepsis or disseminated infections, particularly neisserial or pneumococcal infections, suggest the possibility of complement deficiency or a phagocytic defect. Skin infections, such as furunculosis, cellulitis, or subcutaneous abscesses, could result from impaired phagocytic function, whereas granulomatous lesions and bacterial or fungal infections suggest a killing defect such as in chronic granulomatous disease. Failure to thrive and severe or persistent infections with pathogens such as *C. albicans, P. carinii,* respiratory syncytial virus, parainfluenza virus, or protozoa are suggestive of a defect in cellular immunity. The presence of a positive delayed hypersensitivity skin test rules out major defects in cellular immunity, but more sophisticated tests are needed to evaluate for more subtle abnormalities.

Evaluation of Humoral Immunity

Determination of serum immunoglobulins is adequate for screening purposes, but measurement of specific antibody is necessary to fully evaluate humoral immunity. Antibodies to common vaccines, including tetanus, diphtheria, *H. influenzae,* and *Pneumococcus,* can be obtained through many commercial laboratories. However, the "normal" values reported by most laboratories are the levels thought to be protective, not necessarily the levels achieved by the majority of normal individuals. Unfortunately, there are few data on the normal ranges for adults or children. Comparison of antibody levels pre- and post-immunization allows a better determination of the antibody-forming capacity, but it is crucial that both assays be performed in the same laboratory, preferably at the same time. Determination of antibody titers to measles can be useful, but anti-poliovirus antibodies are difficult to measure, and these determinations are not reliable unless done in a laboratory capable of measuring neutralization. Measurement of isohemagglutinins to ABO blood group antigens, which are natural IgM antibodies to polysaccharide antigens, is useful in older children and adults.

Evaluation of humoral immunity beyond these assays requires access to a sophisticated immunology laboratory and is important for making a specific diagnosis beyond merely identifying the patient as being immunodeficient. IgG subclasses were not listed in the screening or intermediate tests because an abnormality in subclasses alone, in the absence of functional abnormalities, is not of clinical importance. Measurement of subclasses often is technically unreliable, with significant inter-laboratory variability. Determination of subclasses may be of interest, but only in the context of the other immunologic studies and is best left to the immunologist. It is possible to order B cell enumeration studies through hospital laboratories, but interpretation may require considerable expertise. Other studies, such as *in vitro* immunoglobulin production or evaluation of suppressor T cells, are done only in research laboratories.

Evaluation of Cellular Immunity

The absolute lymphocyte count is an important indicator of cellular immunity since the majority of lymphocytes are T cells. However, some patients with significant T cell defects have normal lymphocyte counts due to elevated numbers of B cells or NK cells. Thus, it is important to specifically measure the lymphocyte subsets, and this is usually done using monoclonal antibodies and flow cytometry. A complete absence of one or more subsets may lead to easy interpretation, but generally considerable expertise is required to evaluate the results of such studies. Most hospital and commercial laboratories evaluate only the basic B, T, and NK cell markers, and more extensive evaluation is necessary to fully characterize immune defects. Functional assays, such as lymphoblastic responses to mitogens phytohemagglutinin, concanavalin A, or pokeweed mitogen are useful as screening tests of T cell function. Additional evaluation should include blastogenic responses to specific antigens and allogeneic cells, NK activity, cytokine production, and lymphocytotoxic responses. Measurement of the enzymes adenosine deaminase and purinenucleoside phosphorylase in RBC lysates or in white blood cells can confirm the diagnosis of a purine salvage pathway defect in a patient known to have a cellular immune defect.

Evaluation of Phagocytosis and Complement

Only limited assays of phagocytic function or complement are available outside of medical centers. If CGD is suspected, the hexose monophosphate shunt activity can be determined by the nitrotetrazolium blue assay or by chemiluminescence. The presence of the adhesion molecules CD18, CD11a, CD11b, and CD11c can be measured by flow cytometry using specific monoclonal antibodies. Abnormalities in any of these assays should be confirmed by more specific studies. Some specific components of the complement system, especially C3, C4, and C1 esterase inhibitor, can be readily determined, but assays of function require access to one of only a few laboratories interested in the sophisticated study of the complement system.

Special Considerations for the Evaluation of Children

The incidence of infections, particularly respiratory infections, is much higher in children than in adults. Preschool children or those in elementary school have an average of six infections per year, and as many as 12 per year is within 2 standard deviations of normal. Children in day care or otherwise exposed to a large number of other children are more likely to have a higher incidence of infections. Despite the infections, immunologically normal children will grow and gain weight appropriately. The majority of these children will prove to be immunologically normal and do not need to be evaluated unless the infections have been unusually severe, have been caused by opportunistic organisms, or have led to growth retardation.

Most of the assays available for the study of adults and older children are applicable for the evaluation of the neonate, including premature infants. Unfortunately, there are limited reports of normal values for young children. Most commercial laboratories report age-appropriate ranges, but often these are not developed in their laboratory and may have been generated using a different assay. This is particularly important for IgG subclasses. The ranges of normal immunoglobulins (Buckley et al, 1968) were developed from the study of a limited number of children and may not be entirely applicable to another population of different ethnic or racial background. Similarly, it is important to be aware of the variations in the percentages and absolute numbers of lymphocytes and neutrophils throughout development (Xanthou, 1970; Manroe et al, 1979; Weinberg et al, 1985). It is common to forget that a neonate with a lymphocyte count of $1000/mm^3$ is lymphopenic and should be evaluated. There is even less information on the normal values for T cells and T cell subsets in neonates and infants, but as a result of the study of children for HIV, some data do exist (Yanase et al, 1986). However, these data are difficult to evaluate, and few laboratories report age-adjusted interpretations. Therefore, if such studies are ordered, an immunology consult should be obtained to assist in their interpretation.

The evaluation of antibody formation also must consider the age of the patient. Most children, including premature infants, are able to respond to protein antigens such as tetanus and diphtheria and to the protein-conjugated *Haemophilus influenzae* vaccine (Cates et al, 1988). Children under the age of 2 years have limited ability to respond to the pneumococcal polysaccharide antigens (Sell et al, 1981), but by 5 years of age the response is nearly that of an adult (Paton et al, 1986). Unfortunately, little is known of the response between 2 and 5 years of age, and most commercial laboratories report normal ranges that were developed using assays other than the one used in that laboratory and often done on a limited number of children. Thus, these studies must be interpreted with caution, and it is important to have a good understanding of the laboratory assay being used and how the normal ranges were generated.

THERAPY OF THE PRIMARY IMMUNODEFICIENCY DISEASES

The principal modes of therapy for these disorders are reduction of exposure to infectious agents; aggressive use of antibacterial, antifungal, and antiviral antibiotics; replacement of antibody deficiency with infusions of gamma globulin; and, for the cellular immune defects, reconstitution with immunocompetent tissue. Despite these measures, many patients will continue to suffer from chronic infections and autoimmune diseases. Early diagnosis and prompt institution of therapy are vital, because once chronic infection and tissue damage occur, not even complete immune reconstitution can restore the patient to health.

Therapy of Antibody Deficiency

The majority of infections in patients with antibody deficiency are caused by pyogenic bacteria. Prompt and aggressive therapy with antibiotics is essential. Many patients will require chronic or prophylactic antibiotics, especially if chronic infections such as sinusitis, bronchitis, or otitis are present. In general these patients do not have to be isolated, but consideration should be given to removing young children from day care since the incidence of respiratory infections is high and exposure will result in frequent illness.

All patients with a significant defect in antibody-forming capacity should be treated with gamma globulin replacement (Schiff, 1994a; 1994b). Patients with low immunoglobulin levels but good antibody responses, as is the case with the majority of patients with IgG subclass deficiency and transient hypogammaglobulinemia of infancy, should not be treated. Conversely, those with normal levels but poor responses, as in Wiskott-Aldrich syndrome and hyper-IgE syndrome, should be treated. The initially recommended dose of 100 mg/kg/month effected a marked reduction in the incidence of infection. However, the levels of specific antibody achieved with that dose were low, and a number of studies suggested that higher doses were more effective. Current recommendations are 200 to 400 mg/kg given monthly, or more often if clinically indicated. It must be remembered that the amount of specific antibody to any given organism is low since the plasma is pooled from normal donors. Therefore, in the face of an infection it may be necessary to give frequent infusions in order to provide a constant supply of the relevant antibody.

All of the products currently licensed in the United States are relatively well tolerated. The majority of patients, especially children, experience no adverse reactions. Some patients complain of fever, chills, muscle aches, flushing, chest tightness, or wheezing. These reactions are thought to be due to aggregates of IgG in the infusions or to antigen-antibody reactions. Reactions are more common early in therapy and may actually decrease as higher doses of gamma globulin are used. Most reactions can be treated by decreasing the rate of infusion. In patients with persistent reactions, pretreatment with salicylates or, for more profound reactions, corticosteroids can be beneficial. Antihistamines are useful for treating reactions but should be used judiciously before infusions since they may mask the onset of more serious allergic reactions. More severe reactions are rare but can be life-threatening. A small subset of patients with common variable immune deficiency and complete IgA deficiency can form IgE anti-IgA antibodies (Burks et al, 1986). In these patients even a few milliliters of an IgA-containing product can evoke a life-threatening anaphylactic reaction. Most of these patients can be successfully treated with carefully screened lots of Gammagard, which is the only product with a sufficiently low content of IgA.

Human immunodeficiency virus is destroyed during the preparation of intravenous gamma globulin, and so there has never been a documented instance of transmission of HIV by any gamma globulin product. The intravenous gamma globulin preparations have been relatively free of other infectious agents, but in early 1994 there was an outbreak of hepatitis C involving multiple lots of Gammagard throughout the world. The Gammagard has now been replaced by Gammagard-SD, which is treated with solvent and detergent to destroy enveloped viruses. All other products include a viral-inactivation step, and new processes are being introduced to make the product even safer. However, no process can completely ensure that all viral agents are eliminated. The small risk of transmitting infection must be weighed against the high risk of life-threatening infections in patients unable to make antibody. For patients with low levels of immunoglobulins but good antibody-forming capacity, it is difficult to justify even a small risk of serious infection.

Therapy of Cellular Immune Defects

Early recognition and diagnosis are vital to the treatment of patients with cellular immune defects. Most bacterial and protozoal infections can be treated successfully, but many of the viral infections such as CMV and EBV can result in fatal infections. Thus, once the diagnosis is suspected the child should be placed into protective isolation. All blood products must be irradiated with a minimum of 1500 rads, and 3000 rads are preferable. It is also beneficial to use CMV-negative donors; if no CMV-negative blood is available, the use of frozen deglycerinated blood or blood put through Leukopac filters to remove white cells will reduce the risk of transmitting CMV.

Bone marrow transplantation is the therapy of choice for patients with severe defects in cellular immunity. Patients with complete forms of SCID can undergo transplantation without any form of cytoreductive or ablative therapy, but all other patients must be conditioned to reduce residual cellular immunity. MHC-compatible marrow from an HLA-identical sibling is clearly the preferred source, but techniques utilizing monoclonal antibodies or soy lectin combined with sheep red blood cell rosetting can remove sufficient numbers of T cells to allow transplantation of haploidentical marrow without significant risk of graft-versus-host disease. The ability to use haploidentical donors is of great importance since the majority of infants with T cell disorders do not have HLA-identical donors. Unfortunately, there is a higher rate of graft failure using T-depleted marrow transplants, which may be due to the importance of cytokines derived from mature T cells on marrow growth. Because there are no T lymphocytes in the graft to provide adoptive immunity in the immediate post-transplant period, infants receiving T-depleted marrow transplants remain severely immunodeficient for 90 to 120 days after transplant (Buckley et al, 1993). T cell function, numbers, and mitogen responses usually develop rapidly after that point, but B cell function develops more slowly; some patients require several years for antibody formation to develop and some remain hypogammaglobulinemic.

Before the advent of reliable techniques to remove T cells and permit transplantation of non-HLA-identical marrow, transplantation was done with immunocompetent tissue from other sources. Fetal liver was used for several years, but there are only a few patients who showed any improvement, and for many of these the effects were transient. Fetal thymus and thymic epithelium were also used, especially for DiGeorge anomaly. However, since there is a high incidence of spontaneous improvement, it is not clear that the thymic transplants were efficacious. Various thymic hormones including thymosin fraction 5, thymopoietin, and thymosin pentapeptide have been used with some anecdotal success. An extract made from the lysate of lymphocytes known as transfer factor has been used to treat CMC, and at least transient improvement has been noted.

Patients with ADA deficiency can be treated by enzyme replacement. Initially red blood cell transfusions were used as a source of enzyme, but the enzyme levels achieved were modest, and complications of hypertransfusion were common. Bovine ADA, especially that linked to polyethylene glycol to prolong its half-life, has resulted in good serum levels of ADA and, more importantly, reduction in the toxic levels of deoxyadenosine (Hershfield et al, 1987). There has been significant clinical improvement in many of the patients treated, but immunologic reconstitution has been variable. At best, PEG-ADA is only a temporary measure and should be used only for those patients for whom bone marrow transplant is not an option or who have failed transplant. ADA deficiency is the first disease to be treated with gene therapy, and two patients were being treated with ADA gene inserted into peripheral white blood cells that were infused at regular intervals. More recently the ADA gene was inserted into stem cells of two neonates, but it is still too early to know whether durable reconstitution has occurred.

Genetic engineering techniques have permitted the production of large quantities of cytokines, which has led to therapeutic trials with IL-2, α-interferon, γ-interferon, and granulocyte colony stimulating factor (G-CSF). IL-2 has been used to treat a small number of children who lacked the ability to produce IL-2 and whose *in vitro* lymphocyte proliferation improved in the presence of recombinant IL-2. There was some clinical and immunologic improvement, but unfortunately, a trial of IL-2 linked to PEG had to be suspended because of cerebral vascular accidents in two patients. This problem was not seen with the native IL-2 and has not occurred in patients receiving PEG-ADA, and so the significance of the observation is not clear. Controlled trials are needed for each of these agents before their usefulness can be determined.

REFERENCES

Ambrosino DM, Umetsu DT, Siber GR, et al. Selective defect in the antibody response to *Haemophilus influenzae* type b in children with recurrent infections and normal serum IgG subclass levels. J Allergy Clin Immunol 81:1175–1179, 1988.

Aucouturier P, Lacombe C, Bremard C, et al. Serum IgG

subclass levels in patients with primary immunodeficiency syndromes or abnormal susceptibility to infections. Clin Immunol Immunopath 51:22–37, 1989.
Bastian J, Law S, Vogler L, et al. Prediction of persistent immunodeficiency in the DiGeorge anomaly. J Pediatr 115:391–396, 1989.
Buckley RH, Dees SC, O'Fallon WM. Serum immunoglobulins I. Levels in normal children and in uncomplicated childhood allergy. Pediatrics 41:600, 1968.
Buckley RH, Sampson HA. The hyperimmunoglobulinemia E syndrome. In Franklin EC (ed). Clinical Immunology Update. New York, Elsevier North-Holland, 1981, pp 47–67.
Buckley RH, Schiff SE, Schiff RI, Roberts JL, Markert ML, Peters W, Williams LW, Ward FE. Haploidentical bone marrow stem cell transplantation in human severe combined immunodeficiency. Semin Hematol 30:92–104, 1993.
Burks AW, Sampson HA, Buckley RH. Anaphylactic reactions after gamma globulin administration in patients with hypogammaglobulinemia. N Engl J Med 314:560–564, 1986.
Businco L, Di Fazio A, Ziruolo G, et al. Clinical and immunological findings in four infants with Omenn's syndrome: A form of severe combined immunodeficiency with phenotypically normal T cells, elevated IgE, and eosinophilia. Clin Immunol Immunopath 44:123–133, 1987.
Cates KL, Goetz C, Rosenberg N, Pantschenko A, Rowe JC, Ballow M. Longitudinal development of specific and functional antibody in very-low-birth-weight premature infants. Pediatr Res 23:14–22, 1988.
Cunningham-Rundles C. Clinical and immunologic analyses of 103 patients with common variable immunodeficiency. J Clin Immunol 9:22–33, 1989.
Fischer A, Lisowska-Grospierre B, Anderson DC, Springer TA. Leukocyte adhesion deficiency: Molecular basis and functional consequences. Immunodeficiency Rev 1:39–54, 1990.
Frank MD. Complement in the pathophysiology of human disease. N Engl J Med 316:1565, 1987.
Goodwin SD, Shipp KW. Criteria for use of zidovudine in adult and pediatric inpatients and outpatients. Clin Pharmacy 11:63–68, 1992.
Gutman LT, Herman-Giddens ME, McKinney RE Jr. Pediatric acquired immunodeficiency syndrome. Barriers to recognizing the role of child sexual abuse. Am J Dis Child 147:711–712, 1993.
Herrod HG. Chronic mucocutaneous candidiasis in childhood and complications of non-*Candida* infection: A report of the Pediatric Immunodeficiency Collaborative Study Group. J Pediatr 116:377–382, 1990.
Hershfield MS, Buckley RH, Greenberg ML, et al. Treatment of adenosine deaminase deficiency with polyethylene glycol-modified adenosine deaminase. N Engl J Med 316:589–596, 1987.
Hirshhorn R. Adenosine deaminase deficiency. Immunodeficiency Rev 2:175–198, 1990.
International Chronic Granulomatous Disease Cooperative Study Group. A controlled trial of interferon gamma to prevent infection in chronic granulomatous disease. N Engl J Med 324:509–516, 1991.
Jones D, Adinolfi A, Gallis H (eds). Care of the Patient with HIV Infection. Chapel Hill, Health Sciences Consortium, 1989.
Kersey JH, Shapiro RS, Filipovich AH. Relationship of immunodeficiency to lymphoid malignancy. Pediatr Infect Dis J 7:S10–S12, 1988.

Kirkpatrick CH. Chronic mucocutaneous candidiasis. Antibiotic and immunologic therapy. Ann N Y Acad Sci 544:471–480, 1988.
Kishimoto TK, Springer TA. Human leukocyte adhesion deficiency: Molecular basis for a defective immune response to infections of the skin. Curr Probl Dermatol 18:106–115, 1989.
Lomax KJ, Makech HL, Gallin JI. The molecular biology of selected phagocytic defects. Blood Reviews 3:94–104, 1989.
Malech HL, Gallin JI. Neutrophils in human disease. N Engl J Med 317:867, 1987.
Manroe BL, Weinberg AG, Rosenfeld CR, Browne R. The neonatal blood count in health and disease. I. Neutrophilic cells. J Pediatr 95:89, 1979.
Markert ML. Purine nucleoside phosphorylase deficiency. Immunodeficiency 3:45–81, 1991.
MaWhinney S, Pagano M, Thomas P. Age at AIDS diagnosis for children with perinatally acquired HIV. J Acquired Immune Defic Synd 6:1139–1144, 1993.
McKinney RE, Katz SI, Wilfert CM. Chronic enteroviral meningoencephalitis in agammaglobulinemic patients. Rev Infect Dis 9:334–356, 1987.
Mouy R, Fischer A, Vilmer E, Seger R, Griscelli C. Incidence, severity, and prevention of infections in chronic granulomatous disease. J Pediatr 114:555–560, 1989.
Nauseef WM. Myeloperoxidase deficiency. Hematol Pathol 4:165–178, 1990.
Paton JC, Toogood IR, Cockington RA, Hansman D. Antibody response to pneumococcal vaccine in children aged 5 to 15 years. Am J Dis Child 140:135–138, 1986.
Pizzo PA, Wilfert CM (eds). Pediatric AIDS. Baltimore, Williams & Wilkins, 1991.
Preud'Homme J-L, Hanson LÅ. IgG subclass deficiency. Immunodeficiency Rev 2:129–149, 1990.
Remold-O'Donnell E, Rosen FS. Sialophorin (CD43) and the Wiskott-Aldrich syndrome. Immunodeficiency Rev 2:151–174, 1990.
Roberts R, Gallin JI. The phagocytic cell and its disorders. Ann Allergy 51:330–344, 1983.
Ross SC, Densen P. Complement deficiency states and infection: Epidemiology, pathogenesis, and consequences of neisserial and other infections in an immune deficiency. Medicine 63:243–273, 1984.
Segal AW. The electron transport chain of the microbicidal oxidase of phagocytic cells and its involvement in the molecular pathology of chronic granulomatous disease. J Clin Invest 83:1785–1793, 1989.
Schiff RI. Intravenous gamma globulin: Pharmacology, clinical uses, and mechanisms of action. Pediatr Allergy Immunol 5:63–87, 1994a.
Schiff RI. Intravenous gamma globulin, 2: Pharmacology, clinical uses, and mechanisms of action. Pediatr Allergy Immunol 5:127–156, 1994b.
Sell SH, Wright PF, Vaughn WK, Thompson J, Schiffman G. Clinical studies of pneumococcal vaccines in infants. I. Reactogenicity and immunogenicity of two polyvalent polysaccharide vaccines. Rev Infect Dis 3:S97–107, 1981.
Stoltz W, Graubner U, Gerstmeier J, Burg G, Belohradsky BH. Chediak-Higashi syndrome: Approaches in diagnosis and treatment. Curr Probl Dermatol 18:93–100, 1989.
Sullivan JL. X-linked lymphoproliferative syndrome. Immunodeficiency Rev 1:325, 1989.
Swift M. Genetic aspects of ataxia-telangiectasia. Immunodeficiency Rev 2:67–81, 1990.
Tiller TL, Buckley RH. Transient hypogammaglobuli-

nemia of infancy: Review of the literature, clinical and immunologic features of 11 new cases, and long-term follow-up. Pediatrics 92:347, 1978.

Weinberg AG, Rosenfeld CR, Manroe BL, Browne R. Neonatal blood cell count in health and disease. II. Values for lymphocytes, monocytes, and eosinophils. J Pediatr 106:462–466, 1985.

WHO Scientific Group. Primary immunodeficiency diseases: Report of a WHO scientific group. Immunodeficiency Rev 3:195–236, 1992.

Xanthou M. Leucocyte blood picture in healthy full-term and premature babies during neonatal period. Arch Dis Child 45:242–249, 1970.

Yanase Y, Tango T, Okumura K, Tada T, Kawasaki T. Lymphocyte subsets identified by monoclonal antibodies in healthy children. Pediatr Res 20:1147–1151, 1986.

Yang KD, Hill HR. Neutrophil function disorders: Pathophysiology, prevention, and therapy. J Pediatr 119:343–354, 1991.

Chapter 3
Autoimmune Diseases

JoAnne Kriege, M.D., and Frank M. Graziano, M.D., Ph.D.

Fortunately for us, we possess a tightly regulated and powerfully protective system in our body. This system, collectively designated our host defense system or immune system, includes lymphocytes, macrophages, polymorphonuclear leukocytes, and other amplifying substances such as complement and cytokines. Recognition of nonself by this closely regulated system is beneficial to the host in eliminating infection and cancerous cells. Imagine, then, the destructive consequences of the immune response when its regulation is broken and the response is directed against one's own tissue. The result of this process is autoimmune injury and disease.

Autoreactivity does not always result in a state of disease, however. We are increasingly realizing the essential role that self-recognition plays in the normal immune response. Communication between lymphocytes depends on recognition of self major histocompatibility antigens. In addition, antibody to one's own antibodies (anti-idiotypic antibodies) is part of the normal immune response and forms a network of self recognition necessary for fine regulation of this response. Research into the pathophysiology of autoimmune diseases, with their myriad manifestations of altered immunoregulation, offers valuable opportunities to understand these diseases and to increase our knowledge of the normal immune response.

Autoimmune diseases are multifactorial, with genetic predisposition, hormones, and numerous environmental agents implicated to varying degrees as causal factors. What initiates and maintains autoimmune responses is unclear. Proposed mechanisms for autoimmunity range from nonspecific polyclonal B cell activation, to the targeting of common structures shared by infectious agents (molecular mimicry), to a primary or intrinsic generalized defect in immune regulation. The spectrum of autoimmune disease includes those with single target organs (such as Hashimoto's thyroiditis and type I diabetes mellitus) and those with multi-organ involvement (systemic lupus erythematosus and rheumatoid arthritis). The organ-specific autoimmune diseases are characterized by autoantibodies directed to that single organ. In contrast, systemic autoimmune diseases typically demonstrate a variety of autoantibodies against ubiquitous cellular components (e.g., DNA and RNA).

Many of these diseases are associated with specific HLA haplotypes, and an understanding of the major histocompatibility complex is essential to an appreciation of autoimmunity. The major histocompatibility complex is located on chromosome 6 and is made up of three groups of genes: class I, class II, and class III. The class I genes encode HLA-A, HLA-B, and HLA-C antigens, which are present on all nucleated cells and are important for the recognition of encapsulated viruses and tumor cells by $CD8^+$ (T cytotoxic) cells. Class II genes encode HLA-DR, HLA-DQ, and HLA-DP molecules. Like the class I antigens, these are also cell surface glycoproteins, but they are found only on macrophages, monocytes, dendritic cells, and B and T lymphocytes. These cell surface antigens are important in the interaction between the antigen-presenting cells, such as macrophages, and $CD4^+$ (T helper) cells. The class II molecules are made up of alpha and beta chains, which form an antigen-binding cleft on the cell's surface. An antigen is only recognized by a $CD4^+$ T cell when it is presented in association with the HLA-D antigen to which it is bound (Fig. 3-1) (Johnson et al, 1992). The class III genes encode for various components of the complement cascade.

One inviting explanation for autoimmune phenomena is cross-reactivity. An example of this is rheumatic fever, a condition following group A streptococcal infection in which antibodies directed against the bacteria cross-react with cardiac antigens, resulting in valvular heart disease. The idea of molecular mimicry takes this a step further and postulates that amino acid sequence homology or tertiary structure homology between an antigen (such as a virus) and various cell components may be sufficient for autoreactivity to occur. Many autoimmune diseases are associated with specific HLA haplotypes (Table 3-1). For some of these diseases, homology has been found between the HLA amino acid sequence and that of various infectious agents believed to play a role in inciting the disease. Thus, a susceptible host, when exposed to the inciting antigen, has a disregulated immune response, and autoimmunity occurs.

TABLE 3-1. ASSOCIATION OF MAJOR HISTOCOMPATIBILITY COMPLEX CLASS I AND CLASS II ALLELES WITH RHEUMATIC DISEASES

Ankylosing spondylitis	B27
Reiter's syndrome	B27
Systemic lupus erythematosus	DR2, DR3, B8
Rheumatoid arthritis	DR1, DR4
Sjögren's syndrome	DR2, DR3

In the discussion that follows, we will examine a number of autoimmune diseases that are relatively commonly encountered. Our primary goal is to discuss various aspects of these diseases and relate these to the immunologic concepts that are suggested to be critical to their pathogenesis. Although this discussion will not include all diseases suggested to have an autoimmune basis, it will focus on diseases for which studies have increased our understanding of the immunologic aspects of the processes.

SYSTEMIC AUTOIMMUNE DISEASES

These diseases affect multiple organs to varying degrees. They are often associated with numerous autoantibodies to ubiquitous cell components, such as antinuclear antibodies. Many affect primarily connective tissue and blood vessels; hence, another name for them is the collagen vascular diseases.

Systemic Lupus Erythematosus

Systemic lupus erythematosus (SLE) is a chronic multisystem disorder considered to be the prototype autoimmune disease because of the many autoantibodies associated with it. The disease affects predominantly females of all races in a 4:1 ratio. The incidence among black females, however, is higher than that in white females.

ETIOLOGY AND PATHOGENESIS. The etiology of SLE is not known. Multiple factors appear to play a role: genetic, hormonal, and environmental. Genetic susceptibility is suggested by the high concordance rate in monozygotic twins. In addition, specific histocompatibility antigens have been associated with disease susceptibility as well as the production of various autoantibodies. The observation that SLE in whites is associated with both HLA-B8 and

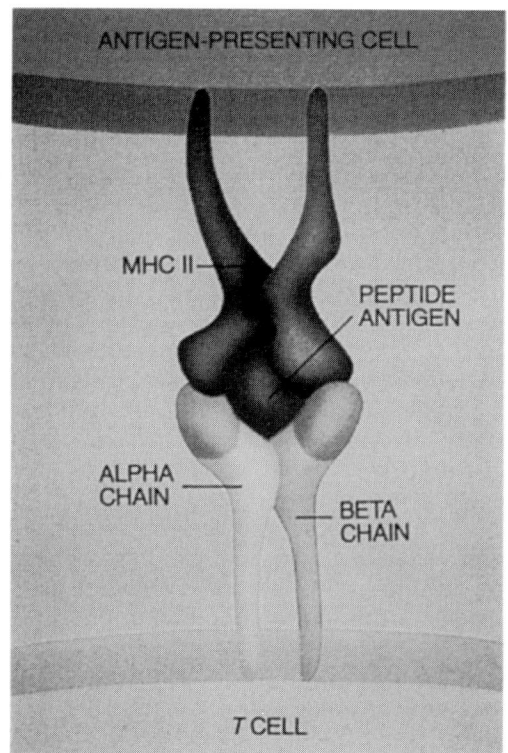

FIGURE 3-1. Interaction between T cell and antigen-presenting cell. (From Johnson HM, Russell JK, Pontzer CH. Superantigens in human disease. Scientific Amer Apr; 266:92-95, 98-101, 1992.)

HLA-DR3 haplotypes may possibly be explained by the common underlying association with C4A null genes (Kemp et al, 1987). The C4A gene is one of two alleles coding for the production of the C4 component of complement. Complement is important in clearing immune complexes. It has been shown that the C4A gene product binds immune complexes more efficiently than the C4B isotype. Therefore patients who are homozygous for C4A null alleles might be at a disadvantage in clearing immune complexes, which then can cause tissue damage (Reveille, 1991). In addition to disease susceptibility, specific HLA haplotypes are associated with autoantibody production in SLE. HLA-DR2 and HLA-DR3 are associated with high titers of antibodies to double-stranded DNA (Alvarellos et al, 1983). HLA-DR4 and HLA-DR5 are associated with the production of Smith and ribonuclear protein (RNP) antibodies, respectively (Condemi, 1992). Hormonal factors presumably play a role, since women are more susceptible to the disease. In addition, approximately 30 percent undergo exacerbation during pregnancy or the postpartum period. Animal studies suggest that female sex hormones facilitate immune responses in susceptible individuals. Environmental factors are also important because SLE may flare after viral infection, ultraviolet light exposure, surgery, stress, and exposure to certain drugs, such as the sulfonamides.

The immunologic abnormalities seen in SLE include antinuclear antibodies (ANAs), immune complexes, complement level depression, tissue deposition of immunoglobulins and complement, circulating anticoagulants, and other autoantibodies (Table 3–2). Antinuclear antibodies are highly sensitive but not specific for the diagnosis of SLE. High titers are most often associated with SLE, and a negative test is strong evidence against a diagnosis of SLE. High titers of antibody to double-stranded DNA (dsDNA) are expressed almost exclusively by patients with SLE (Pisetsky, 1992). Antibodies to the Smith (Sm) antigen are not sensitive (30 percent) but are specific for the diagnosis of SLE and are associated with more severe disease. Antibodies to the Robert (Ro) soluble substance antigen and the Lane (La) soluble substance antigen, also known as SS-A and SS-B, respectively, are associated with the subacute cutaneous lupus (Sontheimer et al, 1982), neonatal lupus (Watson et al, 1984), and secondary Sjögren's syndromes. In SLE, SS-A antibodies indicate milder disease. In some individuals, elevated levels of anti-DNA antibodies and depressed levels of complement are associated with active disease and return to normal with successful treatment (Lloyd and Schur, 1981). Immune complex deposition at various sites initiates complement-mediated tissue injury in SLE. This has been best described in the kidney, where immune complexes are observed by immunofluorescent staining. Measurement of serum immune complexes as a monitor of disease progress or to gauge therapy, however, has been controversial.

Antiphospholipid antibodies develop in as many as 20 percent of patients with SLE. This

TABLE 3–2. SEROLOGIC TEST IN SYSTEMIC LUPUS ERYTHEMATOSUS (SLE)

Test*	Disease Association	Significance
ANA	SLE—>90%	Highly sensitive but not specific
		High titer most often associated with SLE
		Negative test strong evidence against SLE
Anti-dsDNA	SLE—60–70%	High titers almost exclusively expressed in SLE
Anti-Sm	SLE—30%	Poor sensitivity; specificity high for SLE
Anti-Ro (SS-A)	Sjögren's—60%	Neonatal lupus—found in mother and child
	SLE—30%	Mother may not have disease
	Subacute cutaneous lupus—60%	Associated with complete heart block and rash in the child
	Neonatal lupus—90%	
Anti-La (SS-B)	Sjögren's—50%	May be the important antibody in the complete heart block found in neonatal lupus
	SLE—10%	
	Neonatal lupus—?	
Antiphospholipid Antibodies (ACA,LA)	SLE—20–40%	May have increased risk of thrombotic disease
		Some women have an increased risk of spontaneous abortion

*ANA = Antinuclear antibodies; dsDNA = double stranded DNA; Sm = Smith antigen; Ro = Robert antigen; SS-A, SS-B = soluble substance A or B; La = Lane antigen; ACA = anticardiolipin antibody; LA = lupus anticoagulant.

group of antibodies is detected by tests for the lupus anticoagulant and anticardiolipin antibodies. Patients with antiphospholipid antibodies may also have a false-positive VDRL and prolonged partial thromboplastin and prothrombin times. In the laboratory, these antibodies prolong coagulation. Paradoxically, patients with these antibodies may have increased thrombotic events, such as deep venous thromboses, pulmonary emboli, and cardiovascular accidents. In some women, an increased risk of spontaneous abortion has been observed. Additional features of the syndrome include livedo reticularis and thrombocytopenia, which occur secondary to destruction of antiphospholipid antibody coated platelets (Bowles, 1990).

CLINICAL MANIFESTATIONS. The clinical manifestations of SLE are protean. The American College of Rheumatology 1982 revised criteria for the classification of SLE (Table 3–3) focuses on signs and symptoms that, in constellation, distinguish this disorder from other connective tissue diseases (Cervera et al, 1993; Tan, 1982). Many other disease manifestations may be present, such as fever, weight loss, and Raynaud's phenomenon. These features do not distinguish SLE from other conditions, however. In an individual patient, not all systems are affected simultaneously, and the disease is characterized by remissions and exacerbations.

Many drugs can cause a lupus-like syndrome (Table 3–4) (Hess and Mongey, 1991). The most commonly implicated are procainamide, hydralazine, anticonvulsants, and chlorpromazine. Clinically, these patients have symptoms similar to those with idiopathic SLE but typically without renal or CNS involvement. These drugs may also induce serum ANAs without symptoms. Patients with drug-induced lupus have a higher frequency of antihistone antibodies, whereas only 30 percent of those with idiopathic SLE do. The disease usually remits when the drug is discontinued.

TREATMENT. Treatment of SLE is based on severity of disease. Arthritis alone, without significant internal organ involvement, is treated symptomatically with aspirin or nonsteroidal anti-inflammatory drugs. Skin disease often responds to the anti-malarial hydroxychloroquine or chloroquine. High-dose corticosteroids (e.g., prednisone, 1 mg/kg/day) are usually reserved for life-threatening internal organ involvement such as acute lupus nephritis, central nervous system lupus, or severe cytopenias. Cytotoxic agents such as cyclophosphamide and azathioprine are used in the setting of life-threatening disease that is not responding to high-dose corticosteroids alone or is associated with significant steroid toxicity. These drugs have potential for serious complications (marrow suppression, cancer, infection) and should be used cautiously.

TABLE 3–3. THE 1982 REVISED CRITERIA FOR CLASSIFICATION OF SYSTEMIC LUPUS ERYTHEMATOSUS*

CLINICAL MANIFESTATION	FREQUENCY (%)
1. Malar rash	58
2. Discoid rash	10
3. Photosensitivity	45
4. Oral ulcers	24
5. Arthritis	84
6. Serositis	36
7. Renal disorder	39
8. Neurologic disorder	27
9. Hematologic disorder	22
10. Immunologic disorder	78†
11. Antinuclear antibody	96

*The proposed classification is based on 11 criteria. For the purpose of identifying patients in clinical studies, a person shall be said to have systemic lupus erythematosus if any four or more of the 11 criteria are present, serially or simultaneously, during any interval of observation.
†Anti-ds DNA antibodies.

TABLE 3–4. MEDICATIONS IMPLICATED IN THE "DRUG INDUCED LUPUS SYNDROME"

DEFINITE	POSSIBLE	UNLIKELY
Procainamide	Phenytoin	Phenylbutazone
Hydralazine	Carbamazepine	Griseofulvin
Isoniazid	Ethosuximide	Oral contraceptives
Methyldopa	Trimethadione	Gold salts
Quinidine	Mephenytoin	Penicillin
Chlorpromazine	Propylthiouracil	Hydrazine
	Methimazole	L-canavaline
	Beta blockers	Streptomycin
	Penicillamine	Tetracyclines
	Captopril	Methysergide
	Sulfonamides	Allopurinol
	Levodopa	Reserpine
	Nitrofurantoin	
	Tartrazine	
	Lithium	
	Phenelzine	
	Cimetidine	

Modified from Hess EV, Mongey AB. Drug-related lupus. Bull Rheum Dis 40:1–8, 1991.

Rheumatoid Arthritis

Rheumatoid arthritis (RA) is a chronic relapsing inflammatory arthritis affecting multiple synovial joints with varying degrees of systemic involvement. It affects about 1 percent of the population worldwide and is more common in women than men (3:1 ratio).

ETIOLOGY AND PATHOGENESIS. The etiology of rheumatoid arthritis is unknown. Evidence that it is an autoimmune disease includes the presence of rheumatoid factors (80 percent of patients), antinuclear antibodies (30 percent), immune complexes, and occasionally depressed complement levels (usually when the disease is associated with vasculitis). Rheumatoid factors are immunoglobulins directed against the Fc portion of IgG. They may be any immunoglobulin class (G, M, A, E), but the most commonly seen are IgM, and these form the basis for the laboratory detection of rheumatoid factors. Eighty percent of patients who meet the American College of Rheumatology criteria for RA have a positive latex agglutination test for rheumatoid factor. Rheumatoid factors are not specific for RA. They may be detected in chronic infection and other collagen vascular diseases, for example. It is not known whether the autosensitization responsible for the production of rheumatoid factor has a causative role in the pathogenesis of RA or is merely an epiphenomenon.

The presentation of a relevant antigen to an immunogenetically susceptible host is believed to trigger rheumatoid arthritis. More is known about immunogenetics than about specific agents. A majority of patients with rheumatoid arthritis carry HLA-DR4, HLA-DR1, or both (McDermott and McDevitt, 1988). How can we explain the association of two different HLA haplotypes with susceptibility to one disease? An intriguing observation is that these two HLA haplotypes share amino acid sequences, also known as epitopes (Gregersen et al, 1987). Perhaps it is this common epitope, then, that confers susceptibility to rheumatoid arthritis. There is increasing evidence that subtypes of HLA-DR4 and HLA-DR1 are related to the disease severity as well (Calin et al, 1989; Weyand et al, 1992). Proposed triggers in susceptible patients include infectious agents (Phillips, 1988; Venables, 1989), endogenous substances such as collagen (Stuart et al, 1984), and altered immunoglobulins. Of the proposed infectious agents, interest has been renewed in the Epstein-Barr virus. Studies have shown that molecular mimicry between viral glycoprotein (gp110) and the beta chain of the HLA molecules may be associated with susceptibility to rheumatoid arthritis (Roudier et al, 1988, 1989).

CLINICAL MANIFESTATIONS. Clinical features include nonspecific constitutional symptoms such as low grade fever, fatigue, and weight loss. The American College of Rheumatology 1987 revised criteria for the classification of RA are listed in Table 3–5 (Arnett et al, 1988). For criteria 1 to 5, symptoms or signs must be present for at least six weeks. These criteria were designed principally for disease classification for epidemiologic and research purposes. Individual cases must be judged on clinical grounds.

Rheumatoid arthritis is truly a systemic illness, and the term "rheumatoid disease" may be more appropriate. Extra-articular manifestations include rheumatoid nodules, pulmonary disease (nodules, pleuritis, interstitial lung disease), erythema nodosum, and secondary Sjögren's syndrome. Felty's syndrome is the triad of rheumatoid arthritis, splenomegaly, and leukopenia in a patient with rheumatoid arthritis. It is associated with high-titer rheumatoid factor, rheumatoid nodules, and rheumatoid vasculitis (Thorne and Urowitz, 1982).

TREATMENT. Therapy of RA is directed at maintaining muscle strength and joint mobility. The traditional treatment pyramid progresses from aspirin and other NSAIDs to the so-called slow-acting antirheumatic drugs

TABLE 3–5. 1987 REVISED AMERICAN RHEUMATISM ASSOCIATION CRITERIA FOR RHEUMATOID ARTHRITIS*

1. Morning stiffness for at least one hour
2. Swelling of three or more joints observed by a physician
3. Swelling of wrist, metacarpophalangeal or proximal interphalangeal joints
4. Symmetric joint swelling
5. Hand roentgenogram changes typical of rheumatoid arthritis
6. Rheumatoid nodules
7. Serum rheumatoid factor

Four or more criteria must be present to diagnose rheumatoid arthritis.
Criteria 1–4 must be present for at least 6 weeks.

*From Arnett FC et al: The American Rheumatism Association 1987 revised criteria for the classification of rheumatoid arthritis. Arthritis Rheum 31:315–324, 1988.

(SAARDs) (Table 3–6). More recently this rationale has been challenged. Since erosive joint findings occur early in the course of the disease and appear to be irreversible, patients may benefit from early and aggressive use of the SAARDs. The slow-acting agents include anti-malarials (hydroxychloroquine and chloroquine), organic gold compounds (oral or injectable), penicillamine, methotrexate, azathioprine, and cyclophosphamide. Of these, the last two are considered cytotoxic, with potential to induce neoplasia. Systemic corticosteroids, although effective in ameliorating symptoms, have no long-term benefit in preventing disease progression and can cause serious short- and long-term side effects. A severe polyarticular flare or life-threatening extra-articular disease warrants its use. Intra-articular steroids are useful for isolated joint flares, but should be limited to not more than three or four times per year in a given joint since more frequent use may result in joint destruction.

Juvenile Rheumatoid Arthritis

By definition, juvenile rheumatoid arthritis occurs before the age of 16. It is not a single entity but rather a group of arthritides that are classified by their mode of onset and joint distribution (Table 3–7). Twenty percent of patients present with a systemic onset syndrome called Still's disease, characterized by high fever, rash, serositis, lymphadenopathy, hepatosplenomegaly, leukocytosis, and anemia. Arthritis occurs but does not persist. Forty percent of patients present with polyarticular onset, defined as involvement of five or more joints. Twenty-five percent of this group are rheumatoid factor positive, and their disease resembles adult RA. The remaining 40 percent of patients have a pauciarticular onset, involving four or fewer joints. Two subgroups of the pauciarticular group are an antinuclear antibodies (ANA)-positive group with iridocyclitis, which is more common in girls, and an HLA-B27-positive group with bilateral sacroiliitis, more common in boys.

ETIOLOGY AND PATHOGENESIS. Like adult rheumatoid arthritis, the etiology is not known, but is suspected to be multifactorial. Immunologic features include ANAs, rheumatoid factor, and immune complexes. Antinuclear antibodies are detected in 13 percent of all patients with juvenile rheumatoid arthritis. Most patients with a positive rheumatoid factor resemble those with adult-onset RA. Immune complexes may be detected in some patients with Still's disease.

TREATMENT. Treatment is similar to that for RA, with anti-inflammatory drugs, physical therapy, and judicious use of intra-articular steroids forming the mainstay. Use of the so-called slow-acting antirheumatic drugs (SAARDs) is not as well studied in children. Methotrexate in low doses has been shown to be effective.

Sjögren's Syndrome

Sjögren's syndrome is a chronic inflammatory disease of unknown etiology characterized by decreased function of the lacrimal and salivary glands. Clinically this results in keratoconjunctivitis sicca and xerostomia.

TABLE 3–7. JUVENILE ARTHRITIS

Disease Pattern	Female: Male Ratio	Relative Frequency (%)	Clinical Course
Systemic (Still's)	1:1	20	High fever Rash Lymphadenopathy Arthritis
Polyarticular (≥5 joints)	1:2	40	If RF positive, arthritis worse
Pauciarticular (≤4 joints)	6:1	40	Girls: ANA (+) often iridocyclitis Boys: ANA (−), HLA-B27 (+), bilateral sacroiliitis

TABLE 3–6. TREATMENT MODALITIES FOR RHEUMATOID ARTHRITIS

First-line agents
  Aspirin
  Nonsteroidal anti-inflammatory agents
Second-line agents, or slow-acting antirheumatic drugs (SAARDs)
  Antimalarials
  Penicillamine
  Gold
  Sulfasalazine
  Methotrexate
Cytotoxic agents
  Cyclophosphamide
  Azathioprine
Experimental immunologic agents
  Cytokines
  Monoclonal antibodies to T cell subsets or cytokines

The disease is primary in 50 percent of patients and occurs in association with rheumatoid arthritis or other connective tissue diseases in the rest. It affects predominantly females (90 percent).

ETIOLOGY AND PATHOGENESIS. Histologically, the lacrimal and salivary glands show infiltration with lymphocytes, leading ultimately to destruction of the gland. Immunologic features of this disease include abnormal humoral and cell-mediated immunity, as well as HLA associations. Hypergammaglobulinemia is seen in 50 percent of patients and is usually of a polyclonal type. Occasionally patients develop a monoclonal gammopathy. Rheumatoid factors occur in 90 percent of patients, and this is higher than the 80 percent frequency in rheumatoid arthritis. A positive ANA occurs in 70 percent. Antibodies directed against SS-B are relatively specific for primary Sjögren's syndrome. SS-A is found in primary Sjögren's syndrome as well as Sjögren's syndrome associated with SLE. Decreased lymphocyte responses to mitogenic stimulation have been described. There is increased prevalence of HLA-DR3 and HLA-B8 in patients with Sjögren's syndrome.

CLINICAL MANIFESTATIONS. Clinically these patients complain of dry or irritated eyes and dry mouth (sicca symptoms). Vaginal dryness may cause dyspareunia. Physical examination may reveal dry mucous membranes with fissuring of the tongue. Fifty percent of patients have parotid gland enlargement. The Schirmer test reveals decreased tear production. Slit-lamp examination shows abnormal rose bengal or fluorescein staining of the conjunctiva and cornea. Extraglandular lymphocytic infiltration occurs in 10 percent of patients and is observed primarily in the kidneys, lungs, lymph nodes, and muscles. Rarely, patients with Sjögren's syndrome develop lymphoma or Waldenstrom's macroglobulinemia. The lymphoma is often a monoclonal B cell neoplasm.

TREATMENT. Treatment is usually symptomatic, consisting of careful oral hygiene to prevent cavities, artificial saliva, and artificial tears. Corticosteroids and immunosuppressive drugs are reserved for life-threatening extraglandular disease and lymphoma.

Systemic Sclerosis

Systemic sclerosis is a generalized disorder of connective tissue characterized clinically by thickening and fibrosis of the skin (scleroderma) and by fibrosis and arterial occlusions affecting internal organs, including the heart, lungs, kidneys, and gastrointestinal tract.

ETIOLOGY AND PATHOGENESIS. Autoimmunity in idiopathic scleroderma is evidenced by the presence of antinuclear antibodies, mixed cryoglobulins, and rheumatoid factor. In addition, scleroderma is associated with other autoimmune diseases to form overlap syndromes. Mixed connective tissue disease is a particular overlap syndrome with elements of scleroderma, SLE, and polymyositis, together with high-titer antibodies to ribonucleoproteins (RNPs). The particular ANAs found in scleroderma are antibodies to extractable nuclear antigens (ENAs), the nucleus, the centromere, and Scl-70 (Reimer, 1990). In patients with both limited and diffuse scleroderma, the presence of anti-Scl-70 gives a relative risk of 16.7 for the development of pulmonary fibrosis (Briggs et al, 1991).

Scleroderma is one of the few connective tissue diseases in which specific environmental agents are purported to have an etiologic role. These include silica, vinyl chloride, L-tryptophan, bleomycin, and carbidopa.

CLINICAL MANIFESTATIONS. Clinical involvement ranges from limited skin thickening of the distal extremities and face (limited scleroderma) to severe skin thickening including the proximal extremities and trunk (diffuse scleroderma), plus or minus internal organ involvement (systemic sclerosis). The most frequent clinical manifestation (in more than 90 percent of patients) is Raynaud's phenomenon. Dilated and distorted nail-fold capillary loops occur in about 90 percent of patients with systemic sclerosis but are not specific for the disease, since they may also occur in dermatomyositis, mixed connective tissue disease, or Raynaud's phenomenon alone. The most common gastrointestinal tract involvement is impaired esophageal motility. Less commonly seen are malabsorption and intestinal pseudo-obstruction from small bowel involvement, and wide-mouth diverticula in the colon. Pulmonary disease includes pulmonary hypertension, diffuse interstitial lung disease, and pleurisy. Renal involvement is rare but can be fatal due to acute hypertension and oliguric renal failure. Joint contractures, inflammatory myopathy, pericarditis, and myocardial fibrosis may all occur. A subset of patients with calcinosis, Raynaud's phenomenon, esophageal dysfunction, sclerodactyly, and telangiectasias (CREST syndrome) have limited disease with a slower rate of progression. This syndrome is associated with anticentromere antibodies in over 50 percent of patients.

TREATMENT. No agent has proved totally effective in arresting or reversing the fibrosis in this disease. Equally unsatisfactory has been treatment of the pulmonary vasculopathy. Variable results have been observed with D-penicillamine and colchicine in the cutaneous manifestations of the disease. Aggressive treatment of renal crisis with angiotensin-converting enzyme (ACE) inhibitors has improved survival of patients with this complication (Steen and Medsger, 1988).

Inflammatory Myopathy

The inflammatory myopathies have been classified into 6 subtypes: (1) primary idiopathic polymyositis, (2) primary idiopathic dermatomyositis, (3) polymyositis or dermatomyositis associated with malignancy, (4) childhood polymyositis or dermatomyositis, (5) myositis associated with other connective tissue disease, and (6) inclusion body myositis (Bohan et al, 1977). The annual incidence has been estimated at more than 10 cases per million population (Oddis et al, 1990). There are two peaks in incidence, one in childhood, the other in the fifth decade. They are all more common in females than males, with the exception of inclusion body myositis. They have in common inflammation of skeletal muscle with symmetric weakness, usually of the proximal muscles. Diagnosis of myositis is based on measurement of serum muscle enzymes, electromyography, and muscle biopsy. The most sensitive enzyme is creatine kinase, but lactate dehydrogenase, aspartate aminotransferase, alanine aminotransferase, aldolase, myoglobin, and creatine may also be elevated. Muscle biopsy shows inflammatory mononuclear cell infiltrates.

ETIOLOGY AND PATHOGENESIS. An autoimmune etiology is supported by the presence of autoantibodies, the association with other connective tissue diseases, and lymphocyte and plasma cell infiltration in involved muscle. ANAs are the most common autoantibodies in inflammatory myopathy, being present in over half of these patients. Other autoantibodies include anti-SS-A, anti-SS-B, rheumatoid factor, anti-RNP, and antithyroglobulin. In addition, about one third of all patients have autoantibodies specific for myositis. These antibodies are directed against cytoplasmic ribonucleoproteins involved in protein synthesis (Miller, 1991). There is evidence accumulating that these myositis-specific antibodies may define subsets of patients with distinct clinical courses and response to therapy. For example, patients with one type, the antisynthetase antibody, have moderately severe myositis, a high incidence of interstitial lung disease, symmetric polyarthritis, fever, and Raynaud's phenomenon. They also have a moderately good response to therapy but flare with tapering of therapy, and they have a poor prognosis because of their often fatal acute pulmonary events (Love et al, 1991). Defining subsets of more homogeneous patients may lead to better therapy and a more complete understanding of the etiology and pathogenesis of these diseases.

CLINICAL MANIFESTATIONS. Insidious onset of weakness in the proximal muscles of the upper and lower extremities characterizes primary idiopathic polymyositis. Dermatomyositis is similar, with the addition of a characteristic heliotrope rash that sometimes involves only the eyelids and knuckles, but may cover more extensive areas of the body. Inclusion body myositis is distinguished from the two disorders above by characteristic histologic features. Clinically these patients are more likely to have distal weakness and fail to respond to therapy.

Extramuscular manifestations include dysphagia, which is secondary to esophageal striated muscle involvement, and cardiac abnormalities (atrioventricular conduction defects, tachyarrhythmias, low ejection fracture, and dilated cardiomyopathy). Interstitial lung disease develops in up to 10 percent of patients with polymyositis, half of whom have anti-JO-1 antibodies (Bernstein et al, 1984). Skin manifestations, in addition to the heliotrope rash, include subcutaneous calcifications. The association of malignancy with dermatomyositis or polymyositis is controversial (Callen, 1982, 1988; Lakhanpal et al, 1986; Manchal et al, 1985; Richardson and Callen, 1989).

TREATMENT. There are no large, well-controlled, double-blind trials comparing the various methods of treatment. Prednisone is the drug of choice for polymyositis and dermatomyositis. Long-term high-dose prednisone may itself cause a proximal muscle weakness. Differentiating between steroid myopathy and flare of myositis is difficult. The serum muscle enzyme (CK) levels and the relationship between the prednisone dose and the occurrence of weakness may help. Arbitrary adjustment of the steroid dose with careful observation of muscle strength may provide the answer. Methotrexate or azathioprine is advocated for patients with steroid complications, steroid unresponsiveness, or severe disease with respiratory muscle weakness (Bunch, 1981; Dalakas, 1989).

Seronegative Spondyloarthropathies

The seronegative spondyloarthropathies include ankylosing spondylitis, reactive arthritis, psoriatic arthritis, and arthritis associated with inflammatory bowel disease. As the name implies, all of these diseases may affect the spine. Sacroiliitis, ligamentous ossification of the spine, and an asymmetric peripheral oligoarthritis are seen to varying degrees. Enthesopathies, inflammation of soft tissue insertions on bone, are also noted in these conditions. The term seronegative refers to the absence of autoantibodies in these patients.

ETIOLOGY AND PATHOGENESIS. The primary autoimmune aspect of the seronegative spondyloarthropathies is the association with HLA-B27 (see Table 3–1). This allele is found in 95 percent of patients with ankylosing spondylitis and 80 percent with reactive arthritis. It is present in only 7 percent of the general population (Table 3–8). The relevant question is whether HLA-B27 is simply a genetic marker that is closely linked to a causative gene or whether it plays an active role in inciting the disease. HLA-B27 is a class I major histocompatibility antigen and therefore functions in binding extracellular antigens at the cell surface and targeting the cell for destruction by T cytotoxic cells. It has been postulated that certain bacterial or viral infections produce peptides that elicit a T cytotoxic response and later cross-react with self antigens when presented by HLA-B27. This could occur if there were significant homology between the foreign antigen and the HLA-B27 molecule. This has been an inviting hypothesis, especially in explaining the phenomenon of reactive arthritis, which occurs after documented bacterial or viral infections. This molecular mimicry theory is supported by cross-reactivity between gram-negative bacteria—such as *Klebsiella, Shigella,* and *Yersinia*—and the HLA-B27 molecule (Welsh et al, 1980). In addition, amino acid sequence homology has been demonstrated between a *Klebsiella pneumoniae* enzyme and one subtype of the HLA-B27 molecule (Schwimmbeck et al, 1987). Others have argued that these findings are coincidental, or perhaps the result of B27-associated disease and not the cause of it (Russel and Almazor, 1992).

Ankylosing Spondylitis

The incidence of this disease is about 0.1 percent with a 9:1 predominance of males over females. The most common symptom is low back pain, which is frequently worse in the morning and improves with activity. Physical examination may reveal tenderness over the sacroiliac joints and limited motion of the spine on forward flexion. In later stages of the disease marked fusion of the spine with kyphosis and loss of lumbar lordosis may be seen. Radiographs show symmetric sacroiliitis and variable amounts of ankylosis of the posterior longitudinal ligament of the spine, which ascends from the lumbar area proximally. Peripheral joint involvement, when present, most commonly involves the shoulders and hips. Additional features include iritis, iridocyclitis, and carditis. The diagnosis is a clinical one supported by the characteristic x-ray findings. Testing for HLA-B27 is not helpful, since this may be present in 7 percent of the normal population and 80 percent of positive individuals do not get ankylosing spondylitis. Primary treatment consists of nonsteroidal anti-inflammatory agents, such as indomethacin or naproxen, and exercise programs to maintain mobility and posture.

Reactive Arthritis

Noninfectious inflammatory arthritis following an infection is termed reactive arthri-

TABLE 3–8. FREQUENCY OF HLA-B27 IN SERONEGATIVE RHEUMATIC DISEASES AND HEALTHY ADULTS (%)

Ankylosing spondylitis	89
Reiter's syndrome	80
Reactive arthritis	71–85
Inflammatory bowel disease	52
Psoriatic arthritis	
Axial arthropathy	47
Peripheral arthropathy	14
Healthy whites	5–14
Healthy blacks	3–4

tis. One subtype of this is Reiter's syndrome, which is the triad of arthritis, conjunctivitis, and nongonococcal urethritis. Originally described after a *Shigella* epidemic, it has since been seen after infection with other diarrheal pathogens as well as sexually transmitted diseases such as caused by *Chlamydia*. The sacroiliitis may be asymmetric, and the spine involvement often skips areas, rather than ascending in an orderly fashion as in ankylosing spondylitis. Other features include circinate balanitis, keratodermia blennorrhagica (a characteristic scaling rash on the feet), aortitis, and uveitis. For spinal disease, treatment is similar to that of ankylosing spondylitis. The peripheral arthritis and enthesopathies are frustrating to treat, and many of the drugs used in rheumatoid arthritis have been tried with variable success.

Psoriatic Arthritis

Psoriatic arthritis occurs in 6 percent of patients with psoriasis. It may precede, follow, or coincide with onset of the skin disease. There is poor correlation between the severity of the skin disease and that of the joint disease. Five to 15 percent of patients have exclusively distal interphalangeal joint involvement. Seventy percent have an oligoasymmetric illness. About 15 percent have a symmetric arthritis resembling RA, often with a positive rheumatoid factor, probably representing the occurrence of skin psoriasis and RA together. Additional features include aortitis and iritis. Treatment is similar to the management of RA, although antimalarials may cause a severe flare of skin disease and should be used cautiously.

Arthritis and Inflammatory Bowel Disease

Peripheral arthritis is seen in 12 percent of patients with ulcerative colitis and 20 percent of those with Crohn's disease. It typically involves the large joints of the lower extremities. There is a good correlation between the activity of the bowel disease and the peripheral arthritis. About 7 percent have ankylosing spondylitis, with little correlation between the activity of the bowel disease and the spondylitis. Therapy directed at the underlying bowel disease helps the peripheral arthritis, whereas the spinal disease treatment is the same as for ankylosing spondylitis.

ORGAN-SPECIFIC AUTOIMMUNE DISEASES

An autoimmune etiology has been proposed for numerous diseases involving every organ system. Three commonly cited diseases are type I diabetes mellitus, autoimmune thyroiditis, and myasthenia gravis.

Type I Diabetes Mellitus

Type I diabetes mellitus (DM) is a disease of insulin deficiency caused by autoimmune destruction of pancreatic beta cells. It is likely that progressive beta cell destruction develops over years, as demonstrated by subclinical evidence of autoimmunity seven to ten years prior to clinical presentation (Srikanta et al, 1983). Evidence for an autoimmune etiology includes infiltration of the pancreatic islets with lymphocytes and macrophages (Gepts and Lecompte, 1981). Additional evidence for an autoimmune etiology lies in the association of type I diabetes mellitus with other autoimmune diseases. The disease is associated with the HLA-D antigens DR3 and DR4. Interestingly, there is only a 15 percent concordance of disease expression in HLA identical siblings and 50 percent concordance in identical twins, suggesting that environmental factors also play a role.

Primary treatment of type I DM is aimed at insulin replacement. Newer approaches include pancreatic transplantation, novel ways of delivering insulin via pumps, implantation of protected islet cells, and immunotherapy for prediabetics or newly diagnosed patients. By altering or suppressing the immune response, immunotherapy may mitigate beta cell destruction (Winter and Maclaren, 1985). Newer immunotherapies directed specifically at the cells responsible for islet destruction are needed (Herold and Rubenstein, 1992).

Autoimmune Thyroid Disease

Hashimoto's thyroiditis and Graves' disease are two clinical manifestations of autoimmune thyroid disease. They may represent different ends of a continuous spectrum. Hashimoto's thyroiditis is a disease caused by immune destruction of the thyroid gland. Patients have serologic evidence of antibodies directed against the thyroid: anti-thyroglobulin and antimicrosomal antibodies. Further evidence of autoimmunity is shown by the association of the disease with HLA types DR4 and DR5. Histologically, there is infiltration of the gland with T cells, B cells, and macrophages; thus it is likely that both cellular and humoral immunity play a role in gland destruction. With initial destruction of thyroid follicles, increased amounts of thyroid hormone are released and patients may become hyperthyroid. With progressive destruction of the gland, however, thyroid hormone production decreases and the patient becomes hypothyroid. Diagnosis is based on serologic evidence of antithyroid antibodies in the setting of hypo- or hyperthyroidism. Treatment is directed at thyroid hormone replacement to prevent clinical hypothyroidism.

Graves' disease is hyperthyroidism resulting from thyroid-stimulating antibodies. In addition to this humoral response, cell-mediated autoimmunity is suggested by studies showing a defect in suppressor T lymphocyte function in these patients (Volpe, 1991). Graves' disease is highly associated with HLA-DR3 and, like Hashimoto's thyroiditis, is often associated with other autoimmune diseases.

Clinically, patients manifest symptoms of hyperthyroidism: tachycardia, sweating, diarrhea, weight loss, and insomnia. In addition, patients may manifest exophthalmos, which may be secondary to accumulation of immune complexes in the retro-orbital extraocular muscles (Doniach and Florin-Christensen, 1975). Diagnosis of Graves' disease is based on evidence of hyperthyroidism (symptoms and signs above, as well as elevated thyroid hormones), and demonstration of thyroid autoimmunity. Treatment is with antithyroid drug therapy, propylthiouracil or methimazole, to induce a clinical remission. In the setting of persistent disease activity, thyroid ablation with surgery or radioiodine is indicated.

Myasthenia Gravis

Myasthenia gravis is a neuromuscular disorder associated with antibodies directed against the acetylcholine receptor. It is not clear what role these antibodies play in the pathogenesis of this disease, since there is not a strong correlation between serum titers of anti-acetylcholine antibodies and disease severity (Drachman et al, 1982). Other abnormalities found in these patients, which may be relevant, include reduced numbers of acetylcholine receptors, wider postsynaptic clefts, and distorted postsynaptic membranes. An immunologic mechanism is suggested further by the association of the disease with thymic hyperplasia in 70 percent of patients and thymomas in 10 percent. There is also an increased frequency of myasthenia gravis in association with other autoimmune diseases.

Clinically, patients develop weakness, which is exacerbated by repetitive use of muscles. Involvement of muscles innervated by cranial nerves is common, resulting in ptosis, diplopia, dysarthria, and dysphagia. The diagnosis is based on the clinical picture, electrodiagnostic testing, and serologic findings. Treatment with anticholinesterase agents is the mainstay. These drugs increase the amount of acetylcholine at the motor end plate sufficiently to overcome the reduced numbers of available acetylcholine receptors. Data on the use of immunosuppressive agents are limited. Uncontrolled studies suggest that intravenous immunoglobulin may be beneficial. Thymectomy is beneficial in about 70 percent of patients.

SUMMARY

In this chapter we have tried to review the clinical aspects and the underlying immunopathogenesis for diseases in which autoimmunity appears to play a prominent role. We have discussed systemic and organ-specific autoimmune diseases for which we have some understanding of pathogenic processes. The immunopathogenesis of these diseases and autoimmunity in general appear to have the following features in common: (1) genetic susceptibility, (2) an initial insult from an environmental agent, and (3) factors that allow perpetuation of this initial insult, including impaired immune regulation, an excessive inflammatory response, and impaired degradation or clearance of foreign antigens. While we do not understand all the mechanisms underlying autoimmunity, the various diseases that have characteristic autoimmune concomitants are forming the basis for a greater understanding of the mechanism of these disordered immune processes.

REFERENCES

Alvarellos A, Ahearn JM, Provost TT, Dorsch CA, Stevens MB, Bias WB, et al. Relationships of HLA-DR and MT antigens to autoantibody expression in SLE. Arthritis Rheum 26:1533–1535, 1983.

Arnett FC, Edworthy SM, Bloch DA, et al. The American Rheumatism Association 1987 revised criteria for the classification of rheumatoid arthritis. Arthritis Rheum 38:315–324, 1988.

Bernstein RM, Morgan SH, Chapman J, et al. Anti-Jo-1 antibody: A marker for myositis and interstitial lung disease. Br Med J 289:151–152, 1984.

Bohan A, Peter JB, Bowman RL, Pearson CM. A computer-assisted analysis of 153 patients with polymyositis and dermatomyositis. Medicine 56:255–286, 1977.

Bowles CA. Vasculopathy associated with the antiphospholipid syndrome. Rheum Dis Clin North Am 16:471–490, 1990.

Briggs DC, Vaughan RW, Welsh KI, Myers AR, DuBois RM, Black CM. Immunogenetic prediction of pulmonary fibrosis in systemic sclerosis. Lancet 338:661–662, 1991.

Bunch TW. Prednisone and azathioprine for polymyositis: A long-term follow-up. Arthritis Rheum 24:45–48, 1981.

Calin A, Elswood J, Kloud PT. Destructive arthritis, rheumatoid factor, and HLA-DR4: susceptibility versus severity. A case-control study. Arthritis Rheum 32:1251–1255, 1989.

Callen JP. The value of malignancy evaluation in patients with dermatomyositis. J Am Acad Dermatol 6:253–259, 1982.

Callen JP. Malignancy in polymyositis/dermatomyositis. Clin Dermatol 2:55–63, 1988.

Cervera R, Khamashta MA, Font J, Sebastiani GD, Gil A, Lavilla P, Domenech I, Aydintug AO, Jedryka-Goral A, De Ramon E, Galeazzi M, Haga HJ, Mathieu A, Houssiau F, Ingelmo M, Hughes GRV, European Working Party on Systemic Lupus Erythematosus. Systemic lupus erythematosus: Clinical and immunologic patterns of disease expression in a cohort of 1,000 patients. Medicine 72:113–124, 1993.

Condemi JJ. The autoimmune diseases. JAMA 268:2882–2892, 1992.

Dalakas MC. Treatment of polymyositis and dermatomyositis. Curr Opin Rheum 1:443–449, 1989.

Doniach D, Florin-Christensen A. Autoimmunity in the pathogenesis of endocrine exophthalmos. Med Clin North Am 4:341–350, 1975.

Drachman DB, Adams RN, Josifek LF, Self SG. Functional activities of autoantibodies to acetylcholine receptors and the clinical severity of myasthenia gravis. N Engl J Med 307:769, 1982.

Gepts W, Lecompte PM. The pancreatic islets in diabetes. Am J Med 70:105–115, 1981.

Gregersen PK, Silver J, Winchester RJ. The shared epitope hypothesis: An approach to understanding the molecular genetics of susceptibility to rheumatoid arthritis. Arthritis Rheum 30:1205–1213, 1987.

Herold KC, Rubenstein AH. New directions in the immunology of autoimmune diabetes. Editorial. Ann Intern Med 117:436–438, 1992.

Hess EV, Mongey AB. Drug-related lupus. Bull Rheum Dis 40:1–8, 1991.

Johnson HM, Russell JK, Pontzer CH. Superantigens in human disease. Scientific Amer Apr; 266:92–95, 98–101, 1992.

Kemp ME, Atkinson JP, Skanes VM, Levine RP, Chaplin PD. Deletion of C4A genes in patients with systemic lupus erythematosus. Arthritis Rheum 30:1015–1022, 1987.

Lakhanpal S, Bunch TW, Ilstrup DM, et al. Polymyositis-dermatomyositis and malignant lesions: does an association exist? Mayo Clin Proc 61:645–653, 1986.

Lloyd W, Schur PH. Immune complexes, complement and anti-DNA in exacerbations of systemic lupus erythematosus. Medicine 60:208–217, 1981.

Love LA, Leff RL, Fraser DD, Targoff IN, Dalaka M, Plotz P, Miller FW. A new approach to the classification of idiopathic inflammatory myopathy: Myositis-specific autoantibodies define useful homogeneous groups. Medicine 70:360–374, 1991.

Manchal LA, Jin A, Pritchard KI, et al. The frequency of malignant neoplasms in patients with polymyositis-dermatomyositis: A controlled study. Arch Intern Med 145:1835–1839, 1985.

McDermott M, McDevitt H. The immunogenetics of rheumatic diseases. Bull Rheum Dis 38:1–10, 1988.

Miller FW. Humoral immunity and immunogenetics in the idiopathic inflammatory myopathies. Curr Opin Rheum 3:902–910, 1991.

Oddis CV, Conte C, Steen VD, Medsger TA Jr. Incidence of polymyositis-dermatomyositis (PM-DM): A 20-year study of hospital-diagnosed cases. J Rheumatol 17:1329–1334, 1990.

Phillips PE. Evidence implicating infectious agents in rheumatoid arthritis and juvenile rheumatoid arthritis. Clin Exp Rheumatol 6:87–94, 1988.

Pisetsky DS. Anti-DNA antibodies in systemic lupus erythematosus. Rheum Dis Clin North Am 18:437–454, 1992.

Reimer G. Autoantibodies against nuclear, nucleolar, and mitochondrial antigens in systemic sclerosis (scleroderma). Rheum Dis Clin North Am 16:109–184, 1990.

Reveille JD. The molecular genetics of systemic lupus erythematosus and Sjögren's syndrome. Curr Opin Rheum 3:722–730, 1991.

Richardson JB, Callen JP. Dermatomyositis and malignancy. Med Clin North Am 73:1211–1220, 1989.

Roudier J, Peterson J, Rhodes GH, et al. Susceptibility to rheumatoid arthritis maps to a T-cell epitope shared by the HLA-Dw4 DR beta-1 chain and the Epstein-Barr virus glycoprotein gp110. Proc Natl Acad Sci USA 86:104–108, 1989.

Roudier J, Rhodes G, Peterson J, Vaughan JM, Carson DA. The Epstein-Barr virus glycoprotein gp110, a molecular link between HLA-DR4, HLA-DR1, and rheumatoid arthritis. Scand J Immunol 27:367–371, 1988.

Russel AS, Almazor MES. Ankylosing spondylitis is not caused by *Klebsiella*. Rheum Dis Clin North Am 18:95–104, 1992.

Schwimmbeck PL, Yu DTY, Oldstone MBA. Autoantibodies to HLA-B27 in the sera of HLA-B27 patients with ankylosing spondylitis and Reiter's syndrome: Molecular mimicry with *Klebsiella pneumoniae* as potential mechanism of autoimmune disease. J Exp Med 166:173–181, 1987.

Sontheimer RD, Maddison PJ, Reichlin M, Jordon RE, Stasny P, Gilliam JN. Serologic and HLA associations in subacute cutaneous lupus erythematosus: A clinical subset of lupus erythematosus. Ann Intern Med 97:664–671, 1982.

Srikanta S, Ganda OP, Eisenbarth GS, Soeldner JS. Islet-cell antibodies and beta-cell function in monozygotic twins initially discordant for type I diabetes mellitus. N Engl J Med 308:322–325, 1983.

Steen VS, Medsger TA Jr. Outcome of scleroderma renal crisis in the pre- and post-captopril eras. Arthritis Rheum 31:521, 1988.

Stuart JM, Townes AS, Kang AH. Collagen autoimmune arthritis. Annu Rev Immunol 2:199–218, 1984.

Tan EM. The 1982 revised criteria for the classification of systemic lupus erythematosus. Arthritis Rheum 25:1271–1272, 1982.

Thorne C, Urowitz MB. Long-term outcome in Felty's syndrome. Ann Rheum Dis 41:489–492, 1982.

Venables PJW. Infection and rheumatoid arthritis. Curr Opin Rheumatol 1:15–20, 1989.

Volpe R. Autoimmunity causing thyroid dysfunction. Endocrin Metab Clin North Am 20:565–587, 1991.

Watson RM, Lane AT, Barnett NK, Bias WB, Arnett FC, Provost TT. Neonatal lupus erythematosus: A clinical serological and immunogenetic study with review of the literature. Medicine 63:362–378, 1984.

Welsh J, Avakian H, Cowling P, et al. Ankylosing spondylitis, HLA-B27 and *Klebsiella*. I: Cross reactivity studies with rabbit antisera. Br J Exp Pathol 61:85–91, 1980.

Weyand CM, Hicok KC, Conn DL, Goronzy JJ. The influence of HLA-DRB1 genes on disease severity in rheumatoid arthritis. Ann Intern Med 117:801–806, 1992.

Winter WE, Maclaren NK. Type I insulin dependent diabetes: An autoimmune disease that can be arrested or prevented with immunotherapy? *In* Barnes L (ed). Advances in Pediatrics. Chicago, Year Book Medical Publishers, 1985, Vol 32, p. 262.

Chapter 4

Allergic Immune Response

Donald Y. M. Leung, M.D., Ph.D.

ABBREVIATIONS

AD = atopic dermatitis
EBV = Epstein-Barr virus
ELAM-1 = endothelial leukocyte adhesion molecule-1
FcεRI = high affinity IgE receptor
GM-CSF = granulocyte-macrophage colony-stimulating factor
ICAM-1 = intercellular adhesion molecule-1
IFN-α = interferon-alpha
IFN-γ = interferon-gamma
IgE = immunoglobulin E
IL = interleukin
LT = leukotriene
LPR = late phase response
mAb = monoclonal antibody
PAF = platelet activating factor
PBMC = peripheral blood mononuclear cells
r = recombinant
TGF-β = transforming growth factor-beta
TNF-α = tumor necrosis factor-alpha

Our present understanding of allergic immune responses originated with the observations by Prausnitz and Küstner, in 1921, that the intradermal injection of fish extract into a fish-sensitive individual elicited an immediate wheal and flare reaction. Of equal importance, immediate reactivity to the fish allergen could be passively transferred to non-atopic subjects by intradermal injection of their skin with sera from fish-sensitive individuals. Subsequently, the passive transfer of hypersensitivity to other allergens was also observed. The nature of these reaginic antibodies remained unknown for more than 40 years until the Ishizakas identified IgE as the carrier of reaginic activity in the sera of hay fever patients (Ishizaka and Ishizaka, 1967).

The discovery of IgE antibody has provided the basis for immunochemical approaches to the study of mechanisms underlying immediate hypersensitivity reactions. It is now well recognized that the major feature distinguishing atopic individuals from non-atopic individuals is their capacity to develop a sustained IgE response to environmental allergens. IgE has the unique property of binding to high-affinity receptors on basophils and mast cells. The cross-linking of specific membrane-bound IgE with allergen triggers the release of vasoactive mediators, leukocyte chemotactic factors, and cytokines responsible for the clinical manifestations of immediate hypersensitivity reactions.

During the past 10 years, however, it has become increasingly clear that allergic reactions are more than just IgE-mediated immediate responses. Clinically significant allergen-induced reactions are generally characterized by an IgE-dependent biphasic response. In particular, the late phase response (LPR), which is associated with the infiltration of inflammatory cells, is thought to play a critical role in the pathogenesis of chronic allergic diseases. The current review will focus on recent advances in our knowledge regarding the regulation of IgE synthesis and the mechanisms by which mast cells and cytokines participate in the accumulation of inflammatory cells at the site of allergen-induced LPR. In this regard, T cells have recently emerged as important participants in the control of chronic allergic inflammatory responses. A detailed understanding of these processes will

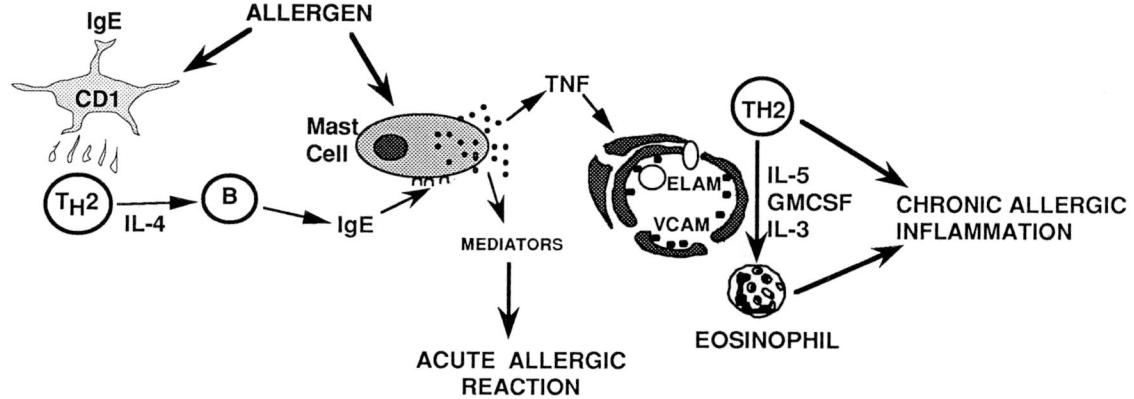

FIGURE 4–1. Schematic diagram of the cellular interactions during the allergic immune response.

have significant implications for the development of new strategies for the treatment of allergic diseases (Fig 4–1).

BIOLOGY AND STRUCTURE OF IMMUNOGLOBULIN E

IgE has a molecular weight of approximately 190 kilodaltons, of which 12 percent is carbohydrate (Ishizaka and Ishizaka, 1967) (Table 4–1). It has the same basic four-chain structure found in other immunoglobulins, that is, two light and two heavy (epsilon) chains. However, the molecular size of the ε polypeptide chain is 11 kilodaltons more than the gamma, delta, or alpha polypeptide chains. This is because the ε chain has five domains (one variable and four constant region domains).

IgE is present in serum as a monomer but is normally found in very low concentrations. As a result of its unique property to bind with high affinity to FcεRI on mast cells, basophils, and Langerhans cells, normal serum IgE levels are sufficient to sensitize these cells (Bieber et al, 1992; Ishizaka and Ishizaka, 1975). Recent studies using genetic engineering techniques have allowed mapping of the IgE binding site for FcεRI to a 76-amino-acid peptide that spans the C-terminal portion of the Cε2 domain and the N-terminal portion of the Cε3 domain in the native IgE molecule (Helm et al, 1988). The IgE molecule can also bind to low-affinity IgE receptors (FcεRII or CD23) on lymphocytes, monocyte/macrophages, eosinophils, and platelets. The binding site for FcεRII has been localized to the N-terminal region of the Cε3 domain proximal to the FcεRI binding site (Vercelli et al, 1989a).

Interaction of IgE with Cellular FcεRI Receptors

The high-affinity FcεRI mediates mast cell and basophil degranulation. Thus it is a major determinant in the development of immediate hypersensitivity reactions. The binding of IgE to FcεRI, however, is not sufficient to activate mast cells and basophils. Exposure of receptor-bound IgE to a multivalent allergen is necessary to initiate cell activation (Ishizaka and Ishizaka, 1975). The FcεRI is a tetrameric complex composed of one α chain, one β chain, and one dimer of identical γ chains (Kinet, 1990). The α chain is predominantly extracellular and is the part of the FcεRI that interacts with IgE. The β and γ chains are hydrophobic membrane proteins that are not

TABLE 4–1. PROPERTIES OF IMMUNOGLOBULIN E

Molecular weight	190 Kd
Carbohydrate content	12%
No. of heavy chain constant region domains	4
Concentration in normal sera	<450 ng/ml
Binds to mast cells, basophils, Langerhans cells via FcεRI	+
Binds to macrophages, lymphocytes, platelets, and eosinophils via FcεRII (CD23)	+

involved in the IgE binding reaction. Transfection studies indicate that efficient surface expression of the IgE-binding α chain requires the co-transfection of the γ cDNA and, to a lesser extent, the β cDNA. The β chain has homology to the CD20 molecule, a protein found on B cells that has ion channel properties. The γ chain has been found in FcεRI(−) cells. This has led to the interesting observation that other Fc receptors also use the γ chain. Recent studies indicate that phosphorylation of the γ chain may be a critical step involved in the activation of mast cells.

It has been known for many years that allergen-induced cross-linking of IgE antibodies on mast cell and basophil surfaces can trigger the release of preformed mediators such as histamine, proteases, heparin proteoglycans, eosinophil chemotactic factors, and neutrophil chemotactic factors (Serafin and Austen, 1987). Later it was recognized that the stimulation of these cells can also lead to the generation of newly formed, cell membrane–derived, lipid breakdown products such as leukotrienes C_4, D_4, E_4, prostaglandin D_2, and platelet activating factor. Each of these preformed or newly formed mediators has been shown to have potent pro-inflammatory effects *in vivo*. These effects include increased vascular permeability and vasodilation, bronchial smooth-muscle contraction, increased mucus production, as well as increased chemotaxis of eosinophils, neutrophils, and mononuclear cells. Thus many of the signs and symptoms of allergic responses can be attributed to these specific mast cell and basophil products, with the particular clinical manifestations of a given hypersensitivity reaction depending on the anatomic location of mediator release.

Recently, it has also been found that cross-linking of IgE on these same cells results in the synthesis and release of a variety of cytokines including IL-1, IL-3, IL-4, IL-5, IL-6, granulocyte-macrophage colony-stimulatory factor (GM-CSF), and tumor necrosis factor-alpha (TNF-α) (Galli et al, 1991). As will be discussed later in this chapter, these cytokines play a critical role in the induction of late-phase allergic responses, regulation of IgE synthesis, promotion of mast cell differentiation and survival, and the sustaining of chronic allergic inflammation by modulating leukocyte effector function and expression of cellular adhesion molecules.

Finally, it has also been shown that human epidermal Langerhans cells bear IgE on their cell surface in disease states associated with hyperimmunoglobulinemia E. This observation has led several investigators to examine the possibility that Langerhans cells may bind IgE via FcεRI. Indeed, recent studies have demonstrated by immunohistochemical staining, as well as by analysis of gene transcripts for the α, β, and γ chains of FcεRI, that Langerhans cells can express FcεRI (Ishizaka and Ishizaka, 1975). The demonstration of this receptor on epidermal Langerhans cells is likely to have important implications for our understanding of allergic reactions after epicutaneous contact with allergens. In this regard, it is of interest that *in vitro* IgE-bearing Langerhans cells from atopic dermatitis patients are able to capture house dust mites for allergen presentation, whereas IgE-negative Langerhans cells are unable to stimulate mite-specific T cells (Mudde et al, 1990).

Interaction of IgE with Cellular FcεRII Receptors

Unlike FcεRI, the low-affinity IgE receptor (FcεRII or CD23) is widely distributed on a variety of cell types (Conrad et al, 1991). There are two forms of the receptor, which differ by only a few amino acids in the terminal portion of the cytoplasmic domains (Yokota et al, 1988). The FcεRIIa form is observed only in B cells, whereas the FcεRIIb form is observed on B lymphocytes, macrophages, platelets, and activated T cells. It remains controversial whether FcεRII is present on eosinophils. There is no structural homology between FcεRI and FcεRII. The FcεRII is a member of the calcium-dependent animal lectin family. Allergic diseases are associated with increased expression of FcεRII on B lymphocytes, macrophages, platelets, and activated T cells. This may reflect, at least in part, the increased synthesis of IL-4 in allergic diseases, and the capacity of IL-4 to up-regulate expression of FcεRII.

The exact function of FcεRII is unclear. Since its discovery, the FcεRII has been proposed to have a role in IgE regulation, either as the intact molecule or as a proteolytically cleaved soluble form (termed sFcεRII or sCD23). This will be discussed later in this chapter. It has also been proposed that FcεRII may be involved in the endocytosis of IgE complexes (Pirron et al, 1990). This results in highly efficient antigen presentation by the respective FcεRII⁺ B cells. More direct roles for FcεRII in the pathogenesis of chronic inflammatory allergic reactions are suggested by the observation that interaction of allergens with IgE bound to FcεRII on monocyte/macrophages, eosinophils, and platelets results in the release of a variety of inflammatory mediators (Rouzer et al, 1982).

REGULATION OF THE HUMAN IMMUNOGLOBULIN E RESPONSE

Since the IgE molecule is the predominant antibody involved in human allergic disease, there has been considerable interest in the study of basic mechanisms involved in its control (Sears et al, 1991). During the past five years, there have been major breakthroughs in our understanding of the cellular and molecular mechanisms underlying the regulation of human IgE synthesis.

Requirements for the Induction of IgE Synthesis

The induction of IgE synthesis requires two signals (Geha, 1992). The *first signal* is delivered by IL-4, which provides the signal for isotype switching to IgE (Finkelman et al, 1988; Lebman and Coffman, 1988). Incubation of B cells with rIL-4 induces a 1.8-Kb germline Cε RNA transcript but not the productive 2.2-Kb ε-mRNA (Gauchat et al, 1990). In murine models, it has been demonstrated that immunoglobulin heavy-chain switch recombination is preceded by expression of the corresponding germline transcript (Berton et al, 1989). These data support the concept that IL-4 controls IgE isotype switching by modulating the accessibility of the ε switch region to a putative common switch recombinase.

IL-4 is necessary but not sufficient for the induction of IgE synthesis. Addition of rIL-4 alone or in combination with a variety of other cytokines, including IL-5 and IL-6, is ineffective in inducing IgE synthesis in highly purified B cell suspensions (Vercelli et al, 1989c). Additional signals are required for switch recombination and expression of productive ε RNA transcripts to occur. These *second signals* can be provided by T cells or a variety of B cell activators including Epstein-Barr virus (EBV) infection, mAb to the B cell antigen CD40, and hydrocortisone.

Induction of IgE Synthesis by T Cells

T cells play two important roles in the induction of IgE synthesis. First, they can provide IL-4. Second, physical contact between T and B cells provides a second signal, which in combination with IL-4 results in the induction of IgE synthesis (Vercelli et al, 1989c). Mixtures of T and B cells synthesize IgE upon incubation with IL-4 only when the T and B cells are cultured in the same well, but not when they are separated by a semipermeable membrane. Furthermore, IL-4–induced IgE synthesis is strongly inhibited by monoclonal antibodies directed against cell adhesion molecules.

Although initial studies focused on the requirement for cognate interaction between T and B cells (recognition by the TCR/CD3 complex on CD4⁺ T cells of MHC class II antigen plus peptide on B cells) as a prerequisite for the induction of IgE synthesis, more recent studies indicate that noncognate interaction between T and B cells, in which the TCR does not recognize the B cell MHC class II antigen plus peptide complex, can also support IL-4–dependent IgE synthesis (Parronchi et al, 1990). Recent studies indicate that these T and B cell interactions are mediated by the B cell antigen CD40 and its ligand expressed on activated, but not on resting, T cells. The importance of this interaction is supported by the observations that soluble CD40 inhibits T cell–dependent IgE synthesis and that peripheral blood mononuclear cells from patients with hyper-IgM syndrome, whose T cells lack the CD40 ligand, are unable to synthesize IgE in the presence of IL-4 (Fuleihan et al, 1986).

T Cell–Independent Systems of IgE Induction

Aside from T cells, there are a number of direct (T cell–independent) B cell activators that can act in combination with IL-4 to induce IgE synthesis. In this regard, it has been shown that stimulation with IL-4 and EBV induces T cell–independent IgE synthesis in human B cells (Thyphronitis et al, 1989). IgE production in this system was shown to be due to *de novo* induction of isotype switching, rather than from expansion of a precommitted sIgE+ B cell population, which has undergone Cε switching *in vivo*, because sIgE-negative B cell precursors could be stimulated by EBV and IL-4 to produce IgE.

More recently, several investigators have reported that highly purified B cells co-stimulated with rIL-4 and various mAbs directed against the B cell antigen, CD40, induce the synthesis of high levels of IgE antibody (Jabara et al, 1991; Ke et al, 1991). Stimulation of B cells from non-atopic donors with anti-CD40 mAb, in the absence of IL-4, results in a small increase of IgG synthesis but no IgE or IgM synthesis. When both anti-CD40 and rIL-4 are added, however, large amounts of IgE are synthesized.

CD40 stimulation alone, however, can enhance IgE production by *in vivo* driven IgE-producing cells from atopic patients (Ke et al, 1991). It is of interest that rIL-4 has been demonstrated to up-regulate CD40 expression on B cells. B cells from atopic donors have been found to have increased expression of CD40 on their cell surface (Renz et al, 1994). Thus, the capacity of anti-CD40 alone to enhance IgE production by B cells from atopic donors may reflect *in vivo* exposure to IL-4. These data suggest that the signals delivered for IgE production by IL4 and CD40 stimulation could serve as a model for activation of IgE synthesis seen *in vivo* in human allergic disease. More importantly, as noted above, the CD40/CD40 ligand interaction appears to be critical for IL-4–induced T cell–dependent IgE synthesis.

Hydrocortisone has also been found to up-regulate IL-4–dependent IgE synthesis by normal unfractionated mononuclear cells (Jabara et al, 1990). These observations have been extended to demonstrate that sIgE-negative B cells from non-atopic donors can be induced to synthesize IgE when incubated with a combination of hydrocortisone and rIL-4. The mechanisms by which hydrocortisone synergizes with IL-4 are unknown. However, these *in vitro* observations provide an immunologic basis for *in vivo* studies, which have demonstrated that during the first two weeks after systemic steroid therapy, atopic individuals frequently have a rise in serum IgE (Settipane et al, 1978).

Taken together, these data indicate that the second signal(s) required for IgE production can be delivered to B cells through different activation pathways. It is likely, however, that these different pathways will share the ability to activate switch recombination in B cells that have been incubated with IL-4 to render the Cε locus accessible.

Modulation of IgE synthesis by Cytokines

Although IL-4 is the only cytokine known to cause isotype switching to IgE synthesis, other cytokines and mediators have been found to modulate IL-4–induced IgE synthesis (Table 4–2). IL-5, a non–isotype-specific B cell growth factor (Pène et al, 1989), and IL-6, a non–isotype-specific late B cell differentiation factor, both up-regulate IgE synthesis induced by IL-4 in PBMC (Vercelli et al, 1989b). Endogenous IL-6, in particular, is critical for IL-4–induced IgE synthesis in PBMC, since anti–IL-6 antibody strongly inhibits the production of IgE in such cultures. TNF-α has also been reported to enhance IgE production, both in T cell–dependent and in T cell–independent systems (Gauchat et al, 1990).

Interferon-gamma (IFN-γ), IFN-α, transforming growth factor-β (TGF-β), IL-8, PAF-acether, prostaglandin E_2 and the neuropeptides, vasoactive intestinal peptide (VIP), and somatostatin have all been reported to inhibit IL-4–induced IgE synthesis in experimental animals and humans. Of all these molecules, IFN-γ has been most extensively studied for its capacity to inhibit IgE synthesis *in vitro* and *in vivo* (Snapper and Paul, 1987). The capacity of human and mouse T cell clones to induce IgE synthesis has been found to be directly correlated with the ratio of secreted IL-4 to IFN-γ. IFN-γ also antagonizes the effects of

TABLE 4–2. IMMUNOREGULATORY EFFECTS OF CYTOKINES ON IgE SYNTHESIS

Induces or Up-regulates	Inhibits or Suppresses
Interleukin-4	Interferon gamma
Interleukin-5	Interferon alpha
Interleukin-6	Tumor necrosis factor-beta
Tumor necrosis factor-alpha	Transforming growth factor-beta
	Interleukin 8
	Prostaglandin E_2
	PAF-acether
	Vasoactive intestinal peptide
	Somatostatin

IL-4 in other systems, e.g., IFN-γ has been reported to inhibit the IL-4–dependent induction of CD23 on B cells (DeFrance et al, 1987).

These various cytokines appear to inhibit IgE synthesis via a variety of mechanisms. Thus, IFN-γ, IFN-α, IL-12, VIP, and somatostatin inhibit IgE synthesis only in the presence of T cells (Finkelman et al, 1991; Kimata et al, 1993; Kiniwa et al, 1992). These data suggest that the mechanism for inhibition of IgE synthesis is indirect and is likely to be mediated through other cell types and/or factors produced upon incubation with these cytokines. It should be noted that IL-12–induced IgE inhibition seems to be mediated at least in part by the release of IFN-γ (Kiniwa et al, 1992). Nevertheless, the mechanisms by which these cytokines act are likely to differ because IFN-γ and IFN-α, but not IL-12, inhibit the expression of ε germline transcripts in PBMC cultures (Kiniwa et al, 1992).

TGF-β and IL-8 inhibit IgE synthesis in both T cell–dependent and T cell–independent systems (Kimata et al, 1992). Thus, these cytokines are likely to act directly on B cells. It is noteworthy that TGF-β acts at the transcriptional level, inhibiting the expression of ε germline transcripts. Inhibition by IL-8, but not by TGF-β, is IgE isotype-specific. Finally, PAF-acether inhibits IgE synthesis in T cell–dependent systems by blocking the expression of both germline and mature Cε transcripts (Deryckx et al, 1992).

Compartmentalization of T Cells by Cytokine Secretion Patterns

In 1986, Mosmann and co-workers described two distinct types of cloned mouse helper T cell lines that were defined primarily by differences in the pattern of lymphokines synthesized (Mosmann et al, 1986). T_{H1}, but not T_{H2}, cells produce IL-2, IFN-γ, and lymphotoxin, whereas T_{H2}, but not T_{H1}, cells produce IL-4, IL-5, IL-6, and IL-10 (Mosmann and Coffman, 1989). IL-3 and GM-CSF were secreted by both types. Although both T_{H1} and T_{H2} cells can enhance B cell proliferation, T_{H2} cells, but not T_{H1} cells, support B cell antibody secretion (Mosmann et al, 1986). This may be due to the ability of T_{H1} cells to kill B cells, probably via IFN-γ and lymphotoxin production, as well as the capacity of T_{H2}, but not T_{H1}, cells to produce IL-6, a B cell differentiation factor. T_{H1} cells appear to be primarily involved in delayed type hypersensitivity responses (Cher and Mosmann, 1987).

The selective expansion of T_{H2} cells is thought to play a critical role in inducing IgE synthesis because of the selective ability of IL-4 secreted by T_{H2} cells to induce immunoglobulin gene switching to the ε locus. In addition to stimulating IgE synthesis via IL-4, T_{H2} cells also enhance two other features of allergic responses. First, at least in mice, IL-3 and IL-4 are mast cell growth factors. Second, IL-5 induces the proliferation and differentiation of eosinophils both *in vitro* and *in vivo* (Yamaguchi et al, 1991).

The mechanisms that regulate the differentiation of resting T cells into T_{H1} versus T_{H2} cytokine secretion phenotypes are an active area of investigation. The nature of the antigen used for cellular activation, the cytokine milieu, and the origin of the antigen-presenting cell, as well as the genetic background of the host, all appear to be important. For example, parasites can induce the expansion of T_{H2} cells in atopic and nonatopic individuals (Mosmann and Coffman, 1989). In mice, the cytokine environment has also been identified as having an important influence on the type of helper T cell generated. T_{H1} cells are preferentially generated when CD4+ cells are cloned in the presence of IFN-γ or IL-12 (Gajewski and Fitch, 1988; Manetti et al, 1993). Conversely, Swain and co-workers (Swain et al, 1990) have reported that the presence of IL-4 during helper T cell effector generation *in vitro* enhances the development of IL-4 and IL-5 secreting effectors while suppressing the development of T cells that secrete IL-2 and IFN-γ.

Allergen-specific CD4+ T cell clones established from atopic patients have a T_{H2} lymphokine profile, provide help for IgE synthesis, and enhance eosinophil differentiation, whereas helper T cell clones from the same patients, specific for nonallergenic antigens, have a T_{H1} profile (Parronchi et al, 1991; Wierenga et al, 1990). Furthermore, CD4+ clones from non-atopic individuals, specific for the same allergens, have a T_{H1} profile (Wierenga et al, 1990). Antigens such as those expressed on parasites seem to be able to evoke a T_{H2} response regardless of the genetic background. In contrast, the genetic background seems to be critical for the generation of a T_{H2} response against allergens. It is also likely that the antigen-presenting cell itself can regulate the differentiation of helper

T cells. In this regard, Finkelman (Finkelman et al, 1988) has reported that antigen-presenting cells, by secreting IFN-α early in the course of an immune response (e.g., to an infectious agent), can down-regulate the IgE response but enhance IgG2a synthesis in mice.

Role of T_{H1}/T_{H2} Cells in Human Allergic Disease

Although mouse T cell clones can frequently be classified into either the T_{H1} or the T_{H2} cell pattern of cytokine secretion, a number of laboratories have shown that other cytokine secretion patterns can be observed (Firestein et al, 1989). Such patterns include the T_{H0} cell pattern in which IL-2, IFN-γ, IL-4, and IL-5 are present. Other intermediate patterns have been seen, particularly when unimmunized mice are used as donors for T cell cloning. Repeated antigen stimulation, however, results in T cells that predominantly produce IL-4 or IFN-γ. These experiments provide evidence for the hypothesis that there are precursor T cells which differentiate into T_{H1} versus T_{H2} cells (Swain et al, 1990).

These results also fit well with data obtained with many human T cell clones. In this regard, most alloreactive or PHA-induced human T cell clones derived from the peripheral blood of normal donors have intermediate patterns of cytokine production that do not fit clearly into T_{H1} or T_{H2} cells. However, T cells isolated from diseased tissues or peripheral blood of patients with active disease have been found to exhibit T_{H1} or T_{H2} type cytokine profiles. Thus, $CD4^+$ T cells isolated from thyroid glands of patients with autoimmune thyroiditis develop into T cell clones that produce IFN-γ but not IL-4. In contrast, most T cells infiltrating the conjunctiva of patients with vernal conjunctivitis develop into T cell clones producing high levels of IL-4 but not IFN-γ (Maggi et al, 1991). Using *in situ* hybridization, Kay and co-workers have also reported increased mRNA expression of IL-3, IL-4, IL-5, and GM-CSF, but no IFN-γ mRNA, expression in skin biopsies of allergen-induced late-phase reactions in atopic subjects (Kay et al, 1991) and asthmatic airways (Robinson et al, 1992).

The potential importance of a dysregulation of IL-4 and IFN-γ production in allergic diseases is further supported by immunologic characterization of PBMC from patients with atopic dermatitis (AD) and marked elevated serum IgE levels (Leung, 1992). B cells and monocytes from AD patients express increased levels of the CD23 (low-affinity IgE receptor) surface antigen. Since IL-4 plays an important role in the induction of IgE synthesis as well as CD23 expression on B cells (DeFrance et al, 1987) and monocytes (Vercelli et al, 1988), these observations suggest that AD is associated with increased secretion of IL-4 *in vivo*. In this regard, several investigators have reported that the increased spontaneous production of IgE *in vitro* by PBMC from AD patients can be inhibited by the addition of anti–IL-4 (Vollenweider et al, 1991). Furthermore, allergen-specific T cells cloned from AD skin lesions and AD peripheral blood demonstrate an increased frequency of T_{H2} cells (Wierenga et al, 1990).

PBMC from AD patients have also been found to have a decreased capacity to produce IFN-γ in response to a number of stimuli (Jujo et al, 1992; Reinhold et al, 1988). A significant inverse correlation has been reported between IFN-γ generation *in vitro* and IgE serum concentrations *in vivo* in AD (Reinhold et al, 1988). Spontaneous IgE production by PBMC from AD patients can also be suppressed by the addition of IFN-γ. Taken together, these data suggest that an imbalance of IL-4 and IFN-γ production may account for many of the immunologic features found in patients with allergic disease and elevated IgE levels. The recent observation that mast cells also produce cytokines such as IL-4 provide a T cell–independent mechanism as well, by which IgE synthesis may be enhanced following exposure of an individual to allergen.

PATHOPHYSIOLOGY OF ALLERGIC REACTIONS

Immediate and Late-Phase Tissue Responses

Following exposure to a relevant allergen, most patients with allergic diseases have an immediate reaction, which is caused by the acute degranulation of mast cells. It is generally clinically evident within 15 to 60 minutes of allergen challenge and subsides within 30 to 90 minutes. During such reactions, elevated levels of plasma histamine and local secretion of histamine and mast cell-derived tryptase can be measured in either the bronchoalveolar lavage fluid of asthmatics challenged with allergen or in skin chamber fluids of atopic individuals undergoing skin allergen challenges.

Three to four hours after the immediate reaction begins to subside, there is frequently the onset of an intense inflammatory reaction, termed the LPR. This is associated with the concomitant infiltration of eosinophils, neutrophils, and mononuclear cells. During this reaction, neutrophils and eosinophils reach their maximum cell accumulation at six to eight hours. In humans, it appears that the eosinophil is the dominant inflammatory cell during LPR. Following a single experimental allergen challenge, the cellular infiltrate consists predominantly of T cells and monocyte/macrophages 24 to 48 hours after allergen exposure. Using *in situ* hybridization, Kay (Kay et al, 1991) has demonstrated that the T cell infiltrate in allergen-induced late-phase skin reactions contains increased mRNA for IL-3, IL-4, IL-5, and granulocyte-macrophage colony-stimulating factor, but no mRNA for IFN-γ. These results suggest that the T cells infiltrating into the allergen-induced LPR are equivalent to the murine T helper type 2 (T_{H2}) subset.

It has become increasingly appreciated that the IgE-mediated LPR plays an important role in the pathogenesis of chronic allergic diseases such as asthma, atopic dermatitis (AD), and allergic rhinitis. For example, it is thought that the local deposition of eosinophil-derived major basic protein during the LPR contributes to the respiratory epithelial damage and lung inflammation found in asthma. The importance of the LPR is further supported by the observation that the intensity of nonspecific bronchial hyperreactivity in asthmatic reactions following allergen broncho-provocation is proportional to the intensity of the LPR (Cartier et al, 1982). Furthermore, clinical improvement in asthmatic symptoms following allergen immunotherapy correlates with an attenuation of the LPR following broncho-provocation challenge (Warner et al, 1978).

The mechanism(s) by which inflammatory cells localize to late-phase reactions have recently been the subject of intense investigation. Leukocyte adhesion molecules in allergen-stimulated skin explants are associated with the release of cytokines such as IL-1 and TNF (Leung et al, 1991). These cytokines have been demonstrated to play an important role in the induction of leukocyte adhesion molecules (Cotran and Pober, 1988). In this regard, the LPR is associated with the induction of leukocyte adhesion molecules such as ELAM-1, VCAM-1, and ICAM-1. Thus, the release of such cytokines may represent an important regulatory event in the local accumulation of inflammatory cells at the site of allergic reactions.

The cytokines secreted during the course of an allergic reaction are likely to be derived from a number of different cell types. Activation of mast cells, following allergen challenge, can result in the early secretion of a number of cytokines relevant to allergic inflammation (Durham et al, 1992). These include IL-1 and TNF-α, which increase expression of endothelial-leukocyte adhesion molecules (Bochner et al, 1990, 1991). The production of IL-4 by mast cells and infiltrating T_{H2} cells can result in the selective expression of VCAM-1 (Schleimer et al, 1992). Since eosinophils, but not neutrophils, express VLA-4, the ligand for VCAM-1, the local secretion of IL-4 in allergic reactions may account for the preferential infiltration of eosinophils, but not neutrophils, into sites of allergic inflammation (Bochner et al, 1991; Walsh et al, 1991). Once eosinophils are activated, they can also produce IL-3, GM-CSF, and IL-5 (Moqbel et al, 1991). These cytokines, which are also produced by T cells and mast cells, promote the proliferation, differentiation, and survival of eosinophils.

Other mechanisms are also likely to contribute to the chronic mast cell activation and tissue inflammation found in chronic allergic diseases. For example, histamine-releasing factors secreted by activated lymphocytes and monocytes during LPR have been reported to induce the degranulation of mast cells and basophils by binding to surface-bound IgE molecules (Lichtenstein, 1988). Langerhans cells in the atopic dermatitis skin lesion and macrophages infiltrating into the asthmatic airways bear IgE antibody on their cell surface (Leung, 1992). Human epidermal Langerhans cells have recently been found to express the high-affinity receptor for IgE (FcεRI) (Bieber et al, 1992). Allergens have also been demonstrated to activate IgE-bearing macrophages in an IgE-dependent manner to synthesize and secrete leukotrienes, PAF, IL-1, and TNF (Rouzer et al, 1982). Patients with atopic dermatitis and asthma contain circulating autoantibodies to IgE, which can also activate macrophages bearing IgE (Quinti et al, 1986). The activation of IgE-bearing Langerhans cells and macrophages by allergens and autoantibodies to IgE could thus contribute to the tissue inflammation.

In summary, the immediate response and LPR following allergen challenge represent a complex sequence of events. Although both responses require mast cell activation, the magnitude and duration of the LPR is dependent on the interaction of a number of different cell types, mediators, and cytokines. In humans, the eosinophil appears to be the most critical cell in mediating the inflammatory responses associated with the LPR and ultimately plays a critical role in the pathogenesis of chronic allergic diseases, particularly asthma.

Role of T Cells and Cytokines in Chronic Allergic Inflammation

A critical issue of great importance to the clinician caring for patients with chronic allergic diseases such as atopic dermatitis or asthma is the elucidation of the factors responsible for the persistence of local tissue immune activation and allergic inflammation. Several factors may contribute to the chronic inflammation: (1) these patients are frequently being continuously exposed to environmental allergens and thus are repeatedly triggering allergic responses and T_{H2} cell expansion; (2) some patients with allergic diseases, such as atopic dermatitis, may have a regulatory T cell defect involving the production of cytokines required to terminate immune responses (in this regard, the observation that patients with severe AD are deficient in their capacity to produce IFN-γ may be relevant because IFN-γ has been found to inhibit IgE synthesis and CD23 expression); (3) once a T_{H2} cell response is established, it may antagonize the function and activation of T_{H1} cells. In this regard, T_{H2} cells produce IL-4 and IL-10. Both these cytokines are known to reduce cytokine production (e.g., IFN-γ secretion by T_{H1} cells). Recent data also suggest that cytokines can induce prolonged survival of inflammatory effector cells and thus contribute to chronic inflammation. Of particular importance, is the observation that T cells from patients with chronic allergic diseases have increased numbers of T_{H2} cells and therefore, following exposure to allergen, secrete cytokines (i.e., IL-3, IL-4, IL-5, IL-6, and GM-CSF), which promote the migration, differentiation, and survival of the two major cellular components of allergic disease: IgE B cells and eosinophils.

CONCLUDING REMARKS

During the past decade there has been considerable progress in our understanding of the cellular and molecular basis of the allergic immune responses. In particular, cytokines such as IL-4 and IL-5 involved in the regulation of IgE synthesis have now been demonstrated to play an important role in the differentiation and survival of eosinophils, a critical effector cell in allergic inflammation (Lopez et al, 1988). This accounts for the frequent observation that atopic individuals have both elevated IgE levels and eosinophilia.

New immunologic therapies in the future are likely to focus on the modulation of T_{H2} cells and their cytokines. Indeed, several recent studies have demonstrated that treatment with cyclosporin results in significant improvement of clinical symptoms due to severe asthma and atopic dermatitis (Alexander et al, 1992; Sowden et al, 1991). It should be noted that cyclosporin therapy has resulted in some liver and renal toxicity and is therefore an unlikely candidate for ongoing treatment of allergic diseases. Nevertheless, these observations serve as a proof of concept, demonstrating that a drug that down-regulates T cell function and cytokine secretion can be effective in reducing the clinical severity of allergic diseases, and give credence to the concept that manipulation of the allergic immune response is likely to be a productive avenue of investigation in the future.

REFERENCES

Alexander AG, Barnes NC, Kay AB. Trial of cyclosporin in corticosteroid-dependent chronic severe asthma. Lancet 339:324, 1992.

Berton MT, Uhr JW, Vitetta ES. Synthesis of germline $\gamma1$ immunoglobulin heavy-chain transcripts in resting B cells: Induction by interleukin-4 and inhibition by interferon-γ. Proc Natl Acad Sci USA 86:2829, 1989.

Bieber T, de la Salle H, Wollenberg A, et al. Human epidermal Langerhans cells express the high affinity receptor for immunoglobulin E. J Exp Med 175:1285, 1992.

Bochner BS, Luscinskas FW, Gimbrone MA Jr, et al. Adherence of human basophils, eosinophils and neutrophils to interleukin 1-activated human vascular endothelial cells: Contributions of endothelial cell adhesion molecules. J Exp Med 173:1553, 1991.

Bochner B, Charlesworth E, Lichtenstein L, et al. Interleukin-1 is released at sites of human cutaneous allergic reactions. J Allergy Clin Immunol 86:830, 1990.

Cartier A, Thomson NC, Frith PA, et al. Allergen-induced increase in bronchial responsiveness to histamine: Relationship to the late asthmatic response and change in airway caliber. J Allergy Clin Immunol 70:170, 1982.

Cher DJ, Mosmann TR. Two types of murine helper T cell clones: 2. Delayed-type hypersensitivity is mediated by T_{H1} clones. J Immunol 138:3688, 1987.

Conrad DH, Squire CM, Barlett WC, et al. Fcε receptors. Curr Opin Immunol 3:859, 1991.

Cotran R, Pober J. Endothelial activation: its role in inflammatory and immune reactions. In Simionescu N, Simionescu M (eds). Endothelial Cell Biology. New York, Plenum, 1988, p 335.

DeFrance T, Aubry J, Rousset F, et al. Human recombinant interleukin-4 induces Fcε receptors (CD23) on B lymphocytes. Proc Natl Acad Sci USA 165:1459, 1987.

Deryckx S, de Waal Malefyt R, Gauchet J-F, et al. Immunoregulatory functions of PAF-acether. VIII. Inhibition of IL-4-induced human IgE synthesis in vitro. J Immunol 148:1465, 1992.

Durham SR, Ying S, Varney VA, et al. Cytokine messenger RNA expression for IL-3, IL-4, IL-5 and granulocyte/macrophage colony-stimulating factor in the nasal mucosa after local allergen provocation: relationship to tissue eosinophilia. J Immunol 148:2390, 1992.

Finkelman FD, Katona IM, Urban JF, et al. IL-4 is required to generate and sustain in vivo IgE responses. J Immunol 141:2335, 1988.

Finkelman FD, Svetic A, Gresser I, et al. Regulation by interferon-α of immunoglobulin isotype selection and lymphokine production in mice. J Exp Med 174:1179, 1991.

Firestein GS, Roder WD, Laxer JA, et al. A new murine CD4⁺ T cell subset with an unrestricted cytokine profile. J Immunol 143:518, 1989.

Fuleihan R, Ramesh N, Loh R, et al. Defective expression of the CD40 ligand in X chromosome–linked immunoglobulin deficiency with normal or elevated IgM. Proc Natl Acad Sci USA 90:2170, 1986.

Gajewski TF, Fitch FW. Anti-proliferative effect of IFN-γ in immune regulation. I. IFN-γ inhibits the proliferation of T_{H2} but not T_{H1} murine helper T cell clones. J Immunol 140:4245, 1988.

Galli SJ, Gordon JR, Wershil BK. Cytokine production by mast cells and basophils. Current Opin Immunol 3:865, 1991.

Gauchat J-F, Lebman DA, Coffman RL, et al. Structure and expression of germline ε transcripts in human B cells induced by interleukin-4 to switch to IgE production. J Exp Med 172:463, 1990.

Geha RS. Regulation of IgE synthesis in humans. J Allergy Clin Immunol 90:143, 1992.

Helm B, Marsh P, Vercelli D, et al. The mast cell binding site on human immunoglobulin E. Nature 331:180, 1988.

Ishizaka K, Ishizaka T. Identification of IgE antibodies as a carrier of reaginic activity. J Immunol 99:1187, 1967.

Ishizaka T, Ishizaka K. Biology of immunoglobulin E. Prog Allergy. 19:60, 1975.

Jabara HH, Ahern DJ, Vercelli D, et al. Hydrocortisone and IL-4 induce IgE isotype switching in human B cells. J Immunol 147:1557, 1991.

Jabara HH, Fu SM, Geha RS, et al. CD40 and IgE. Synergism between anti-CD40 mAb and IL-4 in the induction of IgE synthesis by highly purified human B cells. J Exp Med 172:1861, 1990.

Jujo K, Renz H, Abe J, et al. Decreased gamma interferon and increased interleukin-4 production promote IgE synthesis in atopic dermatitis. J Allergy Clin Immunol. 90:323, 1992.

Kay AB, Ying S, Varney V, et al. Messenger RNA expression of the cytokine gene cluster, interleukin 3(IL-3), IL-4, IL-5, and granulocyte/macrophage colony-stimulating factor, in allergen-induced late-phase cutaneous reactions in atopic subjects. J Exp Med 173:775, 1991.

Ke Z, Clark EA, Saxon A. CD40 stimulation provides an IFN-γ independent and IL4-dependent differentiation signal directly to human B cells for IgE production. J Immunol 146:1836, 1991.

Kimata H, Yoshida A, Fujimoto M, et al. Effect of vasoactive intestinal peptide, somatostatin, and substance P on spontaneous IgE and IgG4 production in atopic patients. J Immunol 150;4630, 1993.

Kimata H, Yoshida A, Ishioka C, et al. Interleukin-8 selectively inhibits immunoglobulin E production induced by IL-4 in human B cells. J Exp Med 176:1227, 1992.

Kinet J-P. The high affinity receptor for immunoglobulin E. Curr Opin Immunol 2:499, 1990.

Kiniwa M, Gately M, Gubier U, et al. Recombinant interleukin-12 suppresses the synthesis of immunoglobulin E by interleukin-4 stimulated human lymphocytes. J Clin Invest 90:262, 1992.

Lebman DA, Coffman RL. Interleukin-4 causes isotype switching to IgE in T cell-stimulated clonal B cell cultures. J Exp Med 168:853, 1988.

Leung DYM. Immunopathology of atopic dermatitis. Semin Immunopath (Springer) 13:427, 1992.

Leung DYM, Cotran RS, Pober JS. Expression of an endothelial leukocyte adhesion molecule (ELAM-1) in elicited late phase allergic skin reactions. J Clin Invest 87:1805, 1991.

Lichtenstein L. Histamine-releasing factors and IgE heterogeneity. J Allergy Clin Immunol 81:814, 1988.

Lopez AF, Sanderson CJ, Gamble JR, et al. Recombinant human interleukin-5 is a selective activator of human eosinophil function. J Exp Med 167:219, 1988.

Maggi E, Biswas P, Del Prete GF, et al. Accumulation of T_{H2}-like helper T cells in the conjunctiva of patients with vernal conjunctivitis. J Immunol 146:1169, 1991.

Manetti R, Parronchi P, Giudizi MG, et al. Natural killer cell stimulatory factor (interleukin-12 [IL-12]) induces T helper type 1 (T_{H1})-specific immune responses and inhibits the development of IL-4-producing T_H cells. J Exp Med 177:1199, 1993.

Moqbel R, Hamid Q, Ying S, et al. Expression of mRNA and immunoreactivity for the granulocyte/macrophage colony-stimulating factor in activated human eosinophils. J Exp Med 174:749, 1991.

Mosmann TR, Cherwinski H, Bond MW, et al. Two types of murine helper T cell clones. I. Definition according to profiles of lymphokine activities and secretory proteins. J Immunol 136:2348, 1986.

Mosmann TR, Coffman RL: T_{H1} and T_{H2} cells: Different patterns of lymphokine secretion lead to different functional properties. Ann Rev Immunol 7:145, 1989.

Mudde GC, Van Reijsen FC, Boland GJ, et al. Allergen presentation by epidermal Langerhans cells from patients with atopic dermatitis is mediated by IgE. Immunology 69:335, 1990.

Parronchi P, Macchia D, Piccinni M-P, et al. Allergen- and bacterial antigen-specific T-cell clone established from atopic donors shows a different profile of cytokine production. Proc Natl Acad Sci USA 88:4538, 1991.

Parronchi P, Tiri A, Macchia D, et al. Noncognate contact-dependent B cell activation can promote IL-4 dependent *in vitro* human IgE synthesis. 144:2102, 1990.

Pène J, Rousset F, Brìere F, et al. Interleukin-5 enhances interleukin-4 induced IgE production by normal human B cells: The role of soluble CD23 antigen. Eur J Immunol 18:929, 1989.

Pirron U, Schlunck T, Prinz JC, et al. IgE-dependent antigen focusing by human B lymphocytes can also be mediated by the low-affinity receptor for IgE. Eur J Immunol 20:1547, 1990.

Quinti I, Brozek C, Geha RS, et al. Circulating IgG antibodies to IgE in atopic syndromes. J Allergy Clin Immunol 77:586, 1986.

Reinhold U, Pawelec G, Wehrmann W, et al. Immunoglobulin E and immunoglobulin G subclass distribution *in vivo* and relationship to *in vitro* generation of interferon-gamma and neopterin in patients with severe atopic dermatitis. Int Arch Allergy Appl Immunol 87:120, 1988.

Renz H, Brodie C, Bradley KL, et al. Anti-CD40 stimulates IgE production in peripheral blood mononuclear cells from patients with atopic dermatitis. J Allergy Clin Immunol 93:658, 1994.

Robinson DS, Hamid Q, Ying S, et al. Predominant T_{H2}-like bronchoalveolar T-lymphocyte population in atopic asthma. N Engl J Med 326:298, 1992.

Rouzer CA, Scott WA, Hamill AL, et al. Secretion of leukotriene C and other arachidonic acid metabolites by macrophages challenged with immunoglobulin E immune complexes. J Exp Med 156:1077, 1982.

Schleimer RP, Sterbinsky SA, Kaiser J, et al. Interleukin-4 induces adherence of human eosinophils and basophils but not neutrophil to endothelium: association with expression of VCAM-1. J Immunol 148:1086, 1992.

Sears MR, Burrows B, Flannery EM, et al. Relation between airway responsiveness and serum IgE in children with asthma and in apparently normal children. N Engl J Med 325:1067, 1991.

Serafin WE, Austen KF. Current concepts: Mediators of immediate hypersensitivity reactions. N Engl J Med 317:30, 1987.

Settipane GA, Pudupakkam RK, McGowan JH. Corticosteroid effect on immunoglobulins. J Allergy Clin Immunol 62:162, 1978.

Snapper CM, Paul WE. Interferon-γ and B cell stimulatory factor-1 reciprocally regulate Ig isotype production. Science 236:944, 1987.

Sowden JM, Berth-Jones J, Ross JS, et al. Double-blind, controlled, crossover study of cyclosporin in adults with severe refractory atopic dermatitis. Lancet 338:137, 1991.

Swain SL, Weinberg AD, English M. CD4+ T cell subsets: lymphokine secretion of memory cells and of effector cells which develop from precursors *in vitro*. J Immunol 144:1788, 1990.

Swain SL, Weinberg AD, English M, et al. Il-4 directs the development of T_{H2}-like helper effectors. J Immunol 145:3796, 1990.

Thyphronitis G, Tsokos GC, June CH, et al. IgE secretion by Epstein-Barr virus-infected purified human B lymphocytes is stimulated by interleukin 4 and suppressed by interferon-γ. Proc Natl Acad Sci USA 86:5580, 1989.

Vercelli D, Helm B, Marsh P, et al. The B cell binding site on human immunoglobulin E. Nature 338:649, 1989a.

Vercelli D, Jabara HH, Arai K, et al. Induction of human IgE synthesis requires interleukin-4 and T-B cell interaction involving the T cell receptor/CD3 complex and MHC class II antigens. J Exp Med 169:1295, 1989b.

Vercelli D, Jabara HH, Arai K, et al. Endogenous IL-6 plays an obligatory role in IL-4 induced human IgE synthesis. Eur J Immunol 19:1419, 1989c.

Vercelli D, Jabara HH, Lee BW, et al. Human recombinant interleukin-4 induces FcεR2/CD23 on normal human monocytes. J Exp Med 167:1406, 1988.

Vollenweider S, Saurat J-H, Rocken M, et al. Evidence suggesting involvement of interleukin-4 (IL-4) production in spontaneous *in vitro* IgE synthesis in patients with atopic dermatitis. J Allergy Clin Immunol 87:1088, 1991.

Walsh GM, Mermod J, Harnell A, et al. Human eosinophil, but not neutrophil, adherence to IL-1-stimulated human unbilical vascular endothelial cells is α4β1 dependent. J Immunol 146:3419, 1991.

Warner JO, Soothill JF, Price JF, et al. Controlled trial of hyposensitization with *Dermatophagoides pteronyssinus* antigen in children with asthma. Lancet 2:912, 1978.

Wierenga EA, Snoek M, deGroot C, et al. Evidence for compartmentalization of functional subsets of CD4+ T lymphocytes in atopic patients. J Immunol 144:4651, 1990.

Yamaguchi Y, Suda T, Suda J, et al. Purified interleukin 5 supports the terminal differentiation and proliferation of murine eosinophilic precursors. J Exp Med 167:43, 1991.

Yokota A, Kikutani H, Tanaka T, et al. Two species of human Fcε receptor II (FcεRII/CD23): tissue-specific and interleukin 4-specific regulation of the gene expression. Cell 55:611, 1988.

Section Two
ETIOLOGY AND PATHOGENETIC FACTORS IN ALLERGY AND ASTHMA

Chapter 5
Epidemiology of Allergy and Asthma

Richard Evans III, M.D., M.P.H., and
Peter J. Gergen, M.D., M.P.H.

Environment and heredity are both involved in the development of allergic disease. Genetically, allergy is clearly associated with IgE antibody production and atopy, that is, the hereditary predisposition to develop these IgE antibodies. We are still learning about the relationship of one allergic disease to another, but there is substantial evidence that all allergic diseases have some connection with one another. The evidence that environmental factors play a part is fairly clear for allergens but less so for pollutants, and even less so for socioeconomic and social variables.

ALLERGIC RHINITIS

Allergic rhinitis represents an IgE-mediated reaction to an allergen. Allergic rhinitis can be seasonal, perennial, or perennial with seasonal exacerbation. In seasonal rhinitis, which is often called hay fever, the specific season of the year during which symptoms occur depends upon the etiologic agent—usually trees in spring, grasses in summer, and weeds in the fall. Perennial rhinitis has many of the same symptoms but without seasonal variation. Not all perennial rhinitis has an allergic basis.

The prevalence of allergic rhinitis in the population is approximately 9 percent to 10 percent (Adams and Benson, 1991; Turkeltaub and Gergen, 1991). Allergic rhinitis is most common in people aged 20 to 40 years and in females and whites, while the risk is somewhat reduced in smokers (Adams and Benson, 1991; Turkeltaub and Gergen, 1991). In the United States, allergic rhinitis is reported to be highest in the West and lowest in the Midwest (Adams and Benson, 1990). Reporting on the 1976–1980 National Health and Nutrition Examination Survey (NHANES II), Turkeltaub and Gergen (1991) found an increase in allergic rhinitis in urban areas, but in their evaluation of data from the National Health Interview Survey (NHIS), Adams and Benson (1991) found no increase in urban areas.

The prevalence of allergic rhinitis appears to be increasing. The NHIS reported that hay fever increased from 7.7 percent in 1979–1981 (Collins, 1986) to 9 percent in 1990 (Adams and Benson, 1991). In Aberdeen, Scotland, surveys of 8- to 13-year-old school children reported that hay fever increased from 3.2 percent in 1964 to 11.9 percent in 1989 (Ninan and Russell, 1992). In England, Fleming and Crombie (1987) found that both men and women consulted general practitioners for allergic rhinitis almost twice as frequently in 1981–1982 as they had a decade earlier.

Natural History

Symptoms of allergic rhinitis may increase over time. In most patients, McKnee (1966) found that symptoms had gotten worse after 10 years, but in more than one third, they had improved. Less than 10 percent of patients have remissions of any substantial duration, but the likelihood of remission is greater in seasonal allergic rhinitis and in patients with a disease duration of less than 5 years (Broder et al, 1974).

Patients with allergic rhinitis may have associated symptoms of either asthma or eczema or both, but it is more common for the diseases to appear concurrently or for asthma and/or eczema to develop first. Åberg and Engström (1990) found this to be the case in 88 percent of 14-year-old children studied.

Chronic nasal inflammation associated with allergic rhinitis may lead to complications, such as sinusitis, nasal or sinus polyps, or even recurrent otitis media with hearing loss. Especially in young children, the latter complication can have adverse effects on speech development, cognition, or both.

ECZEMA

It is difficult to estimate accurately the prevalence of atopic dermatitis (eczema). Mild disease may be overlooked, and in older children, it may be mistaken for other skin conditions. Nevertheless, it is apparent that eczema is more prevalent in some parts of the world than in others. Fergusson et al (1982) reported that 20.4 percent of 3-year-old New Zealanders had histories of eczema. More recently, Ninan and Russell (1992) found that 12 percent of Scottish 8- to 13-year-olds had eczema by history, whereas Burr et al (1989) found that 16 percent of 12-year-olds in South Wales had eczema histories. However, Golding and Peters (1987) found a much lower incidence when they considered only *current* eczema: this British study found only 5 percent of 5-year-olds had histories of eczema during the previous 12 months. Prevalence of eczema in the United States is thought to be 1 percent to 3 percent of the general population (Smith and Slavin, 1988), but prevalence is higher in atopic individuals.

Epidemiologists report an increase in eczema prevalence. In the 1946 British birth cohort, prevalence was 5.1 percent at 6 years of age. The 1958 birth cohort had an eczema prevalence of 7.3 percent at 7 years of age, and by the time the 1970 birth cohort reached age 5 years, prevalence was up to 12.2 percent (Taylor et al, 1984). Between 1973 and 1988, the prevalence of ever having eczema rose from 5 percent to 16 percent among children in South Wales (Burr et al, 1989). Similarly, Ninan and Russell (1992) reported that eczema spiraled up from 5.3 percent to 12 percent in Aberdeen, Scotland, between 1964 and 1989. These findings are in line with reported increases in asthma and allergic rhinitis, which are other atopic diseases, but the cause of the increase has not been clearly defined.

Eczema typically begins in the first few years of life. In early life, eczema is about twice as common in boys as in girls (Smith and Slavin, 1988). In a study of Swiss children with eczema, Queille-Roussel et al (1985) found that 81.5 percent developed eczema before their first birthday, 91.1 percent developed it before 24 months, and nearly all (96.7 percent) had developed it before 36 months. Mild eczema accounts for 22 percent of cases; moderate, 44.5 percent of cases; and severe, 33.5 percent of cases.

Influences on Development

FAMILY HISTORY. Queille-Roussel et al (1985) noted an association between family history of atopy and eczema. A parental history of eczema is an even stronger predictor that a child will develop eczema. A family history of asthma is also predictive but less so (Fergusson et al, 1982).

DIET. Early infant diet may play a major role in the development of eczema. In the Queille-Roussel study, dietary factors were involved in the onset of eczema in 27 percent of cases. Cow's milk is the most common food allergen implicated in infants. Some studies indicate that breast-feeding provides protective effects against eczema, whereas others do not. Van Asperen et al (1984), for example, found no protective effect for exclusive breast-feeding for 4 months in children up to 20 months of age. Part of the reason for these contradictions may be that breast-feeding without eliminating potential allergens from the mother's diet may not be enough to reduce the risk of developing eczema (Kramer and Moroz, 1981).

Solid foods may play a role, but here again there is disagreement. Fergusson et al (1982) reported an association between early exposure to a variety of foods and eczema, but Kramer and Moroz (1981) found no association. In a study of 135 infants of atopic parents, babies fed only breast milk for 6 months had a prevalence of atopic dermatitis of 14 percent at 1 year of age. In a similar breast-fed group, who had solid foods introduced at 3 months, prevalence at one year was 35 percent (Saarinen, 1984). On balance, it would appear that breast-feeding, along with maternal avoidance of allergens, may *postpone* the onset of eczema in high-risk children but may not prevent its eventual development.

Usually atopic dermatitis is mild in adolescents and adults, but occasionally the adult stage produces severe symptoms. At all stages, patients are at risk for *Staphylococcus aureus* infection. Patients may also develop cutaneous viral infections.

ALLERGEN SKIN-TEST REACTIVITY

Positive allergen skin tests are often used to confirm atopy. Although skin tests can be positive in the absence of symptoms of atopic disease, strongly positive skin tests in symptomatic patients do provide presumptive evidence of allergic disease. Gergen et al (1987) reported that 20.2 percent of the general population in the United States have skin-test reactivity to allergens. Regional studies report even higher rates: from 24 percent to 51 percent (Freidhoff et al, 1981; Barbee et al, 1987). In general, grass and weed pollens are associated with the highest rates of reactivity. The rate of allergen skin-test reactivity varies markedly with age. Peak reactivity occurs somewhere between the late teens and early thirties and then drops to less than half the peak in people in their sixties and older (Gergen et al, 1987; Freidhoff et al, 1981; Barbee et al, 1987). Gergen (1987) found increased reactivity in males, in blacks, in those with higher levels of income or education, and in people living in urban areas.

Young children with skin-test positivity tend to retain positivity for years, while the rate of conversion to negativity increases in older age groups. Barbee et al (1987) found that slightly more than a quarter of individuals aged 65 to 74 years at the start of 8-year follow-up converted to negativity during that period.

FOOD ALLERGY

The prevalence of food allergy is difficult to determine because less than one third of reported food allergies can be confirmed by challenge. Food *intolerance* is often mistaken for true food allergy. Food intolerance produces adverse but not immunologic effects, whereas true food allergy is an immunoreaction. In a prospective study of 480 children under 3 years of age enrolled in a private pediatric practice, Bock (1987) found that 28 percent reported "food allergies." Challenge confirmed reactions to fruit and fruit juices in 12 percent but could confirm reactions to other foods in only 8 percent of children. Høst and Halken (1990) prospectively studied 1749 newborns in Denmark and confirmed that 2.2 percent had cow's milk allergy during the first year of life.

Natural History

Immunoreactions to food are usually immediate and may be precipitated by ingesting only minute amounts of the offending food. Høst and Halken (1990) reported that children allergic to cow's milk became sensitized within 1 month after the introduction of milk into the diet. Milk is the most common food to which children are allergic, but egg, soy, peanut, fish, wheat, chicken, and chocolate allergies are not uncommon. The most likely fruits to cause reactions are oranges, tomatoes, apples, and grapes.

Food allergies tend to occur in infancy, with about 80 percent developing within the first year, 16 percent in the second year, and 4 percent in the third year (Bock, 1987). Reaction to fruits and juices often develops later (mean age of onset 15 months) and persists longer than other food allergies.

Most food allergies disappear within the first 3 years of life. Bock (1987) found that most foods could be reintroduced within 9 months. Even children with severe reactions to foods can lose their sensitivity. Bock (1985) reported that about 44 percent of children severely reactive to foods could tolerate at least small amounts of the culprit food 3 to 9 years later, and a third had lost their intolerance altogether.

Influences on Development

Family history of atopy is associated with the development of food allergies. Patients with high levels of IgE are at greater risk for persistence of the allergy. Sampson and Scanlon (1989) reported that individuals who develop skin symptoms alone at initial challenge are most likely to lose their sensitivity. Patients with asthma who develop generalized allergic reactions are at greater risk of developing life-threatening anaphylaxis. Sampson et al (1992) studied 13 patients with severe anaphylactic reactions to food. All patients were highly atopic, with current or previous symptoms of asthma, allergic rhinitis, and atopic dermatitis. Six of the 13 died, and the other seven required intubation.

Skin tests by themselves are not reliable for determining clinical sensitivity. Patients may test positive without any clinical symptoms (Sampson and Albergo, 1984). Accurate diagnosis of food allergy involves both repeated specific food challenges and the demonstration of IgE antibodies to food substances.

INSECT ALLERGY

Yellow jacket, bee, wasp, or hornet stings can cause allergic reactions in sensitized people. Possible reactions to insect stings include severe local reaction, toxic reaction, and generalized allergic reaction. The reported frequency of insect-sting allergy in a given population varies, depending on the criteria used—history, skin test, or RAST—and the age group of the population, but generalized allergic reaction occurs relatively infrequently. Settipane and Boyd (1989) found a frequency of systemic allergic reactions of under 1 percent in 11- to 16-year-old children. There was no difference in frequency between boys and girls with similar life styles. Golden et al (1989) reported that about 3 percent of adults have had systemic sting reactions, and 26 percent show venom sensitivity on RAST or skin test. Sensitization is relatively common after a sting, but it is transient in about half the cases.

Fifteen percent of those with positive skin tests/RAST have negative histories for reaction to insect stings (Golden et al, 1989). Golden and his colleagues found that positive skin tests/RAST correlated, though not closely, with symptoms. Fifty-six percent of those who had had previous systemic reactions had positive tests. Venom sensitivity on skin tests seemed to occur more often in persons who also had skin-test sensitivity to inhalant allergens.

A history of allergic reaction to insect stings may not accurately predict reactions to future stings. Settipane and Boyd (1989) found that 37 percent of untreated sting-sensitive patients had less severe reactions to repeated stings; 42 percent had the same reaction, and 21 percent had worse reactions. Three fourths of children less than 16 years old who had cardiovascular/respiratory responses on initial sting had less severe responses to repeated stings. Of these, 63 percent had no systemic reactions at all to repeated stings, and 25 percent had the same type of reaction when stung again. The interval between stings apparently affects the severity of the reaction. Those experiencing a repeated sting after 5 years are less likely to have systemic reactions to the sting (Settipane and Boyd, 1989). Severe reactions are manifested primarily by the additional symptom of acute dyspnea.

Even though a large percentage of sting-sensitive patients—particularly those under the age of 16 years—improve without venom desensitization, it is prudent to evaluate all sting-sensitive patients for possible immunotherapy. Follow-up of children who have undergone venom therapy demonstrates the effectiveness of treatment in reducing reaction rates (Valentine et al, 1990). Sting-sensitive patients with cardiovascular/respiratory symptoms and positive skin/RAST tests to venom are particularly likely candidates for venom therapy (Settipane and Boyd, 1989).

DRUG ALLERGY

Allergic reactions to drugs occur infrequently and are unrelated to the pharmacologic action of the drug. True drug allergy is the result of an immunologic mechanism. Only a few drugs currently in use are known to have the requisite properties to produce an immune response.

There are three types of allergic reactions to drugs: immediate (within the first hour), accelerated (between 1 and 72 hours), and late (after 72 hours). Immediate reactions include urticaria, which is the most common, and anaphylaxis, which is the most serious. Most reactions consist of urticaria, pruritus, and angioedema, but hypotension and death can occur without the development of other symptoms.

Accelerated reactions usually consist of urticaria or angioedema; hypotension and death are rare. Delayed reactions often present as benign skin eruptions or, occasionally, urticaria. Noncutaneous late reactions include drug fever and serum sickness–like reactions.

In a multinational follow-up of 1790 patients treated with monthly intramuscular benzathine penicillin injections to prevent the recurrence of rheumatic fever, the International Rheumatic Fever Study Group (1991) reported that 3.2 percent had reactions to penicillin. Four patients had immediate reactions (anaphylaxis); 37 had accelerated reactions; and 16 had late reactions.

Penicillin

Many studies have investigated the prevalence of penicillin reaction. In a series of studies in Baltimore, Maryland, the incidence of post-treatment allergic reactions was 1.45 percent in 8000 patients without prior histories of penicillin allergy and 0.45 percent in 3996 patients who had both negative histories of penicillin allergy and negative penicillin skin tests (Adkinson, 1984).

The International Rheumatic Fever Study Group (1991) reported a rate of anaphylaxis of 0.2 percent (1.2 anaphylactic reactions per 10,000 injections) and a death rate of 0.05 percent (0.31 deaths per 10,000 injections) in penicillin-treated patients.

Although penicillin allergy is IgE-mediated, it is generally accepted that there is no increased prevalence of atopic disease in individuals sensitized to penicillin; however, atopic individuals are at greater risk for anaphylaxis if they do have a reaction. Also, patients with histories of prior reactions to penicillin are much more likely to experience another reaction on subsequent exposure than are those without previous histories. In general, pediatric patients have fewer reactions to penicillin than do adults.

The route of administration may influence the rate of penicillin reaction. Patients receiving penicillin parenterally are more likely to react than those receiving it orally, possibly because parenteral doses are higher (see Chapter 22).

Other Drug Allergies

Other drugs capable of producing a true allergic reaction include papain, streptokinase, and insulin and other organ extracts. Approximately 0.4 percent to 4.2 percent of patients treated with chymopapain are allergic to the drug; about 0.4 percent to 0.8 percent of patients experience anaphylactic reaction. About 0.1 percent to 0.2 percent of patients receiving insulin experience systemic reactions, and about 1.7 percent of patients experience reactions to hyperosmolar radiocontrast media. Typically, these reactions are generalized anaphylactoid reactions (Anderson and Adkinson, 1987).

Currently our diagnostic abilities are limited, but it is likely that there are immunologic reactions to other families of drugs (see Chapter 22).

ASTHMA

Asthma is a major public health problem. Costs for asthma care now exceed six billion dollars (Weiss et al, 1992). Asthma is the most common chronic childhood disease, and asthma and wheezing are among the most frequent reasons for visits to the pediatrician. Unfortunately, the study of asthma is hampered by a lack of a universally accepted definition of the disease, which might be more appropriately termed a syndrome. The National Asthma Education Program Expert Panel Report (Sheffer, 1991) recommends the following be used as a working clinical definition:

Asthma is a lung disease with the following characteristics: (1) airway obstruction that is reversible (but not completely so in some patients) either spontaneously or with treatment; (2) airway inflammation; and (3) increased airway response to a variety of stimuli.

Prevalence

Estimates of the prevalence of asthma vary, principally because the definition of asthma and survey questions differ among researchers. Estimated prevalence of childhood asthma in the United States ranges from 3.6 percent to 9.5 percent, depending on the definition/questions used (Table 5–1) (Gergen et al, 1988). Table 5–2 presents asthma prevalence data from NHANES II (1976–1980).

AGE-RELATED FACTORS. Asthma most commonly begins in early childhood, but onset can also occur later in life. Prevalence is highest in childhood and among older adults. The incidence of asthma decreases with age, with the highest rates among infants less than one year old and the lowest among adults (Yunginger et al, 1992).

Childhood asthma usually begins before the age of 5 years and occurs about twice as often in boys as in girls. However, during adolescence, prevalence of asthma among girls equals or exceeds that among boys. In adulthood, rates among men and women are similar (Gergen et al, 1988; Evans et al, 1987). About 50 percent of childhood asthmatics become symptom-free when they reach their teens or twenties (Åberg and Engstrom, 1991). However, follow-up has shown recurrence of wheezing among some of these quiescent asthmatics.

RACIAL/ETHNIC FACTORS. Prevalence varies among racial and ethnic groups in the United States. At all ages, African-Americans have more asthma than whites (Turkeltaub and Gergen, 1991; Gergen et al, 1988). Some Hispanic groups have high prevalence rates, while others do not. Puerto Rican children living in New York City have some of the highest rates of asthma in the United States, while Mexican-American children in the Southwest have among the lowest (Carter-Pokras and Gergen, 1993).

SOCIOECONOMIC STATUS. The effect of socioeconomic status (SES) on the black-white differences in asthma prevalence is not clear.

TABLE 5–1. REPORTED ASTHMA IN THE UNITED STATES BY VARIOUS DEFINITIONS IN CHILDREN 3 TO 17 YEARS OF AGE*

		SEX		RACE	
DEFINITION	TOTAL	Male	Female	White	Black
Ever diagnosed by physician	7.0 (0.49)	8.3 (0.67)	5.5 (0.55)	6.4 (0.54)	10.1 (1.3)
Currently diagnosed by physician	3.6 (0.31)	4.3 (0.41)	2.9 (0.41)	3.3 (0.33)	5.6 (0.76)
Wheezing †	5.3 (0.37)	6.2 (0.44)	4.5 (0.55)	5.0 (0.45)	7.3 (1.0)
Ever diagnosed by physician or wheezing†	9.5 (0.54)	11.2 (0.69)	7.8 (0.72)	8.9 (0.62)	13.1 (1.5)
Now diagnosed by physician or wheezing†	6.7 (0.39)	7.8 (0.43)	5.5 (0.60)	6.2 (0.48)	9.4 (1.1)

*Data from National Center for Health Statistics, Second National Health and Nutrition Examination Survey, 1976 to 1980. Results are mean percentages (±SE).
†During the past 12 months, not counting colds or the flu, frequent trouble with wheezing.

TABLE 5–2. CUMULATIVE PREVALENCE OF ASTHMA* BY SELECTED DEMOGRAPHIC CHARACTERISTICS IN THE UNITED STATES POPULATION AGED 3 TO 74 YEARS

		AGE (YEARS)			
	ALL AGES	3–11	12–44	45–64	65–74
Estimated population with asthma	20,673,000	3,070,000	10,702,000	5,108,000	1,793,000
Sample size with asthma	2512	474	935	637	466
Total†	10.6	10.2	9.9	11.8	12.4
Sex‡					
Male†	11.4	12.0	10.2	12.9	15.5
Female†	9.7	8.3	9.7	10.8	9.9
Race					
White†	10.4	9.7	9.7	11.8	12.4
Black†	12.2	13.4	12.0	11.5	11.8
Region‡					
Northeast†	9.1	9.8	9.4	8.0	8.8
Midwest†	8.6	8.3	7.9	10.1	9.9
South†	12.7	11.8	11.3	15.5	15.6
West†	11.6	10.7	11.0	13.0	14.8
Poverty level‡					
Below†	13.1	9.3	11.7	20.6	20.0
At or above†	10.3	10.4	9.7	11.1	11.4
Residence‡					
Urban†	10.7	10.7	10.5	10.9	11.6
Rural†	10.2	9.2	8.6	13.6	14.1

*Defined as ever been told by a physician that he/she had asthma and/or frequent problems with wheezing in the previous 12 months.
†Rate per 100 persons.
‡Includes all other races not shown separately.
Data from the Second National Health and Nutrition Examination Survey, 1976 to 1980.

In the 1981 NHIS Child Health Supplement, the black-white prevalence difference among children in the United States was virtually eliminated when the study was controlled for SES (Weitzman et al, 1990). In contrast, increased asthma prevalence among African-American children and adults reported in NHANES II (1976–1980) could not be explained by SES factors (Turkeltaub and Gergen, 1991; Schwartz et al, 1990).

Children in urban areas are more likely to have asthma than those in rural areas, but this same trend has not been found in adults (Turkeltaub and Gergen, 1991; Gergen et al, 1988).

REPORTED INCREASES IN PREVALENCE. Many studies report a seemingly increased prevalence of asthma. Is the amount of asthma actually changing in the population? This is a difficult question to assess because there are many confounding factors. It is generally acknowledged that changes in medical labeling have had at least some effect. Other factors often cited include greater awareness of the disease and access to medical care. These and other variables undoubtedly affect prevalence rates, but whether they account for the entirety of the increase is problematic.

Part of the difficulty is that we know little about trends in the occurrence of asthma. Yunginger et al (1992) studied the population of Rochester, Minnesota, from the beginning of 1964 to the end of 1983. During that period, the annual age- and sex-adjusted incidence of definite and probable asthma increased from 183 to 284 persons per 100,000 population. However, the increase occurred only in the 1- to 14-year-old age group.

A number of reports show increases in prevalence during the 1970s and 1980s. For 6- to 11-year-old children, the 1976–1980 NHANES II found a 58 percent increase in affirmative responses to "ever having asthma" since the 1971–1974 NHANES I. The prevalence in this age group was 4.8 percent in NHANES I and 7.6 percent in NHANES II. Prevalence increased in both African-American and white children (Gergen et al, 1988).

The NHIS is another nationwide survey of health data. Evans et al (1987) compared NHIS data from the early and late 1970s, and they also found an increased prevalence of asthma during the decade. More recent NHIS analyses comparing the 1981 and 1988 Child Health Supplement show a continuation of the trend: among 0- to 17-year-olds, asthma increased from 3.1 percent to 4.3 percent (Weitzman et al, 1992).

Morbidity and Mortality

HOSPITALIZATION. In the United States in 1990, approximately 476,000 persons were discharged from the hospital with asthma as their first-listed diagnosis (Graves, 1992). Of these, 40 percent were male; 36 percent were less than 15 years old; and 21 percent were 65 years old or older. From 1979 to 1987, asthma hospitalizations increased 4.5 percent per year among 0- to 17-year-olds. Infants and children up to the age of 4 years had the greatest increase (Gergen and Weiss, 1990). Also, the rate of increase was 1.8 times higher for African-American children than for white children.

POVERTY. Poverty is a factor in differences in hospitalization rates. For example, in Maryland, Wissow et al (1988) found that an excess of asthma hospitalizations among African-Americans might be virtually eliminated by adjusting for poverty.

DEATH. Although relatively few people die from asthma, the death rate is increasing. Weiss and Wagener (1990) reported that asthma deaths among 5- to 34-year-olds increased by 6.2 percent annually during the 1980s. In 1989, there were 4869 asthma deaths in the United States. This represents a death rate of two per 100,000 population. The death rate for African-Americans was nearly twice as high as that for whites: 3.2 versus 1.8 per 100,000. Death rates are also disproportionately high for urban dwellers and those with lower SES (Evans et al, 1987; Weiss and Wagener, 1990).

Strunk et al (1985) identified a variety of individual risk factors that may place an asthmatic at high risk for death. These include: a history of severe disease, lack of access to care, suboptimal pharmacotherapy, depression, and family disturbances.

Allergy and Asthma

Allergy plays an important role in asthma. Asthmatics tend to be more atopic and thus have more allergen skin-test reactivity, allergic rhinitis, and atopic dermatitis than nonasthmatics. In all age groups, asthma increases with increasing IgE levels and/or skin-test reactivity (Sears et al, 1991; Burrows et al, 1989; Gergen and Turkeltaub, 1991). Zimmerman et al (1988) found that atopic children had more severe asthma, but Inouye et al (1985) did not find increased severity of disease among atopic adults. Murray et al (1990), Jonsson et al (1987), and many others have noted an association between eczema and both the development and persistence of asthma.

Asthma often clusters in families, but the precise genetic basis for asthma is still unknown. Parents of asthmatic children are three times more likely to also have asthma than are parents of nonasthmatic children (Sibbald et al, 1980). This family clustering remains after asthmatics are divided into extrinsic and intrinsic groups based on allergen skin-test reactivity. Asthma is more common among the siblings of both extrinsic and intrinsic asthmatics than among controls (Pirson et al, 1991).

Asthma Triggers

ALLERGENS. Allergens that are known to trigger asthma symptoms include house dust mite, alternaria, cockroach, cat dander, and ragweed and rye grass pollens. Prolonged exposure to many of these may be a risk factor for the development of asthma (see Chapters 7 and 8). Higher levels of exposure to house dust mite in infancy may play a role in earlier onset of asthma (Sporik et al, 1990). Tobacco smoke is a well-recognized respiratory irritant, and there are many studies that corroborate its adverse effects in the development and exacerbation of asthma symptoms. For example, Martinez et al (1992) found that children of mothers with high school educations or less who smoked 10 or more cigarettes per day had a 2.5 times increased risk of developing asthma before they were 12 years old. This relationship was absent when mothers had higher educational levels, however.

POLLUTION. Pollution may be a factor in the aggravation of asthma. Pope (1989) implicated fine particulate pollution as a cause for increased hospitalizations for asthma and bronchitis. Bronchial reactivity may be increased by a variety of different pollutants, such as sulfur dioxide and ozone (Pierson et al, 1984).

VIRAL AGENTS. More often in children than in adults, viral agents are associated with exacerbations of asthma. The viral agents implicated include respiratory syncytial virus, parainfluenza, and rhinoviruses (Busse, 1990). Most authorities discount a connection between bacterial infections and asthma. However, coexisting sinusitis makes asthma difficult to control until the sinusitis is adequately treated (Rachelefsky and Spector, 1990).

SUMMARY

Allergic diseases are multifactorial and complex. They are linked together by a perplexing combination of hereditary and environmental factors. Unraveling the relationship would be difficult at best, but the problem is compounded by a lack of universally accepted definitions, diagnostic criteria, and study methodology. At present, we cannot accurately determine the relative importance of genetic and environmental influences, but genetic factors may be more important in determining the overall risk of developing allergy. Environmental factors then may determine the specific allergens to which a person will develop sensitivity. We do know with some certainty, however, that (1) atopy, i.e., the propensity to develop IgE antibody, places a person at greater risk of developing an allergic disease; (2) people with one allergic disease are more likely to have another; and (3) environmental exposure to allergens in risk-prone individuals increases the likelihood of their developing allergic disease.

REFERENCES

Åberg N, Engstrom I. Natural history of allergic disease in children. Acta Paediatr Scand 79:206–211, 1990.

Adams PF, Benson V. Current estimates from the National Health Interview Survey, 1990. National Center for Health Statistics. Vital Health Stat 10(181), 1991.

Adkinson NF Jr. Risk factors for drug allergy. J Allergy Clin Immunol 74:567–572, 1984.

Anderson JA, Adkinson NF Jr. Allergic reactions to drugs and biologic agents. JAMA 258:2891–2899, 1987.

Barbee RA, Kaltenborn W, Lebowitz MD, et al. Longitudinal changes in allergen skin test reactivity in a community population sample. J Allergy Clin Immunol 79:16–24, 1987.

Bock SA. Natural history of severe reactions to foods in young children. J Pediatr 107:676–680, 1985.

Bock SA. Prospective appraisal of complaints of adverse reactions to foods in children during the first 3 years of life. Pediatrics 79:683–688, 1987.

Broder I, Higgins MN, Matthews KP, et al. The epidemiology of asthma and hayfever in a total community, Tecumseh, Michigan. IV. Natural history. J Allergy Clin Immunology 54:10, 1974.

Burr ML, Butland BK, King S, Vaughan-Williams E. Changes in asthma prevalence: two surveys 15 years apart. Arch Dis Child 64:1452–1456, 1989.

Burrows B, Martinez FD, Halonen M, et al. Association of asthma with serum IgE levels and skin-test reactivity to allergens. N Engl J Med 320:271–277, 1989.

Busse WW. Respiratory infections: Their role in airway responsiveness and the pathogenesis of asthma. J Allergy Clin Immunol 85:671–683, 1990.

Carter-Pokras OD, Gergen PJ. Reported asthma among Puerto Rican, Mexican-American, and Cuban-American children: 1982 through 1984. Am J Public Health 83:580–582, 1993.

Collins JG. Prevalence of selected chronic conditions, United States, 1979–1981. Vital Health Stat 10(155), 1986.

Evans R III, Mullally DI, Wilson RW, et al. National trends in the morbidity and mortality of asthma in the US. Prevalence, hospitalization and death from asthma over two decades: 1965–1984. Chest 91:65S–74S, 1987.

Fergusson DM, Horwood LJ, Shannon FT. Risk factors in childhood eczema. J Epidemiol Community Health 36:118–122, 1982.

Fleming DM, Crombie DL. Prevalence of asthma and hay fever in England and Wales. Br Med J 294:279–283, 1987.

Freidhoff LR, Meyers DA, Bias WB, et al. A genetic-epidemiologic study of human immune responsiveness to allergens in an industrial population. I. Epidemiology of reported allergy and skin-test positivity. Am J Med Genet 9:323–340, 1981.

Gergen PJ, Mullally DI, Evans R III. National survey of prevalence of asthma among children in the United States, 1976 to 1980. Pediatrics 81:1–7, 1988.

Gergen PJ, Turkeltaub PC. The association of allergen skin test reactivity and respiratory disease among whites in the U.S. population: Data from the second National Health and Nutrition Examination Survey 1976 to 1980. Arch Intern Med 151:487–492, 1991.

Gergen PJ, Turkeltaub PC, Kovar MG. The prevalence of allergic skin test reactivity to eight common aeroallergens in the U.S. population: Results from the second National Health and Nutrition Examination Survey. J Allergy Clin Immunol 80:669–679, 1987.

Gergen PJ, Weiss KB. Changing patterns of asthma hospitalization among children: 1979 to 1987. JAMA 264:1688–1692, 1990.

Golden DBK, Marsh DG, Kagey-Sobotka A, et al. Epidemiology of insect venom sensitivity. JAMA 262:240–244, 1989.

Golding J, Peters TJ. The epidemiology of childhood eczema: I. A population based study of associations. Paediatr Perinat Epidemiol 1:67–79, 1987.

Graves EJ. Detailed diagnoses and procedures, National Hospital Discharge Survey, 1990. National Center for Health Statistics. Vital Health Stat 13(113), 1992.

Høst A, Halken S. A prospective study of cow milk allergy in Danish infants during the first 3 years of life. Allergy 45:587–596, 1990.

Inouye T, Tarlo S, Broder I, et al. Severity of asthma in skin test-negative and skin test-positive patients. J Allergy Clin Immunol 75:313–319, 1985.

International Rheumatic Fever Study Group. Allergic reactions to long-term benzathine penicillin prophylaxis for rheumatic fever. Lancet 337:1308–1310, 1991.

Jonsson JA, Boe J, Berlin E. The long-term prognosis of childhood asthma in a predominantly rural Swedish county. Acta Paediatr Scand 76:950–954, 1987.

Kramer MS, Moroz B. Do breast-feeding and delayed introduction of solid foods protect against subsequent atopic eczema? J Pediatr 98:546–550, 1981.

Martinez FD, Cline M, Burrows B. Increased incidence of asthma in children of smoking mothers. Pediatrics 89:21–26, 1992.

McKnee WD. The incidence and familial occurrence of allergy. J Allergy 38:226, 1966.

Murray AB, Morrison BJ. It is children with atopic dermatitis who develop asthma more frequently if the mother smokes. J Allergy Clin Immunol 86:732–739, 1990.

National Center for Health Statistics. Vital Statistics of the United States, 1989, vol II, mortality, parts A and B. Washington, D.C. Public Health Service, 1994.

Ninan TK, Russell G. Respiratory symptoms and atopy in Aberdeen schoolchildren: evidence from two surveys 25 years apart. Br Med J 304:873–875, 1992.

Pierson WE, Covert DS, Koenig JQ. Air pollutants, bronchial hyperreactivity, and exercise. J Allergy Clin Immunol 73:717–721, 1984.

Pirson F, Charpin D, Sansonetti M, et al. Is intrinsic asthma a heredity disease? Allergy 46:367–371, 1991.

Pope CA III. Respiratory disease associated with community air pollution and a steel mill, Utah valley. Am J Public Health 79:623–628, 1989.

Queille-Roussel C, Raynaud F, Saurat J-H. A prospective computerized study of 500 cases of atopic dermatitis in childhood. I. Initial analysis of 250 parameters. Acta Derm Venereol (Stockh) 114:87–92, 1985.

Rachelefsky GS, Spector SL. Sinusitis and asthma. J Asthma 27:1–3, 1990.

Saarinan UM. Prophylaxis for atopic disease: Role of infant feeding. Clin Rev Allergy 2:151–167, 1984.

Sampson HA, Albergo R. Comparison of results of skin tests, RAST, and double-blind, placebo-controlled food challenges in children with atopic dermatitis. J Allergy Clin Immunol 74:26–33, 1984.

Sampson HA, Mendelson L, Rosen JP. Fatal and near-fatal anaphylactic reactions to food in children and adolescents. N Engl J Med 327:380–384, 1992.

Sampson HA, Scanlon SM. Natural history of food hypersensitivity in children with atopic dermatitis. J Pediatr 115:23–27, 1989.

Schwartz J, Gold D, Dockery DW, et al. Predictors of asthma and persistent wheeze in a national sample of children in the United States. Association with social class, perinatal events, and race. Am Rev Respir Dis 142:555–562, 1990.

Sears MR, Burrows B, Flannery EM, et al. Relation between airway responsiveness and serum IgE in children with asthma and in apparently normal children. N Engl J Med 325:1067–1071, 1991.

Settipane GA, Boyd GK. Natural history of insect sting allergy: The Rhode Island experience. Allergy Proc 10(2):109–113, 1989.

Sheffer AL. Guidelines for the diagnosis and management of asthma. National Heart, Lung, and Blood Institute National Asthma Education Program Expert Panel Report. J Allergy Clin Immunol 88:425–534, 1991.

Sibbald B, Horn MEC, Brain EA, et al. Genetic factors in childhood asthma. Thorax 35:671–674, 1980.

Smith LJ, Slavin RG. Etiologic and pathogenetic factors in allergic diseases. In Bierman CW, Pearlman DS (eds). Allergic Diseases from Infancy to Adulthood. 2nd ed. Philadelphia, WB Saunders Co, 1988, p 128.

Sporik R, Holgate ST, Platts-Mills TAE, et al. Exposure to house-dust mite allergen (Der P I) and the development of asthma in childhood. N Engl J Med 323:502–507, 1990.

Strunk RC, Mrazek DA, Wolfson-Fuhrmann GS, et al. Physiologic and psychological characteristics associated with deaths due to asthma in childhood. A case-controlled study. JAMA 254:1193–1198, 1985.

Taylor B, Wadsworth J, Wadsworth M, et al. Changes in the reported prevalence of childhood eczema since the 1939–1945 war. Lancet ii:1255–1257, 1984.

Turkeltaub PC, Gergen PJ. Prevalence of upper and lower respiratory conditions in the U.S. population by social and environmental factors: Data from the second National Health and Nutrition Examination Survey, 1976–80 (NHANES II). Ann Allergy 67:147–154, 1991.

Valentine MD, Schuberth KC, Kagey-Sobotka A, et al. The value of immunotherapy with venom in children with allergy to insect stings. N Engl J Med 323:1601–1603, 1990.

Van Asperen PP, Kemp AS, Mellis CM. Relationship of diet in the development of atopy in infancy. Clin Allergy 14:525–532, 1984.

Weiss KB, Gergen PJ, Hodgson TA. An economic evaluation of asthma in the United States. N Engl J Med 326:862–866, 1992.

Weiss KB, Wagener DK. Changing patterns of asthma mortality. Identifying target populations at high risk. JAMA 264:1683–1687, 1990.

Weitzman M, Gortmaker S, Sobol A. Racial, social, and environmental risk factors for childhood asthma. Am J Dis Child 144:1189–1194, 1990.

Weitzman M, Gortmaker SL, Sobol AM, et al. Recent trends in the prevalence and severity of childhood asthma. JAMA 268:2673–2677, 1992.

Wissow LS, Gittelsohn AM, Szklo M, et al. Poverty, race, and hospitalization for childhood asthma. Am J Public Health 78:777–782, 1988.

Yunginger JW, Reed CE, O'Connell EJ, et al. A community-based study of the epidemiology of asthma. I. Incidence rates, 1964–84. Am Rev Respir Dis 146:888–894, 1992.

Zimmerman B, Feanny S, Reisman J, et al. Allergy in asthma. I. The dose relationship of allergy to severity of childhood asthma. J Allergy Clin Immunol 81:63–70, 1988.

Chapter 6
Biology of Allergens

John W. Yunginger, M.D.

Allergens are macromolecular compounds, usually proteins or glycoproteins but occasionally polysaccharides, that are capable of inducing human IgE antibody responses. Haptens are low-molecular-weight materials that by themselves are incapable of inducing a human IgE antibody response, but when combined with host proteins can become immunogenic; an example would be penicillin. Sensitized persons usually recognize more than one allergen from a particular source. For a given allergen source, "major" allergens are those recognized by over half of the individuals allergic to that source, whereas "minor" allergens are recognized by fewer sensitized individuals. Although in theory any foreign protein has the potential to be an allergen, relatively few major pollen, dust mite, insect venom, and animal dander allergens have been isolated, purified to homogeneity, and characterized thoroughly.

FACTORS INFLUENCING ALLERGENICITY

Although most major allergens have molecular weights between 10 and 70 kD, there are no unique physicochemical properties that determine whether a particular compound is allergenic. For a compound to be allergenic, it must gain access to the body's immune system by absorption or injection, be soluble in body fluids, be relatively stable in solution, and be recognized as foreign by the immune system (Holgate and Church, 1993).

Host factors are also important determinants of allergenicity. After an allergen gains access to the body's immune system, it undergoes endocytosis and processing by antigen-presenting cells (APC) such as macrophages (Fig. 6–1) (Holgate and Church, 1993). During processing, the allergen is broken down into small peptides; a region on the peptide (agretope) binds to a hypervariable β1 portion (desetope) of newly synthesized human leukocyte antigen (HLA) class II molecules (Inanue and Allen, 1987). The allergen peptide-HLA-II complex is then transported across the cytoplasm and inserted into the APC membrane, where the "free" side of the allergen peptide (epitope) is subsequently bound to a specific portion (paratope) of the T cell receptor on $CD4^+$ T lymphocytes, leading to lymphokine-mediated clonal expansion of the T cells involved. These allergen-specific $CD4^+$ T cell clones produce high levels of IL-4 and IL-5, produce low levels of IFN-γ (Wierenga et al, 1990), and induce IgE synthesis (Parronchi et al, 1991).

Because allelic HLA molecules have different tertiary structures, APC of different HLA phenotypes utilize different desetopes for binding allergens and orient the allergen peptide differently on their cell surfaces (Schwartz, 1985). The orientation differences, in turn, control which epitopes are available for interaction with T cells. For example, the capacity to produce IgE antibodies to certain grass pollen allergens is associated with the HLA haplotypes DR3/Dw3 and B8 (Ansari et al, 1987, 1989; Freidhoff et al, 1988).

ALLERGEN NOMENCLATURE

The Allergen Nomenclature Subcommittee of the International Union of Immunological Societies has introduced a system for the consistent naming of purified allergens (Marsh et al, 1986). Under this system, an allergen is designated by the first three letters of the

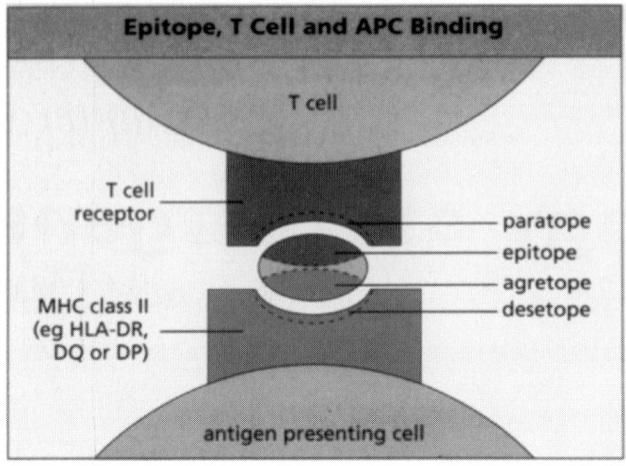

FIGURE 6–1. Interaction between epitope, T cell, and antigen-presenting cell (APC) prior to antibody production. (From Holgate ST, Church MK. Allergens. *In* Holgate ST, Church MK (eds). Allergy. New York, Raven Press Ltd, 1993.)

source genus and the first letter of the species (both italicized), followed by a Roman numeral. Major allergens from the source genus are prioritized to receive lower Roman numerals. Examples would be *Amb a* I from short ragweed pollen *(Ambrosia artemisiaefolia)* and *Der p* I from house dust mite *(Dermatophagoides pteronyssinus)*. Structurally homologous (but not necessarily cross-reactive) components from different species are assigned the same numbers; thus, the *Der p* I-homologous allergen from the house dust mite *Dermatophagoides farinae* is designated *Der f* I. Homologous, closely related components within the same species (isoallergens) are designated by capital letter suffixes in order of decreasing pI. Examples would be short ragweed allergens *Amb a* VA (pI 9.6) and *Amb a* VB (pI 8.5).

ALLERGEN ISOLATION AND CHARACTERIZATION

Allergen isolation and characterization are usually performed by the use of aqueous extracts of source pollens, fungi, mites, foods, and animal pelts or danders. These extracts are complex mixtures of proteins, carbohydrates, enzymes, and pigments, only a portion of which are allergenic. *In vitro* techniques have largely supplanted skin testing as a means of measuring the total allergenicity of an allergenic extract, demonstrating which components of an allergenic extract are allergens, or quantitating individual allergens.

INHIBITION IMMUNOASSAYS

A variety of solid-phase immunoassays are available for measurement of allergen-specific IgE antibodies in sera from individuals suspected of being allergic to that allergen. These assays can be adapted into inhibition immunoassays for quantitation of total allergen (Gleich et al, 1974). To the solid-phase allergen are added fixed quantities of pooled IgE antibody-containing sera from several individuals allergic to the allergen in question, along with varying quantities of either the test extracts or a standard extract of defined allergen content. After incubation, the solid-phase allergen is washed; then radiolabeled or enzyme-labeled anti-human IgE is added. With addition of increasing amounts of fluid-phase allergen in the first stage of the assay, less IgE antibody is available to react with the solid-phase allergen. Dose response inhibition curves can thus be constructed from the test extracts and compared to the dose response inhibition curve of the standard extract.

IMMUNOBLOTTING

When allergenic extracts are separated by polyacrylamide gel electrophoresis (PAGE) in the presence of sodium dodecylsulfate (SDS), the various components migrate in relation to their apparent molecular weight (Weber and Osborn, 1969). Thin-layer isoelectrofocusing (TLIEF) is a related technique in which the components in an allergenic extract are separated according to their isoelectric points (Varga and Ceska, 1972). For immunoblotting, the components of an allergenic extract that have been separated by SDS-PAGE or TLIEF are transferred passively or electrophoretically to nitrocellulose papers, which are subsequently reacted with IgE antibody-containing sera and radiolabeled or enzyme-labeled anti-human IgE to produce autoradiographs or colored banding patterns (Stott, 1989). Only the allergenic (IgE-binding) components of the extract produce visible bands. When performed in this fashion, immunoblotting provides physicochemical data (molecular weights, isoelectric points) on the individual allergens in a crude allergen extract.

IMMUNOELECTROPHORESIS

In crossed immunoelectrophoresis (CIE) the components of the allergenic extract are separated by gel electrophoresis in one direction. The gel is then rotated 90 degrees, and electrophoresis is performed in the second direction into a gel containing rabbit antiserum to the allergen in question (Lowenstein, 1978). The gel containing the precipitin arcs is then reacted sequentially with human IgE antibodies and radiolabeled anti-human IgE, as in the immunoblotting technique described previously, to produce crossed radioimmunoelectrophoresis (CRIE) autoradiographs.

ALLERGEN CLONING

Allergens may also be isolated by recombinant DNA technology (Holgate and Church, 1993). In this technique, messenger RNA is isolated from the allergen source, and complementary DNA prepared by transcribing the RNA using the enzyme reverse transcriptase. The single-stranded copy DNA (cDNA) produced is then converted into double-stranded DNA with the enzyme DNA polymerase and the resulting material inserted into appropriate vectors, such as plasmids, using restriction endonucleases, and cloned. The array of cDNA reflecting the starting RNA represents the library which is then screened to isolate the cDNA coding for the allergens of interest. Screening may be accomplished by hybridization using oligonucleotide probes synthesized on the basis of amino acid sequences obtained by conventional protein sequencing of known allergens or by using sera from allergic individuals. The latter technique is used when direct information of the allergens is unavailable, and use is made of vectors, termed expression vectors, which direct the synthesis of the allergen. The protein produced is detected using anti-IgE reagents as described previously for immunoblotting.

QUANTITATION OF INDIVIDUAL ALLERGENS

In cases where individual allergens have been isolated or cloned, antibodies may be raised to the allergens, permitting subsequent allergen quantitation by immunoassay. Polyclonal antibody-based immunoassays have been used to quantitate major ragweed (*Amb a* I) and cat (*Fel d* I) allergens by single radial immunodiffusion (Mancini et al, 1965). Monoclonal antibody–based assays have also been reported for quantitation of a variety of purified allergens.

MONITORING ALLERGEN EXPOSURE

Exposure to outdoor allergens has traditionally been estimated by use of a variety of air samplers to entrap airborne particulates. Following this, pollen grains and fungal spores are counted by light microscopy. Accurate recognition of these particles requires skill; several reference works are available to assist with the identification (Lewis et al, 1983; Platts-Mills and Solomon, 1993). Viable fungal spores may also be quantitated using a multistage sequential sieve impinger sampler with culture plates positioned beneath each stage.

Exposure to indoor allergens is assessed with greater difficulty. Animal danders and arthropod emanations are amorphous and lack identifiable units. These allergens may be measured immunochemically, however (Swanson et al, 1985). Personal breathing zone air samplers and high-volume area samplers are used to entrap airborne particulates onto filters; eluates from these filters can then be tested for allergen content by the immunoassay techniques described previously. Immunochemical analysis of reservoir household dust also provides an estimate of allergen exposure. For example, the *Der p* I content of household dust has been used to define threshold levels for sensitization to house dust mites (Platts-Mills et al, 1987).

REFERENCES

Ansari AA, Kihara TK, Marsh DG. Immunochemical studies of *Lolium perenne* (rye grass) pollen allergens *Lol p* I, II, and III. J Immunol 139:4034, 1987.

Ansari AA, Shenbagamurthi P, Marsh DG. Complete amino acid sequence of a *Lolium perenne* (perennial rye grass) pollen allergen, *Lol p* II. J Biol Chem 264:11181, 1989.

Freidhoff LR, Ehrlich-Kautzky E, Meyers DA, et al. Association of HLA-DR3 with human immune response to *Lol p* I and *Lol p* II allergens in allergic subjects. Tissue Antigens 31:211, 1988.

Gleich GJ, Larson JB, Jones RT, et al. Measurement of the potency of allergy extracts by their inhibitory capacities in the radioallergosorbent test. J Allergy Clin Immunol 53:158, 1974.

Holgate ST, Church MK. Allergens. *In* Holgate ST, Church MK (eds). Allergy. New York, Raven Press Ltd, 1993, p 1.

Lewis WH, Vinay P, Zenger VE. Airborne and Allergenic Pollen of North America. Baltimore, The Johns Hopkins University Press, 1983.

Løwenstein H. Quantitative immunoelectrophoretic methods as a tool for the analysis and isolation of allergens. Progr Allergy 25:1, 1978.

Mancini G, Carbonara AO, Heremans JF. Immunochemical quantitation of antigens by single radial immunodiffusion. Immunochemistry 2:235, 1965.

Marsh DG, Goodfriend L, King TP, et al. Allergen nomenclature. Bull WHO 64:767, 1986.

Parronchi P, Macchia D, Piccinni M-P, et al. Allergen- and bacterial antigen-specific T-cell clones established from atopic donors show a different profile of cytokine production. Proc Natl Acad Sci USA 88:4538, 1991.

Platts-Mills TAE, Hayden ML, Chapman MD, et al. Seasonal variation in dust mite and grass-pollen allergens in dust from the houses of patients with asthma. J Allergy Clin Immunol 79:781, 1987.

Platts-Mills TAE, Solomon WR. Aerobiology and inhalant allergens. *In* Middleton E Jr, Reed CE, Ellis EF, et al (eds). Allergy Principles and Practice. 4th ed. St. Louis, Mosby–Year Book Inc, 1993, Vol I, p 469.

Schwartz RH. T-lymphocyte recognition of antigen in association with gene products of the major histocompatibility complex. Ann Rev Immunol 3:237, 1985.

Stott DI. Immunoblotting and dot blotting. J Immunol Methods 119:153, 1989.

Swanson MC, Agarwal MK, Reed CE. An immunochemical approach to indoor aeroallergen quantitation with a new volumetric air sampler: Studies with mite, roach, cat, mouse, and guinea pig antigens. J Allergy Clin Immunol 76:724, 1985.

Unanue ER, Allen PM. The basis for the immunoregulatory role of macrophages and other accessory cells. Science 236:551, 1987.

Varga JM, Ceska M. Characterization of allergen extracts by gel isoelectrofocusing and radioimmunosorbent allergen assay. J Allergy Clin Immunol 49:274, 1972.

Weber K, Osborn M. The reliability of molecular weight determinations by dodecyl sulfate-polyacrylamide gel electrophoresis. J Biol Chem 244:4406, 1969.

Wierenga EA, Snoek M, de Groot C, et al. Evidence for compartmentalization of functional subsets of CD4+ T lymphocytes in atopic patients. J Immunol 144:4651, 1990.

Chapter 7

Common Allergenic Pollen and Fungi

William R. Solomon, M.D., Richard W. Weber, M.D., and William K. Dolen, M.D.

POLLEN AND SPORE PREVALENCE

The catalogs of allergen extract manufacturers list a wide range of pollens, fungi, and other substances available for diagnostic testing and specific immunotherapy. Extracts are commercially available for most recognized allergenic materials, although field collection and custom extraction of unusual agents are occasionally indicated. Since keeping every available extract in the office is impractical and testing every patient for every known allergenic substance is inappropriate, the practicing allergist must choose from the variety of available extracts.

It is not possible to devise a universal list of appropriate extracts for testing in all patients presenting with a given symptom complex. For pollens and, to a lesser extent, fungi, regional lists are available, but have generally been unsatisfactory because such lists are too broad for a given area in the region, or they are incomplete or inaccurate, or they fail to reflect *relative* prevalence. Generally, the range of pollen and fungal extracts stocked in the allergy office should reflect (1) results of local and regional botanical surveys conducted with a qualified botanist, (2) knowledge of locally and regionally indigenous allergenic plants, (3) recent aerobiologic data (pollen and fungi) obtained by a qualified local counting station, (4) surveys of fungi prevalent indoors, (5) knowledge of which plants are generally considered clinically significant for the region, and (6) insight into cross-reactivity patterns. Unfortunately, this information is incomplete for many areas, and one must often rely on the opinions and experiences of local colleagues in choosing extracts for clinical use.

For an individual patient, the choice of allergenic extracts for testing is guided primarily by the patient's history and physical examination, and will reflect the physician's knowledge, training, experience, and practice habits. Although exhaustive testing is occasionally indicated, indiscriminate testing is inconvenient to patients and office staff and is an unwise use of health care resources.

Aeroallergen Sampling: Uses and Limitations

Although it is generally assumed that there is a direct relationship between magnitude of pollen or fungal spore exposure and severity of allergic symptoms, neither threshold levels nor dose-response effects have been thoroughly explored. In fact, certain pollens (e.g., pine) are produced in huge quantities but cause little if any symptoms in most individuals with respiratory allergy. British workers have observed that grass pollen-sensitive patients, with few exceptions, develop symptoms when mean 24-hour airborne levels reach 20 grains/m^3. Comparable data for other pollens and fungal spores are not available, although for ragweed a modal value of about 100 grains/m^3 (with considerable intersubject variation in threshold) might be anticipated. In addition, the nasal response appears to be related to total recent allergen exposure as well as to ongoing challenge levels of specific pollen. Previous exposure to sensitizers appears to "prime" the nasal mucosa to react at lower levels of the same or an unrelated pollen allergen (Connell, 1969). Further, there are differences between pollen data obtained at rooftop level (where aeroallergen collection stations are usually located) and ground level (where patients are) and from place to place within a community. For these reasons, the value of "pollen and spore counts" in predicting severity of symptoms is limited, especially when counts are derived from gravity samplers. Optimally performed sampling at a central "station" reveals major aeroallergens generally present in the air but will not reflect true personal levels of exposure, which may differ sharply.

Despite these reservations, aeroallergen data provide, at the least, a qualitative view of exposure for correlation retrospectively with clinical events. Annual dates of pollen and fungal spore appearance and disappearance may be estimated and peak periods identified. For relatively abundant pollens and larger fungus spores, even gravity slides allow prevalence trends to be identified, although their correlative value is limited.

In many areas, pollen and fungal spore counts based on gravity slide data often are announced by news media to an eager public. Unfortunately, the limitations of these data are mentioned only rarely, and patients often are perplexed by apparent discrepancies between their symptoms and published exposure levels. In general, such reports, describing periods one or more days previously, are no more informative than trends derived from several previous pollen seasons. Moreover, patients often are needlessly distressed by minor day-to-day variation in published data, viewing these as predictors of serious discomfort. Physicians should recognize these misunderstandings about the significance of aeroallergen sampling and should try to educate their patients accordingly.

Methods for Aeroallergen Sampling

"GRAVITY" SLIDES AND PLATES. Atmospheric variables that affect particle prevalence also can modify the behavior of pollens and fungal spores with respect to sampling devices. These effects are most troublesome with traditional "fallout" techniques using greased microscope slides (Ogden et al, 1974) or open plates of culture medium. Horizontal surfaces will collect particles, and pollen data have been gathered in this way for decades. In practice, an adhesive-coated, 1- by 3-inch glass slide is exposed for 24 hours in a housing of standard design (Durham, 1946). Particles are deposited from turbulent air flow and, following exposure, are identified microscopically by transmitted light. Data are expressed as "particles per unit area" (usually per cm^2) of slide surface. Viable recoveries have also been studied by substituting plates of nutrient agar in the standard housing (or Durham sampler) for periods of 12 to 60 minutes. Colonies are identified after incubation of the culture plate for 1 to 7 days.

Sampling by fallout is simple and requires inexpensive, readily available materials. Unfortunately, with gravitational techniques, the volume of air from which particles are recovered cannot be determined, adding uncertainty to comparisons of particle prevalence from different dates or locations. Recoveries by gravity slides (and plates) vary with wind speed, wind direction, and turbulence levels. Furthermore, collections are sparse for all but the most abundant pollens and spores, and larger particles are more likely to accumulate than smaller ones. For these reasons, gravitational techniques are useful in identifying prominent pollens qualitatively but do not yield reliable quantitative pollen concentrations.

VOLUMETRIC SAMPLERS. The term "volumetric" denotes the ability to relate recoveries to defined volumes of air; two types of mechanical samplers provide particle data in relation to such units (Fig. 7–1). These are (1) impactors, in which an adhesive-coated sampling surface is whirled in a circular path through particle-bearing air, and (2) suction samplers (spore traps), which aspirate air at fixed rates into flow channels with sharp bends. Particles with too much momentum to follow the angular path strike the walls at predictable points where sampling surfaces are positioned. Both types of devices provide quantitative data as "particles per unit volume of air." Popular impactors include the rotorod family of samplers, while the drum (Burkard) version of the Hirst spore trap is widely used. Suction devices that provide volume-related recoveries on agar media include several slit samplers and the Andersen ("stacked sieve") impinger (Solomon, 1984; Solomon and Platts-Mills, 1993).

FUNGAL CULTURES. Unlike pollens and many other allergenic substances, airborne

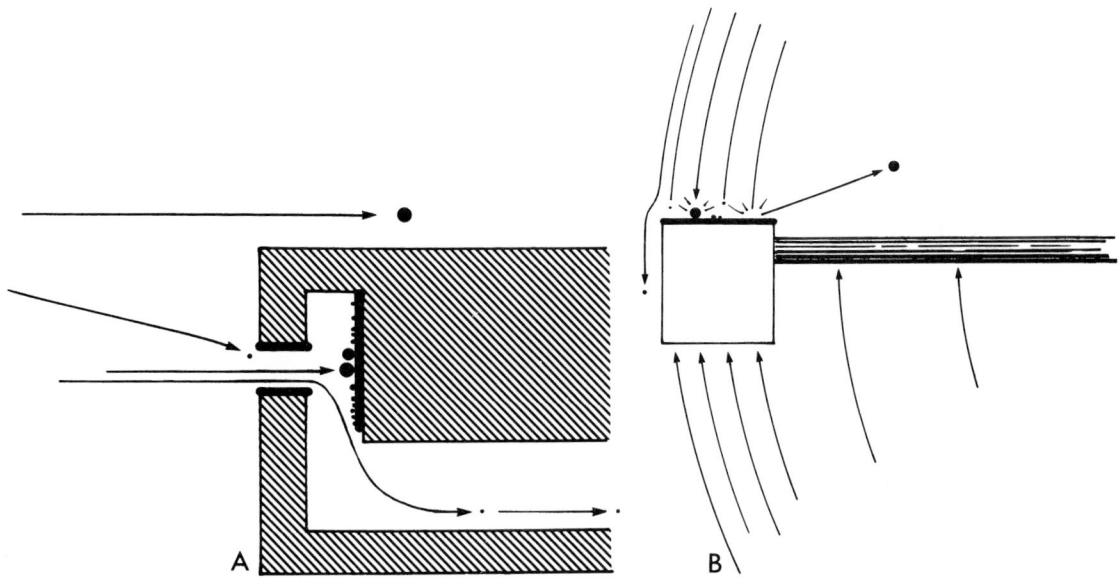

FIGURE 7–1. Collection principles employed by volumetric samplers. *A,* Suction traps (impingers) deposit particles at bends in their internal flow systems. These devices have especially high efficiency for small particles, which readily enter the traps from a moving air stream. *B,* Rotating arm impactors employ rapidly rotated, adhesive-coated, narrow surfaces to intercept particles. The efficiency of impaction varies predictably with increasing particle size. "Bounce-off" can occur, and its frequency defines the "adhesive efficiency" of the collecting surface.

fungi originate largely from inapparent, microscopic growth. Consequently, insight into exposure requires direct air sampling. Collection techniques must be carefully chosen to give a true picture of prevalence. Methods that rely upon growth formed on exposed agar media, for example, indicate the presence of only *viable* particles and exclude possibly significant fungal allergens that fail to grow recognizably. Selective recovery is a limitation common to all known media, although some (e.g., malt extract agar and Sabouraud glucose agar) are less restrictive than others. Prevalence data also are readily biased by collecting particles on greased slides or on open plates of growth media by fallout. Since variations in air speed, direction, and turbulence strongly affect such deposition and the volume of air contributing particles is unknown, resulting data cannot be readily compared sequentially or among sites. Furthermore, particle fallout on collection surfaces is proportional to particle diameter (or, more specifically, to diameter squared) so that larger particles will be overrepresented in collections (Fig. 7–2). Applications of techniques accurate for particles of diverse sizes have emphasized the true abundance of many ascospores and basidiospores as well as of small imperfect fungus spores, which were unnoticed previously (Gregory, 1973).

Growth on semisolid media is essential for determining numerous taxa (e.g., form species of *Penicillium* and *Aspergillus,* yeasts, and zygomycetes) with minute, nondescript, spheroidal spores. The interested reader is referred to the publication by von Arx (1981), which describes identification to genera, and also to Barron (1968), Barnett (1987), Ellis (1971), and Onions (1992) for technical advice on handling fungi in culture.

Recoveries as colonies on growth media considerably underestimate prevalence, as judged by spores in microscopic deposits collected simultaneously. In addition, it is clear that many airborne spore types—especially sexual spores of certain fleshy fungi—still cannot be identified to genus because they are neither distinctive in form nor capable of growing on available media.

Sampling indoor air with open culture dishes ("settling plates") has dubious value in evaluating patients with obscure symptoms. If this method is used, the physician must recognize its relative exclusion of smaller particles (Solomon, 1975), a special concern

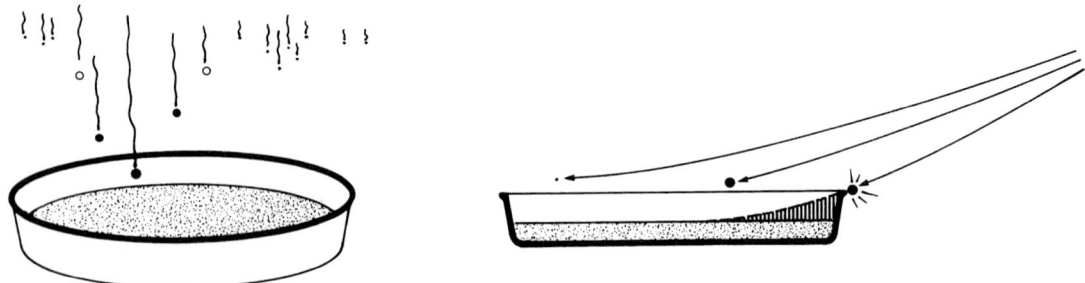

FIGURE 7–2. Problems in particle collection by open culture plates. At left, the markedly greater fallout of larger (than smaller) particles is emphasized using the (unnatural) example of still air. A similar effect is easily observed with normal atmospheric motion (right). Here again, recovery varies with particle size, and in rapidly moving air, deposition may be hindered by the protruding lip of the culture dish.

since small-spored fungi often predominate in indoor air.

ALLERGEN NOMENCLATURE

The term "allergen" here denotes a protein or glycoprotein that can induce a specific IgE response and react with the resulting antibody molecules. Allergenic extracts are complex mixtures of allergens as well as nonallergenic proteins and other substances. Recently, allergens of many plant and animal extracts have been identified and characterized at the molecular level; some (e.g., *Fel d* I, the major cat allergen) have been cloned, sequenced, and synthesized.

An allergen is designated as *major* if it is recognized by the antibodies of a majority of sensitized patients; *minor* allergens are those recognized by somewhat fewer individuals. It is important to note that a given pollen, for example, may contain several major allergens and that an *individual patient* may be sensitized *only* to a minor allergen. By international agreement, biogenic allergens are named using the first three letters of the source's genus name, the first letter of its species name, and a Roman numeral usually assigned in chronologic order of discovery.

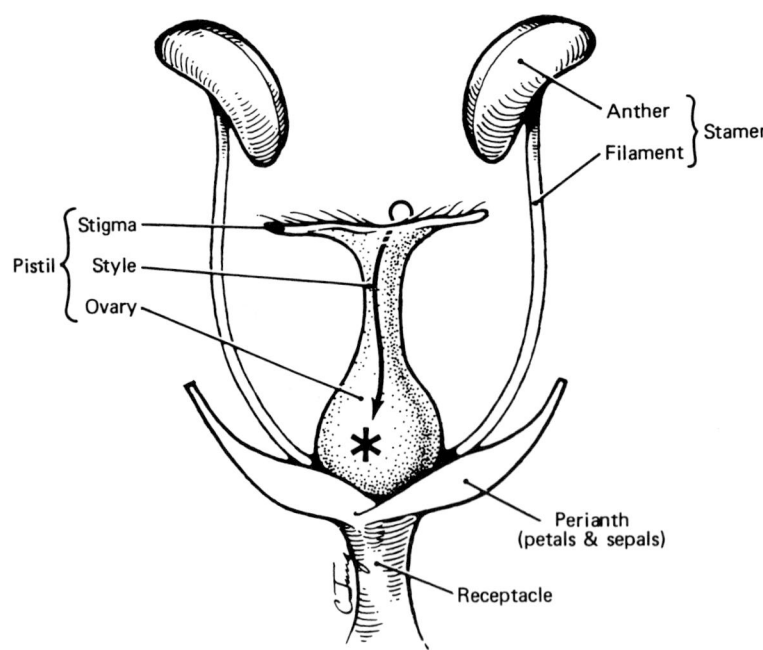

FIGURE 7–3. Structure of a wind-pollinated flower. Note the relatively large anthers, broad stigma, and reduced perianth; no nectaries are present. The arrow indicates the general path of pollen tube growth to effect fertilization (*). Having both male and female organs, this flower is "perfect."

Generally, but not always, lower numerals indicate more major allergens. Thus, a major allergen of Bermuda grass, *Cynodon dactylon*, is designated *Cyn d* I. Allergens generally contain several peptide epitopes capable of recognition by T cells as well as several epitopes recognized by IgE.

MAJOR ALLERGENIC POLLENS

Basic Characteristics of Pollens

POLLENS IN REPRODUCTIVE BIOLOGY. Pollen grains—common to all flowering plants—serve as vectors for male gametes or reproductive cells. Pollens develop in distinctive floral structures (Fig. 7–3), the *anther sacs*. One or more anther sacs with suitable protective coverings (i.e., the anthers) are usually borne on stalks or *filaments*, and termed *stamens*. The developmental phase in which flowers open and release mature pollen grains is called *anthesis*.

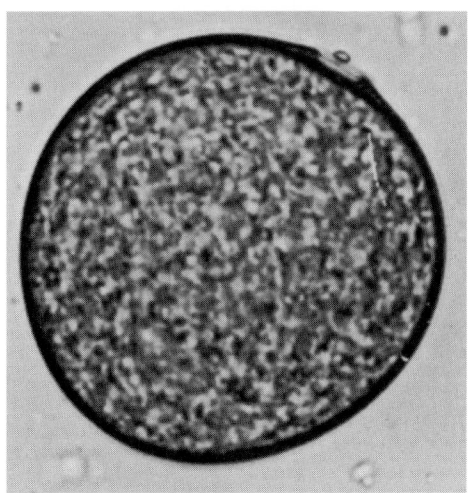

FIGURE 7–5. Pollen grain of a grass. The single pore, with its "operculum" of exine substance, is seen in side view and optical section.

In most flowering plants, pollination is effected by one or more animal vectors, generally insects. Such plants are termed "entemophilous." However, all of the grasses, and many of the trees and "weeds" disperse pollen in the wind, and are termed "anemophilous" (Fig. 7–4). In either case, the goal of pollen transport is of viable grains on a *stigma*, the terminal and most exposed part of the female *pistil*. After this is accomplished, both the pollen grain and the stigmatic surface release recognition substances, some of which (e.g., *Amb a* I of ragweed) are important human allergens. Pollen germination occurs following exchange of compatible chemical signals, and a tubular structure emerges from the grain, penetrates the stigma, and grows down through the subjacent *style*, finally reaching the ovary. Fertilization results in production of both an embryo and nutritive endosperm, the components of the future seed.

Fundamentals of Pollen Structure. Wind-borne pollen grains are usually spheroidal, with limited surface ornamentation, and 20 to 40 microns in size. The pollen wall is comprised of two main layers, the outer *exine* and the inner *intine* (Figs. 7–5, 7–6, and 7–7). The exine stains with basic fuchsin, while the intine does not. The exine is divided into the external *sexine*, which has numerous micropores and substructures, and the internal *nexine*. Most pollen grains have a variable number of apertures in the form of pores or furrows (or both) (Fig. 7–7). These provide access to the outside for substances (including

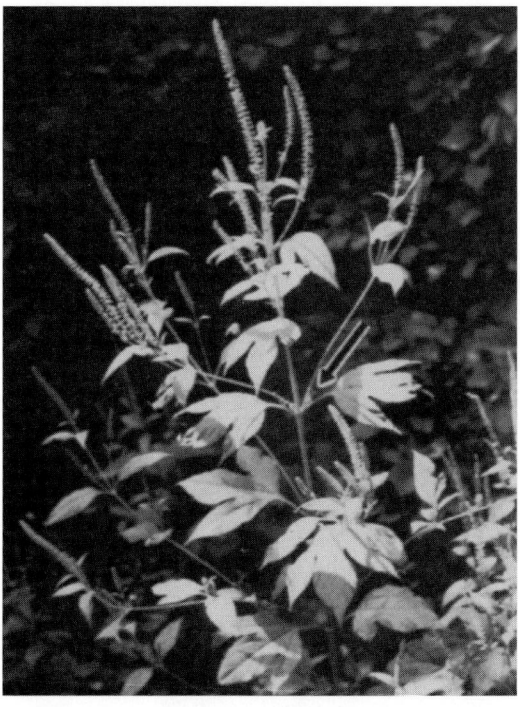

FIGURE 7–4. Giant ragweed, a highly successful wind-pollinated species. Male flowers are produced in crowded terminal spikes, whereas female flowers (arrow) are fewer and occupy the bases of the leaves. The three-lobed leaves are the basis of the Latin name of this plant, *Ambrosia trifida*.

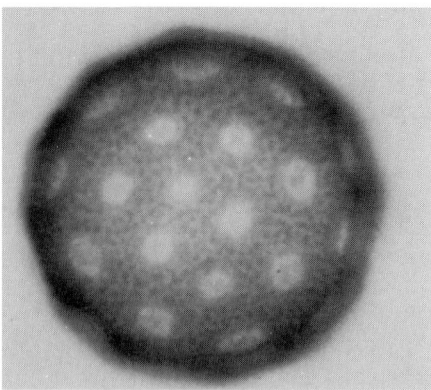

FIGURE 7-6. Pollen grain of lambs quarters, a chenopod. The "golf-ball" appearance, due to numerous regularly spaced pores, is typical of the chenopod-amaranths.

Pollen Sources and Similarities

Pollen sources have traditionally been segregated into grass, weed, and tree groups. While such a classification is easy to conceptualize, it tends to muddy botanical relationships: although grasses are fairly isolated in order and family, various plant families contain members that may be trees, shrubs, or annual weeds. The possible disparity between form and relationships may have a negative impact on understanding cross-reactivity, which furthermore may be important for clinical considerations such as skin test interpretation and allergen immunotherapy. Additionally, one assumes a set sequence of pollination that may not be correct: trees pollinate first, followed by grasses, then weeds. This is roughly true, but numerous trees pollinate in the autumn, and certain weeds in the early spring (Lewis et al, 1983). Despite these concerns, however, it remains easiest to group allergenic plants into these rough categories. Therefore, the following discussion, while organized into the grass, tree, and weed brackets, will nonetheless attempt to reenforce botanical taxonomic relationships. Exceptions to usual pollination patterns will be noted.

allergenic compounds) associated with the intine. Characteristics such as size, shape, and the number and nature of apertures generally allow the recognition of pollen types. Structural features do not usually permit identification at the species level but frequently do allow for genus recognition. Occasionally, grains may only be identifiable to the level of families or orders, as with the grasses or chenopod-amaranth group. Several illustrated references provide detailed information on pollen identification (Ogden et al, 1974; Lewis et al, 1983; Smith, 1984 and 1986).

The older taxonomies were based primarily on sometimes misleading morphologic similarities. Newer classifications, incorporating

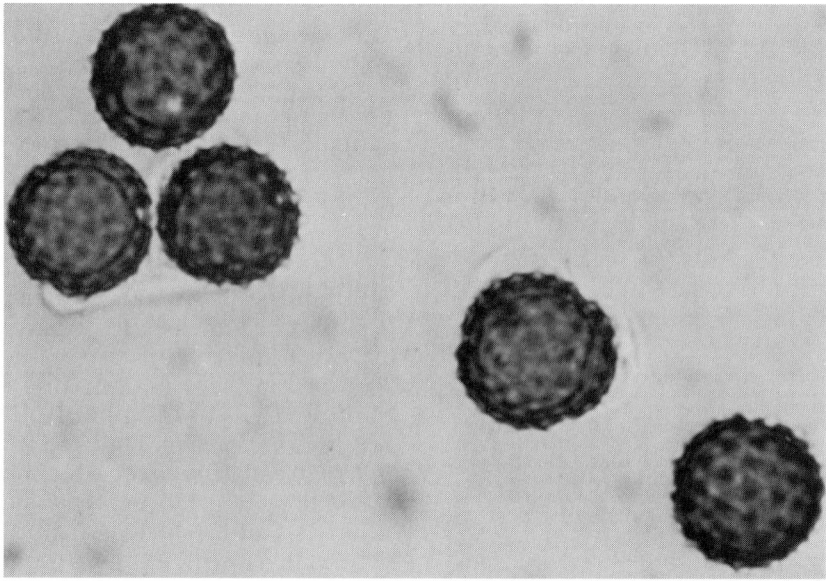

FIGURE 7-7. Short ragweed pollen stained with fuchsin. Spiny grains, each with three pores, are typical of ragweed and of many additional species in the aster family (also called Compositae). Several grains show intramural air spaces between the pores.

group shifts as well as the renaming of genus and species, have followed the development of techniques such as electron microscopy, chemical analyses, and gene sequencing (Gaut and Clegg, 1991). These methods have shed greater light on the probable phylogeny (Martin et al, 1993), the importance of which is that more closely related plants, evolving from more recent common ancestors, could be expected to contain similar allergenic proteins. More distantly related plants would be expected to share fewer proteins and hence demonstrate less cross-reactivity (Weber, 1981). The newer classification will primarily be used, with occasional reference to the older nomenclature for orientation. Botanical relationships of common inducers of pollinosis are depicted in Figures 7–8 through 7–10. There are still differing opinions on the appropriate classification of numerous plants; the taxonomy listed in the figures is that supported by cross-reactivity data and emphasizes relationships. The plant division Pinophyta (old classification Gymnospermae) encompasses the conifers (Fig. 7–8). The division Magnoliophyta (Angiospermae) contains the flowering plants. The class Liliopsida (Monocotyledonae) includes plants such as the grasses, palms, sedges, and rushes (Fig. 7–9). The class Magnoliopsida (Dicotyledonae) comprises the large remainder of a variety of flowering trees and weeds. Figure 7–10 illustrates members that have been incriminated in hayfever; it does not include the great number of other orders and families that are principally insect-pollinated and not factors in pollinosis.

Grasses and Allies

GRASSES. Poaceae (Graminae) is an exceedingly large botanical family. There are thousands of grasses, belonging to several subfamilies, in turn containing a number of tribes (delineated in Fig. 7–9), most of which have members incriminated in pollinosis. The most prominent is Pooideae (or Festucoideae), which includes the temperate climate pasture grasses and most of the cereal grains. Examples include perennial rye *(Lolium perenne)*, orchard *(Dactylis glomerata)*, meadow fescue *(Festuca elatior)*, smooth brome *(Bromus inermus)*, and timothy *(Phleum pratense)*. With only minor exceptions, members of the fescue subfamily strongly cross-react (Leiferman et al, 1976; Martin et al, 1985). Sweet vernal, *Anthoxanthum odoratum*, and timothy may

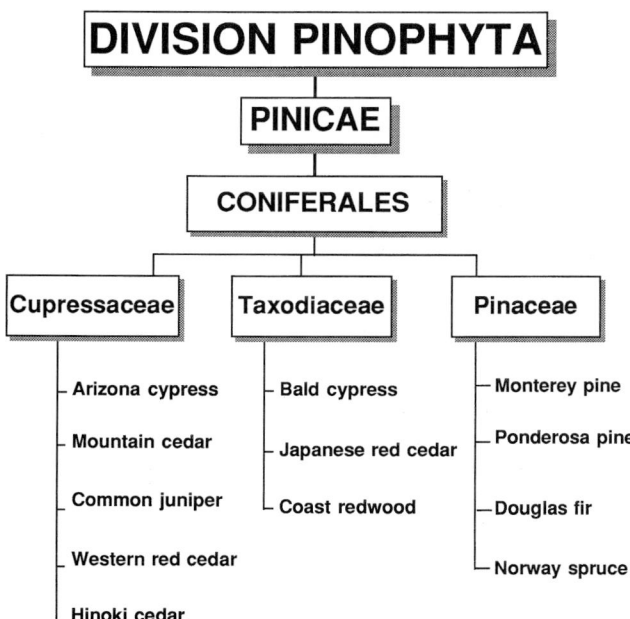

FIGURE 7–8. Taxonomy of representative allergenic trees of three families in the order Coniferales, subclass Pinicae, division Pinophyta. This botanical division has previously been named class Gymnospermae.

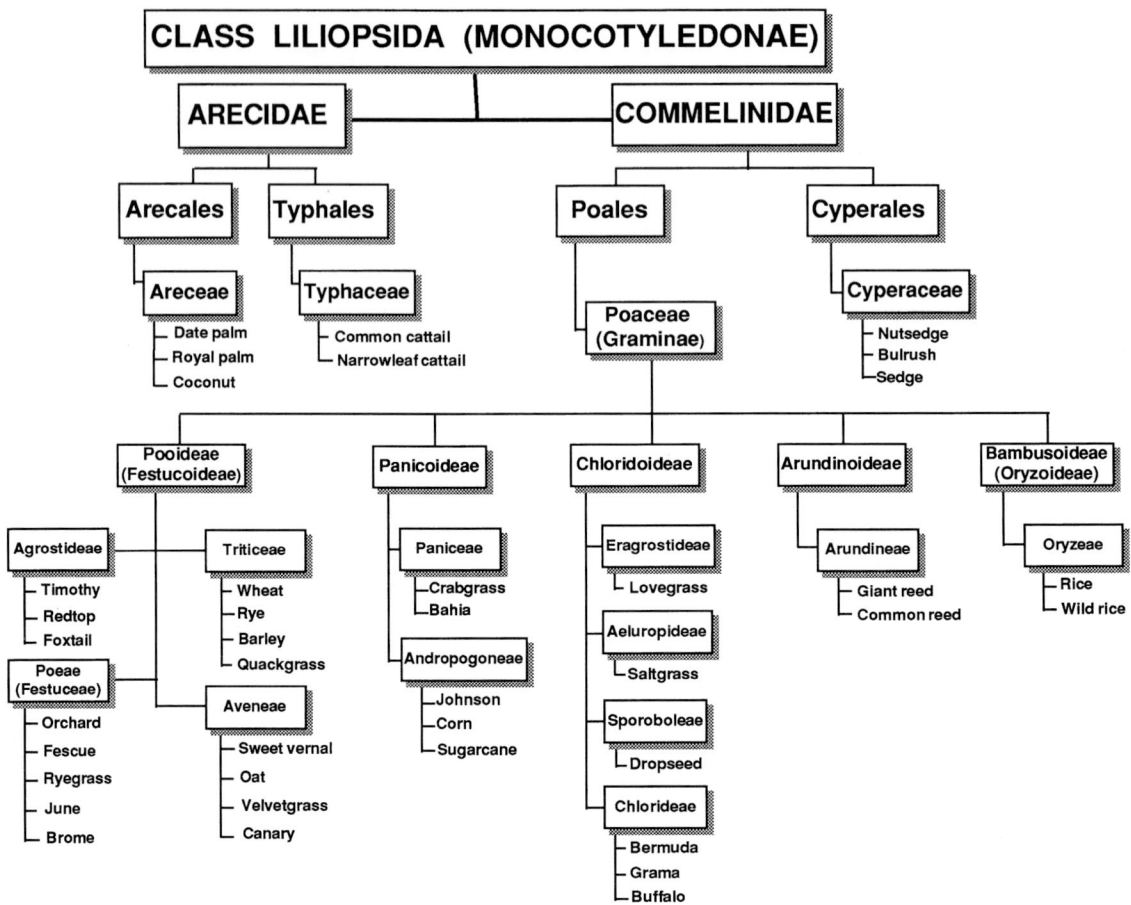

FIGURE 7–9. Taxonomy of representative allergenic members of the class Liliopsida, division Magnoliophyta, previously named subclass Monocotyledonae, class Angiospermae. The grass family, Poaceae, is divided into 5 subfamilies and 12 tribes.

each contain some unique allergens, although this is best substantiated for timothy.

A number of grass allergens have been characterized, with at least partial amino acid sequencing and cloning (Table 7–1). Four groups of perennial ryegrass allergens had been appreciated for a number of years, with group I being the most critical allergen. More recent work has demonstrated additional allergens, group V representing another major allergen. Although sequencing has demonstrated marked homology between a variety of species, this does not always equate with cross-reactivity as delineated by antibody-binding studies (Matthiesen and Løwenstein, 1991; Sivasubramanian et al, 1992).

Southern grasses show greater allergenic diversity. Bermuda *(Cynodon dactylon,* subfamily Eragrostoideae) is a potent sensitizer and is a prevalent grass in the southern states. It appears to contain unique allergens not shared with the fescue northern grasses, although it does demonstrate cross-inhibition of some prairie grasses such as grama *(Bouteloua gracilis)* and salt grass *(Distichlis stricta)* (Martin et al, 1985). The Panicoideae subfamily contains johnson grass *(Sorghum halepense),* bahia *(Paspalum notatum),* and corn *(Zea mays),* the first of moderate importance and the latter of no significance except perhaps for farmers. Cross-reactivity data on johnson grass is conflicting. Rice *(Oryza sativa,* subfamily Oryzoideae) is of minor importance in the United States as an allergen but apparently is a significant inducer of pollinosis in the far east. Very preliminary work with cattails and sedges has not revealed cross-reactivity with grasses.

Timing of grass pollination varies with the

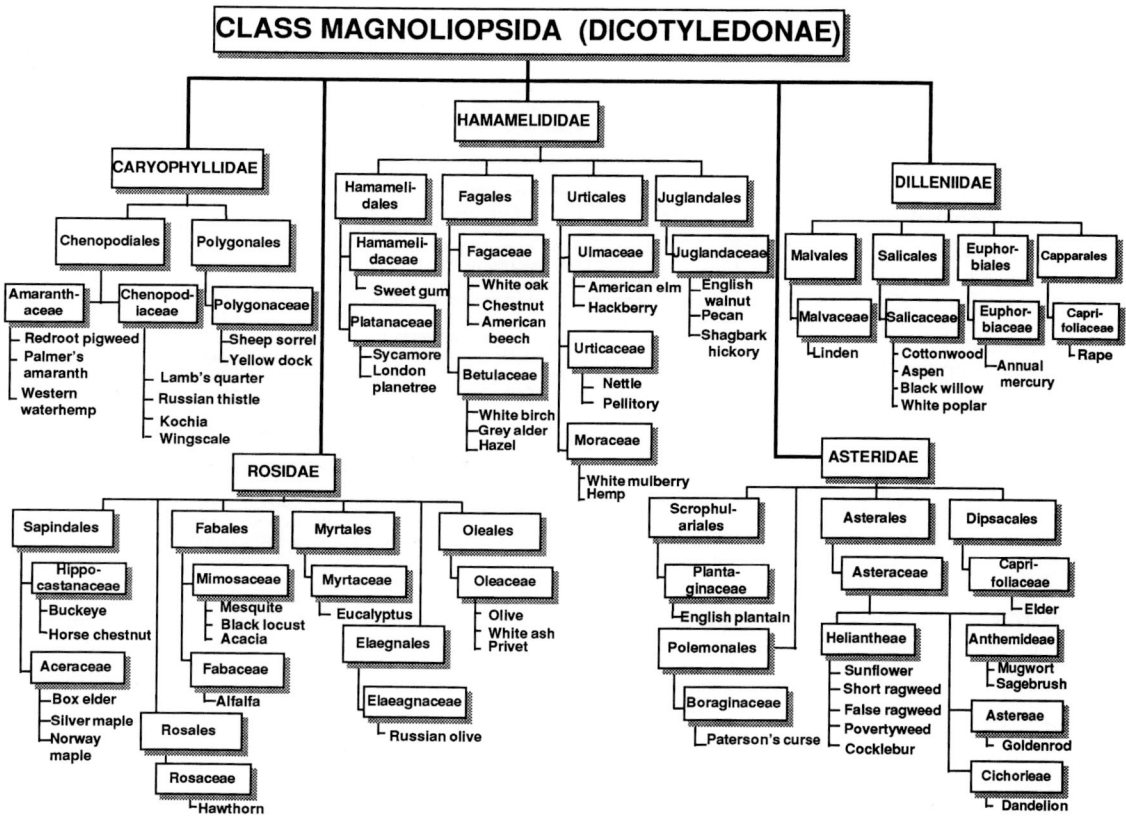

FIGURE 7-10. Taxonomy of representative allergenic members of the class Magnoliopsida, division Magnoliophyta, previously named subclass Dicotyledone, class Angiospermae. Subclasses, orders, families, and individual members are listed, as well as tribes in family Asteraceae.

species as well as the geographic area. Figure 7–11 lists several representative northern and southern grasses and their respective periods of anthesis in sectors of the United States. In the northern states, the major peak of grass pollen is seen in May and June, with certain grasses pollinating later in the summer. As one moves south, the season broadens out; in portions of southern California, Texas, Florida, and Hawaii, grass pollen may be seen the entire year.

Grass pollens (Fig. 7–5) are fairly nondescript, with a single pore, in the range of 20 to 45 microns in diameter (some grains, such

TABLE 7–1. CHARACTERIZED GRASS ALLERGENS

Group	Molecular Weight in Kilodaltons	Comments
I	27–36	Major allergen. High cross-reactivity across species. High homology of COOH terminus with II and III, but no cross-reactivity
II	11	Minor; acidic
III	11	Minor; basic
IV	50–60	Minor; basic
V	32–38	Major
VI	14	No shared cross-reactivity with V
IX	28–34	Minor, basic
X	12	Cytochrome C

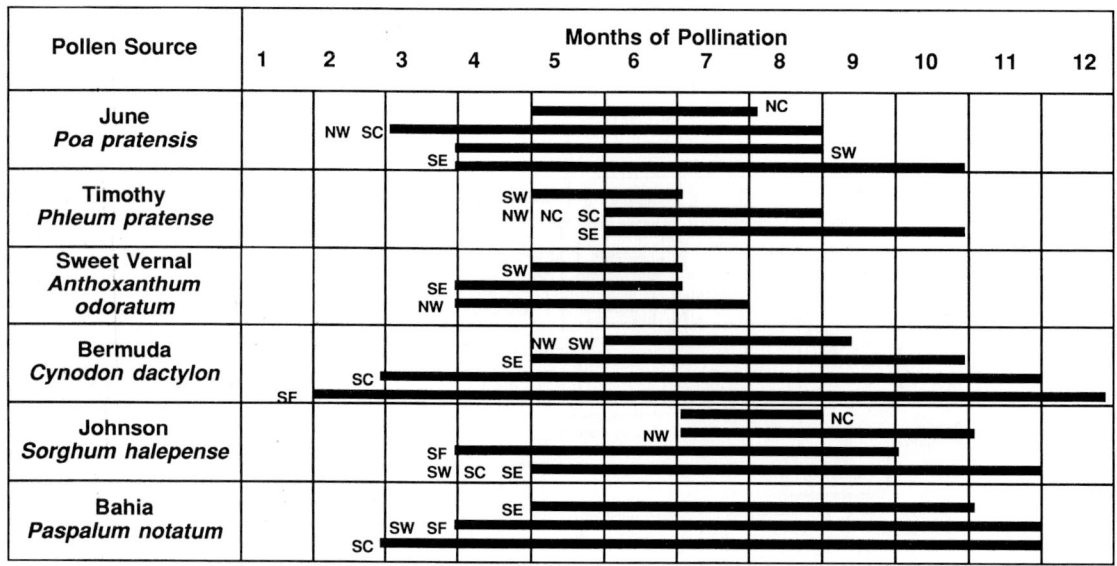

FIGURE 7–11. Periods of anthesis in month of the year by U.S. region for representative northern and southern grasses. NC = north central; NE = northeast; NW = northwest; SC = south central; SE = southeast; SF = south Florida; SW = southwest.

as corn, are much larger). Species are generally indistinguishable from each other. Palm pollens have a single furrow. Cattail pollens are distinctive for being found as tetrads on pollen samplers.

GRASS ALLIES. The class Liliopsida, in addition to the grasses, contains palms, sedges, and cattails (see Fig. 7–9). All of these have been suspected of causing pollinosis, although never to the degree seen with grasses. However, the role of palm pollen in causing symptoms is being looked at again in areas such as southern California and Florida. Preliminary data suggest no cross-reactivity among the sedges, cattails, and grasses. A large assortment of plants belonging to this class are not normally incriminated as aggravants of hay fever. Some, such as the lilies, may sporadically cause difficulty, often in occupational settings.

Trees

CONIFERS. The division Pinophyta is separate from the flowering plants. Most of the plants incriminated in pollinosis are members of the order Coniferales, which has several families of interest (see Fig. 7–8). The most important is Cupressaceae, containing cedars, junipers, pfitzers *(Juniperus spp., Thuja spp.),* and cypresses *(Cupressus spp.).* Exposure comes not only from forest stands, but from the ubiquitous use of a variety of these plants in home landscaping. In semi-arid portions of the western states, scrub junipers cover foothills and lower mountains. Pollen grains are relatively small, are produced in copious amounts, and are potent sensitizers. In central and western Texas, mountain cedar *(Juniperus ashei)* counts may be >5000 grains/m^3, and it is the leading cause of pollinosis. Members of this family are strongly antigenically and allergenically cross-reactive (Yoo et al, 1975). A smaller family, Taxodiaceae, includes bald cypress, redwoods, sequoias, and a very important producer of pollinosis in Japan, Japanese red cedar (sugi, *Cryptomeria japonica*). Studies generally do not show cross-reactivity with the junipers, but there are conflicting reports concerning Japanese red cedar (Yoo et al, 1975; Yasueda et al, 1983).

The pine family, Pinaceae, consists of pines *(Pinus spp.),* spruces *(Picea spp.),* hemlocks *(Tsuga spp.),* and firs *(Abies spp., Pseudotsuga).* Pollens are larger, usually with two prominent air bladders, making these quite distinctive on sampler specimens. Fortunately, despite being produced in copious amounts, pine pollens are weak allergenically and produce little significant hay fever.

NETTLE ORDER (URTICALES). This order contains several families of interest, which have both tree and weed members. Ulmaceae contains elms and hackberries. Although American elm *(Ulmus americana)* has been nearly obliterated by Dutch elm disease, several other elm species such as Chinese, Siberian, and red elms are resistent to the fungal blight. These may be significant pollen producers, although usually in a short pollen season. Most pollinate in the early spring, although some such as Chinese, red, and scrub elm pollinate in the late summer or early fall. Pollination periods of important hay fever trees are illustrated in Figure 7–12. Hackberries *(Celtis spp.)* have also been incriminated as inducers of pollinosis in the early spring. Pollen grains are relatively nondescript, with up to five small pores along the equatorial plane.

The mulberries of the family Moraceae are potent sensitizers. White mulberry *(Morus alba)*, introduced into the larger cities of Arizona, has become such a hay fever nuisance, that further plantings are prohibited by law. Grains are small (14 to 20 microns) and usually two-pored.

WILLOW FAMILY (SALICACEAE). This family possesses two genera: *Populus* (the poplars, cottonwoods, and aspen) and *Salix* (the willows). These are widely distributed trees. Quaking aspen, *Populus tremuloides,* is prevalent in the northern and Rocky Mountain states; in the Great Plains, eastern cottonwood *(Populus deltoides)* is common, especially along river and creek beds. These plants are moderate pollen producers, but because of their prevalence, skin test reactivity is commonly found. Based on skin test correlations and older studies using Prausnitz-Küstner (P-K) neutralization, willows and poplars seem to strongly cross-react. Poplar and cottonwood pollens are fairly large and lack apertures; willow grains are smaller and have three to four furrows. Poplars are wind-pollinated, whereas willows are predominantly insect-pollinated (although appreciable amounts may become airborne). Pollination usually occurs in early to mid spring, followed a month later by large amounts of airborne seed-carrying tufts of cotton. Since in many areas the cotton flies during peak

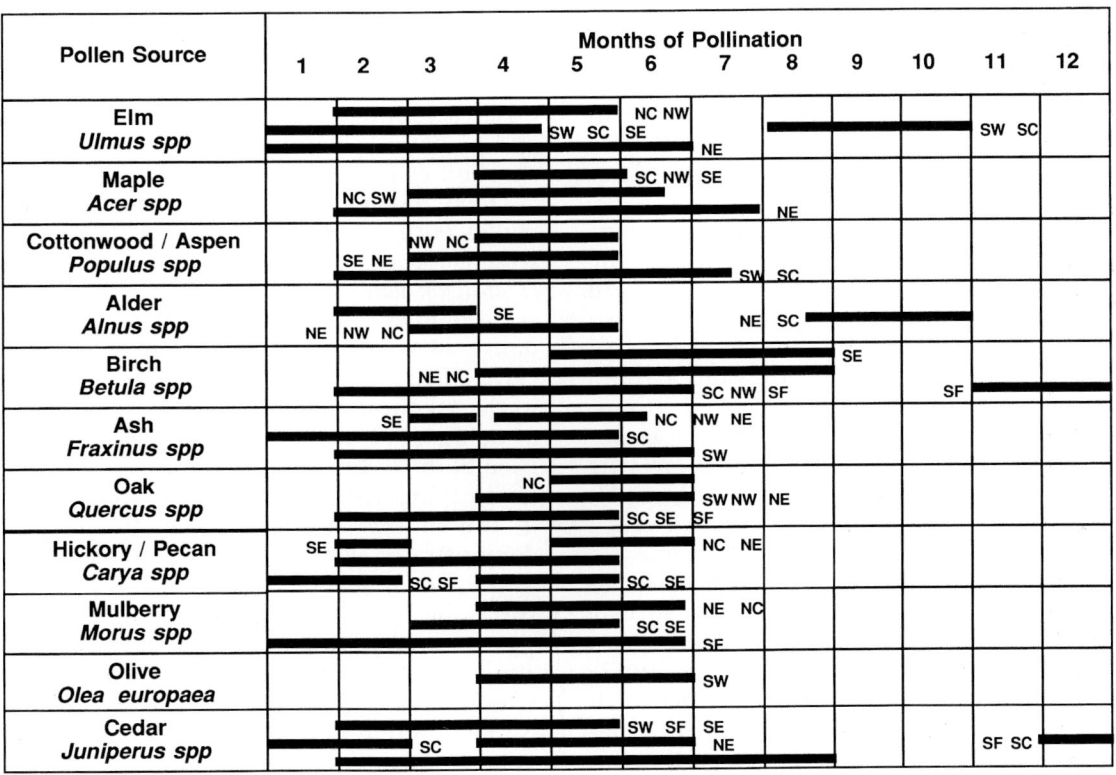

FIGURE 7–12. Periods of anthesis in month of the year by U.S. region for representative allergenic trees. Abbreviations same as in Figure 7–11.

grass pollination, patients erroneously attribute their grass-pollen hay fever to the cottonwood cotton.

BEECH ORDER (FAGALES). While there is some disagreement whether the beech (Fagaceae) and birch (Betulaceae) families should be in the same or different orders, cross-reactivity data support our considering them together (see Fig. 7–10). There is strong cross-allergenicity within the birch family, and this extends across to the beech family as well (Valenta et al, 1992). Amino acid sequencing of the major alder allergen, *Aln g* I, shows partial identity with the corresponding allergens of birch (*Bet v* I), hornbeam (*Car b* I), and oak (*Que a* I) pollens (Ipsen and Hansen, 1991). Fagaceae contains beeches, oaks, and chestnuts. Betulaceae includes birches, alders, hazel, hornbeams, and hophornbeams. Birch *(Betula verrucosa)* is the major cause of pollinosis in Scandinavia, with alder *(Alnus glutinosa)* also a prominent inducer of symptoms. In the United States, birch is more prevalent in the eastern states; alder is more important west of the Rockies and a predominant producer of tree pollinosis in the Pacific northwest.

Alder pollen generally has four to five pores, whereas birch has three very prominent aspidate pores. Oaks are tricolporate, with distinctive pores within furrows. Members of the birch family generally pollinate in April or May; oaks pollinate at the same time in most of the United States, except for a later season in the southwest.

MAPLES (ACERACEAE). This family is comprised of two genera, *Acer* and *Dipteronia*, the latter consisting of trees native to China. All the maples, as well as box elder (ash-leaf maple, *Acer negundo*), are contained in *Acer*. These are prevalent in North America and range from entirely insect-pollinated to amphiphilous (both) to wind-pollinated (especially box elder). Box elder is rapid-growing and is frequently a nuisance, a weed tree. It pollinates in April. Other maples will reach anthesis either earlier or later. In some regions with two predominant species, such as silver maple *(Acer saccharinum)* and Norway maple *(Acer platanoides)*, there may be two distinct pollen peaks, 6 weeks apart. While Norway maple is largely insect-pollinated, it appears to produce enough pollen to be observed on samplers. Maple pollens are tricolporate, with long furrows. In areas where oak and maple pollinate at the same time, it may be difficult to distinguish between these two, especially with the smaller grains and shorter furrows of box elder. Cross-reactivity data in this family are limited. There appears to be both skin test and RAST inhibition disparity between box elder and other maples (Bernstein et al, 1976). Older studies suggested some cross-reactivity between maples and members of Fagales.

WALNUT FAMILY (JUGLANDACEAE). Hickories *(Carya spp.)* and walnuts *(Juglans spp.)* are trees of the northern temperate and subtropical climates and are useful for their edible nuts, oils, and woods, and as street and lawn trees. Hickories are found primarily in the eastern states, with pecans *(C. illinoensis* and *C. texana)* found in the southern states. Pecans are a major cause of tree pollen allergy in the southeast. Walnuts are scattered throughout the northeastern states and are prominent in the southwest, where they may locally be important inducers of hay fever. Skin test correlations are high between hickories and pecans, and preliminary inhibition studies show lesser similarities between *Carya* and *Juglans*. Hickory pollen grains are large (frequently >50 micron), triporate, and circular to rounded-triangular in appearance. *Juglans* pollens are smaller and polyporate, with the pores limited to one hemisphere. Pollination is in May and June in the northern states, onset a month earlier in the middle states, and as early as January and February along the Gulf coast.

OLIVE FAMILY (OLEACEAE). This family includes both trees and shrubs, including olive *(Olea europaea)*, ash *(Fraxinus spp.)*, and privet *(Ligustrum vulgare)*. The latter is primarily insect-pollinated, but the two trees are abundant pollen producers and of significant concern. Olive is an extensively planted crop tree in the Mediterranean basin and a major cause of pollinosis. Native and introduced ashes are used both for lumber and for street and lawn landscaping. Ashes are especially troublesome in the southwest. Cross-reactivity has been demonstrated between olive and ash, as well as between several shrubs in the family (Bousquet et al, 1985). A recent study has shown strong cross-inhibition between olive and Russian olive *(Elaeagnus angustifolia)*, which is somewhat surprising since the latter is in a different family and order (Kernerman et al, 1992).

Olive pollen is light and easily becomes airborne despite extensive insect pollination. Ash frequently appears quadrangular with four pores and furrows. Both have peak pollination in April and May.

Weeds

NETTLE ORDER (URTICALES). This order was also discussed above, under Trees. The nettle family (Urticaceae) contains two members of particular interest. Pellitory *(Parietaria spp.)* is acknowledged as a major producer of hay fever in the Mediterranean basin. It is found in more limited distribution in the United States but appears to be a problem in the California bay area. Nettle produces a small pollen grain in copious amounts and may be a more significant hay fever plant than previously appreciated (Fig. 7–13). There is no allergenic cross-reactivity between nettle and pellitory. Classified either as a separate family or under Moraceae, hemp *(Cannabis sativa)* and hops *(Humulus lupulus)* may be mild hay fever inducers. Grown in the midwest originally for the production of rope, *Cannabis* was most prevalent in Iowa and eastern Nebraska.

GOOSEFOOT ORDER (CHENOPODIALES). Two closely related families are found within this order: Chenopodiaceae and Amaranthaceae. The knotweed family, Polygonaceae, may be classified within this group as well, although some systems place it in a separate order, Polygonales (see Fig. 7–10). The chenopods include the highly significant major tumbleweeds: Russian thistle *(Salsola kali)* and kochia *(Kochia scoparia)*, also known as burning bush or summer cypress. These are aggressive weeds that were introduced into the Great Plains, and over the past 70 years kochia especially has extended its range to stretch into the midwest and northeastern states, southward to the Gulf coast, as well as into southern California. In some parts of the country, kochia has been used as a landscaping ornamental due to its frequently red stems. Russian thistle is a major pollinosis factor in the Middle East. Lamb's quarters *(Chenopodium al-*

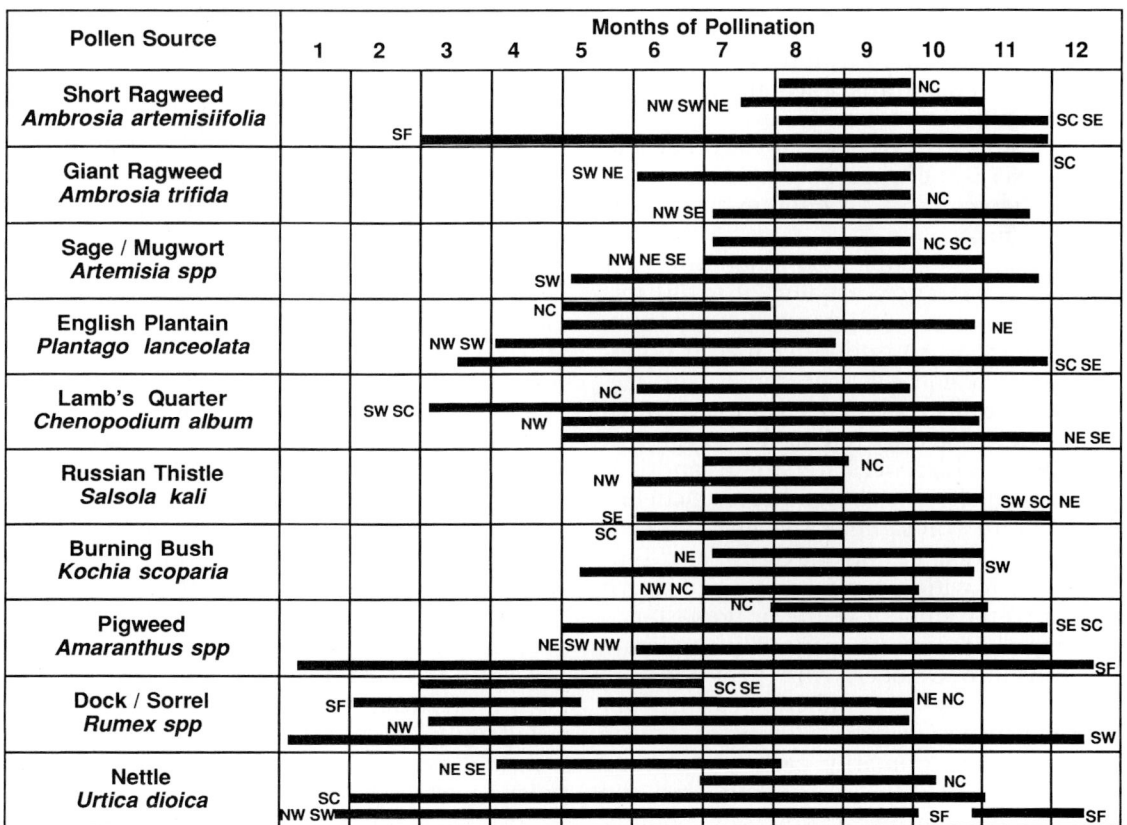

FIGURE 7–13. Periods of anthesis in month of the year by U.S. region for representative weeds. Abbreviations same as in Figure 7–11.

bum) is a ubiquitous plant found throughout North America and Europe. It is a modest pollen producer, however. Scales *(Atriplex spp.)* are well adapted to the arid, alkaline soils of the western states. Cultivated sugar beet *(Beta vulgaris)* was a potent inducer of hay fever until low pollen strains were developed, with propagation primarily by root cuttings. Pigweeds such as *Amaranthus retroflexus* are also prevalent, showing a range similar to that of lamb's quarters. Palmer's amaranth *(Amaranthus palmeri)* is especially common in the southwest, while western water hemp *(Acnida tamariscina)* is common in the midwest and south.

Polygonaceae contains the sorrels and docks. Sheep sorrel *(Rumex acetosella)* is considered a moderate hay fever inducer. Curly or yellow dock *(R. crispus)* is a common weed but a low pollen producer.

Cross-reactivity data support the close relationship between the chenopods and amaranths. There is almost allergenic identity among the *Amaranthus* species and almost as striking similarities among the *Atriplex* species. The other chenopods show varying degrees of cross-inhibition within the family and across to the amaranths; Russian thistle appears to contain some unique allergens (Wodehouse, 1957; Weber, 1981; Weber and Nelson, 1985). There are no data concerning cross-allergenicity of chenopod-amaranths with polygons.

Pollens of the chenopod-amaranths are similar in appearance, usually 20 to 30 microns in diameter. Grains are pantoporate, with as many as 80 uniformly spaced pores, giving them a golfball appearance (see Fig. 7–6). The number of pores varies between species; some have as few as 14 to 20, but generally the differences are subtle, and it is easiest to classify them together as "chenopod-amaranth" on sampler specimens (Lewis et al, 1983). *Rumex* grains have three or four furrows, each with a central pore, and starch granules are prominent in the protoplast.

Chenopod-amaranths generally pollinate from July into October, with peaks in late August to early September. Seasons are longer in southern regions. *Rumex spp*, on the other hand, are primarily early pollinators, in April through June, coinciding with the grasses. In the southwest, however, pollination may occur throughout much of the year (see Fig. 7–13).

ASTER FAMILY (ASTERACEAE). This family (also called Compositae) is the largest among flowering plants. It contains a dozen tribes, most of which contain only insect-pollinated plants of little interest to allergists. The sunflower tribe (Heliantheae), mayweed tribe (Anthemideae), and ragweed tribe (Ambrosieae) are closely related, with newer taxonomies classifying Ambrosieae as a subtribe of Heliantheae (Ambrosiinae; see Fig. 7–10). Ragweeds belong to the genus *Ambrosia*. False and slender ragweeds had previously been classified as a separate genus, *Franseria*, but have now been incorporated into *Ambrosia*. Also within the same (sub)tribe are cocklebur *(Xanthium commune)* and the marsh elders *(Iva spp.)*. The major four ragweeds are short *(A. artemisiifolia)*, giant *(A. trifida)*, western *(A. psilotachya)*, and false *(A. acanthicarpa)*. The former two are most common in the east and midwest and are estimated to cause as much hay fever as all the other ragweeds combined. The mayweed tribe contained the mugworts and sages of the genus *Artemisia*. Mugwort *(A. vulgaris)* is an important allergenic plant, not only in the midwest and east, but in Europe as well. The ragweeds have been viewed as Western Hemisphere plants, but short ragweed has been introduced to several European locations, and other *Ambrosia* exist there as well. Many other members of this family have been incriminated as occasional sources of pollinosis. For the most part, these are either low pollen producers or insect-pollinated, with sporadic quantities of pollen becoming airborne. In the east, goldenrod *(Solidago spp.)* was commonly blamed for the hay fever caused by ragweed. A minority of ragweed-sensitive people will also react to goldenrod. Along the west coast, some species of *Baccharis* are wind-pollinated and have been incriminated as hay fever producers.

At least 9 allergens have been isolated from short ragweed, the most important being *Amb a* I (antigen E). Almost all clinically sensitive ragweed sufferers will react to *Amb a* I and *Amb a* II (AgK). These two allergens show cross-reactivity. Decreasing percentages will respond to *Amb a* III, *Amb a* IV, and *Amb a* V. Most of these allergens have two or more electrophoretically distinct isoallergen forms. Certain patients' antibodies may be able to distinguish the homologous allergens from short and giant ragweed, such as *Amb a* V and *Amb t* V. Although there are some conflicting reports, Yunginger and Gleich (1972) found AgE in short, giant, southern, and false ragweed, with minimal amounts in slender ragweed. No AgE was found in sages, cocklebur, marsh elders, or plantain. RAST inhibition studies by the same group supported these findings, with essentially overlapping inhibition curves from short, giant, western, and false ragweeds; slender and southern ragweeds were less potent, and other members of the family showed no inhibition (Leiferman et al, 1976). Preliminary studies of *Artemisia* extracts by ELISA inhibition reveals strong cross-reactivity between several species.

Ragweed pollen grains are small (about 18 to 22 microns) and tricolporate with frequently inapparent pores and furrows, and they have short broad-based spikes (see Fig. 7–7). Other composites such as *Baccharis* and *Solidago* have longer spikes. *Iva spp.,* like the ragweeds, have shorter spikes. *Artemisia* pollen grains are tricolporate, with more apparent furrows and a thickened exine between the furrows, giving a scalloped appearance in the polar view. *Artemisia* spikes are short and interspersed with granules on the surface, giving a rougher appearance.

Ragweeds and sages pollinate in the late summer, pollen classically beginning in mid-August and peaking in early September. Ragweed pollen onset and peak occur later as one moves south, and along the Gulf coast pollen may be observed for much of the year (see Fig. 7–6). Anthesis usually persists until the first significant frost. Recent evidence indicates that sage is more cold-hardy than ragweed and can continue to produce low levels of pollen into colder weather.

PLANTAINS (FAMILY PLANTAGINACEAE). These plants, while widespread, are generally considered to be of little significance in pollinosis; only the English plantain, *Plantago lanceolata,* produces copious amounts of pollen. However, in areas such as the northwest, plantains may account for a quarter of the airborne pollen in July and August, and skin test positivity is common. Pollination may be prolonged, from May through October (see Fig. 7–13). Pollen grains are of average size, with six to ten pores, and resemble chenopod-amaranth pollens except for the much fewer pores.

Old P-K neutralization data exist (Rackemann and Wagner, 1936) showing inhibition of plantain by both grass and ragweed, but not the converse. This suggests that grass and ragweed possess the relevant allergens of plantain, but not vice versa. As mentioned above, plantain does not contain AgE (*Amb a* I). Work from Australia has suggested similarities between plantain and a common Australian weed, Paterson's curse *(Echium plantagineum),* of the family Boraginaceae (Katelaris et al, 1982).

Distribution of Pollens

Various sources describe the regional distribution of allergenic plants in North America and elsewhere (Lewis et al, 1983; Falagiani, 1990; Solomon and Platts-Mills, 1993). Tabulations of regional airborne pollen surveys are available (Chang, 1980; Samter and Durham, 1955). More current reports of local and regional pollen prevalence are compiled by the American Academy of Allergy and Immunology.

Reducing Pollen Exposure

OUTDOORS. Major allergenic pollens (and fungal spores) are so well mixed throughout the lower atmosphere that avoidance measures can only hope to curtail *excessive* exposure. This goal may be reached by attention to "common sense" considerations, such as not walking through ragweed-infested fields during a symptomatic period. Ambitious programs of urban allergenic plant eradication have not been successful because pollen is carried in the wind for great distances.

INDOORS. Enclosed spaces offer refuges from aeroallergens, although patients' activity patterns limit the benefits of this option. Indoor pollen prevalence may be reduced by closing windows and using central air conditioning or a window unit efficient at particle exclusion. Various devices, including high-efficiency particulate air (HEPA) filters, which produce essentially particle-free air, are available for installation in home or office environments but may not add substantially to the protection from pollen afforded by central air conditioning and should not be recommended automatically.

THE POLLEN REFUGE OPTION. To escape one's allergies through a bold geographic move is a popular fantasy among affected persons and their families. Such relocations can be effective if the offenders are regionally limited and newly encountered allergenic plants are unimportant. Escape often is difficult, however, because of multiple pollen and fungal spore sensitivities, the importance of animal or house dust allergens that travel with the patient, or the presence of other factors unimproved by relocation. In addition, the social disruption, loss of job seniority, and financial hardships involved emphasize the need for *caution in advising or condoning a major family move.* When this option is contemplated seriously, trial periods of at least 4 weeks in the new area (preferably in more than one season) should be employed before a final decision is implemented. Highly ragweed-sensitive persons contemplating several comparable job offers are justified in giving precedence to coastal Pacific Northwest and West Coast opportunities; the wide distribution of grass and tree pollens in North America leaves little hope for completely avoiding these factors in settled areas.

Temporary travel may be used effectively for pollen avoidance. Ragweed-sensitive subjects have long used trips abroad, ocean cruises, or sojourns on the West Coast or in Northern Canada or Alaska to secure late summer relief.

MAJOR ALLERGENIC FUNGI

Basic Characteristics of Fungi

Despite their diversity, fungi as a group differ fundamentally from plants, animals, actinomycetes, and slime molds (Myxomycetes). Fungi have true nuclei and cell walls of chitin or cellulose. Except for unicellular forms, fungi are composed of microscopic strands or "hyphae"; these (Fig. 7–14) proliferate simply, as in "molds," or form specialized fleshy structures, as in mushrooms and sac fungi. In most forms, well-defined septa divide the hyphal strands, and metabolic debris tends to occupy older, more central segments as growth proceeds peripherally.

Most allergenic fungi can grow on nonliving organic matter, while a few (i.e., obligate parasites) require a living host. Both groups need moisture, oxygen, preformed carbohydrate, and occasionally additional growth factors.

Many airborne fungi show a distinctive morphology, which permits identification microscopically. This approach is applicable especially to the dark-spored imperfect fungi (Table 7–2), to many sexual spores of fleshy fungi, and to rust and smut spores. Although there is no comprehensive guide available, illustrations of selected particles have been published (Gregory, 1973; Smith, 1984 and 1986). An extensive set of ascospore drawings (Dennis, 1981) and monographs depicting the spores of imperfect fungus taxa are also available (Barron, 1977; Barnett, 1987; Ellis, 1971; Ellis and Ellis, 1985).

Many familiar fungi grow actively at 20°C and may flourish well above or below this temperature; others require low temperatures, proliferating even under refrigeration. A small group of "thermophilic" fungi grow *only* at temperatures of 50°C or higher, while others (e.g., *Aspergillus fumigatus*) tolerate these temperatures but also grow well at temperatures below 50°C. Given adequate moisture, many fungi grow actively on nutritionally barren man-made substrates (Fig. 7–15).

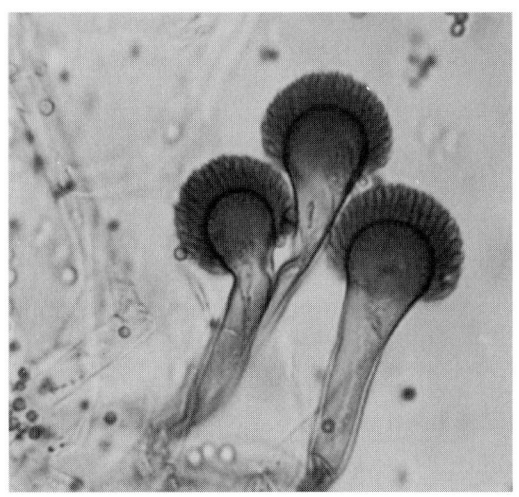

FIGURE 7–14. Photomicrograph of *Aspergillus fumigatus,* a typical filamentous imperfect fungus. Hyphal strands (left) are the basic structural units of these organisms. Spores (conidia) are characteristically borne on specialized hyphae (conidiophores), which, in *Aspergillus* form species, are terminally expanded; three such "vesicles" are shown at the right.

TABLE 7–2. IMPERFECT FUNGI OF SPECIAL INTEREST TO ALLERGISTS

FORM GENUS AND MAJOR FORM SPECIES*	SRR†	NOTEWORTHY CHARACTERISTICS D = DARK GRAY OR BLACK COLONIES ("DEMATIACEOUS")
Alternaria—*A. alternata* = *A. tenuis*	+ + + +	Widespread on vegetation; probably most clinically reactive airborne fungus allergen (D)
Cladosporium—*C. cladosporioides, C. herbarum*	+ +	Formerly termed "Hormodendrum"; highest outdoor spore levels in most regions. Form species' allergens may differ (D)
Epicoccum—*E. purpurascens*	+ +	Especially on grains, grasses; produces orange pigments but sporulates poorly on many agar media
Stemphylium—*S. botryosum*	+ + +	Imperfect form of *Pleospora herbarum*, an ascomycete (D)
Curvularia—*C. lunata*	+ + +	Especially in warmer areas (D)
Helminthosporium—*H. solani*	+ + +	Agriculturally centered, epidemic at times (D) (*Drechslera* and *Bipolaris* are similar form genera)
Fusarium—*F. roseum, F. nivale*	+ +	Imperfect forms of several ascomycete genera: colonies produce slime spores and prominent pigments. Ascospores may produce much *Fusarium* growth
Phoma—*P. herbarum*	+ + +	Sphaeropsid: slime-spored: reactivity said to parallel that to *Alternaria* form species and both may be asexual forms of certain ascomycete species
Penicillium (more than a dozen common types)	+	Often perennially present indoors and outdoors: unrelated to sensitivity to penicillin
Aspergillus—*A. flavus, A. fumigatus, A. amstelodami, A. glaucus,* others	+ +	Indoor and occupational exposures common: *A. fumigatus, A. flavus* also produce allergic aspergillosis
A. niger	(±)	Prominent on wood and paper
Candida—*C. albicans, C. tropicalis*	+ +	*C. albicans* is a common human gut and orificial saprophyte; uncommon in air
Rhodotorula—*R. glutinis*	+	Prominent during wet weather; acid-tolerant red yeast: grows well in indoor fluid reservoirs
Aureobasidium—*A. pullulans*	+ +	Formerly termed "Pullularia"; common soil, leaf saprophyte. Pleomorphic on agar media (D)
Monilia sitophila	+	Prominently associated with milling and bakery trades: extremely rapid grower
Botrytis—*B. cinerea*	+ +	Prevalence regionally variable; prominent plant pathogen
Geotrichum—*G. candidum*	+	Vaguely defined form genus; probably asexual forms of basidiomycetes
Sporobolomyces—*S. roseum*	+ +	Yeast, usually pink, actively discharging spores; suspected autumn allergen in Great Britain
Gliocladium—*G. roseum*	+ +	Slime-spored; young growth Penicillium-like
Trichoderma—*T. viride*	+	Prominent in soil; rapid grower

*Additional form genera including *Cephalosporium, Verticillium, Sporothrix, Pithomyces,* and numerous yeasts are widely encountered but have received little or no clinical evaluation.
†SRR = Estimated relative Skin Reactivity Rate among exposed atopic subjects in North America using available skin testing materials.

Although fungal components may be ingestant allergens, inhaled spores are the major source of exposure. Spores are specialized reproductive structures that usually are resistant to harsh environmental conditions. Depending on the fungus (or even upon a particular growth phase), spores may be asexual (diploid) or sexual (haploid) with dissimilar "mating types." Many fungi may produce sexual *and* asexual spores at different phases of their life cycles. Since these stages may occur separately, they often have been described and named as if they were individual organisms.

Those types that generate asexual spores (i.e., imperfect fungi, deuteromycetes) are classified according to the form of their spore-producing organs. However, it is now clear that biologically dissimilar fungi have evolved imperfect (asexual) stages which are morphologically almost alike. Since the arrangement of the imperfect fungi does not necessarily reflect natural affinities, their taxa are termed "*form* species," and these are grouped in "*form* genera." While the concept of *form* taxa imparts some order to a large and difficult group, members of *form* genera cannot be assumed to contain identical allergens. This limitation has often been overlooked in the past, both by physicians and allergen extract suppliers, in labeling fungus extracts with "generic" names only.

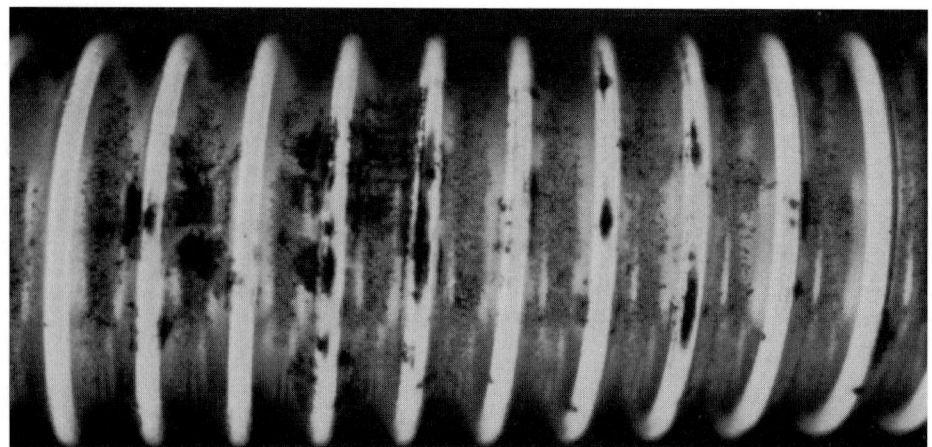

FIGURE 7–15. Fungal growth within the plastic tubing leading to a water-filled spirometer used for ventilatory testing. Airborne dust and droplets of saliva provide the only nutrient source for these organisms. An ample supply of moisture permits fungi to colonize such marginal sites.

Classes of Fungi

The taxonomy of fungi is based largely upon the morphology and mode of development of their spores. They can be classified into the five following principal groups.

FUNGI IMPERFECTI (DEUTEROMYCETES). This *form class* of fungi that reproduce asexually includes most of the currently recognized allergenic fungi (see Table 7–2). With a few exceptions, these form taxa are saprophytic, and spores ("conidia") develop on more or less specialized hyphal structures. In one subclass (Sphaeropsidales), spores arise in flask-shaped organs and are extruded in slimy masses, which are dispersed by dew and raindrops; *Phoma* exemplifies this group. Another distinct subclass (Melanconiales) has spore-forming hyphae in cushion-like masses; some members are plant pathogens but are not recognized as important allergens. Most additional deuteromycetes (Moniliales) lack these specialized structures (e.g., *Alternaria* and *Penicillium* species).

The imperfect fungi bear spores, singly or multiply, on exposed hyphae except for a tiny group (Mycelia Sterilia), which appears to multiply by vegetative appendages alone. Tenuous attachments permit spores of many taxa to be scoured and dispersed readily by air currents; such "dry spore" dispersal is typical of common genera, including *Alternaria* (see Fig. 7–10), *Cladosporium* (formerly termed *Hormodendrum*), and many *Penicillium* species. Out of doors, these types are most prevalent on hot, dry, windy days. By contrast, many fungi (e.g., species of *Phoma, Fusarium,* and *Cephalosporium)* produce mucinous masses of "slime" spores, dispersed during rain and humid periods.

Although allergists are most familiar with imperfect fungi, there remains substantial uncertainty concerning their clinical role for a variety of reasons: gaps in knowledge of their prevalence in many areas of the country and of the amount of exposure in specific environments or with specific activities, a dearth of information on the intensity of exposure necessary to induce symptoms, and unclear antigenic relationships among biologically related taxa.

DOWNY MILDEWS (OÖMYCETES). These relatively primitive fungi include economically important parasites of plants and certain insects. Agricultural exposure to heavily infected crops occasionally provokes allergic respiratory responses.

SUGAR AND BREAD MOLDS (ZYGOMYCETES). The allergic impact of this class is due largely to members of the order Mucorales, including species of *Rhizopus, Mucor,* and *Absidia*. These fungi are prominent saprophytes of biologic debris, including food residues and leaf litter. While ubiquitous in soil, their level in air usually is low. However, with seepage of ground water or soiling of furnishings with food, these organisms may flourish indoors. Close inspection of infected substrates may disclose the globular reproductive structures (sporangia), each containing myriad spores (sporangiospores); microscopically, broad hyphae with few septae are typical.

SAC FUNGI (ASCOMYCETES). These fungi produce sexual spores (ascospores) in a sac-like cell (or "ascus"). Ascospores often are launched into air by processes requiring moisture, reaching greatest abundance in humid or rainy weather. Many familiar imperfect fungi, including *Aspergillus, Fusarium,* and *Helminthosporium* form species, are asexual states of ascomycetes. The yeast used in brewing and baking is an additional member of this class. The few ascospore types evaluated as test allergens have elicited moderate rates of reactivity in exposed atopic subjects (Bruce, 1963).

MUSHROOMS, PUFFBALLS, RUSTS, AND SMUTS (BASIDIOMYCETES). These fungi resemble ascomycetes in producing sexual spores (among other types), which are shot from their points of origin, given adequate moisture, and are abundant at night and during rainy periods. Characteristic spores, "basidiospores," are formed—most commonly in tetrads—on specialized cells or "basidia." Numerous parasitic forms (e.g., smuts, bunts, and rusts) produce additional spores during stages of development, often on a succession of hosts. Heavy agricultural exposures to spores of rusts and grain smuts have produced allergic symptoms, but it is not known whether more casual exposures are harmful. Asthma has been associated with homes containing spores of the dry rot fungus *(Merulius lacrymans),* and skin sensitivity to other basidiospores has been described (Gold et al, 1984; Santilli et al, 1982).

Distribution and Clinical Relevance

FUNGI OUTDOORS. Since fungi grow principally on leaf surfaces and in plant litter and soil, atmospheric spore concentrations vary with local cycles of plant growth and decrease with snow cover. Airborne fungi are prominent throughout the growing season in temperate areas, but peak spore levels occur in late summer and autumn, particularly during hot, breezy periods when "dry-spore" forms abound. Recoveries at these times are dominated by spores of *Alternaria* and *Cladosporium* species, which seem to achieve their highest levels in grassland and cultivated (especially grain-growing) areas. At night and during rain, ascospores and basidiospores reach maximum prevalence along with splash-dispersed spores of imperfect taxa. Whether respiratory symptoms that worsen during humid and rainy weather reflect exposure to these little studied particles is unknown.

Symptoms are induced in fungus-sensitive patients by situations and activities that accentuate exposure to common deuteromycetes. Spore levels are higher close to the ground in natural areas than at urban rooftop sites. Substantial airborne dispersion of fungus particles occurs when plant growth is disturbed (e.g., by traversing vegetated areas). Exposure peaks also occur with mowing lawns or harvesting grains. Composts, in which fungi flourish, pose special hazards for mold-sensitive persons. Symptoms also commonly develop after exposure to hay, ensilage, mulches, dry soil, commercial peat moss, compost piles, and leaf litter. However, there is little objective support for the belief that spore levels are specifically increased in the vicinity of lakes and other surface waters.

FUNGI INDOORS. Occupational contact with plant or animal products—especially in humid interiors—can produce heavy exposure to airborne fungal antigens, and perennial symptoms may result. When spores are numerous outdoors, this source will dominate recoveries made in normally ventilated interiors. Fungi originating indoors are more likely to be evident when buildings are closed (e.g., in winter or with central air conditioning in summer) and especially when levels of outdoor fungi are low. At these times, *Penicillium, Aspergillus,* and *Fusarium* form species and occasionally *Rhodotorula* and other yeasts predominate. This often contrasts sharply with the *"Cladosporium-Alternaria"* pattern so typical of outdoor air in northern states in summer (Solomon, 1975) (see Fig. 7–15).

Outside the growing season, the correlation between relative humidity and indoor fungus level has been strong. This association probably reflects both moisture as a factor promoting fungus growth and colonization of humidifying devices by fungi. "Cool-mist" vaporizers are frequently contaminated and emit fungus-laden aerosols (Solomon, 1974); presumably furnace humidifiers and ultrasonic units pose related risks. Pets and active small children foster increased indoor fungus levels by soiling surfaces with food residues and outside debris. Although house plants and soil harbor fungi, their effect on indoor air levels is often negligible; however, humid conditions and actively disturbed growth will increase indoor exposure risks.

Reduction of indoor mold spore exposure

requires meticulous general hygiene and, often, control of excessive indoor moisture. Central air conditioning will permit window closure during warm periods, thus excluding outdoor particles and also reducing relative humidity. At other times, supplementary humidification should be restrained, with levels of 20 to 25 percent relative humidity viewed as adequate and mechanical dehumidification used freely. Small amounts of natural ventilation will often curtail moisture accumulation in "tight" buildings. Shower curtains and refrigerator drip trays, as well as basements and outside walls where water condenses or seeps, deserve special concern. Cleaning these areas with solutions of sodium hypochlorite, Lysol, or other commercial products such as zephiran (available as Roccal and use 1 ounce in 1 gallon of tap water) will inhibit mold growth, although regrowth occurs all too quickly. Specific indoor antifungal agents have not yet been proved safe and effective. Small moldy objects may be decontaminated by placing them in a plastic bag for 12 to 24 hours with a small amount of paraformaldehyde or propylene oxide. When humidity control alone fails, fungus growth in limited spaces also may be attacked by volatilizing paraformaldehyde; treated areas must be *completely* ventilated before use.

FUNGI IN FOODS. Fungi are important in the production of many foods and industrial chemicals (Onions, 1992). Various yeasts (especially *Saccharomyces cerevisiae*) are employed in the preparation of baked goods, beer, wines, and some liquors as well as vinegar and vinegar products—especially processed meats. Most cheeses result from bacterial fermentations but are readily contaminated in storage; in addition, Camembert and blue-veined cheeses (e.g., Roquefort) utilize specific *Penicillium* species. Commercial mushrooms, the spore-producing organs of basidiomycetes (e.g., *Agaricus bisporis*), are rarely ingestant allergens. Soy and steak sauces are produced using *Aspergillus oryzae*. Fungi are employed in the early stages of chocolate production. In addition, fungi commonly contaminate foodstuffs during extended storage, even at refrigerator temperatures.

Although massive ingestion of yeast- and mold-containing foods (e.g., a wine, cheese, and pizza feast) will, at times, provoke respiratory symptoms in young adults, ingested fungi probably are an infrequent cause of prolonged allergic problems. Highly allergic patients occasionally may benefit from a trial withdrawal of dietary fungi followed by a diagnostic challenge. The "mold-free diet" typically eliminates fresh rolls, coffee cakes, pizza dough, dried yeast, and foods refrigerated over 72 hours as well as fermented beverages and fruits. Fresh fruits and vegetables should be peeled or scrubbed before consumption, but other dietary components, including commercial breads, are acceptable. The duration of such trials should be individualized, and avoidance should be continued only when its favorable effect has been clearly demonstrated.

CLINICAL SIGNIFICANCE OF FUNGUS SENSITIVITY. Sensitivity to inhaled fungal allergens is a common factor in allergic rhinitis and asthma. However, the overall impact of fungi and the role of individual offenders are still debated. Thermotolerant species also may colonize body cavities, producing persistent and distinctive disease in allergic subjects (see Chapter 40). Although associations between asthma and dermatophyte infections have been reported (Ward et al., 1989), their extent and a broader role for fungus materials in urticaria and eczema remain speculative.

Evaluation of sensitivity to fungi is difficult because of their diversity, their uncertain regional distribution, and often prolonged periods of exposure. Plant dusts contain abundant fungi; however, algae, actinomycetes, storage mites, and bacterial endotoxins also may be responsible for observed health effects. Clinical allergy to fungal allergens *alone* is uncommon. However, there is little doubt that IgE-mediated allergy to fungi is widespread, especially to species of *Alternaria* (Fig. 7–16) and other dark deuteromycetes. These may be responsible for symptoms throughout most of a local growing season or, at least, at times different from major pollen peaks.

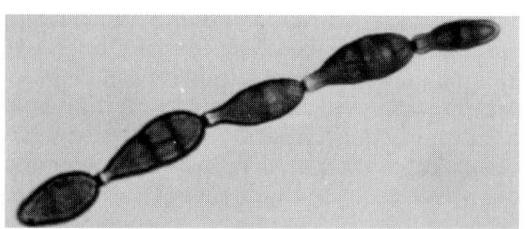

FIGURE 7–16. *Alternaria alternata* spores borne in characteristic chains. These brown, multiseptate particles are widely abundant in outdoor air and are among the most clinically important fungus allergens.

Although many additional molds produce positive skin test reactions, their clinical importance and allergenic similarities, if any, are yet to be fully defined. Determining fungus prevalence in air remains a key to estimating exposure and to setting priorities for clinical evaluation.

REFERENCES

Barnett HL, Hunter BB. Illustrated Genera of Imperfect Fungi. 4th ed. New York, Macmillan, 1987.

Barron GL. The Genera of Hyphomycetes from Soil. Baltimore, Williams & Wilkins, 1968.

Bernstein IL, Perera M, Gallagher J, et al. In vitro cross-allergenicity of major aeroallergenic pollens by the radioallergosorbent technique. J Allergy Clin Immunol 57:141–152, 1976.

Bousquet J, Guerin B, Hewitt B, et al. Allergy in the Mediterranean area. III. Cross-reactivity among Oleaceae pollens. Clin Allergy 15:439–448, 1985.

Bruce RA. Bronchial and skin sensitivity in asthma. Int Arch Allergy Appl Immunol 22:294, 1963.

Burge HA. Fungus allergens. Clin Rev Allergy 3:319, 1985.

Chang WWY. Pollen survey of the United States. In Patterson R (ed). Allergic Diseases—Diagnosis and Management. 2nd ed. Philadelphia, JB Lippincott Co., 1980.

Connell JT. Quantitative intranasal pollen challenges. III. The priming effect in allergic rhinitis. J Allergy 43:33, 1969.

Dennis RWG. British Ascomycetes. 3rd revised and enlarged ed. Forestburg, NY, Lubrecht and Cramer, 1981.

Durham OC. The volumetric incidence of airborne allergens. IV. A proposed standard method of gravity sampling, counting and volumetric interpolation of results. J Allergy 17:79, 1946.

Ellis MB. Dematiaceous Hyphomycetes. Kew, Surrey, Commonwealth Mycol Instit, 1971.

Ellis MB, Ellis JP. Microfungi on Land Plants. An Identification Handbook. New York, Macmillan Publishing Co., 1985.

Falagiani P. Pollinosis, Boca Raton, CRC Press, 1990.

Gaut BS, Clegg MT. Molecular evolution of alcohol dehydrogenase 1 in members of the grass family. Proc Natl Acad Sci USA 88:2060–2064, 1991.

Gold BL, Burge HA, Muilenberg ML, Solomon WR. Epidermal reactivity to basidiospore extracts. J Allergy Clin Immunol 73:113, 1984.

Gregory PH. Microbiology of the Atmosphere. 2nd ed. New York, John Wiley & Sons, 1973.

Ipsen H, Hansen OC. The NH_2-terminal amino acid sequence of the immunochemically partial identical major allergens of alder *(Alnus glutinosa)* Aln g I, birch *(Betula verrucosa)* Bet v I, hornbeam *(Carpinus betulus)* Car b I and oak *(Quercus alba)* Que a I pollens. Mol Immunol 28:1279–1288, 1991.

Katelaris C, Baldo BA, Howden MEH, et al. Investigation of the involvement of *Echium plantagineum* (Paterson's curse) in seasonal allergy. IgE antibodies to *Echium* and other weed pollens. Allergy 37:21–28, 1982.

Kernerman SM, McCullough DR, Green J, et al. Evidence of cross-reactivity between olive, ash, privet and Russian olive tree pollen allergens. Ann Allergy 69:493–496, 1992.

Leiferman KM, Gleich GJ, Jones RT. The cross-reactivity of IgE antibodies with pollen allergens. II. Analysis of various species of ragweed and other fall weed pollens. J Allergy Clin Immunol 58:140–148, 1976.

Lewis WH, Vinay P, Zenger VE. Airborne and Allergenic Pollen of North America. Baltimore, Johns Hopkins University Press, 1983.

Martin BG, Mansfield LE, Nelson HS. Cross-allergenicity among the grasses. Ann Allergy 54:99–104, 1985.

Martin W, Lydiate D, Brinkmann H, et al. Molecular phylogenies in angiosperm evolution. Mol Biol Evol 10:140–162, 1993.

Matthiesen F, Løwenstein H. Group V allergens in grass pollens. II. Investigation of group V allergens in pollens from 10 grasses. Clin Exp Allergy 21:309–320, 1991.

Ogden EC, Raynor GS, Hayes JV, Lewis DM, Haines JH. Manual for Sampling Airborne Pollen. New York, Hafner Press, 1974.

Onions AH, et al. Smith's Introduction to Industrial Mycology, 7th ed., New York, Cambridge Univ. Press, 1992.

Rackemann FM, Wagner HC. The desensitization of skin sites passively sensitized with serum of patients with hay fever. Crossed reactions of different pollens. The variations in the recipient. J Allergy 7:319–332, 1936.

Samter M, Durham OC. Regional Allergy of the United States, Canada, Mexico, and Cuba. Springfield, Charles C Thomas, 1955.

Santilli JJ, Marsh DG, Collins RP, Alexander JF Jr, Norman PS. Basidiospore sensitivity and asthma. J Allergy Clin Immunol 69:98, 1982.

Sivasubramanian B, et al. Human T cell responses to purified pollen allergens of the grass, *Lolium perenne*: Analysis of relationship between structural homology and T cell recognition. J Immunol 148:2378–2383, 1992.

Smith EG. Sampling and Identifying Allergenic Pollens and Molds. San Antonio, Texas, Blewstone Press, Vol. 1, 1984; Vol. 2, 1986.

Solomon WR. Fungus aerosols arising from cold-mist vaporizers. J Allergy Clin Immunol 54:222, 1974.

Solomon WR. Assessing fungus prevalence in domestic interiors. J Allergy Clin Immunol 56:235, 1975.

Solomon WR. Sampling airborne allergens. Ann Allergy 52:140, 1984.

Solomon WR, Platts-Mills TAE. Aerobiology and inhalant allergens. In Middleton E Jr, Reed CE, Ellis EF (eds). Allergy: Principles and Practice. 4th ed. St. Louis, C.V. Mosby Co., 1993.

Valenta R, Duchene M, Ebner C, et al. Profilins constitute a novel family of functional plant pan-allergens. J Exp Med 175:377–385, 1992.

Von Arx JA. The Genera of Fungi Sporulating in Pure Culture. 3rd ed. Forestburg, N.Y., Lubrecht and Cramer, 1981.

Ward GW Jr, Karlsson G, Rose G, Platts-Mills TAE. Trichophyton asthma: sensitization of bronchi and upper airways to dermatophyte antigen. Lancet i:859, 1989.

Weber RW. Cross-reactivity among pollens. Ann Allergy 46:208–215, 1981.

Weber RW, Nelson HS. Pollen allergens and their interrelationships. Clin Rev Allergy 3:291–318, 1985.

Wodehouse RP. Antigenic analysis by gel diffusion. III. Pollens of the Amaranth-Chenopod group. Ann Allergy 15:527–536, 1957.

Yasueda H, Yui Y, Shimizu T, et al. Isolation and partial

characterization of the major allergen from Japanese cedar *(Cryptomeria japonica)* pollen. J Allergy Clin Immunol 71:77–86, 1983.

Yoo T-J, Spitz E, McGerity JL. Conifer pollen allergy: Studies of immunogenicity and cross antigenicity of conifer pollens in rabbit and man. Ann Allergy 34:87–93, 1975.

Yunginger JW, Gleich GJ. Measurement of ragweed antigen E by double antibody radioimmunoassay. J Allergy Clin Immunol 50:326–337, 1972.

Chapter 8

Other Allergenic Plants and Animals

Richard W. Weber, M.D., and William K. Dolen, M.D.

THE INDOOR ENVIRONMENT

That some constituent of the dust in homes could be an aggravant of asthma and rhinitis has been appreciated for over 70 years. It has long been apparent that indoor dust is a heterogeneous mix of items such as mold, animal danders, plant fibers, and other breakdown products of home furnishings. However, results of allergy testing with these products in house dust–sensitive patients indicated the presence of unique but unidentified allergens which were potent sensitizers. Initially, patients were tested and treated with autologous extracts, that is, extracts produced from dust from their own homes. With time, immunotherapy shifted to use of commercially prepared house dust extracts from a variety of sources, many not well characterized. Immunotherapy with crude commercial house dust extracts appeared to be efficacious, despite the lack of identification of the most important allergenic ingredient. It was not until 1967 that the pioneering work of Voorhorst and co-workers identified *Dermatophagoides pteronyssinus* as the major house dust allergen in the Netherlands. The following year, Miyamoto and colleagues working in Japan reported on the role of *Dermatophagoides farinae* in house dust–induced asthma. In retrospect, mites had been reported to cause asthma in Germany in the 1920s. It is now recognized that house dust–mites cause and/or trigger symptoms of asthma, rhinitis, atopic dermatitis, and possibly urticaria and vernal conjunctivitis (Korsgaard and Iversen, 1991; Sporik et al, 1992; Colloff, 1992; Colloff et al, 1992).

House Dust Mites

D. pteronyssinus and *D. farinae* (European and American house dust mites, respectively) are considered the major allergenic dust mites. They may cohabitate the same homes, although *D. farinae* appears to better tolerate lower humidities and therefore will be found in drier areas (Lang and Mulla, 1977). Other dust mites, *D. microceras* and *Euroglyphus maynei,* may be found in homes as well, especially in areas of greater moisture. In tropical and subtropical countries a nonpyroglyphid mite, *Blomia tropicalis,* has been found in significant numbers along with *D. pteronyssinus, D. farinae,* and *E. maynei* (Arlian et al, 1993a). Between 5 and 8 percent of mites may be storage mites which are found primarily in grain and hay, such as *Acarus, Glycyphagus, Lepidoglyphus, Tyrophagus,* and *Tarsonemus.* The latter genus includes predator mites, which feed on *Dermatophagoides.* While sensitization to emanations of these other mites does occur and may also account for some occupational exposures, they are minor factors for the great number of patients (Iverson and Dahl, 1990; Colloff et al, 1992).

Dust mites thrive at temperatures of about 25° to 30°C, and relative humidity (RH) of 75 to 80 percent. Viable *D. pteronyssinus* mites are usually not found with RH below 65 percent, and mites will definitely be eliminated with persistent humidity below 45 percent (Hallas, 1991). *D. farinae* may survive at lower RH at lower temperatures, for example, at humidities of 45 percent RH at 15°C (Colloff et al, 1992). The major food source of dust mites is human skin scales, the digestion of which is facilitated by colonization of the scales by fungi. Therefore, conditions that contribute to mold growth will also augment mite populations. However, at higher humidities, mites are forced out by fungal overgrowth.

House dust mites have five life stages: egg, six-legged larva, eight-legged protonymph, tritonymph, and adult male or female mite. Dust mites cannot regulate body temperature, and so population growth is controlled by ambient temperature (and humidity). At lower temperatures numbers decline, and time necessary for full maturation increases. Under optimal conditions, egg-to-adult metamorphoses take 3 to 4 weeks, with the adult living for 6 weeks. Females will produce between 40 and 80 eggs (Colloff et al, 1992).

Seven groups of house dust mite allergens have been described, and four of these have enzymatic activity (Table 8–1). Group I, the major allergens, are cysteine proteases, group III serine proteases, group IV amylase, and group VI chymotrypsin. These are gut-associated, appear to be digestive enzymes, and are found in larger amounts in mite fecal pellet extracts (Colloff et al, 1992). Group I allergen (*Der p* I, *Der f* I) has been localized to the fecal pellet peritropic membrane. A *D. pteronyssinus* mite produces an average of 20 pellets per day, each fecal ball containing roughly 100 pg of *Der p* I (Tovey et al, 1981). Group II allergens do not appear to be gut related and are not found in increased amount in fecal material. The recently cloned 22 kilodalton group VII allergen has not been localized (Shen et al, 1993).

At least six antigenic sites have been described for *Der p* I and *Der f* I, one of which shows cross-reactivity with monoclonal antibodies. Antibodies to crude extracts have shown at least 21 cross-reacting antigens, half of which are allergens for human antisera (Arlian, 1991). Between 80 and 95 percent of human mite–specific IgE cross-reacts between *D. pteronyssinus* and *D. farinae*. Limited cross-reactivity has been demonstrated in various studies between *Dermatophagoides, Euroglyphus, Blomia,* and the storage mites, as well as with the scabies mite, *Sarcoptes scabiei* (Arlian, 1991; Arlian et al, 1993a; Arlian et al, 1993b).

Cockroaches

Sensitivity to cockroach allergens has been appreciated for over thirty years, but its role as an important factor in asthma has only recently been elucidated (Bernton and Brown, 1967; Pollart et al, 1989; Kang et al, 1993). Prevalence of cockroach allergen is inversely related to socioeconomic status (whereas dust mite allergen is not), although in the southern states cockroach infestation is ubiquitous. It has been reported that cat allergen and cockroach allergen are inversely related: homes with cats have fewer roaches, presumably because cats ingest the roaches. The most cosmopolitan of species is the German cockroach (*Blattella germanica*) found in all 50 states; it is strictly domestic, not surviving outside. Other roaches, such as the American (*Periplaneta americana*) and the oriental (*Blatta orientalis*) will be found both in and around homes. These three cockroaches comprise the greatest indoor burden, but at least a half dozen other species may be clinically relevant in certain locales (Helm et al, 1990; Duff and Platts-Mills, 1992).

The major cockroach allergens primarily originate in the gut epithelium, with lesser contributions from the Malpighian vessels (a kidney equivalent) and ovaries (Zwick et al, 1991). Exposure may come from feces, saliva, or body part fragments. Three allergens have been characterized: *Per a* I, *Bla g* I, and *Bla g* II (Schou et al, 1990; Pollart et al, 1991). The first two are cross-reactive, whereas the latter is species-specific. Molecular weights range from 25 to 36 kilodaltons.

TABLE 8–1. PURIFIED HOUSE DUST MITE ALLERGENS

Group	Molecular Weight in Kilodaltons	Comments
I	24	Cysteine protease, gut-related
II	15	
III		Serine protease (trypsin), gut-related
IV	60	Amylase, gut-related
V	15	
VI		Chymotrypsin
VII	22	Cloned allergen

Animal Danders

Immediate hypersensitivity to animals is common and important at home, in the workplace, and at school. At the time of the initial allergy evaluation, many patients are fully aware of their problem because episodic exposure in the form of domestic airway challenges has produced predictable symptoms. When the history is inconclusive, either because the patient refuses to acknowledge symptoms or because of continuous pet exposure, an avoidance trial may be indicated before a beloved pet is banished from the home or immunotherapy is considered. Clinically significant exposure due to residual animal allergen may persist for weeks to months, however; cat and dog allergens are readily airborne and "sticky" in the sense that they readily adhere to various types of surfaces. As with other allergenic substances, the finding of a positive skin test or *in vitro* test is not in itself indicative of clinically relevant sensitization.

Home or workplace exposure to any nonaquatic mammal might produce allergic sensitization. In North America, the most common mammalian pets are dog and cat, although hamsters, gerbils, and guinea pigs are popular, and even rabbits and pigs have been domesticated. The major dog and cat allergens are present at high levels in house dust and in the air in relatively undisturbed domestic environments (Sakaguchi et al, 1993). Additionally, children from homes with pets bring allergens to school on clothing, producing allergen levels which could be high enough to produce symptoms in some sensitized children (Munir et al, 1993).

Dogs. All canine breeds can cause allergy, and several dog allergens can be clinically important. A 23-kilodalton major allergen, *Can f* I is found in dog hair and saliva; a 19-kilodalton major allergen is found in saliva and skin (Spitzauer et al, 1993). Urinary allergens have been described, and dog serum albumin is also allergenic. The various breeds can differ in their expression of allergens (Moore and Hyde, 1980), and the use of extracts obtained from different breed sources may be advantageous in testing.

Cats. Humans recognize at least seven cat allergens that are carried on respirable particles the same size as those produced by therapeutic nebulizers (Platts-Mills et al, 1991). Once thought to be a salivary allergen, the 36-kilodalton heterodimer allergen *Fel d* I is found in skin sebaceous glands and dermis (Charpin et al, 1991). Other members of the cat family possess an analogous, cross-reacting protein (de Groot et al, 1990). Cat albumin is also allergenic, and cat extracts contain small amounts of a protein sufficiently similar to *Can f* I to be cross-reactive, a phenomenon Aalberse has termed "Dog in Cat." In addition to the cat itself, furniture and walls (Wood et al, 1992) are major reservoirs for cat allergens, which remain detectable for a considerable time after the pet has been removed. Thus, simple pet removal will be ineffective unless the household is completely cleaned.

Farm Animals. Horses, cattle, hogs, sheep, reindeer, and other farm animals may sensitize both the farmer and family members. Horse hair, once thought to be an important cause of indoor allergic symptoms, is no longer used as a stuffing for upholstered furniture and mattresses.

Rodents. Although the role of domestic exposure cannot be completely ignored, rodent allergy is primarily an occupational disorder that may be prevalent in nearly a third of exposed laboratory workers. Sensitized workers typically report onset of symptoms within minutes of entering the animal room. In rats, mice, and guinea pigs, the major allergens are in urine, which, as an aerosol with particle sizes 5 to 10 μm in diameter, permits efficient distribution, airway penetration, and prolonged airborne time (Platts-Mills et al, 1986). Urinary allergens are less important in rabbits (Warner and Longbottom, 1991). When total avoidance is not practical, modifications of the animal housing area will reduce airborne allergen concentration (Gordon et al, 1992).

Birds and Feathers. Aged feather extracts sometimes used for diagnostic testing are probably contaminated with mite and other allergenic substances found in house dust, but IgE-mediated inhalant allergy (as distinguished from extrinsic allergic alveolitis) to fresh bird feathers has also been described (van Toorenenbergen et al, 1985). Egg allergy is not necessarily associated with feather allergy, although sensitization to both is reported (Anibarro Bausela et al, 1991).

Human Dander. House dust contains many proteins of human origin, including blood group antigens, IgA and IgG (Kifuji et al, 1993), and human hair and dander. Humans shed several grams of skin per week, providing a major food source for house dust mites, and human dander has long been thought to be allergenic (reviewed by Berrens, 1970). Voorhorst demonstrated skin test reactivity to a human dander extract in hairdressers and reported nearly a 50 percent prevalence of substantial reactivity in a general allergy clinic population, noting prior reports of a high prevalence of dander allergy in atopic dermatitis patients (Voorhorst, 1977). The question whether human skin contains unique, clinically important allergens warrants reexamination.

Indoor Environmental Control

A great deal of attention has been raised recently to the relationship between asthma and exposure to indoor allergens such as dust mite, cat, and cockroach. Correlations can be made with both emergency room visits for acute asthma and sensitization, and with sensitization in asthmatics versus control subjects (Pollart et al, 1989; Platts-Mills et al, 1991; Call et al, 1992). In 1990, Sporik and colleagues were able to show the impact of exposure to high levels of *Der p* I in infancy and the subsequent development of asthma. It now appears that levels of >2 µg group I mite allergen per gram of house dust leads to sensitization, and that levels >10 µg/gm are likely to be associated with increased risk of asthma (Platts-Mills et al, 1991). It may be expected that similar threshold level determinations for the other major indoor allergens, *Fel d* I and *Bla g* I, will be forthcoming.

Considering then the relationship of indoor exposure to disease, it seems important to decrease exposure as much as possible. With pets, this would be best achieved by removal of the animal, although decrease in *Fel d* I has been shown to be quite delayed, even for months (Wood et al, 1989). This in part is due to the carriage of *Fel d* I on a variety of particle sizes, some very small (<0.25 micron), and therefore more difficult to remove. On the other hand, mite allergen is usually associated with fecal pellets, which are larger particles of about 10 microns. The disparity between mite and cat allergen carrier particles also means that cat allergen can easily be found in dust on walls and in air samples of undisturbed rooms, whereas mite allergen is not (Swanson et al, 1989; Wood et al, 1992). This observation has major impact on the utility of air filtration systems in removing these allergens.

Active control of dust mite allergens may be achieved through several mechanisms: conventional cleaning methods for limiting dust and removing allergen; decreasing allergen production by killing mites with acaricides; denaturing allergens; and air-cleaning filtration devices (Pollart et al, 1988; Nelson et al, 1988; Colloff et al, 1992; Fernandez-Caldas and Fox, 1992). Traditional methods include removing carpeting, down comforters and pillows, dust collecting knickknacks, and encasing mattresses, boxsprings, and pillows. Although results are dependent on patient compliance, some studies have shown benefit from these measures (Murray and Ferguson, 1983; Dorward et al, 1988). Vacuuming has been notoriously poor in removing mites from carpeting. Additionally, standard appliances frequently spray allergen into the air (from leaking collection bags).

The acaricide most studied has been benzyl benzoate. This product has been found to have both antimite and antifungal activity (Hart et al, 1992). While some studies have shown dramatic results in decreasing mite allergen concentrations, other have not been so impressive (Bischoff et al, 1990; Colloff et al, 1992). A recent position paper has suggested that acaricides be used in conjunction with thorough post-treatment vacuuming, and that a variety of factors in individual homes will affect efficacy. Additionally, it was suggested that acaricides not be applied to surfaces with which children may have prolonged close contact, such as pillows and mattresses (Colloff et al, 1992).

Tannic acid denatures several allergens such as *Der p* I and *Fel d* I. It may be obtained as a 3 percent solution and applied to carpet. It has also been incorporated into solutions or dry foams with benzyl benzoate. This combination may be more effective than the isolated agents (Hart et al, 1992).

Air-filtration systems for homes, either as free-standing units or attached to furnaces, have been heavily promoted by their manufacturers. Two types include high-efficiency particulate air (HEPA) filters and electrostatic precipitators. Despite the ability to remove particulate matter from rooms very efficiently, clinical improvement in allergic disorders is difficult to show (Nelson et al, 1988; Colloff et al, 1992; Fernandez-Caldas and Fox, 1992). Some studies have shown modest effects, but others have shown no advantage over conventional measures (Reisman et al, 1990; Antonicelli et al, 1991). At present, the consensus appears to be that such systems require more study to demonstrate benefit, and they cannot be recommended in place of conventional control measures.

INHALANT INSECT ALLERGY

A variety of arthropods have been incriminated in inhalant allergy. Compared to the magnitude of pollen and mold spore allergy, and the importance of the major indoor allergens discussed above, these are relatively minor occurrences. The majority of these are occupational exposures: workers exposed to moths raised for larva bait, or grasshoppers and crickets raised for laboratory or school experiments, or *Daphnia* raised as fish food, or occupational asthma from sewer flies. A few, however, may impact on large numbers of patients: specifically, caddis fly and mayfly hatches, and green nimitti midge exposure.

CADDIS FLY AND MAYFLY. Over sixty years ago, separate reports were published from both ends of Lake Erie. To the east, from June to late August, large swarms of adult caddis flies resulted in the release of fine hairs from their bodies and wings into the air. These sensitizing particles were important causes of inhalant allergy. At the west end of Lake Erie, in June and July, large hatches of adult mayflies occurred. The insects would shed a coat, which was light and easily disrupted. These mayfly adults would live for only a few hours, but large amounts of shed skin and dead adults would accumulate, with significant airborne debris.

MOTHS. In the western Great Plains states, similar epidemics of miller moths would occur in sporadic years, causing inhalant allergy. The adult moths would migrate from the plains of Kansas and Nebraska to the alpine meadows of the Rockies, frequently in vast numbers, usually in May through July. Fewer numbers would survive to return to the Great Plains to lay eggs. Scales from the wings would be dispersed in large numbers and reportedly could also be sensitizing. Similarly, in the Pacific northwest, scales from Douglas fir tussock moths could either be primary irritants or stimulate an IgE response. Sensitization has been reported in occupational settings in forest product workers, but Kino and Oshimo reported skin-test positivity to moth and butterfly extracts in over 50 percent of a group of asthma patients who had no obvious exposure (Kino and Oshima, 1978).

CHIRONOMID MIDGES. Along the headwaters of the Nile in northern Sudan, large numbers of the green nimitti midge (*Cladotanytarsus lewisi*) breed. Hypersensitivity has been recognized for over sixty years, manifesting as both asthma and rhinitis (Gad El Rab and Kay, 1980). In 1982, Baur and co-workers were able to show that the allergen in a similar midge, *Chironomus thummi thummi,* resided on a low-molecular-weight (16 kilodaltons) hemoglobin, or erythrocruorin. Cross-reactivity was demonstrated with *C. lewisi*.

OTHER ALLERGENIC SUBSTANCES

A patient with classic allergic symptoms not explained by a routine evaluation presents a supreme challenge to the trained, experienced, and astute clinical allergist. Early reports of allergy to natural latex, a substance once thought inert, were received by the scientific community with a great deal of skepticism, but it soon became obvious that latex is a major cause of inhalant and skin allergy as well as anaphylaxis. Other "new" allergenic substances still await description by teams of clinicians and bench scientists because under the right circumstances, nearly any protein, glycoprotein, or hapten might function as a clinically relevant allergen. It is not surprising that the literature is replete with case reports of patients in whom unusual substances have induced a human allergic response. Understandably, these uncommon sensitizers have received less scientific attention than have major allergenic substances. Many have not been studied in this era of molecular allergy, and some are considered allergenic only on the basis of clinical anecdote.

LATEX. Allergy to latex products, produced from the sap of the rubber tree (*Hevea braziliensis*), has been reported world-wide since 1979 (see Chapter 24). Sensitized individuals have experienced the gamut of allergic reactions, including inhalant allergy, contact dermatitis, urticaria, other skin rashes, angioedema, anaphylaxis, and death. Several major and minor allergens (at least some of which might be altered by processing) have been reported; rubber elongation factor is a major allergen present in natural rubber as well as in finished products (Czuppon et al, 1993). Different products contain very different allergen levels. Latex allergens are absorbed by glove powders and can become airborne. Latex sensitization has also been associated with oral pruritus ("oral allergy syndrome") following ingestion of avocados, bananas, and chestnuts, suggesting at least partial cross-reactivity. At present, no latex extract for skin testing is commercially available; many investigators and clinicians have prepared extracts using commercial latex products, but such preparations vary widely in allergen content and the safety and efficacy of such preparations is unknown. Anaphylaxis from epicutaneous skin testing with nonstandardized materials has been reported (Kelly et al, 1993). Several manufacturers offer materials for *in vitro* testing, but these are also nonstandardized and contain highly variable levels of major and minor allergens.

FICUS TREES. A member of the mulberry family (Moraceae), the weeping fig tree (*Ficus benjamina*) is widely used as an ornamental indoor plant. The tree sap contains at least 11 allergens which, when aerosolized, produce inhalant symptoms in sensitized nursery workers. *Ficus* allergy may affect about 5 percent of a domestic patient population (Axelsson et al, 1990).

ORRIS ROOT. Many years ago, orris root (obtained from the Florentine iris) was used widely in the manufacture of cosmetics. A potent sensitizer, it was such a common cause of inhalant allergy that it is no longer used for this purpose in the United States.

PYRETHRUM. Used for pest control for more than 100 years (Casida, 1980), pyrethrum is derived from the dried flowers of the pyrethrum daisy (*Tanacetum cinerariifolium*), like ragweed a member of the chrysanthemum (composite) family. Early insecticide products were powders produced from ground flowers and contained allergenic proteins clearly implicated in inhalant allergy (Ramirez, 1930). Although pyrethrum powder is still available, most modern preparations contain pyrethrins, six insecticidal esters extracted from pyrethrum flowers, which are not allergenic.

SILK. Silk is a proteinaceous thread obtained from the cocoon produced by the caterpillar of the silkworm moth (*Bombyx mori*). Sericin, a glue-like material that holds the threads together in the cocoon, is allergenic. Silk allergy may present as inhalant allergy, particularly in textile workers, or as urticaria or atopic dermatitis. Generally, finished silk textiles are not allergenic, but silk waste—which is used for producing rugs, certain heavy fabrics, and stuffing material for quilts and mattresses—contains several silk allergens that may be clinically important in the home environment (Johansson et al, 1985).

JUTE, SISAL, HEMP, FLAX, AND COTTON. Jute, sisal, and hemp are vegetable fibers widely used in the manufacture of burlap bags, rugs, carpet pads, twine, rope, and air filters. Inhalation of particles may produce chronic lung disease similar to byssinosis, which is caused by inhalation of cotton and flax. All may be a source of inhalant occupational allergy, and allergic sensitization has been demonstrated in hemp workers (Zuskin et al, 1992). Cotton linters, a component of house dust, have been incriminated in inhalant allergy; although aged cotton linters produce positive skin tests in some individuals (perhaps due to dust mite contamination), the fresh product is not allergenic and substances producing nonspecific histamine release have been described in cotton extracts (Berrens, 1970). The clinical relevance of domestic exposure to these vegetable fibers is unknown.

KAPOK. Closely related to cotton, kapok is a short, buoyant fiber obtained from seed pods of kapok trees in the family Bombacaceae. It is used mainly in upholstery stuffing, but also in sleeping bags, boat cushions, and life preservers. Long thought to be a potent allergenic substance, kapok might merely serve as a substrate for mite or fungal growth (Bunnag and Dhorranintra, 1978). Kapok specific allergens may also exist.

WOOL. Sheep's wool is a potent cutaneous and respiratory irritant. Data conclusively demonstrating that wool is allergenic are lacking.

TOBACCO. While tobacco smoke is clearly and primarily a respiratory irritant, IgE-mediated inhalant allergy and contact urticaria to tobacco leaf have been described. An allergenic 18-kilodalton glycoprotein (tobacco glycoprotein antigen) has been purified both from tobacco leaves and from cigarette smoke condensate, and a similar substance is found in other members of the Solanacea family, which includes eggplant, green pepper, potato, and tomato (Becker et al, 1976). The clinical relevance of this allergen is unknown.

PSYLLIUM. Obtained from the seed husks of

Plantago ovata, psyllium (also called ispaghula) is used as a source of dietary fiber (believed to reduce serum cholesterol levels) and as a bulk laxative. The allergens are probably contained in contaminants from parts of the seed other than the husk. Inhalant psyllium allergy is an occupational disease that can affect health care workers, and ingested psyllium has produced anaphylaxis. Although a member of the same genus, English plantain (*Plantago lanceolata*) does not appear to cross-react with psyllium (James et al, 1991).

FLAXSEED (LINSEED) AND COTTONSEED. Both containing extremely potent allergens, flaxseed (also called linseed) and cottonseed are used in the baking industry and for animal feed. Flaxseed is a component of many health food products, including Roman Meal, and is used in the production of cosmetics, patent leather, and other substances. Cottonseed flour is a component of a wide variety of commercially produced foods, including doughnuts and pizza dough. Both may be inhalant or ingestant allergens. As with all strongly allergenic substances, even epicutaneous skin testing should be performed with extra caution; the clinician may wish to consider *in vitro* testing first when dealing with patients suspected of being highly sensitized.

CASTOR BEAN. In addition to the toxin ricin, castor beans (*Ricinus communis*) contain some of the most potent allergens known, capable of producing sensitization in very low concentrations. The bean is important as a source of castor oil and wax, used both medically and in the cosmetic industry. The hulls are ground and used as animal feed and fertilizer. Castor bean allergy is common both in workers and in persons living in the vicinity of mills. Castor beans contain heat-stabile and heat-labile allergens, which apparently are not present in oil or wax in significant amounts (Lehrer et al, 1980). When sacks used to transport castor beans are reused for transporting other substances (e.g., coffee beans) or are processed into felt, symptoms may occur in a sensitized patient (Topping et al, 1982).

VEGETABLE GUMS. The vegetable gums (karaya, tragacanth, gum arabic or acacia, chicle, carob, carragheen, guar gum) are so prevalent in the environment that daily exposure may be assumed for most patients. They are widely used as excipients in medications, foods, cosmetics, adhesives, printers' inks, and other substances (Sheldon et al, 1967; Lagier et al, 1990). Clearly causes of occupational inhalant allergy, they were at one time also regarded by clinicians as important causes of inhalant or ingestant allergy (manifesting as rhinitis, asthma, urticaria, angioedema) in the general population. Unfortunately, the prevalence of clinically relevant sensitization is unknown, and many clinicians no longer test for these substances. The role of routine testing for vegetable gums in patients with allergic symptoms warrants study. Cross-reactivity between the gums has not been found.

COMMON FOODS. Inhalant allergy to common foods ordinarily occurs in an occupational setting where food workers are exposed to organic dusts (e.g., grain flours, soybeans, tea, coffee) or aerosols. Bakers' asthma results from chronic inhalation of wheat and other flours. Inhalant green coffee bean allergy is prevalent in at least 21 percent of coffee mill workers (Osterman et al, 1982). The several allergens of the green coffee bean do not cross-react with those of the castor bean and fortunately are destroyed in the roasting process (Lehrer et al, 1981).

REFERENCES

Anibarro Bausela B, Martin Esteban M, Martinez Alzamora F, Pascual Marcoes C, Ojeda Casas JA. Egg protein sensitization in patients with bird feather allergy. Allergy 46:614–618, 1991.

Antonicelli L, Bilo MB, Pucci S, et al. Efficacy of an air-cleaning device equipped with a high-efficiency particulate air filter in house dust mite respiratory allergy. Allergy 46:594–600, 1991.

Arlian LG. House-dust-mite allergens: A review. Exp Appl Acarol 10:167–186, 1991.

Arlian LG, Vyszenski-Moher DL, Fernandez-Caldas E. Allergenicity of the mite, *Blomia tropicalis*. J Allergy Clin Immunol 91:1042–1050, 1993a.

Arlian LG, Rapp CM, Fernandez-Caldas E. Allergenicity of *Euroglyphus maynei* and its cross-reactivity with *Dermatophagoides* species. J Allergy Clin Immunol 91:1051–1058, 1993b.

Axelsson IGK, Johansson SGO, Larsson PH, Zetterström O. Characterization of allergenic components in sap extract from the weeping fig (*Ficus benjamina*). Int Arch Allergy Appl Immunol 91:130–135, 1990.

Baur X, Dewair M, Fruhmann G, et al. Hypersensitivity to chironomids (non-biting midges): Localization of the antigenic determinants within certain polypeptide sequences of hemoglobins (erythrocuorins) of *Chironomus thummi thummi* (Diptera). J Allergy Clin Immunol 69:66–76, 1982.

Becker CG, Dubin T, Wiedemann HP. Hypersensitivity to tobacco antigen. Proc Natl Acad Sci USA 73:1712–1716, 1976.

Bernton HS, Brown H. Cockroach allergy. II: The relationship of infestation to sensitization. South Med J 60:852–855, 1967.

Berrens L. The allergens in house dust. Progr Allergy 14:259–339, 1970.

Bischoff E, Fischer A, Liebenberg B. Assessment and control of house dust mite infestation. Clin Ther 12:216–220, 1990.

Bunnag C, Dhorranintra B. A study of the cross antigenicity between long-used kapok and mold extracts. Ann Allergy 40:84–85, 1978.

Call RS, Smith TF, Morris E, et al. Risk factors for asthma in inner city children. J Pediatr 121:862–866, 1992.

Casida JE. Pyrethrum flowers and pyrethroid insecticides. Environ Health Perspect 34:189–202, 1980.

Charpin C, Mata P, Charpin D, Lavaut MN, Allasia C, Vervloet D. *Fel d* I allergen distribution in cat fur and skin. J Allergy Clin Immunol 88:77–82, 1991.

Colloff MJ. Exposure to house dust mites in homes of people with atopic dermatitis. Br J Dermatol 127:322–327, 1992.

Colloff MJ, Ayres J, Carswell F, et al. The control of allergens of dust mites and domestic pets: A position paper. Clin Exp Allergy 22(suppl 2):1–28, 1992.

Czuppon AB, Chen Z, Rennert S, Engelke T, Meyer H, Heber M, Baur X. The rubber elongation factor of rubber trees (*Hevea braziliensis*) is the major allergen in latex. J Allergy Clin Immunol 92:690–697, 1993.

De Groot H, van Swieten P, Aalberse RC. Evidence for a *Fel d* I-like molecule in the "big cats" (Felidae species). J Allergy Clin Immunol 86:107–116, 1990.

Dorward AJ, Colloff MJ, MacKay NS, et al. Effect of house dust mite avoidance measures on adult atopic asthma. Thorax 43:98–102, 1988.

Duff AL, Platts-Mills TAE. Allergens and asthma. Pediatr Clin North Am 39:1277–1291, 1992.

Fernandez-Caldas E, Fox RW. Environmental control of indoor air pollution. Med Clin North Am 76:935–952, 1992.

Gad El Rab MO, Kay AB. Widespread immunoglobulin E-mediated hypersensitivity in the Sudan to the "green nimitti" midge, *Cladotanytarsus lewisi* (dipter: Chironomidae). J Allergy Clin Immunol 66:190–197, 1980.

Gordon S, Tee RD, Lowson D, Wallace J, Taylor AJN. Reduction of airborne allergenic urinary proteins from laboratory rats. Br J Indust Hyg Med 49:416–422, 1992.

Hallas TE. The biology of mites. Allergy 46(suppl 11):6–9, 1991.

Hart BJ, Guerin B, Nolard N. *In vitro* evaluation of acaricidal and fungicidal activity of the house dust mite acaricide, Allerbiocid. Clin Exp Allergy 22:923–928, 1992.

Helm RM, Squillace DL, Jones RT, et al. Shared allergenic activity in Asian (*Blatella asahinai*), German (*Blattella germanica*), American (*Periplaneta americana*), and Oriental (*Blatta orientalis*) cockroach species. Int Arch Allergy Appl Immunol 92:154–161, 1990.

Iverson M, Dahl R. Allergy to storage mites in asthmatic patients and its relation to damp housing conditions. Allergy 45:81–85, 1990.

James JM, Cooke SK, Barnett A, Sampson HA. Anaphylactic reactions to a psyllium-containing cereal. J Allergy Clin Immunol 88:402–408, 1991.

Johansson SGO, Wüthrich B, Zortea-Caflish C. Nightly asthma caused by allergens in silk-filled bed quilts: clinical and immunologic studies. J Allergy Clin Immunol 75:452–459, 1985.

Kang BC, Johnson J, Veres-Thorner C. Atopic profile of inner-city asthma with a comparative analysis on the cockroach-sensitive and ragweed-sensitive subgroups. J Allergy Clin Immunol 92:802–811, 1993.

Kelly KJ, Kurup V, Zacharisen M, Resnick A, Fink JN. Skin and serologic testing in the diagnosis of latex allergy. J Allergy Clin Immunol 91:1140–1145, 1993.

Kifugi K, McCullough J, Ownby DR. Relationship between dust mite allergen and human IgA in house dust samples. Ann Allergy 70:219–224, 1993.

Kino T, Oshima S. Allergy to insects in Japan. I. The reaginic sensitivity to moth and butterfly in patients with bronchial asthma. J Allergy Clin Immunol 61:10–16, 1978.

Korsgaard J, Iversen M. Epidemiology of house dust mite allergy. Allergy 46(suppl 11):14–18, 1991.

Lagier F, Cartier A, Somer J, Dolovich J, Malo J-L. Occupational asthma caused by guar gum. J Allergy Clin Immunol 85:785–790, 1990.

Lang JD, Mulla MS. Distribution and abundance of house dust mites, *Dermatophagoides* spp., in different climatic zones of southern California. Environ Entomol 6:213–216, 1977.

Lehrer SB, Karr RM, Müller DJG, Salvaggio JE. Detection of castor allergens in castor wax. Clin Allergy 10:33–41, 1980.

Lehrer SB, Karr RM, Salvaggio JE. Analysis of green coffee bean and castor bean allergens using RAST inhibition. Clin Allergy 11:357–366, 1981.

Miyamoto T, Oshima S, Ishizaki T, et al. Allergenic identity between the common floor mite (*Dermatophagoides farinae* Hughes, 1961) and house dust as a causative antigen in bronchial asthma. J Allergy 42:14–28, 1968.

Moore BS, Hyde JS. Breed-specific dog hypersensitivity in humans. J Allergy Clin Immunol 66:198, 1980.

Munir AKM, Einarsson R, Schou C, Dreborg SKG. Allergens in school dust. I. The amount of the major cat (*Fel d* I) and dog (*Can f* I) allergens in dust from Swedish schools is high enough to probably cause perennial symptoms in most children with asthma who are sensitized to cat and dog. J Allergy Clin Immunol 91:1067–1074, 1993.

Murray AB, Ferguson AC. Dust-free bedrooms in the treatment of asthmatic children with house or house dust mite allergy: A controlled trial. Pediatrics 71:418–422, 1983.

Osterman K, Zetterström O, Johansson SGO. Coffee worker's allergy. Allergy 37:313–322, 1982.

Nelson HS, Hirsch SR, Ohman JL, et al. Recommendations for the use of residential air-cleaning devices in the treatment of allergic respiratory diseases. J Allergy Clin Immunol 82:661–669, 1988.

Platts-Mills TAE, Heymann PW, Longbottom JL, Wilkins SR. Airborne allergens associated with asthma: particle sizes carrying dust mite and rat allergens measured with a cascade impactor. J Allergy Clin Immunol 77:850–857, 1986.

Platts-Mills TAE, Ward GW, Sporik R, Gelber LE, Chapman MD, Heymann PW. Epidemiology of the relationship between exposure to indoor allergens and asthma. Int Arch Allergy Appl Immunol 94:339–345, 1991.

Pollart S, Chapman MD, Platts-Mills TAE. House dust mite and dust control. Clin Rev Allergy 6:23–33, 1988.

Pollart SM, Chapman MD, Fiocco GP, et al. Epidemiology of acute asthma: IgE antibodies to common inhalant allergens as a risk factor for emergency room visits. J Allergy Clin Immunol 83:875–882, 1989.

Pollart SM, Smith TF, Morris EC, et al. Environment exposure to cockroach allergens: Analysis with monoclonal antibody-based immunoassays. J Allergy Clin Immunol 87:505–510, 1991.

Ramirez MA. Pyrethrum: An etiologic factor in vasomotor rhinitis and asthma. J Allergy 1:149, 1930.

Reisman RE, Mauriello PM, Davis GB, et al. A double-blind study of the effectiveness of a high-efficiency particulate air (HEPA) filter in the treatment of patients with perennial allergic rhinitis and asthma. J Allergy Clin Immunol 85:1050–1057, 1990.

Sakaguchi M, Inouye S, Irie T, Miyazawa H, Watanabe M, Yasueda H, Shida T, Nitta H, Chapman MD, Schou C, Aalberse RC. Airborne cat (*Fel d* I), dog (*Can f* I), and mite (*Der* I and *Der* II) allergen levels in the homes of Japan. J Allergy Clin Immunol 92:797–802, 1993.

Schou C, Lind P, Fernandez-Caldas E, et al. Identification and purification of an important cross-reactive allergen from American (*Periplaneta americana*) and German (*Blattella germanica*) cockroach. J Allergy Clin Immunol 86:935–946, 1990.

Sheldon JM, Lovell RG, Mathews KP. A Manual of Clinical Allergy. 2nd ed. Philadelphia, WB Saunders Company, 1967.

Shen H-D, Chua K-Y, Lin K-L, et al. Molecular cloning of a house dust mite allergen with common antibody binding specificities with multiple components in mite extracts. Clin Exp Allergy 23:934–940, 1993.

Spitzauer S, Schweiger C, Anrather J, Ebner C, Scheiner O, Kraft D, Rumpold H. Characterization of dog allergens by means of immunoblotting. Int Arch Allergy Appl Immunol 100:60–67, 1993.

Sporik R, Chapman MD, Platts-Mills TAE. House dust mite as a cause of asthma. Clin Exp Allergy 22:897–906, 1992.

Sporik R, et al. Exposure to house-dust mite allergen (*Der p* I) and the development of asthma in childhood: A prospective study. N Engl J Med 323:502–507, 1990.

Swanson MC, Campbell AR, Lauck PA-C, et al. Correlations between levels of mite and cat allergens in settled and airborne dust. J Allergy Clin Immunol 83:776–783, 1989.

Topping MD, Henderson RT, Luczynska CM, Woodmass A. Castor bean allergy among workers in the felt industry. Allergy 37:603–608, 1982.

Tovey ER, Chapman MD, Platts-Mills TAE. Mite faeces are a major source of house dust mite allergens. Nature 289:592–593, 1981.

van Toorenenbergen AW, Gerth van Wijk R, van Dooremalen G, Dieges PH. Immunoglobulin E antibodies against budgerigar and canary feathers. Int Arch Allergy Appl Immunol 77:433–437, 1985.

Voorhorst R, Spieksma FTM, Varekamp H, et al. The house-dust mite (*Dermatophagoides pteronyssinus*) and the allergens it produces. Identity with the house-dust allergen. J Allergy 39:325–339, 1967.

Voorhorst R. The human dander atopy. I. The prototype of auto-atopy. Ann Allergy 39:205–212, 1977.

Warner JA, Longbottom JL. Allergy to rabbits. III. Further identification and characterization of rabbit allergens. Allergy 46:481–491, 1991.

Wood RA, Chapman MD, Adkinson NF Jr, et al. The effect of cat removal on allergen content in household-dust samples. J Allergy Clin Immunol 83:730–734, 1989.

Wood RA, Mudd KE, Eggleston PA. The distribution of cat and dust mite allergens on wall surfaces. J Allergy Clin Immunol 89:126–130, 1992.

Zuskin E, Kanceljak B, Schachter EN, Witek TJ, Maayani S, Goswami S, Marom Z, Rienzi N. Immunological findings in hemp workers. Environ Res 59:350–361, 1992.

Zwick H, Popp W, Sertl K, et al. Allergenic structures in cockroach hypersensitivity. J Allergy Clin Immunol 87:626–630, 1991.

Chapter 9

Nonallergenic Environmental Factors

Jane Q. Koenig, Ph.D., and Paul V. Williams, M.D.

Outdoor air pollution in the United States was first regulated at the national level by the Clean Air Act (CAA) of 1970. Actions authorized by the CAA have led to reductions of sulfur dioxide (SO_2) and total suspended particulate matter. At the same time, however, the population of the United States has grown substantially, with the attendant growth of automobiles and other vehicles producing troublesome concentrations of nitrogen oxide, ozone, fine particles, and other toxic emissions in many urban (and suburban) areas. In 1989, over 85 million individuals in the United States lived in counties exceeding the National Ambient Air Quality Standards (NAAQS) for at least one air pollutant (EPA, 1991) (Fig. 9–1).

The 1980s saw an increase in the prevalence, mortality, and morbidity of asthma (Fig. 9–2). This was manifested by an increase in hospitalizations for asthma, particularly in children less than 15 years old. In 1993, the Centers for Disease Control and Prevention issued statistics on the estimated populations at risk residing in communities that did not attain one or more of the national air quality standards in 1991 (Table 9–1). There is great concern that the changing patterns of air pollution exposure in the United States are partially responsible for the discouraging and alarming asthma statistics (Scott, 1990; Molfino et al, 1992). The increases in morbidity and mortality mentioned above have been more marked in blacks and other inner-city residents. Exposure to outdoor and indoor air pollutants may be greater for minority children, since they tend to live closer to pollutant sources such as freeways, industrial sites, and disposal sites. This is particularly true in the bigger cities, where asthma mortality rates are among the highest (Evans, 1992; Weiss et al, 1992a).

This chapter will summarize the known relationships between air pollution and allergic disease, relying on a review of human laboratory and epidemiologic studies. The outdoor pollutants of concern are the "criteria pollutants" regulated by the U.S. Environmental Protection Agency (EPA) and the source-dependent "air toxics." Indoor air man-made pollutants include many of the same chemicals, although the pattern of exposure differs from that of outdoor exposures.

OUTDOOR AIR POLLUTANTS

The six air pollutants regulated by the NAAQS are SO_2, ozone (O_3), nitrogen dioxide (NO_2), particulate matter equal to or less than 10 micrometers in diameter (PM_{10}), carbon monoxide (CO), and airborne lead. Since both CO and lead affect organ systems other than the respiratory system, they are not discussed here. Table 9–2 lists the concentration and averaging time for the six criteria pollutants. Each of the four pollutants of concern for respiratory risk has been shown to aggravate allergic diseases.

Sulfur Dioxide (SO_2)

CONTROLLED LABORATORY STUDIES. Sulfur dioxide is a primary pollutant emitted from coal-fired power plants, smelters, refineries, paper and pulp mills, and food processing.

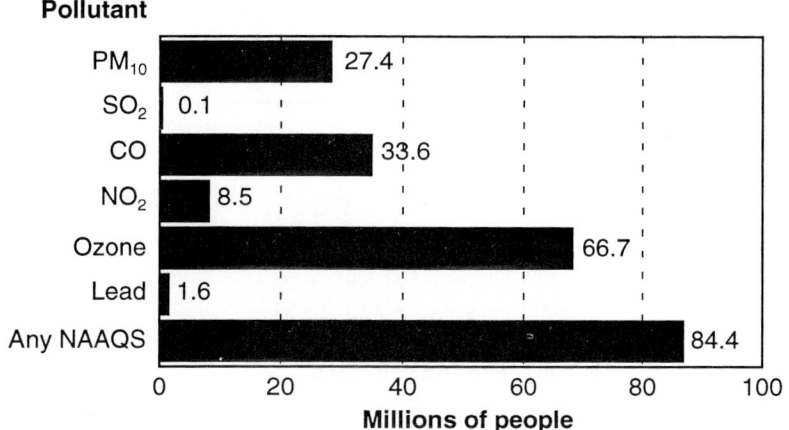

FIGURE 9–1. Populations in countries with measured air pollutant concentrations above primary National Ambient Air Quality Standards (1989). (From National Air Quality and Emissions Trends Report, 1989. EPA-450/4-91-003, Feb 1991.)

Exposure to SO_2 is associated with exaggerated decrements in pulmonary function in subjects with asthma (Koenig et al, 1981, 1983a; Sheppard et al, 1981). For instance, Koenig et al (1981) exposed nine adolescent subjects (aged 14 to 18 years)—all of whom had allergic asthma as well as exercise-induced bronchospasm (EIB)—to 1.0 ppm SO_2 during moderate exercise. Pulmonary function was measured before, during, and after the exposures. The combination of exercise and SO_2 elicited large changes in all the pulmonary function measurements (Table 9–3).

In general, subjects with asthma experience significant decrements in pulmonary function at concentrations of SO_2 (0.5 ppm) that are at least an order of magnitude lower than the levels affecting individuals without asthma (5.0 ppm). Some studies indicate that only 2.5 minutes of exposure to 0.25 ppm SO_2 is an adequate stimulus to produce significant SO_2-induced bronchoconstriction (Horstman et al, 1988). The effects of inhaled SO_2 in asthmatic patients have been shown to be exaggerated by combination of SO_2 with cold air (Linn et al, 1984; Bethel et al, 1984) and by prior exposure to ozone (Koenig et al, 1990).

SO_2 affects the upper respiratory tract as well. SO_2 is a highly water-soluble gas and has been shown to be taken up readily in the nasal passages during quiet breathing (Speizer and Frank, 1966). Exposure to 1.0 ppm SO_2 increased the work of breathing through the nose in a group of adolescent subjects with asthma (Koenig et al, 1985).

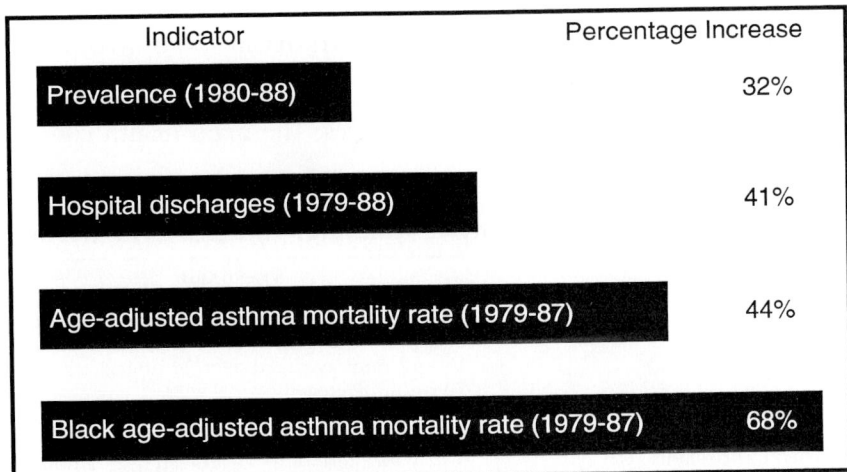

FIGURE 9–2. Asthma on the rise. For reasons that remain unclear, the number of deaths due to asthma and the number of people with asthma appear to be rising throughout the United States. (Source: American Lung Association, 1990.)

TABLE 9–1. ESTIMATED POPULATIONS AT RISK RESIDING IN COMMUNITIES THAT HAVE NOT ATTAINED ONE OR MORE NATIONAL AMBIENT AIR QUALITY STANDARD—UNITED STATES, 1991

Population Subgroup at Risk	Pollutant	At-Risk Population Living in Nonattainment Areas	
		No.	(%)
Preadolescent children (aged ≤13 yrs)	PM_{10}, SO_2, O_3, NO_2	31,528,939	(63)
Elderly (aged ≥65 yrs)	PM_{10}, SO_2, O_3	18,846,666	(60)
Persons with pediatric asthma	PM_{10}, SO_2, O_3, NO_2	2,285,061	(61)
Adults (aged ≥18 yrs) with asthma	PM_{10}, SO_2, O_3, NO_2	4,279,413	(65)
Persons with chronic obstructive pulmonary disease	PM_{10}, SO_2, O_3, NO_2	8,831,970	(64)
Persons with coronary heart disease	CO	3,493,847	(33)
Pregnant women	CO, Pb	1,602,045	(38)
Children aged ≤5 yrs	Pb	74,312	(3)

Morb and Mortal Wkly Rep, 42:302, 1993.

EPIDEMIOLOGIC STUDIES. Cross-sectional epidemiologic studies have noted decreased pulmonary function (Stern et al, 1989) and increased rates of respiratory illness, cough, wheeze, and lower respiratory infection (Ware et al, 1986; Dockery et al, 1989) in large groups of children living in areas with high concentrations of ambient sulfates, including SO_2, and other fine particulate matter. A recent study in Vancouver, British Columbia, found a significant association between visits to hospital emergency departments for asthma and ambient levels of SO_2 and sulfuric acid (Bates et al, 1990). Sulfur dioxide concentrations in community air tend to be highly correlated with levels of fine particles. As discussed later in this chapter, fine particles have been associated with a number of adverse respiratory outcomes. It is difficult to differentiate between the effects of SO_2 and the effects of particles in the statistical models used to test for respiratory effects.

However, it appears that the particles are more important in the equation than the SO_2. Therefore it is hard to describe the exact effect of airborne SO_2 on respiratory morbidity and mortality.

There have been two reports of SO_2 morbidity after accidental exposures in the workplace. In one study, seven workers were followed for 4 years (Harkonen et al, 1993). A reversible obstruction of the bronchi was still observable 3 years after the accidental exposure. A retrospective study of accidental SO_2 exposures in 230 workers found an average change of -291.9 ml in FEV_1 (Henneberger et al, 1993).

Nitrogen Dioxide (NO_2)

CONTROLLED LABORATORY STUDIES. Nitrogen dioxide is primarily a combustion pollutant emitted from mobile and stationary sources. The main health concerns regarding

TABLE 9–2. UNITED STATES NATIONAL AMBIENT AIR QUALITY STANDARDS

Pollutant	Standard
Sulfur dioxide (SO_2)	0.14 ppm (365 $\mu g/m^3$) averaged over 24 hours*
	0.03 ppm (80 $\mu g/m^3$*) averaged over 1 year
Total particulates (PM_{10})	150 $\mu g/mm^3$ averaged over 24 hours*
	50 $\mu g/m^3$ averaged over 1 year
Carbon monoxide (CO)	35 ppm (40 $\mu g/m^3$) averaged over 1 hour*
	9 ppm (10 $\mu g/m^3$) averaged over 8 hours
Photochemical oxidants (O_3)	0.12 ppm (240 $\mu g/m^3$) averaged over 1 hour*
Nitrogen dioxide (NO_2)	0.05 ppm (100 $\mu g/m^3$) averaged over 1 year
Airborne lead	1.5 $\mu g/m^3$ averaged over 24 hours

*May be exceeded once per year.

TABLE 9–3. PERCENTAGE CHANGE IN PULMONARY FUNCTION MEASUREMENTS AFTER EXPOSURE TO SO₂ OR AIR IN NINE ADOLESCENT ASTHMATIC SUBJECTS

MEASUREMENT	CHANGE FROM BASELINE	
	With SO$_2$	With Air
FEV$_1$	23% decrease	0% change
Resp resistance	67% increase	13% decrease
Maximal flow (50)	44% decrease	9% increase
Maximal flow (75)	50% decrease	24% increase

NO$_2$ exposure are (1) increased bronchial hyperresponsiveness after exposure in controlled settings and (2) possible increased infectivity in human subjects similar to that clearly seen in animal toxicologic studies.

Although controlled exposures to ambient level concentrations of NO$_2$ have not resulted in significant, consistent decrements in pulmonary function measurements, such exposures have been associated with increased airway hyperresponsiveness. Folinsbee (1992) recently published the results of a meta-analysis of 25 studies evaluating the relationship between controlled inhalation of NO$_2$ and enhanced bronchial hyperresponsiveness (BHR). The sample included 20 studies with asthmatic subjects and five with healthy subjects. The NO$_2$ concentrations ranged from as low as 0.1 ppm in the studies with asthmatic subjects and reached as high as 7.5 ppm in studies with healthy subjects. A variety of stimuli were used to test for BHR, including methacholine, histamine, SO$_2$, cold air, and allergens. The conclusion from this analysis was that there was an overall trend toward increased BHR (+60 percent) after NO$_2$ stimuli among subjects with asthma.

Three studies using controlled laboratory protocols have investigated markers of infectivity in healthy human subjects. Two studies found no evidence for increased infectivity (Pinkston et al, 1988; Rubinstein et al, 1991). On the other hand, Frampton et al (1989) reported evidence of increased susceptibility to infections in human subjects exposed to NO$_2$. They found that alveolar macrophages (AM) retrieved from subjects after exposure to NO$_2$ were deficient in their virus inactivation compared to AMs from air-exposed subjects. Another study looked directly at the effect of NO$_2$ exposure on infectivity in healthy adult subjects by instilling attenuated cold-adapted viruses into the nostrils of subjects exposed to either air or 1-, 2-, or 3-ppm NO$_2$ (Goings et al, 1989). A total of 152 subjects were studied over the 3-year period of this study. Infection was determined by virus recovery or by a fourfold or greater increase in serum or nasal wash influenza-specific antibody titers, or by both. Although the differences between air and NO$_2$ treatment were not statistically significant, 91 percent of the subjects became infected after NO$_2$ exposure compared to 71 percent after air. Unfortunately, no research evaluating changes in susceptibility to infection after NO$_2$ exposure in subjects with allergy and/or asthma has been reported.

EPIDEMIOLOGIC STUDIES. Epidemiologic studies suggest that indoor exposure of children to NO$_2$ from combustion sources is the major health risk from this pollutant at this time. Although the results of individual studies are inconclusive, a recent meta-analysis of epidemiologic studies of exposure in children to indoor concentrations of NO$_2$ found an odds ratio of 1.2 for increased respiratory illness associated with long-term exposure to 30 µg/m^3 NO$_2$ (~15 ppb) (Hasselblad et al, 1992). None of the studies in the data base was designed to test the sensitivity of susceptible populations such as children with asthma. Also, actual concentrations of indoor NO$_2$ were not measured in most studies. As part of the Harvard Six-City Study, Neas and co-workers (1991) reported in a sample of 1500+ children aged 7 to 11 that annual exposure to NO$_2$ was positively associated with increased chronic respiratory symptoms. The symptoms recorded were shortness of breath with wheeze, chronic wheeze, chronic cough, and chronic phlegm. In general, a 15 ppb increase in the annual NO$_2$ levels within households was significantly associated with the cumulative incidence of these lower respiratory tract symptoms. The overall odds ratio was 1.4 (95 percent CI, 1.1 to 1.7). Girls had a stronger association than boys (odds ratio of 1.7 vs 1.2). There was no association with standard pulmonary function measurements. These results could be interpreted as showing an adverse respiratory effect from NO$_2$ at concentrations found indoors.

Ozone (O$_3$)

Ozone is the most ubiquitous air pollutant in the United States. It is a secondary pollutant produced by the interaction of sunlight and chemical precursors (nitrogen oxides and volatile hydrocarbons). Over 66 million individuals live in areas where the ozone concentration exceeds the NAAQS set by the EPA (EPA, 1991). Two excellent reviews of the respiratory effects of ozone are available (Lippmann, 1992; Beckett, 1991).

CONTROLLED LABORATORY STUDIES. Careful dose-response relationships between ozone concentrations and durations of exposure in healthy subjects have shown that 10 to 20 percent of subjects are unusually sensitive (McDonnell et al, 1983) and that FEV_1 values continue to decrease with length of exposure up to 6 hours (Horstman and Folinsbee, 1990). The primary effects of ozone exposure are reduced lung function, pain upon deep inspiration (believed to be the mechanism for the lung function decrements), and cough.

There is controversy regarding the population most sensitive to ozone. One impacted group consists of individuals who exercise vigorously outdoors in urban areas with elevated concentrations of ozone. Reviews often conclude that asthmatic subjects are no more sensitive to ozone than healthy subjects. However, at least four studies indicate that asthmatics show an increased sensitivity to ozone. Silverman (1979) found consistent decreases in the maximal expiratory flow rate in asthmatic subjects exposed to 0.25 ppm O_3 for 2 hours. Kreit and co-workers (1989) reported greater pulmonary function changes in asthmatic subjects than in healthy subjects after exposure to 0.40 ppm O_3. (Peak concentrations of O_3 in Los Angeles are now in the range of 0.30 to 0.35 ppm). Hackney and co-workers reported that more subjects who showed sensitivity to O_3 exposure had bronchial hyperresponsiveness than did a group of ozone nonresponders (1989). Additional evidence comes from a study by Aris et al (1991), who found that ozone-sensitive subjects had positive responses to a methacholine challenge whereas matched ozone-insensitive subjects did not. One controlled laboratory study was conducted with young children aged 8 to 11 years, evaluating the effects of exposure to 0.12 ppm O_3 during vigorous exercise (McDonnell, 1985). Although the children were healthy, the study is of interest because, unlike studies with adults, which find decrements in pulmonary function and increases in symptoms, the young children reported no symptoms. This finding may be a matter of concern, since symptoms of respiratory distress can serve as a defense mechanism to stop or slow exertion. There is also concern about interactions between outdoor air pollutants and allergens in sensitized individuals. Molfino et al (1991) compared the effects of ragweed allergen with and without exposure to 0.12 ppm O_3 in seven asthmatic subjects. Ozone exposure halved the amount of allergen required to reduce FEV_1 by 15 percent.

Two important questions for research in the field of health effects of air pollution—ethnic and gender diversity—have been broached in studies of ozone. Early findings of enhanced effects of ozone in women were criticized as confounded by lung size. Messineo and Adams (1990) studied two groups of women, one with an average vital capacity of 3.7 liters and the other with an average of 5.1 liters. Both groups showed equal decrements in FVC and FEV_1 after exposure to both 0.18 and 0.30 ppm O_3. In a comparison of the potential effects of ethnicity, separate groups of male and female African-American and Caucasian young healthy adult subjects were exposed to six concentrations of ozone ranging from 0 to 0.40 ppm (Seal et al, 1993). Although the analysis of variance for all groups combined did not find a significant interaction between ozone and race, black males had significant pulmonary function decrements compared to white males after ozone exposure. Since many areas with elevated air pollution also have high minority populations, additional research into ethnic variations in this field is needed.

Another area of increasing interest is the search for biomarkers of effects or exposure in bronchoalveolar lavage fluid. Several studies have demonstrated increased inflammatory mediators, such as histamine and fibronectin, as well as markers of increased permeability, such as albumin, after O_3 exposure in healthy subjects (Koren et al, 1989; Graham and Koren, 1990); however, no studies of subjects with asthma have been reported.

The upper respiratory tract does not receive nearly as much attention as the lung in studies of air pollution effects. Bascom and associates evaluated the effects of O_3 inhalation in a group of subjects with allergic rhinitis using a nasal lavage procedure (1990). One purpose of the study was to detect O_3-enhanced responses to allergens. Although none was seen, several markers of O_3-induced tissue damage were seen; increased concentrations of histamine and albumin were detected in nasal lavage fluid. Also a recent study in our laboratory compared ozone exposures (0.120 and 0.240 ppm) in asthmatic and healthy subjects and found increased neutrophils in nasal lavage fluid only in the asthmatics (Williams et al, 1992; McBride et al, 1994).

EPIDEMIOLOGIC STUDIES. Ozone exposure has not been convincingly associated with increased mortality, but it has been tied to increases in respiratory morbidity. Kinney et al (1989) conducted repeated measurements of lung function on 154 elementary school children in Tennessee and found that decrements in FVC, FEV_1, and maximal flow were associated with daily O_3 concentrations. The maximal hourly O_3 level was 78 ppb which is considerably below the NAAQS for O_3 (120 ppb). Both emergency room visits in New Jersey (Cody et al, 1992) and hospital admissions in Southern Ontario, Canada (Bates and Sizto, 1987) have been associated with elevated concentrations of O_3. The latter study concluded that some other atmospheric condition in the summer was affecting respiratory disease and suggested that it might be an "acid summer haze." In a study designed to investigate the lasting effects of elevated ozone concentrations in children, Zwick et al (1991) examined pulmonary function, bronchial hyperresponsiveness, allergic sensitization, and serum lymphocyte subpopulations in 10- to 14-year-old children in Austria. Children were recruited from an area with high ozone concentrations (group A) and also from an area with lower ozone concentrations (group B). There were no differences in respiratory symptoms or lung function between groups, but the children in group A had more frequent and more severe bronchial hyperresponsiveness tested with methacholine challenges. Also in group A, the numbers of helper T cells were decreased and those of suppressor T cells were increased, which resulted in a significantly low helper/suppressor cell index. These findings suggest a relationship between elevated ozone and a worsening of asthma.

Particulate Matter Less than 10 Micrometers in Diameter (PM_{10})

CONTROLLED LABORATORY STUDIES. It is not possible to accurately reproduce in a laboratory exposure system the complex atmospheric nature of community PM_{10}. However, one form of PM_{10}, sulfuric acid (H_2SO_4), has been shown in laboratory experiments in subjects with asthma to decrease pulmonary function (Koenig et al, 1983b; Hanley et al, 1992) and may aid in the interpretation of the effects of acid summer haze.

EPIDEMIOLOGIC STUDIES. In the last 5 years, a handful of studies have brought attention to the harmful effects of fine particles on the respiratory system. Several of these studies were conducted by Pope and associates in the Salt Lake City area where a steel mill is the primary emitter of the fine particles. These studies have associated PM_{10} with increased medication use in both children and adults with asthma and peak flow decrements and increased respiratory symptoms in nonasthmatic subjects (Pope et al, 1991). Elementary school absences in this community were reported in a separate study; the children were not screened for asthma (Ransom and Pope, 1992).

The most alarming association between health and PM_{10} comes from a series of studies conducted by Schwartz and co-workers, which have been reviewed recently (1991/92). In summary, these studies find a consistent 6 to 7 percent increase in mortality associated with an average 100 $\mu g/m^3$ increase in daily PM_{10} levels in several communities of diverse meteorologic conditions. A glance at Table 9–2 reveals that the EPA standard for PM_{10} for a 24-hour period is 150 $\mu g/m^3$. When these investigators performed an analysis on individuals tracked for 14 to 16 years, the increased risk of death was even higher (26 percent) (Dockery et al, 1993). The deaths are from both respiratory and cardiac causes; asthma was not reported as a single item. However, a recent study in Seattle found a significant association ($p < 0.005$) between emergency department visits for asthma and PM_{10} concentrations in persons under the age of 65 years (Schwartz et al, 1993). The PM_{10} level in Seattle during the study period (1989 to 1990) did not exceed 103 $\mu g/m^3$, raising concern that the current standard of 150 $\mu g/m^3$ is not sufficiently protective.

Wood Smoke

Wood smoke is a special category of PM_{10}. In some communities where wood is burned frequently during the winter months, wood smoke is responsible for as much as 80 percent of PM_{10} in residential neighborhoods. Epidemiologic research has shown that wood smoke is a risk factor for increased respiratory symptoms, increased lower respiratory tract disease, and decreased pulmonary function in young children. These data have been reviewed recently (Larson and Koenig, 1994). Other forms of burning can also affect patients with asthma. One study demonstrated a decrease in pulmonary function in individuals with asthma exposed to open leaf burning during low-level exercise such as walking (From et al, 1992).

INDOOR AIR POLLUTION

As the quality of our outdoor air improves with enforcement of air pollution guidelines, the quality of indoor air becomes more important. This is particularly true since people spend the majority of their time indoors.

Epidemiologic studies have shown a significant association between the physician's diagnosis of asthma and a variety of indoor air pollutants (Dekker et al, 1991). Two common forms of indoor air pollution have been covered as outdoor pollutants, NO_2 and wood smoke. Wood smoke concentrations outdoors are predictive of indoor concentrations since the fine particles (in general less than 1 μg/m³) readily penetrate indoors. In fact, this penetration is true of most PM_{10} from other combustion sources as well, since these particles are also extremely small. This outdoor-indoor ratio of PM_{10}, ranging from 0.55 to 0.70, may help to explain the PM_{10}-mortality associations, which seem counterintuitive if people actually spend only 5 to 10 percent of their time outdoors.

Environmental Tobacco Smoke (ETS)

Data concerning the relationship between exposure to ETS and respiratory health were reviewed by a National Research Council committee in 1986 (National Academy Press, 1986). Children with asthma who live with a mother who smokes have significantly more symptoms, lower FEV_1 values, and a greater responsiveness to a histamine challenge test than children with asthma whose mother does not smoke (Murray and Morrison, 1986). In a study of 9-year-old school children, boys who lived with parents who smoked had increased bronchial hyperresponsiveness compared to boys who lived with parents who did not smoke (odds ratio = 4.3, p = 0.009) (Martinez et al, 1988). The effect was not significant in girls. The authors conclude that the increased frequency of bronchial hyperresponsiveness may increase the risk of development of asthma. There also is evidence that ETS can cause asthma. Weitzman et al (1990), using National Health Interview Survey data, found asthma to be present in 2.3 percent of children of nonsmoking mothers, 2.6 percent of children whose mothers smoked less than 0.5 packs per day, and 4.8 percent of children whose mothers smoked more than 0.5 packs per day. Seventy percent of children in the United States live in houses where at least one adult smokes (Weiss et al, 1983). With respect to adverse respiratory outcomes and ETS, it is not always clear whether the harmful exposure occurred postnatally or *in utero*. The American Academy of Pediatrics found that 26 percent of children in the United States live in a household with a mother who reported smoking during pregnancy (1986).

Sick Building Syndrome

A combination of synthetic chemicals in construction products and tightening of buildings for energy conservation has created residences and workplaces where occupants complain of myriad symptoms. These symptoms—which include headache; eye, nose, and throat irritation; fatigue; dizziness; and nausea (Stolwijk, 1991)—are often attributed to "sick building syndrome." Unfortunately, because these symptoms are commonly caused by conditions other than indoor air pollution and because they are difficult to quantify, attempts to evaluate this syndrome have not been successful. Some of these symptoms are present in individuals with allergic disease.

Several years ago, EPA conducted a survey of agents found indoors that had toxic potential. That study, called the Total Exposure Assessment Methodology (TEAM), concluded that exposures to volatile compounds, including toluene, benzene, chloroform, tetrachloroethylene, and p-dichlorobenzene, were significantly higher in indoor air than in outdoor air (Wallace et al, 1986). However, it is extremely difficult to connect symptoms of ill ease with a particular chemical exposure. Formaldehyde is often considered as a cause of irritation from indoor air due to its presence in building materials. Controlled laboratory studies of subjects with asthma exposed to 1 to 3 ppm formaldehyde have found no effect on pulmonary function tests (Sheppard et al, 1984; Witek et al, 1987). In retrospect, these findings are not surprising since formaldehyde is extremely water-soluble and would be taken up by the nasal mucosa under normal breathing conditions. In fact, it is the nose that has been shown to be a target organ for formaldehyde exposure predisposing to nasal cancer in rodents (Kerns et al, 1983). A recent review of the immunologic effects of formaldehyde concluded that there were no conclusive studies showing the development of IgE-mediated respiratory tract symptoms secondary to inhalation of formaldehyde (Bardana and Montanaro, 1991).

THE ECONOMIC BURDEN OF AIR POLLUTION

One study attempted an analysis of the economic value of health benefits of clean air. In the Los Angeles area, it is estimated that PM_{10} causes an increased risk of death in any year of 1 person per 10,000, and O_3 causes up to 17 days of adverse respiratory symptoms (Hall et al, 1992). Specifically for asthma, Weiss et al (1992b) found the cost of illness related to asthma in 1990 to be approximately $6.2 billion. Since air pollution has been significantly associated with emergency department visits for asthma, some percentage of the $6.2 billion is due to air pollution. In the Schwartz et al (1993) study in Seattle, we found that 12 percent of asthma visits were associated with PM_{10}. If that holds for the entire United States (Seattle is not an especially polluted city), the cost of PM_{10} alone for asthma would be over $7 million.

SUMMARY

The preponderance of scientific evidence from epidemiologic surveys and controlled exposure studies indicates that both indoor and outdoor pollutants, at levels of current exposure, are associated with an increase in respiratory symptoms and even mortality. Furthermore, patients with asthma are particularly sensitive to ambient levels of these pollutants, which are becoming increasingly important triggers of airway obstruction and inflammation.

REFERENCES

American Academy of Pediatrics Committee on Environmental Hazards. Involuntary smoking. A hazard to children. Pediatrics 77:755–757, 1986.

Aris R, Christian D, Sheppard D, Balmes JR. The effects of sequential exposure to acidic fog and ozone on pulmonary function in exercising subjects. Am Rev Respir Dis 143:85–91, 1991.

Bardana EJ Jr, Montanaro A. Formaldehyde: An analysis of its respiratory, cutaneous, and immunologic effects. Ann Allergy 66:441–452, 1991.

Bascom R, Naclerio RM, Fitzgerald TK, Kagey-Sobotka A, Proud D. Effect of ozone inhalation on the response to nasal challenge with antigen of allergic subjects. Am Rev Respir Dis 142:594–601, 1990.

Bates DV, Baker-Anderson M, Sizto R. Asthma attack periodicity: A study of hospital emergency visits in Vancouver. Environ Res 51:51–70, 1990.

Bates DV, Sizto R. Air pollution and hospital admissions in Southern Ontario: The acid summer haze effect. Environ Res 43:317–331, 1987.

Beckett WS. Ozone, air pollution, and respiratory health. Yale J Biol Med 64:167–175, 1991.

Bethel RA, Sheppard D, Epstein J. Interaction of sulfur dioxide and cold dry air in causing bronchoconstriction in asthmatic subjects. J Appl Physiol 57:491–423, 1984.

Cody RP, Weisel CP, Birnbaum G, Lioy PJ. The effect of ozone associated with summertime photochemical smog on the frequency of asthma visits to hospital emergency departments. Environ Res 58:184–194, 1992.

Dekker C, Dales R, Bartlett S, Brunekreef B, Zwanenberg H. Childhood asthma and the indoor environment. Chest 100:922–926, 1991.

Dockery DW, Pope CA III. Acute respiratory effects of particulate air pollution. Am Rev Public Health 15:107–132, 1994.

Dockery DW, Speizer FE, Stram DO, Ware JH, Spengler JD, Ferris Jr BG. Effects of inhalable particles on respiratory health of children. Am Rev Respir Dis 139:587–594, 1989.

EPA. National Air Quality and Emissions Trends Report, 1989. EPA-450/4-91-003, Feb 1991.

Evans R. Asthma among minority children. A growing problem. Chest 101:368S–371S, 1992.

Folinsbee LJ. Does nitrogen dioxide exposure increase airways responsiveness? Toxicol Indust Health 8:273–283, 1992.

Frampton MW, Smeglin AM, Roberts NJ Jr, Finkelstein JN, Morrow PE, Utell MJ. Nitrogen dioxide exposure in vivo and human alveolar macrophage inactivation of influenza virus in vitro. Environ Res 48:179–192, 1989.

From LJ, Bergen LC, Humlie CJ. The effects of open leaf burning on spirometric measurements in asthma. Chest 101:1236–1239, 1992.

Goings SA, Kulle TJ, Bascom R, Sauder LR. Effects of nitrogen dioxide exposure on susceptibility to influenza A virus infection in healthy adults. Am Rev Respir Dis 139:1075–1081, 1989.

Graham DE, Koren HS. Biomarkers of inflammation in ozone-exposed humans: Comparison of the nasal and

bronchoalveolar lavage. Am Rev Respir Dis 142:152–156, 1990.
Hackney JD, Linn WS, Shamoo DA, Avol EL. Responses of selected reactive and nonreactive volunteers to ozone exposure in high and low pollution seasons. *In* Schneider T, et al (eds). Atmospheric Ozone Research and Its Policy Implications. Amsterdam, The Netherlands, Elsevier, 1989, pp 311–318.
Hall JV, Winer AM, Kleinman MT, Lurmann FW, Brajer V, Colome SD. Valuing the health benefits of clean air. Science 255:812–817, 1992.
Hanley QS, Koenig JQ, Larson TV, Anderson TL, van Belle G, Rebolledo V, Covert DS, Pierson WE. Response of young asthmatics to inhaled sulfuric acid. Am Rev Respir Dis 145:326–331, 1992.
Harkonen H, Nordman H, Korhonen, Winblad I. Long-term effects of exposure to sulfur dioxide. Am Rev Respir Dis 128:890–893, 1983.
Hasselblad V, Eddy DM, Kotchmar DJ. Synthesis of environmental evidence; Nitrogen dioxide epidemiology studies. J Air Waste Manage Assoc 42:662–671, 1992.
Henneberger PK, Ferris BG Jr, Sheehe PR. Accidental gassing incidents and the pulmonary function of pulp mill workers. Am Rev Respir Dis 148:63–67, 1993.
Horstman DH, Folinsbee LJ. Ozone concentration and pulmonary response relationships for 6.6 hour exposures with five hours of moderate exercise to 0.08, 0.10, and 0.12 ppm. Am Rev Respir Dis 142:1158–1163, 1990.
Horstman DH, Seal L Jr, Folinsbee LJ, Ives P, Roger LJ. The relationship between exposure duration and sulfur dioxide-induced bronchoconstriction in asthmatic subjects. Am Ind Hyg Assoc J 49:38–47, 1988.
Kerns WD, Pavkov KL, Donofrio DJ, Gralla EJ, Swenbery JA. Of formaldehyde in rats and mice after long-term inhalation exposure. Cancer Res 43:4382–4392, 1983.
Kinney PL, Ware JH, Spengler JD, Dockery DW, Speizer FE, Ferris BG Jr. Short-term pulmonary function change in association with ozone levels. Am Rev Respir Dis 139:56–61, 1989.
Koenig JQ, Pierson WE, Horike M, Frank R. Effects of SO_2 plus NaCl aerosol combined with moderate exercise on pulmonary function in asthmatic adolescents. Environ Res 25:340–348, 1981.
Koenig JQ, Pierson WE, Horike M, Frank R. A comparison of the pulmonary effects of 0.5 ppm versus 1.0 ppm sulfur dioxide plus sodium chloride droplets in asthmatic adolescents. J Toxicol Environ Health 11:129–139, 1983a.
Koenig JQ, Pierson WE, Horike M. The effects of inhaled sulfuric acid on pulmonary function in adolescent asthmatics. Am Rev Respir Dis 128:221–225, 1983b.
Koenig JQ, Morgan MS, Horike M, Pierson WE. The effects of sulfur oxides on nasal and lung function in adolescents with extrinsic asthma. J Allergy Clin Immunol 76:813–818, 1985.
Koenig JQ, Covert DS, Hanley Q, van Belle G, Pierson WE. Prior exposure to ozone potentiates subsequent response to sulfur dioxide in adolescent asthmatic subjects. Am Rev Respir Dis 141:377–380, 1990.
Koren HS, Devlin RB, Graham DE et al. Ozone-induced inflammation in the lower airways of human subjects. Am Rev Respir Dis 139:407–415, 1989.
Kreit JW, Gross KB, Moore TB, Lorenzen TJ, D'Arcy J, Eschenbacher WL. Ozone-induced changes in pulmonary function and bronchial responsiveness in asthmatics. J Appl Physiol. 66:217–222, 1989.
Larson TV, Koenig JQ. Wood smoke: Emissions and non-cancer respiratory effects. Ann Rev Public Health 15:133–156, 1994.
Linn WS, Shamoo DA, Venet TG, Bailey RM, Wightman LH, Hackney JD. Comparative effects of sulfur dioxide exposures at 5°C and 25°C in exercising asthmatics. Am Rev Respir Dis 129:234–239, 1984.
Lippmann M. Environmental Toxicants: Human Exposures and Their Health Effects. New York, Van Nostrand Reinhold, 1992.
Martinez FD, Guiseppina A, Macri F, Conci E, Midulla F, De Castro G, Ronchetti R. Parental smoking enhances bronchial responsiveness in nine-year-old children. Am Rev Respir Dis 138:518–523, 1988.
McBride DE, Koenig JQ, Luchtel DL, Williams PV, Henderson WR Jr. Inflammatory effects of ozone in the upper airways of subjects with asthma. Am Rev Respir Crit Care Med 149:1192–1197, 1994.
McDonnell WF, Chapman RS, Leigh MW, Strope GL, Collier AM. Respiratory responses of vigorously exercising children to 0.12 ppm ozone exposure. Am Rev Respir Dis 132:875–879, 1985.
McDonnell WF, Horstman DH, Hazucha MJ, Seal E Jr. The pulmonary effects of ozone exposure: Dose-response characteristics. J Appl Physiol 54:1345–1352, 1983.
Messineo TD, Adams WC. Ozone inhalation effects in females varying widely in lung size: Comparison with males. J Appl Physiol 69:96–103, 1990.
Molfino NA, Slutsky AS, Zamel N. The effects of air pollution on allergic bronchial responsiveness. Clin Exp Allergy 22:667–672, 1992.
Molfino NA, Wright SC, Katz I, Tarlo S, Silverman F, McClean PA, et al. Effect of low concentrations of ozone on inhaled allergen responses in asthmatic subjects. Lancet 338:199–203, 1991.
Murray AB, Morrison BJ. The effect of cigarette smoke from the other on bronchial responsiveness and severity of symptoms in children with asthma. J Allergy Clin Immunol 77:575–581, 1986.
National Academy of Science, Environmental tobacco smoke. National Research Council. Washington, DC. National Academy Press, 1986.
Neas LM, Dockery DW, Ware JH, Spengler JD, Speizer FE, Ferris BG Jr. Association of indoor nitrogen dioxide with respiratory symptoms and pulmonary function in children. Am J Epidemiol 134:204–219, 1991.
Pinkston P, Smeglin A, Roberts NJ Jr, Gibb FR, Morrow PE, Utell MJ. Effects of in vitro exposure to nitrogen dioxide on human alveolar macrophage release of neutrophil chemotactic factor and interleukin-1. Environ Res 47:48–58, 1988.
Pope CA III, Dockery DW, Spengler JD, Raizenne ME. Respiratory health and PM_{10} pollution: A daily time series analysis. Am Rev Respir Dis 144:668–674, 1991.
Ransom MR, Pope CA III. Elementary school absences and PM_{10} pollution in Utah Valley. Environ Res 58:204–219, 1992.
Rubinstein I, Reiss TF, Bigby BG, Stities DP, Boushey HA Jr. Effects of 0.60 ppm nitrogen dioxide on circulating and bronchoalveolar lavage lymphocyte phenotypes in healthy subjects. Environ Res 55:18–30, 1991.
Schwartz J, Slater D, Larson TV, Pierson WE, Koenig JQ. Particulate air pollution and hospital emergency room visits for asthma in Seattle. 147:826–831, 1993.
Schwartz J. Particulate air pollution and daily mortality: A synthesis. Public Health Rev 19:39–60, 1991/92.
Scott M. Study links pollution with increase in asthma. Environ Health Newsletter 29:184, 1990.

Seal E Jr, McDonnell WF, House DE, Salaam SA, DeWitt PJ, Butler SO, Green J, Raggio L. The pulmonary response of white and black adults to six concentrations of ozone. Am Rev Respir Dis 147:804–810, 1993.

Sheppard D, Saisho A, Nadel JA, Boushey HA. Exercise increases sulfur dioxide-induced bronchoconstriction in asthmatic subjects. Am Rev Respir Dis 123:483–491, 1981.

Sheppard E, Eschenbacher WL, Epstein J. Lack of bronchomotor response in up to 3 ppm formaldehyde in subjects with asthma. Environ Res 35:133–139, 1984.

Silverman F. Asthma and respiratory irritants (ozone). Environ Health Perspect 29:131–136, 1979.

Speizer FE, Frank R. The uptake and release of SO_2 by the human nose. Arch Environ Health 12:725–728, 1966.

Stern B, Jones L, Raizenne M, Burnett R, Meranger JC, Franklin CA. Respiratory health effects associated with ambient sulfates and ozone in two rural Canadian communities. Environ Res 49:20–39, 1989.

Stolwijk JAJ. Sick building syndrome. Environ Health Perspect 95:99–100, 1991.

Wallace LA, Pellizzari ED, Hartwell TD, Whitmore R, Sparacino C, Zelon H. Total exposure assessment methodology (TEAM) study: Personal exposures, indoor-outdoor relationships, and breath levels of volatile organic compounds in New Jersey. Environ Int 12:369–387, 1986.

Ware JH, Ferris Jr BG, Dockery DW, Spengler JD, Stram DO, Speizer FE. Effects of ambient sulfur oxides and suspended particles on respiratory health of preadolescent children. Am Rev Respir Dis 133:834–842, 1986.

Weiss ST, Tager IB, Schenker M, Speizer FE. The health effects of involuntary smoking. Am Rev Respir Dis 128:933–942, 1983.

Weiss KB, Gergen PJ, Crain EF. Inner city asthma. The epidemiology of an emerging US public health concern. Chest 101:362S–371S, 1992a.

Weiss KB, Gergen PJ, Hodgson TA. An economic evaluation of asthma in the United States. N Engl J Med 326:862–866, 1992b.

Weitzman M, Gortmaker S, Walker DK, Sobol A. Maternal smoking and childhood asthma. Pediatrics 85:505–511, 1990.

Williams PV, McBride DE, Koenig JQ, Henderson WR, Pierson WE. Effect of ozone on the upper and lower respiratory tract. J Allergy Clin Immunol 89:230, 1992.

Witek TJ, Schacher EN, Tosun T, et al. An evaluation of respiratory effects following exposure to 2 ppm formaldehyde in asthmatics; lung function symptoms and airway reactivity. Arch Environ Health 41:230–237, 1987.

Zwick H, Popp W, Wagner C, Reiser K, Schmoger J, Bock A, Herkner K, Radunsky K. Effects of ozone on the respiratory health, allergic sensitization, and cellular immune system in children. Am Rev Respir Dis 144:1075–1079, 1991.

Section Three
PRINCIPLES OF DIAGNOSIS AND MANAGEMENT

Chapter 10
Evaluation of the Patient with Chronic Respiratory Symptoms

David G. Tinkelman, M.D.

Allergic, respiratory, and immunologic problems are among the most common complaints of children and adults presenting to the clinician, comprising almost 25% of the caseload in a busy pediatric practice. In most instances, these patients present with acute respiratory problems. However, chronic respiratory complaints also contribute significantly to the number of patients seen by the primary care clinician and the specialist. These complaints are primarily restricted to the upper airway, but to a lesser though significant degree, they also involve the lower airways. It is not always simple to identify the source of the problem from the history and physical examination alone. Often, further testing is necessary to determine the source of the problem (the upper or lower airway or both) as well as etiologic factors (allergic, nonallergic including infection, or immunologic). This chapter will focus on the tools available to the physician for the evaluation of the patient presenting with chronic respiratory symptoms and recurrent infections relating to dysfunction of the immune system.

HISTORY

As in most areas in medicine, the history is essential in making the diagnosis and defining the scope of the problem. The history-taker should search for information to define the symptoms and their severity and for related information that will help in the diagnosis and staging of the problem.

CHIEF COMPLAINT. What is the problem that actually brought the patient to see the clinician? This is usually a short statement regarding some type of respiratory complaint, for example, rhinorrhea, nasal congestion (stuffiness), sneezing, ear or eye problems, coughing, wheezing, or shortness of breath. "I can't breathe" is a fairly frequent complaint that does not necessarily implicate either the upper or lower airway as the cause of the problem. Occasionally the chief complaint may simply be "I am sick all the time!"

HISTORY OF PRESENT ILLNESS. This will define the aspects of the chief complaint that may give clues as to the etiology. Asking the key questions is like investigating a crime! When did it start? What sites of the body are involved? How long does it last? Is there a diurnal, weekly, or seasonal pattern? Are the symptoms related to particular locations? What makes it better, including specific kinds of medications, or what makes it worse? Does activity make a difference? What happens when you laugh? What do you do to make the symptoms feel better? Often this characterization of the symptoms will lead to the diagnosis or to a strong suspicion of the diagnosis.

Cough is one of the most frequent complaints presented to the physician. This can be due to the upper airway or lower airway exclusively, or can involve both. Information regarding temporal relationships and precipitating events is important. Trying to characterize what the cough "sounds like" is often difficult and misleading. A night cough or a cough with exercise or laughing may be different from a cough that occurs only when the patient eats. The presence of coughing should lead to a series of questions related to possible sinus involvement. For example, does the cough increase when the patient is lying down or appears to have drainage? The relationship of chronic sinus involvement to the lower airways has been strongly implicated, particularly in children (Rachelefsky et al, 1984). This may be related to different factors including postnasal drainage and sinobronchial reflex.

Another common etiology of coughing is exercise-induced bronchospasm. This may not be apparent to the clinician at the time of the examination, or even to the parent or patient in many cases. Since most of the symptoms in school-age children occur only at school or when playing with peers, specific questioning is required related to this possibility. Wheezing may or may not accompany the cough. It is a good principle for the clinician to ask for teacher input regarding the symptoms that may occur at school. Often teachers observe symptoms of disease or side effects of medications that are not present later in the day when the child comes home.

Other possible etiologies for chronic cough in both children and adults must be carefully considered. These include foreign body ingestion, chronic bronchitis, and cancer. Specific questioning and radiographic examination will help to evaluate the patient for these possibilities.

PAST MEDICAL HISTORY. The past medical history can give information directly related to the presenting symptom in response to the question: Has this been a problem in the past? The recurrence of symptoms of prolonged coughing or of wheezing should suggest the possibility of asthma. The finding or suggestion of exercise-induced asthma can be found in patients with documented asthma as well as in a high percentage of patients with allergic symptoms involving primarily the upper airways (Pierson, 1988). The complaint of "many colds" might suggest a chronic sinus involvement that has never been totally resolved. This is not an unusual event in patients suffering immunologic problems; neither is it unusual for this to be the case in patients with normal immunologic function who suffer from allergic rhinitis. It is fairly common for normal preschool-age children to have "frequent" upper respiratory tract infections throughout the winter months.

Involvement of related allergy problems should also be investigated thoroughly. Allergy symptoms often have a defined progression through the early years of life. It is common to see a young child have eczema, followed by chronic upper airway symptoms such as drainage and recurrent ear, nose, and throat infections, and ending with a chronic cough of occult asthma or frank asthma.

It is essential to gather information from the patient or parent about a history of symptoms that might suggest gastroesophageal reflux or aspiration. These are problems that the patient might not think are related and fail to offer spontaneously. Questions about a possible foreign body aspiration should also be included in this part of the history. A sudden onset of coughing that might actually get better for a while is a common history for foreign body aspiration in children.

FAMILY HISTORY. Allergy, asthma, and certain immunodeficiency diseases are often inherited, at least in part. Any information regarding allergy symptoms or diagnoses in the family may lead to a greater suspicion for an allergic etiology of the presenting problem (Horwood et al, 1985). Sometimes the diagnosis may be unclear. Questions should be asked about previous diagnoses of hay fever, rose fever, allergy, sinus problems, sinusitis, bronchitis, wheezy bronchitis, chronic bronchitis, asthma, and recurrent pneumonia. Questions should be posed regarding the presence of cystic fibrosis in the family. There might also be a history of the death of an infant or a small child that might, in some way, be related to the present problem.

ENVIRONMENTAL HISTORY. Perhaps in no other situation in medicine is the environmental history more important than in the patient with respiratory symptoms (Table 10–1). The respiratory tract is exquisitely sensitive and reactive to environmental exposure, both on an allergic and irritant basis. Questions should be asked about the home environment with special emphasis on the bedroom. Are there stuffed animals? What kind of pillow, carpet, and bedding are present? Are there pets in the house and are they allowed in the bedroom? Does anyone smoke in the house? Questions regarding the environment outside the house are also important, such as at school, at work, or in daycare settings.

Sometimes it is exposure to an irritant or allergen involved with some type of hobby that creates the problem environment. It is a good idea to question whether the patient or anyone in the house has any particular hobby that might be associated with an increased exposure to a particular chemical, dust, animal, or other substance (see also Chapter 7).

TABLE 10–1. ELEMENTS OF THE HISTORY

Temporal relationships
Environmental relationships
Family history
Smoking history
Drug abuse

CIGARETTE SMOKE EXPOSURE. Smoke exposure is of such importance to the respiratory tract that special emphasis must be placed on it in the history. In addition to active smoking, exposure to passive smoke may predispose an individual to an increase in upper and lower airway disease. There may be exposures that the family or patient does not want to discuss. One of the parents or the patient may be a smoker, or grandparents or friends may smoke.

DRUG ABUSE. Unfortunately, even young children may have become abusers of recreational drugs that may affect the respiratory tract. Questions regarding illicit drug use should be put to the patient discreetly. In children this requires a setting where the parents are not present. It is unlikely that the child will admit to use of these drugs with a parent in the room.

It is a good idea to obtain information about any prescribed and nonprescribed medication use at this time. It is useful information to learn about all medications that have been used for this problem and their success or failure rate as well as observed adverse effects. Sometimes patients and parents do not equate inhaler preparations with "medications" and fail to mention these in the history. Parents may forget to tell about use of medication for other medical problems. Patients may feel that the physician is only interested in respiratory-related medications and may be selective in offering information unless encouraged by specific questions.

PHYSICAL EXAMINATION

The initial general observations should impress the physician as to the patient's level of distress and need for immediate attention. Spasmodic cough, throat clearing, rhinorrhea or hypernasality of voice, color, and work of breathing can be observed with the first greetings. The patient's general state of nutrition should be observed (emaciated, normal, or obese).

It is essential to weigh and measure children periodically. This will provide the physician with an early assessment of the pattern of growth, which could be affected both by disease and by medication. Children with chronic disease or recurrent infections often exhibit a failure to grow appropriately and appear malnourished.

CUTANEOUS EXAMINATION. This includes an examination of the skin, hair, and nails. Does the patient have dry, scaly skin? Are there cutaneous lesions, such as areas of eczema, that suggest allergic diathesis? Are there signs of recurrent infection, e.g., scabbed papules consistent with impetigo? Are there petechiae on the face consistent with severe spasmodic cough? Does the patient appear jaundiced, consistent with hepatitis from disease or medication? Are there areas of contact dermatitis?

THE EYES. An external assessment may reveal darkening of the skin below the eyes, called allergic "shiners." This condition usually reflects altered blood flow in the plexus of vessels below the eyes in the paranasal sinus region with exudation of fluid and edema. This may result from a variety of causes including allergic rhinitis, infections, and noninfectious sinusitis. An examination of the eyes generally includes an examination of the lens, conjunctiva, and lids. Many of these patients will undergo steroid therapy of one type or another in the future. Therefore, an examination of the lens for opacities and the fundus for lesions should be performed and recorded as a baseline measurement. Conjunctival inflammation is a common finding in allergic individuals, particularly during the pollen seasons.

THE EARS. The child with respiratory symptoms often has involvement of the middle ear, and a good tympanic membrane examination utilizing a pneumatic otoscope is essential. Many patients with a history of recurrent infections will have grossly abnormal-appearing tympanic membranes or chronic fungal infections of the external ear canal. The appearance of middle ear fluid suggests secondary eustachian tube dysfunction, as does the finding of a retracted tympanic membrane due to negative middle ear pressure.

THE NOSE. An external examination may reveal a transnasal crease, which is due to the upward rubbing of the nose over a substantial period of time. It is most often associated with itching of the nose found in allergic rhinitis, although it can be congenital. A thorough examination of the nasal passages evaluating the turbinates and septum can be informative. The secretions should also be noted, although there is a great deal of variability in the secretions at different times of day. Discolored secretions are not unusual for the normal child and do not necessarily indicate an infectious process of the nose or sinus.

The examination of the infant often demonstrates marked narrowing of the nasal passages in the presence of secretions or edema. It is difficult to examine the nose of an infant that is crying. Patience and a small speculum or earpiece are essential to an examination for the color of the membranes and the degree of obstruction.

Examination for polyps or foreign body (in children with appropriate history) and tumors should be performed to explain nasal obstruction or other symptoms.

MOUTH AND THROAT. Open-mouth breathing is common in both children and adults. This may be due to an acute situation with obstruction of the nasal passages, or it may represent a more chronic obstruction with secondary mandibular malocclusion. This characteristic appearance is often termed "adenoidal facies." When examining the inside of the mouth, one should note lesions on the tongue, such as a geographic tongue, as well as the condition of the oropharynx and the tonsils. Some children with chronic infections have a partial or complete cleft palate or have a cleft palate repair that continues to be a problem for normal drainage of the sinuses. Tonsillar size varies with age. It is normal for the tonsils to increase in size with age through puberty and then begin to shrink in size. Children and young adults who have experienced several upper respiratory tract infections in the past may have gross swelling of the tonsils, either unilaterally or bilaterally. In fact, in some cases the degree of swelling of the tonsils may be so great as to partially occlude the oropharyngeal passage.

An examination of the neck for lymph gland hypertrophy may suggest chronicity of the problem and the presence of continuous secretions. An assessment of the size of the thyroid as well as the positioning of the trachea is important. An external compression of the airway can lead to significant wheezing and airway obstruction.

THE CHEST. This examination includes a general assessment of (1) the symmetry of the thoracic cage at rest, with inspiration, and with expiration, (2) the anteroposterior diameter of the chest cavity, and (3) general diaphragmatic movement. Always evaluate for the presence of digital clubbing, which is specific for cyanotic cardiac disease or cystic fibrosis and is rarely seen in uncomplicated asthma. These observations often give information about chronicity and severity of obstruction of airflow. There should be a general assessment of the ability to move air and the effort required to do so. In some children and, to a lesser degree, in adults, aberrations in the formation of the chest wall can create a protuberance of the sternum (pectus carinatum or pigeon breast) or a concavity of the chest with the sternum bending inward (pectus excavatum). Usually these rib problems are primarily of a cosmetic nature and do not impinge on the development or function of the lungs. In extreme cases, however, there can be compression of the lung, causing the developing lung to grow asymmetrically to areas of less compression.

Auscultation should be performed to evaluate the movement of air to all lung fields, the nature and characteristics of breath sounds, and the presence or absence of adventitial sounds. It is common for a foreign body to initially increase, and then later decrease, the breath sounds in a localized area. Careful examination for the presence or absence of sounds is important.

Examination of the young child can be difficult. It is difficult to assess the lungs in a child who is screaming, although the air movement from the act of screaming does offer an opportunity for assessment of airflow and respiratory effort. Tricks are often helpful in the case of the toddler, who might be induced to blow out a light or a party favor.

CARDIOVASCULAR SYSTEM. A general assessment evaluates the presence and character of peripheral pulses and the presence or absence of central and peripheral cyanosis. Auscultation of the heart evaluates heart rate and rhythm as well as the presence of any abnormal sounds. The presence of a murmur in a patient with diminished exercise tolerance may require a more sophisticated evaluation. Especially in children, it must be determined whether the murmur is functional in nature or is playing a role in the patient's dyspnea with activity. A quick assessment of peripheral edema or hepatomegaly will also be helpful in the assessment of cardiac function. Not all wheezing is asthma. Cardiac wheezing can be present even in a child and usually is associated with other signs of congestive heart failure, such as edema.

GASTROINTESTINAL SYSTEM. This part of the examination focuses on the presence or absence of organ enlargement or masses. A child with rectal prolapse should be suspected of having cystic fibrosis.

MUSCULOSKELETAL SYSTEM. This examination determines the presence of clubbing.

NEUROLOGIC SYSTEM. This assessment, at the minimum, evaluates the level of alertness and irritability of the child. Patients, both children and adults, receiving certain medications may have altered states of alertness and irritability. A patient who is experiencing reduced oxygenation to the brain may also have altered central nervous system functioning.

DIAGNOSTIC TESTING

A variety of diagnostic tests is available to help the clinician in the diagnosis and management of the patient with chronic respiratory tract symptoms and recurrent infections. (Table 10–2). The following describes the most common office tests, including tests for the presence or absence of upper or lower airway inflammatory disease and tests for the presence or absence of allergy or immunologic dysfunction, which may be playing an etiologic role. Although it is possible to perform all of these tests in the primary care physician's office, many are best reserved for the specialist, who can provide optimal technique and data interpretation.

Tests for Upper Airway Disease

NASAL CYTOLOGY. Nasal cytology can give information regarding the etiology of upper airway symptoms. Often it is difficult to determine whether secretions are due to allergic, infectious, or nonspecific inflammatory etiol-

TABLE 10–2. DIAGNOSTIC TESTING

Tests for upper airway disease
  Nasal cytology
  Sinus radiograph
  Fiberoptic rhinoscopy
Tests for lower airway disease
  Sputum cytology
  Chest radiograph
  Sweat test
  Pulmonary function evaluation
  Determination of nonspecific bronchial hyperactivity
    Methacholine or histamine challenges
    Exercise challenges
Determination of nonspecific and specific allergy
  Total eosinophil count
  Total IgE level determination
  In vivo determination of specific allergy
  In vitro determination of specific allergy

ogy. The type and quantity of cells present in the nasal passage may point to a diagnosis. Obtaining cells for cytology is a simple office procedure in which a nasal specimen is obtained and stained, and a quantitative and qualitative cell count is made. The patient can supply the specimen by blowing nasal secretions into a sheet of waxed paper, but the best method is to scrape along the inferior turbinate with a small spoon-shaped curette, made for such a purpose. The specimen is then stained with Hansel's stain and examined under a microscope. The presence of a preponderance of polymorphonucleated white blood cells usually suggests an infectious rather than an allergic process. When there is a large quantity of eosinophils, the suggestion is that allergy may be an important etiologic factor. However, neither the presence of nasal eosinophils (e.g., nonallergic rhinitis with eosinophils) nor their absence (particularly with concomitant infection) makes or excludes an etiologic diagnosis.

SINUS RADIOGRAPH. It is almost impossible to accurately assess the presence of a sinus infection or inflammation on physical examination. Limited anterior rhinoscopy generally does not permit visualization of sinus ostia; a simple viral URI can often mimic acute bacterial sinusitis on physical examination. A sinus radiographic series can help to differentiate these entities and is an important consideration in the evaluation of the patient with chronic respiratory tract symptoms of the upper and lower airways, as well as the patient with chronic or recurrent infections. It has been suggested that the value of this procedure is less in a child less than one year old. However, in children over this age a sinus radiographic evaluation is of significant benefit. One should remember that simple edema of the respiratory tract that extends from the turbinates to the sinus lining does not always imply a bacterial infection of the sinuses. This can be seen in the patient with allergic rhinitis during the height of the symptoms (Harlin et al, 1988). It is sometimes necessary to obtain a CT scan of the sinuses (a limited coronal scan may be sufficient) to confirm the diagnosis, particularly when the patient with a normal sinus radiograph has failed to respond to appropriate therapy. A more detailed explanation of the evaluation of the sinuses can be found in Chapter 30, Sinusitis.

FIBEROPTIC RHINOSCOPY. As described above, the history and gross examination may not be sufficient to determine the etiology of the chronic symptoms being described. Visualization of the nasal passages and sinus ostia may permit an immediate diagnosis. This procedure requires training in the use of this equipment, a thorough understanding of the anatomy of the nasal and sinus passages, and the equipment and space to perform this procedure effectively. It is not to be performed by the untrained and unskilled clinician as there are potential risks involved in the procedure, particularly in the small child. With rhinoscopy it is possible to determine whether there is significant inflammation and edema of the mucosa, to visualize polyps, to observe the types of drainage coming from the sinus ostia, and to identify structural abnormalities (including tumors) that were otherwise inapparent. Rhinoscopy can delay or eliminate the need for radiographic evaluation in many cases. The procedure requires the patient to be somewhat cooperative and thus is only recommended in older children and adults when performed as a routine office procedure.

Tests for Lower Airway Disease

SPUTUM CYTOLOGY. This often performed test is of limited benefit in most patients, particularly in children who will give saliva specimens in the vast majority of cases. It is best reserved for the older child or adult who is able to understand the procedure and who has chronic lung symptoms. The cytologic evaluation may be of some benefit to differentiate an infectious from a noninfectious process. An eosinophil-laden specimen may confirm a noninfectious inflammatory problem. Cultures of the sputum have proved to be of little benefit.

CHEST RADIOGRAPH. PA and lateral radiographs of the chest are essential for the proper evaluation of the patient with chronic chest symptoms. Therefore, any patient with chronic cough that is not directly demonstrated to be a symptom of uncomplicated reversible airway obstruction, with or without wheezing, should have an initial chest radiograph. In the vast majority of children with chronic cough, including those with asthma, the chest radiograph is usually normal. It can provide important information about many of the chronic lung diseases of children including immunodeficiencies, tuberculosis, and cystic fibrosis. In the adult, the films can give information regarding infiltrates, scarring, asymmetry, and masses. The contour of the lung, the presence or absence of vascular engorgement, and adenopathy are all useful for assessing lung health.

SWEAT TEST. Children under 4 years of age who have chronic chest symptoms—such as chronic cough, wheezing, or recurrent bronchitis or pneumonia—that are not attributable to completely reversible airway obstruction should be evaluated by a sweat test to rule out cystic fibrosis. This disease can present in many ways, and it can become apparent at different ages in different children. A sweat test performed by iontophoresis has significant diagnostic value and is easily obtained in most urban areas of the country. A sweat test is not indicated in a child with recent onset of respiratory symptoms.

PULMONARY FUNCTION EVALUATION. It is impossible to diagnose and manage hypertension without using a sphygmomanometer to measure blood pressure. It is similarly impossible to evaluate and manage chronic lung disease without spirometry to measure and assess lung function (Pratter et al, 1983). Spirometry can give information about lung volumes as well as flow of air through the large and small airways of the lung. Measurement of peak flow, although useful in the management of asthma (particularly over long periods of time), does not reflect the status of the small airways of the lung and is totally effort-dependent (Guidelines for the Diagnosis and Management of Asthma, 1991).

The importance of pulmonary function testing cannot be overemphasized in the diagnosis and management of asthma. It is essential for clinicians to establish a baseline level of function from which to monitor long-term lung function and the effect of various therapeutic endeavors. Spirometry can be useful in the management of the acute attack as well as longitudinally over years. These tests can be performed and compared to standardized tables of normal predicted values or to the patient's own values.

There are several standardized tables of predicted normal values for older children (generally 6 years old and older) and adults. Thus there is significant variation in ranges of normal for children of different body sizes of the same height. Since "predicted normal" values for a particular individual may be abnormally low, it is a good idea to perform spirometry both before and after administration of an aerosol bronchodilator to gain a better assessment of possible airflow limitation and immediate reversibility by bronchodilator. Proper interpretation of pulmonary function tests must be made within the context of historical and physical findings. For more information regarding the specifics of pulmonary function testing, see Chapter 12.

Measurement of the peak expiratory flow rate at home has been proved to be a useful tool for following the course of patients with asthma. This is a totally effort-dependent test which requires the patient to blow forcefully for a very short period of time. It is therefore easier for young children to perform than spirometry. When the test is performed reliably by the patient, it can serve as an important tool to learn more about the day-to-day variation of the clinical state, as an indicator of trouble ahead because of falling levels, as a guide to the effect of and indication for medication, and as a barometer of bronchial hyperresponsiveness (Cross and Nelson, 1991).

DETERMINATION OF NONSPECIFIC BRONCHIAL HYPERRESPONSIVENESS. Asthma is an inflammatory lung disease that is manifested by increased nonspecific bronchial hyperresponsiveness. Generally, children with asthma have completely normal airway function measurements on spirometry. Despite this finding, however, there is a measurable increase in bronchial airway responsiveness (Hopp, 1984). In order to make the diagnosis or to quantify the degree of airway responsiveness, it is necessary to perform a bronchial challenge with nonspecific airway stimuli, such as methacholine or histamine (Pattemore et al, 1990), or with an exercise challenge (Anderson, 1985). These tests are generally safe and relatively easy to perform in the proper setting and with properly trained personnel to administer the challenge and monitor the results. For a complete description of these measurements of bronchial responsiveness, see Chapter 13.

Measurement of bronchial hyperresponsiveness has been found to be a good correlate with the clinical severity of asthma. It also can be useful to confirm the diagnosis of mild forms of reactive airway disease, such as cough variant asthma, or when an exercise challenge is difficult to perform. The clinician should be aware of the risks involved with challenge procedures, and they probably are best reserved for the specialist to perform.

Determination of Suggestive and Specific Allergy

TOTAL EOSINOPHIL COUNT. The total eosinophil count in the circulating blood can be an indicator of an allergic reaction. There may also be some correlation between elevated total eosinophil counts and basic control of asthma, which may or may not be related to allergy. It does not correlate directly with any particular symptom or severity of symptom. It is often simply a measurement derived from the total white blood cell count multiplied by the percent eosinophils found on the differential count. The presence or absence of eosinophils does not allow for a diagnosis to be made. For all these reasons, the total eosinophil count has little significant usefulness in the diagnosis or management of most respiratory problems.

TOTAL IgE LEVEL DETERMINATION. The total IgE level is a nonspecific test that may give circumstantial evidence suggesting the presence of allergy. In most clinical situations it does not correlate directly with any specific disease state. The two exceptions to this statement are allergic bronchopulmonary aspergillosis (ABPA) (see Chapter 40) and atopic dermatitis, in which there appears to be a correlation between the severity of the clinical state and the IgE level.

An elevated IgE level gives the presumption that the patient is atopic, but the lack of an elevation does not preclude this state (Burrows et al, 1989). The level does not correlate at all with atopic sensitivity to any particular antigen, other than, perhaps, *Aspergillus* antigens.

The total IgE level can be assessed by several methodologies such as those employing radiologic and fluorometric assessments and newer techniques such as nephalometry. Obtaining this level is not recommended in the standard evaluation of allergic disease.

IN VIVO DETERMINATION OF ALLERGEN-SPECIFIC IgE. Currently, *in vivo* determination of specific allergy is best accomplished by skin testing to a variety of antigens. This method of testing introduces a small amount of antigenic material into the skin and depends on the recognition of the antigen by IgE and the presence of mediators in the skin for a positive test. Skin testing can be performed in a variety of ways with varying degrees of sensitivity and specificity, depending on the technique, the concentration of antigen, and the technician performing the test. These tests can be performed in patients of all ages, including infants if necessary, with some degree of reliability. However, it is essential to have appropriate positive and negative controls placed on the skin of each patient.

IN VITRO DETERMINATION OF ALLERGEN-SPECIFIC IgE. Determining specific IgE reactivity to antigens can be performed by several tests, classically represented by the radioallergosorbent test (RAST) and variations utilizing radioactive or enzymatic assays. *In vitro* testing offers a less traumatic test that is not dependent on a technician's application or interpretation of results; however, it does generally cost more per test than skin testing, does not give immediate results, and is less sensitive than skin testing (Berg and Johansson, 1974). There is little information regarding the reliability of these tests in infants.

Tests of Immunologic Function

QUANTITATIVE IMMUNOGLOBULINS. Measuring the total amount of circulating antibodies may prove useful in the patient with recurrent infections. In infants less than 9 months of age, it may be difficult to distinguish between the contribution of passive maternal antibodies and the antibodies produced by the infant. Many infants have relatively low levels of circulating antibodies during the first 2 years of life and experience an increased frequency of infections (McGeady, 1987). The absence of circulating IgA is a fairly common disorder associated with individuals with recurrent respiratory tract infections. Therefore, in the evaluation of a patient with frequent infections, particularly one with frequent respiratory tract infections, the determination of quantitative immunoglobulins may prove to be useful.

MEASUREMENT OF QUALITATIVE FUNCTION OF THE ANTIBODY SYSTEM. Some patients may have normal quantitative levels of immunoglobulins, yet fail to mount a normal antibody response to specific infectious agents. This type of response can be measured by assessing the specific antibody formation following certain vaccinations. The most commonly measured antibody levels follow immunization with tetanus, diphtheria, and pneumococcal vaccines (Ferrante et al, 1990). In order to be confident in the immunologic competency of the antibody system, a qualitative assessment is indicated in the patient with recurrent infections and normal (or near normal) quantitative immunoglobulin levels. For more information regarding the immunologic evaluation, refer to the Chapters in Section One.

CONCLUSION

The patient with chronic respiratory tract symptoms may have a variety of well-defined problems involving either the upper or lower respiratory tract or a combination of both. It is the role of the clinician to identify the organs involved and to define the pathologic mechanism responsible for the symptoms. It is through a thorough history, physical examination, and appropriate laboratory studies that such information is obtained. This information allows a progression of appropriate therapy not only to control the presenting symptoms, but to prevent their ongoing nature and recurrence. Often there is a combination of allergic and nonallergic factors involved, and a thorough understanding of the role of each is necessary to be successful in the total management of chronic symptoms.

REFERENCES

Anderson SD. Issues in exercise-induced asthma. J Allerg Clin Immunol 76:763–771, 1985.

Berg TLO, Johansson SGO. Allergy diagnosis with the radioallergosorbent test: A comparison with the results of skin and provocation tests in an unselected group of children with asthma and hay fever. J Allerg Clin Immunol 54:209, 1974.

Burrows B, Martinez FD, Halonen M, et al. Association of asthma with serum IgE levels and skin test reactivity to allergens. N Engl J Med. 320:271–277, 1989.

Cross D, Nelson HS. The role of the peak flow meter in the diagnosis and management of asthma. J Allerg Clin Immunol 87:120–128, 1991.

Ferrante A, Beard L, Feldman R. IgG subclass distribution of antibodies to bacterial and viral antigens. J Pediatr Infec Dis 9:S16, 1990.

Guidelines for the Diagnosis and Management of Asthma. National Asthma Educational Program. National Heart Lung Blood Institute. National Institute of Health. Publication No. 91-3042, 1991.

Harlin SL, Ansel DG, Lane SR, et al. A clinical and pathologic study of chronic sinusitis: The role of the eosinophil. J Clin Allerg Immunol 81:867–875, 1988.

Hopp J, Bewtra AJ, Nair NM, et al. Specificity and sensitivity of methacholine inhalation challenge in normal and asthmatic children. J Allerg Clin Immunol 74:154, 1984.

Horwood LJ, Furgusson DM, Hons BA, Shannon FT. Social and familial factors in the development of early childhood asthma. Pediatrics 75:859, 1985.

McGeady S. Transient hypogammaglobulinemia of infancy: Need to reconsider name and definition. J Pediatr 110:47, 1987.

Pattemore PK, Asher MI, Harrison AC, et al. The interrelationship among bronchial hyperresponsiveness and the diagnosis of asthma and asthma symptoms. Am Rev Resp Dis 142:549–554, 1990.

Pierson WE. Exercise-induced bronchospasm in children and adolescents. Pediatr Clin North Am 35:1031, 1988.

Pratter MR, Hingston DM, Irwin RS. Diagnosis of bronchial asthma by clinical evaluation. Chest 84:42, 1983.

Rachelefsky GS, Katz RM, Siegel SC. Chronic sinus disease with associated reactive airway disease in children. Pediatrics 73:526, 1984.

Chapter 11
Tests for IgE Antibody

Dennis R. Ownby, M.D.

Tests for allergen-specific IgE were performed as aids to the diagnosis of allergic disease long before IgE was discovered as a distinct class of immunoglobulin. In 1873, Blackley first described the local cutaneous itching, swelling, and erythema that occurred when grass pollen was rubbed into a scarification on a sensitive person. The scratch test was redescribed as a test related to immediate-type allergic disease by Smith in 1909. Later, the intradermal test and the prick test were described. The first explanations for the cutaneous reactions elicited by pollens or pollen extracts involved the concept that the pollens contained a "toxin" to which some persons were sensitive.

A major milestone in the understanding of allergic disease was the discovery by Prausnitz and Kustner that human serum could transfer the skin sensitizing factor from an allergic to a nonallergic individual (P-K reaction). Years of investigation were ultimately rewarded with the discovery that the skin sensitizing, or reaginic, component of human serum resided in a unique class of immunoglobulin, which was termed immunoglobulin E or IgE. Shortly after the discovery of IgE by the Ishizakas (1967), a unique myeloma was reported by Johansson and Bennich (1967), which was also determined to be of the IgE class. The relatively large quantities of IgE protein obtained from the myeloma made it possible to produce antibodies to IgE and subsequently to develop immunoassays for total and antigen-specific IgE.

SKIN TESTING

With the advent of immunoassays for allergen-specific IgE, there were predictions that skin testing would rapidly be phased out of clinical practice in favor of immunoassays (Lichtenstein et al, 1973). Over 20 years later, skin tests are still the major method for detecting allergen-specific IgE used in clinical practice. There are multiple reasons for the continued clinical use of skin tests. Among the most important reasons are: the high sensitivity, ease of performance, rapid results, and low cost per skin test (Council on Scientific Affairs, 1987). As with any other test, skin tests can yield false-negative or false-positive results because of inadequacies of the tests, or because they are poorly performed or interpreted.

PHYSIOLOGY OF SKIN-TEST REACTIONS. Skin tests are performed by introducing a small quantity of allergen into the epidermis by pricking, puncturing, or scratching the skin or by intradermal injection. The immediate wheal and flare response resulting from a skin test is the result of a complex series of interactions. After the allergen has been introduced into the skin, the allergen diffuses through the skin and interacts with IgE antibody bound to mast cells. If the allergen binds to two or more IgE antibody molecules bound to a mast cell bridging the IgE molecules, a signal is generated initiating mediator release from the cell. IgE binds to mast cells and basophils via a high-affinity receptor, FcεRI.

Most of the immediate skin response is due to the release of histamine (Smith et al, 1980). The central wheal of the skin response is due to histamine-induced vasopermeability and secondary edema. The central erythema results from histamine-induced arteriolar vasodilation and the circumferential erythema results from the stimulation of nerve receptors and a resulting axon reflex vasodilation.

Most of the visible skin response to an allergen can be blocked by H_1-receptor antagonist, but complete inhibition requires both H_1 and H_2 antagonists (Smith et al, 1980). In addition to the release of histamine, a variety of other preformed and newly synthesized mediators are released.

Following the immediate skin response, there may be a late-phase reaction, which begins 3 to 5 hours, peaks at 6 to 12 hours, and resolves approximately 24 hours after the immediate response. The late-phase reaction is an edematous reaction resulting from the local influx of inflammatory cells including mononuclear cells, eosinophils, basophils, and neutrophils. The reaction is accompanied by the deposition of fibrin. Clinically, the likelihood of a late-phase reaction and the size of the reaction are related to (1) the sensitivity of the person, (2) the quantity of the allergen introduced, and (3) other poorly defined influences (Frew and Kay, 1988).

Skin tests can also be performed with vasoactive agents such as histamine or with mast cell secretagogues such as compound 48/80, codeine, and morphine. Histamine induces an immediate cutaneous response only while some of the mast cell secretagogues may induce both immediate and late-phase reactions. These results suggest that mediators other than histamine are responsible for late-phase reactions.

The ideal skin test method should (1) provide high sensitivity for detecting specific IgE, (2) provide minimal risk of inducing a systemic reaction in the patient, (3) be easy to perform and reproduce, and (4) be inexpensive (Bousquet and Michel, 1993). Unfortunately, no single method of skin testing completely meets all of these requirements. Current skin testing techniques can be divided into two general categories: epicutaneous and intradermal. The major difference between the two categories is that epicutaneous tests rely on allowing a small quantity of allergen extract to penetrate the skin as a result of a small prick or puncture, whereas intradermal tests are performed by directly injecting extract into the skin. Epicutaneous tests tend to be less likely to provoke systemic allergic reactions but are also less sensitive at detecting specific IgE than are intradermal tests. Although intradermal tests have exquisite sensitivity, they are more likely to be falsely positive than epicutaneous tests. For these reasons, epicutaneous tests are typically performed before intradermal tests, especially with allergens that are associated with a high risk of systemic reactions such as penicillin or insect venoms. An alternative is to start skin testing with very weak dilutions of the allergen.

EVALUATION OF PATIENTS PRIOR TO SKIN TESTING. Before any patient is skin tested, the patient's history should be evaluated by an experienced physician and the patient should be examined. Beyond establishing the likelihood of allergic disease, the history and physical examination should alert the physician to any unusual risks of skin testing for the patient. Skin testing is generally safe but always carries a small risk of inducing a systemic allergic reaction or anaphylaxis. Treatment of major systemic allergic reactions and anaphylaxis requires the use of epinephrine. Anything that might increase a patient's risk of anaphylaxis or alter their response to epinephrine should be discovered and evaluated prior to skin testing. In patients with histories of unusually severe allergic reactions or reactions resulting from minimal allergen exposure, the physician ordering the skin tests may wish to start the skin tests with more dilute extracts than normal or with a limited number of tests. Patients on medications, such as beta blocking agents, may not respond normally to treatment with epinephrine, therefore, beta blockers should normally be discontinued prior to skin testing (Hepner et al, 1990). Pregnancy is another relative contraindication to skin testing, because the fetus *in utero* may be highly vulnerable to hypoxia resulting from a systemic reaction in the mother. It is also possible that mediators liberated during systemic reactions may induce uterine contractions leading to premature labor or other complications. The potential risks and benefits of skin testing must also be weighed carefully in patients with chronic medical problems, which might compromise their ability to recover from a systemic reaction. Examples of compromised individuals include individuals with severe lung disease or unstable angina. Finally, patients with current, severe, allergic symptoms, especially unstable asthma, should not be skin tested until after their symptoms have been stabilized, because these patients appear to have a greater risk of systemic reactions (Lockey et al, 1987). The patient's history may also suggest that he or she should be evaluated for dermatographism before being skin tested.

SKIN-TESTING TECHNIQUES

PERCUTANEOUS OR EPICUTANEOUS TESTING. Percutaneous or epicutaneous tests may be performed by a variety of methods, but the most common methods are the prick or puncture techniques. The modified prick test, which was popularized by Pepys (1975), is performed on previously cleansed skin by passing a small needle (e.g., 25- or 26-gauge) through a drop of allergen extract at approximately a 45-degree angle to the surface of the skin. The needle is lightly pressed into the epidermis, and the tip of the needle is then lifted up, producing a pricking sensation. The prick of the skin should not be deep enough to produce visible bleeding. After the prick has been made through the drop of extract, the extract can be blotted from the skin since there is no evidence that leaving the extract on the skin results in a significantly larger reaction (Ownby and Anderson, 1982). The technique for the prick test is illustrated in Figure 11–1.

Another popular method of epicutaneous testing is the puncture technique. Briefly, a drop of allergen extract is placed on cleansed skin. A puncture device is then pushed into the skin through the drop of extract. Commonly used puncture devices are constructed to allow a small point to penetrate 1 to 1.5 mm into the skin. Further penetration of the point is prevented by a collar or flare of the instrument's diameter. The bifurcated needle, originally designed for smallpox vaccination, can also be used for puncture testing. The bifurcated needle is pressed firmly against the skin, through a drop of extract, and the needle is rocked back and forth and side to side (Fig. 11–2).

A single needle or puncture device can be used for multiple prick skin tests on the same patient if all residual extract is cleaned from the needle between tests. Adequate cleaning can usually be accomplished by wiping the needle with an alcohol-soaked pledget or by briefly swirling the device in a container of alcohol. On completion of the tests on an individual patient, the device should be discarded. The tests can be applied to any area of normal skin, but the most common sites used for testing are the back, volar forearms, and the anterior aspect of the thighs. Each test should be placed a minimum of 4 cm from other tests, and care should be taken to avoid smearing or mixing the extracts. In highly sensitive patients, or with some devices producing larger reactions, the distance between tests may need to be increased because large reactions may obscure reactions in adjacent tests.

Several studies have evaluated the relative size and consistency of cutaneous reactions resulting from use of various devices (Adinoff et al, 1989; Demoly et al, 1991). Not all studies evaluated the same devices, and even when the same devices are evaluated, the results are not always consistent. In general, devices made of metal seem to produce more consistent results than do devices made of plastic. Devices that automatically limit the depth of penetration into the skin also tend to produce more consistent results than do devices with which the depth of skin penetration is dependent on the person performing

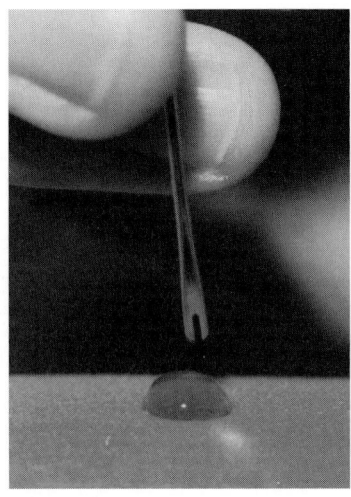

FIGURE 11–2. Puncture skin testing using a bifurcated needle. The needle will be firmly pressed down onto the skin through the drop of extract and then the needle will be rocked back and forth before being lifted.

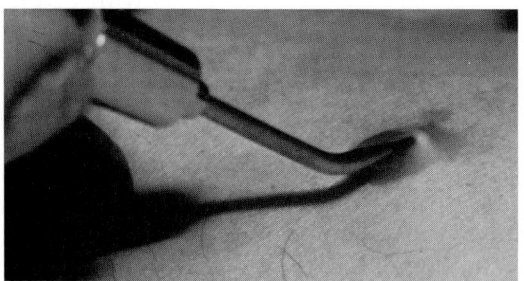

FIGURE 11–1. Prick skin testing using a bent needle in a holder. Note that the skin is slightly tented as the needle is being lifted upward after having been passed lightly into the skin.

the test (Adinoff et al, 1989; Demoly et al, 1991). When selecting a skin-test device, the physician may also wish to consider the availability and ease of use of the device.

INTRADERMAL SKIN TESTS. Intradermal tests provide the ultimate in skin-test sensitivity, but they are technically more difficult to apply properly. Intradermal tests are typically performed using a 25-, 26-, or 27-gauge needle. Some manufacturers provide needles with a special intradermal bevel, which helps to limit the depth of needle penetration. After the allergen extract is drawn into the syringe, the tip of the needle is inserted into the superficial dermis and a small volume of extract (approximately 0.02 ml) is injected. If the injection is performed properly, a distinct bleb, 2 to 3 mm in diameter, will be present (Fig. 11–3). As with prick-puncture tests, intradermal tests should be placed 4 to 6 cm apart to prevent interference.

The most common errors with intradermal tests are injecting the extract too deeply, injecting too large a volume, and inducing excess bleeding. If the extract is injected too deeply, little or no reaction will be visible on the surface of the skin even if the individual is sensitive. Injecting too large a volume may lead to false-positive reactions because of irritation, and a large volume increases the risk of a systemic reaction (Bousquet and Michel, 1993). Inducing bleeding while trying to properly inject the extract into the epidermis is a problem, especially with struggling subjects such as children. Bleeding at the site may induce more local irritation, leading to false-positive reactions.

POSITIVE AND NEGATIVE CONTROLS FOR SKIN TESTING. Because of the many variables present when performing skin testing, positive and negative controls must be included to allow accurate interpretation of test results. The negative control is usually normal saline or the same buffer that has been used to dilute the allergen extracts used for testing. There should be minimal or no reaction to the negative control. Erythema of less than 5 mm in diameter is a common response to the slight trauma of the test, while a larger response suggests inadequate cleaning of the device between tests or dermatographism. The negative control must be applied in the same fashion as all the other tests. There may be a tendency on the part of persons performing the tests to use less vigor in applying the negative control since they know that the control should not produce any response. If the negative control is not placed with the same effort as that applied to the other tests, problems such as dermatographism may be missed.

Positive controls for skin testing are usually either histamine or a mast cell secretagogue, such as codeine. For epicutaneous tests, histamine is usually used at a concentration of 1 mg/ml, although some have recommended a concentration of 10 mg/ml because some normal individuals do not respond to the 1 mg/ml concentration (Bernstein, 1988). For intradermal testing, histamine is most often used at a concentration of 0.01 mg/ml. Some allergists believe that a mast cell secretagogue is a more appropriate positive control than a direct agonist like histamine, because a positive response to a secretagogue indicates that the cutaneous mast cells are fully functional (Bernstein, 1988). Failure to respond to the positive control suggests that there is some interference with skin testing, such as the patient failing to discontinue antihistamine drugs before testing. One problem associated with the use of codeine or morphine as a positive control is that of stocking a controlled substance.

RECORDING AND SCORING SKIN TEST RE-

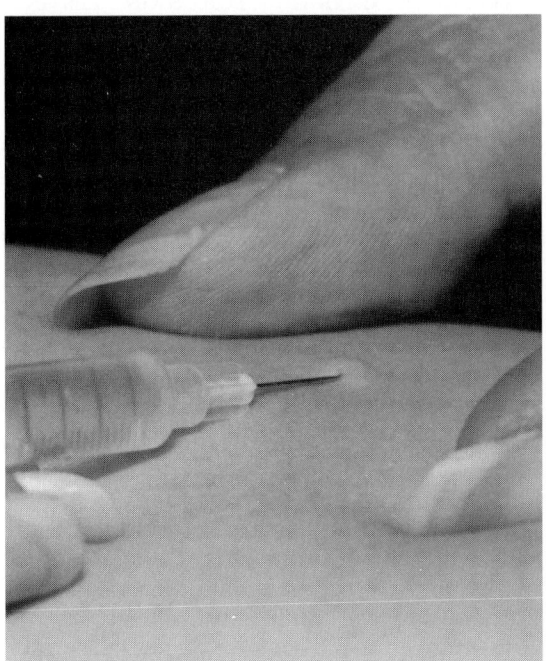

FIGURE 11–3. Intradermal skin testing using a 26-gauge needle and disposable syringe. Correct technique should result in a distinct bleb 2 to 3 mm in diameter, as shown.

sults. Despite many years of use and many investigations (Bernstein, 1988), there is still little consensus concerning the scoring and recording of skin test results. The most commonly used system grades both epicutaneous and intradermal tests on a five-point scale whereby 0 is a negative test and increasing degrees of reaction are graded from 1+ to 4+. A commonly used scoring system for intradermal tests is presented in Table 11–1. In terms of patient management, the actual size or grade of the skin test reaction is less important than the physician's criteria for determining whether the test is positive or negative. A negative test means that the patient does not have allergen-specific IgE; a positive test means that the patient has produced IgE specific for the allergen. Most investigators consider an epicutaneous test positive when the wheal of the test is 2 or 3 mm larger than the wheal produced by the negative control and the wheal is surrounded by erythema.

Many studies performed over several decades have shown that reactions on the skin of infants can be similar to those on the skin of older children and adults if specific IgE is present (Menardo et al, 1985; VanAsperen et al, 1984; Skassa-Brociek et al, 1987). The intensity of the skin reaction of infants is less than that of older children. A study evaluating the changes in skin reactivity with age found that the mean wheal diameter produced by a 1 mg/ml concentration of histamine was 1.3 mm in infants less than 2 years of age and 2.6 mm in children 4 to 6 years of age (Skassa-Brociek et al, 1987). The results of this and other studies suggest that the criteria for a positive skin test must be reduced for infants. Thus, in infants less than 2 years of age, a prick-puncture skin test with a wheal of 1 mm or more, with erythema, is probably a true positive in the presence of a nonreactive negative control. The popular notion that infants cannot be skin tested is based mostly on the fact that infants rarely produce detectable quantities of allergen-specific IgE (Van-Asperen et al, 1984).

The results of skin tests, like the results of other diagnostic tests, should become part of the patient's medical record. Since patients frequently relocate, the results of skin tests performed by one physician should be interpretable by another knowledgeable physician. To be interpretable by another physician, several items of information need to be included with the skin test results. Necessary information includes: identification of the allergens tested, the method of testing (prick-puncture or intradermal) for each allergen, the device used for testing, the source of the allergen extracts, the concentration of extracts used for testing, the identity and concentration of the positive control, and either the measured diameters of the skin tests or the criteria used for grading the skin tests. This information is easily placed at the bottom or on the back of sheets designed for recording skin tests (Nelson, 1993).

Allergen Extracts for Skin Testing. The quality of the allergen extracts is one of the most important variables determining the value of skin tests (Bousquet and Michel, 1993). Highly potent and standardized extracts produce skin tests with fewer false-positive and false-negative reactions. Standardized skin test extracts should contain adequate quantities of all relevant allergens and have consistent compositions. The biologic potency of a standardized extract should be directly related to the units used to express the extract's concentration. Whenever possible, standardized extracts should be used for testing, and all diagnostic extracts should be obtained from commercial manufacturers who have reputations for producing high-quality extracts. Current exceptions to the use of commercial extracts are some foods, especially fruits, where the allergens appear to be highly labile. If important allergens are labile, testing using fresh juice from the fruit may be more accurate than a commercial extract. The Scandinavians have proposed the "prick and prick" technique whereby the fresh fruit is first pricked and then the patient is pricked

TABLE 11–1. GRADING SYSTEM FOR SKIN REACTIONS TO INTRADERMAL TESTS

Grade	Erythema	Wheal
0+	<5 mm	<5 mm
±	5–10 mm	5–10 mm
1+	11–20 mm	5–10 mm
2+	21–30 mm	5–10 mm
3+	31–40 mm	5–10 mm or with pseudopods
4+	>40 mm	>15 mm or with many pseudopods

From Norman PS. Skin testing. In Rose NR, DeMacario EC, Fahey JL, et al (eds). Manual of Clinical Laboratory Immunology. 4th ed. Washington, DC, American Society for Microbiology, 1992.

(Dreborg, 1988). The major problem with this form of testing is that it is difficult to standardize and it is difficult to control for nonspecific irritation, which can produce false-positive reactions.

QUALITY CONTROL OF SKIN TESTING. Skin tests are diagnostic tests and all diagnostic tests should be subject to certain standards and quality controls. The ease with which skin tests are performed has led many to neglect the quality control of skin testing. Quality control of skin testing should include testing (1) the knowledge of the person performing the tests, (2) inter- and intra-operator reproducibility of tests, (3) consistency of procedures, (4) control of extract quality, and (5) consistent recording of test results. The person performing the tests must know how to apply the tests and factors that may affect the results of the tests, such as interfering drugs and skin abnormalities. The inter- and intra-operator reproducibility should also be known. The long-term stability of testing extracts is more difficult to control; therefore, prevention is the best choice. Extracts should be purchased in buffers providing maximum stability (e.g., 50 percent glycerin) (Nelson, 1979; Nelson, 1981). Low temperatures also help to preserve extract potency, and so extracts should be kept refrigerated except when they are actually being used for testing. It is good office practice to periodically check extract expiration dates so that extracts that have expired can be discarded. The persons scoring the skin test responses should follow specific criteria for scoring test results.

DIAGNOSTIC VALUE OF SKIN TESTS. Several task force reports and position papers have concluded that, when properly performed, prick-puncture tests are the most convenient and cost-effective method for detecting allergen-specific IgE in patients (Bernstein, 1988; Dreborg et al, 1989). The value of prick-puncture tests is greatest when high-potency, standardized extracts are used (Bernstein, 1988; Dreborg et al, 1989). In situations in which the risk of a false-negative test is high (as with insect venom and drugs), negative prick-puncture tests should be confirmed with intradermal tests. Scratch tests are not recommended because of the difficulty in producing consistent results (Nelson, 1983; Dreborg et al, 1989).

Even when false-positive and false-negative tests are excluded from consideration, the problem of clinical interpretation of test results remains. Skin test results must be interpreted in light of the clinical history and relative risks to the patient. When the patient's history strongly suggests that the patient is symptomatic following exposure to an allergen, and the patient has a positive skin test to the allergen, the probability that the patient suffers from an allergic disease caused by the allergen is very high. Conversely, when the patient's history does not suggest the presence of allergic disease and skin tests are negative, the probability of allergic disease is very low.

The most difficult clinical situations are when there is little or no apparent correlation between the patient's history and the results of skin tests. It is not uncommon to see a patient with symptoms typical of seasonal allergic rhinitis occurring in the late summer and fall who has positive skin tests not only to late summer pollens, but also to spring or early summer pollens. In this situation, it is easy to attribute the allergic rhinitis to a sensitivity to the late summer or fall pollens. The difficulty is in deciding on the significance of the sensitivity to the spring and early summer pollens. Studies have shown that about half the asymptomatic individuals who have positive skin tests to seasonal pollens will develop symptoms that will correspond to the positive skin tests over an interval of a few years (Hagy and Settipane, 1976). This observation demonstrates that the presence of IgE alone does not provide an adequate basis for the diagnosis of allergic disease. The observation also suggests that with allergen exposure, some persons will respond by producing specific IgE antibodies; following IgE antibody production many, but not all, persons will develop allergic symptoms if allergen exposure continues. Some studies have also suggested that patients may develop symptoms before specific IgE antibody is detectable. One of the challenging aspects about the diagnosis of allergic disease is that knowledge of the presence or the quantity of allergen-specific IgE does not point to information about the presence or type of allergic disease in the patient (Ownby, 1988).

NUMBER OF SKIN TESTS. A frequently discussed question is the number of skin tests that need to be performed to adequately evaluate a patient. Several workshop reports and position papers have stated that the majority of allergic individuals can be adequately evaluated with less than 50 tests for specific IgE

150—PRINCIPLES OF DIAGNOSIS AND MANAGEMENT

(Council on Scientific Affairs, 1987; Bernstein, 1988), but this is controversial (Chin et al, 1993). The choice of allergens for testing should be based on the patient's history, the geographic area of the country, and in some cases special considerations. Special considerations may include the patient's occupation, hobbies, or other environmental factors.

IN VITRO TESTS FOR ALLERGEN-SPECIFIC IgE ANTIBODIES

PRINCIPLES OF *IN VITRO* ASSAYS. Most available assays for allergen-specific IgE antibodies utilize the principle of immunoabsorption illustrated in Figure 11–4 (Ownby, 1988; Homburger and Katzmann, 1993). The allergen of interest is bound to a solid-phase support. The solid-phase support can be any of a variety of materials such as a paper disc, a plastic microtiter well, or cellulose particles. After the solid phase has been prepared, the patient's serum is incubated with the solid phase. If the patient has antibodies specific for the allergen on the solid phase, the antibodies will become bound to the allergen, and the remaining serum proteins, including unbound antibodies, can be washed away from the solid phase. A labeled anti–human IgE antibody is then incubated with the solid phase. If allergen-specific IgE antibodies have bound to the solid phase, there will be a proportionate binding of the anti-IgE antibody. After washing, the quantity of anti-IgE

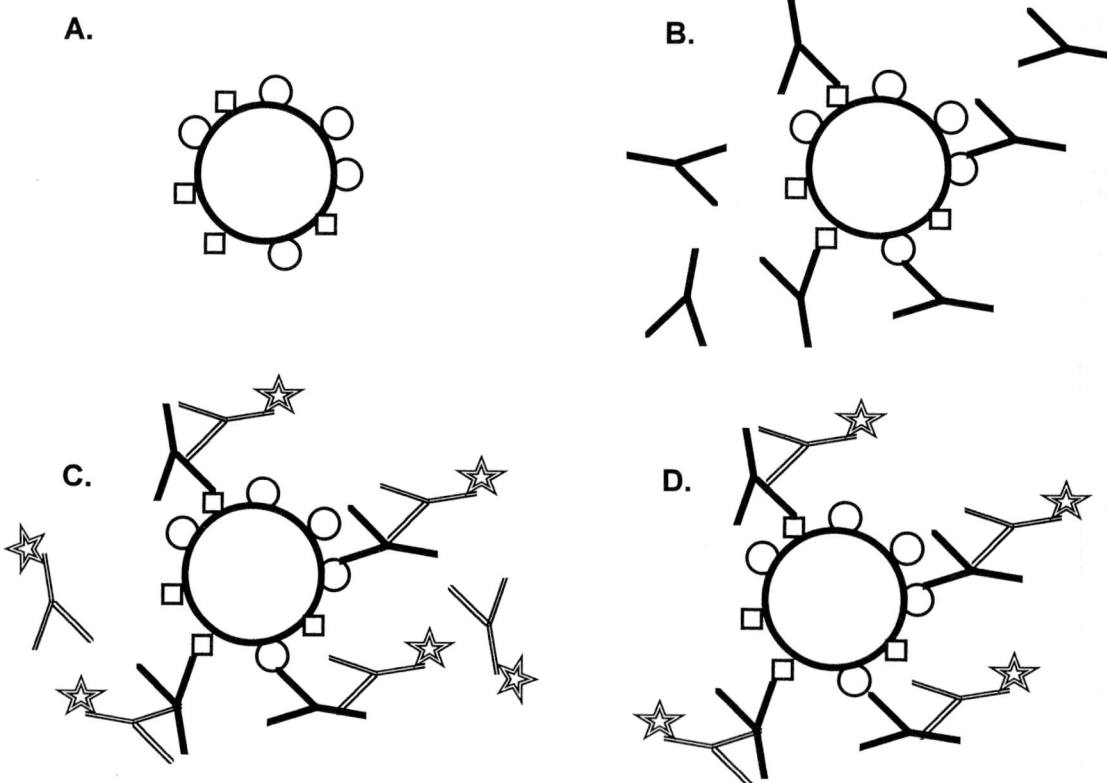

FIGURE 11–4. Schematic presentation of an immunosorbent assay for allergen-specific IgE antibody. *A,* Allergen represented by small circles and squares has been bound to solid phase. *B,* Serum that may contain IgE antibodies specific for the allergen is incubated with the solid phase. Specific antibodies bind to the allergen and nonbound antibodies are removed by washing. *C,* Labeled anti-human IgE antibody is incubated with the solid phase and the anti-IgE antibody binds to the immobilized IgE. Nonbound anti-IgE is washed away. *D,* The amount of anti-IgE antibody on the solid phase is proportional to the concentration of allergen-specific IgE in the serum tested.

antibody bound to the solid phase can be converted either into a class score or into some unit of IgE antibody by comparison to a standard curve. Initial tests for IgE antibodies used radiolabeled anti-IgE antibodies, but in recent years there has been a trend toward using enzyme-labeled antibodies. The primary advantages of enzyme labels are longer shelf life, freedom from the problems of handling radioisotopes, and the ability to use less expensive detection equipment.

Scoring Test Results. Currently, there is no universally agreed upon standard for reporting the results of tests for allergen-specific IgE antibodies. The most commonly used method consists of class scores based on the scoring used in the first commercially available assay. The radioallergosorbent test (RAST), originally marketed by Pharmacia Diagnostics (Phadebus, RAST), related all allergen-specific IgE values to a standard curve divided into five classes from 0 to 4. This scoring system provided results in terms of Phadebus RAST units (PRU). Class 0 indicated undetectable IgE, while classes 1 to 4 represented increasing quantities of IgE.

The scoring system used by Pharmacia was relatively conservative. To increase the sensitivity of the assay, the scoring system was modified and became known as the modified RAST scoring system (Williams et al, 1992). In the modified RAST system, a single quantity of IgE is used to calibrate the counting of the radioisotope, and all classes are linearly related to this standard. The modified scoring system does increase the sensitivity of the test, but at the expense of specificity, since only the scoring system and not the actual detection limit of the assay has been changed (Practice Standard Committee, 1983; Williams et al, 1992; Bernstein, 1988). Owing in large part to the way diagnostic tests are licensed by the Food and Drug Administration (FDA) in the United States, most companies marketing tests for IgE have adopted scoring systems that mimic the Pharmacia scoring system. Alternative methods to obtain results consistent with modified RAST scores are also typically given.

A third scoring system, used by some laboratories, relates the results of assays for a given allergen to the results obtained when sera from known nonallergic individuals are tested in the same assay. The mean and standard deviation of the negative sera results are computed, and sera producing results greater than the mean plus three standard deviations are scored as positive. Test results can also be expressed as the ratio or percentage of the results of the test serum to the results of a negative control serum pool. In most RAST type assays, a value of more than three times the negative control is positive (Homburger and Katzmann, 1993). Recently, some manufacturers have begun to produce assays that provide results in terms of mass units of IgE (e.g., nanograms or international units of IgE per ml). The accuracy of the mass units for these new assays has not been independently confirmed. The critical question for clinicians is which class score or value of IgE is considered positive evidence of the definite presence of specific IgE.

Quality of Test Results. Most clinicians are not directly involved with the laboratory performing tests for allergen-specific IgE, but they should assure themselves that the results they are obtaining are of high quality by obtaining the answers to several questions. The first question is where the test is actually performed. Many local laboratories send infrequently ordered tests, such as test for IgE, to outside reference laboratories. The second question is what method is used for the assay? Is it a commercially available assay or has the laboratory constructed its own assay, which has not been subjected to FDA evaluation? If a commercial assay is being used, is it being performed according to the manufacturer's directions or has it been modified by the laboratory? Next, who are the people actually performing the tests, what are their qualifications, and who is the laboratory director? Has the laboratory director had any special experience with IgE testing? Most importantly, what kind of quality control does the laboratory use for IgE tests? Does the laboratory participate in blinded proficiency testing? If so, the laboratory should be willing to provide a summary of the proficiency test results. Does the laboratory have positive control sera for the allergens being tested? If the laboratory has never had a positive test result for a particular allergen, how valid are negative results with the allergen?

Diagnostic Value of *In Vitro* Test Results. Studies of the diagnostic value of *in vitro* tests are often confusing because the distinction between the detection of allergen-specific IgE antibody and the diagnosis of allergic disease is often blurred (Ownby, 1988). If an *in vitro* test fails to detect specific IgE antibody when the antibody is truly present, the test lacks sensitivity (Table 11–2). The problem is how to determine whether IgE antibody is present. In most studies, skin tests are taken as the true indicators of the presence or absence of IgE antibody, but how is the accuracy of the skin tests confirmed? Skin tests usually are not performed in replicates, and as already discussed, prick-puncture skin tests and intradermal skin tests may yield different results. If the patient with a positive skin or *in vitro* test does not develop symptoms when exposed to the allergen, does this mean that the patient does not have IgE specific for the allergen or that the patient is not clinically sensitive, that is, not allergic to the allergen? If the *in vitro* test is positive and the sample does not have specific IgE, the test lacks specificity. Thus, the sensitivity of a test is the probability of obtaining a positive test result when the patient truly has allergen-specific IgE and the specificity of a test is the probability of obtaining a negative test when the patient truly does not have specific IgE antibodies (Table 11–2).

Many studies have compared the results of *in vitro* tests to the results of skin tests (Bernstein, 1988). In most studies, *in vitro* tests have a sensitivity of 60 percent to 80 percent and a specificity of 90+ percent when compared to skin tests (Ownby, 1988; Bernstein, 1988; Practice Standard Committee, 1983). The sensitivity and specificity can markedly vary, depending on the specific allergen being tested, the test system employed, and the scoring system used (Bernstein, 1988; Practice Standard Committee, 1983). In clinical terms, a well-performed *in vitro* test should rarely be falsely positive, but *in vitro* tests may be falsely negative in 20 percent to 40 percent of patients. Therefore, a negative *in vitro* test should not be used to conclusively rule out the possibility of allergic sensitivity.

ADVANTAGES AND DISADVANTAGES OF SKIN TESTS AND *IN VITRO* TESTS. Depending on the clinical situation, either skin tests or *in vitro* tests may be used to evaluate a patient for allergen-specific IgE. As listed in Table 11–3, there are certain advantages to each testing method. The most important advantage of skin testing is the high degree of sensitivity (Bernstein, 1988). When an intradermal skin test is properly performed, the risk of failing to detect allergic sensitization is extremely low. This degree of sensitivity is important when the risk of failing to detect specific IgE is great for the patient, as when patients are being tested for sensitivity to stinging insects and to drugs such as penicillin. In these situations, the risk of a false-positive reaction for the patient may be added inconvenience and expense, but the risk of a false-negative test may be a life-threatening allergic reaction.

The most important advantage of *in vitro* tests is their safety. If an individual has had a life-threatening reaction to an allergen, espe-

TABLE 11–2. INDICES OF DIAGNOSTIC TEST PERFORMANCE

1. *Sensitivity:* The percentage of positive test results in all patients having the disease.

$$\text{Sensitivity} = \frac{\text{True Positive}}{\text{True Positives} + \text{False Negatives}} \times 100$$

2. *Specificity:* The percentage of negative test results in all patients free of the disease.

$$\text{Specificity} = \frac{\text{True Negatives}}{\text{True Negatives} + \text{False Positives}} \times 100$$

3. *Efficiency:* The percentage of patients correctly classified as having or as free of disease.

$$\text{Efficiency} = \frac{\text{True Positives} + \text{True Negatives}}{\text{Total Positives} + \text{Total Negatives}} \times 100$$

4. *Predictive value of a positive test (positive predictive value):* The percentage of positive tests that correctly predict disease.

$$\text{Positive predictive value} = \frac{\text{True Positives}}{\text{True Positives} + \text{False Positives}} \times 100$$

5. *Predictive value of a negative test (negative predictive value):* The percentage of negative tests that correctly predict the absence of disease.

$$\text{Negative predictive value} = \frac{\text{True Negatives}}{\text{True Negatives} + \text{False Negatives}} \times 100$$

Adapted from Galen RS, Gambino SR. Beyond Normality: The Predictive Values and Efficiency of Medical Diagnosis. New York, John Wiley & Sons, 1975.

TABLE 11–3. IMPORTANT DIFFERENCES BETWEEN SKIN TESTS AND *IN VITRO* TESTS FOR DETECTING ALLERGEN-SPECIFIC IgE ANTIBODIES

ADVANTAGES OF SKIN TESTS	ADVANTAGES OF *IN VITRO* TESTS
Most sensitive type of test	No risk of inducing anaphylaxis
Results available in minutes	Results not affected by medications
Greater selection of allergens for testing	Condition of skin does not influence test results
Less personnel and reagent expense per test	Better documentation of quality control
Minimal equipment is required	May be more convenient for patients

cially an allergen for which there is little prior experience with skin testing or no standardized skin test extract, an *in vitro* test offers the possibility of detecting specific IgE without subjecting the patient to the risk of an allergic reaction during skin testing. The patient should understand that if the *in vitro* test is positive and consistent with the patient's history, the diagnosis is relatively assured, but a negative *in vitro* test does not exclude the possibility of sensitivity. In the face of a suggestive history and a negative *in vitro* test, the patient should still be skin tested before a final clinical judgment is made.

In routine allergy practice, skin testing has been found to be more cost-effective than *in vitro* testing. The cost-effectiveness is more pronounced as multiple allergens are tested. There are also the advantages of allowing the patient to see the immediate allergic reaction on his or her own skin and the immediate availability of results. In comparison, *in vitro* tests offer the ability to test patients whose skin is overtly reactive (extreme dermatographism) or who cannot be adequately skin tested because of extensive dermatitis, other skin disease, or because of interfering drugs. It may also be more convenient for both the patient and the physician to send blood samples to reference laboratories for testing with rare allergens than for the physician to obtain appropriate allergen extracts for testing, or for the patient to travel to another location for the testing.

OTHER USES FOR *IN VITRO* TESTS. A unique advantage of *in vitro* tests in some clinical situations is the ability to modify the test to evaluate allergen cross-reactivity. Hamilton et al (1993) have recently reported that allergen inhibition of *in vitro* tests was a cost-effective technique in the evaluation of patients allergic to hymenoptera stings. Hymenoptera-sensitive patients often react to multiple venoms, and the question is whether the patient is sensitive to each venom or whether the reactions are due to cross-reactive allergens. To answer this question, Hamilton et al (1993) evaluated the ability of individual venoms to inhibit IgE binding to other venoms. For example, a patient may have a history consistent with anaphylaxis following an insect sting and the most likely insect was a yellow jacket. When the patient is skin tested, there are positive reactions to both yellow jacket and white-faced hornet. Should the patient be treated with both yellow jacket and hornet venom or will yellow jacket venom alone be adequate treatment? If the binding of the patient's IgE to hornet venom can be inhibited by 90 percent by preincubation with yellow jacket venom, it is highly likely that the reaction to hornet venom was the result of cross-reactivity and not the result of sensitivity to both venoms. By reducing the number of venoms needed for treatment, substantial cost savings can be obtained.

TOTAL SERUM IgE

METHODS FOR MEASURING TOTAL IgE CONCENTRATIONS. Although a variety of assays have been used to measure the small concentrations of IgE normally present in human serum, the most frequently used current method is a two-site immunometric assay (Homburger and Katzmann, 1993). Two-site immunometric assays are sometimes referred to as "sandwich" assays because the substance being measured is sandwiched between two antibodies. The first antibody, either a polyclonal or monoclonal anti–human IgE antibody, is attached to a solid phase such as a paper disc or plastic well in a microtiter plate. After appropriate steps are taken to prevent the nonspecific binding of other proteins to the solid phase, the solid phase is incubated with an appropriate dilution of the serum to be tested. IgE in the serum becomes bound to the solid-phase anti-IgE in proportion to the concentration of IgE in the serum sample. After the nonbound proteins are washed away, the quantity of IgE bound to the solid phase is determined by reacting the solid phase with a second soluble anti-IgE antibody. The second anti-IgE antibody is labeled either with a radionuclide or with an enzyme. Following washing to remove the unbound labeled anti-IgE, the amount of radioactivity or the amount of enzymatic activity in the sample is measured and converted into units of IgE by comparison to a standard curve. A variety of commercial assays are available and most are accurate to a concentration of approximately 1 IU/ml of IgE. Modifications of these assays can increase sensitivity to approximately 0.1 IU/ml.

Serum concentrations of IgE vary widely in normal individuals. IgE levels are very low at birth and gradually rise, peaking in the second decade of life and then declining slowly into old age. Representative data on IgE levels in a skin-test negative population of children and adults are shown in Table 11–4. Although the geometric mean values are relatively low, there is a 95 percent confidence interval at all ages.

Most laboratories and publications currently present IgE concentrations as international units (IU) or nanograms per milliliter. One IU is generally believed to equal 2.4 ng of IgE. The new Systeme International (SI) specifies that IgE be reported as micrograms per liter (μg/L) with two significant digits (XX $\times$ 10^n) (Lundberg et al, 1986).

TOTAL SERUM IgE IN ALLERGIC DISEASE. Most studies have consistently shown that total serum IgE concentrations tend to be higher in allergic adults and children than in nonallergic individuals of similar ages. Unfortunately, there is a relatively large overlap between serum IgE concentrations in allergic and nonallergic individuals, and this overlap limits the diagnostic value of total IgE measurements. Wittig et al (1978) calculated the diagnostic sensitivity and specificity of total serum IgE determination using three cutoff levels in 570 asthmatic and 244 rhinitic individuals. When a high IgE value of 320 IU/ml was chosen, the specificity of the IgE was 98 percent in both the rhinitis and asthma groups, but the sensitivity was only 55 percent for asthma and 30 percent for rhinitis. If the level was reduced to 100 IU/ml, the sensitivity increased to 78 percent and 60 percent for asthma and rhinitis, but the specificity fell to 80 percent in both groups. Other studies have found that the optimal IgE concentration for distinguishing allergic from nonallergic individuals varied from 50 IU/ml to 100 IU/ml. Klink et al (1990) studied serum IgE levels in 2657 individuals including nonallergic, rhinitic, and asthmatic individuals and concluded that there was no IgE concentration which distinguished allergic from nonallergic groups in a clinically meaningful way.

Although measurements of total serum IgE concentrations are not generally useful in individuals with possible allergic disease, total serum IgE measurements are valuable in the diagnosis and management of allergic bronchopulmonary aspergillosis (ABPA). Patients with ABPA typically have serum IgE levels higher than 500 IU/ml. With adequate glucocorticoid therapy, total serum IgE levels tend to fall. A sudden increase in serum IgE may herald a disease exacerbation (Leser et al, 1992).

IgE IN CORD BLOOD. The availability of

TABLE 11–4. TOTAL SERUM IgE LEVELS IN SKIN TEST–NEGATIVE CHILDREN AND ADULTS (IU/ml)

AGE (YEARS)	N	SEX	GEOMETRIC MEAN	GEOMETRIC MEAN $\pm$ 2 S.D.
6–14	69	M	40.9	2.0–824.1
	71	F	40.7	3.4–452.9
15–34	213	M	23.3	0.9–635.3
	201	F	16.5	0.8–349.1
35–54	145	M	20.4	0.9–443.6
	154	F	14.6	0.7–286.4
55–74	224	M	19.8	0.8–484.2
	348	F	10.7	0.6–198.6
75+	61	M	17.8	0.8–387.3
	83	F	8.9	0.4–208.9

Modified from Klink M, Cline MG, Halonen M, et al. Problems in defining normal limits for serum IgE. J Allergy Clin Immunol 85:440, 1990.

IgE assays with greater analytic sensitivity has made it possible to measure the usually very small concentrations of IgE found in the cord blood of infants. It was hoped that the concentration of IgE in cord blood would represent the infant's basal genetic propensity toward IgE production and hence be a useful predictor of the infant's genetic risk of allergic disease. A number of studies have now evaluated the predictive value of cord blood IgE levels with variable results. The largest study and the study with the longest follow-up interval was originally reported by Croner et al (1982). At 7 years of age, children born with IgE concentrations of >1.3 IU/ml had a 57.5 percent risk of allergy compared to a risk of only 12.5 percent in children with IgE levels of ≤1.3 IU/ml (Croner et al, 1982; Kjellman and Croner, 1984; Croner and Kjellman, 1990). Although the majority of studies have shown that cord blood IgE concentrations were prognostically significant, several studies have not found that cord blood IgE concentrations were significantly related to allergic risk (Ownby, 1993). Unfortunately, many of the studies evaluating the prognostic value of cord blood IgE measurements have followed infants for only a few years after birth.

TOTAL SERUM IgE IN NONALLERGIC DISEASES. Total serum IgE concentrations have been measured in many nonallergic diseases including parasitic, infectious, neoplastic, HIV, and renal diseases. Serum IgE has also been studied in cigarette smokers and bone marrow transplant recipients. While statistically significant differences have been found in many of these conditions, the clinical value of measuring IgE in these conditions is small. The principal value of these studies has been to learn more about the normal physiology of IgE (Ownby, 1993).

During metazoan parasitic infections, serum IgE levels increase, and there is usually an association between increasing levels of tissue invasion and increasing levels of IgE. Most of the serum IgE is not directed toward parasitic antigens. The parasitic infection appears to result in an increase in total IgE antibody production, probably by stimulating an increase in the cytokines, which promote IgE production. With effective treatment of the parasitic infection, IgE levels usually fall. The value of IgE production during parasitic infections is still being investigated, but there is a growing consensus that IgE antiparasite antibodies probably play a role in host defense against parasites.

Total IgE concentrations are also of diagnostic value in two relatively rare conditions. The first condition is the hyper IgE, recurrent infection syndrome originally described by Buckley et al (1972). In this condition, serum IgE concentrations typically exceed 1000 IU/ml, and concentrations above 10,000 IU/ml are relatively common. This is the one condition in which antistaphylococcal IgE antibodies are usually detectable. The second rare condition is IgE myeloma (Allevato et al, 1984). Patients with symptoms suggestive of myeloma and with laboratory findings suggestive of light-chain disease should have IgE measured. The relatively small quantities of IgE present, even in myelomas, may be missed by the methods usually used for evaluation of myelomas. The distinction between light-chain disease and IgE myeloma is important because of the different prognoses (Allevato et al, 1984).

REFERENCES

Adinoff AD, Rosloniec DM, McCall LL, et al. A comparison of six epicutaneous devices in the performance of immediate hypersensitivity skin testing. J Allergy Clin Immunol 84:168–174, 1989.

Allevato PA, Deegan MJ, Chu J-W, et al. A case of IgE myeloma: Methodology and review of the literature. Henry Ford Hospital Med J 32:134–141, 1984.

Bernstein IL. The proceedings of the task force on guidelines for standardizing old and new technologies used for the diagnosis and treatment of allergic diseases. J Allergy Clin Immunol 82:487–526, 1988.

Bousquet J, Michel F-B. In vivo methods for study of allergy. Skin tests, techniques, and interpretation. In Middleton E Jr, Reed CE, Ellis EF, et al. (eds). Allergy Principles and Practice. 4th ed. St. Louis, Mosby-Year Book, 1993, p 573.

Buckley RH, Wray BB, Belmaker EZ. Extreme hyperimmunoglobulinemia E and undue susceptibility to infection. Pediatrics 49:59–70, 1972.

Chin JT, Nelson B, Sokol W, et al. Extended evaluation of diagnostic skin-testing practices in Orange County, California. Allergy Proc 14:283–286, 1993.

Council on Scientific Affairs. In vivo diagnostic testing and immunotherapy for allergy. Report I, part II, of the allergy panel. JAMA 258:1505–1508, 1987a.

Council on Scientific Affairs. In vivo diagnostic testing and immunotherapy for allergy. Report I, part I, of the allergy panel. JAMA 258:1363–1367, 1987b.

Croner S, Kjellman NIM, Eriksson B, et al. IgE screening in 1701 newborn infants and the development of atopic disease during infancy. Arch Dis Child 57:364–368, 1982.

Croner S, Kjellman NIM. Development of atopic disease in relation to family history and cord blood IgE levels. Eleven-year follow-up in 1654 children. Pediatr Allergy Immunol 1:14–20, 1990.

Demoly P, Bosquet J, Manderscheid JC, et al. Precision of skin prick and puncture tests with nine methods. J Allergy Clin Immunol 88:758–762, 1991.

Dreborg S. Food allergy in pollen sensitive patients. Ann Allergy 61:41, 1988.

Dreborg S, Backman A, Basomba A, et al. Skin tests used in type I allergy testing. Position paper. Allergy 44(suppl 10):1–44. 1989.

Frew AJ, Kay AB. The pattern of human late-phase skin reactions to extracts of aeroallergens. J Allergy Clin Immunol 81:1117–1121, 1988.

Hagy GW, Settipane GA. Risk factors for developing asthma and allergic rhinitis. A 7-year follow-up of college students. J Allergy Clin Immunol 58:330–336, 1976.

Hamilton RG, Wisenauer JA, Golden DBK, et al. Selection of Hymenoptera venoms for immunotherapy on the basis of patient's IgE antibody cross-reactivity. J Allergy Clin Immunol 92:651–659, 1993.

Hepner MJ, Ownby DR, Anderson JA, et al. Risk of systemic reactions in patients taking beta-blocker drugs receiving allergen immunotherapy injections. J Allergy Clin Immunol 86:407–411, 1990.

Homburger HA, Katzmann JA. Methods in laboratory immunology. Principles and interpretation of laboratory tests for allergy. In Middleton E Jr, Reed CE, Ellis EF, et al. (eds). Allergy Principles and Practice. 4th ed. St. Louis, Mosby-Year Book, 1993, p 554.

Ishizaka K, Ishizaka T. Identification of γE-antibodies as a carrier of reaginic activity. J Immunol 99:1187–1198, 1967.

Johansson SGO, Bennich H. Immunologic studies of an atypical (myeloma) immunoglobulin. Immunol 13:381–394, 1967.

Kjellman NIM, Croner S. Cord blood IgE determination for allergy prediction—a follow-up to seven years of age in 1,651 children. Ann Allergy 53:167–171, 1984.

Klink M, Cline MG, Halonen M, et al. Problems in defining normal limits for serum IgE. J Allergy Clin Immunol 85:440–444, 1990.

Leser C, Kauffman HF, Virchow C Sr, et al. Specific serum immunopatterns in clinical phases of allergic bronchopulmonary aspergillosis. J Allergy Clin Immunol 90:589–599, 1992.

Lichtenstein LM, Ishizaka K, Norman PS, et al. IgE antibody measurements in ragweed hay fever. J Clin Invest 52:472–482, 1973.

Lockey RF, Benedict LM, Turkeltaub PC, et al. Fatalities from immunotherapy and skin testing. J Allergy Clin Immunol 79:660–677, 1987.

Lundberg GD, Iverson C, Radulescu G. Now read this: The SI units are here. JAMA 255:2329–2339, 1986.

Menardo JL, Bosquet J, Rodiere M, et al. Skin test reactivity in infancy. J Allergy Clin Immunol 75:646–651, 1985.

Nelson HS. The effect of preservatives and dilution on the deterioration of Russian thistle (*Salsola pestifer*), a pollen extract. J Allergy Clin Immunol 63:417–425, 1979.

Nelson HS. Effect of preservatives and conditions of storage on the potency of allergy extracts. J Allergy Clin Immunol 67:64–69, 1981.

Nelson HS. Diagnostic procedures in allergy. I. Allergy skin testing. Ann Allergy 51:411–417, 1983.

Nelson HS. Allergen skin testing. AAAI, News and Notes 1:15–16, 1993.

Ownby DR, Anderson JA. An improved prick skin-test procedure for young children. J Allergy Clin Immunol 69:533–535, 1982.

Ownby DR. Allergy testing: *In vivo* versus *in vitro*. Pediatr Clin North Am 35:995–1009, 1988.

Ownby DR. Clinical significance of IgE. In Middleton E Jr, Reed CE, Ellis EF, et al. (eds). Allergy Principles and Practice. 4th ed. St. Louis, Mosby-Year Book, 1993, p 1059.

Pepys J. Skin testing. Br J Hosp Med 14:412, 1975.

Practice Standard Committee. Skin testing and radioallergosorbent testing (RAST) for diagnosis of specific allergens responsible for IgE-mediated diseases. J Allergy Clin Immunol 72:515–517, 1983.

Skassa-Brociek W, Manderscheid JC, Michel FB, et al. Skin test reactivity to histamine from infancy to elderly. J Allergy Clin Immunol 80:711–716, 1987.

Smith JA, Mansfield LE, deShazo R. An evaluation of the pharmacologic inhibition of immediate and late cutaneous effect to allergen. J Allergy Clin Immunol 65:118, 1980.

VanAsperen PP, Kemp AS, Mellis CM. Skin test reactivity and clinical allergen sensitivity in infancy. J Allergy Clin Immunol 73:381–386, 1984.

Williams PB, Dolen WK, Koepke JW, et al. Immunoassay of specific IgE: Use of a single point calibration curve in the modified radioallergosorbent test. Ann Allergy 69:48–52, 1992.

Wittig HJ, McLaughlin ET, Leifer KL, et al. Risk factors for the development of allergic disease: Analysis of 2,190 patient records. Ann Allergy 41:84–88, 1978.

Chapter 12

Assessment of Lung Function: Pulmonary Function Testing

Sally E. Wenzel, M.D., and Gary L. Larsen, M.D.

There are many ways to assess the lung in the patient with pulmonary-related complaints. After a detailed history and physical examination, with particular emphasis on the respiratory tract, it is a common procedure to obtain a chest roentgenogram and, occasionally, an arterial blood gas determination to further this assessment. However, these offer very little data regarding the functional capacity of the lungs. Various measurements of pulmonary function are also available and important in the evaluation and management of respiratory disease, and some tests can be performed by children as young as 5 or 6 years of age. Pulmonary function tests can assist patient evaluation and serve as important and indispensable aids in the care of many acute and chronic pulmonary disorders. This is especially true in the diagnosis and care of patients with asthma and other obstructive airway disorders, because wheezing, often used as an index of airflow limitation, does not occur in the smaller airways. Auscultation also is a grossly imperfect way of assessing obstruction to airflow. This chapter will review common tests of lung function and particularly those that can be performed and interpreted in the physician's office or other clinical setting. Table 12–1 indicates the clinical applications and limitations of these tests that aid in the diagnosis, evaluate precipitants of the symptoms, assess the effects of therapy, and follow the course of the disease. Although many of the examples in the figures are from the assessment of pediatric patients, the general principles apply to adults as well. The emphasis of this chapter is on asthma, but the physiology of diseases that may be mistaken for asthma will be presented as well.

PULMONARY FUNCTION TESTS

Tests of lung function most easily conducted and interpreted within the physician's office may be grouped into two broad categories: lung volumes (or capacities) and flow rates (volume per unit of time).

DEFINITION OF LUNG VOLUMES AND CAPACITIES. Air within the lung is partitioned into various functional compartments called volumes. Sums of volumes are termed capacities. The proportion of these compartments is similar among healthy individuals. The absolute values of these subdivisions change with age

TABLE 12–1. PULMONARY FUNCTION TESTS: CLINICAL APPLICATIONS AND LIMITATIONS

Applications
  Aid in diagnosis
  Quantitate disease severity
  Define precipitants of symptoms
  Evaluate therapy
  Follow the disease course
Limitations
  Wide range of normal values
  Dynamic changes with age
  Variable patient cooperation
  Lack of tests for infants, small children

and body size (primarily height) and may differ among races and sexes. Various lung volumes and capacities are displayed in Figure 12–1. The volume of air that is inspired and expired during normal, quiet breathing is the tidal volume (V_T) and normally equals approximately 10 percent of the maximum amount of air contained within the lung. The maximal volume of air that can be inhaled over and above the tidal volume is the inspiratory reserve volume (IRV); the maximal volume of air that can be exhaled from normal breathing is the expiratory reserve volume (ERV). The air in the lung that cannot be expelled with maximal effort is termed the residual volume (RV).

As noted, the sums of the volumes in the lung make up various functional components termed capacities. Thus, the sum of all of the volumes (RV + ERV + V_T + IRV) is the total lung capacity (TLC). The total amount of air that can be exhaled (from the point of maximum inspiration) is the vital capacity (VC) and is thus the sum of the IRV, the V_T, and the ERV. The functional residual capacity (FRC) is composed of the ERV and the RV. Normally, the VC equals approximately 75 percent of the TLC, with the RV accounting for the remaining 25 percent. The FRC is approximately 40 percent of the TLC in healthy individuals. These relationships may be altered in obstructive airways diseases, such as asthma, in which the absolute values of the RV and FRC increase, as does the ratio of either to the TLC (see the right side of Fig. 12–1 and Fig. 12–2A).

MEASUREMENTS OF LUNG VOLUMES AND CAPACITIES. Many of the volumes and the VC discussed previously can be measured with the use of a simple spirometer as displayed in Figure 12–1. The maximal expiratory vital capacity maneuver is employed to measure these functions. The subject is instructed to perform a slow, full inhalation of air to maximum inflation, hold his or her breath for a brief period of time, and then perform a sudden, sustained maximal exhalation to RV that lasts a minimum of 3 seconds. From the volume-time tracing produced (spirogram) shown in Figure 12–1, the VC plus all lung volumes except the RV can be calculated. It is important to stress, however, that the RV (and thus the FRC and TLC, both of which include the residual volume) cannot be calculated from this record. Other methods must be employed to measure these compartments. Although the techniques used in these assessments are more complicated than simple spi-

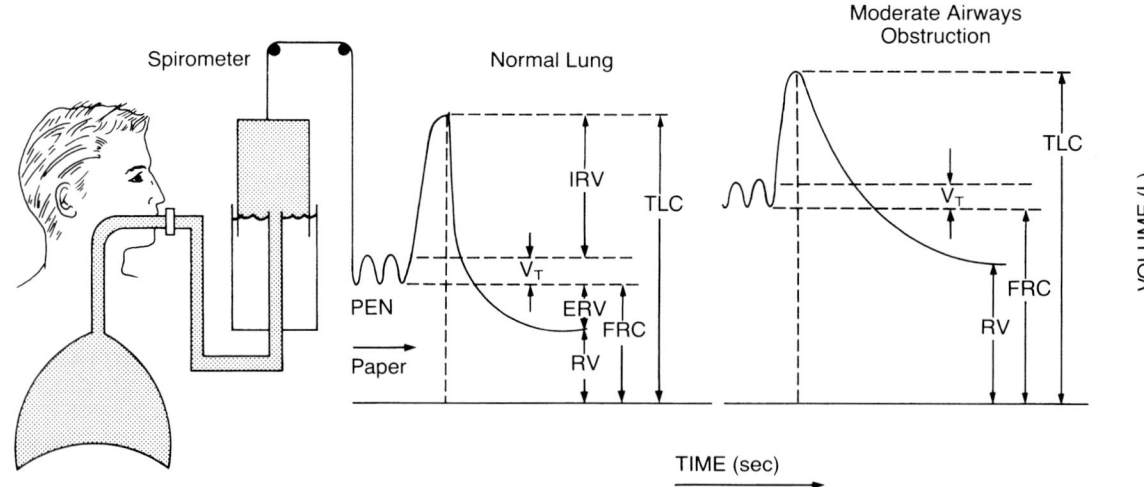

FIGURE 12–1. Normal lung volumes and capacities and an example of those found with moderate airway obstruction are displayed as a spirogram (volume versus time tracing). The volumes and capacities include tidal volume (V_T), inspiratory reserve volume (IRV), expiratory reserve volume (ERV), residual volume (RV), vital capacity (VC), functional residual capacity (FRC), and total lung capacity (TLC). The VC and all volumes except the RV can be measured with a simple spirometer, as displayed. To assess RV as well as TLC and FRC, spirometry has to be combined with either body plethysmography or a gas dilution technique (see text). With moderate airways obstruction, expiratory airflow is decreased, as represented by less volume of air exhaled per unit of time; lung volumes (RV, FRC) are increased.

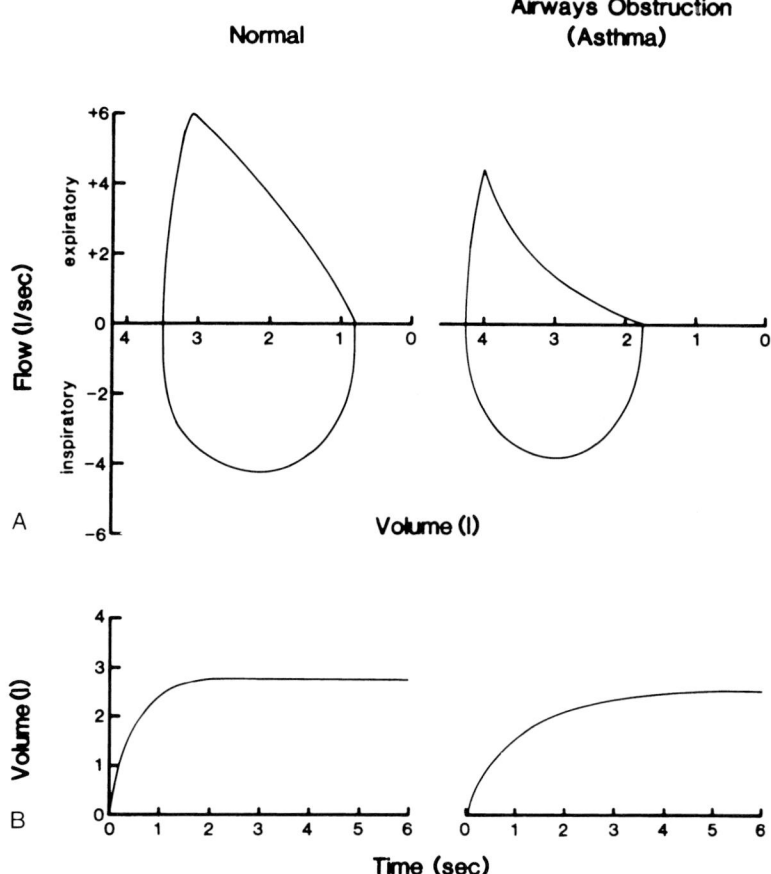

FIGURE 12–2. Flow-volume loops are compared with volume-time tracings (spirograms) in a patient with asthma at two time points. Pulmonary functions displayed on the left, when disease is well controlled (Normal), are compared with a time when the patient is unstable (Airways Obstruction). In *A*, flow is on the y-axis, and volume on the x-axis. Normal maximal inspiratory and expiratory curves that constitute the flow-volume loop are shown on the left. (Maximal inspiration (total lung capacity) is the point of zero flow on the left side of the loop (approximately 3.5 L); maximal exhalation (residual volume) is at the point of zero flow at the right side of the loop (0.8 L in this example). With a forced vital capacity maneuver, expiratory flow reaches a maximum value soon after the onset of effort and then decreases to zero flow as a straight line or with some convexity. With airways obstruction (right), hyperinflation is noted (increase in residual volume), and flow rates decrease as manifest in the curve that becomes concave. Note that the inspiratory loop is relatively preserved with moderate lower airway obstruction (compare with Fig. 12–5). In *B*, volume is plotted on the y-axis against time on the x-axis. A normal expiratory curve is shown on the left. With a forced vital capacity maneuver, volume reaches a plateau within 2 seconds (approximately 2.7 L). Forced expiratory volume at 1 second (FEV_1) is read from the y-axis, where the 1-second time mark intersects the curve (approximately 2.4 L). With airways obstruction on the right, the volume-time curve is less steep. The FEV_1 is therefore decreased, and a longer period of time is required for the curve to plateau at vital capacity. Although minimally diminished in this example, forced vital capacity may be more decreased, especially with more severe obstruction.

rometry, and the equipment needed is not usually found within the physician's office or a clinic, it is important to review briefly the principles involved in the determination of these compartments that may be useful clinically.

The TLC and the RV both can be computed if the FRC is known. The FRC usually is determined by one of two techniques, i.e., gas dilution or body plethysmography. With gas dilution, the changes in concentration of a relatively insoluble gas (helium or nitrogen) are monitored as the subject breathes either single or multiple breaths in a closed (re-breathing) or an open (nonbreathing) system. In most laboratories where this principle is applied, helium is utilized as the reference gas in a closed-circuit technique. The subject breathes from a spirometer containing a mixture of helium and air until the concentration of helium is the same in both the lungs and the spirometer. The volume of gas in the system is noted before the test begins, and the helium concentration is noted once equilibration occurs; a simple formula can then be used to calculate the volume of air in the lung at the initiation of inspiration (FRC) from the spirometer (Cherniack, 1992). With this method of assessing FRC, all areas of the lung must communicate with the airways to be measured. Thus, if some air-containing units do not communicate with the central airways because of complete airways obstruction, the FRC may be underestimated.

The other method employed to assess the FRC is body plethysmography. A plethysmograph is an airtight chamber in which the subject sits and performs various respiratory maneuvers through a mouthpiece. This application takes advantage of Boyle's law, which states that the volume of a gas in a container varies inversely with the pressure to which it is subjected. For measuring lung volume in the plethysmograph, the airway is occluded at the end of a quiet expiration (at FRC). Through continued respiratory efforts against an occluded airway, the subject compresses and decompresses the gas within the chest. By measuring pressure and volume changes in the plethysmograph produced by this maneuver, the FRC may be determined, again through use of a simple formula (Cherniack, 1992). With this technique, air-containing units do not need to communicate with airways to be measured; thus, lung volume assessed by this method will not be underestimated in the presence of severe or complete obstruction of airways. The RV and TLC may be calculated from the FRC, as determined by either method.

DEFINITION AND MEASUREMENT OF FLOW RATES. By analyzing the volume of air that can be expired from the lung in a defined period of time, various flow rates can be derived. Because maximal flow rates reflect the degree of resistance to airflow or airways obstruction, they are useful measurements of lung function that are commonly assessed in diseases such as asthma.

Flow rates vary with lung size, lung volume, and patient effort. Airway caliber increases with age and height, leading to a decrease in the resistance to airflow and the ability to produce higher flow rates. At any given age and height, the flow rate also depends on the lung volume at which it is measured; one reason for this is that the elastic recoil pressure is greater at higher lung volumes. As discussed in more detail elsewhere (Cherniack, 1992), recoil pressure is one of the major determinants of flow rates generated during maximal expiratory maneuvers.

The most common measurements of flow include the peak expiratory flow rate (PEFR) and the forced expiratory volume at one second (FEV_1). The PEFR is the maximal flow recorded during a forced expiratory maneuver from TLC and is expressed in L/sec. This test of lung function, which correlates with FEV_1 is simple to perform, easily learned, and reproducible. In addition, PEFR may be assessed by a number of hand-held devices specifically made for this one pulmonary function. These devices include a sturdy professional model (Wright peak-flow meter) as well as less durable plastic models (Mini-Wright peak-flow meter, Vitalograph Pulmonary Monitor, Assess Peak Florometer and others) suited for monitoring of PEFR in the home and at work.

FEV_1 is the most sensitive and reproducible measured flow rate within a physician's office or clinic and is easily determined from a spirogram (see Fig. 12–1 and Fig. 12–2B) or from flow-volume curves. It is extremely helpful in disease diagnosis and management. This function is obtained from a recording of a maximal forced expiratory maneuver that goes from full inspiration to full expiration. It is often compared with the forced vital capacity as a ratio (FEV_1/FVC). A value greater than 0.80 in children and young adults is consistent with normal airflow, without limitation (Polgar and Promadhat, 1971) (Fig. 12–3 and Fig. 12–4). The ratio may decrease with age but should remain greater than 70 percent.

Aside from the spirogram (volume-time tracing), flow rates may also be determined from flow-volume curves (Fig. 12–2A). Instead of displaying volume and time, flow and volume are exhibited. The maneuver employed to generate the expiratory flows is the same (maximal FVC), but in many instances, the maximal expiratory maneuver is followed by a maximal inspiratory maneuver so that

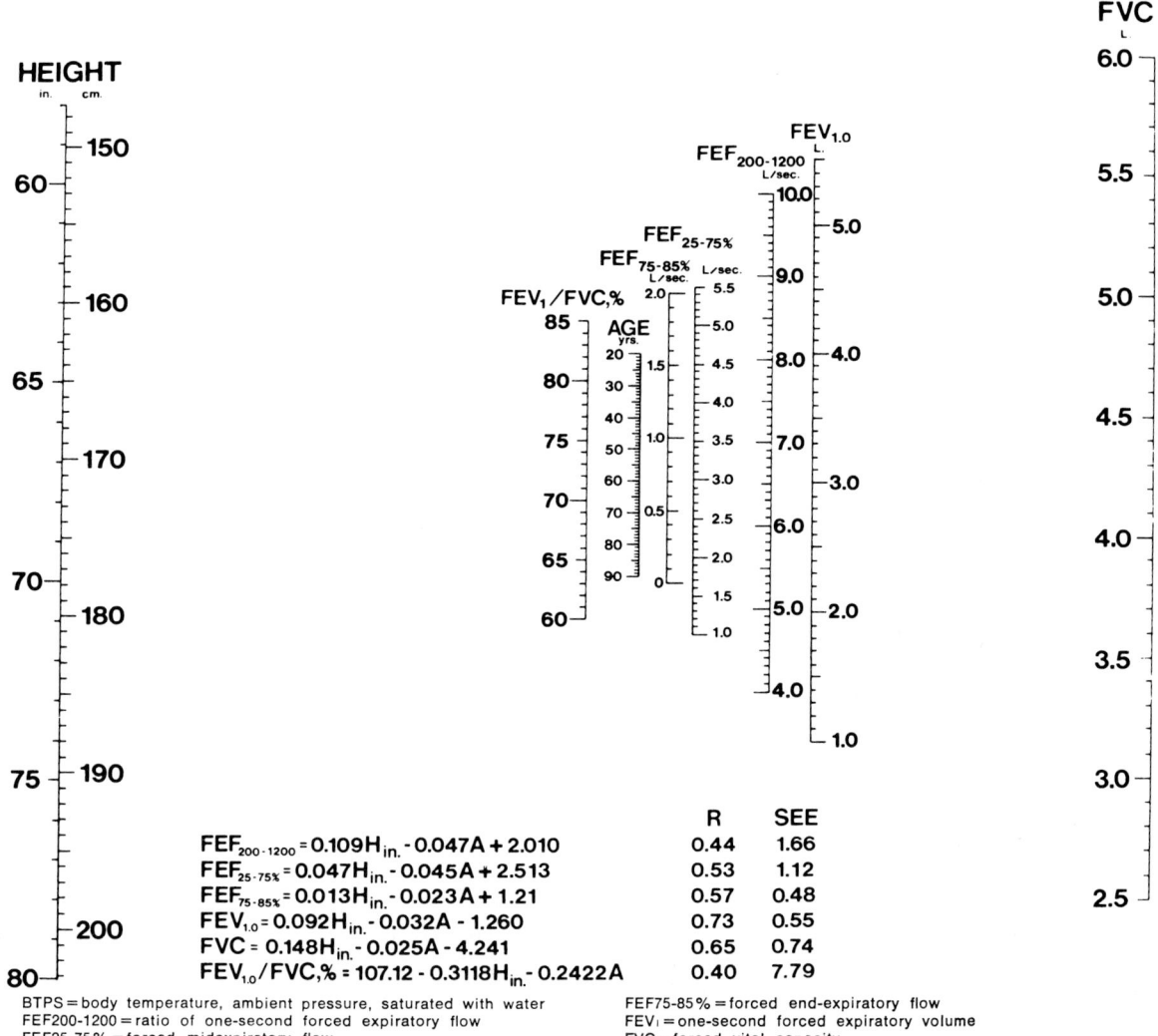

FIGURE 12–3. Spirometry in the evaluation of pulmonary function. Shown are normal predicted values for males. (From Morris et al. West J Med 125:110–118, 1976.)

both inspiratory and expiratory flows can be assessed. One consequence of this method of recording is that instantaneous flow rates at any point in the maneuver may be read directly from the curves. Thus, the highest flow generated after the onset of the expiratory maneuver is the PEFR. On some equipment, a small deflection of the expiratory limb of the flow-volume loop signifies 1 second has elapsed since expiration began, allowing computation of the FEV_1 (not shown in Fig. 12–2A).

SPIROGRAMS VERSUS FLOW-VOLUME CURVES. Both methods of recording forced expiratory maneuvers can be employed alone or in combination with a complete assessment of lung volumes and capacities (via a gas dilution technique or body plethysmography) to obtain a more complete picture of pulmonary physiology. There are differences, however, between the two tracings that should be pointed out. As mentioned, flow rates from a spirogram reflect mean flows, whereas flows from a flow-volume curve represent instantaneous flows. Thus, it is easier by visual inspection to examine the expiratory portion of the flow-volume curve and, from the shape of the curve alone, to determine whether airflow limitation exists (Hyatt and Black, 1973). For example, on the normal curve depicted

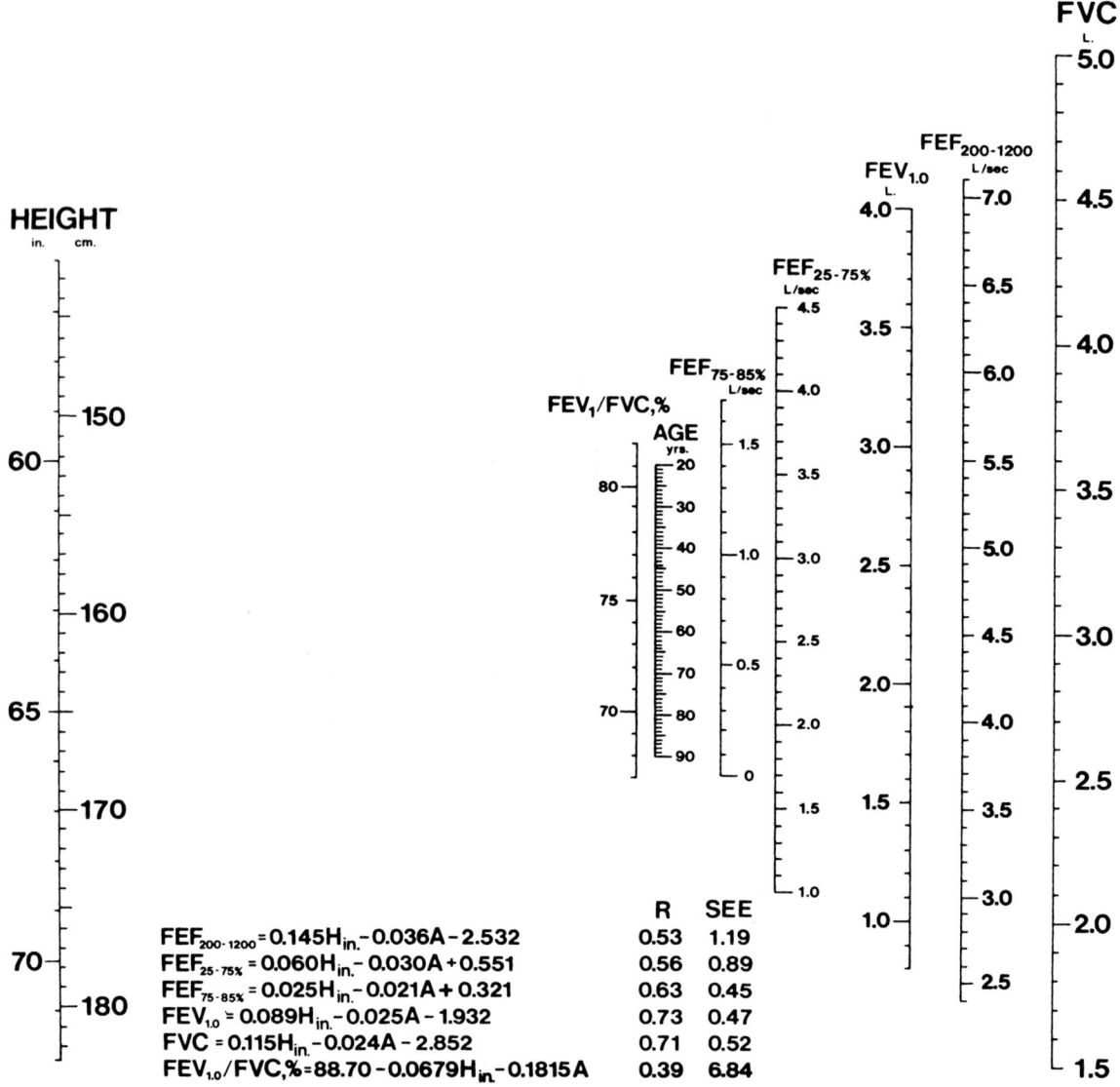

FIGURE 12–4. Spirometry in the evaluation of pulmonary function. Shown are normal predicted values for females. (From Morris et al. West J Med 125:110–118, 1976.)

in Figure 12–2A, the descending limb of the expiratory portion of the flow-volume loop is straight or slightly convex. However, when airways obstruction exists, as shown in the right-hand portion of Figure 12–2A, the descending curve becomes "scooped out" and is concave. Mild degrees of airways obstruction are harder to identify by inspection of the spirogram and are more obvious on the flow-volume curve. Artifacts also are easier to identify when instantaneous flow is displayed. Common artifacts include less than maximal effort in the initiation of the forced expiratory maneuver, premature termination of the test (not blowing completely to residual volume), and coughing during the expiratory maneuver. On the flow-volume curve flow does not increase to a maximum value within the first 25 percent of the VC when the initial effort is suboptimal, and flow precipitously returns to the point of zero flow when effort is terminated prematurely. Coughing during the maneuver leads to very uneven flow rates.

Another advantage of a flow-volume analysis is that both inspiratory and expiratory curves can be examined. The contour of a normal inspiratory curve is shown in Figure 12–2A, and as can be seen, the inspiratory flow rate is roughly equivalent to the expiratory flow rate at 50 percent of VC. With diffuse airways obstruction, such as that observed with mild to moderate asthma (right portion of Fig. 12–2A), the expiratory curve is more abnormal than the inspiratory curve. This differential effect of diffuse lower airways obstruction on the inspiratory and expiratory curves is due partly to transmural pressures generated by these maneuvers. In cases of lower airways obstruction (during expiration) external positive pressures from the thoracic cage exceed pressures in the airways, so that flow in these airways is limited. In contrast, during inspiration, the negative pressures generated by the outward expansion of the thoracic cage and diaphragm produce a type of "vacuum" effect, pulling the airways open.

Other types of pathology within the airways may result in different patterns on the flow-volume loop (Miller and Hyatt, 1973). As shown in Figure 12–5, with fixed airways obstruction within the central airways (larynx, trachea) that is either intrathoracic or extrathoracic, truncation of both the inspiratory and expiratory limbs of the flow-volume loop occurs. This type of abnormality can be seen in a patient with subglottic stenosis, in whom the pathology involves the total circumference of the airway. Tumors invading the walls of the airways may also produce such a pattern. With an extrathoracic lesion that is variable, the lower airways still undergo dilatation and compression during the respiratory cycle. In these types of obstruction, the lack of a surrounding thoracic cage eliminates the development of negative pressure surrounding the airway so that the negative pressure in the airways on inspiration causes collapse and/or a decrease in flow. Laryngomalacia produces this type of pattern. When a lesion affects a major intrathoracic airway (trachea or main stem bronchus) and dynamic movements with respiration still occur, a variable intrathoracic pattern is seen in which flow limitation is greatest on expiration. Certain types of vascular rings as well as other masses compressing the airways can produce this pattern. The configuration of the flow-volume loop found with a diffuse disease (asthma, COPD) within the intrathoracic airways (right side of Fig. 12–2A) should be contrasted to the configuration found with a more localized lesion within the major airways that produces variable compression during expiration (right side of Fig. 12–5). In the latter, there is more truncation of the expiratory flow at high lung volumes.

OTHER TESTS. In addition to spirometry performed in the physician's office, an occasional patient may require more sophisticated tests that are performed only in a well-equipped pulmonary function laboratory. The techniques of assessing absolute lung volumes (TLC, FRC, RV) are but some examples and have been discussed previously. These tests are useful in discriminating between an *obstructive* process associated with air-trapping and increased lung volumes and a *restrictive* process, such as interstitial lung disease (ILD), which limits or "restricts" lung volume.

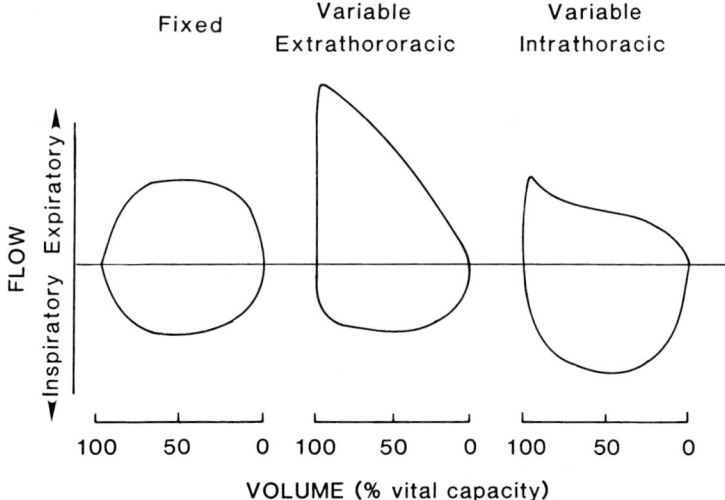

FIGURE 12–5. Flow-volume loops are displayed for various types of obstructing lesions of the proximal airways (trachea and larynx) that may present as wheezing. For comparison, the normal configuration of a flow-volume loop is shown on the left side of Figure 12–2A. With a lesion that is circumferential, preventing either compression or dilation of the airway with respiratory efforts, a "fixed" pattern is seen with truncation of both the inspiratory and expiratory curves. If a lesion permits compression or dilation with respiration, the pattern will depend on whether the lesion is extrathoracic or intrathoracic. With the extrathoracic lesion, the inspiratory curve is more affected. The intrathoracic lesion will have more of an effect on expiratory airflow.

In addition, measurement of the more detailed mechanical properties of the lung by obtaining a pressure-volume curve may aid in the diagnosis of a patient with a confusing clinical picture or spirometric values or both. For example, in a patient with emphysema, a marked loss of elastic recoil pressure (increased compliance) is noted on a pressure-volume curve, whereas in a patient with a disease, such as interstitial fibrosis, an increase in elastic recoil (decreased compliance) is noted. When a defect in gas diffusion is suspected, the diffusing capacity of carbon monoxide (DL_{CO}) across the alveolar-capillary membrane can be assessed. Low DL_{CO} values are found in diseases characterized by loss of gas exchange units (alveolar destruction, i.e., emphysema) or interstitial processes within the lung which produce an increase in parenchymal tissue, with a relative loss of alveolar units. Lastly, simple measurement of pressure changes generated at the mouth on inspiration and expiration can be helpful in determining whether a decrease in lung volumes (as one might see in a "restrictive" process) is due to a defect in the lung tissue (ILD; normal to high pressures), due to an alteration in an element of the thoracic cage (muscles, ribs, nerves; decreased pressures), or due to reduced effort (decreased pressures).

INDICATIONS FOR USE OF PULMONARY FUNCTION TESTS

Pulmonary function tests may be used for many purposes. However, they are invaluable tools in the diagnosis and management of patients with lung disease. In the initial assessment of a patient, they can help in the evaluation of complaints, often aiding in the differential diagnosis. For those patients with asthma, tests of lung function may be especially helpful in identifying specific precipitants of airways obstruction. With the institution of therapy, the assessment of pulmonary function may indicate the efficacy of acute therapy and also offer an objective means for following the course of a patient's disease over time.

AID IN DIAGNOSIS. Assessment of pulmonary physiology can help to define diagnostic possibilities when history and physical findings are not enlightening. An important diagnostic consideration, for example, relates to whether the pulmonary problem is based on an obstructive or a restrictive process. Examples of obstructive problems include asthma, chronic bronchitis, emphysema, and cystic fibrosis; restrictive problems include chest wall deformities limiting lung expansion as well as interstitial disorders due to collagen vascular diseases, hypersensitivity pneumonitis, sarcoidosis, and interstitial fibrosis. It is important to recognize that certain diseases may produce both obstruction and restriction. Thus, the distinction between obstructive and restrictive disorders may not be as clear as the example that follows.

Physiologically, the characteristics of obstructive and restrictive disorders are compared in Figure 12–6. In an obstructive disorder, there is airflow limitation with decrease in maximal expiratory flows, as demonstrated by the concave characteristics of the flow-volume curve as well as decrease in the FEV_1/FVC ratio. In addition, there commonly is evidence of hyperinflation with an increase in RV and FRC. In a restrictive disorder, on the other hand, lung volumes, including TLC, VC, and RV, all tend to be low. Although the FEV_1 may be less than predicted, the FEV_1/FVC ratio is normal to high, indicating a lack of airflow limitation. Also, flow related to volume is not subnormal but higher than predicted. This fact can be appreciated by plotting flows on an absolute lung volume axis, as in Figure 12–6. An important feature of this type of pulmonary problem is that flow corrected for lung volume often is elevated, which may be due to interstitial fibrosis produced by the disease process, causing the lung to become "stiffer" with greater elastic recoil. Since this recoil is one of the determinants of maximal expiratory flow rates, flows can be supernormal.

Pulmonary function tests are used commonly to confirm the presence of reversible airway obstruction in patients suspected of having asthma (Fig. 12–7). This confirmation is most often accomplished by performing lung functions before and after the administration of an inhaled bronchodilator. In standard spirometry, the FEV_1 must improve greater than 15 percent from baseline for "reversible" obstruction to be termed present. Other measures are considerably less specific.

Other studies are capable of demonstrating airways hyperreactivity and can be employed as diagnostic aids in patients suspected of having asthma. However, because these studies

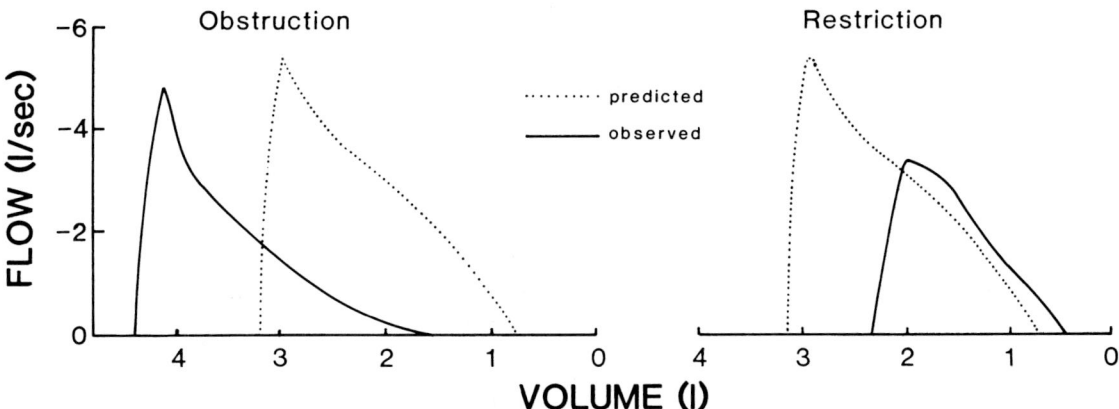

FIGURE 12–6. Expiratory flow-volume curves demonstrate the findings in an obstructive versus a restrictive pulmonary disease. The patient on the left had asthma and demonstrated gas trapping (increased RV) as well as a decrease in flow rates. On the right, the child with a restrictive disorder (idiopathic interstitial pneumonia) had low lung volumes and no evidence of obstruction to airflow, as defined by a normal FEV_1/FVC ratio and above normal flow rates when corrected for lung volumes. This patient was thought to have asthma until tests of lung function pointed to a restrictive process.

by nature are intended to assess the production of bronchoconstriction, it is of utmost importance to know the degree of impairment present before challenge is undertaken. In general, subjects who undergo such challenges should be symptom-free at the time of study and have lung functions of at least 80 percent of their best previous efforts. The procedures must be conducted in a standardized fashion by personnel well versed in the performance of provocation tests as well as assessments of pulmonary function. Equipment and medications always must be on hand to reverse severe airways obstruction that can develop over a short period of time.

A common physiologic method to demonstrate airways lability is the exercise challenge. Exercise is a frequent precipitant of airways obstruction in patients with asthma. Documenting the presence of exercise-induced bronchoconstriction not only helps to establish the diagnosis of asthma but also pinpoints a precipitant in an individual patient that can be approached through therapy (see further discussion in Chapter 26).

Normal lung functions with flow rates and volumes that do not change appreciably with administration of bronchodilators do not in themselves preclude the existence or diagnosis of asthma. In addition to the quiescent phase of this disorder, this finding occurs in patients in whom chronic cough is the only manifestation of reactive airways disease (Cloutier and Loughlin, 1981). An exercise

FIGURE 12–7. The expiratory flow-volume curve for a child with asthma is shown before and after administration of an inhaled adrenergic drug. For comparison, the predicted values are also shown. Lung function is only mildly abnormal before administration of the bronchodilator, with only mild concavity of the descending portion of the curve, and no significant increase in residual volume. Following treatment, lung function improves significantly; the curve is now convex, with flows greater than predicted values. The test results confirmed reactivity of the airways and helped define the optimal lung function for the patient.

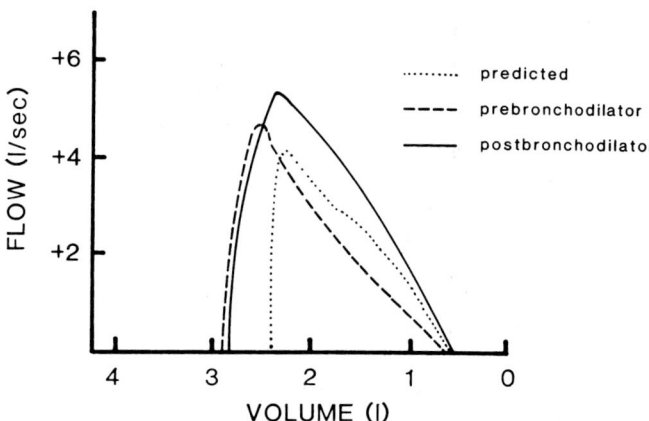

test, however, may demonstrate airways lability. A bronchial challenge with either histamine or methacholine is a diagnostic study that may be employed to determine whether airways hyperreactivity exists. In this test, serial lung functions are performed before and successively after increasing doses of one of these bronchoconstricting drugs. The objective of the challenge is to determine whether airways obstruction will occur at concentrations of a drug that do not lead to airways obstruction in normal subjects. It is a potentially dangerous procedure; the test must be performed in a standardized fashion with a medical and technical staff well versed in procedure and interpretation of a challenge (Cropp et al, 1980). In general, a 20 percent decrease in the FEV_1, following a dose of drug of <8 mg/ml, is considered a positive response. Normal subjects and many subjects with fixed (nonreversible) obstruction will not exhibit significant declines in lung functions in response to the maximally selected doses of either drug employed for challenges.

Asthma differs from other forms of obstructive lung disease on the basis of the largely reversible nature of the disease. However, many obstructive processes may have some degree of reversibility (i.e., cystic fibrosis and chronic bronchitis). In these cases, the clinical history may be important in determining the disease process. In adults, the history of significant cigarette smoking, onset later in life, and lack of an allergic component make the diagnosis of a form of COPD (with a bronchospastic component) much more likely. Chronic bronchitis–predominant forms of COPD are much more likely to have a reversible component than are emphysema-predominant syndromes. Although a provocational challenge may be helpful in sorting out these diseases, chronic bronchitis and cystic fibrosis patients may also have a mild to moderate degree of hyperresponsiveness (usually >1 mg/ml) to methacholine or histamine.

It is important to bear in mind that many types of lung disease may appear with dyspnea, or other respiratory symptoms, not due to asthma. The patient whose pulmonary functions are displayed as the example of restriction in Figure 12–6 presented with a diagnosis of "asthma" because of vague symptoms she experienced with exercise. Her evaluation included the flow-volume curve shown as well as an evaluation of the pressure-volume characteristics of her lung (Macklem, 1975). The last evaluation demonstrated noncompliant or "stiff" lungs, consistent with a restrictive and not an obstructive process. A subsequent lung biopsy specimen demonstrated an interstitial process of undefined etiology. It is stressed that patients who present or are referred for evaluation of asthma may not have evidence of reversible airways obstruction. A thorough evaluation of any pulmonary problem is dependent on acquiring information on the physiology of the underlying process. Table 12–2 presents several diseases that may become confused with asthma and their distinct pulmonary function characteristics. Lastly, it is important to emphasize that disorders that lead to abnormalities in the flow-volume loop (as already discussed, see Fig. 12–5) may appear with wheezing, which is interpreted by patients or medical personnel to be due to asthma.

THE EVALUATION OF PRECIPITANTS. Pulmonary function tests also can facilitate the evaluation of precipitants that can lead to airways obstruction. One example mentioned is exercise as a trigger in asthma. As with some other precipitants, when exercise is recognized as a factor, therapy can be directed at preventing this problem.

Pulmonary function tests also can be used to assess other potential triggers. For example, antigens to which an asthmatic has IgE antibody may or may not be triggers for disease. Even though the probable importance of a particular antigen may be gauged by the history and the degree of the positive skin test reaction (Cavanaugh et al, 1977), these relationships often are unclear. In certain instances, it may be important clinically to determine whether exposure to a particular allergen can induce respiratory symptoms in the patient. The simplest and possibly the safest approach to this problem may be to measure PEFR in the home or work environment after natural exposure of the patient to the antigen in question. This also may be a critical diagnostic tool in evaluating adults when there is concern about occupational lung disease. At other times, especially if considering an antigen that is perennial or for which the intensity of natural exposure is hard to gauge, bronchial challenge with antigen may be indicated (Fig. 12–8). It is important to stress that this is not a routine office procedure and, if contemplated, should be cause for referral to a hospital or clinic where the procedure is

TABLE 12–2. PULMONARY FUNCTION ABNORMALITIES ASSOCIATED WITH DIFFERENT DISEASE STATES

			PULMONARY FUNCTION TEST				
DISEASE	FEV_1	FEV_1/FVC	Bronchodilator Response	Total Lung Capacity	Airways Reactivity	D_LCO	COMMENTS
Asthma	↓ or nl	↓ or nl	+	↑ or nl	↑	↑ or nl	Results may vary from day to day
Emphysema	↓	↓	−	↑	nl or sl ↑	↓	↑ compliance on p-v curve
Cystic fibrosis	↓	↓	+ or −	↑	↑ or nl	nl	
Vocal cord dysfunction	↓ or nl	↓ or nl	+ or −	nl	nl	nl	Flattened inspiratory loop
Interstitial lung disease	↓ or nl	↑ or nl	−	↓	nl	↓	↓ compliance on p-v curve

p-v, pressure-volume

carried out frequently. A major reason for this precaution is that severe airways obstruction to inhaled antigen may be precipitated immediately after antigen challenge (immediate asthmatic response) or hours after exposure (late asthmatic response). The time course of both the immediate and late responses is shown in Figure 12–8.

The immediate asthmatic response occurs within minutes of the exposure, peaks within 15 to 30 minutes, and resolves over 1 to 2 hours. The late response has an onset 2 to 4 hours after challenge and usually peaks within 8 to 12 hours, but may take several

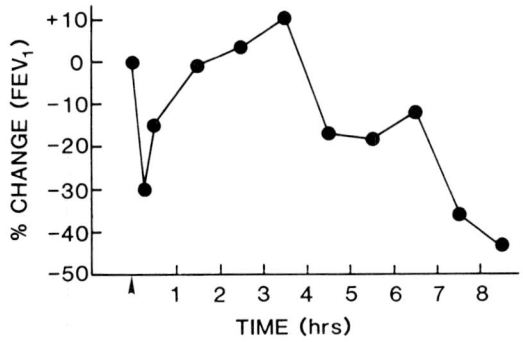

FIGURE 12–8. Changes in lung function (FEV_1) from baseline values versus time after antigen challenge (*arrowhead*) are shown for a patient with both an immediate and a late asthmatic response after antigen challenge. While the immediate response is easily reversed with inhaled or injected adrenergic agents, the late response may be more resistant to therapy and require steroids for early resolution.

days to resolve. Patients who respond to antigen challenge may have an immediate reaction, an immediate and late reaction, or an isolated late reaction. The first two patterns are the most frequent. Whereas the immediate response is reversed easily with inhaled or injected adrenergic drugs, the late response may be incompletely or only temporarily reversed with adrenergic drugs and may require steroids for resolution. Thus, observation of a subject for a minimum of 12 hours after antigen challenge is recommended to document the response and to treat appropriately. Another potential sequela of bronchial challenge is that nonspecific airways reactivity may increase after a late asthmatic response (and possibly after an isolated immediate reaction), making the airways of the patient more susceptible to other triggers and possibly intensifying the problem of asthma. This is usually a short-lived problem, however. These potential problems underscore the importance of performing antigen challenges only when clinically indicated and in a proper setting. The reader is referred to Bhagat et al (1985) and Cropp et al (1980) for more extensive discussions of antigen challenges in asthma.

Other potential triggers also can be assessed with the aid of pulmonary function tests. The responses to ingested substances, such as aspirin, tartrazine, and metabisulfite, are common concerns in patients with asthma (Mathison and Stevenson, 1979; Stevenson and Simon, 1981). Pulmonary function tests help quantitate the patient's response to these agents and define the time course. As with bronchial challenges, these challenges are not without risks and should be performed cautiously only in a setting where deterioration in lung function can be controlled and treated appropriately.

EVALUATION OF THERAPY. Pulmonary function tests are an important aid in evaluating both acute and chronic effects of treatment in patients with various lung diseases (Table 12–2). An example of their usefulness in the initial care of a child with severe asthma is demonstrated in Figure 12–9. On patient presentation (left side of figure), the flow-volume curve demonstrated evidence of significant obstruction with marked increase in the residual volume, a descending limb of the expiratory curve that was concave, and flow rates that were depressed. After inhalation of a bronchodilator, no significant change in lung function was noted. Because of a history compatible with asthma that was poorly controlled over the recent past, oral corticosteroids were started. After several days of therapy, the response to repeat administration of inhaled bronchodilator is seen. Although pretreatment lung functions did not improve measurably from those performed earlier, there was a significant response to inhaled drug with a decrease in RV, an increase in the FVC, and increases in flow rates. This pattern (no initial objective response to adrenergic agents until institution of steroid therapy) is not uncommon in children or adults with severe asthma and persistent wheezing (Ellul-Micallef and Fenech, 1975).

The benefit of assessing lung function in the emergency treatment of asthma in children (Guidelines, 1991) and adults (Fanta et al, 1982) has been documented. While there is little doubt that these objective measures can be of assistance in assessing the degree to which the acute airways obstruction is reversed, it is important to stress that pulmonary function tests should supplement and not replace a careful history and serial examination of the patient with acute wheezing.

An evaluation of the effectiveness of therapy also is frequently undertaken before elective surgery in patients with asthma or other chronic lung diseases. The indications for such assessments, the tests employed, and the benefits that can be derived have been reviewed recently (Zibrak et al, 1990).

FOLLOWING THE COURSE OF A DISEASE. Assessment of pulmonary function is helpful in charting the course of a disease. This is especially true when dealing with a process that is progressive, such as cystic fibrosis or interstitial lung disease, or intermittent, such as asthma. The assessment provides an objective means for measuring the effectiveness of therapy in delaying the progression of the disease and also allows realistic counseling of the patient and family about prognosis.

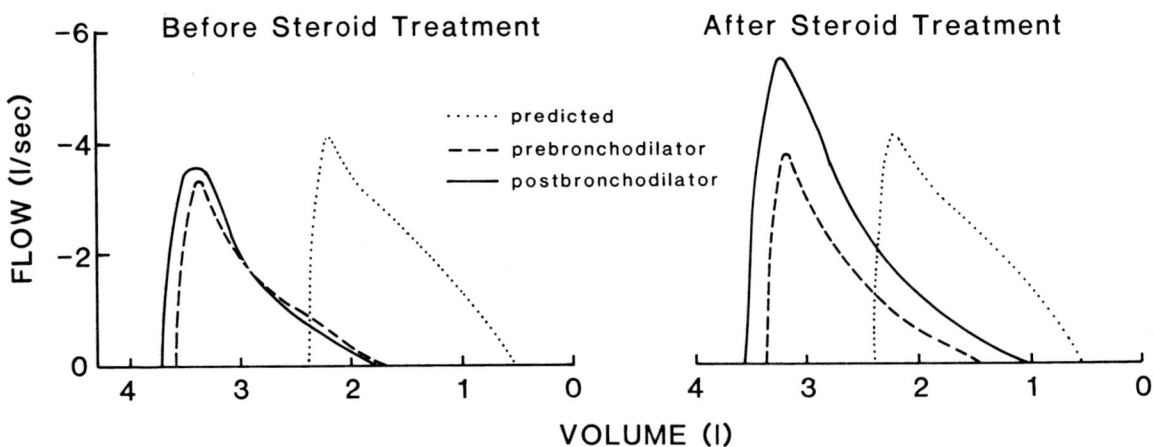

FIGURE 12–9. The response to inhaled bronchodilator is shown in a child with asthma before and after a course of oral steroids. As shown on the left, the functions reveal a marked increase in residual volume as well as significant airflow limitation. Inhaled adrenergic drugs are ineffective in reversing this obstruction. After administration of oral steroids, as shown on the right, the same inhaled bronchodilator leads to a marked increase in flow and a decrease in residual volume. Despite this beneficial response, lung function never completely normalized in the patient.

Although asthma generally is thought of as a disease in which irreversible damage does not occur, it is evident that many patients with severe disease do, in fact, have irreversible damage, limiting airflow (Loren et al, 1978). Whether this represents a sequela of poorly controlled asthma or is the result of a separate insult to the airways (e.g., viral illness in childhood) often is not apparent. Close observation of alterations in physiology over time is likely to provide useful information concerning factors that predispose the patient to irreversible obstruction.

Recently, the regular use of home or work place peak flow measurements by the patient has been determined to be helpful to the physician and the patient in following the course of asthma. Peak flow measurements can give the patient and physician an objective measure of pulmonary function on a daily basis, over time, as well as provide an indicator of response to treatment. Rational approaches to therapy, based on an objective measure, the peak flow, can then be undertaken. Using one of the home peak flow devices (mentioned previously) and charting the measurements can offer a guide to the judicious use of drugs on an outpatient basis, especially in the patient requiring multiple medications. Peak-flow devices also can be employed to give a patient with a poor perception of the disease an awareness of a decrease in lung function, thus allowing earlier therapeutic intervention.

CAVEATS IN PULMONARY FUNCTION TESTS

As with any laboratory tests, limitations of pulmonary function tests must be appreciated in order to utilize them appropriately. Major limitations of clinical importance are summarized next.

WIDE RANGE OF NORMAL VALUES. Ranges of normal are defined by an analysis of large groups of subjects who are free of obvious disease when tested. Numerous different indices are published and utilized by various spirometry programs and may vary somewhat. Normal pulmonary function values are based primarily on height, sex, and race (Polgar and Promadhat, 1971). Despite the ability to form subgroups of individuals in these categories, there is a wide range of normal values, and there are many practical applications of this point. First, the physician must have a knowledge of the magnitude of change necessary for an alteration in lung function to be of clinical significance. As noted previously, some tests are more reproducible than others. This topic is dealt with in more detail in other discussions of pulmonary function tests (Lemen, 1990). Second, values within a normal range may not be normal for the patient. For example, note the change in lung function in the case of the asthmatic patient illustrated in Figure 12–7. Lung function varied from a normal range before therapy to an above "predicted" range, with bronchodilator treatment. Also, a single determination may not give an accurate picture of the patient's overall lung function. Serial measurements in the physician's office or at the patient's home (e.g., with a peak flow meter) over time will be more enlightening in this regard than measurements obtained only during visits to the physician's office.

DYNAMIC CHANGES WITH AGE. In contrast to arterial blood gas tensions, which are fairly constant throughout life, major physiologic alterations take place in lung volumes and flows with growth and aging (Knudson et al, 1983). Consequently, serial determinations of lung functions tend to be much more informative than isolated tests. This is especially true for children and adults with chronic diseases that may be progressive; both the lung function at a point in time and the overall pattern of change in volumes and flows with time are critical to their care. Employing graphs that demonstrate plots of functions versus time (similar to plots of height, weight, and head circumference in the growing infant and child) should enhance our ability to detect problems at an earlier time in the course of the disease (Lemen, 1990).

PATIENT COOPERATION. In all tests of lung function performed in a physician's office or a clinic, the cooperation of the patient is paramount. Pulmonary function tests, although not especially difficult or unpleasant to perform, do rely on a certain level of psychomotor maturation. Thus, it is possible to test lung function in children less than 5 years of age only with special techniques. There also is a learning effect associated with repeated testing; as the subject becomes more comfortable with the equipment and individuals conducting the tests, the reproducibility of results generally improves. This effect applies to adults as well as children and must be taken into consideration in interpreting the results of the test. Some children and adults have a great deal of difficulty in performing lung function tests properly and may require an unusual amount of repeated efforts in order to obtain valid and reproducible information. Lastly, there may, on occasion, be a concern with patient effort. Spirometric measurements will be uniformly decreased if the patient does not, for whatever reason, give maximal effort. Close observation by the pulmonary function technician may help to determine whether patient effort is optimal.

LACK OF AVAILABLE TESTS FOR INFANTS AND SMALL CHILDREN

Although various methods have been and are being developed and employed for assessment of lung function in preschool children, these remain research tools not available for routine office use. The inability to assess lung function in preschool children is a serious drawback in assessing their pulmonary status. Many respiratory illnesses (asthma, cystic fibrosis) may first manifest symptoms within children of this age group. The airways during this period of rapid growth may be subjected also to significant insults, such as viral infections, that can have lifelong consequences. Reliable tests of lung functions in this preschool group will be essential to measure more precisely the degree of impairment caused by these diseases and to assess objectively effectiveness of therapy. One hopes that specialized techniques now limited to research laboratories will become available for general clinical use in the near future.

EQUIPMENT FOR ASSESSMENT OF PULMONARY FUNCTION TESTS

A number of pieces of equipment are available for the routine assessment of lung function. Every primary care office should have a peak-flow meter. In addition, inexpensive peak-flow meters may be used in the home. Spirometers analyze either volume or time, with measurement of FEV_1, FVC, flow and volume signals, depiction of maximal inspiratory and expiratory maneuvers, and generation of flow-volume loops. Several spirometers have been reviewed recently and are acceptable for primary care office use (Nelson et al, 1990). In considering various pieces of equipment, aside from expense, a desirable feature is a permanent copy of the spirogram or the flow-volume curve so that this record can be reviewed to ensure that the maneuver is technically acceptable. Whereas a direct readout of the numeric results is convenient, the ability to inspect the test visually will decrease errors in assessment. The decision to purchase a unit that provides test results from a volume-time tracing versus a flow-volume curve or a unit that provides information from both types of analysis must be based on cost and preference for viewing the data. Although most offices will not have (and will not need) equipment to measure lung volumes by gas dilution or body plethysmography, the value of assessing lung volumes for certain clinical problems must be borne in mind. This ordinarily can be accomplished through referral to medical centers where equipment and those with expertise for such measurements are available.

Ideally, normal data should be generated for each practice setting, thereby standardizing a local healthy population with specific equipment and technicians, for comparison with patients with pulmonary complaints. Since this is impractical in a busy office or clinic, the use of either published normal values or standards furnished by the manufacturer ordinarily will suffice. When employing a new machine for testing lung functions, it is helpful to test several normal subjects and to compare their values to values obtained in older equipment that has been standardized through past use and maintenance. The need to maintain and calibrate equipment routinely before use is critical to accurate acquisition of data. Reference to standards of spirometry is recommended for all those who employ tests of lung function (see Figs. 12–3 and 12–4; Table 12–3) (Nelson et al, 1990, Taussig et al, 1980).

PERSONNEL AND ENVIRONMENT FOR CONDUCTING PULMONARY FUNCTION TESTS

The need for a motivated office nurse or assistant who is knowledgeable about pulmonary functions, who can teach and coach pa-

TABLE 12-3. AVERAGE (50 PERCENT) PULMONARY FUNCTION VALUES IN CHILDREN

Height		FVC (L)			$FEF_{25-75\%}$		PEFR	
Cm	In	Boys	Girls	$FEV_1(L)$	L/min	L/sec	L/min	L/sec
100	39.4	1.00	1.00	.70	55	.91	100	1.67
102	40.2	1.03	1.00	.75	60	1.00	110	1.83
104	40.9	1.08	1.07	.82	64	1.06	120	2.00
106	41.7	1.14	1.10	.89	70	1.17	130	2.17
108	42.5	1.19	1.19	.97	75	1.25	140	2.33
110	43.3	1.27	1.24	1.01	80	1.33	150	2.50
112	44.1	1.32	1.30	1.10	86	1.43	160	2.67
114	44.9	1.40	1.36	1.17	90	1.50	174	2.90
116	45.7	1.47	1.41	1.23	96	1.60	185	3.08
118	46.5	1.52	1.49	1.30	100	1.67	195	3.25
120	47.2	1.60	1.55	1.39	105	1.75	204	3.40
122	48.0	1.69	1.62	1.45	110	1.83	215	3.58
124	48.8	1.75	1.70	1.53	118	1.97	226	3.77
126	49.6	1.82	1.77	1.59	121	2.01	236	3.93
128	50.4	1.90	1.84	1.67	127	2.12	247	4.11
130	51.2	1.99	1.90	1.72	132	2.20	256	4.27
132	52.0	2.07	2.00	1.80	139	2.32	267	4.45
134	52.8	2.15	2.06	1.89	142	2.37	278	4.63
136	53.5	2.24	2.15	1.98	149	2.48	289	4.82
138	54.3	2.35	2.24	2.06	153	2.55	299	4.98
140	55.1	2.40	2.32	2.11	159	2.65	310	5.17
142	55.9	2.50	2.40	2.20	163	2.72	320	5.33
144	56.7	2.60	2.50	2.30	170	2.83	330	5.50
146	57.5	2.70	2.59	2.39	173	2.88	340	5.67
148	58.3	2.79	2.68	2.48	180	3.00	351	5.85
150	59.1	2.88	2.78	2.57	183	3.05	362	6.03
152	59.8	2.97	2.88	2.66	190	3.17	373	6.22
154	60.6	3.09	2.98	2.75	195	3.25	384	6.40
156	61.4	3.20	3.09	2.88	200	3.33	394	6.57
158	62.2	3.30	3.18	2.98	205	3.42	404	6.73
160	63.0	3.40	3.27	3.06	210	3.50	415	6.92
162	63.8	3.52	3.40	3.18	215	3.58	425	7.08
164	64.6	3.64	3.50	3.29	220	3.67	436	7.28
166	65.4	3.78	3.60	3.40	225	3.75	446	7.43
168	66.1	3.90	3.72	3.50	230	3.83	457	7.62
170	66.9	4.00	3.83	3.65	236	3.93	467	7.78
172	67.7	4.20	3.83	3.80	241	4.01	477	7.95
174	68.5	4.20	3.83	3.80	246	4.10	488	8.13
176	69.3	4.20	3.83	3.80	251	4.18	498	8.30

Data from Polgar G, Promadhat V. Pulmonary Function Testing in Children: Techniques and Standards. Philadelphia, WB Saunders Co., 1971.

tients patiently through new procedures, and who can recognize technical problems that interfere with accurate assessments cannot be overstated. This person also should be responsible for assuring routine calibration of the equipment.

In the testing of children, the environment should be friendly, free of distractions, and removed from areas where painful procedures take place. When the same child-oriented technician helps the patient during each visit to perform the test in an unhurried, nonthreatening setting, more consistent results are insured. Time should be allowed for the child to become comfortable with the equipment and to practice blowing through the unattached disposable mouthpiece or other similar devices (Fig. 12–10). An opportunity to see the curve simultaneously develop on the spirometer paper or screen may serve visually to reinforce better effort. Even if their trials are suboptimal, familiarity with staff and equipment will foster a willingness to correctly perform the test during subsequent visits. The same principles can apply to older patients, who may have equal difficulties in performing these effort-dependent tests.

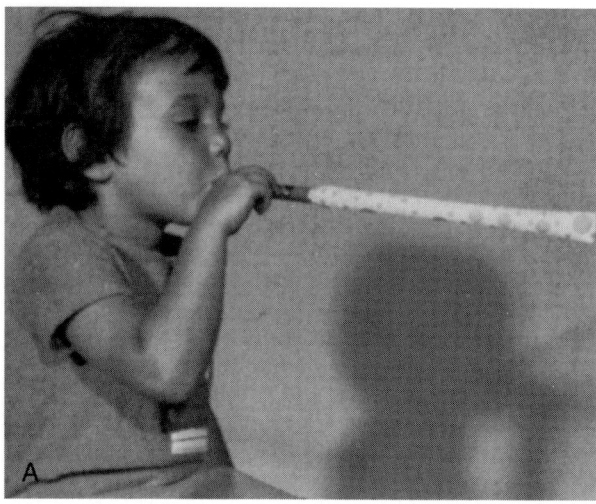 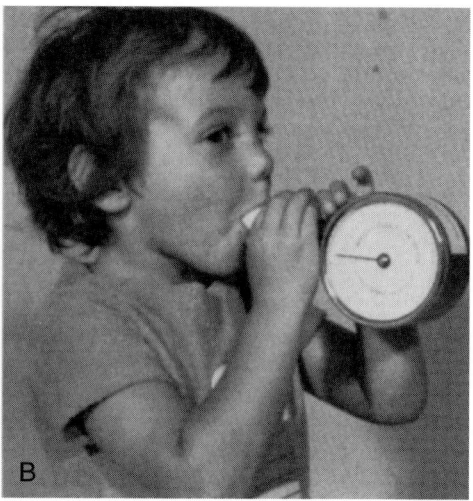

FIGURE 12–10. Use of a party favor (*A*) to teach lung function maneuver (*B*) to small children.

REFERENCES

Bhagat RJ, Strunk RC, Larsen GL. The late asthmatic response. Ann Allergy 54:272, 297–301, 1985.

Cavanaugh MJ, Bronsky EA, Buckley JM. Clinical value of bronchial provocation testing in childhood asthma. J Allergy Clin Immmunol 59:41–47, 1977.

Cherniack RM. Pulmonary Function Testing. 2nd ed. Philadelphia WB Saunders Co, 1992.

Cloutier MM, Loughlin GM. Chronic cough in children: A manifestation of airway hyperreactivity. Pediatrics 67:6–12, 1981.

Cropp GJA, Berstein IL, Boushey HA, Hyde RW, Rosenthal RR, Spector SL, Townley RG. Guidelines for bronchial inhalation challenges with pharmacologic and antigenic agents. Am Thor Soc News 6:11–19, 1980.

Ellul-Micallef R, Fenech FF. Effect of intravenous prednisolone in asthmatics with diminished adrenergic responsiveness. Lancet ii: 1269–1271, 1975.

Fanta CH, Rossing TH, McFadden ER. Emergency room treatment of asthma. Relationships among therapeutic combinations, severity of obstruction and time course of response. Am J Med 72:416–422, 1982.

Guidelines for the diagnosis and management of asthma. National Heart, Lung and Blood Institute, National Asthma Education Program Expert Panel Report. J Allergy Clin Immunol 88:425–534, 1991.

Hyatt RE, Black LF. The flow-volume curve. A current perspective. Am Rev Respir Dis 107:191–199, 1973.

Knudson RJ, Lebowitz MD, Holberg CJ, Burrows B. Changes in the normal maximal expiratory flow-volume curve with growth and aging. Am Rev Respir Dis 127:725–734, 1983.

Lemen RJ. Pulmonary function testing in the office, clinic and home. *In* Chernick V (ed). Kendig's Disorders of the Respiratory Tract in Children. Philadelphia, WB Saunders Co, 1990.

Loren ML, Leung PK, Cooley RL, Chai H, Bell TD, Buck VM. Irreversibility of obstructive changes in severe asthma in childhood. Chest 74:126–129, 1978.

Macklem PT. New tests to assess lung function. N Engl J Med 293:339–342, 1975.

Mathison DA, Stevenson DD. Hypersensitivity to nonsteroidal anti-inflammatory drugs: indications and methods for oral challenges. J Allergy Clin Immunol 64:669–674, 1979.

Miller RD, Hyatt RE. Evaluation of obstructive lesions of the trachea and larynx by flow-volume loops. Am Rev Respir Dis 108:475–481, 1973.

Nelson SB, Gardner RM, Crapo RO, Jensen RL. Performance evaluation of contemporary spirometers. Chest 97:288–297, 1990.

Polgar G, Promadhat V (eds). Pulmonary Function Testing in Children. Philadelphia, WB Saunders Co, 1971.

Stevenson DD, Simon RA. Sensitivity to ingested metabisulfites in asthmatic subjects. J Allergy Clin Immunol 68:26–32, 1981.

Taussig LM, Chernick V, Wood R, Farrell P, Mellins RB. Standardization of lung function testing in children. Proceedings and recommendations of the GAP Conference Committee, Cystic Fibrosis Foundation. J Pediatr 97:668–676, 1980.

Zibrak JD, O'Donnell CR, Marton K. Preoperative pulmonary function testing. Ann Intern Med 112:763–771, 1990.

Chapter 13

Inhalation Bronchoprovocation

Gail G. Shapiro, M.D., Paul V. Williams, M.D., and Sheldon Spector, M.D.

Airway hyperresponsiveness refers to the characteristic of the airways of patients with asthma to constrict after exposure to stimuli that do not affect the airways of most normal individuals. This is a key feature of asthma, the degree of hyperresponsiveness relating more closely to the severity of asthma than resting lung function (Juniper et al, 1981; Murray et al, 1981). Within a sample of patients with asthma, there is a correlation between reactivity or responsiveness and clinical disease, so that greater airway responsiveness is associated with more symptoms, lower AM peak flow rates, greater diurnal variation in peak flow, greater response to bronchoconstricting stimuli, and a more intense level of treatment. In a given population, however, an individual may show extreme bronchial hyperresponsiveness but have mild disease, and vice versa. In addition, some individuals manifest hyperresponsiveness, usually to a mild degree, without showing clinical evidence of asthma. These individuals may have residual responsiveness years after the cessation of clinical asthma or may have it transiently following a respiratory infection, or associated with allergic rhinitis. Because of this, hyperresponsiveness as measured with bronchoprovocative challenges cannot be considered synonymous with asthma. Rather, these challenges are diagnostic techniques used to verify impressions derived from a history and physical examination.

There are both genetically determined and acquired factors contributing to airway hyperresponsiveness. Population studies, done with a variety of bronchoprovocation challenges, have demonstrated a unimodal distribution of reactivity, confirming that both genetic and environmental factors play a role. Another indicator of genetic and environmental factors is the fact that responsiveness varies in different populations and different environments (Turner et al, 1986). In twin studies, concordance for bronchial hyperresponsiveness is greater for identical than for non-identical twins. However, concordance is less than 50 percent (Bias, 1973). Studies of siblings and parents of asthmatic children demonstrate that 39 percent have abnormal bronchial lability (Godfrey and Konig, 1975). Age also appears to be a significant factor in airway reactivity (Hopp et al, 1985). Several studies have noted a high incidence of airway reactivity in infants. Normal healthy patients younger than 21 years and older than 60 years have higher bronchial responsiveness than those aged 21 to 60 (Fig. 13–1) (Juniper et al, 1981).

Recent findings suggest that allergic sensitization and the eosinophilic inflammatory reaction in children are major factors contributing to acquired bronchial hyperresponsiveness. House dust mite exposure can affect airway hyperresponsiveness, and seasonal variations in hyperresponsiveness correspond to mite antigen levels (Van Der Heide et al, 1994). In addition to allergens, environmental factors causing bronchial hyperresponsiveness include infections and contaminants. A history of croup or more than two lower respiratory infections in early childhood is associated with bronchial hyperresponsiveness as

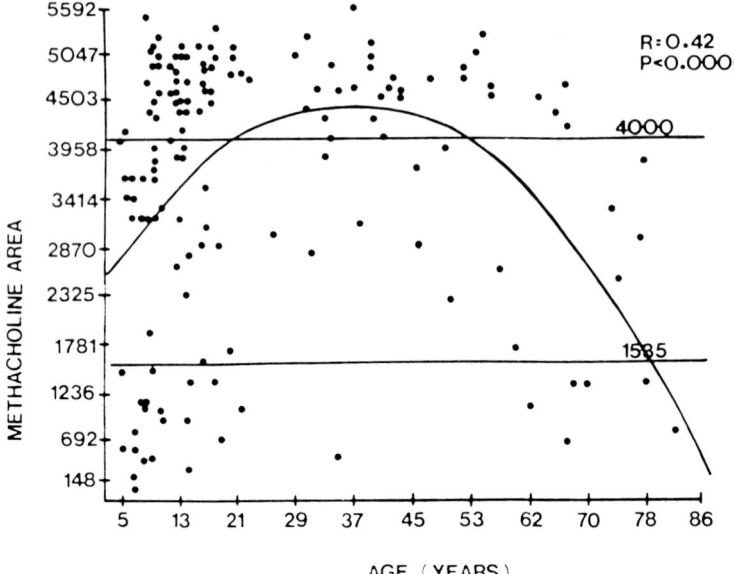

FIGURE 13–1. Methacholine responses in unselected patients, showing differences in reactivity with age. Results >4000 indicate normal responses. Values <1535 indicate methacholine responses that are <250 breath units of methacholine. (From Hopp RJ, Bewtra A, Nair NM, Townley RG. The effect of age on methacholine challenge. J Allergy Clin Immunol 76:609–613, 1985.)

late as 10 years after infection. Pertussis may evoke a first episode of bronchospasm in children. Individuals recovering from pertussis may have persistent bronchial hyperresponsiveness for months or for years, or permanently. Respiratory syncytial virus (RSV) infection in children may be the precursor of subsequent asthma, children with a history of bronchiolitis in infancy showing a high frequency of abnormal bronchial lability later in childhood (Pullan and Hey, 1982; McConnochie and Roghmann, 1984). Interestingly, Welliver et al (1981) have shown the association between RSV-specific IgE in nasopharyngeal secretions of children who wheeze with the infection. Increased bronchial lability may also be seen after rhinovirus infection. Environmental pollutants such as SO_2, NO_2, and O_3 may transiently enhance bronchial hyperresponsiveness; passive smoking may also contribute to bronchial hyperresponsiveness. More persistently harmful are low–molecular-weight chemicals encountered in occupational settings.

WHY PERFORM BRONCHOPROVOCATION CHALLENGES?

The reasons for applying challenge techniques to children and adults are noted in Table 13–1. A variety of methods have been used to determine the presence and severity of airway hyperresponsiveness. These include both pharmacologic (methacholine and histamine) and nonpharmacologic (exercise, nonisotonic aerosol, or cold air hyperventilation) methods. These bronchoprovocation challenges are important clinically as methods to help clarify whether symptoms that suggest a diagnosis of asthma are indeed due to this condition. For example, patients sometimes present after having received an assortment of anti-asthma medications for cough or recurrent bronchitis, yet no physician has ever documented reversible obstruction after bronchodilator inhalation. If baseline pulmonary function is normal in the face of such a history, bronchoprovocation challenge may be valuable. At times a challenge test may be used to help judge the severity of a patient's asthma and possibly response to therapy. In

TABLE 13–1. PURPOSES FOR BRONCHOPROVOCATION CHALLENGES IN CHILDREN

Clarify diagnosis of asthma suggested by history
Quantify severity of disease
Determine and compare utility of drugs for asthma control
Determine and compare duration of action drugs
Understand asthma mechanisms
Epidemiologic studies of airway responsiveness

Modified from Shapiro GG, Bierman CW. Inhalation bronchoprovocation in children. In Spector SL (ed). Provocative Challenge Procedures: Background and Methodology. New York, Futura Publishing, 1989, pp 395–416.

the research setting, bronchoprovocation challenges provide a method for studying pharmacologic modulation of asthma, e.g., the ability of a drug to diminish airway reactivity suggests clinical usefulness. The degree to which this reactivity can be modified can be used as a means to compare the antiasthma characteristics of drugs. Bronchoprovocation challenges have also been used in epidemiologic studies of large groups of healthy as well as asthmatic children. These studies have helped clarify the role of airway reactivity in asthmatic and normal children by showing the similarities and differences between these groups.

Bronchoprovocation challenge does not discriminate well between patients with COPD and asthma. A large segment of the COPD population also has bronchial hyperresponsiveness.

PHARMACOLOGIC CHALLENGES

Bronchoprovocation challenges with the chemicals methacholine and histamine measure smooth muscle responsiveness. These chemical challenges depend on the ability of these agents to affect bronchial smooth muscle receptors in such a way as to produce bronchoconstriction in individuals with reactive airways at concentrations that have little or no effect on normal subjects.

Much of the data of the 1960s and 1970s expounds the usefulness of chemical bronchoprovocation. Both methacholine and histamine emerged as useful agents for eliciting bronchial hyperresponsiveness, their inhalation in graded doses producing similar dose-response curves capable of sorting subjects with reactive airways from normals. Most of these studies, however, were done in patients who were either clearly asthmatic or clearly normal. Several recent epidemiologic studies of large numbers of unselected children (Peat et al, 1991; Backer et al, 1991a; 1991b; Pattemore et al, 1990; Burrows et al, 1992) have shown that not all asthmatics have positive challenge tests at all times, and asymptomatic patients may have airway reactivity (Fig. 13–2). Thus, as mentioned above, airway reactivity cannot be considered synonymous with asthma, and these challenges are not particularly useful as screening tests for asthma in unselected populations. The probability of asthma in patients with a positive provocative

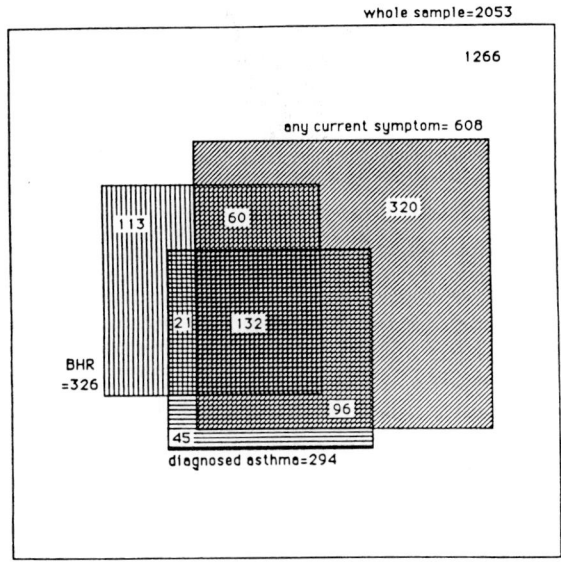

FIGURE 13–2. Proportionate Venn diagram showing combined overlap of children with "any current symptom," those with diagnosed asthma, and those with BHR in a group of 2053 children. Numbers of children in each category are shown. (From Pattemore PK, Asher MI, Harrison AC, Mitchell EA, Rea HH, Steward AW. The interrelationship among bronchial hyperresponsiveness, the diagnosis of asthma, and asthma symptoms. Am Rev Respir Dis 142:549–554, 1990.)

challenge is largely influenced by the history, physical examination, and clinical impression of the likelihood of asthma. A decrease of FEV_1 greater than 20 percent is generally accepted as a discriminating end point to separate the normal and hyperresponsive groups; the terms PD_{20} or PC_{20}, provocative dose, or provocative concentration of test agent causing a 20 percent decline in FEV_1 are current measures of bronchoprovocation. Hopp et al (1987) have suggested that the area under the dose-response curve plotted with methacholine concentration versus the drop in FEV_1 is a more discriminating method for quantifying airway reactivity. Other methods of expressing the response to challenge include the slope of the dose-response curve (DRS), defined as the percentage fall in FEV_1 at the last dose divided by the total dose administered (Peat et al, 1991), and the bronchial responsiveness index (BRindex), defined as the log of the slope of the percent decline from baseline FEV_1 after the last dose per unit dose of methacholine (Burrows et al, 1992). These latter two methods may be more useful in epidemiologic studies, because a value that related well to symptom history can be calculated for the entire sample, even if the patient does not experience a 20 percent drop in FEV_1. For clinical use, however, the PD_{20} or PC_{20} remains the simplest method of recording the response.

Challenge techniques with histamine and methacholine have been well standardized and are easily applied to children and adults. They involve having the subject inhale increasing amounts of drug until the protocol is completed or a drop in FEV_1 greater than 20 percent has occurred. By 20 to 30 minutes following this induction of bronchospasm, there will usually be spontaneous recovery. If the patient becomes uncomfortable, bronchodilator inhalation will rapidly return pulmonary function to normal. The short duration of bronchoconstriction, the ability to control the dose of bronchoconstrictive stimuli, and the lack of a late-phase response are positive features of these challenges.

The two widely used techniques for administering methacholine and histamine challenges to adults are also applicable to children. One of these involves tidal volume breathing of aerosol that is generated continuously by a nebulizer and delivered directly into a face mask. This technique has an advantage for the testing of children since little patient cooperation is required. The second method involves intermittent generation of aerosol by a nebulizer with a mouthpiece connected to a Rosenthal-French dosimeter, a solenoid valve device that allows aerosol to be generated for a specified time interval. The patient can initiate nebulization by pressing a button or spontaneously with inspiration.

A number of factors must be standardized to allow for comparisons between different challenges of the same individual and for comparisons between different centers. With the continuous generation method, nebulizer output needs to be regulated. If a Wright nebulizer is used, output should be 0.13 to 0.16 ml/min. Since Wright nebulizers have been difficult to obtain at times, other nebulizers are often used. Some of these have been characterized so that the output, which appears to give results comparable to those of the Wright standard, is known. It is important to use these data or create one's own equivalency data if one is to characterize the patient's sensitivity with relation to scales established with the Wright nebulizer (Juniper and Hargreave, 1986). Although the nebulizer output is an important technical variable, it is also important to consider the effect of evaporation on the test parameters. Evaporative losses have been shown to decrease the temperature of the solution by as much as 11°C, most of which occurs in the first 2 minutes. There will be a decrease in output with time and an increase in solute concentration over time. As a consequence, the use of the total output to determine the dose could overestimate the amount of agonist delivered. Also, these findings suggest that the nebulizer solutions should be changed after each test, and nebulizers should be calibrated under the exact parameters of the test. Particle size generated should be between 1 and 4 µ aerodynamic mass median diameter, and time of inhalation must be 2 minutes.

With the dosimeter method, a DeVilbiss 42 or 646 nebulizer has generally been used. Output per inhalation and the number of inhalations must be standardized. Also, patients must consistently start at the same lung volume, attempt to inhale at the same rate, and hold their breath for the same amount of time with each inspiration. These requirements may be difficult for younger children, in which case the continuous (tidal volume) method should be utilized. When these guidelines have been followed, the continuous method and intermittent method result in similar levels of sensitivity to chemical challenge and good reproducibility (Ryan et al, 1981).

To summarize the dosimeter method, compressed air at 20 psi is connected to the input value of the dosimeter, which is set at 0.6 sec per inhalation. A DeVilbiss 42 or 646 nebulizer is also connected to the dosimeter. The patient inhales from a mouthpiece attached to the nebulizer containing the methacholine solution. Each respiration begins from functional residual capacity. With each inspiration, methacholine or histamine is delivered for 0.6 second. According to the protocol established by the Bronchoprovocation Committee of the American Academy of Allergy and Immunology in 1975 (Chai, et al, 1975), after an initial inhalation of five breaths of normal saline, five breaths each of nine increasing concentrations of drug are delivered with no breath-holding between inspirations (9 mg of aerosol being generated per inhalation). FEV_1 is measured at 1 1/2 and 3 minutes after each concentration with two expiratory efforts (the best being taken) until the FEV_1

drops by 20 percent or more or until all nine concentrations have been delivered. Failure to obtain a 20 percent decline in FEV_1 makes the diagnosis of hyperreactive airways unlikely at that point in time.

With the continuous generation method, aerosol is generated by a Wright nebulizer and delivered directly into a face mask. The subject has a nose clip in place and breathes with tidal breathing through the mouth for 2 minutes. Nebulizer output is kept constant. The subject inhales saline followed by increasing doses of methacholine or histamine. Again, the challenge is discontinued if there is a drop in FEV_1 of 20 percent or more below the value after saline inhalation.

Since baseline airway caliber can influence methacholine results, and patients with moderate airway obstruction are more susceptible to bronchoconstricting stimuli, it is usually recommended that the FEV_1 be greater than the 70 percent predicted in order to perform the challenge. This can be difficult in moderate-to-severe asthmatics, who cannot maintain stable airways if they have to stop their medications as usually recommended. Weiss et al (1989) have devised a three-tiered medication regimen that allows for maintenance of FEV_1 >70 percent in most asthmatic children and still maintains reproducibility. It is unlikely, however, that children with a low FEV_1 would be challenged with methacholine or histamine unless participating in a research protocol. They also noted that methacholine challenge in children is reproducible within one doubling concentration for at least 1 month (Fig. 13–3).

The dosage schedules often used for methacholine and histamine are, in general, increasing twofold increments (Table 13–2). Results are expressed in terms of the concentration required to cause a 20 percent drop in FEV_1 or the number of breath units required, where 1 breath unit equals 1 breath of 1 mg/ml of methacholine or histamine. A truncated methacholine protocol (Table 13–3) has been useful clinically for adults and children, since it decreases the number of inhaled concentrations from nine to five, thus shortening the procedure (LaBraico et al, 1984). This is especially helpful for children whose attention span may be shorter than one expects for adults. An abbreviated histamine protocol, using fewer doses and a shorter time interval for measuring FEV_1, also compares favorably with the standard protocol (Table 13–4).

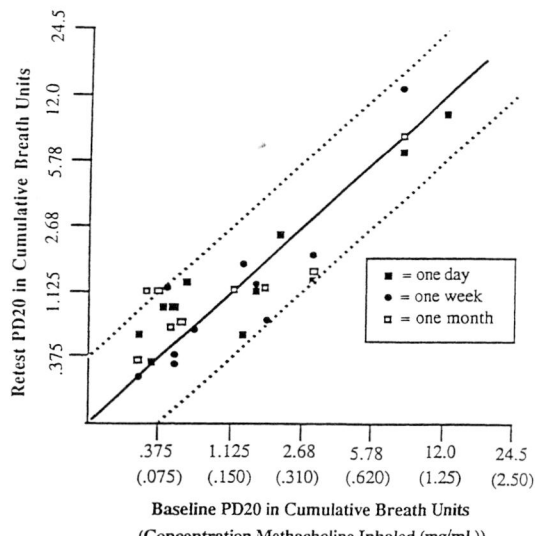

FIGURE 13–3. Comparison of responses to inhaled methacholine. Individual data points plotting the FEV_1 in cumulative breath units are shown for the baseline test in comparison to tests done 1 day later ($r = 0.98$, $p < 0.0001$), 1 week later ($r = 0.95$, $p < 0.0001$), and 1 month later ($r = 0.98$, $p < 0.0001$). The inner solid line is the line of identity and the outer dashed lines delimit the region of one doubling concentration difference. The intervals on the x and y axis are doubling cumulative breath units of methacholine. Noncumulative doubling concentrations of inhaled methacholine are also shown in parentheses on the abscissa. (From Weiss ME, Wheeler B, Eggleston P, Adkinson NF. A protocol for performing reproducible methacholine inhalation tests in children with moderate to severe asthma. Am Rev Respir Dis 139:67–72, 1989.)

Analysis of the responses in asthmatics compared with those of normals has also suggested that the PD_{12} may be sufficient for methacholine challenge (Eliasson et al, 1992), and the PC_{10} or PC_{15} correlate well with the PC_{20} in histamine challenge (van Aalderen et al, 1989). One small study suggested that the response that best separates asthmatics from normals may differ for each type of challenge (Eliasson et al, 1992). These findings require further confirmation, but if true could enable one to shorten the challenges even further.

Methacholine challenge has been applied to the detection of bronchial hyperresponsiveness in children under 5 years of age, the production of cough and/or wheezing being the criteria for a positive challenge (Adinoff and Strunk, 1984). This technique may be extremely useful in clinical settings and may be made more objective with the addition of peak-flow measurements before challenge

TABLE 13–2. BREATH UNITS FOR METHACHOLINE AND HISTAMINE CHALLENGE ON A MG/ML BASIS*

Methacholine Concentrations (mg/ml)	Cumulative No. Breaths	Units/ Breath	Units/5 Breaths	Cumulative Units/5 Breath†
0.075	5	0.075	0.375	0.375
0.15	10	0.15	0.750	1.125
0.31	15	0.31	1.55	2.68
0.62	20	0.62	3.10	5.78
1.25	25	1.25	6.25	12.0
2.50	30	2.50	12.50	24.5
5.00	35	5.00	25.00	49.5
10.00	40	10.00	50.00	99.5
25.00	45	25.00	125.00	225.0
Histamine Base Concentrations (mg/ml)	**Cumulative No. Breaths**	**Units/ Breath**	**Units/5 Breaths**	**Cumulative Units/5 Breath†**
0.03	5	0.03	0.15	0.15
0.06	10	0.06	0.30	0.45
0.12	15	0.12	0.60	1.05
0.25	20	0.25	1.25	2.30
0.50	25	0.50	2.50	4.80
1.00	30	1.00	5.00	9.80
2.50	35	2.50	12.00	22.30
5.00	40	5.00	25.00	47.30
10.00	45	10.00	50.00	97.30

*One breath unit = 1 inhalation of 1 mg/ml histamine base.
†If final FEV_1 test is performed at other than a 5-breath interval (i.e., 23 breaths), the cumulative units are calculated by adding 3 × 0.25 = 0.75 to 2.30 = 3.05.
Modified from Chai H, Farr RS, Froehlich LA, Mathison DA, McLean JA, Rosenthal RR, Sheffer AL, Spector SL, Townley RG. Standardization of bronchial inhalation challenge procedures. J Allergy Clin Immunol 56:323–327, 1975.

and after delivery of each concentration. Avital and co-workers (1988) used the production of tracheal wheezing as an end point in defining bronchial hyperresponsiveness in a pediatric sample. Among older children who could perform spirometry, the agreement between the two methods was 80 percent. They recommend this method as being simpler and as efficacious as an alternative method of looking at a drop in transcutaneous oxygen tension, studied by Mochizuki et al (1985) and Murakami et al (1990) (Fig. 13–4). Computerized lung sound analysis has also been used in histamine challenge in young children and found to be as sensitive, or more sensitive, than conventional PC_{20} or tracheal auscultation (Beck et al, 1992).

Histamine and methacholine challenges are extremely valuable in clinical situations. Both safety and clinical utility have been docu-

TABLE 13–3. TRUNCATED METHACHOLINE PROTOCOL

Methacholine Concentrations (mg/ml)	Cumulative Breaths	Units/5 Breaths	Cumulative Units/5 Breaths
0.025	5	0.13	0.13
0.25	10	1.25	1.38
2.50	15	12.50	13.88
10.00	20	50.00	63.88
25.00	25	125.00	188.88

From Shapiro GG, Bierman CW. Inhalation bronchoprovocation in children. In Spector SL (ed). Provocative Challenge Procedures: Background and Methodology. New York, Futura Publishing, 1989, pp 395–416.

TABLE 13–4. DOSING AND CUMULATIVE BREATH UNITS FOR THE STANDARD HISTAMINE PROTOCOL AND THE ABBREVIATED HISTAMINE PROTOCOL

STANDARD HISTAMINE PROTOCOL			ABBREVIATED HISTAMINE PROTOCOL		
Concentration (mg/ml)	Inhalations	Cumulative Breath Units (mg/ml)	Concentration (mg/ml)	Inhalations	Cumulative Breath Units (mg/ml)
0.03	5	0.15	.06	1	0.16
0.06	5	0.45	.16	3	0.64
0.12	5	1.05	2.12	1	2.76
0.25	5	2.3	2.12	4	11.24
0.5	5	4.8	10.6	3	43.04
1.0	5	9.8	10.6	4	85.44
2.5	5	22.3			
5.0	5	47.3			
10.0	5	97.3			

From Schmidt LE, Thorne PS, Watt JL, Schwartz DA. Is an abbreviated bronchial challenge with histamine valid? Chest 101:141–145, 1992.

mented (Shapiro and Simon, 1992). It has been documented that they are more sensitive than a history and physical examination in the diagnosis of asthma (Pratter et al, 1983). Cough may be the only manifestation of asthma, and chemical challenge may be uniquely capable of confirming this diagnosis. Shapiro et al (1982) studied 166 children to clarify the etiology of their chronic cough or other undiagnosed pulmonary symptomatology. Methacholine challenge was negative in 58 (35 percent), in whom, therefore, the diagnosis of asthma was considered improbable. Forty-one patients (25 percent) had mild methacholine sensitivity, 49 (30 percent) had moderate sensitivity, and 18 (11 percent) had extreme sensitivity. Many of these patients had chief complaints of cough or bronchitis

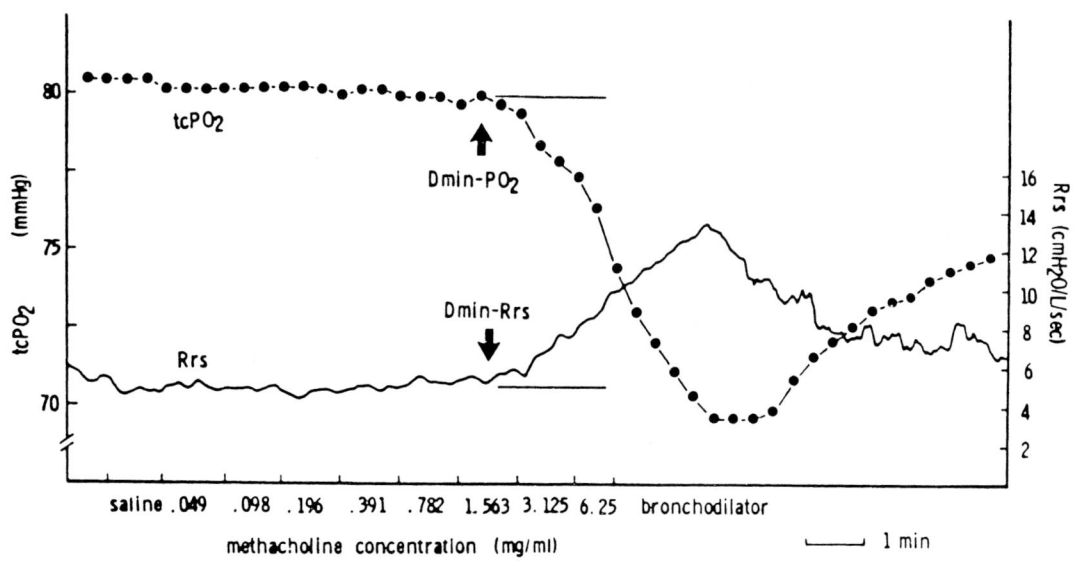

FIGURE 13–4. Typical methacholine inhalation challenge with monitoring of respiratory resistance (Rrs) by the oscillation method and transcutaneous PO_2 ($tcPO_2$). The Dmin-PO_2 indicates the inflection point where the $tcPO_2$ changed linearly and denotes the bronchial sensitivity. The Dmin-Rrs indicates the point of change of respiratory resistance. (From Mochizuki H, Mitsuhashi M, Tokuyama K, Tajima K, Morikawa A, Kuroume T. Bronchial hyperresponsiveness in younger children with asthma. Ann Allergy 60:103–106, 1988.)

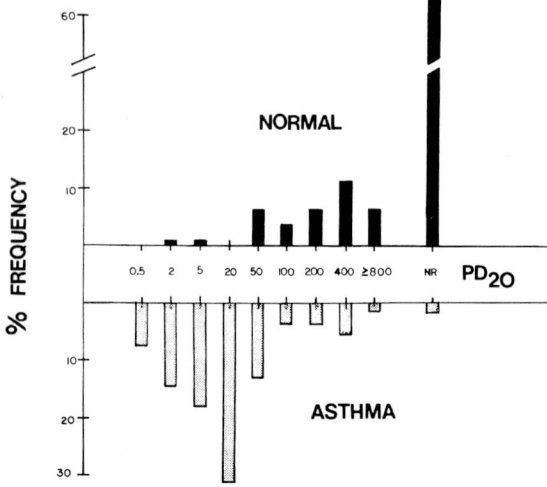

FIGURE 13–5. Percent of normal and asthmatic individuals responding at each PD_{20} concentration. (From Hopp RJ, Bewtra A, Nair NM, Townley RG. Specificity and sensitivity of methacholine inhalation challenge in normal and asthmatic children. J Allergy Clin Immunol 74:154–158, 1984.)

and did not complain of wheezing. Methacholine challenge helped to clarify appropriate therapy in these individuals.

Numerous evaluations of pharmacologic modulation of asthma include chemical challenge as a means of showing whether a drug can alter airway responsiveness and, subsequently, asthma symptomatology. Furukawa and co-workers (1988) studied theophylline compared to cromolyn for control of mild-to-moderate chronic asthma in children. Although asthma symptoms and pulmonary function were similar with the two drugs, only cromolyn diminished bronchial reactivity measured with methacholine challenge. A pediatric study comparing chronic therapy with the beta agonist terbutaline alone, cromolyn alone, or the two combined showed a reduction in methacholine sensitivity with the regimens that included cromolyn and an increase with terbutaline alone (Shapiro et al, 1988).

The amount of time that a drug protects against a bronchoconstriction challenge can be measured by chemical bronchoprovocation challenge, which is thus a useful means of establishing duration of action of the drug. It is also possible to determine whether tachyphylaxis develops to the protective qualities of a bronchodilator by doing repeated challenges over time. Chemical challenges are also used in epidemiologic research to define the proportion of subjects with reactive airways as well as to classify their characteristics. Hopp and co-workers (1984) compared methacholine sensitivity in a nonatopic pediatric population and a population of current asthmatic children. The best specificity and sensitivity of the challenge occurred at a provocative dose of 100 breath units of methacholine (Figs. 13–5 and 13–6). Challenges may be useful for discerning asthma mechanisms. Bhagat and Grunstein (1984) found marked methacholine sensitivity among patients with extremely labile asthma characterized by rapid deterioration, though this group's histamine sensitivity was not clustered in the extreme range. Provocative testing can also be useful in discerning severity of asthma, as a guide to patient management of children and adults. Murray et al (1981) evaluated a population of children with asthma who were symptom-free. The correlation between asthma history score and provocative histamine dose was stronger than that between asthma score and any spirometric test, suggesting that the histamine test more accu-

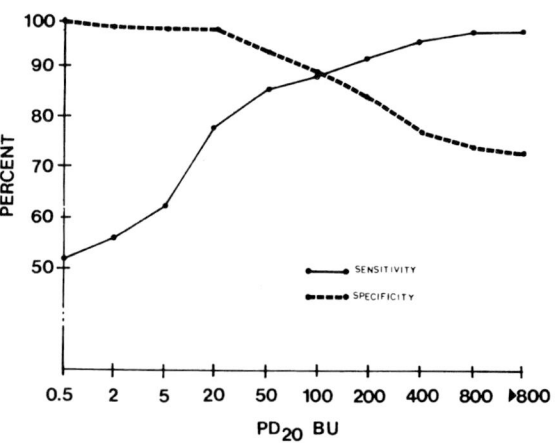

FIGURE 13–6. Patients with a clinical diagnosis of asthma will generally show a PD_{20} less than 100 breath units of methacholine. Below this point, one achieves more specificity in identifying those with clinical asthma. Above this point, one improves sensitivity in identifying asthmatics but loses specificity and will include many who do not have clinical asthma. (From Hopp RJ, Bewtra A, Nair NM, Townley RG. Specificity and sensitivity of methacholine inhalation challenge in normal and asthmatic children. J Allergy Clin Immunol 74:154–158, 1984.)

rately assessed the overall severity of the asthma.

NONPHARMACOLOGIC CHALLENGES

Bronchoprovocation challenges involving inhalation of cold air, water, and saline seem to elicit bronchial hyperresponsiveness by altering temperature, salt, and fluid homeostasis in the airways and thus changing airway osmolarity. A change in airway osmolarity is also believed to be at least part of the mechanism of exercise-induced asthma. Whereas the response to methacholine and histamine are limited to transient smooth muscle effects, osmotic challenges can produce sequelae such as a refractory period, late-phase reaction, and heightened responsiveness to a subsequent methacholine or histamine challenge. These alterations suggest that in contrast to chemical challenges, which directly and transiently affect smooth muscle, osmotic challenges affect the epithelium and may stimulate nervous and inflammatory excitation that either causes or occurs concurrently with bronchoconstriction.

Cold air hyperventilation provides an alternative to chemical bronchoprovocation for children and adults. While there is the advantage that cold air is a "natural" stimulus, there are disadvantages to this technique compared to chemical challenge. Although recent data suggest that there is a dose-response relationship, and that a dose-response curve can be plotted by interrupting the cold air challenge at minute intervals and performing pulmonary function tests, most studies have used a single period of stimulus delivery after which pulmonary function is measured, and this does not allow one to establish a dose-response curve. The equipment needed for air cooling and maintaining the patient in a eucapneic state is more expensive than the apparatus for chemical challenge. Finally, protocols have not been standardized among centers.

The equipment for isocapneic hyperventilation of cold air involves a source of compressed air delivered to a heat exchanger that can bring the temperature to $-15°C$ or $-10°C$. Most studies have used a 5 to 7 L target balloon as a visual cue to regulate the patient's breathing. The patient is coached to hyperventilate at a minute ventilation of about 25 times FEV_1, which compares to that of moderately strenuous activity. The patient can learn to breathe at this rate by keeping the target balloon inflated while it is being evacuated at the required rate by a vacuum pump. Alternatively, some protocols provide audible recorded breathing sounds to the subject and train him or her to breathe at this rate. Hypocapnia is avoided by use of a compressed air mixture of 5 percent CO_2, 21 percent O_2, 74 percent N_2, or by adding a constant stream of 5 percent CO_2 at 2 L/min into the inspiratory line (Townley and Hopp, 1987; Reisman et al, 1987; Heaton et al, 1984; McLaughlin and Doyor, 1983).

Hyperventilation has generally been for a 4-minute period. Spirometry is performed every few minutes after challenge for 15 to 20 minutes, the best FEV_1 of several trials being used. A drop in FEV_1 of 10 percent or more has been considered positive (Reisman et al, 1987). It appears that maximal falls in FEV_1 occur at 3 to 4 minutes and that recovery to <10 percent drop in FEV_1 occurs by 11 minutes (Tal et al, 1984). Reisman et al (1987) suggest spirometry at 4, 6, and 8 minutes after challenge. Considering a drop in FEV_1 >10 percent as a positive test, they claim sensitivity of cold challenge of 95 percent and specificity of 89 percent, results similar to those of methacholine challenge. This differs from earlier work from the same center, in which a somewhat different protocol yielded 100 percent specificity but only 57 percent sensitivity (Galdes-Sebaldt et al, 1985).

Ultrasonically nebulized water challenge is another bronchoprovocative technique that lacks a standardized protocol. It appears to be highly specific for diagnosing airway hyperresponsiveness but is much less sensitive than chemical challenge (Table 13-5). Ultrasonically nebulized distilled water (UNDW) challenge requires minimal equipment and little extra effort from the patient, since tidal breathing is used (Hopp et al, 1988). A dose-response curve is generated since patients begin by breathing a low dose of water, and this dose is gradually increased.

During a typical procedure, ultrasonically nebulized distilled water is generated at a known rate, allowing inspired volume to be recorded. For precision, the delivered dose should be checked by weighing the cannister and tubing before and after each interval of the challenge. Hopp et al (1988) have used a system generating approximately 8 cc of

TABLE 13-5. SENSITIVITY OF DISTILLED WATER CHALLENGES IN DIFFERENT STUDIES

CLINICAL STUDIES	SAMPLE SIZE/ AGE RANGE (Y)	AMOUNT INHALED (ML)	DECREASE IN FEV_1 TO DEFINE RESPONSE (%)	SENSITIVITY TO ASTHMA (%)	TYPE OF NEBULIZER
Galdes-Sebalt et al	21/7-16	—	10	71	DeVilbiss model 65
Lemire et al	11/20-43	44	20	91	DeVilbiss ultra neb 100
Bascom and Bleecker	15/28-40	38	20	53	DeVilbiss model 65
Anderson et al	55/11-56	33	20	100	Mist O2 Gen EN 143a
Black et al	12/20-41	33	20	73	Mist O2 Gen EN 143a
Hopp et al	66/21-37	82	10	76	DeVilbiss model 646
Epidemiologic study, present report	446/7-10	20	10	36	Habel m608

From Frischer T, Studnicka M, Neumann M, Götz M. Determinants of airway response to challenge with distilled water in a population sample of children aged 7 to 10 years old. Chest 102:764–770, 1992.

water per minute. Subjects inhale nebulized water for 15 seconds, 30 seconds, and then 1, 2, and 4 minutes. For each of these intervals the subject tidal breathes with a nose clip in place through a mouthpiece connected to a Hans-Rudolph nonrebreathing valve (#2700), which is attached to the nebulizer. Three minutes after each step above, subjects perform two or three forced expiratory maneuvers, the highest being recorded. The test is stopped when the subject's FEV_1 drops 20 percent or more compared to baseline or the second 4-minute step is completed. UNDW is not a useful screening test for asthma owing to its lack of sensitivity but remains an interesting research tool. Comparing UNDW challenge to methacholine challenge in children, Galdes-Sebaldt and co-workers found 100 percent specificity for the former compared to 83 percent for the latter, but only 71 percent sensitivity with ultrasonic mist compared to 95 percent with methacholine (Galdes-Sebaldt et al, 1985). In a study by Eichler et al in children (1992), up to 100 percent of their patients had significant falls in small airway function, suggesting a peripheral airway effect. They suggested that the mid-expiratory flow rate at 25 percent of vital capacity (MEF25) and at 50 percent of vital capacity (MEF50) might be better variables to evaluate in UNDW challenges. Bronchoconstriction persisted for 10 minutes after their challenges, and so a bronchodilator may be indicated to reduce airflow obstruction. In addition, UNDW challenges have been associated with increases in bronchial hyperresponsiveness, and late reactions have been described (Mattioli et al, 1986).

Anderson (1985) initiated interest in ultrasonic saline as a bronchoprovocation challenge. Patients inspire increasing volumes of 4.5 percent NaCl, though for patients suspected of being highly sensitive, a solution of 2.7 percent NaCl is used. Spirometry is performed after incremental volumes of saline are inspired, the challenge being completed when there is a reduction of more than 20 percent in FEV_1 or a total of 33 ml has been administered. Continued experience with the test suggests that the total volume to be administered can be reduced to as little as 15 ml, with only a minor decrease in sensitivity (Smith and Anderson, 1990). Furthermore, since normal patients do not decrease their FEV_1 more than 10 percent, a change in FEV_1 of 15 percent after hypertonic saline challenge may be sufficient, increasing the sensitivity to over 92 percent in one study (Smith and Anderson, 1990). Fifty percent of asthmatics tested with hypertonic saline have a 20 percent reduction in FEV_1 after inhaling less than 2 ml. Others have modified this protocol using water of increasing salinity for 2-minute increments and recording pulmonary function after each concentration is inhaled. There is currently no accepted standardized hypertonic saline protocol. In contrast to UNDW challenges, neither increases in methacholine reactivity nor late responses have been observed after hypertonic saline challenges (Smith et al, 1987). Both UNDW and hypertonic saline challenges are likely to identify asthmatics with moderate-to-severe airway hyperreactivity, with less sensitivity for identifying milder asthmatics. Hypertonic saline challenges have been shown to be reproducible to within 1.5 doubling volumes over a period of several weeks (Smith and Anderson, 1990). Both UNDW and hypertonic saline challenges have been shown to produce a refractory period (O'Callaghan et al, 1991; Belcher et al, 1987) and, in the case of hypertonic saline, a cross-refractoriness with exercise (Belcher et al, 1987).

Antigen challenges are less frequently used than chemical and nonpharmacologic challenge. They may be used to document environmental antigens as a course of asthma. For example, crab workers may wheeze due to crab aerosol inhalation. These challenges are potentially dangerous since late responses, which may be severe, are common. Also, there is an overlap in response by subjects whose allergic sensitivity to an antigen is manifested clinically as rhinitis only and those who also have bronchospasm. Thus, the occurrence of bronchospasm during a challenge is not specific for clinically significant disease (Bruce et al, 1975).

Antigen provocation can be performed with dust mite, mold, animal, pollen, and other environmental antigens. Lyophilized antigens that have been reconstituted within several days of challenge should be used. Prick testing followed by serial dilutions of intradermal skin testing should be done to establish the initial concentration for challenge, the weakest concentration producing a 5-mm wheal greater than control on intradermal test being a proper starting point. The challenge procedure resembles the dosimeter method of chemical provocation. First five inhalations of saline are delivered, and spirometry is performed, the best of two or three expiratory efforts being taken as baseline. At 10-minute intervals, five inhalations of increasing concentrations of antigen are delivered unless there is a drop of >15 percent in FEV_1. For a decrease of 15 to 19 percent, the same dose is repeated, and fewer inhalations may be given at the physician's discretion. The challenge is complete after there has been a decrease of >20 percent in FEV_1 or the entire sequence of dilutions is administered. Since late reactions may occur for up to 12 hours after challenge, the patient should be studied at hourly intervals, at least with peak flow determinations. Corticosteroid therapy may be necessary to treat the increased bronchial hyperresponsiveness that may result from a positive challenge. In certain instances, fresh materials may reveal positive results and extracts may be imperfect. In other instances, provocative chemicals may not be antigens involved in immunologic reactions but provoke bronchospasm nevertheless, (e.g., plicatic acid causes red cedar workers' asthma).

OTHER RESEARCH AVENUES

Bronchial challenges with mast cell products and other naturally occurring molecules that appear to be important modifying factors of airway stability have provided insight into airway hyperresponsiveness. Challenges with leukotrienes show that asthmatics have a marked and selective hyperresponsiveness to LTE_4 (O'Hickey et al, 1988). Prostaglandins are also products of arachidonic acid metabolism that stimulate bronchoconstriction. There is a correlation between airway responsiveness to $PGF_{2\alpha}$ and methacholine, both being reproducible and having a cumulative dose effect (Thomson et al, 1981). The potency of PGD_2 is approximately 3.5 greater than that of $PGF_{2\alpha}$ and 10 times that of histamine (Spector et al, 1993). The effect of platelet activating factor, another phospholipid mediator, on airway hyperresponsiveness in humans is unclear and highly variable between studies. Bronchial challenges with adenosine, a naturally occurring purine nucleoside formed from adenosine monophosphate (AMP), show that smooth muscle of asthmatic individuals *in vitro* is more responsive than that of nonasthmatic individuals (Bjorck et al, 1992). These challenge studies involving mediators of inflammation and airway homeostasis add to our knowledge of asthma pathophysiology and give clues to possible therapeutic interventions such as the production of antagonists to naturally occurring bronchoprovocative agents in asthmatics.

COMPARISONS OF CHALLENGES

Methacholine and histamine challenges are extremely sensitive indicators of airway hyperresponsiveness. Their advantage is their diagnostic thoroughness. Epidemiologic surveys have assessed the methacholine responsiveness of asthmatic and normal children in order to determine a reasonable discriminating point between these groups. When one administers a challenge that incorporates dosing up to 800 breath units (BU) of methacholine, in contrast to the typical challenge of up to 200 breath units, a fascinating relationship is revealed. Ninety-eight percent of asthmatic subjects respond with a 20 percent or greater drop in FEV_1 and 87 percent have a PD_{20} of 100 BU or less. Among normals, 12 percent have a PD_{20} under 100 BU, 25 percent have a PD_{20} over 100 BU, and 63 percent do not have a fall in FEV_1 of 20 percent. The best sensitivity and specificity (89 percent for each) occurs at a PD_{20} of 100 BU. This cut-off gives a false-positive rate of 19 percent and a false-negative rate of 6 percent. Using a 200-BU methacholine cut-off decreases the false-negative rate to 4 percent, but the false-positive rate increases to 27 percent (Hopp et al, 1984). Backer and co-workers examined the sensitivity and specificity of histamine challenge in an unselected population of children and adolescents and found the best results occurred at a PC_{20} of <2.4 mg/ml (Backer et al, 1991b). For clinical studies, however, they found that a PC_{20} of <8 mg/ml was best, although the positive predictive value was low.

Those patients who are apparently normal but have positive methacholine challenge may be a group earmarked for future asthma. A significant number of these individuals may develop clinical asthma in subsequent years (Table 13–6), particularly if they have a positive family history of asthma. Alternatively, they may have residual reactivity, which may continue to wane with time, or reactivity that is genetically predetermined but will never be of clinical consequence. Since the future for any particular individual is unpredictable, an isolated methacholine challenge that is positive is of no clinical value. Rather, chemical challenges take on validity when they are used to clarify and corroborate information derived from the history and physical examination.

Bronchial responsiveness to histamine and methacholine correlate fairly well. However, histamine may be less reliable for distinguishing normals from asthmatics, and it may cause headaches and facial flushing at higher concentrations.

Exercise challenge is less sensitive than chemical challenge and is a poorer screening test for airway hyperresponsiveness. Chatham et al (1982) noted that six of 15 asthmatics did not respond to maximal exercise challenge with a 10 percent fall in FEV_1, while one of ten normal subjects did. Comparisons of cold air, ultrasonic mist, and methacholine inhalation tests in normal and asthmatic children (Galdes-Sebaldt et al, 1985) reiterated the increased sensitivity of methacholine, 95 percent versus 57 percent for cold air and 71 percent for UNDW. However, cold air challenge with 4 minutes of cold air hyperventilation at $25 \times FEV_1$ rather than at four levels of ventilation (2, 5, 10, and $20 \times FEV_1$) showed similar sensitivity and specificity for methacholine and cold air challenge in children (Reisman et al, 1987). Cold air challenge was equivalent to methacholine in distinguishing adult asthmatics from normals (O'Byrne et al, 1982).

Smith and co-workers (Smith and Anderson, 1986) have shown similar responses of asthmatics to isocapneic hyperventilation and ultrasonically nebulized 4.5 percent NaCl. They hypothesized that the parallel PD_{20}s and slopes of water loss compared to drop in FEV_1 attest to airway hyperosmolarity being the mechanism for isocapneic hyperventilation-induced bronchospasm, hypertonic inhalation-induced bronchospasm and inferentially, exercise-induced bronchospasm.

From these comparisons it appears that methacholine, histamine, and isocapneic hyperventilation of cold air are sensitive indicators of bronchial hyperresponsiveness. Hypertonic saline challenge, though less well studied, is also sensitive. Exercise challenge and ultrasonically nebulized hypotonic solutions are less sensitive for separating asthmatic and normal subjects.

The challenge that one chooses will largely

TABLE 13–6. DEVELOPMENT OF ASTHMA IN RELATION TO THE SEVERITY OF BRONCHIAL HYPERRESPONSIVENESS*

Severity of Bronchial Hyperresponsiveness	No.	No. of Cases of Asthma	%
Moderate or severe	1	1	100
Mild	10	4	40
Slight	47	4	8.2
Undetectable	88	2	2.2

From Zhong NS, Chan RC, Yang MO, Wu ZY, Zheng JP, Li YF. Is asymptomatic bronchial hyperresponsiveness an indication of potential asthma? A two-year follow-up of young students with bronchial hyperresponsiveness. Chest 102:1104–1109, 1992.

depend on one's goals. If one seeks to define a level of physical disability from exercise-induced bronchospasm, an exercise challenge will obviously be most helpful. There may on occasion be a need to confirm that a particular antigen is asthma producing. For most purposes, chemical challenge with methacholine or histamine will be most valuable. These agents promise excellent sensitivity, fairly good specificity, short duration of action, simplicity, and standardized protocols.

REFERENCES

Adinoff A, Strunk R. Methacholine inhalation challenge (MC) in young children: Results of testing and follow-up. J Allergy Clin Immunol 73:124, 1984. (Abstract)

Anderson SD. Bronchial challenge by ultrasonically nebulized aerosols. Clin Rev Allergy 3:427–439, 1985.

Avital A, Bar-Yishay E, Springer C, Godfrey S. Bronchial provocation tests in young children using tracheal auscultation. J Pediatr 112:591–594, 1988.

Backer V, Dirksen A, Bach-Mortensen N, Hansen KK, Laursen EM, Wendelboe D. The distribution of bronchial responsiveness to histamine and exercise in 527 children and adolescents. J Allergy Clin Immunol 88:68–76, 1991a.

Backer V, Groth S, Dirksen A, Bach-Mortensen N, Hansen KK, Laursen EM, Wendelboe D. Sensitivity and specificity of the histamine challenge test for the diagnosis of asthma in an unselected sample of children and adolescents. Eur Respir J 4:1093–1100, 1991b.

Beck R, Dickson U, Montgomery MD, Mitchell I. Histamine challenge in young children using computerized lung sound analysis. Chest 102:759–763, 1992.

Belcher NG, Rees PJ, Clark TJH, Lee TH. A comparison of the refractory periods induced by hypertonic airway challenge and exercise in bronchial asthma. Am Rev Respir Dis 135:822–825, 1987.

Bhagat RG, Grunstein MM. Comparison of responsiveness to methacholine, histamine and exercise in subgroups of asthmatic children. Am Rev Respir Dis 129:224, 1984.

Bias WB. The genetic basis of asthma. In Austen KF, Lichtenstein LM (eds.) Asthma. New York, Academic Press, 1973.

Bjorck T, Gustafsson LE, Dahlen SE. Isolated bronchi from asthmatics are hyperresponsive to adenosine, which apparently acts indirectly by liberation of leukotrienes and histamine. Am Rev Respir Dis 145:1087–1091, 1992.

Bruce CA, Rosenthal RR, Lichtenstein LM, Norman PS. Quantitative inhalation bronchial challenge in ragweed hay fever patients: A comparison with ragweed-allergic asthmatics. J Allergy Clin Immunol 56:331, 1975.

Burrows B, Sears MR, Flannery EM, Herbison GP, Holdaway MD. Relationships of bronchial responsiveness assessed by methacholine to serum IgE, lung function, symptoms and diagnoses in 11-year-old New Zealand children. J Allergy Clin Immunol 90:376–385, 1992.

Chai H, Farr RS, Roehlich LA, Mathison DA, McLean JA, Rosenthal RR, Sheffer AL, Spector SL, Townley RG. Standardization of bronchial inhalation challenge procedures. J Allergy Clin Immunol 56:323–327, 1975.

Chatham M, Bleecker ER, Smith PL, Rosenthal RR, Mason P, Norman PS. A comparison of histamine, methacholine, and exercise airway reactivity in normal and asthmatic subjects. Am Rev Respir Dis 126:235–240, 1982.

Eichler I, Gotz M, Zarbovic JJ, Kofinger A. Distilled water challenges in asthmatic children: Comparison of different protocols. Chest 102:753–758, 1992.

Eliasson AH, Phillips YY, Rajagopal KR, Howard RS. Sensitivity and specificity of bronchial provocation testing. An evaluation of four techniques in exercise-induced bronchospasm. Chest 102:347–355, 1992.

Furukawa CT, DuHamel TR, Weimer L, Shapiro GG, Pierson WE, Bierman CW. Cognitive and behavioral findings in children taking theophylline. J Allergy Clin Immunol 81:83–88, 1988.

Galdes-Sebaldt M, McLaughlin FJ, Levison H. Comparison of cold air ultrasonic mist and methacholine inhalation as tests of bronchial reactivity in normal and asthmatic children. J Pediatr 107:526–530, 1985.

Godfrey S, Konig P. Exercise-induced bronchial liability in wheezy children and their families. Pediatrics 56(suppl):851–855, 1975.

Heaton RW, Henderson AF, Costello JF. Cold air as a bronchial provocation technique. Chest 86:810–814, 1984.

Hopp RJ, Bewtra A, Nair NM, Townley RG. The effect of age on methacholine response. J Allergy Clin Immunol 76:609–613, 1985.

Hopp RJ, Bewtra AK, Nair NM, Townley RG. Specificity and sensitivity of methacholine inhalation challenge in normal and asthmatic children. J Allergy Clin Immunol 74:154–158, 1984.

Hopp RJ, Christy J, Brewtra A, Nair NM, Townley RG. Incorporation and analysis of ultrasonically nebulized distilled water challenges in an epidemiologic study of asthma and bronchial reactivity. Ann Allergy 60:129–133, 1988.

Hopp RJ, Weiss SJ, Nair MN, Bewtra AK, Townley RG. Interpretation of the results of methacholine inhalation challenge tests. J Allergy Clin Immunol 80:821–830, 1987.

Juniper EF, Frith PA, Hargreave FE. Airways responsiveness to histamine and methacholine; relationship to minimum treatment to control symptoms of asthma. Thorax 36:575–579, 1981.

Juniper EF, Hargreave FE. Airway responsiveness by aerosol inhalation tests: Variability in results due to unexpected differences between calibrated nebulizers [abstract]. Bull Eur Physiopathol Respir 22:165S, 1986.

LaBraico JM, Reed CE, Rosenthal RR, Shapiro GG, Spector SL, Townley RG. Multicenter evaluation of airways hyperreactivity using a standardized methacholine challenge. (Abstract) J Allergy Clin Immunol 73:124, 1984.

Mattioli S, Foresi A, Corbo GM, Valente S, Patalano F, Clappi G. Increase in bronchial responsiveness to methacholine and late response after the inhalation of ultrasonically nebulized distilled water. Chest 90:726–732, 1986.

McConnochie KM, Roghmann KJ. Bronchiolitis as a possible cause of wheezing in childhood: New evidence. Pediatrics 74:1, 1984.

McLaughlin FJ, Dozor AJ. Cold air inhalation challenge in the diagnosis of asthma in children. Pediatrics 72:503–509, 1983.

Mochizuki H, Mitsuhashi M, Tokuyame K, Tajima K, Morikawa A, Kuroume T. A new method of estimating bronchial hyperresponsiveness in younger children. Ann Allergy 55:162, 1985.

Murakami G, Igarashi T, Adachi Y, Matsuno M, Adachi Y, Sawai M, Yoshizumi A, Okada T. Measurement of bronchial hyperreactivity in infants and preschool children using a new method. Ann Allergy 64:383–387, 1990.

Murray AB, Fergusun AC, Morrison B. Airway responsiveness to histamine as a test for overall severity of asthma in children. J Allergy Clin Immunol 68:119, 1981.

O'Byrne PM, Ryan G, Morris M, McCormach D, Jones NL, Morse JL, Hargreave FE. Asthma induced by cold air and its relation to nonspecific bronchial responsiveness to methacholine. Am Rev Respir Dis 125:281–285, 1982.

O'Callaghan C, Milner AD, Swarbick A. Nebulized water as a bronchoconstricting challenge in infancy. Arch Dis Child 66:948–951, 1991.

O'Hickey SP, Arm JP, Rees PJ, Spur B, Lee TH. The relative responsiveness to inhaled leukotriene E4, methacholine and histamine in normal and asthmatic subjects. Eur Respir J 1:913–7, 1988.

Pattemore PK, Asher MI, Harrison AC, Mitchell EA, Rea HH, Stewart AW. The interrelationships among bronchial hyperresponsiveness, the diagnosis of asthma, and asthma symptoms. Am Rev Respir Dis 142:549–554, 1990.

Peat JK, Salome CM, Berry G, Woolcock AJ. Relation of dose-response slope to respiratory symptoms in a population of Australian school children. Am Rev Respir Dis 144:663–667, 1991.

Pratter MR, Hingston DM, Irwin RS. Diagnosis of bronchial asthma by clinical evaluation. Chest 84:42–47, 1983.

Pullan CR, Hey EN. Wheezing, asthma and pulmonary dysfunction 10 years after infection with respiratory syncytial virus in infancy. Br Med J 284:1665, 1982.

Reisman J, Mappa L, de Benedictis F, McLaughlin J, Levison H. Cold air challenge in children with asthma. Pediatr Pulmonol 3:251–254, 1987.

Ryan G, Dolovich MB, Roberts RS, Frith PA, Juniper EF, Hargreave FE, Newhouse MT. Standardization of inhalation provocation tests: Two techniques of aerosol generation and inhalation compared. Am Rev Respir Dis 123:195–199, 1981.

Shapiro GG, Furukawa CT, Pierson WE, Bierman CW. Methacholine bronchial challenge in children. J Allergy Clin Immunol 69:365, 1982.

Shapiro GG, Furukawa CT, Pierson WE, Sharpe MJ, Menendez R, Bierman CW. Double-blind evaluation of nebulized cromolyn, terbutaline and the combination for childhood asthma. J Allergy Clin Immunol 81:449–454, 1988.

Shapiro GG, Simon RA. Bronchoprovocation Committee Report. J Allergy Clin Immunol 89:775–778, 1992.

Smith CM, Anderson SD, Black JL. Methacholine responsiveness increases after ultrasonically nebulized water but not after ultrasonically nebulized hypertonic saline in patients with asthma. J Allergy Clin Immunol 79:85–92, 1987.

Smith CM, Anderson SD. Hyperosmolarity as the stimulus to asthma induced by hyperventilation? J Allergy Clin Immunol 77:729–736, 1986.

Smith CM, Anderson SD. Inhalation challenges using hypertonic saline in asthmatic subjects: A comparison with responses to hyperpnea, methacholine and water. Eur Respir J 3:144–151, 1990.

Spector SL, Smith LJ, Glass M, et al. The effects of six weeks of therapy with oral doses of ICI, 204, 219, a leukotriene D4 receptor antagonist, in subjects with bronchial asthma. Am J Respir Crit Care Med 150:618–623, 1994.

Tal A, Pasterkamp H, Serrette C, Leahy F, Chernick V. Response to cold air hyperventilation in normal and in asthmatic children. J Pediatr 104:516–521, 1984.

Thomson NC, Roberts R, Bandouvakis J, Newball H, Hargreave FE. Comparison of bronchial responses to prostaglandin $F_{2\alpha}$ and methacholine. J Allergy Clin Immunol 68:392–398, 1981.

Townley RJ, Hopp RJ. Inhalation methods for the study of airway responsiveness. J Allergy Clin Immunol 80:111–124, 1987.

Turner KJ, Dowse GK, Stewart GA, Alpers MP. Studies on bronchial hyperreactivity, allergic responsiveness and asthma in rural and urban children of the highlands of Papua, New Guinea. J Allergy Clin Immunol 77:558–566, 1986.

Van Aalderen WMC, Gerritsen J, Koeter GH, van der Weele LT, Postma DS, Knol K. The reproducibility and agreement of three indices of airway responsiveness to histamine in asthmatic children. Pediatr Pulmonol 6:113–117, 1989.

Van Der Heide S, de Monchy JG, de Vries K, et al. Seasonal variation in airway hyperresponsiveness and natural exposure to house dust mite allergens in patients with asthma. J Allergy Clin Immunol 93:470–475, 1994.

Weiss ME, Wheeler B, Eggleston P, Adkinson NF. A protocol for performing reproducible methacholine inhalation tests in children with moderate to severe asthma. Am Rev Respir Dis 139:67–72, 1989.

Welliver RC, Wong DT, Sun M, Middleton E Jr, Vaughan RS, Ogra PL. The development of respiratory syncytial virus-specific IgE and the release of histamine in nasopharyngeal secretions after infection. N Engl J Med 305:841, 1981.

Chapter 14

Diagnostic Challenges

Ronald A. Simon, M.D.

This chapter will discuss both general and specific measures and procedures in order to accomplish diagnostic ingestion challenges in almost any situation involving virtually any substance. Techniques for bronchoprovocation and food challenges are described in other chapters. For other issues pertaining to the design and evaluation of clinical trials, the reader is referred to Metcalfe (1990).

GENERAL PRINCIPLES

DIETARY AVOIDANCE. When applicable, the offending/suspect substance should be avoided for 24 hours. This will already be the case for subjects who believe that certain substances are the cause of their medical problems. Some investigators have suggested avoiding the challenge substance for as long as 2 weeks. There are no data to suggest that this is necessary (Stevenson, 1993; Simon, 1993). In fact, if one has not been avoiding the substance and remains asymptomatic, then there is no need to suspect that agent. Furthermore, if the subject is symptomatic and not avoiding the substance that is purported to be the cause of his problems, one should be able to produce symptoms and signs during the challenge.

SITE OF CHALLENGE. Challenges are performed in the fasting patient and usually begin in the morning. Thus, should a reaction occur, proper personnel should be available to treat the reaction. Whether challenges should be performed in the office or in a hospital requires some individual decision-making. Wherever the challenge is performed, emergency resuscitative equipment should be available and trained personnel must be present. These personnel must be well qualified both to perform the challenge itself and to administer emergency treatment. In addition, the office staff must be committed to provide individual attention to the subject who is reacting. The physician must also be available to spend the time to supervise the treatment of reactions. Allergists who do skin tests and give immunotherapy take upon themselves the burden of treating severe anaphylaxis. The same guidelines and procedures for treating anaphylaxis should be operable if one performs diagnostic challenges in the office. If that is not the case or if the occurrence would prove too disruptive to the office schedule or if the patient's history of reaction is severe, one may wish to perform the challenge in the hospital. The response time to obtain the paramedic help and the distance to the closest hospital should also be taken into account when one is deciding where to perform diagnostic challenges.

DOSAGE. Suggested dosages for specific common challenges are listed on Table 14–1. In these cases and for those in which proto-

TABLE 14–1. DOSES FOR COMMON ADDITIVES USED IN CHALLENGE PROTOCOLS

ADDITIVE	DOSE (mg)
Tartrazine	25, 50
Sulfites (potassium, metabisulfite)	1, 5, 10, 25, 50, 100, 200
MSG (monosodium glutamate)	250, 500, 1,000, 2,500, 5,000
Aspartase (Nutrasweet)	25, 75, 150
Parabens (ethylprobomethyl)	25, 50, 100
Benzoates (sodium)	25, 50, 100
BHA (butylated hydroxy anisole/BHT)	25, 50, 100

cols have not been established, the starting dose for challenge should be individualized, depending on the severity of the subject's reaction and the estimated dose that was consumed.

Much detective work may be involved in determining the amount of the substance ingested. However, one can usually make some estimate by obtaining recipes from restaurants or by reading package labels for home-cooked meals. When one has an idea of the relative concentration of the offending substance, one then needs to assess the *amount* of the substance-containing food that has been ingested. When no estimate can be determined, it is usually prudent to begin with a 1-mg dose. Then increases (doubling, 10-fold, or some combination thereof) can be employed. When the ingested dose has been estimated, one tenth, one hundredth, or less of that dose can be administered, depending on the firmness of the estimate and the severity of the reaction.

The final dose to be administered should be at least equal to the estimated historical exposure or to a maximal natural exposure, if known.

TIMING. Where standardized protocols are nonexistent, the interval between doses depends on the patient's history. Usually the time described by the patient is doubled for safety reasons. However, one must also consider the half-life of the substance, if known. This would increase the safety of the challenge procedure because by challenging beyond the half-life one would avoid an accumulating dosage effect. For example, we now recommend a 3-hour interval between aspirin challenge doses. Otherwise, with shorter intervals one may have a reaction to the dose previously administered, which begins shortly after the dose just administered. This could lead to a more severe reaction representing the summation of both doses. If time permits, using the example of reports of monosodium glutamate–provoked asthma (Allen et al, 1987), one should wait 12 to 24 hours to see whether there are any delayed reactions before proceeding to a different substance. If more than one substance is used for challenge purposes on one day and the reaction ensues, one may have to repeat the challenges on separate days in order to be sure that the reaction was an immediate reaction to the last substance administered rather than a delayed reaction to an earlier challenge.

SUBSTANCE VEHICLES. Generally, challenges should be performed utilizing opaque capsules. One exception to this in the past was with sulfites when they were being applied as a liquid to fresh fruits and vegetables. We then utilized a solution challenge, which was swished around the mouth and then swallowed. Since this application to foods served as fresh was banned by the FDA in 1986, we currently use capsule challenges for sulfites as well.

We have switched from lactose to sucrose placebos because if multiple lactose placebos are given to a lactose-deficient subject, gastrointestinal symptoms may ensue. At best, these would be uncomfortable; at worst, they might be interpreted as a false-positive reaction or unblind the study.

CHALLENGES IN URTICARIA/ ANGIOEDEMA PATIENTS

The incidence of reactions to any food and drug additives in patients with chronic urticaria and angioedema is unknown. This is not because of an inadequate number of studies, but rather because of the lack of properly and vigorously controlled studies and inherent problems in challenging with chronic urticaria. These issues will be discussed below.

Challenges in urticaria patients can be a difficult problem. There are many factors that may be related to the outcome of the challenge. One of these is patient selection. This is particularly important for research studies in which the prevalence of reaction to a particular substance and a population of patients with urticaria is being studied.

PATIENT SELECTION. Selection of patients for study may include (1) all available patients with chronic urticaria or only those with chronic idiopathic urticaria, (2) only those with a history suggestive of additive-provoked urticaria, or (3) only those whose urticaria improved after a diet free of commonly implicated additives. Depending on the group selected and the challenge protocol, different percentages of chronic urticaria patients have been reported as additive-sensitive. These and other variables to follow are often omitted or poorly stated in published reports and only add more confusion to the already difficult task of comparing results of different studies.

ACTIVITY OF URTICARIA AT THE TIME OF THE STUDY. The relative degree of activity or inactivity of urticaria or angioedema at the time of challenge appears to be important in determining the ability of the skin to respond during subsequent challenges. Patients with active urticaria are more likely to develop further urticaria; the challenges performed on patients whose urticaria is in remission are more likely to yield negative results. In one study by Lumry et al (1982), only one in 15 patients whose urticaria was in remission experienced a reaction to aspirin, whereas 7 of 10 patients whose urticaria was active at the time of challenge reacted to the aspirin.

In order to reach a "happy medium" for this criterion, we suggest tapering antihistamines to the "lowest effective dose" in subjects who have chronic idiopathic urticaria as their primary diagnosis. This allows some disease activity but in a controlled sense, both in terms of the patient's symptoms and to establish a stable baseline urticaria from which a reaction can be discerned. For subjects with acute urticaria, the activity of their urticaria would obviously not be an issue.

MEDICATIONS. Medication usage is also an important variable in urticaria challenges. In several studies regarding the incidence of food additives in urticaria, no reference is made to whether medications, particularly antihistamines, are withheld or continued during challenges (Simon, 1993). There are important caveats to bear in mind while performing or interpreting challenge studies that do mention details of medication withdrawal: (1) discontinuation of antihistamines immediately before or within 24 hours of challenge is likely to induce false-positive reactions, (2) continuation of antihistamines during challenges may block some of the milder reactions and thereby promote false-negative results, and (3) subjects are also more likely to experience breakthrough urticaria the longer the interval from the last antihistamine dose to the test substance associated with a "positive challenge." This phenomenon is accentuated if placebo control challenges are given first before the additive challenge and in close proximity to the protective effect of the last antihistamine tablet. Then, as the day wears on, breakthrough urticaria is more likely to occur following one of the additive doses, and this is construed as a positive challenge.

A good time to perform a challenge without persistent antihistamine effect would be when the histamine skin test is no longer suppressed (Bosso and Simon, 1993). The effects of newer, long-acting H_1 antihistamine-blocking reactions would be expected to be prolonged. Therefore, medications such as astemizole, terfenadine, and loratadine should be withheld until positive histamine and codeine skin tests are elicited.

REACTION CRITERIA. In most studies in the literature, loosely defined and sometimes even subjective criteria are utilized for defining a positive urticarial response. The reaction criteria simply consist of "clear signs of urticaria developing within 24 hours." However, reaction criteria should be as objective as possible. The studies by Simon and Stevenson (1993) and by Lumry et al (1982) represent the only reported challenge studies that utilize an objective system for scoring urticarial responses.

In these studies, the "rule of nines" used for assessing thermal burns is a useful method for semiquantitative skin scoring. For each of the nine equally divided surface areas of the body, a score of 0 to 4 may be assigned and a total score derived (0 to 36 points) (Fig. 14–1). A score of 0 is assigned a particular area where no urticaria is seen. A score of 1 represents urticaria estimated to cover <25 percent of that particular body surface area. A score of 2 represents ≥25 but <50 percent; a score of 3 is ≥50 but <75 percent; and a score of 4 indicates anywhere from ≥75 percent to complete coverage with hives. A positive urticarial response may be defined as either an absolute increase in the total score of 9 points or an increase of more than 300 percent from the baseline score determined before challenge.

For angioedema patients, a positive response may be defined as a relative increase in the size of the affected body part by more than 50 percent. This can often be assessed by a water displacement method whereby measurements of each extremity and/or the total body are determined by immersion before and after challenge. Symptoms should always reproduce the patient's history. Studies in the literature actually will report subjective symptoms as a positive response to a substance when the patient's primary diagnosis is urticaria.

BASELINE OBSERVATION. Prior to *any* challenges in urticaria patients, there should be a baseline period of observation during which

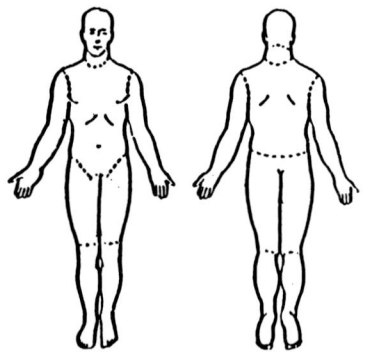

0 - No lesions

1 - Isolated urticarial lesions

2 - Urticaria involving less than 25% of area

3 - Urticaria involving less than 50% of area

4 - Diffuse urticaria - more than 50% of area

NOTE: When recording the TRUNK, which includes BACK and CHEST/ABDOMEN, multiply score by 2 and record.

FIGURE 14–1. Each of the nine thermal injury zones is approximately 11 percent of the cutaneous surface. Each area is surveyed for urticarial lesions. The sum of scores from all nine areas is the total score.

skin scores are recorded at the same intervals as during the subsequent challenges (Bosso and Simon, 1993). The appropriate length of the baseline observation period depends on various factors such as the activity of the patient's urticaria, the interval of time between discontinuation of antihistamines and the challenges, and the length of the challenge protocol.

In general, one day of pure observation with skin scoring followed by one day of single-blind placebo challenge with skin scoring should be performed.

One might elect not to observe patients who are completely free of hives at the time of the challenge. In this instance, a one-day placebo challenge should suffice. Skin scores on those 2 days should not vary by more than three points or 30 percent, whichever is greater, before one proceeds to the placebo-controlled additive challenges.

PLACEBOS. The importance of placebo control studies in additive challenges for urticaria cannot be overemphasized. Studies that do not utilize placebo controls are useless in specifically linking urticarial responses to a challenge substance. There is a surprising number of published studies of additive challenges that did not employ placebo controls. When placebos are properly utilized, the incidence of "reactions" approaches 30 to 40 percent. However, even in most of the placebo-controlled studies, the placebo is usually the first challenge substance, often followed by aspirin and then additives. Thus, a spontaneous flare of urticaria was least likely to coincide with the first "placebo" challenge, particularly if antihistamines were withheld just prior to the challenge. This emphasizes the need for the baseline observation period described above, as well as a tapering of the antihistamine dose to the "most effective" dose, also described above.

The use of an all-day placebo challenge after the baseline period is also helpful in determining the spontaneous variability in the urticaria under a challenge setting. Then, the use of multiple placebos at least equal to the number of additive dosages and by random distribution enhances the design of the placebo control challenge and eliminates the bias of the negative first challenge of placebo protocol.

It should be emphasized, however, that for patients in whom one believes suggestion may play a role in a positive response, a placebo should always be administered first even if this is a single-blind challenge. In such patients, the last dose should also be a placebo administered in single-blind fashion.

CONTROLS. It appears from our data that reactions to food additives and other substances previously believed to be important factors in the causation of chronic idiopathic urticaria are unusual, even rare. Therefore, we suggest a screening open challenge protocol. The contents of the Scripps Clinic Multiple Additive Challenge for chronic idiopathic urticaria and angioedema is listed in Table 14–2.

If the Multiple Additive Challenge is not warranted because a particular substance has been implicated, one may wish to proceed with a single-blind challenge. This would allow individualization of the dosages or administration of additional placebos during the course of the challenge. However, the only way to confirm that a particular substance is

TABLE 14–2. THE SCRIPPS CLINIC MULTIPLE ADDITIVE CHALLENGE

Additive	Dose (mg)
Tartrazine	50
Sulfites	200
MSG	2500
Aspartase	150
Parabens	100
Benzoates	100
BHA	100

the cause of urticaria (or for that matter, any other reaction) is by a double-blind placebo-controlled challenge protocol. Also, this is obviously the case for any published research studies.

Because exacerbations of urticaria may be stress-provoked, it is necessary to blind the study subjects. Furthermore, particular subjects who believe that additives in general or a specific substance in particular may be provoking their urticaria may have a positive response by suggestion. Double-blinding ensures that nurses and physicians do not transmit unspoken signals of concern or apprehension when the "real" test subject is administered. In addition, it is important to eliminate observer bias, whenever possible, because positive responses may simply consist of the appearance of hives or an increase in the number of hives compared to those observed at baseline.

CHALLENGES IN ASTHMATIC PATIENTS

SAFETY. For reasons of patient safety, challenges should be performed only when the forced expiratory volume in 1 second (FEV_1) is >70 percent of the predicted normal values or the patient's prior best. In addition, for adults, the FEV_1 should be >1.5 liters in absolute value. We also continue all oral bronchodilators during the challenges. In addition, we continue (often increase) corticosteroids (both inhaled and oral) in order to have a stable tracheobronchial tree, particularly in view of the medications that have to be discontinued.

MEDICATIONS. Inhaled bronchodilators, including ipatropium, should be discontinued the morning of the study. Cromolyn and nedocromil should be discontinued 48 hours prior to the challenge (Simon, 1990). Likewise, traditional antihistamines should be withdrawn 24 hours prior to challenge. There are no data on which to base the discontinuation of long-acting antihistamines such as astemizole or loratadine. It is also unclear whether at least some of the protective effects of antihistamines seen in aspirin and sulfite challenges have been due to anticholinergic side effects or to H_1 antihistamine effect. In any case, antihistamines might at most modify reactions and usually have not been shown to make the difference between a positive and negative challenge. As already noted, we continue theophylline at therapeutic levels, as well as corticosteroids. In our experience, theophylline and steroids do not interfere with ingestive challenges, although a study of aspirin-sensitive asthmatics suggested that corticosteroids may increase the threshold reaction dose (Nizankowska and Szczeklik, 1989). We believe that withholding the theophylline and steroids is much more likely to lead to a false-positive challenge in an unstable asthmatic patient. Several examples of this phenomenon are illustrated in Figure 14–2.

CONTROLS. The same controls used for the challenges in urticaria patients should be employed here. For asthmatic challenges it is probably a more important safety requirement to use single-blind challenges to individualized doses. At each successive step in the challenge protocol, dosages increase at least twofold. After the patient has experienced a 10 to 15 percent drop in the FEV_1 value after a particular dose, one may wish to add a dose at half the usual increment of increase in an effort to prevent a precipitous fall in FEV_1 value at a higher dose challenge. This would obviously not be possible with an initial double-blind challenge protocol. For asthmatic subjects, the additional variables of proper patient training and coaching have become important.

CRITERIA FOR POSITIVE REACTION. False-positive challenges in unstable asthmatic patients are always a concern. To help control for this variable and to establish the stability of a subject's bronchial airways, we recommend that patients undergo a single-blind straight placebo challenge for a length of time equal to that of the proposed challenge. During this period of time, the FEV_1 value should not fall by more than 10 percent of baseline. Pulmonary function is measured at baseline

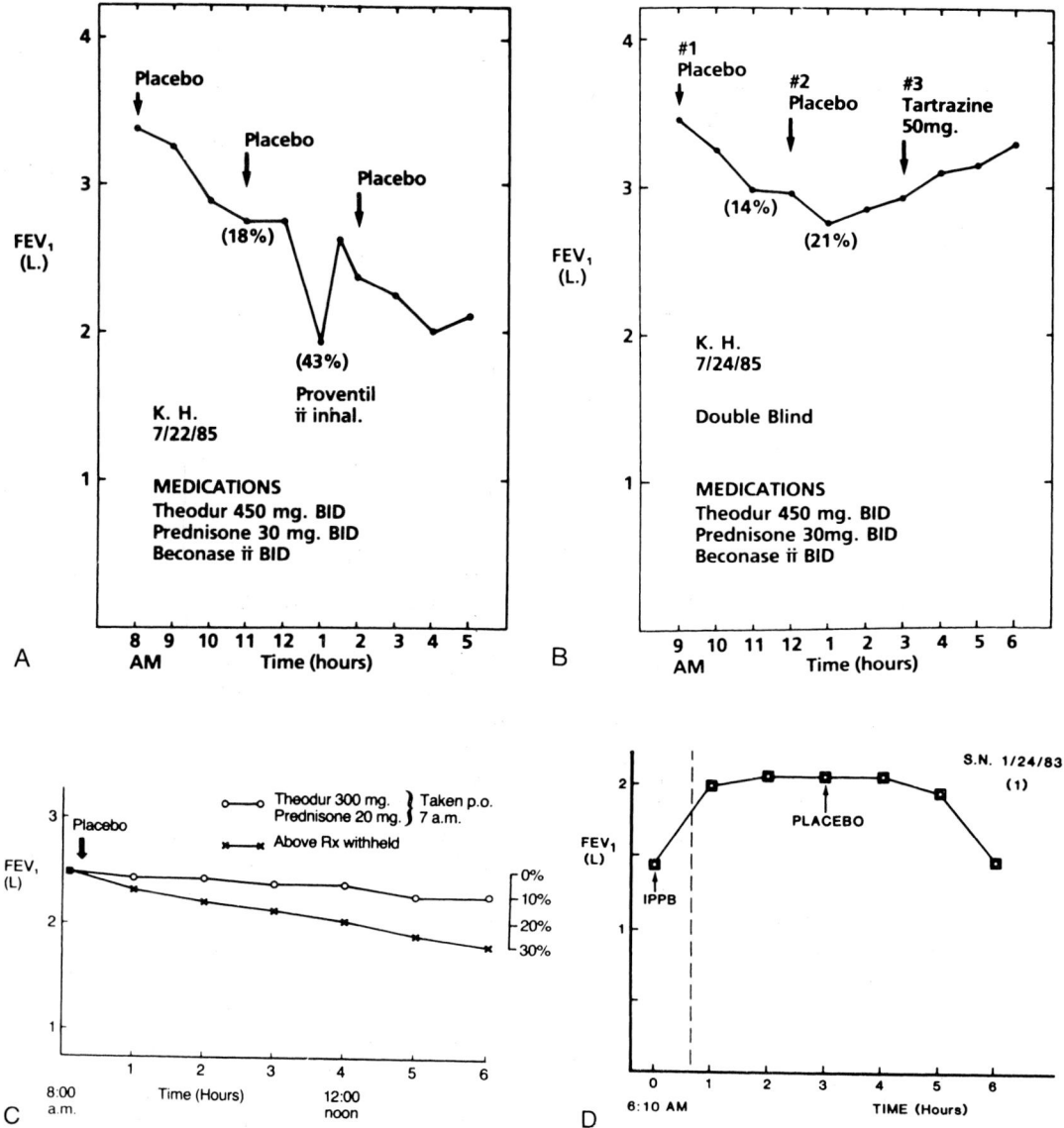

FIGURE 14–2. *A,* Normal baseline FEV$_1$, which declined by 43 percent over the next 9 hours following placebo challenges (even despite a burst of prednisone). *B,* Same subject 2 days later following additional treatment. Airways more stable; however, if dose 2 had been tartrazine, the subject may have been labeled "tartrazine-sensitive" and an uncontrolled study yielding a false-positive would have resulted. *C,* Effect on lung function of withholding theophylline and prednisone in a steroid-dependent asthmatic (30 percent spontaneous fall in FEV$_1$) versus continuation of medication (<10 percent fall). *D,* Effect of administration of isoproterenol by IPPB. Baseline FEV$_1$ increases from 1.5 to 2 liters. Spontaneous decline 5 hours later to pretreatment baseline. Had an active agent rather than placebo been administered, the spontaneous decline may have been misinterpreted as a "reaction."

and then before each challenge dose (sooner if symptoms occur). A 20 percent drop in the FEV$_1$ from baseline is considered a positive challenge (Stevenson and Simon, 1993; Simon and Stevenson, 1993).

No late-phase reactions have been described following challenges with ASA or food and drug additives. However, one case of a delayed asthmatic reaction to monosodium glutamate has been reported (Allen et al, 1987). If the history warrants, pulmonary function can be tested 6 to 8 hours after the early-phase reaction, following the conclusion of the challenge, or whenever relevant.

CHALLENGES IN PATIENTS WITH ANAPHYLAXIS

CONTROLS. The same controls as described for urticaria and asthmatic patients are applicable for anaphylaxis patients.

MEDICATIONS. It would be difficult to withdraw medications from patients who have recurring anaphylaxis. However, if the medications appear to be completely effective in preventing anaphylaxis, this may in fact be necessary. Whether or not hospitalization would be required needs to be considered on an individual basis. This would not be the problem for patients who have episodic anaphylaxis and are not on a regular medication program. For them the effects of H_1 antihistamines and blocking reactions would be expected to be more profound and therefore medications such as astemizole, terfenadine, and loratadine should be withheld until a positive histamine skin test and a positive codeine skin test are elicited.

CRITERIA FOR POSITIVE REACTION. As in the other categories of patients described above, a negative, straight, single-blind placebo challenge for the same period of time that one is planning for the active substance challenge should be performed. In addition, whatever symptoms are produced during the challenge should reproduce the signs and symptoms described by the patients in their history. Finally, symptoms should be objective, such as changes in vital signs. Both blood pressure and pulse need to be measured to differentiate a vasovagal (decreased pulse and blood pressure) from a truly anaphylactic (increased pulse and blood pressure) type of reaction. An urticarial response can be scored as described in the section above. Asthmatic responses can be recorded as described in the asthma section.

CHALLENGES IN PATIENTS WITH OTHER SYMPTOMS

Any variety of symptoms, even subjective signs such as headache or fatigue, can be amenable to challenge testing. The general criteria described for urticaria, asthma, and anaphylaxis challenges might be applicable here. The criteria for judging the positive reaction are particularly crucial. A baseline evaluation (time to be individualized) is important when dealing with subjective complaints. Establishing a negative straight placebo challenge is at least equally important. One needs to reproduce the patient's historical signs and symptoms utilizing a dosage equivalent to that of the natural exposure and in a time frame that mimics the patient's history. When possible, any objective signs and symptoms should also be noted.

In general, one can perform a challenge with virtually any substance in virtually any subject as long as the subject can provide a consistent scenario, including a single substance that, at a particular threshold dose, reproducibly provokes the same set of symptoms and signs in the same time frame. By utilizing the suggestions made above, one usually finds that there is no reaction to the offending substance or placebo in the confines of the allergy laboratory. This can be extremely helpful in dissuading a patient from his or her previously held misconceptions and misattributions. Other times patients react to the placebo, which again can be equally effective in further patient management. As described in other sections, because of the possibility of a placebo response in such patients, I always give, in single-blind manner, a placebo as the first and last challenge doses of any single- or double-blind challenge.

Some subjects may still be unwilling to consume the previously considered offending substance on their own. If that is the case, I will have the patient consume the substance in an open manner in the controlled allergy laboratory environment. This is usually negative but when "positive" produces vague subjective symptoms or objective signs of a cholinergic nature.

REFERENCES

Allen DH, Delohery J, Baker G. Monosodium L-glutamate-induced asthma. J Allergy Clin Immunol 80:530–537, 1987.

Bosso JV, Simon RA. Urticaria, angioedema, and anaphylaxis provoked by food additives. *In* Schocket AL (ed). Clinical Management of Urticaria and Anaphylaxis. New York, Marcel Dekker Inc, 1993.

Lumry WR, Mathison DA, Stevenson DD, et al. Aspirin

in chronic urticaria and/or angioedema: Studies of sensitivity and desensitization. J Allergy Clin Immunol 69 (Suppl):135, 1982.
Metcalfe DD, Sampson KA. Experimental methodology for clinical studies on adverse reactions to foods and food additives. J Allergy Clin Immunol 86:421, 1990.
Nizankowska E, Szczeklik A. Glucocorticoids attenuate aspirin-precipitated adverse reactions in aspirin-intolerant patients with asthma. Ann Allergy 63:159, 1989. (Abstract)
Simon RA. Specific challenge procedures. Workshop on experimental methodology studies of adverse reactions to foods and food additives. J Allergy Clin Immunol 86:428, 1990.
Simon RA, Stevenson DD. Adverse reactions to food and drug additives. *In* Middleton E Jr, Reed CE, Ellis EF, Adkinson NF Jr, Yunginer JW, Busse WW (eds). Allergy Principles and Practice. St. Louis, Mosby-Year Book, 1993, pp 1687–1704.
Stevenson DD, Simon RA. Sensitivity to aspirin and nonsteroidal anti-inflammatory drugs. *In* Middleton E Jr, Reed CE, Ellis EF, Adkinson NF Jr, Yunginer JW, Busse W (eds). Allergy Principles and Practice. St. Louis, Mosby-Year Book, 1993, pp 1747–1766.

Chapter 15

Principles of Avoidance

Gary P. Rakes, M.D., and Thomas A. Platts-Mills, M.D., Ph.D

The concept that one should avoid that which makes an illness worse is intuitive—prevention is better than trying to cure. Allergic disease is dependent on allergen sensitization, continued allergen exposure, and environmental trigger factors. Each mechanism is a potential target for avoidance (Fig. 15–1), and the evaluation of any patient with asthma or other allergic disease should be designed to evaluate allergen sensitization (skin tests), present allergen exposure (history, inspection and/or measurement), and environmental precipitants. Once identified, avoidance of these factors can prevent or improve the symptoms of atopic illnesses.

The term avoidance, as used here and elsewhere, refers to any means of decreasing exposure to a harmful situation. This can be accomplished using two very different strategies. 1. Remove the patient from exposure. The patient goes out of his or her way to avoid symptoms with the help of time (i.e., going out only during times of low pollen counts), of place (staying inside, moving to a different area), or of barriers (face masks). 2. Remove the offending agent. A patient can be instructed how to banish, evict, or contain allergens, allergen sources, and environmental precipitants. As a call to arms, the latter approach does not concede life style and is favored by most patients.

Avoidance techniques have lagged, by necessity, behind the evolving skills of identifying and measuring allergens and environmental precipitants. Recommending an avoidance protocol requires an understanding that it will be effective, that is, exposure is reduced and symptoms can improve as a result. It follows that unless there are reproducible ways of measuring environmental exposure and patient response, these conditions of effectiveness cannot be met or studied. For many years, exposure to allergens and environmental precipitants was understood only in gross, semiquantitative terms. Two cats comprise more exposure than one cat, which comprises more exposure than no cats. Visible mold growth indoors was considered significant exposure to fungi. Dust was anathema to asthmatics. For most seasonal allergens, pollen counts and identification under the microscope generally correlated well with seasonal allergic symptoms. In the last 25 years,

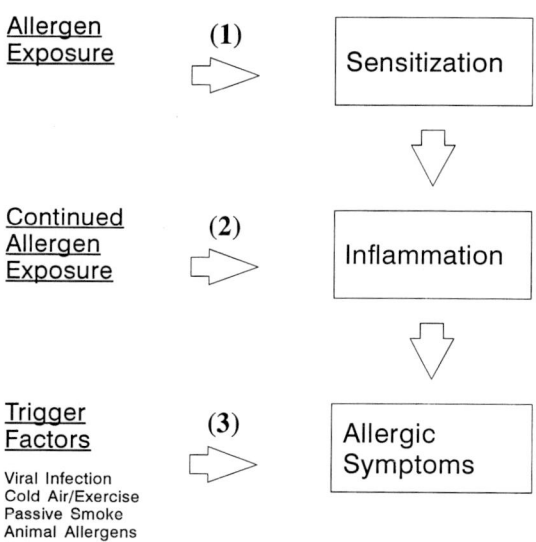

FIGURE 15–1. Targets of avoidance. (1) Is it possible to prevent allergen sensitization? If so, which infants need avoidance intervention? (2) Reduction of ongoing allergen exposure is the main focus of most avoidance research and protocols. (3) Some of the triggering factors that influence expression of allergic symptoms can be avoided.

however, allergen and environmental research has made great progress. The development of monoclonal antibodies has allowed purification and measurement of many of the molecules that provoke IgE-related illnesses. Technical sophistication has allowed better analysis of environmental factors and how they relate to allergic illnesses. As a result, air and dust can be sampled and allergen or chemical concentration can be consistently quantitated—before and after avoidance interventions. In particular, allergens not appreciated on a macroscopic level, such as those produced by mites or cockroaches, can now be identified and studied.

ALLERGEN AVOIDANCE

In general, patients and their physicians concentrate on the home as a battleground for avoidance. This is not just a decision of convenience and control; it has become clear that indoor allergens are very important causes of sensitization, bronchial hyperreactivity, and symptoms. This was first suggested in the early twentieth century after patients with asthma (Storm van Leeuwen et al, 1927) and atopic dermatitis (Rost, 1932) found relief in a dust-free environment, only to have their condition worsen when they returned home. House dust was proposed as a domestic culprit because skin testing with dust extracts revealed wheal and flare responses in many patients with rhinitis, asthma (Kern, 1921), and atopic dermatitis (Tuft, 1947). As a result, it became normal practice among allergists to recommend avoidance of dust, but specific refinements beyond this general admonishment awaited a better understanding of its composition. Dust from each home is a heterogeneous mixture that can combine ubiquitous outdoor allergens, such as pollens and molds, with residues derived from humans, pets, pests, and microscopic animals (Table 15–1). The components of the mixture vary according to the inhabitants and the location. The conclusion of studies in many different environments is that almost any foreign protein that accumulates in house dust can become an allergen. The development of methods to identify and quantify most of these proteins has clarified the relationship between allergen exposure and atopic disease. The same techniques have been used to analyze the efficacy of avoidance techniques and have resulted in specific recommendations for each of the major allergens.

TABLE 15–1. INDOOR ALLERGEN SOURCES

Acarids	*Pets*	*Outdoor pollens, including:*
Dust mites	Cats	Trees
Spiders	Dogs	Grasses
Pests	Rabbits	Ragweeds
Cockroaches	Pet mice and rats	*Fungi, including:*
Other insects	Gerbils	Aspergillus
Wild rats and mice	Hamsters	Penicillium
	Guinea pigs	Cladosporium
	Ferrets	Outdoor species

The importance of outdoor allergens such as molds and pollens has been historically easier to conceive: allergic symptoms worsened during times of increased exposure measured by environmental sampling of pollen counts and mold spores. Unfortunately, avoidance of outdoor allergen exposure generally means retreat behind face masks and behind doors. Inside the home, outdoor allergens in house dust can become a significant cause of indoor exposure.

Dust Mites: A Model for Allergen Avoidance

The best studied indoor allergens are those generated by dust mites, which are widely considered the most important source of house dust allergen in temperate and subtropical climates. In some areas, up to 80 percent of allergic asthmatics are sensitive to dust mite allergens (Sporik et al, 1990; Sears et al, 1989; Platts-Mills and Chapman, 1987). Patients and physicians have not always readily understood that such sensitization is clinically important. Patient histories often do not reflect an immediate association between flares of symptoms (wheezing, rhinorrhea, itching) and dust exposure. It is also difficult to convince patients of the importance of microscopic and "invisible" dust mites without the visual evidence that cats, cockroaches, or mold growth offer. However, once methods were developed to count dust mites or quantitate dust mite allergen in house dust, it became clear that mites were often present in large numbers and that their avoidance resulted in symptomatic improvement of the sensitized atopic patient. Thus this process has served as a model for investigating other indoor allergens.

Studies beginning in the early 1970s demonstrated that patients with asthmatic symptoms improved when removed from their homes to hospitals, sanatoriums, or locales with low levels of mites or mite allergens (Platts-Mills et al, 1982; Platts-Mills et al, 1983; Charpin et al, 1991). Controlled studies in houses employing methods that can effect a >90 percent reduction in mite allergen levels resulted in significant reduction of asthma symptoms and bronchial hyperreactivity (Walshaw and Evans, 1986; Murray and Ferguson, 1983; Ehnert et al, 1991). An association between sensitivity and exposure to dust mite allergen and atopic dermatitis has also been demonstrated; however, the causal role of dust mite exposure and the role of specific IgE antibodies in the pathology is not clear. None the less, mite avoidance studies in atopic dermatitis have demonstrated symptomatic improvement (Platts-Mills et al, 1985). There is also growing evidence that sensitization and development of atopic illnesses (asthma, rhinitis, atopic dermatitis) can be delayed, attenuated, or halted by preventing high-level exposure in childhood (Arshad et al, 1992; Sporik et al, 1990).

Avoidance measures for dust mites depend on a knowledge of the mite's biology and of the nature of its allergens. Dust mites are microscopic, feed on skin scales, and thrive only with adequate warmth and humidity. Therefore, mite populations are highest in human bedding, but in a house with a humidity of >65 percent and a temperature of >65°F, any dust repository such as carpeting or upholstered furniture is an attractive niche for mites. Many dust mite proteins have been identified, most as elutable constituents of mite fecal pellets. The pellets are large compared to particles carrying other indoor allergens (cats, molds), and are approximately the size of pollen grains (10 to 35 microns). In keeping with their size, mite fecal pellets only stay airborne for a few minutes; exposure depends on proximity and disturbance. Because the fecal pellets fall rapidly, it is difficult to standardize airborne measurements. Therefore, exposure is best studied by measuring mite allergen or dust mites in dust vacuumed from home surfaces. The allergens persist for many months after eradication of live mites (Platts-Mills et al, 1982).

Given the relevance of temperature and humidity to mite growth, it is no surprise that different localities and climates have varying levels of infestation (Table 15–2). Studies on the relationship between exposure (mites or micrograms of allergen per gram of house dust) and sensitization have demonstrated a consistent relationship. Threshold levels of exposure have been proposed (Platts-Mills and de Weck, 1989; Pope et al, 1993). The first level proposed was 2 µg of $Der\ p$ I allergen per gram of dust as a risk factor for sensitization. This level has now been supported by a series of studies. The implication is that fewer than 10 percent of genetically atopic children raised in houses with less than this level will become sensitized. Indeed, recent studies in the "mite-free" city of Los Alamos, New Mexico (altitude 7200 feet) show that mite sensitization is unusual and is not a significant risk factor for asthma (Sporik et al, 1994). By contrast, sensitization to mite allergens is common and is strongly associated with asthma in areas with high levels of mite allergen. Indeed, some studies suggest that

TABLE 15–2. PREVALENCE OF HOUSEHOLD DUST MITE, CAT AND COCKROACH ALLERGEN GREATER THAN PROPOSED THRESHOLD VALUES FOR SENSITIZATION IN THREE DIFFERENT AREAS IN THE UNITED STATES

		Los Alamos* New Mexico n ≅ 100	Albemarle Co.* Virginia n ≅ 70	Atlanta Georgia n ≅ 60
Dust Mite				
Group 1	>2 µg/g	5%	90%	79%
	>10 µg/g†	0%	80%	30%
Cat				
$Fel\ d$ I	>8 µg/g	50%	50%	4%
Cockroach				
$Bla\ g$ II	>2 units/gm	2%	4%	85%

*Provisional values
†Proposed threshold for symptoms

exposure to high levels of mite allergen in the first 2 years can lead to early onset and increased severity of asthma (Sporik et al, 1990). The level of exposure necessary to exacerbate asthma is not well defined and probably varies greatly among patients. However, 10 μg/gm of dust is a level that has been associated with an increased risk of acute asthma attacks. There is a common misconception that patients with allergic diseases are exposed to much higher levels of mite allergens. In most studies this is not true; the levels of dust mite allergen in houses of the majority of patients are in a range similar to those in their neighbors' houses.

Dust Mite Avoidance Techniques

Complete eradication of dust mites in indiginous areas is not attainable, but a 90 percent reduction can be achieved. The following techniques (Table 15–3) are meant to be combined in a protocol of dust mite avoidance.

THE BEDROOM. Most avoidance strategies for dust mites focus on the bedroom. Adults and children spend approximately 8 hours a day in bed with nose and mouth close to a source of dust mite allergens. Mattress and pillow covers impervious to mites and skin scales (using vinyl or special vapor permeable fabrics) have clearly been shown to be effective in reducing allergen levels and asthma symptoms in mite-sensitive patients (Ehnert et al, 1991; Owen et al, 1990). Hot water (>130°F) kills mites, and the bedding should be washed every 1 to 2 weeks (McDonald and Tovey, 1992). Cool water does not kill mites and detergents appear to protect mites, possibly because of their salt content. Washable polyester pillows may be used if covers are not tolerated. Nonwashable items such as comforters can be fitted with impervious covers. Water beds are generally a poor mite habitat, but some contain integrated padding and should be covered. Surface vacuuming of uncovered mattresses reduces dust but not live mite counts, and has to be repeated at least every week.

CARPETING AND UPHOLSTERY. Carpeting, as a morass of debris and humidity, offers an ideal habitat for dust mite growth and accumulation of other allergens. Upholstered furniture is also a dust mite refuge; sofas sometimes contain the highest concentration of live mites in the house. Vacuum cleaning regularly is helpful in removing surface dust but does not impact significantly on the embedded mite and allergen concentrations. Indeed, airborne allergen levels usually increase during vacuuming owing to agitation of surface dust and to leakage of the usual single layer bags. Double-thickness "allergy" vacuum cleaner bags should be recommended, and sensitive patients should avoid operating the vacuum cleaner or wear masks while doing so. Steam or hot shampooing of carpeting and upholstery may reduce mite allergen levels for as long as a month but does not reduce mite numbers deep in the carpeting. Cool shampooing is not of benefit and may actually increase mite populations by providing moisture. The most effective method is to eradicate

TABLE 15–3. DUST MITE AVOIDANCE INSTRUCTIONS

Bedding:
    Encase mattresses, box springs, pillows with zippered covers made of plastic or impermeable fabric.
    Wash bedding (sheets, pillow cases, mattress pads, blankets) in hot (130° F) water weekly. Nonwashable items such as comforters should be used only if covered.
Carpets and Upholstery
    Remove carpets and upholstered furniture, especially those in bedrooms and basements.
    If left in place, then:
        1. Carpets and upholstered furniture should be vacuumed weekly using a machine with double or leak-proof filter bag. Patients should avoid vacuuming, or wear a mask while doing so.
        2. Regular treatment with acaracides or tannic acid may offer additional benefit.
Dust Collectors
    Items such as knickknacks, books, and stuffed animals should be either removed from the bedroom or kept in closed cabinets or drawers.
    Fabric curtains should be replaced with wipable shades or venetian blinds.
    Heating and air conditioning filters should be changed or cleaned regularly.
Humidity and Temperature
    Control humidity (<50%) and temperature with air conditioning in hot and humid climates. Dehumidifiers may be helpful in basement areas.
    Increased indoor ventilation in cold, dry climates.

the habitat by removing carpeting in favor of hard floors and to replace cloth furniture with vinyl or leather sofa and chairs.

Acaricides are topical chemicals that kill mites. Their use is an attractive concept if carpets and upholstery are to be left in place. Those studied include benzyl benzoate, pirimiphos methyl, pyrethroids, and natamycin (an antifungal). Most have been shown to be effective *in vitro* with mite cultures and as agricultural pesticides. Less clear is the optimal preparation and means of application for reducing allergen exposure in the home. Again, mites dwell deep within bedding, carpeting, and upholstery; any topical preparation must work deeply to be of use. Pirimiphos methyl, a chemical used to kill mites in stored grain, has been shown to reduce mite levels in carpeting for as long as 6 weeks, but it is not available in the United States for domestic use. Benzyl benzoate (Acarosan) is a scabicide used on humans and is available in the form of a powder in the United States. The moist powder has been shown to reduce mite allergen levels for over 2 months when applied over a 12- to 18-hour period with repeated brushing (Hayden et al, 1992). The powder may enhance removal of dust particles from the carpet during vacuuming.

Another carpet and upholstery treatment available in the United States is 3 percent tannic acid solution. This acid denatures mite allergen and has been shown to reduce mite allergen levels, even when inhibition of the assay by the tannic acid is prevented by using bovine serum albumin in the extracting fluid (Woodfolk et al, 1994). The live dust mites are uneffected, necessitating frequent applications. No chemical treatment should be recommended as superior to carpet removal or as the sole avoidance measure adopted.

DUST COLLECTORS. For any indoor allergen sensitivity, steps should be taken to facilitate cleaning in the bedroom and throughout the house. Shelves, stuffed animals, fabric curtains, and bric-a-brac all collect dust and make cleaning difficult. Washable (certain stuffed animals) and wipable (vinyl lamp and window shades) items should be encouraged. Clothing that may be washed infrequently, such as woolens and winter coats, can sustain mites and should be stored in drawers or other closed compartments.

TEMPERATURE AND HUMIDITY. Dust mites are rare or absent in climates with low humidity and temperatures, and their growth and numbers can be suppressed if indoor humidity and temperature are controlled (Fig. 15–2). Mites are exquisitely sensitive to drying because they have to absorb water from the air. If possible, absolute humidity should be kept below 45 percent. In dry climates and seasons, this can be done by improving ventilation and air exchange with the outside. In more humid areas and times, air conditioning can lower indoor moisture. Attention to decreasing sources of humidity (e.g., basement leaks, condensation) is important. A particular problem is basement or ground floor carpeting that becomes or stays damp, making an ideal environment for mites and fungi. Humidifiers and vaporizers should be used with caution. The ideal temperature for dust mite growth in culture is between 70°F and 80°F, causing the rate of egg production to increase and the time from egg to adulthood to shorten. Therefore, cooler indoor temperatures should reduce mite numbers. This leads to major differences within the United States, and there is a generally negative correlation with average temperature.

Dust Mite Avoidance from Birth

Of present and future interest is the question whether avoidance of dust mites from birth in "susceptible" children can affect the expression of atopic diseases. If the answer is "yes," then atopic illnesses should be rarer in populations that live in areas with low mite numbers. Three such native-born populations (In Alaska; Papua, New Guinea; and Briancon, France) show a lower prevalence of asthma (Platts-Mills and de Weck, 1989). Indeed, the Highland Natives of New Guinea experienced an increase in asthma cases after contact with western civilization, a change attributed to the introduction of blankets that subsequently became mite infested. However, factors other than mite exposure might affect asthma expression; besides differences in climate, the small sample populations are isolated by both geography and genetics. Prospective studies to judge whether dust mite allergen avoidance decreases the expression of allergic diseases might answer these questions. Unfortunately, these are difficult to perform and interpret. Dust mite avoidance is hard to control for and may also reduce other allergens, introducing many potential variables. It is also difficult to define with enough sensitivity the population at risk for allergic

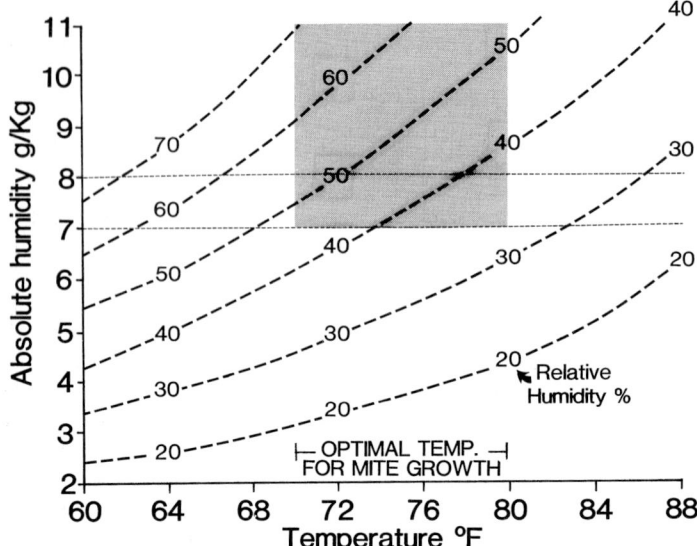

FIGURE 15–2. Optimal humidity and temperature for mite growth.

disease, even using markers such as family history and cord blood IgE. Recognizing this, Arshad et al (1992) demonstrated a reduction of allergic disorders in "at risk" infants and toddlers when dust mite and common food allergens were avoided from birth. Despite the incomplete evidence, many physicians prescribe dust mite and other allergen avoidance for infants of atopic patients.

Pets and Laboratory Animals

CATS. Domestic cats are common as pets or household members and are found in approximately 50 percent of homes in the United States. Unfortunately, cat allergy is also commonplace, and is found in as many as 3 percent of Americans. Unlike those with mite allergy, most cat-sensitive patients who live in a home without a cat are acutely aware of the symptomatic relationship; they wheeze or have rhinitis symptoms immediately (i.e., within 15 minutes) on any exposure to cats. On the other hand, this immediate relationship is generally not apparent to allergic patients living in a house with a cat. The proper avoidance recommendation seems obvious: remove the cat or cats from the home. This simple solution, however, often becomes complicated because of the nature of the allergen and because of the nature of some pet owners.

The major cat allergen is *Fel d* I, a well-characterized 37 kD protein produced by both sebaceous and salivary glands (Chapman et al, 1988; DeBlay et al, 1991). It becomes airborne on small particles of varying sizes and, unlike dust mite allergen, can stay afloat for hours indoors. The particles saturate carpeting, seem to adhere well to any surface, and can be measured on walls and clothing. It is present in concentrations much higher than dust mite, reaching values as high as 1 mg/gm of dust. Levels of allergen similar to that found in some houses with resident cats have been measured in houses without cats (Gelber et al, 1993), presumably carried in on clothing. Because of this pervasiveness, removal of a cat is likely to take over 3 months to effect low levels (<8 μg/gm) (Fig. 15–3). This decline in concentration can be enhanced by aggressive cleaning techniques, such as carpet removal and washing of all surfaces (e.g., walls, furniture). Minimum thresholds of exposure have not been settled, but levels of more than 8 μg/gm of house dust are associated with sensitization and symptoms.

Pet owners are often loath to surrender their cats (or any pet), even when suffering severe symptoms attributable to the animals. Despite enthusiastic and repeated advice, a patient may either deny that there is a problem or refuse to cooperate. Even when the cat is relegated to the outdoors, the patient often invites excessive contact and resulting exposure. As an alternative to abandoning these patients, cat allergen abatement techniques have been studied and can be offered (Table 15–4). The regimen of hard floors,

PRINCIPLES OF AVOIDANCE—201

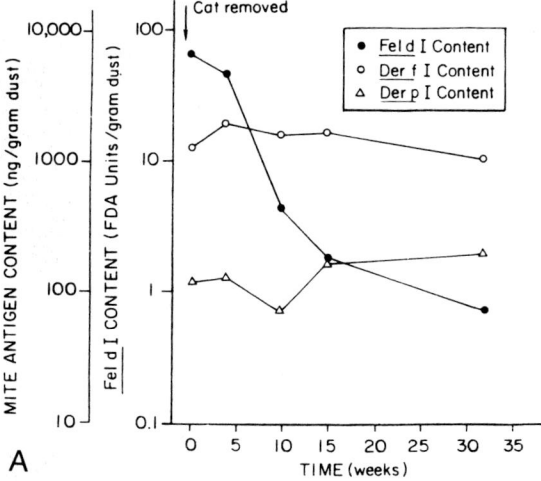

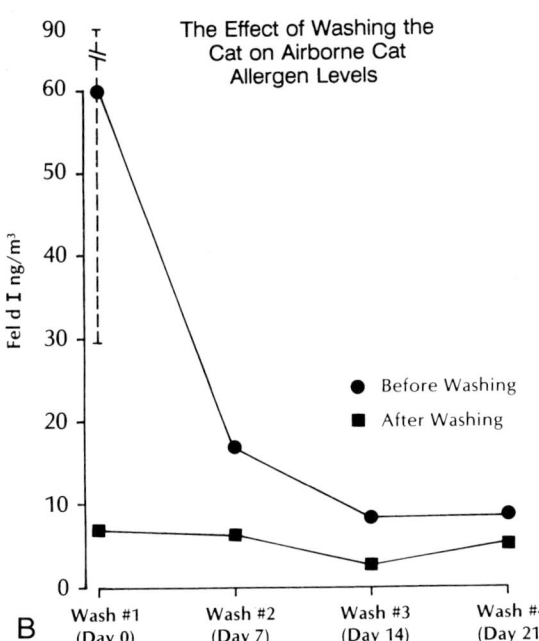

FIGURE 15–3. Effect of cat removal (*A*) and washing (*B*) on reduction of allergen levels. (*A* is from Wood et al. The effect of cat removal on allergen content in household dust samples. J Allergy Clin Immunol 83:730, 1989; *B* is from De Blay et al. Airborne cat allergen *(Fel d I).* Am Rev Respir Dis 143:1334, 1991.)

high-energy particulate air (HEPA) filters, aggressive cleaning (no carpets), and regular cat washing was found to be effective in reducing airborne cat allergen levels by ≥90 percent in a model apartment. Cat washing may be difficult, but the animals become accustomed to this treatment if exposed to water and bathing as a kitten. HEPA filters are effective devices for removing small airborne particles but work best to lower cat allergen levels only in combination with bare floors and aggressive cleaning. Whether this regimen can be of practical benefit for the average cat-allergic patient is yet to be determined. Indeed, recent evidence has suggested that weekly distilled water washes alone are not effective in reducing airborne cat allergen levels (Klucka et al, 1994). However, some patients maintain that *in situ* avoidance techniques have allowed them to become symptom-free co-inhabitants with cats.

Dogs. Unlike cats, domesticated dogs are not as commonly recognized for provoking acute allergic responses. One theory is that most dogs are outdoors and/or regularly washed. However, some patients are clearly allergic and improve with the animal's removal. There have been many different allergens identified from dander, hair, saliva, and serum extracts. Some patients have breed-specific atopy upon skin testing, supporting the long-held concept that some patients are allergic to only certain breeds of dog. Research has been hampered by the wide array of identified allergens, but in the last 3 years, a major allergen present in saliva and dander, *Can f* I, has been purified (Schou et al, 1991; De Groot et al, 1991). Studies are currently under way to characterize its role indoors. In some locales (Los Alamos, New Mexico) with low dust mite and cockroach populations, dog is clearly the predominant indoor sensitization (Sporik et al, 1994). The avoidance recommendation should be removal. Whether relegation to the outdoors is adequate for symptomatic relief is unknown. Allergen re-

TABLE 15–4. PROCEDURES FOR REDUCING AIRBORNE CAT ALLERGEN LEVELS

Remove cat from the home or relegate to the outdoors. It will take up to 4 months for allergen levels to subside.

If cannot or will not remove cat, then:
Banish cat from bedroom
Wash cat weekly
Remove carpeting in favor of polished floors
Minimize upholstered furniture
Vacuum with high-efficiency filter
HEPA air filters (effective only if no carpeting)
Wash or wet-wipe walls regularly

duction techniques for dogs remaining inside the home have not been published.

OTHER ANIMALS. Many different pets have been identified as allergy-provoking. Other than cats and dogs, the most common include rabbits, rodents, guinea pigs, and ferrets. Allergens derived from pet birds or feather-filled items can sometimes be of importance, but down pillows and comforters are usually more important as allergen sources because they offer excellent refuge for dust mites. Cage bird proteins can induce hypersensitivity pneumonitis. Testing, namely skin tests for pet allergens and serologic tests for suspected hypersensitivity, can prompt the animal's removal from the home. Because research is driven by the number of cases, allergens derived from pets other than dogs and cats have not been studied. An exception is that urinary proteins have been identified as the major allergens generated by mice and rats; these are important as allergens for many laboratory workers and residents of rodent-infested housing. Significant reduction of airborne rat urinary allergen has been accomplished in laboratory vivariums with the combination of rapid room air exchanges and high-efficiency filters. By law, laboratory animals are kept in rooms with over 10 air changes per hour. Specific abatement procedures for pets such as rodents and rabbits are not defined and perhaps not necessary, because patients seem more willing to give up pets other than dogs or cats. The patient must be warned that the indoor allergen may persist at symptomatic levels for months after removal of the animal, especially without aggressive cleaning.

Indoor Pests

COCKROACHES. Cockroaches are an important source of indoor allergen, especially in multi-unit housing and in urban areas (Call et al, 1992) (see Table 15–1). Infestation is common, though many patients are reluctant to tell physicians. Therefore, many clinicians include cockroaches as a part of a skin test battery for indoor inhalants. Three species account for most infestations in the United States: German (*Blatella germanica*), American (*Periplaneta americana*), and Oriental (*Blatella orientalis*). Skin testing can be carried out with a mixture of the three species. Specific allergens have been purified for the first two and are thought to be associated with their feces or saliva (Pollart et al, 1991). Highest concentrations of their allergens are found in food areas. Extermination is the obvious recommendation, but many patients find it difficult to completely eradicate the insects. Professional extermination is often hampered by the rapid repopulation from other roach colonies elsewhere in multi-unit housing. The apparent solution is relocation to a cockroach-free single dwelling, but the insects will move with furniture and other household items. Unfortunately, professional extermination and moving are both expensive options, especially for the segment of the population most affected. At present, there are no studies that define the quantitative reduction in exposure that needs to be achieved for symptomatic improvment.

OTHER PESTS. Wild rats and mice are a significant health problem for people living in infested dwellings. As mentioned previously, the major allergens are urinary proteins that become part of the house dust. As with cockroaches, many patients are reluctant to admit their presence, and so clinical suspicion and skin testing are appropriate. Eradication in multi-unit housing is a problem. Spiders and insects (e.g., crickets, flies, and moths) are potential allergen producers, but any significance is unclear. If there is any question of a relationship to illness and symptoms, eradication is the obvious recommendation.

Pollens

Weed, tree, and grass pollens are familiar as seasonal causes of allergic symptoms. Wind-borne pollen grains are highly effective at carrying allergens. They stay aloft even in light winds, despite being relatively heavy. Pollen counts, using a variety of mechanical samplers, reflect availability for inhalation and correlate well with symptoms. Any avoidance recommendation concedes stalemate: if the patient goes outdoors during the relevant season of pollination, exposure is *fait accompli* unless measures such as masks and respirators are adopted. Since indoor seclusion and face gear are usually unacceptable to patients who have pharmacologic options, advice is gauged to limit exposure with minimal disruption to life style. Patients should receive precise information about the sensitizing plant and relevant pollination dates. This allows institution of a prophylactic medication regimen, and it gives each patient a chance to plan events and trips by location and time of year (i.e., camping trips, outdoor sports, outdoor weddings). If outside activities at peak times of pollination are unavoidable, filter masks may be an option, especially for those who work outdoors.

If the dwelling is air conditioned with adequate filters, the indoors can be an acceptable refuge from pollens. Windows should remain closed, and under no circumstance should window fans be allowed to blow outdoor air inward. If these conditions are met, indoor air filters (HEPA filters are highly effective in removing particles the size of pollen grains) offer little in addition. Routine dust control measures indoors would theoretically help to remove settled pollens.

Molds

Many patients are sensitized to molds, but the importance of this relationship is not well characterized. Any investigation in the home has been limited by the lack of simple and reproducible allergen assays and inability to quantify exposure to the relevant mold proteins. Some allergens are not present in spores (e.g., *Asp f* I), and some spores (e.g., *Penicillium* and *Aspergillus*) cannot be distinguished. Culture results are highly dependent on conditions. As a result, avoidance methods are difficult to evaluate, and efforts to control molds in the home depend on general measures known to inhibit their growth.

Fungi need adequate moisture and organic nutrients. Basements and ground floors are often high humidity areas suitable for mold growth, and if relocation is not feasible, other measures need to be taken to compromise their growth. Carpeting and other ceiling or wall coverings offer a reservoir for any moisture and should be removed. Dehumidifiers can reduce ambient humidity but have little effect on surface moisture from underground walls and floors. Surface treatments with waterproofing coating can reduce ground-water weeping. Growth on wet surfaces can be controlled by regular treatments with fungicidal chemicals such as a bleach solution. Air conditioning systems can support fungal growth, especially large building ductwork. Organic material such as papers, vegetable matter, firewood, and old books that harbor mold should be stored in living areas.

Unlike pollens, outdoor molds are present nearly year-round in temperate climates. They go through seasonal cycles in abundance, dependent on humidity, temperature, and availability of decaying organic matter. For example, in the Mid-Atlantic region of the United States, *Alternaria* is at its highest levels in late fall. In the same region, airborne fungal spores are at their nadir during the cold and dry months of winter. As with indoor molds, it is hard to quantify exposure, because spore counts may not correlate well with allergen exposure, but the patient can attempt avoidance during times of optimal growth. It is possible to identify and avoid areas of high exposure such as the vicinity of decaying leaves, mown grass, and barns. Other recommendations are similar to those for outdoor pollens, that is, stay indoors with air conditioning and no open windows during the summer. Because of the lack of true seasonality, compliance is difficult with these year-round restrictions.

THE ENVIRONMENT

Allergic illnesses emerge from the interaction of atopic predisposition (read genetics), allergen exposure, and "other factors." As one part of this equation, the discrete pathway connecting allergens and immediate reactions has been well studied since the discovery of IgE by Ishizaka in 1967; although complicated, immediate hypersensitivity offers the reassurance of the familiar class-specific antibody reaction. Less understood are the mechanisms at work behind the many environmental "triggers." The limited ability to measure and relate exposure to many of the proposed precipitants has sometimes allowed speculation instead of science to determine avoidance advice.

HOME AND OFFICE CONSTRUCTION. The same years that produced the growth in knowledge about allergens also accommodated a change in home construction techniques and life style in most industrialized countries. Energy efficiency became a primary goal, and as a result many houses suffer poor ventilation and air exchange. Indoor allergens, particulates, and gases concentrate within the house instead of exchanging with outside air. Most poorly ventilated homes also allow the accumulation of indoor humidity.

At the same time, homes are maintained at warm temperatures through all seasons. Both factors favor dust mite and mold growth. Another, older, trend in home decorating and design equates affluence with wall-to-wall carpeting and sumptuous furniture, items that offer safe harbor for dust mites and a reservoir for allergens. The antithesis of this description—a cold, breezy house with polished floors and wooden furniture—should not be offered as the ideal, but simple design and maintenance decisions for homes can offer a much improved habitat for those with allergic diseases.

Many of the steps already discussed for dust mite avoidance help to control humidity and facilitate dust and allergen removal. In addition, special attention to heating and air conditioning systems and to sources of humidity is important (Pope et al, 1993). In-line high-efficiency air filters can remove the majority of bioaerosols, but any filter needs regular maintenance. Ductwork should remain dry and be kept free of accumulated dust and debris. Sources of moisture such as clothes driers should be vented outside. Humidifiers may cause excessive indoor humidity and can aerosolize fungal and bacterial growth. Another area of concern is that many types of new building materials and carpeting can release volatile organic gases such as formaldehyde; the health consequences are not completely understood but at least merit particular concern for ventilation.

INFECTIONS. Viral infection of the respiratory tract is associated with wheezing and has been identified in 10 to 50 percent of asthma attacks (Pattemore et al, 1992) This finding is even more common in wheezing children less than 2 years of age, when viral infection (predominately by respiratory syncytial virus) can be demonstrated in 70 percent of cases (Duff et al, 1993). In older children and adults, rhinovirus is the primary infection seen, but other seasonal agents include influenza A, coronavirus, and parainfluenza. Infection with *Mycoplasma pneumoniae* is sometimes associated with this older age group as well. The mechanism of this triggering is not well defined. Any airway infection can compromise pulmonary mechanical reserve, but lower respiratory tract agents such as influenza A and respiratory syncytial virus can cause small airway inflammation and obstruction. Other mechanisms are needed to explain why pathogens with little or no lower respiratory tract effect (i.e., rhinovirus) can provoke wheezing or allergic illnesses. Published theories include humoral and cell-mediated mechanisms, generation of bronchial hyperreactivity, and immune (IgE) potentiation (Bardin et al, 1992). By contrast, there is no association between bacterial infection of the respiratory tract and wheezing—except for the important exception of sinusitis.

An understanding of how, and when, most viruses are spread is important for those with asthma and other respiratory illnesses. It is reasonable to recommend hand washing and hygiene (no fingers to eyes and nose), simple methods that work for nosocomial illnesses. This becomes especially important for caretakers of infants and toddlers in day care centers. Seasonal anticipation of many viruses justifies a reluctance to withdraw medications in asthmatics who are doing well. It is the recommendation of several American and Canadian groups that the influenza A vaccine be given to anyone with chronic respiratory illnesses (Prevention and control of influenza, 1991), and many physicians include asthma within that definition. The Committee on Infectious Diseases of the American Academy of Pediatrics specifically recommends that all children with moderate and severe asthma older than 6 months be immunized yearly against influenza. There is concern that influenza immunizations may incite asthma exacerbations, causing some physicians to specifically avoid immunizing severe asthmatics (Correspondence, 1992).

TOBACCO SMOKE. Advice to stop tobacco smoking by and around patients is a normal part of health education. The health risks for the tobacco smoker are well defined, and exposure to secondhand smoke is an increasing source of concern. Several investigations have reported increased airway reactivity, diminished pulmonary function, and presentation with wheezing among young children exposed to environmental tobacco smoke (Murray and Morrison, 1989; Evans et al, 1987; Martinez et al, 1992). It is important that physicians be consistent in their recommendations to stop, "if not for yourself, then for your child (family member or housemate)." Patients who have a physician recommend smoking cessation are more likely to be successful. Family members who do not stop smoking should be advised to avoid smoking around the patients. This should include explicit instructions to avoid smoking anywhere inside the home because many wrongly consider smoking in another room to be adequate protection. Every room shares the same atmosphere, especially in constructions with poor ventilation. The same attention should be given to other shared spaces, such as automobiles and workplaces. Indoor air filters are not adequate as the only means of tobacco smoke avoidance. Small and inexpensive models only remove larger, odor-causing particles in the small air sample they process. HEPA filters can effectively rid room-sized environments from particulate byproducts of smoke but do not contain the wide variety of combustion gases.

OTHER COMBUSTION BYPRODUCTS. The burning of any organic fuel generates particulate and gaseous pollutants. Many, such as carbon monoxide and nitrogen dioxide, have well-defined health consequences at high concentrations, but these are unusual in the home. At "normal" indoor levels, nitrogen dioxide has been associated with respiratory symptoms in children, but other studies have been inconclusive (Gold, 1992). Of more practical concern is the combined effect of different fuel byproducts at "normal" indoor and outdoor levels, but any impact is difficult to describe because of the many different variables involved (e.g., type of combustion, temperature, ventilation, filters). Prospective studies are prohibitively complicated (i.e., changing heating systems in a large population). Wood stoves have been associated with a higher incidence of respiratory symptoms and asthma in some studies (Honicky et al, 1986) but not in others. Outdoors, air pollution indexes and smog alerts in metropolitan areas have been linked to an increase in respiratory symptoms.

Clearly, one can advise against wood stoves that are not airtight and open fireplaces that do not "draw" well. They generate unacceptable levels of indoor pollutants that can cause respiratory symptoms even in those without allergic illness. Because of the economic consequences, however, specific avoidance recommendations concerning other methods of heating and geographic (urban exposure) location are difficult to justify without consistent evidence of allergic and respiratory morbidity. On an individual basis, a change in locale or heating system may be justified, especially if symptoms seem to worsen on exposure to the indoor or outdoor environment of concern. As with tobacco smoke, indoor air filters at best only remove particulate pollutants, not gases.

CONCLUSIONS

Considerable good will and confidence go into avoidance advice for the patient with asthma or allergic disease. Never too late, the "at-risk" patient is identified by wheezing, or a runny nose, or by eczema. Standardized tests and historical clues can identify allergens and environmental precipitants; then allergen-specific avoidance advice detailed in this chapter can be given.

Unfortunately, this ideal often breaks down when faced with the many variables involved in the expression of each individual's illness. Effective avoidance protocols and instructions are for naught if the patient cannot or will not comply. Frequent problems include:

1. *Information overload.* Skin tests can generate a long menu of allergens to be avoided. For example, a patient can be confronted with advice about dust mites, cats, ragweed, three molds, and four tree pollens. Too often, the details most important to that patient are diluted and forgotten in a barrage of instructions.

2. *Money.* Recommendations, for example, that patients pull up their wall-to-wall carpeting, change heating systems, or change jobs are doomed to failure because of the expense.

3. *Life style.* Habits (smoking, carpeted floors, foods) and hobbies are difficult to give up.

4. *Relevance.* Avoidance advice should be strictly tailored to the identified allergens and precipitants only—a particular problem with prepared handouts that discuss all aeroallergens.

5. *Sentimental attachment.* Many patients will not conceive of giving up a pet or stuffed animal.

6. *Wolf crying.* When giving avoidance advice, it is a temptation to employ scare tactics and predict dire consequences if advice is not followed (i.e., "if you don't give up your cat, you'll end up in the intensive care unit"). When the forewarned outcome fails to occur, a patient may conclude that avoidance is unnecessary.

Problems such as these can be anticipated and addressed with careful planning and education. It is helpful to assign priorities to avoidance recommendations by deciding which factors are most important for each patient. Primary goals should be clearly discussed in person, then additional information can be given through handouts or other media. Some of the mystique of "allergies" should be addressed by explaining how allergens induce inflammation and allergic symptoms. Regular visits allow completion of short-term goals and reiteration of ongoing avoidance concerns. Finally, chastisement for lack of compliance with avoidance instructions is rarely helpful. Treatment plans should evolve with each visit and allow compromises (e.g., an *in situ* cat allergen reduction protocol for someone who will not give up a pet).

REFERENCES

Arshad SH, Matthews S, Gant C, Hide D. Effect of allergen avoidance on development of allergic disorders in infancy. Lancet 339:1493, 1992.

Bardin PG, Johnston SL, Pattemore PK. Viruses as precipitants of asthma symptoms, II. Physiology and mechanisms. Clin Exp Allergy 22:809, 1992.

Call RS, Smith TF, Morris E, Chapman MD, Platts-Mills TAE. Risk factors for asthma in inner city children. J Pediatr 121:862, 1992.

Chapman MD, Aalberse RC, Brown MJ, et al. Monoclonal antibodies to the major feline allergen *Fel d I*. II. Single step affinity purification of *Fel d I*. N-terminal sequence analysis, and development of a sensitive two-site immunoassay to assess *Fel d I* exposure. J Immunol 140:812, 1988.

Charpin D, Birnbaum J, Haddi E, et al. Altitude and allergy to house-dust mites: A paradigm of the influence of environmental exposure on allergen sensitization. Am Rev Respir Dis 143:983, 1991.

Correspondence. Influenza and asthma. Lancet 339:194, 367,741, 1992.

De Blay F, Chapman MD, Platts-Mills TAE. Airborne cat allergen (*Fel d I*). Am Rev Respir Dis 143:1334, 1991.

De Groot H, Goei K, VAn Swicter P, et al. Affinity purification of a major and minor allergen from dog extract: Serologic activity of affinity-purified *Can f I* and *Can f I*-depleted extract. J Allergy Clin Immunol 87:1056, 1991.

Duff Al, Pomeranz ES, Gelber LE, et al. Risk factors for acute wheezing in infants and children: Viruses, passive smoke, and IgE antibodies to inhalant allergens. Pediatrics 92:535, 1993.

Ehnert B, Lau S, Weber A, et al. Reduction of mite allergen exposure and bronchial hyperreactivity. J Allergy Clin Immunol 87:320, 1991.

Gelber LE, Seltzer LH, Bouzoukis JK, et al. Sensitization and exposure to indoor allergens as risk factors for asthma among patients presenting to hospital. Amer Rev Resp Dis 147:573, 1993.

Evans D, Levison MJ, Feldman CH, et al. The impact of passive smoking on emergency room visits of urban children with asthma. Am Rev Resp Dis 135:567, 1987.

Gold DR. Indoor air pollution. Clin Chest Med 13:215, 1992.

Hayden ML, Rose G, Kiduch KB, et al. Benzyl benzoate moist powder: investigation of acarical activity in cultures and reduction of dust mite allergens in carpets. J Allergy Clin Immunol 89:536, 1992.

Honicky RE, Osborne Js, Akpom CA. Symptoms of respiratory illness in young children and the use of wood-burning stoves for indoor heating. Pediatrics 75:587, 1986.

Kern RA. Dust sensitization in bronchial asthma. Med Clin North Am 5:751, 1921.

Klucka CV, Ownby DR, Green J, et al. Cat washings, Allerpet or acepromazine do not diminish Fel d I shedding. J Allergy Clin Immunol 93:180, 1994. (Abstract)

Martinez FD, Cline M, Burrows B. Increased incidence of asthma in children of smoking mothers. Pediatrics 89:21, 1992.

McDonald LG, Tovey E. The role of water temperature and laundry procedures in reducing house dust mite populations and allergen content of bedding. J Allergy Clin Immunol 90:599, 1992.

Murray A, Morrison B. Passive smoking by asthmatics: Its greater effect on boys than on girls and on older than younger children. Pediatrics 84:451, 1989.

Murray AB, Ferguson AC. Dust-free bedrooms in the treatment of asthmatic children with house dust or house dust mite allergy: A controlled trial. Pediatrics 71:418, 1983.

Owen S, Morgtanstern M, Hepworth J, et al. Control of house dust mite antigen in bedding. Lancet 335:396, 1990.

Pattemore PK, Johnston SL, Bardin PG. Viruses as precipitants of asthma symptoms, I: epidemiology. Clin Exp Allergy 22:325, 1992.

Platts-Mills TAE, Chapman MD. Dust mites: Immunology, allergic disease, and environmental control. J Allergy Clin Immunol 80:755, 1987. (Review)

Platts-Mills TAE, de Weck AL. Dust mite allergens and asthma: A world-wide problem. J Allergy Clin Immunol 83:416, 1989.

Platts-Mills TAE, Tovey ER, Mitchell EB, et al. Reduction of bronchial hyperreactivity during prolonged allergen avoidance. Lancet 2:675, 1982.

Platts-Mills TAE, Mitchell EB, Rowntree S, et al. The relevance of inhalant and food allergens to the etiology and management of patients with atopic dermatitis. N Engl Reg Allergy Proc 6:255, 1985.

Platts-Mills TAE, Tovey ER, Mitchell EB, et al. Long-term effects of living in a dust-free room on patients with allergic asthma: reversal of bronchial hyperreactivity. Monographs In Allergy 18:153, 1983. (Review)

Pollart S, Smith TF, Morris EC, et al. Environmental exposure to cockroach allergens: Analysis with monoclonal antibody-based enzyme immunoassays. J Allergy Clin Immunol 87:505, 1991.

Pope AM, Patterson R, Burge H (eds). Indoor Allergens: Assessing and Controlling Adverse Health Effects. Washington, D.C., National Academy Press, 1993.

Prevention and control of influenza. Mort Morb Weekly Report 40 No rr-6, 1991.

Rost GA. Uber Erfagrungen mit der allergenfreien Kammer nach Storm van Leeuwen: Insbesondere in der Spatperiode der exsudativen Diathese. Arch Derm Syphillis 155:297, 1932.

Sears MR, Hervison GP, Holdaway MD, et al. The relative risks of sensitivity to grass pollen, house dust mite, and cat dander in the development of childhood asthma. Clin Exp Allergy 19:419–424, 1989.

Schou C, Hansen G, Linter T, et al. Assay for the major dog allergen, *Can f I*: Investigation of house dust samples and commercial dog extracts. J Allergy Clin Immunol 88:847, 1991.

Sporik R, Holgate ST, Platts-Mills TAE, et al. Exposure to house dust mite allergen (*Der p* I) and the development of asthma in childhood: A prospective study. N Engl J Med 323:502, 1990.

Sporik R, Rose G, Honsinger R, et al. Sensitization to dog allergen (*Can f* I) as a risk factor for asthma in New Mexico: Relationship to allergen exposure in houses. J Allergy Clin Immunol 93:229, 1994. (Abstract)

Storm van Leeuwen W, Einthoven W, Kremer W. The allergen proof chamber in the treatment of bronchial asthma and other respiratory diseases. Lancet i:1287, 1927.

Tuft LA. Importance of inhalant allergen in atopic dermatitis. J Invest Derm 12:211, 1947.

Walshaw MJ, Evans CC. Allergen avoidance in house dust mite sensitive adult asthma. Q J Med 58:199, 1986.

Wood R, Chapman M, Atkinson N, et al. The effect of cat removal on allergen content in household dust samples. J Allergy Clin Immun 83:730, 1989.

Woodfolk JA, Hayden ML, Miller JD, et al. Chemical treatment of carpets to reduce allergens: A detailed study of the effects of tannic acid on indoor allergens. J Allergy Clin Immunol 94:19, 1994.

ACKNOWLEDGMENT: Supported by Grants No. IU01 A1-34607 and AI-20565.

Chapter 16
Pharmacology and Therapeutics

F. Estelle R. Simons, M.D.

The pharmacologic treatment of asthma, rhinitis, and other allergic disorders continues to evolve rapidly. As a result of recent advances in our understanding of the pathophysiology of allergic disease, there is now increased emphasis on use of medications with anti-inflammatory, anti-allergic, or immunomodulatory effects.

This chapter will address the benefits and risks of medications currently in use, with emphasis on newer anti-allergics, glucocorticoids, adrenergic agonists, methylxanthines, anticholinergics, and H_1-receptor antagonists. It will focus primarily on medications used for prevention and relief of chronic asthma or allergic rhinitis symptoms. It will emphasize medications given by inhalation, the rationale being that when medications are directed to the relevant site of action, rapid onset of effect and maximum benefit are obtained with minimum risk to other tissues.

ANTI-ALLERGICS: CROMOLYN, NEDOCROMIL

Structure and Activity

Cromolyn has a double bicyclic ring structure and nedocromil sodium has a tricyclic structure (Fig. 16–1).

Mechanism of Action

Cromolyn inhibits antigen-induced release of histamine and other mediators of inflammation from sensitized connective tissue–type mast cells, but not from basophils *in vitro*. Its actions are species- and tissue-specific. It is active on mast cells obtained from human bronchoalveolar lavage fluid and, to a lesser extent, on mast cells from fragments of human lung tissue or from enzymatically dispersed human lung *in vitro*. It also suppresses mediator release induced by nonimmune substances such as chemicals, drugs, and biologicals. It inhibits chemotaxis of eosinophils and neutrophils. It suppresses the appearance of activated monocytes and neutrophils in the

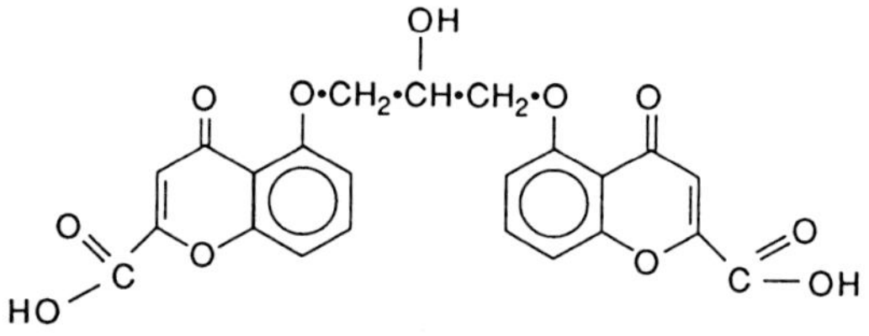

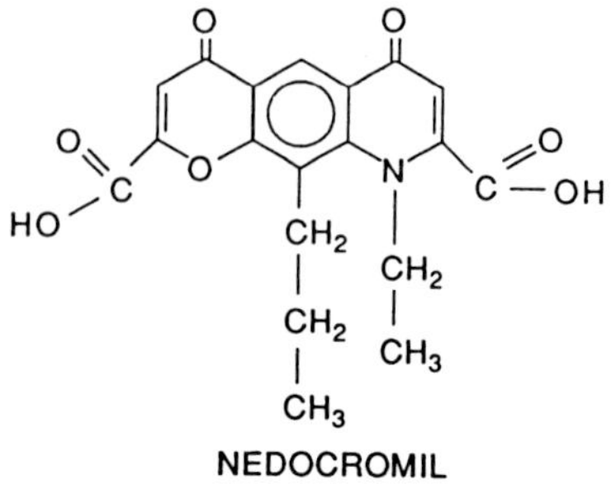

FIGURE 16–1. Chemical structure of cromolyn and nedocromil.

circulation that accompanies increases in airway resistance when asthmatics are challenged with antigen or exercise. It is not an antagonist of any chemical mediator. It may have neurophysiologic effects in the airways.

Cromolyn blocks both the early and late responses to allergen if given before challenge and prevents the development of associated airway hyperresponsiveness. If given after allergen challenge and after the early asthmatic response develops, it shifts the early part (3 to 5 hours) of the late allergic response curve to the right significantly, but does not affect the maximal late response or the associated increase in airway hyperresponsiveness (Cockcroft et al, 1993) (Fig. 16–2).

If given before challenge, it also blocks exercise- and cold, dry air-induced asthma and the response to nonimmune bronchoconstrictor stimuli such as histamine, methacholine, and adenosine, although it is not as effective as β_2-adrenergic agonists in this regard.

Nedocromil, a topically active pyranoquinolone dicarboxylic acid derivative (Fig. 16–1), has a broader spectrum of anti-allergic and anti-inflammatory effects than cromolyn *in vitro*. In addition to inhibiting antigen or anti–human IgE-induced mediator release from mucosal and connective tissue mast cells, including bronchoalveolar lavage mast cells, it inhibits eosinophil and neutrophil chemotaxis. It produces dose-dependent inhibition of human eosinophil activation and mediator release, and dose-dependent inhibition of human neutrophil-derived histamine-releasing factor. It inhibits cytokine production: interleukin-6 production by alveolar macrophages from patients with asthma, interleukin-1–induced production of interleukin-8 by cultured human bronchoepithelial cells, and synthesis and release of granulocyte-macrophage colony-stimulating factor from human bronchial epithelium. It downregulates alveolar macrophages from patients with asthma. It also inhibits IgE-mediated activation of platelets and inhibits the cytotoxic response to aspirin found in the platelets of patients with aspirin-induced asthma (Brogden and Sorkin, 1993).

In single-dose studies, nedocromil, 4 mg, protects against bronchospasm induced by neurokinin A, bradykinin, substance P, aden-

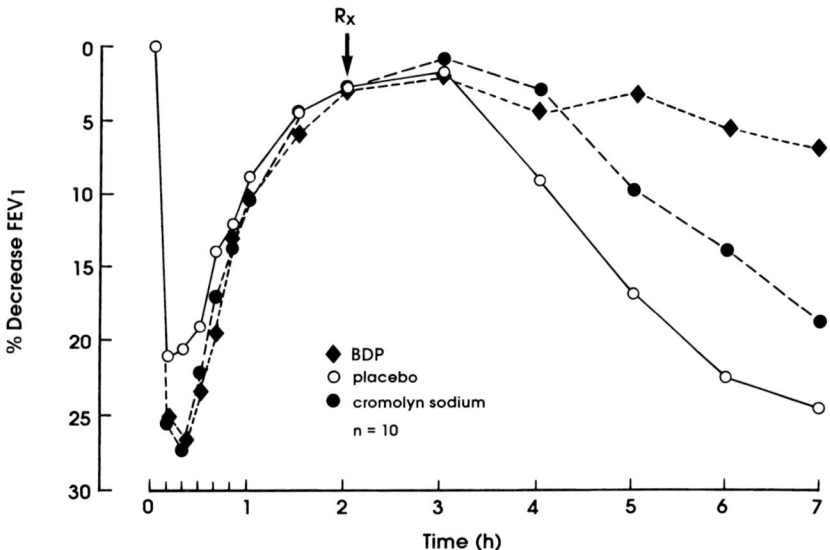

FIGURE 16–2. In a double-blind, double-dummy, random-order study in 10 atopic patients with mild, stable asthma, beclomethasone dipropionate (BDP), 500 μg, *or* cromolyn, 20 mg, *or* placebo was administered 2 hours *after* allergen challenge and after the early allergic response. BDP reduced the late allergic response significantly, in contrast to cromolyn or placebo, which did not differ in efficacy. BDP also had a small effect on the allergen-induced increase in airway responsiveness to methacholine. Cromolyn shifted the early part (3 to 5 hours) of the late allergic response curve to the right significantly, but did not affect the maximal late allergic response or the associated increased responsiveness to methacholine. (From Cockcroft DW, et al. Beclomethasone given after the early asthmatic response inhibits the late response and the increased methacholine responsiveness and cromolyn does not. J Allergy Clin Immunol 91:1163, 1993.)

osine monophosphate, ultrasonically nebulized distilled water, sodium metabisulfite, and exercise. It is more effective than cromolyn in preventing bronchospasm induced by adenosine monophosphate, fog, metabisulfite, and possibly exercise. Nedocromil inhibits both the early and the late response to allergen; however, like cromolyn, if given after the occurrence of the early response, it is unable to interrupt the ongoing cascade of inflammatory events leading to the late response and the associated increase in airways responsiveness (Crimi et al, 1993).

Pharmacokinetics

After topical administration of cromolyn, about 7 percent of the dose is absorbed and rapidly excreted unchanged in the bile and urine. The remainder is expelled, or swallowed and excreted via the gastrointestinal tract, from which only 1 percent is absorbed.

After nedocromil inhalation by normal volunteers, plasma concentrations reach a maximum of 3.3 µg/L at 20 minutes and bioavailability is 9.2 percent; absorption is increased by exercise. Regardless of the experimental route of administration, nedocromil is cleared rapidly from the body, with a serum elimination half-life of 2.3 hours. It is not metabolized.

Clinical Use in Asthma

Regular preventative treatment with cromolyn results in decreased asthma symptoms, improved lung function, and decreased need for bronchodilator treatment (Murphy and Kelly, 1987). A trial of cromolyn inhaled four times daily for 4 to 6 weeks is necessary in order to determine whether or not a patient will respond to it. It is most likely to be effective in atopic patients with mild seasonal or perennial asthma. As severity of asthma increases, the benefits of cromolyn are less apparent. Regular use of a concentrated (5 mg/actuation) cromolyn formulation decreases baseline bronchial hyperreactivity (Hoag and McFadden, 1991), but unfortunately, in North America, only the low dose, 1 mg/actuation cromolyn formulation or 1.8 mg/2 ml ampule cromolyn formulation are available. There is little rationale for combining cromolyn treatment with inhaled glucocorticoid treatment.

Nedocromil, like cromolyn, is intended for prevention rather than relief of chronic asthma symptoms. In double-blind studies 6 to 12 weeks in duration, nedocromil, 4 mg, inhaled four times daily is significantly more effective than placebo in reducing asthma symptoms, despite decreased concomitant bronchodilator use, and in improving morning and evening peak expiratory flow rates (Ruggieri and Patalano, 1989). In children, nedocromil is significantly better than placebo in reducing asthma symptoms when used in a dose of 4 mg four times daily via metered-dose inhaler (1.75 mg/actuation). In some studies, it has been demonstrated to be effective in a dose of 4 mg twice daily.

In patients with mild or moderate asthma, nedocromil may be as effective as low-dose inhaled glucocorticoids (400 µg/day) in reducing bronchial hyperresponsiveness and decreasing symptoms, although not in improving FEV_1 (Bel et al, 1990) (Fig. 16–3). In chronic asthma management, nedocromil is positioned as being intermediate in efficacy between cromolyn and inhaled glucocorticoids; time and additional placebo-controlled studies comparing it to these medications will tell if this is justified.

Clinical Use in Allergic Rhinitis

In patients with seasonal or perennial allergic rhinitis, cromolyn is more effective than placebo in prevention of sneezing, rhinorrhea, and nasal itching. The degree of improvement is modest, and not all patients have a favorable response. It has maximal efficacy when used prophylactically before the onset of seasonal symptoms or before episodic allergen exposure. It is administered intranasally as a 2 percent spray via a metered-dose mist in a dose of two inhalations (2.6 mg each) or as a dry powder (10 mg/inhalation) four to six times daily. The frequency of administration required probably leads to lack of compliance. In allergic rhinitis, cromolyn is as effective as the H_1-antagonist terfenadine, but possibly less effective than the topical intranasal H_1-antagonist levocabastine (not available in the United States), and definitely less effective than intranasal glucocorticoids.

In patients with seasonal allergic rhinitis, nedocromil 1 percent solution, usually administered four times daily, is more effective than placebo in suppressing sneezing, nasal itching, discharge, and blockage. In some

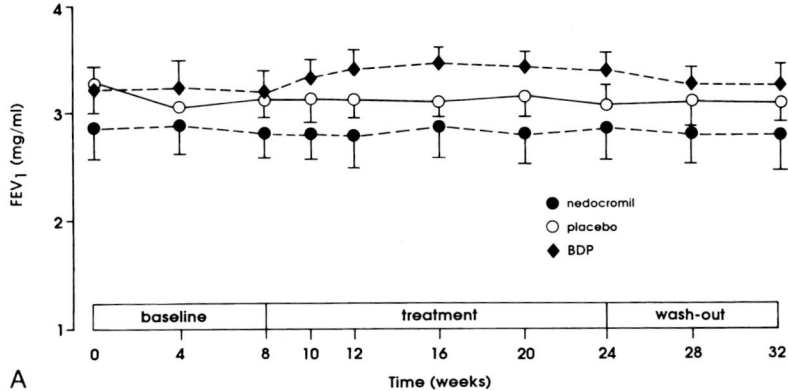
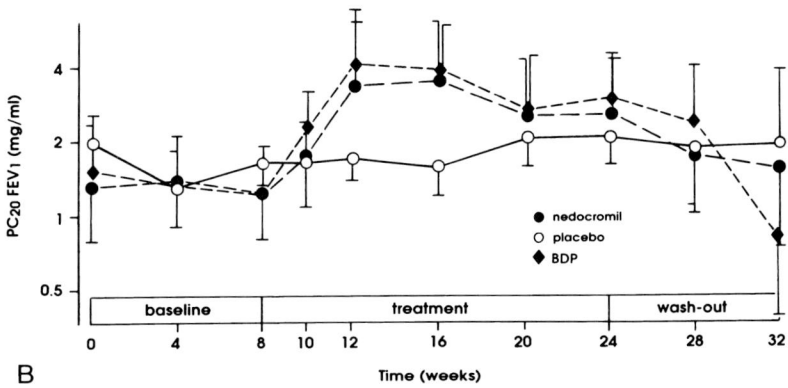

FIGURE 16–3. In 25 non-steroid-dependent, non-atopic asthmatic adults, the effect of nedocromil, 4 mg, or beclomethasone dipropionate (BDP), 100 μg, or placebo four times daily for 4 months was investigated in a double-blind, parallel-group study. *A,* Symptom scores (not shown) and FEV_1 did not change significantly after treatment with nedocromil or placebo, but improved after 4 weeks of treatment with BDP ($p<0.05$). *B,* Symptom scores and PC_{20} did not change in the placebo group, but improved threefold after 8 weeks of treatment with nedocromil or BDP ($p<0.001$). (From Bel EH, et al. The long-term effects of nedocromil sodium and beclomethasone dipropionate on bronchial responsiveness to methacholine in nonatopic asthmatic subjects. Am Rev Respir Dis 141:21, 1990.)

studies, it has been slightly more effective than cromolyn, although the difference has not been statistically or clinically significant (Schuller et al, 1990). More information is needed about the comparative efficacy and safety of nedocromil versus H_1-antagonist or topical glucocorticoid treatment in allergic rhinitis.

Adverse Effects

Cromolyn is the least toxic of all the medications used for chronic asthma or rhinitis treatment and rarely produces any adverse effects.

Nedocromil does not cause any serious adverse effects. After intrapulmonary or intranasal administration, up to 13 percent of patients complain of a bitter taste in the mouth. This problem is noted less frequently when the newer mint-flavored metered-dose inhaler formulation is used. Cough, mild headache, nausea, vomiting, and throat irritation have also been reported. After intranasal administration, epistaxis, sneezing, and nasal burning are noted occasionally.

GLUCOCORTICOIDS

Chronic asthma and rhinitis treatment has been revolutionized by inhaled glucocorticoids such as triamcinolone acetonide, flunisolide, beclomethasone dipropionate (BDP), budesonide, and fluticasone propionate, which have low systemic activity and high topical anti-inflammatory activity in comparison to older glucocorticoids such as dexamethasone (Fig. 16–4). Their relative binding affinity for the human lung glucocorticoid receptor and topical blanching potency in human skin are listed in Table 16–1. BDP and budesonide are the most extensively studied of these medications (Barnes and Pedersen, 1993; Brogden and McTavish, 1992; Holliday et al, 1994).

Mechanism of Action

Glucocorticoids act by regulating gene expression. When they combine with the cytosolic steroid receptor, they form a complex that interacts with DNA, generates messenger RNA, and produces proteins and other factors

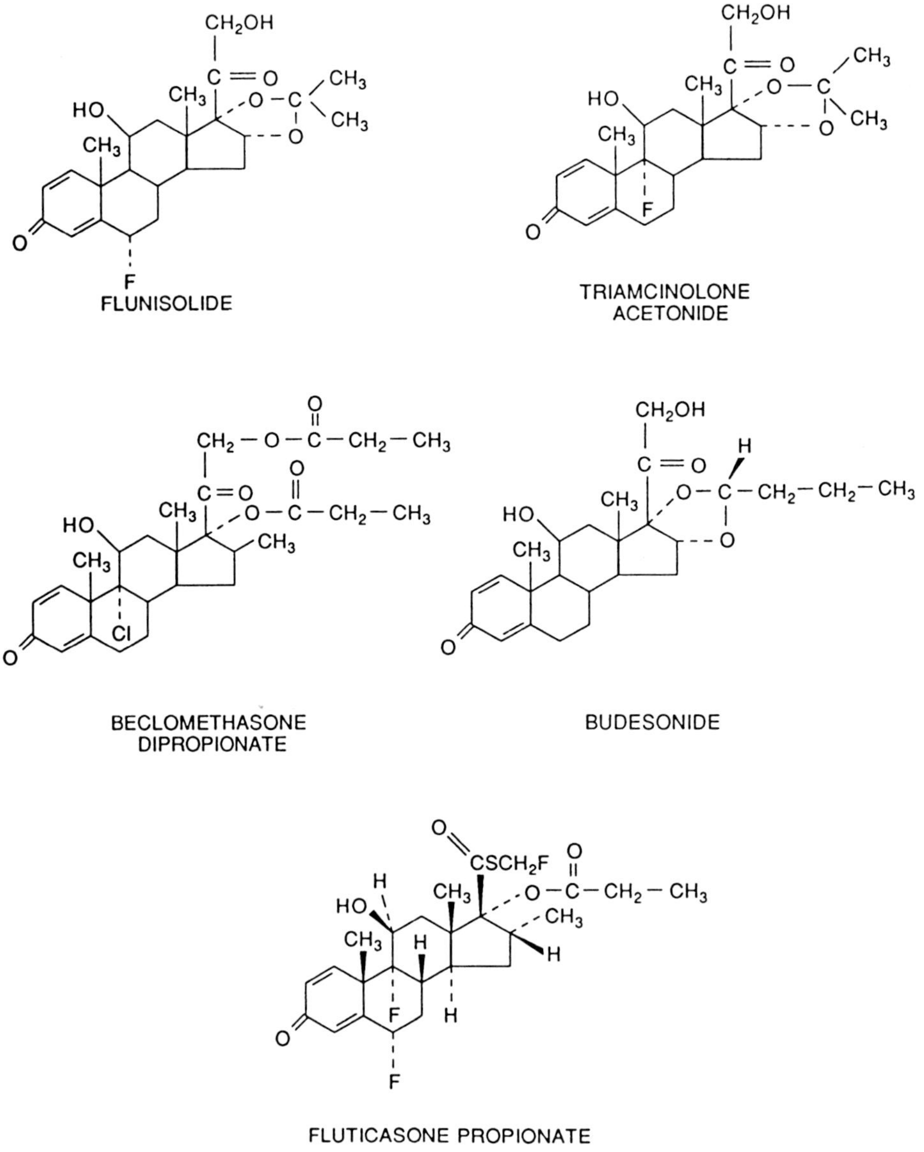

FIGURE 16–4. Chemical structure of glucocorticoids administered by inhalation to prevent asthma or allergic rhinitis symptoms.

TABLE 16–1. RELATIVE BINDING AFFINITY FOR HUMAN LUNG GLUCOCORTICOID RECEPTOR AND TOPICAL BLANCHING POTENCY IN HUMAN SKIN

GLUCOCORTICOID	BINDING AFFINITY	BLANCHING POTENCY
Dexamethasone	1.0	1
Triamcinolone acetonide	3.6	330
Flunisolide	1.8	330
BDP/BMP	0.4/13.5	600/450
Budesonide	9.4	980
Fluticasone propionate	18.0	1200

From Barnes PJ, Pedersen D. Efficacy and safety of inhaled corticosteroids in asthma. Am Rev Respir Dis 148:S1–S26, 1993.
BDP = beclomethasone dipropionate; BMP = beclomethasone monopropionate

that have regulatory effects on the cell producing them as well as on the function of other cells.

Glucocorticoids have a variety of important, multifaceted anti-inflammatory actions in the airways (Schleimer, 1993). These include inhibition of secretion of cytokines and other mediators, inhibition of leukocyte priming, inhibition of arachidonic acid metabolite and platelet activating factor (PAF) release, synergism or permissive effects on responses to catecholamines and other hormones, and modulation of enzyme systems. They restore the integrity of the epithelium, with normalization of the ratio of ciliated cells to goblet cells, an increase in the number of intraepithelial nerves, and a decrease in the number of endothelial gaps in the postcapillary veins. Most importantly, they decrease inflammation in the epithelium and submucosa (Holgate et al, 1991) (Fig. 16–5). These effects occur at concentrations in the airways of 10^{-4} to 10^{-3} M, which can be achieved after inhalation of a 400-μg dose. They correlate with reduction in asthma symptoms, improvement in pulmonary function, and a significant decrease in airway responsiveness to methacholine.

In a sensitized patient, when inhaled glucocorticoids are administered before antigen challenge, they block the immediate and late responses to the antigen and protect against the antigen-induced increase in nonspecific bronchial hyperresponsiveness. Even when inhaled after antigen challenge, they block the late response (Cockcroft et al, 1993) (see Fig. 16–2). Regular inhalation of glucocorticoids also decreases bronchial hyperresponsiveness to nonimmune challenges of all kinds, including exercise, in a time- and dose-dependent manner.

In allergic rhinitis, glucocorticoids reduce mast cells, basophils, eosinophils, neutrophils, and other inflammatory cells in the nasal mucosa and in nasal secretions. They also inhibit basophil histamine release. Patients with allergic rhinitis who are treated with a topical intranasal glucocorticoid for 1 week, then challenged intranasally outof season with antigen to which they are naturally sensitized, have a reduced early- and late-phase response to antigen, as evidenced by fewer symptoms and by decreased levels of mediators and eosinophils, mast cell progenitors, and neutrophils in the nasal lavage fluid. The augmentation of the response to a second antigen challenge or to a histamine challenge is also reduced (Mygind, 1993). In contrast, even high-dose systemic corticosteroid treatment (e.g., oral prednisone, 60 mg daily for 2 days) does not inhibit influx of neutrophils or reduce the early response to nasal provocation with antigen, although it does ameliorate eosinophil influx and other aspects of the late-phase reaction, and subsequent nasal mucosal hyperresponsiveness.

Pharmacokinetics

Most of the pharmacokinetic studies on inhaled glucocorticoids have been conducted in healthy volunteers. The effect of disease and of concomitant inhalation of other medications has not been investigated.

Flunisolide undergoes rapid first-pass metabolism in the liver to 6-β-hydroxyflunisolide, which is metabolically active. When flunisolide is given by inhalation, peak plasma levels of approximately 1.4 ng occur, and the plasma elimination half-life is 1.6 to 2 hours. The systemic bioavailability of any swallowed flunisolide that is absorbed from the gastrointestinal tract is about 20 percent.

The pharmacokinetics of triamcinolone acetonide and of BDP have not been studied in detail in humans, although it is known

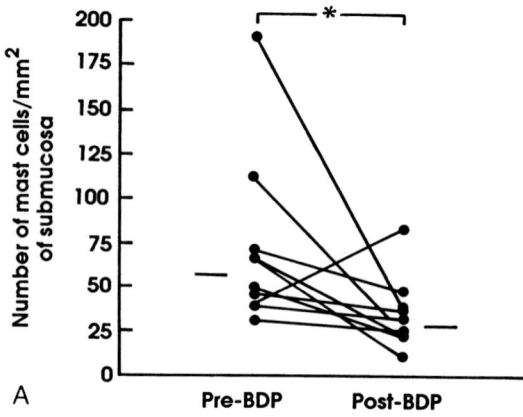
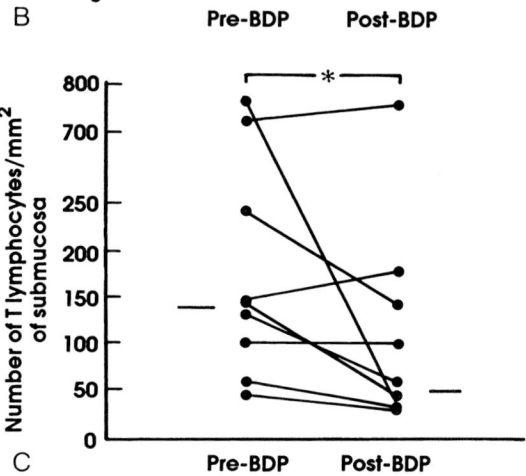

FIGURE 16–5. Numbers of mast cells (A), eosinophils (B), and T lymphocytes (C) in the submucosa of endobronchial biopsy tissue obtained by fiberoptic bronchoscopy before and after 6 weeks of treatment with inhaled beclomethasone dipropionate (BDP), 2000 μg/day for 2 weeks, followed by 1000 μg/day for 4 weeks. The investigators noted a similar significant decrease in epithelial mast cells, eosinophils, and T lymphocytes (not shown). The significant decrease in inflammation was accompanied by decreased asthma symptoms, albuterol usage, peak expiratory flow variation, and airway responsiveness (sevenfold). The beneficial effects of inhaled glucocorticoids in asthma are attributed to their anti-inflammatory action in the airways. (From Holgate ST, et al. Allergic inflammation and its pharmacological modulation in asthma. Int Arch Allergy Appl Immunol 94:210, 1991.)

that BDP is metabolized to beclomethasone monopropionate, a potent active compound which itself is metabolized to beclomethasone, an inactive compound (Szefler, 1991).

Budesonide is a 1:1 mixture of two epimers, with the 22R epimer being twice as active as the 22S epimer. The elimination of budesonide has been well studied following intravenous administration in healthy male volunteers. The plasma half-life is 2.8 hours. Plasma protein binding is 88.3 percent, with negligible binding to transcortin. Ninety percent of budesonide absorbed from the gastrointestinal tract is inactivated on first pass through the liver. From *in vitro* studies with human liver, two major metabolites with 1 to 10 percent of the biologic activity of budesonide have been identified: 6-β-hydroxybudesonide and 16-α-hydroxyprednisolone. In *in vitro* studies in human liver, budesonide is metabolized about three times faster than triamcinolone and four times faster than BDP, suggesting that it has an extremely advantageous therapeutic index.

Fluticasone propionate has a plasma half-life of 3.1 hours after intravenous administration and undergoes virtually complete first-pass extraction by the liver, with total body clearance equivalent to hepatic blood flow. In addition to its lack of bioavailability, its principal metabolite, a 17-carboxylic acid derivative, has negligible glucocorticoid activity.

Clinical Use in Asthma

Inhaled glucocorticoids are more effective than β_2-adrenergic agonists (Van Essen-Zandvliet et al, 1992; Haahtela et al, 1991) for suppressing chronic inflammation in asthma and thus for the long-term prevention and control of asthma symptoms. This is evidenced by freedom from symptoms, asthma exacerbations, and need to use "rescue" medications, objectively documented by improved pulmonary function and reduced bronchial hyperresponsiveness (Barnes and Pedersen, 1993; Hargreave et al, 1990). In mild or moderate asthma, their efficacy is similar to or slightly greater than that of theophylline (Tinkelman et al, 1993), cromolyn (Shapiro et al,

1991), and nedocromil (Bel et al, 1990). In severe chronic asthma, they are likely to be more effective than theophylline or anti-allergics, although for obvious reasons, there are few long-term studies in this population.

They are recommended as first-line treatment of chronic asthma in adults. They are being positioned increasingly early in the treatment of chronic asthma in children and are now recommended for any child who requires an inhaled β_2-agonist more than three or four times daily or who has not responded to a 6-week trial of cromolyn or equivalent nonglucocorticoid treatment (Dukes et al, 1994).

The onset of action of glucocorticoids requires several days, and the maximum bronchoprotective effect may be seen only after many months of therapy (Van Essen-Zandvliet et al, 1992) (Fig. 16–6). The principles of use of inhaled glucocorticoids for chronic asthma are: achieve control of symptoms and then use the lowest dose possible to prevent recurrence of symptoms. Symptom diaries and/or peak expiratory flow monitoring at home will ensure that optimal benefit is obtained and risk is minimized. Normalization of pulmonary function and bronchial responsiveness may require unacceptably high doses of inhaled glucocorticoids in some subgroups of patients (e.g., children and postmenopausal women).

A wide variety of inhalation devices for administration of glucocorticoids permits their use in patients of all ages and with all degrees of obstruction to airflow and levels of ability to perform maximal inspiratory maneuvers. Glucocorticoids can be administered to infants via metered-dose inhaler, face mask and spacer, or, in the case of budesonide, via face mask and wet nebulization (not available in the United States); the latter route has the disadvantages of being inefficient, cumbersome, and time-consuming. The Turbuhaler device seems to be particularly efficient in delivery of medications to the airway; patients who receive budesonide via Turbuhaler after obtaining it via metered-dose inhaler experience improved asthma control despite a 50 percent decrease in budesonide dose (Agertoft and Pedersen, 1994). Additional comprehensive clinical comparisons of the various inhalation devices and, indeed, of the glucocorticoids themselves should be performed in patients with asthma.

Information on prednisolone or methylprednisolone equivalents of inhaled glucocorticoids is still incomplete. Some investigators have reported that very high doses of inhaled glucocorticoids (BDP 1500 µg/day) may not have any greater oral glucocorticoid-sparing effects than low doses (BDP 300 µg/day) (Hummel and Lehtonen, 1992).

Although inhaled glucocorticoids are extremely effective in suppressing the pathophysiologic changes underlying asthma and may even prevent progression of asthma to chronic irreversible airflow obstruction, they do not cure the disorder. Patients with asthma who discontinue regular inhaled glucocorticoid treatment develop increased symptoms, more asthma exacerbations, greater need for "rescue" medications, increased bronchial hyperreactivity, and decreased pulmonary function within weeks or months, depending on the length of their previous course of treatment.

Apparent failure of glucocorticoid treatment in chronic asthma is seldom due to actual lack of effectiveness of the medication. More likely, it is due to (1) lack of compliance with medications that are not perceived to be immediately effective by the patients and are more expensive than bronchodilators, or (2) continued exposure to asthmagenic stimuli such as house pets or cigarette smoke. True glucocorticoid resistance is rare and may be due to relative insensitivity of T lymphocytes to glucocorticoid effects (Cypcar and Busse, 1993). It is diagnosed when inhaled and oral glucocorticoids fail to improve the patient's asthma, although the patient remains responsive to bronchodilators.

Clinical Use in Rhinitis

Chronic allergic rhinitis treatment has been revolutionized by glucocorticoids such as triamcinolone acetonide, flunisolide, BDP, budesonide, and fluticasone propionate. Although these intranasal glucocorticoids are reported to have similar efficacy in allergic rhinitis treatment, some, such as BDP and budesonide, are much more comprehensively studied than others (Bryson and Faulds, 1992).

Glucocorticoids are more effective when given by intranasal inhalation in rhinitis than when given by mouth or by injection. In patients with seasonal allergic rhinitis, intranasal glucocorticoids should be started several days before the pollen season begins and

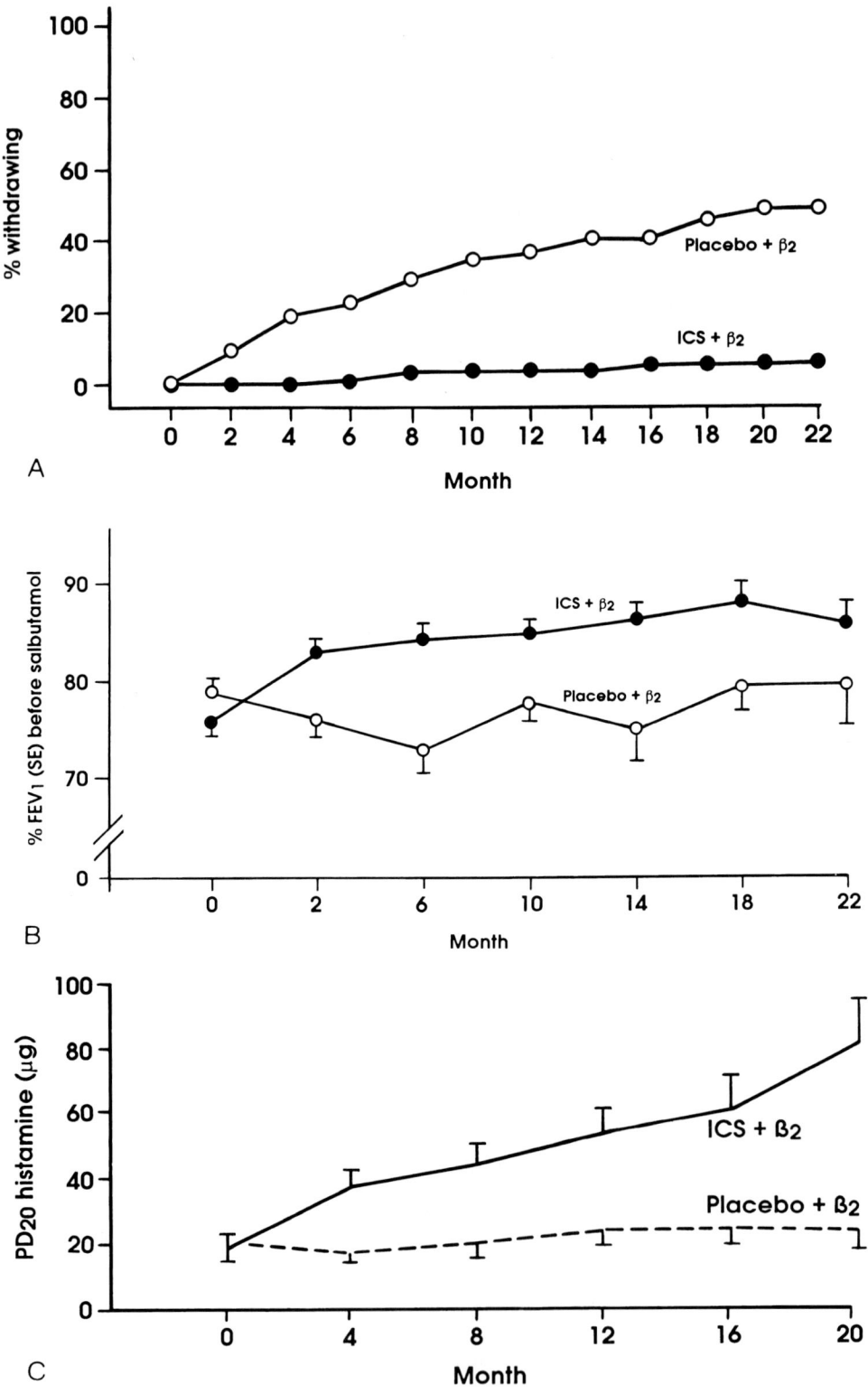

FIGURE 16–6 *See legend on opposite page*

should be used regularly rather than on an "as needed" basis. In patients with severe nasal blockage, inhalation of a decongestant immediately before inhalation of the glucocorticoid may be helpful during the first few days of glucocorticoid treatment. The maximum recommended doses required to achieve control of symptoms initially should be reduced once this goal has been reached. Glucocorticoids are more effective than H_1-antagonists or cromolyn in allergic rhinitis treatment.

Adverse Effects

Inhaled glucocorticoids are relatively safe compared to oral glucocorticoids, the only other medications that are as effective in reducing chronic inflammation of the airways (Barnes and Pedersen, 1993). To date, the adverse effects of inhaled glucocorticoids have been comprehensively studied only for BDP and budesonide. Clinical toxicity is extremely rare during long-term trials in which manufacturers' recommended doses have been administered; however, dose-related, reversible biochemical abnormalities of hypothalamic-pituitary-adrenal axis function, bone metabolism, growth, and lipid/carbohydrate metabolism may occur, especially when these recommendations are exceeded.

Treatment with inhaled glucocorticoids may cause dose-dependent hypothalamic-pituitary-adrenal (HPA) axis suppression by reducing corticotropin (ACTH) production leading to reduced cortisol secretion by the adrenal glands. HPA axis function can be assessed by means of tests for basal adrenal activity (e.g., single morning plasma cortisol levels, 24-hour integrated plasma cortisol, or 24-hour urinary free cortisol) or HPA response after stimulation (e.g., the short tetracosactrin or metyrapone tests). BDP may have a greater suppressive effect than budesonide, especially at high daily doses (>1600 μg in adults and ≥800 μg in children). The clinical importance of small but statistically significant reduction and responses in these tests is not known, as the reduced responses are often within the normal range of the tests. Improvement in HPA axis function is repeatedly and consistently shown in adreno-suppressed glucocorticoid-dependent patients whose oral glucocorticoid dose is reduced after introduction of inhaled glucocorticoids in doses as great as 2000 μg/day.

Long-term treatment with inhaled glucocorticoids does not seem to be associated with increased risk of osteoporosis or vertebrae and rib fractures, in contrast to long-term treatment with systemic steroids. Using bone densitometry measurements, no reduction in bone density has been found during 3 years of budesonide treatment. Inhaled glucocorticoids can sometimes be shown to interfere with markers of bone turnover in a dose-dependent manner. The magnitude of the changes is extremely small and is significantly less than the changes produced by systemic glucocorticoids. BDP and budesonide can affect serum osteocalcin levels, an index of bone protein, but only BDP increases urinary hydroxyproline excretion, an index of collagen degradation. Other markers that may be affected include bone-specific serum alkaline phosphatase, an index of osteoblast activity, and urinary calcium excretion, which reflects the difference between bone mineralization and resorption (Barnes and Pedersen, 1993).

The benefit/risk ratio of inhaled glucocorticoids in children must be examined critically, as these medications are now being used in

---

FIGURE 16–6. In a double-blind study, 116 children with asthma were randomly assigned to treatment with albuterol, 200 μg, plus budesonide, 200 μg, three times daily (BA + CS) *or* to albuterol, 200 μg, plus placebo three times daily (BA + PL). *A*, After a median follow-up time of 22 months, 26 patients receiving BA + PL (45 percent) had withdrawn from randomized treatment because of asthma symptoms, compared with three patients receiving BA + CS (p<0.0001). *B*, The FEV_1 showed an absolute increase of 7 percent after 2 months of BA + CS compared with a decrease of 4 percent after 2 months of BA + PL. This 11 percent difference (p<0.0001) was then maintained after a median follow-up of 22 months. *C*, Mean airway responsiveness expressed as provocative dose of histamine required to give a 20 percent fall in FEV_1 increased from baseline to 4 months by 0.98 doubling doses in children receiving BA + CS, compared with a decrease of 0.42 doubling doses in patients receiving BA + PL. This difference of 1.4 doubling doses (p<0.0001) did not reach a plateau even after 22 months. This study provides strong evidence that inhaled glucocorticoids are important in the long-term management of asthma. (From Van Essen-Zandvliet EE, et al. Effects of 22 months of treatment with inhaled corticosteroids and/or beta-2-agonists on lung function, airway responsiveness, and symptoms in children with asthma. Am Rev Respir Dis 146:457, 1992.)

milder asthma, at an increasingly young age, and in larger doses in this population. Knemometry, a sensitive measure of short-term growth of the lower leg, has been found to be abnormal in children taking 2.5 mg prednisolone/day or in children inhaling BDP, 400 or 800 μg/day, and budesonide, 800 μg/day, by metered-dose inhaler and Nebuhaler (large-volume spacer), but not budesonide, 400 μg/day by metered-dose inhaler and Nebuhaler, or fluticasone propionate, 200 μg/day, by Diskhaler. Such studies have not been performed in children inhaling flunisolide or triamcinolone acetonide. The clinical relevance of the knemometry studies is unclear, as treatment with budesonide up to 710 μg by metered-dose inhaler and Nebuhaler or Turbuhaler for 3 to 6 years has not been associated with growth suppression (Agertoft and Pedersen, 1994). Asthma itself can lead to growth delay or impairment, as can use of systemic steroids.

Concerns about posterior subcapsular cataracts have not been substantiated in patients on inhaled glucocorticoids (Simons et al, 1993), although they remain a concern in patients receiving high-dose oral glucocorticoids for prolonged periods of time.

Easy bruising and skin thinning may be noted in patients receiving high-dose inhaled glucocorticoids for years.

Metabolic effects on glucose metabolism (e.g., increase in fasting insulin, peak glucose, and insulin/glucose ratio during glucose tolerance tests) and on lipid metabolism (e.g., increase in high-density lipoprotein cholesterol) have also been reported after high-dose inhaled glucocorticoids, but not after usual therapeutic doses.

FDA labelings warn that use of inhaled glucocorticoids could be associated with increased severity of varicella and other viral infections; however, this link is not firmly established by currently available data.

Inhaled glucocorticoids may have local effects on the upper airways. Oropharyngeal candidiasis may be related to local deposition and to total daily dose and dose frequency. Reversible hoarseness of the voice may be due to local steroid myopathy of the laryngeal muscles and is related to total dose but not dose frequency. Cough and throat irritation may occur owing to additives in metered-dose inhaler formulations. The use of large-volume spacers with metered-dose inhalers appears to protect against candidiasis but not dysphonia. Rinsing and expectoration after inhaling any formulation of any glucocorticoid leads to improvement of the benefit/risk ratio of the medication (Toogood, 1990).

The most common adverse effects of the intranasal glucocorticoids are local nasal irritation (especially after flunisolide use), burning, sneezing, and rarely, bloody nasal discharge. Patients with perennial allergic rhinitis who have used BDP or budesonide intranasally regularly for 5 years have had no evidence of atrophy of the nasal mucosa in biopsy specimens. Rarely, nasal septal perforation has been reported in patients using intranasal glucocorticoids. Cause and effect has not been proved; nevertheless, patients should be instructed to direct glucocorticoid inhalations away from the nasal septum. An increased incidence of nasopharyngeal infection, including *Candida* infection, has not been noted.

β-ADRENERGIC AGONISTS

Structure and Activity

All β-adrenergic agonists contain a catechol moiety, consisting of 3,4-hydroxyl groups on the benzene ring. The catechol moiety is subject to rapid inactivation by the action of catechol 3-O-methyltransferase. Repositioning of the hydroxyl groups, as in metaproterenol or terbutaline, or substituting another group for the 3-hydroxyl group, as in albuterol, salmeterol, and formoterol, results in prolongation of the bronchodilator action. Increased selectivity for the β_2-adrenergic receptor can be achieved by increasing the bulk of the side chain (Fig. 16–7).

The new β_2-adrenergic agonists, salmeterol and formoterol, have an extremely prolonged effect. The long nonpolar tail of the salmeterol molecule is anchored to an exoreceptor site adjacent to the β_2-adrenergic agonist in the cell membrane pocket, allowing the phenylethanolamine "head" of the molecule to rebound readily to the β_2-receptor. Formoterol also has the ability to rebound readily to the β_2-receptor (Brogden and Faulds, 1991; Faulds et al, 1991).

Mechanism of Action

Beta-adrenergic agonists bind directly to beta-receptors on the cell surface. The recep-

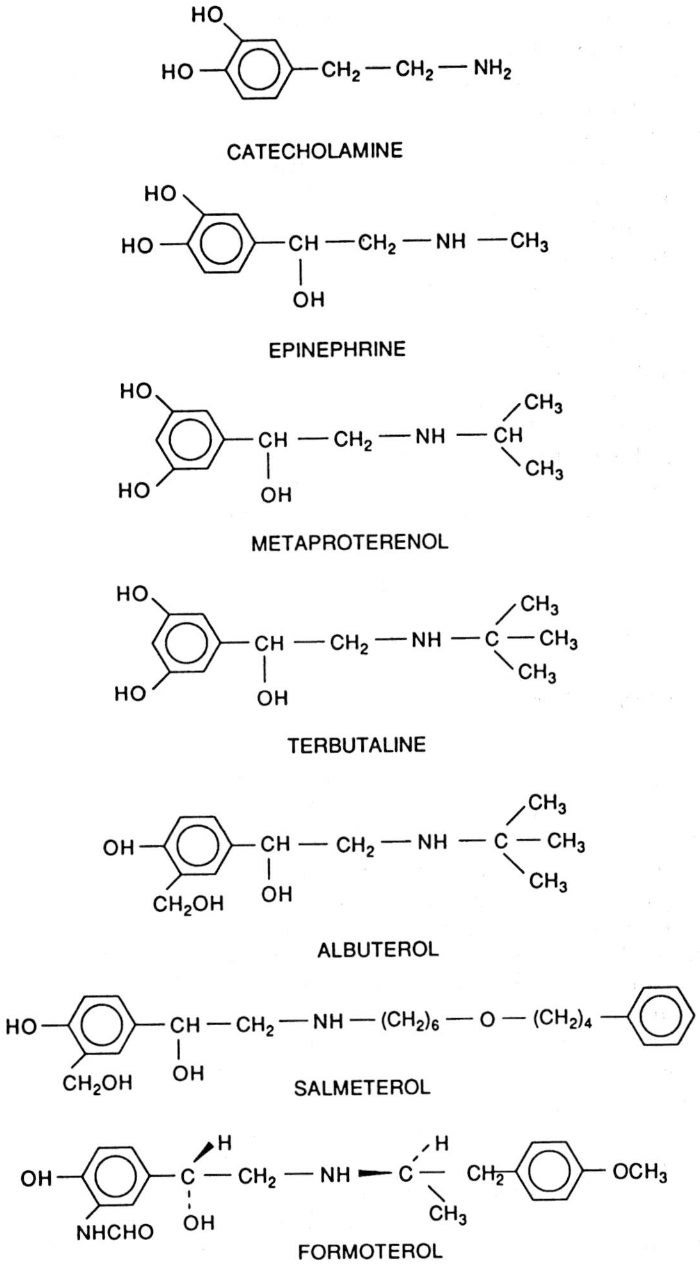

FIGURE 16–7. Catecholamine structure; epinephrine, a catecholamine which has α-adrenergic and β-adrenergic properties; and some selective β$_2$-adrenergic agonists (not catecholamines by virtue of repositioning or substitution of the para-hydroxy groups on the benzene ring), including the very long-acting β$_2$-adrenergic agonists salmeterol and formoterol.

tors link to the adenylate cyclase catalytic unit, leading to stimulation of adenylate cyclase and conversion of adenosine triphosphate (ATP) to cyclic 3',5'-adenosine monophosphate (cyclic AMP). Cyclic AMP binds to specific protein kinases; for example, in smooth muscle, it phosphorylates myosin light-chain kinase, causing relaxation.

In addition to bronchial smooth muscle relaxation, β$_2$-adrenergic agonists increase ion and water secretion and increase ciliary beat frequency, resulting in improved mucociliary clearance, and inhibit release of mediators of inflammation from human basophils and lung mast cells *in vitro*. The relative clinical significance of these effects is unknown.

β$_2$-receptors are present on airway smooth muscle throughout the respiratory tract and are especially dense in the distal airways. Beta-adrenergic agonists cause dose-dependent bronchodilation in large and small airways in normal and asthmatic subjects. They are functional antagonists of smooth muscle constriction produced by all contractile stimuli. They are effective inhibitors of exercise- and allergen-induced early asthmatic responses. If used in a single dose before allergen challenge or as long-term treatment, they do not block the late asthmatic response or its accompanying increase in airway responsiveness.

Most β_2-adrenergic agonists used currently for asthma treatment are highly selective for β_2-receptors and have little affinity for α- or β_1-receptors. This β_2 selectivity may be lost if high doses are administered or if the medications are given by mouth or by injection, rather than by inhalation. β_2 selectivity varies from one agent to another, and there is some evidence that albuterol, terbutaline, and metaproterenol are more β_2-selective than fenoterol (Wong et al, 1990).

Clinical Effects

Epinephrine has α_1-, β_1-, and β_2-adrenergic actions. Injected intramuscularly or subcutaneously, it remains the medication of first choice for the treatment of anaphylaxis. The α_1 activity results in vasoconstriction and decreased mucosal edema, and the β_2 activity relieves bronchoconstriction and prevents additional release of mediators of inflammation.

Short-acting β_2-adrenergic agonists such as albuterol or terbutaline are useful medications for prevention of exercise-induced asthma and for "rescue" treatment of "breakthrough" asthma symptoms. They have a more rapid onset of action and are more effective bronchodilators than methylxanthines such as theophylline or anticholinergics such as ipratropium bromide. They provide dose-related relief of wheezing, coughing, and shortness of breath. In hospitalized patients with acute asthma, frequent or semicontinuous nebulization of albuterol is becoming common practice.

In chronic asthma treatment, frequent use or overuse of β_2-adrenergic agonists serves as an important indicator that asthma is not optimally controlled. In retrospective pharmacoepidemiology studies, overuse of β_2-adrenergic agonists has been strongly linked with asthma deaths, although a cause and effect relationship has not been established (Suissa et al, 1994).

Administration of β_2-adrenergic agonists such as albuterol on a regular basis three or four times daily is no longer recommended. These medications do not provide relief of chronic inflammation in the airways. Short-acting β_2-adrenergic agonists used regularly for weeks or years may increase bronchial hyperresponsiveness slightly (Sears et al, 1990; Van Schayck et al, 1990). This increase is not progressive. It is not necessarily accompanied by increased symptoms or a decline in pulmonary function; in one recent large crossover study in 341 people with moderate asthma, albuterol, 200 μg four times daily regularly did not produce lower peak flows and was associated with less frequent asthma symptoms than "as needed" albuterol (Chapman et al, 1994).

The subsensitivity to β_2-adrenergic agonists that may develop over days or weeks is related to a down-regulation of the β receptors or decreased efficiency of the coupling mechanism of the β receptors to adenylate cyclase (Snell, 1994). Glucocorticoids are capable of markedly enhancing the responses to β-adrenergic agonists by increasing the number of β receptors.

Lack of compliance with β_2-adrenergic agonists is generally evidenced as overuse or as lack of flexibility in usage, rather than as underuse. Assessment of compliance with these medications is generally made indirectly using history, diary cards, and peak expiratory flow monitoring records. Cannisters or dry powder formulation containers can be weighed, and Rotacaps or discs can be counted. Rarely, MDI Chronologs are used to record the precise times of inhalations, or serum β_2-agonist concentrations are measured.

The very long-acting inhaled β_2-adrenergic agonists salmeterol and formoterol have recently been introduced. Single doses of these medications have a duration of action of at least 12 hours, not only for bronchodilation, but also for protection against bronchoconstrictive stimuli such as exercise, or inhalation of cold, dry air, methacholine, histamine, or allergen (Simons et al, 1992) (Fig. 16–8). Administered twice daily, these medications are significantly more effective than placebo or albuterol administered four times daily in preventing daytime and nighttime wheezing, coughing, and shortness of breath; they are also more effective in improving peak expiratory flow rates, decreasing variability in peak expiratory flows, decreasing the need for sup-

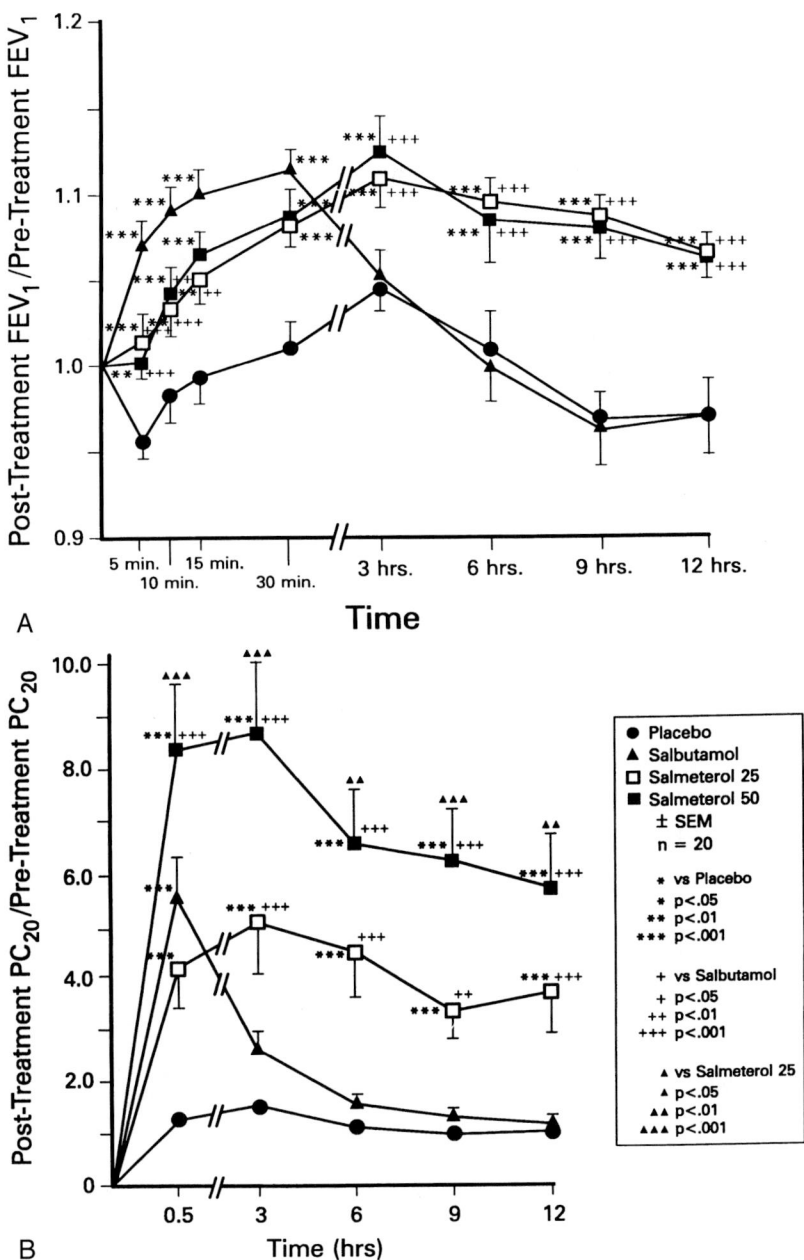

FIGURE 16–8. The bronchodilator and bronchoprotective effects of salmeterol, 25 (21) and 50 (42) μg, albuterol, 200 (180) μg, and placebo were compared in a double-blind, within-patient four-way crossover, single-dose study in 20 subjects. *A,* FEV_1 increased significantly from 5 to 30 minutes after albuterol, and from 5 minutes to 12 hours after salmeterol, 25 or 50 μg, compared with placebo. FEV_1 was significantly lower after salmeterol at 5 and 10 minutes than after albuterol, but was significantly greater after salmeterol than after albuterol from 2 to 12 hours. *B,* After albuterol, there was a significant increase in the PC_{20} only at 30 minutes. After salmeterol, 25 or 50 μg, the PC_{20} increased significantly from 30 minutes to 12 hours. Salmeterol has a significantly longer bronchodilator and bronchoprotective effect than albuterol. (From Simons FER, et al. Bronchodilator and bronchoprotective effects of salmeterol in young patients with asthma. J Allergy Clin Immunol 90:840, 1992.)

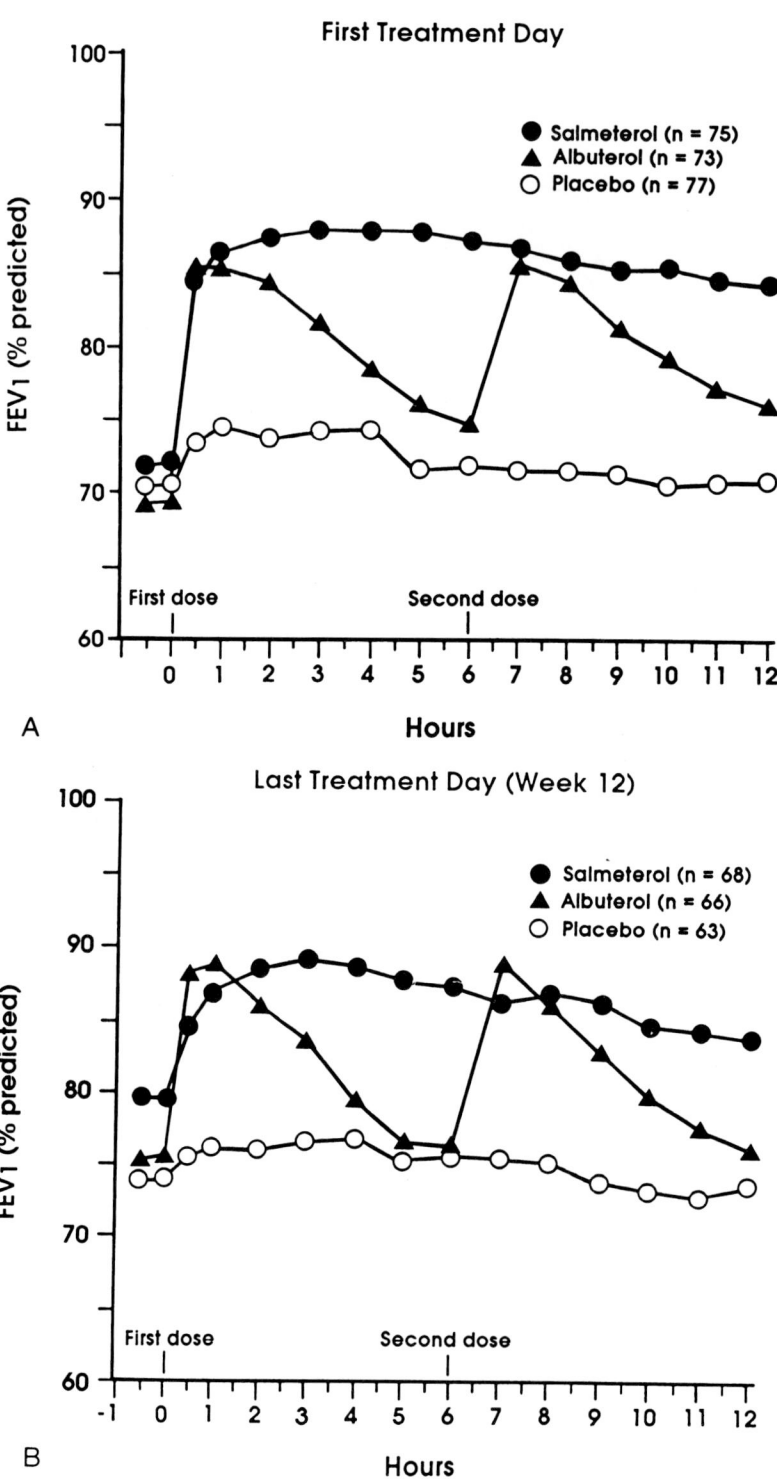

FIGURE 16–9 *See legend on opposite page*

plementary albuterol, and improving quality of life. Their bronchodilator effect does not wane with time (Fig. 16–9) (Pearlman et al, 1992), although a decrease in bronchoprotective effect has been found after 1 or 2 months of regular salmeterol treatment (Cheung et al, 1992; Ramage et al, 1994). After cessation of treatment, there is no sustained improvement in lung function or airway hyperresponsiveness; nor has a rebound increase in bronchial hyperresponsiveness been found. These medications are particularly useful in prevention of nocturnal asthma symptoms and in prolonged prevention (up to 12 hours) of exercise-induced bronchospasm. Some physicians believe they should always be used in conjunction with inhaled glucocorticoids.

Adverse Effects

Adverse effects from β-adrenergic agonists occur as a result of extrapulmonary β-adrenoreceptor stimulation. When these medications are given by the inhaled route, fewer adverse effects for comparable pulmonary efficacy are achieved than when they are given orally or by injection.

Skeletal muscle fibers, like bronchial smooth muscle fibers, contain β_2-receptors. Individuals have varying degrees of susceptibility to tremor from β_2-adrenergic agonists. The tremor is dose-related and tolerance to it may occur. Rarely, patients complain of insomnia or other central nervous system adverse effects associated with β_2-agonist use.

Some β-adrenergic agonists such as epinephrine and isoproterenol have a high affinity for β_1-receptors as well as for β_2-receptors, and cause an increase in heart rate, cardiac output, and palpitations. Selective β_2-adrenergic agonists inhaled in high doses or given systemically may cause adverse cardiac symptoms via direct stimulation of the β_2-receptors in the heart or via reflex changes following β_2-agonist–induced peripheral vasodilation, decreased peripheral vascular resistance, and reflex sympathetic cardiac stimulation.

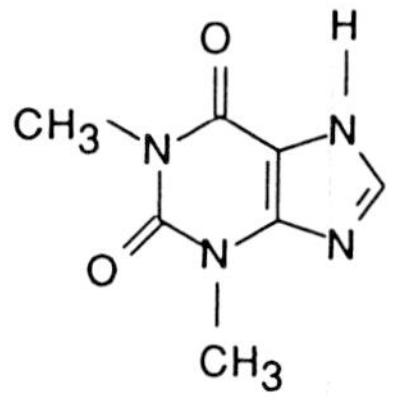

Administration of selective β_2-agonists in large amounts, even by inhalation, and administration of less β_2-selective agents may be associated with transient reduction in plasma potassium, calcium, and magnesium concentrations; an increase in glycogenolysis; and hyperglycemia. Tolerance to the metabolic effects occurs rapidly.

FIGURE 16–10. The chemical structure of theophylline, the prototype methylxanthine.

METHYLXANTHINES

Structure and Activity

Theophylline, the best-studied of the methylxanthines (Weinberger and Hendeles, 1993) (Fig. 16–10), will be the main focus of this section, as other medications in this class—such as dihydroxypropyl-theophylline (dyphylline), profylline, and enprofylline—are infrequently used. Until the late 1980s, theophylline was widely prescribed for both acute and chronic asthma management. Its role has subsequently declined in importance as, in addition to concerns over its narrow therapeutic index and potential to cause serious adverse reactions, it lacks the rapid bronchodilator effect of selective β_2-adrenergic ag-

---

FIGURE 16–9. In a double-blind, parallel study, 234 patients were assigned to receive either 42 μg salmeterol twice daily *or* 180 μg albuterol four times daily, *or* placebo. All patients could use supplemental inhaled albuterol as needed. A single dose of salmeterol produced a greater increase in FEV_1 (mean AUC) than two doses of albuterol taken 6 hours apart. *A*, The difference was significant on day 1 and at week 4 of the study, but not at week 8 or (*B*) week 12. Salmeterol also improved peak expiratory flow and mean overall symptom score better than albuterol or placebo (not shown). There was no evidence of tolerance to the bronchodilating effects of salmeterol. In mild-to-moderate asthma, salmeterol twice daily was superior to albuterol four times daily or as needed. (From Pearlman DS, et al. A comparison of salmeterol with albuterol in the treatment of mild-to-moderate asthma. N Engl J Med 327:1420, 1992.)

onists. It is useful as ancillary treatment in patients with severe chronic asthma requiring high-dose inhaled glucocorticoids (Brenner et al, 1988).

Mechanism of Action

The mechanisms of action of theophylline, while still not fully understood, extend beyond smooth muscle relaxation and bronchodilation. Other pharmacologic effects include improved mucociliary clearance, reduced microvascular permeability, improved contractility of the fatigued diaphragm, decreased systemic and pulmonary vascular resistance, enhanced cardiac output and diuresis, stimulation of endogenous catecholamine release, and stimulation of respiratory drive.

Theophylline has immunomodulatory effects in patients with chronic asthma. It attenuates the early and late response to allergen, and at doses too low to have a significant bronchodilator effect, it has been reported to reduce the number of activated eosinophils beneath the epithelial basement membrane in bronchial biopsy tissue (Sullivan et al, 1994).

Theophylline nonspecifically inhibits all five isoenzymes of phosphodiesterase including type III, involved in bronchoconstriction, and type IV, which is pro-inflammatory. It is not known whether the theophylline concentrations usually achieved *in vivo* are high enough to have a significant phosphodiesterase inhibition effect. Adenosine antagonism was formerly thought to contribute to the anti-asthmatic action of theophylline, as administration of aerosolized adenosine produces bronchoconstriction that can be antagonized by theophylline, but enprofylline, a methylxanthine that does not antagonize adenosine, is a more effective bronchodilator, on a molar basis, than theophylline (Persson, 1988).

Theophylline has some protective effect against exercise-induced bronchospasm, against many different chemical constrictors including histamine or methacholine, and against the immediate response to allergen, but regardless of the stimulus for bronchoconstriction, it provides less protection than β_2-adrenergic agonists. The late response to allergen and concomitant increase in airways responsiveness is significantly decreased in the presence of serum theophylline concentrations greater than 10 mg/L.

Pharmacokinetics

Theophylline is rapidly and completely absorbed after oral administration, although sporadic absorption and "dose dumping" have been noted with some formulations taken with food, particularly high-fat meals. Theophylline is metabolized by the hepatic cytochrome P_{450} system, predominantly by oxidation, and little is excreted unchanged in the urine. Individuals vary considerably in their ability to metabolize this medication (Weinberger and Hendeles, 1993; Snell, 1994). Infants under age 6 months and elderly patients may be slow metabolizers and therefore at high risk of toxicity unless timely, appropriate adjustments in dose and dose interval are made. Concomitant administration of other medications metabolized in the cytochrome P_{450} system, for example, antibiotics (some quinolones such as ciprofloxacin and macrolides such as erythromycin), or H_2-antagonists such as cimetidine, and other drugs such as methotrexate may impair theophylline elimination, increase theophylline levels, and increase potential toxicity. Hepatic dysfunction, heart failure, or febrile illness may also impair theophylline elimination. Smoking, on the other hand, results in more rapid biotransformation of theophylline. Enprofylline, unlike theophylline, is excreted almost unchanged via the renal route.

Clinical Effects

The degree of bronchodilation produced by methylxanthines is directly proportional to the logarithm of the plasma concentration. Theophylline is the only medication used in asthma and allergy treatment for which the therapeutic range is defined quantitatively by plasma concentrations, and for which monitoring of plasma concentrations is required for optimal therapy. The currently recommended "therapeutic range" of concentrations is 5 to 15 mg/L.

A wide selection of sustained-release theophylline formulations is available. Some of these formulations have a duration of action of 24 hours and are useful ancillary medications in the management of nocturnal asthma. At the onset of treatment, one half to two thirds of the initial whole daily dose (generally no more than 600 mg/day in an adult) should be administered, and serum concentrations should be monitored within 48 to 72 hours.

Adverse Effects

Adverse effects following theophylline administration are related to dose and plasma theophylline concentration, and are especially likely to occur when concentrations exceed 15 to 20 mg/L (Weinberger and Hendeles, 1993). Gastrointestinal effects such as anorexia, nausea, and vomiting may be troublesome, particularly during initiation of theophylline treatment. Theophylline causes relaxation of the esophageal sphincter and may contribute to gastroesophageal reflux. It may cause adverse central nervous system effects such as nervousness and headache. It has been blamed for causing behavioral problems, poor classroom adaptation, and poor school performance, but these adverse effects have been difficult to prove objectively in rigorously controlled double-blind studies. Where they have been documented, they seem to be more common in children already predisposed to learning problems, depression, and anxiety. Although insomnia is often attributed to theophylline, objective studies in children and adults with asthma have not confirmed significant disruption of sleep or significant impairment of sleep quality. Theophylline may also cause subclinical tremor and, occasionally, adverse metabolic effects (Milgrom and Bender, 1993).

Theophylline overdose may result in nausea, vomiting, tachycardia, and other cardiac arrhythmias due to inotropic effects, and in seizures and other signs of central nervous system toxicity. This problem is not uncommon; 2.8 percent of 5557 consecutive serum theophylline concentrations measured in two emergency departments during a 2-year period were greater than 30 mg/L. In this population, 88 percent of the patients had been chronically overdosed, primarily as a result of physician or patient errors. Charcoal hemoperfusion is the treatment of choice for severe theophylline toxicity (Sessler, 1990).

CHOLINERGIC (MUSCARINIC) ANTAGONISTS

Structure and Activity

Anticholinergic medications include atropine, ipratropium bromide, oxitropium bromide, thiazinamium chloride, and glycopyrrolate. These compounds, which have very different chemical structures, are competitive antagonists of the muscarinic actions of acetylcholine, inhibiting its effects on postganglionic efferent parasympathetic receptors and on some effector cells that are not directly innervated by the parasympathetic system. Atropine, the prototype anticholinergic medication, is a tertiary amine. It crosses the blood-brain barrier easily, is well absorbed from the gastrointestinal tract, lungs and nasal mucosa, and is consequently prone to cause systemic adverse effects.

Ipratropium bromide is now the most commonly used anticholinergic and will be discussed as the prototype anticholinergic agent (Gross, 1988) (Fig. 16-11). It is a topically active synthetic quaternary derivative of *n*-isopropyl noratropine. Unlike atropine, it has low lipid solubility, does not cross the blood-brain barrier, and is poorly absorbed from the gastrointestinal tract and nasal mucosa. Tissue selectivity can therefore be achieved by ad-

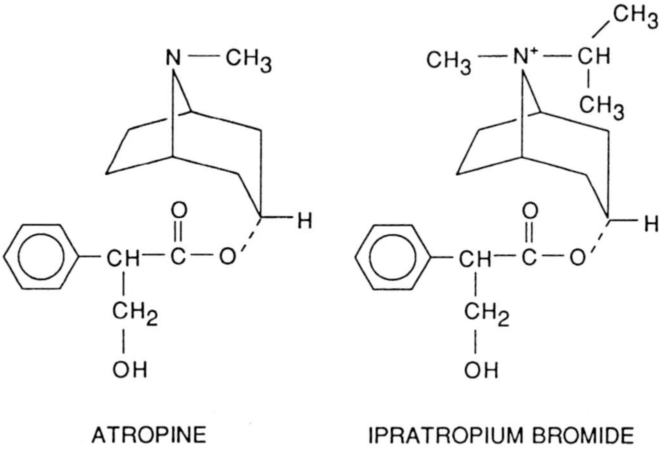

FIGURE 16-11. The chemical structure of atropine and ipratropium bromide.

ATROPINE

IPRATROPIUM BROMIDE

ministration of quaternary amines via the inhaled route.

Mechanisms of Action

Muscarinic receptors, more plentiful in the proximal than the distal airways, are present on bronchial smooth muscle, submucosal glands, mast cells, and prejunctional postganglionic nerves. At least five subtypes have been cloned and nine genes for subtype receptors have been identified. Subtypes M_1, M_2, and M_3 exist in the airways. M_1 receptors facilitate neurotransmission in parasympathetic ganglia; M_2 receptors are autoreceptors on postganglionic nerves where they provide feedback inhibition of acetylcholine release. M_3 receptors are present on the smooth muscle cells and submucosal glands, and mediate the classic muscarinic effects in the airways. None of the antimuscarinic medications available for clinical use is selective for receptor subtypes.

The airways are tonically constricted by vagal efferent nervous activity, and administration of aerosolized antimuscarinics to healthy volunteers causes bronchodilation, principally of the large central airways (Barnes, 1990). In asthma, anticholinergic medications protect against methacholine challenge and against the effects of gases and dust. They also prevent and reverse bronchoconstriction induced by psychogenic stimuli and by β-adrenergic antagonists such as propranolol. Ipratropium bromide, in contrast to atropine, may protect against allergen-induced bronchoconstriction. The bronchodilator effect of ipratropium bromide peaks at 30 to 60 minutes and lasts for 6 hours. The peak is lower, and the effect is slower in onset but longer lasting than that produced by albuterol or other short-acting $β_2$-adrenergic agonists.

In the nasal mucosa, ipratropium bromide prevents and relieves rhinorrhea by interfering with parasympathetic transmission to the submucosal glands. It does not relieve itching or sneezing, which occurs reflexly when sensory nerves in the nasal mucosa are stimulated; nor does it relieve nasal blockage, which is due to engorgement of the mucosal capacitance vessels. In patients with allergic or nonallergic rhinitis challenged intranasally with methacholine, ipratropium bromide significantly administered before challenge reduces nasal discharge.

Pharmacokinetics

Ipratropium bromide is poorly absorbed by the oropharyngeal and nasal mucosa, and the swallowed drug is poorly absorbed from the gastrointestinal tract. Serum ipratropium bromide concentrations are extremely low after inhalation, with peak concentrations being achieved at approximately 3 hours. The elimination half-life is 3.2 to 3.8 hours. Ipratropium bromide metabolites have little or no anticholinergic activity.

Clinical Use

Anticholinergic medications such as ipratropium bromide play an adjuvant role in asthma treatment. Certain subgroups of patients with chronic asthma, for example, older, non-atopic patients, benefit particularly from the addition of ipratropium bromide to $β_2$-adrenergic agonist treatment, and ipratropium bromide is first-line treatment in adults with chronic obstructive pulmonary disease. Long-term administration is well tolerated. Subsensitivity or tachyphylaxis has not been found; nor have unfavorable interactions with other drugs been reported. In acute asthma, ipratropium bromide, although not helpful when used alone, is sometimes administered concomitantly with a short-acting $β_2$-adrenergic agonist such as albuterol to enhance and prolong bronchodilation.

In chronic rhinitis, ipratropium bromide is useful for treatment in patients whose predominant symptom is rhinorrhea (Meltzer et al, 1992) (Fig. 16–12), and for those with paroxysmal rhinorrhea induced by hot or spicy liquids ("gustatory rhinitis" or "salsa snuffles"), by cold air ("skiers' nose"), or by irritants. It is administered in a dose of 320 μg/day (40 μg in each nostril four times daily); in some patients with profuse nasal discharge, higher doses are required. It is effective within minutes and has a duration of action of at least 4 hours (Meltzer, 1991).

Adverse Effects

Atropine potentially causes many dose-related systemic adverse effects, including reduction in glandular secretions, dryness of the mouth, thirst, dilation of the pupils, blurred vision, and difficulty in urinating. Very high doses may result in bradycardia followed by tachycardia; increased intraocular pressure

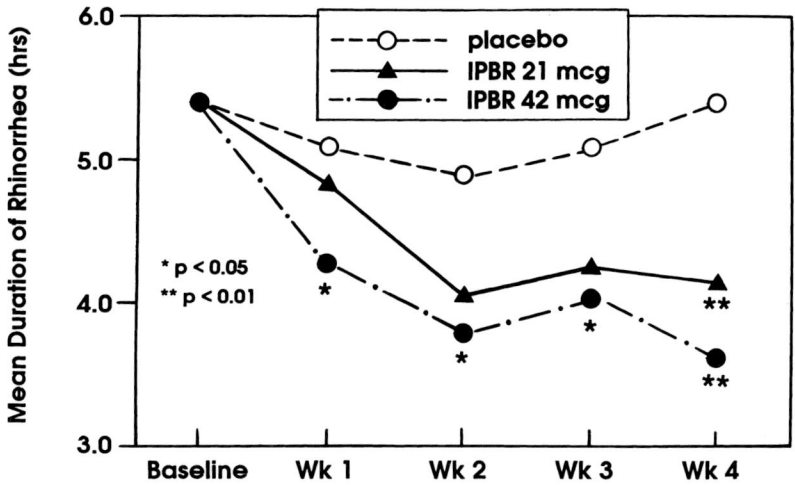

FIGURE 16–12. In a double-blind, parallel study of 123 patients with perennial allergic rhinitis, ipratropium bromide, 21 or 42 μg, *or* placebo, 1 spray/nostril, was given three times daily for 4 weeks. Mean duration and severity of rhinorrhea was decreased in both ipratropium bromide treatment groups by comparison with placebo, with greatest improvement in the group treated with the higher ipratropium bromide dose. No significant differences occurred among the treatment groups in duration or severity of postnasal drip, congestion, or sneezing. No changes in nasal cytology were noted. (From Meltzer EO, et al. Ipratropium bromide aqueous nasal spray for patients with perennial allergic rhinitis. J Allergy Clin Immunol 90:242, 1992.)

and glaucoma; decreased intestinal motility; hot, flushed dry skin; and restlessness and coma.

Inhalation of ipratropium bromide in recommended doses does not produce tremor, nervousness, excitation, or any other central nervous system effects. It does not inhibit salivation, impair urinary flow, or cause tachycardia or other significant cardiovascular effects. It does not cause dilation of the pupils, loss of visual acuity, or other ocular adverse effects unless it contacts the eye directly. Paradoxical bronchoconstriction has occurred in asthma chiefly after inhalation of ipratropium bromide via wet nebulization and has been attributed to hypotonicity of the nebulizer solution, presence of preservatives, or blockade of postganglionic, presynaptic M_1 receptors.

Following intranasal inhalation of ipratropium bromide, local or systemic adverse effects are extremely infrequent. In the recommended dose of 320 μg/day, it seldom even produces dryness of the nasal mucosa, although elderly patients may be more prone to this effect and patients of any age given very high doses (e.g., 1600 μg/day) may experience it. It has no rebound effect, does not decrease olfactory sensitivity, and does not impair mucociliary transport.

H_1-RECEPTOR ANTAGONISTS (ANTIHISTAMINES)

Structure and Activity

H_1-receptor antagonists, commonly used for symptomatic treatment of allergic rhinitis and urticaria, are highly selective for histamine H_1-receptors and have no activity at histamine H_2- or H_3-receptors. In addition, most second-generation H_1-antagonists have minimal activity at muscarinic cholinergic, 5-OH-tryptaminergic, or α-adrenergic receptors. The relative lack of central nervous system effects of the second-generation H_1-antagonists is attributable chiefly to their relative inability to cross the tightly fused outer membranes of the endothelial cells lining the brain capillaries.

H_1-antagonists contain an ethylamine group and have some structural resemblance to histamine (Fig. 16–13). Their traditional classification into six major groups—ethanolamines, ethylenediamines, alkylamines, piperazines, piperidines, and phenothiazines—is less helpful than it was years ago, as many of the second-generation H_1-antagonists do not fit readily into this system. For example, although terfenadine, astemizole, levocabas-

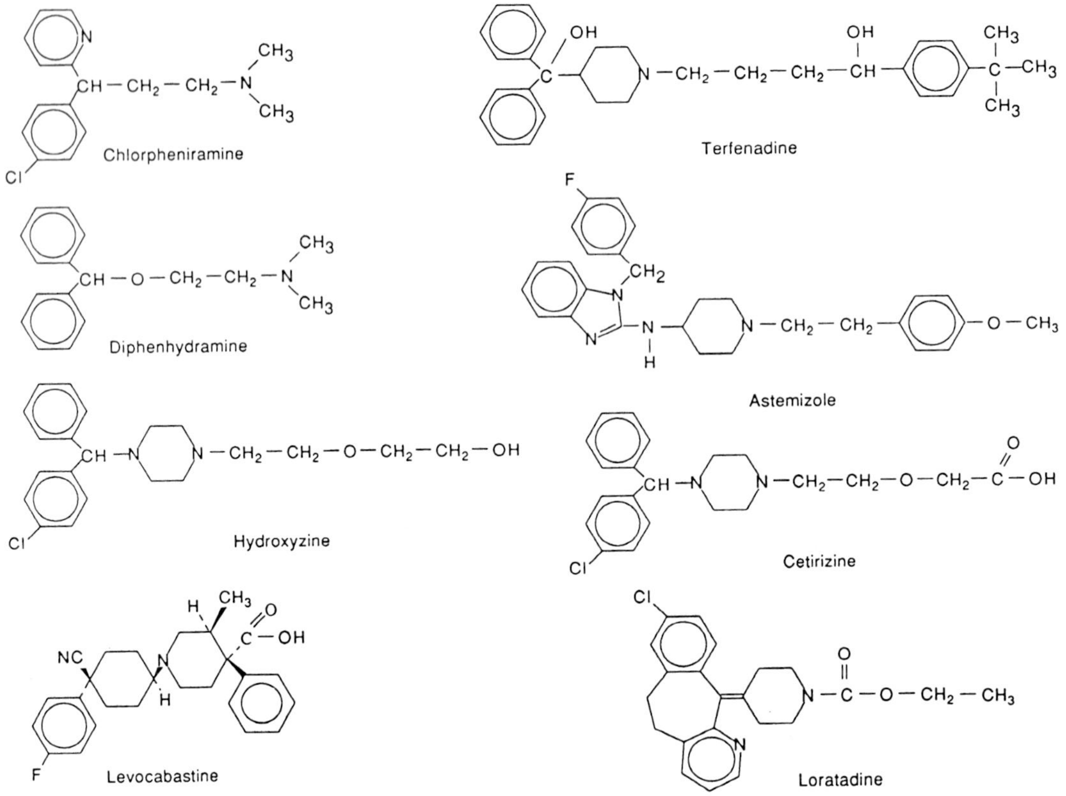

FIGURE 16–13. The chemical structure of some commonly used H_1-receptor antagonists.

tine, and ketotifen each contain a piperidine group, they have diverse chemical structures.

Mechanisms of Action

At low concentrations, H_1-antagonists are competitive antagonists of histamine and bind to H_1-receptors, thus preventing histamine from binding. At higher concentrations, some second-generation H_1-antagonists such as terfenadine, astemizole, and loratadine also decrease the maximum response to histamine and depress the slope of the dose-response curve, effects which are more characteristic of a noncompetitive type of inhibition. These H_1-antagonists also dissociate less readily from the H_1-receptor site than other H_1-antagonists. For many H_1-antagonists, tissue concentrations of active H_1-antagonist metabolite(s) at the H_1-receptor site may be more relevant than tissue concentrations of the parent compound.

In vitro, many H_1-antagonists have anti-allergic effects on human basophils and mast cells. These effects vary with the H_1-antagonist concentration, the stimulus for mediator release, and the chemical mediator of inflammation being measured. For some H_1-antagonists, the anti-allergic effects are of little clinical importance, as the concentrations required for suppression of histamine release are up to 1000 times higher than those achieved *in vivo* after usual doses. Others administered in recommended doses before antigen challenge on the nasal mucosa or skin of patients naturally sensitized to the antigen being tested, decrease release of histamine or prostaglandin D_2 (PGD_2). Although a few, such as ketotifen, are promulgated for their anti-allergic effects, the relative contribution of anti-allergic effects to the overall clinical effectiveness of H_1-antagonists is unknown. Some H_1-antagonists also attenuate migration of eosinophils and other inflammatory cells (Rimmer and Church, 1990).

Pharmacokinetics/Pharmacodynamics

H_1-antagonists are well absorbed when administered orally, with peak serum concentrations being reached approximately 2 hours after dosing in fasting patients. All the first-generation H_1-antagonists and most of the second-generation H_1-antagonists currently available, with the exception of cetirizine, acrivastine, and levocabastine, are metabolized by the hepatic cytochrome P_{450} system. Serum elimination half-life values range from less than 24 hours for medications such as terfenadine, loratadine, and cetirizine, to approximately 24 hours for chlorpheniramine, astemizole and azelastine, to 9.5 days for as-temizole active metabolites. Serum elimination half-life values for H_1-antagonists may be prolonged in elderly patients, in patients with hepatic dysfunction, and in patients concomitantly receiving hepatic mixed-function oxygenase inhibitors such as ketoconazole or other imidazole antifungals, and erythromycin or other macrolide antibiotics.

Peak effect of H_1-antagonists generally occurs 5 to 7 hours after oral dosing and 3 to 5 hours after peak serum concentrations are achieved (Fig. 16–14). Effectiveness persists even when serum concentrations of the parent compound have declined to the lowest limits of analytic detection, because of the presence of active metabolites and/or high tissue/serum concentration ratios. H_1-antago-

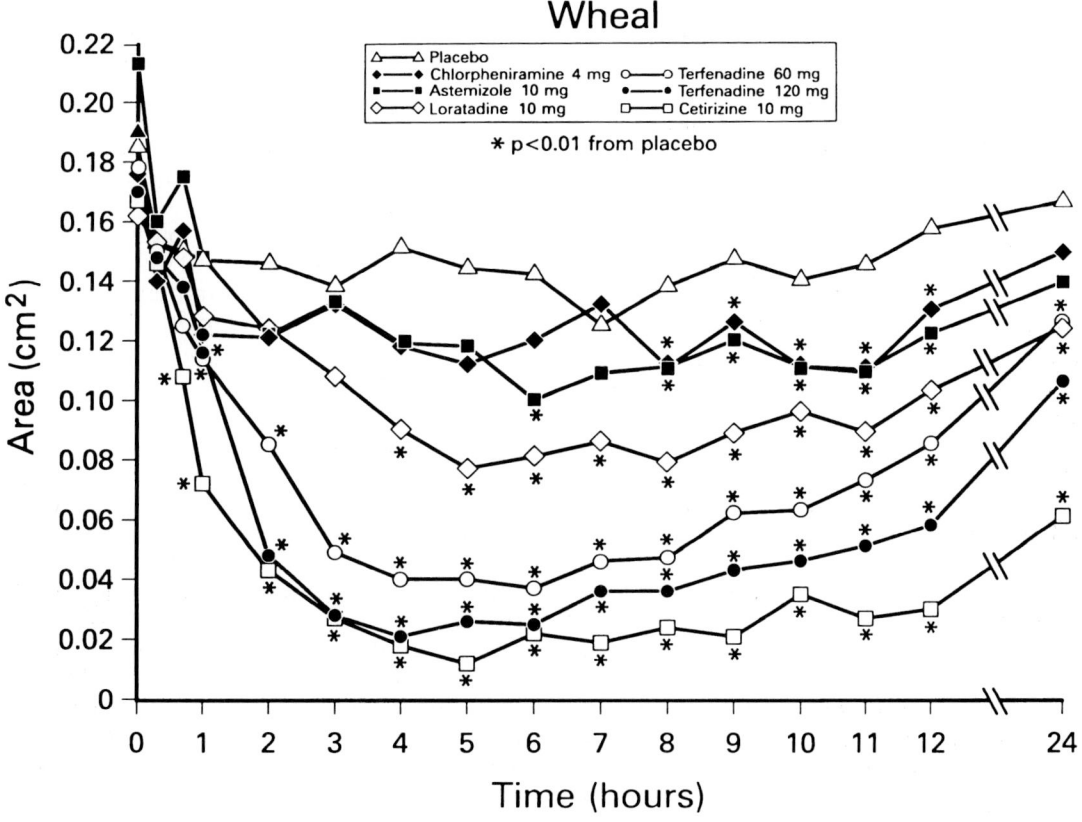

FIGURE 16–14. In a single-dose, double-blind, seven-way crossover study in 20 healthy male subjects, mean wheal areas were measured after epicutaneous histamine phosphate, 1 mg/mL, before and up to 24 hours after a single oral dose of placebo or H_1-receptor antagonist. The rank order of suppression was, from most effective to least effective: cetirizine 10 mg >terfenadine 120 mg >terfenadine 60 mg >loratadine 10 mg >astemizole 10 mg >chlorpheniramine 4 mg >placebo. (From Simons FER, et al. A double-blind, single-dose, crossover comparison of cetirizine, terfenadine, loratadine, astemizole, and chlorpheniramine versus placebo: Suppressive effects on histamine-induced wheals and flares during 24 hours in normal subjects. J Allergy Clin Immunol 86:540, 1990.)

nists, though commonly used as "rescue" medications, should, if possible, be given before exposure to allergen in order to achieve maximum efficacy (Simons and Simons, 1994).

The pharmacokinetics of terfenadine and cetirizine do not change during chronic administration. Subsensitivity (tachyphylaxis) to the peripheral H_1-receptor blocking activity of terfenadine, loratadine, and cetirizine has generally not been found in wheal and flare studies or in allergic rhinitis studies conducted over 5 to 12 weeks during which compliance has been closely monitored.

Clinical Use of H_1-Receptor Antagonists

H_1-antagonists provide effective treatment for mild-to-moderate seasonal and perennial allergic rhinoconjunctivitis in which the symptoms of nasal itching, sneezing, watery rhinorrhea, ocular itching, redness, and tearing predominate. They do not relieve nasal blockage effectively, and this is the rationale for marketing them in fixed-dose combination with an oral decongestant, usually pseudoephedrine. The second-generation H_1-antagonists terfenadine, astemizole, loratadine, cetirizine, or acrivastine, administered in manufacturers' recommended doses, provide greater relief of allergic rhinitis symptoms than placebo and are as effective as chlorpheniramine and other first-generation H_1-antagonists. The newer H_1-antagonists are believed to be similar in efficacy to each other, although no comprehensive, direct comparison of all of them exists. Topical H_1-antagonists such as levocabastine and azelastine provide rapid, sustained relief of itching, sneezing, and rhinorrhea.

In allergic rhinoconjunctivitis, second-generation H_1-antagonists such as terfenadine are as effective as cromolyn, but less effective than topical intranasal glucocorticoids; however, patients treated with an H_1-antagonist in combination with a topical intranasal glucocorticoid have better relief of ocular symptoms than patients treated with a glucocorticoid alone.

In chronic urticaria, second-generation H_1-antagonists such as terfenadine, astemizole, loratadine, or cetirizine relieve pruritus and reduce the number, size, and duration of wheals. They are probably as effective as their predecessors, although in one study, terfenadine, 120 mg daily, was less effective than hydroxyzine, 100 mg daily. In some patients with urticaria refractory to treatment with an H_1-antagonist alone, concurrent treatment with an H_2-antagonist such as cimetidine or ranitidine enhances relief of pruritus and wheal formation.

In atopic dermatitis, based on a few short-duration studies in small numbers of patients, the second-generation relatively nonsedating H_1-antagonists in recommended doses may be no more effective than first-generation H_1-antagonists such as diphenhydramine or hydroxyzine for relief of pruritus.

In asthma, pretreatment with H_1-antagonists provides some protection against bronchospasm induced by histamine, exercise, cold dry air, hyperventilation, hypertonic or hypotonic saline, distilled water, adenosine-5-monophosphate, or allergen. The amount of protection varies with the H_1-antagonist, the dose, and the stimulus used for bronchoconstriction. *H_1-antagonists do no harm in asthma and may contribute to symptom relief in mild chronic asthma.* The clinical importance of this effect is probably small and generally occurs at doses higher than those required for relief of allergic rhinitis symptoms (Frew and Holgate, 1993; Simons and Simons, 1994). Ketotifen, which has prominent anti-allergic effects, is used in some countries for treatment of asthma in infancy and early childhood.

Adverse Effects

In manufacturers' recommended doses, the second-generation H_1-antagonists produce the same incidence of central nervous system functional impairment as placebo does, as determined using subjective symptom scores and a variety of objective performance tests and electroencephalographic tests. They produce significantly less impairment than first-generation H_1-antagonists. They do not interact with other central nervous system–active chemicals such as alcohol or diazepam. Lack of central nervous system adverse effects is their major advantage, as they are not necessarily more effective than the first-generation H_1-antagonists.

The second-generation H_1-antagonists do not cause dry mouth, urinary retention, or other anticholinergic effects. Astemizole occasionally causes increased appetite and inappropriate weight gain. Azelastine may cause dysgeusia (metallic taste) when administered orally and, less commonly, when applied topically to the nasal mucosa.

H_1-antagonists may affect cardiac repolarization. Rarely astemizole and terfenadine, administered in overdose or to patients with preexisting hepatic or cardiac disorders, or concomitantly with a cytochrome P_{450} inhibitor such as ketoconazole or erythromycin, may prolong the QTc interval and cause ventricular arrhythmias, including torsade de pointes (Simons, 1994).

DECONGESTANTS (α-ADRENERGIC AGONISTS AND IMIDAZOLINES)

Structure and Activity

The chemical structure of α-adrenergic agonists determines their specificity and efficacy (Fig. 16–15). Phenylephrine is a direct α_1-adrenergic agonist. Phenylpropanolamine has an indirect effect on α_1 receptors. Pseudoephedrine is nonselective, i.e. mediates vasoconstriction via α_1 and α_2 receptors and also has β_1 and β_2 effects. The imidazoline xylometazoline and its hydroxy-derivatives (oxymetazoline, naphazoline, and antazoline), applied topically, stimulate both α_1 and α_2 receptors, especially the latter, causing local vasoconstriction (Brown, 1992).

Mechanism of Action

α-Adrenergic receptors are located in the plasma membrane of many cell types in the body. Two types, α_1 and α_2, have been defined pharmacologically and physiologically, and seven distinct subtypes, α_{1A}, α_{1B}, α_{1C}, and α_{2A}, α_{2B}, α_{2C}, and α_{2D}, have been cloned. α-Adrenergic receptors elicit changes in cellular metabolism by interaction with cell membrane receptors that are coupled to intracellular effector enzymes by guanine nucleotide–binding regulatory proteins (G-proteins) and exert their effect via G-protein-mediated signal transduction.

α_1 Receptors are found on postjunctional (postsynaptic) membranes, in arterioles in the skin, mucosa, viscera, and kidney (resistance vessels), and in veins throughout the body, where response to receptor activation consists of vasoconstriction. α_2 Receptors are found on presynaptic nerve endings, where receptor activation results in inhibition of norepinephrine release, and on postsynaptic membranes in the central nervous system, where response to receptor activation results in decreased sympathetic tone.

Whether administered by mouth or topically, decongestants decrease the volume of blood in the nasal mucosal capacitance vessels (sinusoids), which have a rich sympathetic innervation. They thereby reduce the blood supply to the nasal mucosa, decrease mucosal edema, decrease the amount of fluid on the mucosal surface, and increase nasal patency (Fig. 16–16) (Wight and Cochrane, 1989; Witek et al, 1992).

Pharmacokinetics/Pharmacodynamics

Phenylephrine administered orally has such poor bioavailability that it is of little therapeutic value via this route. Phenylpropanolamine and pseudoephedrine are well absorbed when administered orally and have serum elimination half-life values of approximately 4 and 6 hours, respectively. Phenylpropanolamine is metabolized to an active hydroxylate; however, 63 to 73 percent of a dose is excreted in the urine as unchanged drug. Pseudoephedrine is also largely excreted unchanged in the urine.

Systemic absorption of imidazolines occurs after topical application, but there is little

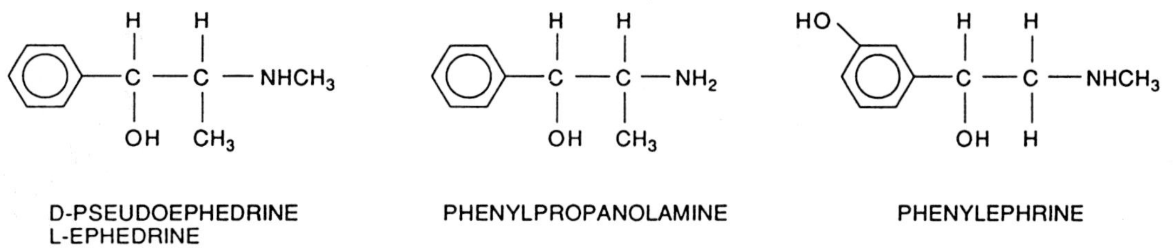

FIGURE 16–15. The chemical structure of α-adrenergic agonists.

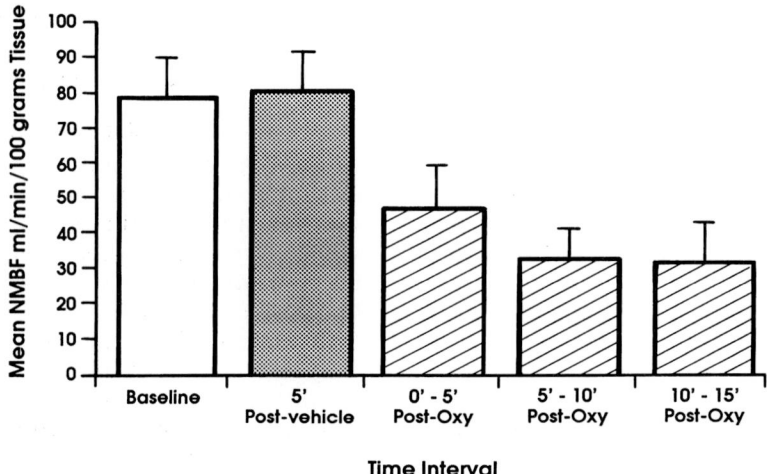

FIGURE 16–16. In seven subjects, the effect of oxymetazoline, 60 μg on nasal mucosal blood flow was measured by laser Doppler velocimetry. Nasal airflow was measured by anterior rhinomanometry, and subjectively perceived airflow was measured by visual analog scales (not shown). A reduction of nasal mucosal blood flow was observed following oxymetazoline, but not after vehicle application at 5, 10, and 15 minutes, and was accompanied by subjective relief of congestion. Nasal airflow did not change significantly. (From Witek RG Jr, et al. Superficial nasal mucosal blood flow and nasal patency following topical oxymetozoline hydrochloride. Ann Allergy 68:165, 1992.)

published information about imidazoline pharmacokinetics and pharmacodynamics.

Clinical Usage

Orally administered α-adrenergic agents are useful in relieving the symptom of nasal congestion or blockage and have been objectively documented to decrease nasal resistance. Phenylpropanolamine, 37.5 mg, or pseudoephedrine, 60 mg, needs to be administered every 6 hours, but long-acting formulations are available, permitting administration of phenylpropanolamine, 75 mg, or pseudoephedrine, 120 mg, every 12 hours. Both these medications are commonly used in fixed-dose combinations with other medications such as an H_1-antagonist.

Topical decongestants such as phenylephrine, xylometazoline, and oxymetazoline have been demonstrated objectively to reduce blood flow in the nasal mucosa and improve nasal airflow, with concomitant, rapid, subjective relief of nasal obstruction. These medications facilitate visualization and rhinoscopic evaluation of the upper airway. They are also useful during initiation of intranasal glucocorticoid treatment in patients with severe nasal blockage, or on a temporary basis during air travel, or for decreasing obstruction of the sinus ostia in patients whose allergic rhinitis is complicated by sinusitis (Wight and Cochrane, 1989; Witek et al, 1992).

Adverse Effects

An overdose of phenylpropanolamine or pseudoephedrine may result in hypertension, cardiac arrhythmias, stroke, seizures, psychosis, renal failure, and fatality. In manufacturers' recommended doses, phenylpropanolamine may cause night terrors in children, insomnia and nervousness in patients of any age, and elevation of blood pressure; pseudoephedrine seems less likely to cause these effects than phenylpropanolamine. There is a relative contraindication to the use of oral decongestants in patients with hypertension, heart disease, seizure disorder, or hyperthyroidism, and in those receiving concomitant treatment with monoamine oxidase inhibitors, tricyclic antidepressants, or methyldopa.

In infants and young children, absorption of topically applied phenylephrine or imidazoline derivatives such as xylometazoline and oxymetazoline may cause systemic adverse effects, including central nervous system depression, coma, reduction in body temperature, and apnea.

Topical decongestants are highly effective and have a rapid onset of action. Repeated use may lead to rebound congestion, and prolonged use may cause chronic rhinitis, secondary hyperemia, tachyphylaxis, and nasal mucosa irritability, the so-called "rhinitis medicamentosa." Relief of this condition can be obtained only by withdrawal of the offending decongestant and treatment with inhaled glucocorticoids. Irreversible nasal changes secondary to the use of imidazoline derivatives have not been documented.

PHARMACOLOGIC MANAGEMENT: THE FUTURE

New classes of anti-inflammatory medications and new bronchodilators will be introduced for the therapy of asthma and other allergic disorders during the next few years (Barnes, 1992; Frew and Holgate, 1993; Morley, 1993).

Mediator Antagonists

While experience with H_1-receptor antagonists suggests that it is unlikely that antagonizing a single mediator will ever be a panacea in the treatment of allergic disorders, development of these specific antagonists teaches us much about the pathophysiology of these disorders.

Several antagonists for lipid mediators are currently undergoing clinical trials (Bjornsdottir and Bush, 1993). Leukotriene D_4 (LTD_4) antagonists such as MK 571, LY 171883, SK&F 104353, and ICI 204, 219 provide significant protection against some bronchoconstrictors such as exercise challenge and inhibit the early and late response to allergen. They offer no protection against histamine or methacholine-induced challenges. They have a modest, dose-related effect in decreasing symptoms and need for "rescue" medication in patients with chronic asthma. Aspirin-sensitive patients may particularly benefit from LTD_4 antagonists.

PAF antagonists have been developed. UK74,505 in a single oral dose inhibits the airway effects of inhaled PAF for up to 24 hours, but is ineffective in allergen challenge tests.

A potent and stable bradykinin (BK2) receptor antagonist, HOE-140, has been developed.

Inhibition of neurogenic inflammation using antagonists of sensory neuropeptides such as substance P, neurokinin A, and calcitonin gene-related peptide are being developed. A potent neurokinin 1 (NK_1) antagonist CP96,345 seems to be effective in blocking the inflammatory effects of tachykinins released endogenously by nerve stimulation. Inhibition of peptide release from C fibers by stable, peripherally active opioid antagonists is also being studied.

Enzyme Inhibitors

Cyclooxygenase inhibitors, which decrease or prevent the formation of prostaglandins and thromboxane, do not seem to be of any therapeutic value in asthma and may actually make aspirin-sensitive asthmatics worse. The 5-lipoxygenase inhibitors such as zileuton or MK-886, which binds to a 5-lipoxygenase–activating protein (FLAP) in the cell membrane, inhibit formation of 5-lipoxygenase products including leukotriene B_4, leukotriene C_4, and leukotriene D_4. Zileuton protects against challenge with leukotrienes, cold air, or allergen and is also effective in chronic asthma when administered orally four times daily.

Chloride Channel Blockers

Inhaled furosemide protects against challenge with exercise, fog, allergen, sodium metabisulfite, and adenosine and also inhibits induced cough, perhaps by blocking a type of chloride channel necessary for the activation of inflammatory cells and sensory nerves. It causes diuresis when inhaled in high concentrations, but derivatives with reduced diuretic potency or other selective chloride channel blockers may be developed in the future.

Immunomodulators

Cyclosporine A inhibits T lymphocyte function. In low doses, it has a steroid-sparing effect in patients with extremely severe asthma.

Medications that block the production or action of cytokines involved in the inflammatory response in asthma may be useful. Studies of human recombinant IL-1 receptor antagonist are under way, and an antibody to IL-5 has been developed. Monoclonal antibodies that inhibit cell adhesion molecules may be useful therapeutically in asthma. A monoclonal antibody to intracellular adhesion molecule 1 on endothelial cells has been studied in primates. IgE synthesis by lymphocytes is dependent on IL-4; thus IL-4 synthesis inhibitors or receptor antagonists might be useful. Peptides that block allergen-induced immune reactions at the level of the interaction between the antigen-presenting cell and the T lymphocyte appear to be promising.

Bronchodilators

Phosphodiesterase isoenzymes involved in human smooth muscle contraction (type III) and inflammation (type IV) comprise a small percentage of total phosphodiesterase activity. A variety of selective phosphodiesterase isoenzyme inhibitors are being developed.

Selective M_3 antagonists, which block only postjunctional receptors on smooth muscle cells, may be more useful than nonselective muscarinic antagonists.

Cyclic guanosine 3'5'-monophosphate (cGMP) stimulators include atrial natriuretic factor and nitro compounds such as isosorbide dinitrate, glyceryl trinitrate, and sodium nitroprusside, which activate soluble guanylate cyclase and cause dose-dependent relaxation of airway smooth muscle.

Medications that block calcium entry through voltage-dependent calcium channels have not been effective in asthma, in contrast to heparin and other medications that inhibit release of calcium from intracellular stores or inhibit phosphoinositide turnover.

Opening of potassium channels results in relaxation of smooth muscle and inhibition of secretions. Potassium channel activators are currently being developed as anti-asthma compounds, with attempts being made to separate the bronchodilator from the hemodynamic effects.

CONCLUSION

The pharmacologic management of asthma, rhinitis, and other allergic disorders has improved remarkably during the past two decades. Further advances are imminent, as several medications in preclinical and clinical development significantly modify the complex inflammatory response that is the hallmark of these disorders.

REFERENCES

Agertoft L, Pedersen S. Effects of long-term treatment with an inhaled corticosteroid on growth and pulmonary function in asthmatic children. Respir Med 88:373–381, 1994.

Barnes PJ. Muscarinic receptors in airways: recent developments. J Appl Physiol 68:1777–1785, 1990.

Barnes PJ. New drugs for asthma. Eur Respir J 5:1126–1136, 1992.

Barnes PJ, Pedersen S. Efficacy and safety of inhaled corticosteroids in asthma. Am Rev Respir Dis 148:S1–S26, 1993.

Bel EH, Timmers MC, Hermans J, Dijkman JH, Sterk PJ. The long-term effects of nedocromil sodium and beclomethasone dipropionate on bronchial responsiveness to methacholine in nonatopic asthmatic subjects. Am Rev Respir Dis 141:21–28, 1990.

Bjornsdottir US, Bush RK. Leukotriene antagonists and inhibitors. Immunol Allergy Clin North Am 13:861–890, 1993.

Brenner M, Berkowitz R, Marshall N, Strunk RC. Need for theophylline in severe steroid-requiring asthmatics. Clin Allergy 18:143–150, 1988.

Brogden RN, Faulds D. Salmeterol xinafoate. A review of its pharmacological properties and therapeutic potential in reversible obstructive airways disease. Drugs 42:895–912, 1991.

Brogden RN, McTavish D. Budesonide. An updated review of its pharmacological properties, and therapeutic efficacy in asthma and rhinitis. Drugs 44:375–407, 1992.

Brogden RN, Sorkin EM. Nedocromil sodium. An updated review of its pharmacological properties and therapeutic efficacy in asthma. Drugs 45:693–715, 1993.

Brown OM. Adrenergic drugs. In Smith CM, Reynard AM (eds). Textbook of Pharmacology. Philadelphia, WB Saunders Company, 141–167, 1992.

Bryson HM, Faulds D. Intranasal fluticasone propionate. A review of its pharmacodynamic and pharmacokinetic properties and therapeutic potential in allergic rhinitis. Drugs 43:760–775, 1992.

Chapman KR, Kesten S, Szalai JP. Regular vs as-needed salbutamol in asthma control. Lancet 343:1379–1382, 1994.

Cheung D, Timmers MC, Zwinderman AH, Bel EH, Dijkman JH, Sterk PJ. Long-term effects of a long-acting β_2-adrenoceptor agonist, salmeterol, on airway hyperresponsiveness in patients with mild asthma. N Engl J Med 327:1198–1203, 1992.

Cockcroft DW, McParland CP, O'Byrne PM, et al. Beclomethasone given after the early asthmatic response inhibits the late response and the increased methacholine responsiveness and cromolyn does not. J Allergy Clin Immunol 91:1163–1168, 1993.

Crimi E, Violante B, Pellegrino R, Brusasco V. Effect of multiple doses of nedocromil sodium given after allergen inhalation in asthma. J Allergy Clin Immunol 92:777–783, 1993.

Cypcar D, Busse WW. Steroid-resistant asthma. J Allergy Clin Immunol 92:362–372, 1993.

Dukes MNG, Holgate ST, Pauwels RA. Report of an international workshop on risk and safety of asthma therapy. Clin Exp Allergy 24:160–165, 1994.

Faulds D, Hollingshead LM, Goa KL. Formoterol. A review of its pharmacological properties and therapeutic potential in reversible obstructive airways disease. Drugs 42:115–137, 1991.

Frew AJ, Holgate ST. Clinical pharmacology of asthma. Implications for treatment. Drugs 46:847–862, 1993.

Gross NJ. Ipratropium bromide. N Engl J Med 319:486–494, 1988.

Haahtela T, Järvinen M, Kava T, et al. Comparison of a β_2-agonist, terbutaline, with an inhaled corticosteroid, budesonide, in newly detected asthma. N Engl J Med 325:388–392, 1991.

Hargreave FE, Dolovich J, Newhouse MT. The assessment and treatment of asthma: A conference report. J Allergy Clin Immunol 85:1098–1111, 1990.

Hoag JE, McFadden ER Jr. Long-term effect of cromolyn sodium on nonspecific bronchial hyperresponsiveness: A review. Ann Allergy 66:53–63, 1991.

Holgate ST, Djukanovic R, Wilson J, Roche W, Britten K, Howarth PH. Allergic inflammation and its pharmacological modulation in asthma. Int Arch Allergy Appl Immunol 94:210–217, 1991.

Holliday SM, Faulds D, Sorkin EM. Inhaled fluticasone propionate. A review of its pharmacodynamic and pharmacokinetic properties, and therapeutic use in asthma. Drugs 47:318–331, 1994.

Hummel S, Lehtonen L, and Study Group. Comparison of oral-steroid sparing by high-dose and low-dose inhaled steroid in maintenance treatment of severe asthma. Lancet 340:1483–1487, 1992.

Meltzer EO. Anticholinergic treatment of nasal disorders. Immunol Allergy Clin North Am 11:35–44, 1991.

Meltzer EO, Orgel HA, Bronsky EA, et al. Ipratropium bromide aqueous nasal spray for patients with perennial allergic rhinitis: A study of its effect on their symptoms, quality of life, and nasal cytology. J Allergy Clin Immunol 90:242–249, 1992.

Milgrom H, Bender B. Current issues in the use of theophylline. Am Rev Respir Dis 147:S33–S39, 1993.

Morley J. Immunopharmacology of asthma. Immunology Today 14:317–322, 1993.

Murphy S, Kelly HW. Cromolyn sodium: a review of mechanisms and clinical use in asthma. DICP 21:22–35, 1987.

Mygind N. Glucocorticosteroids and rhinitis. Allergy 48:476–490, 1993.

Pearlman DS, Chervinsky P, LaForce C, et al. A comparison of salmeterol with albuterol in the treatment of mild-to-moderate asthma. N Engl J Med 327:1420–1425, 1992.

Persson CGA. Xanthines as airway anti-inflammatory drugs. J Allergy Clin Immunol 81:615–617, 1988.

Ramage L, Lipworth BJ, Ingram CG, Cree IA, Dhillon DP. Reduced protection against exercise induced bronchoconstriction after chronic dosing with salmeterol. Respir Med 88:363–368, 1994.

Rimmer SJ, Church MK. The pharmacology and mechanisms of action of histamine H_1-antagonists. Clin Exp Allergy 20:3–17, 1990.

Ruggieri F, Patalano F. Nedocromil sodium: a review of clinical studies. Eur Respir J 2:568s–571s, 1989.

Schleimer RP. Glucocorticosteroids. Their mechanisms of action and use in allergic diseases. In Middleton E Jr, Reed CE, Ellis EF, Adkinson NF Jr, Yunginger JW, Busse WW (eds). Allergy Principles and Practice. St. Louis, Mosby–Year Book, 1993, pp 893–925.

Schuller DE, Selcow JE, Joos TH, et al. A multicenter trial of nedocromil sodium, 1% nasal solution, compared with cromolyn sodium and placebo in ragweed seasonal allergic rhinitis. J Allergy Clin Immunol 86:554–561, 1990.

Sears MR, Taylor DR, Print CG, et al. Regular inhaled beta-agonist treatment in bronchial asthma. Lancet 336:1391–1396, 1990.

Sessler CN. Theophylline toxicity: clinical features of 116 consecutive cases. Am J Med 88:567–576, 1990.

Shapiro GG, Sharpe M, DeRouen TA, et al. Cromolyn versus triamcinolone acetonide for youngsters with moderate asthma. J Allergy Clin Immunol 88:742–748, 1991.

Simons FER. H_1-receptor antagonists. Comparative tolerability and safety. Drug Safety 10:350–380, 1994.

Simons FER, McMillan JL, Simons KJ. A double-blind, single-dose, crossover comparison of cetirizine, terfenadine, loratadine, astemizole, and chlorpheniramine versus placebo: Suppressive effects on histamine-induced wheals and flares during 24 hours in normal subjects. J Allergy Clin Immunol 86:540–547, 1990.

Simons FER, Persaud MP, Gillespie CA, Cheang M, Shuckett EP. Absence of posterior subcapsular cataracts in young patients treated with inhaled glucocorticoids. Lancet 342:776–778, 1993.

Simons FER, Simons KJ. The pharmacology and use of H_1-receptor antagonist drugs. N Engl J Med 330:1663–1670, 1994.

Simons FER, Soni NR, Watson WTA, Becker AB. Bronchodilator and bronchoprotective effects of salmeterol in young patients with asthma. J Allergy Clin Immunol 90:840–846, 1992.

Snell NJC. Drug interactions with anti-asthma medication. Respir Med 88:83–88, 1994.

Suissa S, Ernst P, Boivin J-F, et al. A cohort analysis of excess mortality in asthma and the use of inhaled β-agonists. Am J Respir Crit Care Med 149:604–610, 1994.

Sullivan P, Bekir S, Jaffar Z, Page C, Jeffery P, Costello J. Anti-inflammatory effects of low-dose oral theophylline in atopic asthma. Lancet 343:1006–1008, 1994.

Szefler SJ. Glucocorticoid therapy for asthma: clinical pharmacology. J Allergy Clin Immunol 88:147–165, 1991.

Tinkelman DG, Reed CE, Nelson HS, Offord KP. Aerosol beclomethasone dipropionate compared with theophylline as primary treatment of chronic, mild to moderately severe asthma in children. Pediatrics 92:64–77, 1993.

Toogood JH. Complications of topical steroid therapy for asthma. Am Rev Respir Dis 141:S89–S96, 1990.

Van Essen-Zandvliet EE, Hughes MD, Waalkens HJ, et al. Effects of 22 months of treatment with inhaled corticosteroids and/or beta-2-agonists on lung function, airway responsiveness, and symptoms in children with asthma. Am Rev Respir Dis 146:547–554, 1992.

van Schayck CP, Graafsma SJ, Visch MB, Dompeling E, van Weel C, van Herwaarden CLA. Increased bronchial hyperresponsiveness after inhaling salbutamol during 1 year is not caused by subsensitization to salbutamol. J Allergy Clin Immunol 86:793–800, 1990.

Weinberger M, Hendeles L. Theophylline. *In* Middleton E Jr, Reed CE, Ellis EF, Adkinson NF Jr, Yunginger JW, Busse WW (eds). Allergy Principles and Practice. St. Louis, Mosby-Year Book, 816–855, 1993.

Wight RG, Cochrane T. A comparison of the effects of xylometazoline on nasal airflow, and on blood flux as measured by Laser Doppler flowmetry. Acta Otolaryngol (Stockh) 108:284–289, 1989.

Witek TJ Jr, Canestrari DA, Hernandez JR, Miller RD, Yang JY, Riker DK. Superficial nasal mucosal blood flow and nasal patency following topical oxymetazoline hydrochloride. Ann Allergy 68:165–168, 1992.

Wong CS, Pavord ID, Williams J, Britton JR, Tattersfield AE. Bronchodilator, cardiovascular, and hypokalaemic effects of fenoterol, salbutamol, and terbutaline in asthma. Lancet 336:1396–1399, 1990.

Chapter 17

Immunotherapy for Allergic Disease

Dennis K. Ledford, M.D., and Richard F. Lockey, M.D.

Immunotherapy has its roots in the advances of immunology that occurred at the end of the nineteenth and the beginning of the twentieth century. The initial rationale for immunotherapy was incorrect. The original concept was that allergic rhinitis and conjunctivitis were caused by toxins released by pollen particles. It was thought that protective antibody, or antitoxin, would develop when subjects with this disease were vaccinated, or immunized, with pollen extracts. This approach had been originally used by Behring and Kitasato in 1890 for toxins produced by diphtheria and clostridia bacteria.

The evolving concept of anaphylaxis, beginning with Portier and Richet in 1902, and astute clinical observations of human allergic disease directed investigators to conclude that the mechanism responsible for clinical allergy is a hypersensitivity reaction, not exposure to exogenous toxins. Immunotherapy is a form of immunomodulation that decreases allergen hypersensitivity. During the succeeding decades, the clinical experience and majority of clinical trials have attested to the efficacy of immunotherapy.

IMMUNOLOGIC EFFECTS

Immunotherapy is not desensitization since clinical improvement occurs despite the persistence, and occasional increase, of specific IgE antibody (Creticos et al, 1984). The mechanism by which immunotherapy is effective in allergic disorders remains incompletely defined. The following hypotheses are partially supported by clinical and scientific data.

"BLOCKING ANTIBODY." Immunotherapy induces allergen-specific IgG or "blocking antibody," which competes with IgE for allergen binding (Fig. 17–1) (Løwenstein et al, 1986; Muller et al, 1986; Van Metre et al, 1982). There are a few studies demonstrating clinical improvement in the absence of an increase in allergen-specific IgG, but the bulk of evidence shows a correlation between reduced symptom and medication scores and serum levels of specific IgG (Creticos et al, 1993; Golden et al, 1989; Sadan et al, 1969). However, within study populations there are individuals with a significant increase in allergen-specific IgG without clinical improvement. The role of IgG in affecting allergic symptoms has been better established in insect venom sensitivity than in inhalant allergy (Djurup et al, 1985). This may be due to the other mitigating factors applicable only to inhalant sensitivity.

DECREASE IN IgE. Immunotherapy results in a reduction of allergen-specific IgE (Djurup et al, 1985). The decrease in specific IgE is gradual, although IgE levels increase initially in response to treatment (Creticos et al, 1984; Ewan et al, 1988). Studies with ragweed immunotherapy also show a decrease in the postseasonal rise in IgE (Fig. 17–2) (Van Metre et al, 1982). However, symptoms often improve before the levels of allergen-specific IgE have decreased or even when the levels have increased (Creticos et al, 1984). Thus, since there is no clinical correlation with specific IgE levels, IgE need not be monitored during immunotherapy.

MODULATION OF MAST CELLS AND BASOPHILS. Immunotherapy modulates target cell

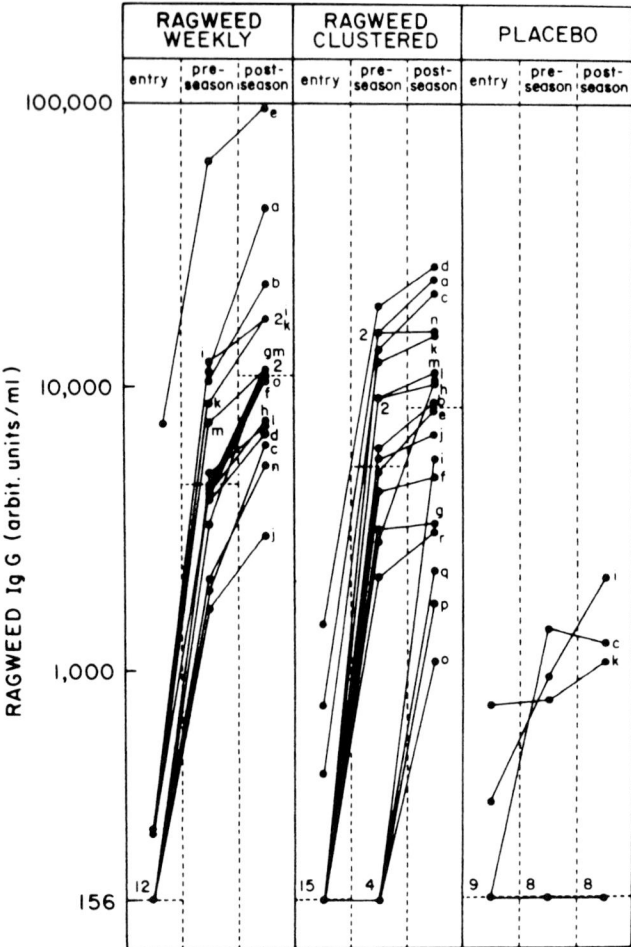

FIGURE 17–1. The levels of serum-specific IgG for ragweed before immunotherapy and during immunotherapy, both prior to the ragweed pollen season and following the season. The amount of ragweed-specific IgG is presented in arbitrary units on the abscissa. The entry levels (before immunotherapy) were assayed on samples collected for February 21 to March 12, the preseason levels (during immunotherapy) July 21 to August 6, and the postseason levels (during immunotherapy), October 10 to October 27. The median levels of ragweed-specific IgG are displayed by the horizontal dashed lines. The lower-case letters and numbers designate the results of individual study subjects and correspond to Figure 17–2. The amount of ragweed-specific IgG increased with immunotherapy and increased further following ragweed pollen exposure during immunotherapy. There was no change in the level of ragweed-specific IgG in a group of ragweed-allergic subjects receiving placebo injections. (From Van Metre TE Jr, Adkinson NF Jr, Amodio FJ, et al. A comparison of immunotherapy schedules for injection treatment of ragweed pollen hay fever. J Allergy Clin Immunol 69:181, 1982.)

function and thereby reduces mediator release from mast cells and basophils, in spite of the presence of specific IgE on their surfaces (Mendoza and Minagawa, 1982). Such an effect has been demonstrated by a post-immunotherapy decrease of histamine release from peripheral blood basophils following *in vitro* allergen challenge, which preceded a decrease in specific IgE or an increase in specific IgG. A decrease in skin test and nasal reactivity prior to changes in IgE and IgG antibody levels probably results from this reduction of mediator release from mast cells and basophils despite allergen-IgE interaction on cell membranes (Creticos et al, 1984; Pienkowski et al, 1985). This is not the final hypothesis. Suppression by immunotherapy of the late-phase allergic response, which is due to inflammatory cells attracted by mast cell and basophil chemoattractants, also suggests that the cellular modulation of IgE-mediated disease is clinically important (Price et al, 1988).

INCREASE IN SUPPRESSOR LYMPHOCYTE ACTIVITY AND MODULATION OF OTHER REGULATORY CELLS. Immunotherapy alters regulatory cellular networks, in part, by increasing T lymphocyte suppressor activity (Rocklin et al, 1980). IgE production, maturation of select mast cell populations, macrophage activation, mediator release from mast cells and basophils, and bone marrow cellular responses are all regulated by T lymphocytes (Tamir et al, 1987). Therefore, alteration in T cell function affects allergic mechanisms. Alteration of T cell function following immunotherapy has only been demonstrated in a few studies (Dominiguez et al, 1983; Fennerty et al, 1988; Hseih, 1989). In addition to lymphocytes, alveolar macrophages, platelets, mononuclear cells, and vascular endothelial cells produce

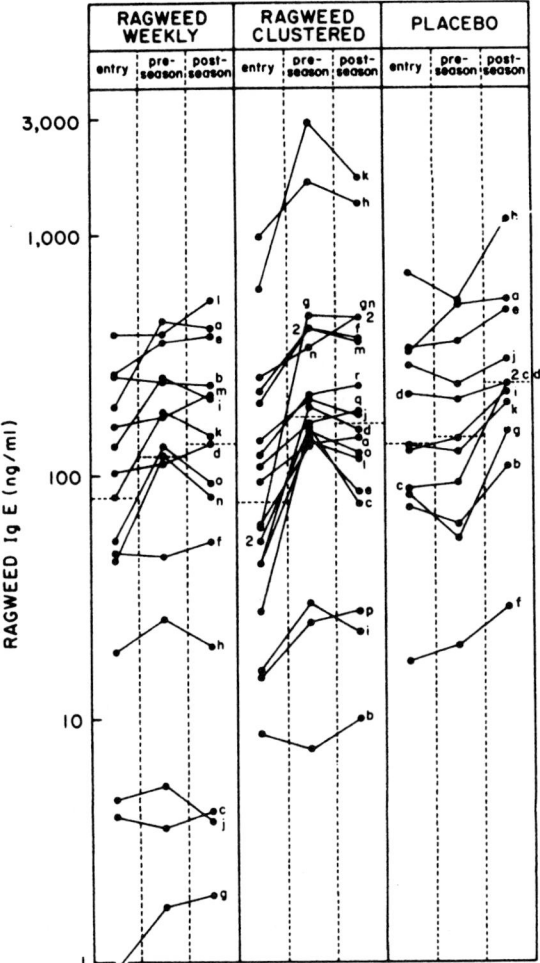

FIGURE 17-2. The levels of serum-specific IgE for ragweed before immunotherapy and during immunotherapy, both prior to the ragweed pollen season and following the season. The amount of allergen-specific IgE is presented in a semilogarithmic plot of ng/ml on the abscissa. The entry levels (before immunotherapy) were assayed on samples collected for February 21 to March 12, the preseason levels (during immunotherapy), July 21 to August 6, and the postseason levels (during immunotherapy), October 10 to October 27. The median levels of ragweed-specific IgE are displayed by the horizontal dashed lines. The lower-case letters and numbers designate the results for individual study subjects and correspond to Figure 17–1. Levels of the placebo group rose from a median of 132 ng/ml at entry to 141 ng/ml before the season and to 243 ng/ml after the season. IgE increase from before to after the season was significant in the placebo-treated group (p = 0.007) but the increase was not significant in the immunotherapy groups. However, the levels of ragweed-specific IgE did not decrease in the immunotherapy groups despite clinical improvement. (From Van Metre TE Jr, Adkinson NF Jr, Amodio FJ, et al. A comparison of immunotherapy schedules for injection treatment of ragweed pollen hay fever. J Allergy Clin Immunol 69:181, 1982.)

factors that release histamine from mast cells and basophils. Severity of asthma and bronchial hyperreactivity correlates with basophil responsiveness to histamine-releasing factors and with the spontaneous production of histamine-releasing factors (Alum et al, 1987). Grass pollen immunotherapy followed by grass pollen challenge results in decreased production of histamine-releasing factors (Kuna et al, 1989). Thus, these intricate cellular networks that regulate allergy may be affected by immunotherapy.

ALLERGEN EXTRACTS

The methods used to manufacture aqueous allergen extracts has not changed appreciably since the initial report of the efficacy of "hypodermic inoculation of pollen vaccine" in 1911. A certain mass of source material, for example a pure pollen, is mixed with a given volume of a buffered solution. The extractable proteins are dissolved, the insoluble material removed, and a preservative added to maintain allergen stability (Van Metre and Adkinson, 1991).

That equipotent, standardized extracts are necessary for immunotherapy has been recognized for years. Physicochemical parameters—such as weight/volume (weight of raw material per volume of buffer) and protein nitrogen units (PNU)—were initially used in an attempt to quantify potency. The complexity of allergenic extracts, containing from 10 to 80 different antigens, resulted in the failure of the physicochemical means described (Løwenstein et al, 1991).

The immunochemical techniques developed following the discovery of IgE permit more precise characterization of the antigenic and allergenic components of available extracts. These techniques include the radioallergosorbent test (RAST), enzyme-linked immunosorbent assay (ELISA), RAST inhibition, ELISA inhibition, crossed radioimmunoelectrophoresis, and immunoblots utilizing electrophoretic separation of components by their isoelectric points or molecular weights (Løwenstein et al, 1991). These procedures demonstrate that 25 to 50 percent of the detectable antigens contained in an extract are allergenic (Weeke et al, 1983). Major allergens are antigens recognized by IgE contained in 50 percent of sera from selected, clinically allergic subjects. Immunochemically pure extracts can be prepared that contain the relevant, specific allergens in appropriate ratios and no irrelevant antigens.

There are two principal methods of standardizing allergen extracts:

1. Measuring potency with bioassays of histamine release, quantitative skin tests and/or challenge studies or with non-bioassays of specific IgE with RAST or ELISA inhibition.
2. Measuring specific allergens by radial immunodiffusion (Mancini technique), crossed immunolectrophoresis and crossed radioimmunoelectrophoresis, rocket immunoelectrophoresis, gel electrophoresis, and immunoblots.

Both *in vivo* and *in vitro* tests are necessary, but their relative importance remains unclear (Løwenstein et al, 1991). *In vivo* assays provide a more direct index of allergen activity but are somewhat impractical for routine commercial use. *In vitro* assays are easier and more readily available, and they do not require selected patient populations on whom the tests are performed.

The formulation of international standards defining the process of allergen standardization has facilitated the production of standardized extracts used to assess uniformity of extracts manufactured world-wide. Standard reference extracts have been quantified, lyophilized, and stored to permit comparison of future extracts with these standards. The World Health Organization has the following standardized allergen extracts: short ragweed pollen, timothy grass pollen, *Dermatophagoides pteronyssinus*, birch pollen, and dog hair/dander. Standardized extracts of Bermuda grass pollen, *Alternaria alternata*, rye grass pollen, *Dermatophagoides farinae*, and cat hair/dander are currently being developed. Ultimately, the ideal is to have all allergen extracts standardized, thus facilitating the comparison of studies world-wide (Løwenstein et al, 1991).

PROOF OF EFFICACY

Rhinoconjunctivitis

Noon and Freeman first reported the efficacy of immunotherapy for hay fever in 1911. The clinical application of immunotherapy grew rapidly during the first half of the twentieth century despite the absence of controlled trials. This may be attributed to the high prevalence of allergic diseases, approximately 20 percent of the population, and the previously limited availability of effective pharmacologic therapy.

CLINICAL TRIALS. A variety of clinical trials, with variable blinding and control groups, have been done for seasonal and perennial allergic rhinitis since 1954 (Bousquet et al, 1990; Brunet et al, 1992; Creticos et al, 1993; D'Souza et al, 1973; Dreborg et al, 1986; Ewan et al, 1988; Franklin and Lowell, 1967; Horst et al, 1990; Meriney et al, 1986; Ortolani et al, 1984; Reid et al, 1986; Van Metre et al, 1982). Twenty-two of the 26 best-designed, double-blind trials demonstrated efficacy; 18 of 21 demonstrated an increase in allergen-specific IgG or a decrease in allergen-specific IgE, or both. Four of the remaining five did not measure humoral responses, and the one study showing clinical benefit without confirmatory humoral changes was of 3 months' duration and measured only antigen-specific IgE. Skin tests with allergens before and after immunotherapy were documented in nine of the 22 beneficial studies. Four showed no change and five demonstrated decreased skin test reactivity. Nasal allergen challenges were performed before and after immunotherapy in seven of the studies showing efficacy. Six of the seven demonstrated decreased nasal or conjunctival reactivity to the allergen used for immunotherapy. Basophil histamine release was decreased in one study following immunotherapy but unchanged in three others in which it was measured.

The four double-blind studies that did not demonstrate clinical improvement were similar in design to the positive trials. Immunologic changes observed in three of these negative studies include increased specific IgG in three and decreased IgE in one. Skin test reactivity decreased in one of the two negative studies in which it was measured, *in vitro* basophil histamine release was unchanged in one study, and nasal provocation with antigen was decreased in the one negative study in which it was measured. Thus, there is no obvious explanation for the negative results in these four trials.

In summary, the majority of the controlled trials with immunotherapy demonstrate beneficial clinical effects in both seasonal and perennial allergic rhinitis. Laboratory tests and challenge studies, in general, correlate with the clinical findings. However, the many exceptions indicate that there is not a specific confirmatory test to demonstrate clinical benefit. Symptom improvement remains the standard response variable.

Asthma

Fifteen of the 21 double-blind, placebo-controlled studies of asthma demonstrated clinical improvement following immunotherapy; three did not report clinical outcome; and three did not show improvement (Bousquet et al, 1990; Bruce et al, 1992; Creticos et al, 1993; Dreborg et al, 1986; Haugaard et al, 1992, 1993; Hedlin et al, 1986; Horst et al, 1990; Malling et al, 1986; Ortolani et al, 1984; Reid et al, 1986; Sundin et al, 1986; Taylor et al, 1974; Van Metre et al, 1988). Twelve of the 15 clinically efficacious studies demonstrated an increase in specific IgG following immunotherapy; only one displayed a decrease in specific IgE. None of the three studies in which *in vitro* release of histamine from basophils was assayed showed a change with immunotherapy. Eleven of the 15 studies showing efficacy measured bronchial responses to allergen challenge before and after immunotherapy. In nine of these, bronchial sensitivity to allergen decreased. Ten of the 15 documented allergen skin test changes; in eight of these, allergen skin test sensitivity decreased. Three of the controlled trials did not document clinical outcomes, but all three showed decreased bronchial sensitivity to allergen and an increase in allergen-specific IgG. Six studies measured bronchial hyperreactivity to methacholine or histamine before and after immunotherapy. In one of these, bronchial hyperreactivity decreased; the other five did not change. One of the three double-blind, controlled studies not showing clinical benefit demonstrated a decrease in skin test reactivity and an increase in specific IgG.

In summary, the majority of controlled trials demonstrated beneficial effects in both seasonal and perennial allergic asthma. Studies in which specific IgG was measured usually demonstrated an increase when clinical improvement was noted, but not always. There are fewer trials showing efficacy with immunotherapy in asthma than with rhinitis. This may be explained by (1) the difficulties of designing and performing such studies in asthma, (2) the lower prevalence of seasonal versus perennial asthma, (3) the effect of nonallergic factors that aggravate asthma (viral infections, sinusitis, pollutants, irritants, air temperature and humidity changes, esophageal reflux), and (4) coexisting diseases, such as chronic obstructive lung disease, which contribute to symptoms.

Insect Sting Anaphylaxis

A double-blind, placebo-controlled trial of venom and whole-body extract immunotherapy in individuals with a history of anaphylactic reactions to Hymenoptera stings demonstrated that only venoms were effective when subjects were tested by sting challenge (Hunt et al, 1978). Previous, uncontrolled trials using whole-body extract suggested effectiveness of such treatment, but this was not confirmed when treated subjects were purposely stung under controlled conditions. The use of venom extracts has facilitated the study of immunologic responses of Hymenoptera-hypersensitive individuals undergoing immunotherapy. Specific IgG usually increased with venom immunotherapy, and the higher maintenance doses were associated with higher levels of specific IgG (Hunt et al, 1978). Specific IgE generally increased initially and decreased after 3 years or more of treatment (Bousquet et al, 1989; Graft et al, 1987). However, use of specific IgG or specific IgE antibody levels did not permit prediction of the risk of anaphylactic reactions to stings in subjects who discontinued immunotherapy (Golden et al, 1989). A large study demonstrated excellent safety for immunotherapy using these standardized venom extracts (Lockey et al, 1990).

The available studies confirm clinical benefit with imported fire ant whole-body extract immunotherapy, which has also been shown to contain the venom-specific allergens (Freeman et al, 1992; Hoffman et al, 1991; Johansson et al, 1985; Reed et al, 1987; Strom et al, 1983; Watkins et al, 1987). However, treatment failures have been reported, and no double-blind trial with whole-body extract, venom, and placebo has been done (Lockey, 1974, 1990; Paull and Coghlan, 1986).

Food Allergy

There are no clinical studies to indicate that food immunotherapy, either oral or by injection, has a role in the management of allergic individuals. One group of investigators demonstrated efficacy with immunotherapy in peanut-sensitive subjects (Oppenheimer et al, 1992). However, more data are needed before such therapy can be recommended for routine clinical use. Food immunotherapy in highly allergic individuals may have a greater risk for severe, life-threatening reactions than inhalant immunotherapy (Oppenheimer et al, 1992).

Ineffective Methods of Immunotherapy

Low-dose immunotherapy, such as that recommended by Rinkel, have been used by some physicians for treatment of allergic disease (Rinkel, 1963). A skin test end-point titration to select a "safe" dose of allergen extract is used for low-dose treatment programs. The skin test end point is defined as the fivefold dilution of allergen extract that induces a positive intradermal skin test reaction sufficient to cause the wheal size to increase by 2 mm. Administration of the determined dose is claimed to relieve symptoms within minutes; the dose is repeated at intervals to maintain improvement, and the prolonged increase of dosage over weeks is allegedly not required. Local and systemic reactions rarely, if ever, occur because of the small amount of allergen administered. A large, placebo-controlled study of low-dose therapy (Rinkel method) utilizing mixed allergens administered over 2 years failed to demonstrate clinical benefit (Hirsch et al, 1981).

The idea that the pathogenesis of rhinitis and sinusitis is caused by bacteria in the nasal pharynx led to the hypothesis that immunization with bacterial extracts, derived from culture of the respiratory tract of the treated subject, would be beneficial (Morrey, 1913). Such bacterial vaccines were advocated for the treatment of recurrent rhinitis and sinusitis during the early part of the twentieth century. Such treatment was also advocated for asthma that was aggravated by respiratory infections. Those vaccines were shown not to be effective for treatment of asthma or any other respiratory tract disease, although they are still widely used (Frankland et al, 1955; Johnstone, 1974).

Dose Dependence of Immunotherapy

Larger amounts of administered allergen generally result in greater clinical and immunologic improvement. A comparison of two doses of allergen extract for treatment of ragweed hay fever demonstrated improvement only with the higher dose (up to 0.5 cc of 1:50 w/v extract) (Franklin and Lowell, 1967). A comparison of high-dose ragweed immunotherapy (11 μg of antigen E) with low-dose Rinkel immunotherapy (0.001 μg of antigen E) demonstrated clinical improvement and immunologic responses only in the high-dose group (Van Metre et al, 1982). Increasing the dose of immunotherapy beyond a certain level does not result in further improvement, as demonstrated by a ragweed study showing improvement with a twofold but not a fivefold increase in dose (Creticos et al, 1984). Studies of immunotherapy for asthma have led to similar conclusions. For example, improvement with immunotherapy in asthma due to cat allergen correlates with the dose of allergen administered (Ohman et al, 1984; Sundin et al, 1986; Taylor et al, 1974; Van Metre et al, 1988). The improvement was assessed both by clinical symptoms and by bronchial challenge with cat allergen. Comparison of several studies with venom immunotherapy demonstrates that a 100-μg maintenance dose is 96 to 100 percent effective following sting challenge, whereas a 50-μg maintenance dose is 79 percent effective (Golden et al, 1981). Thus, the data consistently indicate that clinical improvement following immunotherapy is dependent on the dose administered.

Summary

1. The beneficial effects of immunotherapy are limited to the allergens administered (Norman and Lichtenstein, 1978; Reid et al, 1986). Nonspecific reduction of allergic sensitivity or symptoms does not occur. Conflicting information exists as to whether bronchial hyperreactivity improves with immunotherapy (Hedlin et al, 1986; Malling et al, 1986; Meriney et al, 1986; Sundin et al, 1986; Van Metre et al, 1988). There may be some beneficial effects in decreasing hypersensitivity to allergens that cross-react antigenically with the allergen(s) administered.

2. Improvement is dose-dependent, although most available studies have not addressed this issue. Available data indicate that approximately 4 to 12 μg of an allergen is required for maintenance immunotherapy (Grammer et al, 1991).

3. Immunotherapy is most likely to benefit subjects who are highly sensitive. However, such subjects are at highest risk for anaphylaxis associated with immunotherapy (Lockey, 1974; Reid et al, 1993; Stewart and Lockey, 1992).

Additional studies are needed to address the following issues:

1. Additional standardized allergen extracts should be utilized for immunotherapy trials.
2. The appropriate maintenance dose for all allergens should be determined. Comparisons among studies are possible only if the amount of allergen administered is identified.
3. Multiple-allergen immunotherapy needs additional study since most allergic subjects are sensitive to many allergens, and the general rule is to administer multiple allergens per vial for treatment.
4. Outcome data are needed to compare pharmacologic management with immunotherapy. Such studies should assess the most cost-effective therapy, incorporating the risk/benefit ratios of pharmaco- and immunotherapy, the long-term anatomic and physiologic results, and life style issues. Additional information concerning the natural history of allergic disease, particularly asthma, is needed to make these assessments.
5. Additional studies are needed to explore the efficacy of immunotherapy in populations below 6 and over 50 years of age.
6. The optimal duration for immunotherapy needs to be determined.

CLINICAL APPLICATIONS OF IMMUNOTHERAPY

Indications

Table 17-1 suggests some considerations for utilizing immunotherapy (Bush et al, 1991). The symptoms or disease process should be consistent with known immunologic mechanisms, such as allergic asthma, allergic rhinoconjunctivitis, or insect sting anaphylaxis. Chronic urticaria, eczema, and food allergy have not been consistently benefited by immunotherapy, but treatment of severe atopic dermatitis with immunotherapy is a consideration in selected cases. Specific IgE for appropriate allergens must be documented, and symptoms should correlate with exposure to those specific allergens selected for immunotherapy. An exception to this recommendation, although not accepted by all investigators, is that individuals with anaphylaxis following Hymenoptera envenomation by a species of stinging insect, other than the imported fire ants and harvester ants, should be treated with all venoms against which the individual has specific IgE. The correlation of symptoms with allergen exposure and sensitivity requires a knowledge of the environment of the subject as well as a familiarity with the quality and reliability of allergen testing reagents used to document sensitivity. Quality allergen extracts are a prerequisite for testing and treatment. Progress has been made to improve allergen extracts, but certain extracts, notably molds, have been difficult to standardize (Reed et al, 1989; Salvaggio et al, 1993). The age of the subject is a factor in that studies showing benefits with immunotherapy have been limited, for the most part, to children older than 6 years of age and adults younger than 50 years (Bush et al, 1991). This should not be construed to mean that immunotherapy is not beneficial in older and younger age groups, only that there are limited data proving benefit.

The association of symptoms with exposure may be difficult to document with perennial asthma and rhinitis. The severity and duration of symptoms should be of a degree to justify immunotherapy. Perennial symptoms should be associated with a high degree of allergic sensitivity coupled with a failure of avoidance measures and chronic, safe pharmacologic therapy. Significant seasonal symptoms should be present for at least two seasons despite the appropriate use of safe, pharmacologic therapy and appropriate avoidance measures. Occasionally immunotherapy should be considered earlier if symptoms are particularly severe.

Spontaneous improvement does occur in some allergic individuals of all age groups, but more commonly in younger children—a fact that confuses interpretation of clinical improvement with immunotherapy in this age group. Older adults with asthma may have a component of fixed obstructive lung disease that will not benefit from immunotherapy. Discussions with all candidates for immunotherapy should precede initiation of the treatment. The benefits versus risks, including the potential for anaphylactic reactions with the

TABLE 17–1. CONSIDERATIONS FOR INITIATING IMMUNOTHERAPY

1. Presence of IgE-mediated disease proven to benefit from immunotherapy
    a. Allergic rhinitis
    b. Allergic asthma
    c. Anaphylaxis following Hymenoptera stings
2. Documentation of sensitivity to allergens associated with symptoms
3. Symptoms of sufficient duration and severity
    a. Two seasons of seasonal symptoms despite avoidance measures and pharmacologic therapy
    b. Perennial symptoms failing trials of avoidance measures and chronic pharmacologic therapy
    c. Anaphylaxis following Hymenoptera sting except children with cutaneous anaphylaxis only
4. Availability of allergenic extract of allergen responsible for sensitivity
5. Other considerations
    a. Discussion of long-term nature of treatment and need for compliance
    b. Discussion of risk versus benefit of treatment
    c. Accessibility of facilities and personnel capable of administering treatment and evaluating and treating anaphylaxis
    d. Emphasis of avoidance as treatment of choice

Adapted from Bush RK, Huftel MA, Busse WW. Patient selection. *In* Lockey RF, Bukantz SC (eds). Allergen Immunotherapy. New York, Marcel Dekker Inc, 1991, p 27.

rare occurrence of death, should be reviewed. The treatment should only be administered in facilities capable of treating anaphylaxis, and particular caution should be exercised when treating individuals with chronic asthma, especially when symptomatic.

Allergen Selection

Allergens are selected for immunotherapy when exposure to them results in significant symptoms and when significant sensitivity to them has been documented by the use of available testing and treatment reagents. The treating physician should be knowledgeable concerning the local environment to permit association of symptoms with known allergens. Challenge studies are seldom performed, and allergens for immunotherapy should not be chosen solely on the basis of either skin tests or *in vitro* testing. Potential outdoor allergens consist primarily of plant-derived materials (particularly pollen from wind-pollinated plants), fungal products (particularly mold spores), and airborne wings and body parts from insects (Burge and Solomon, 1991). The seasons for pollen exposure in temperate climates are spring for trees, spring and summer for grasses, and fall for weeds. Numerous exceptions do occur, and in the deep southern regions of North America, there is a great deal of overlap of these seasons. Airborne mold spores generally are detected when temperature and humidity are increased, with very high levels occurring in the Gulf Coast states and associated with farming activities in the Midwest. Indoor allergens are perennial, although there are changes in levels of dust mite allergen that correlate with seasonal environmental changes (Burge and Solomon, 1991; Stewart et al, 1993). Indoor allergens are derived from house dust mites, storage mites, fur-bearing animals, insects, and mold spores. Selected workers are exposed to significant allergen concentrations, as in wood working, certain chemical industries, animal husbandry, animal research and agriculture, and food processing. Heating and air conditioning systems may become contaminated with various potential allergens, most notably mold. Clinical acumen, inspection and knowledge of the environment, and experience are needed to accurately determine the important allergens in a selected environment.

Relative Contraindications to Immunotherapy

Specific clinical circumstances may dissuade the treating physician from utilizing immunotherapy, or at least introduce additional caution due to the potential for increased adverse events.

BETA BLOCKER TREATMENT. It is unclear whether the frequency of adverse reactions to immunotherapy, particularly anaphylaxis, is increased in patients on beta blocker therapy, but the severity of anaphylaxis is potentially much greater (Kaplin et al, 1989; Toogood, 1988). The anaphylaxis of such patients is relatively refractory to treatment with adrenergic agents, such as epinephrine, and is a particular risk for patients with asthma. The

American Academy of Allergy and Immunology has published the following recommendations (Executive Committee, Position Statement, 1989):

1. The concomitant use of beta blocking agents and allergen immunotherapy should be avoided when possible. Potential benefits and risk must be weighed carefully in patients who cannot substitute an alternative drug for their beta blocker. Although systemic reactions following skin testing are rare, special precautions should be observed. RAST testing may be appropriate to avoid reactions in sensitive individuals.

2. A warning label should be placed on both beta blockers and allergen extracts, addressing the potentially severe reactions that may occur during concomitant use of these agents.

PREGNANCY. There is no absolute contraindication for immunotherapy in a pregnant woman (Metzger et al, 1978; Schatz et al, 1993). The principle of *prima non nocere*, first do no harm, would lead a prudent physician to postpone immunotherapy during pregnancy, since this is a long-term treatment modality and could be initiated following delivery (Schatz et al, 1993). Cautious modification of the schedule of administration is advised if a treated subject becomes pregnant while receiving immunotherapy. The dose is not increased and probably should be decreased during the pregnancy, and regular treatment is resumed after delivery. Breastfeeding is not a contraindication to immunotherapy.

HYPERSENSITIVITY CONDITIONS NOT EXCLUSIVELY DEPENDENT ON IgE MECHANISMS. Immunologic diseases, even when associated with IgE antibody, are not improved by immunotherapy unless allergen-specific IgE mast cell and basophil degranulation is the essential and primary pathophysiologic mechanism. Examples of hypersensitivity disorders in which an IgE mechanism is not essential include allergic bronchopulmonary aspergillosis and hypersensitivity pneumonitis. Despite the presence of significant quantities of specific IgE, immunotherapy has no beneficial effect and is relatively contraindicated in such conditions.

IMMUNE COMPLEX AND AUTOIMMUNE DISEASE. There are no prospective studies to demonstrate that immunotherapy causes or aggravates immune complex disease, vasculitis, or autoimmune disease (Katalaris and Walls, 1984). There are case reports of necrotizing vasculitis occurring during immunotherapy, but these are most likely coincidental occurrences (Phanuphak and Kohler, 1980; Yang et al, 1979). Likewise, there is no evidence that immunotherapy adversely affects autoimmune disease, but the common perception is that the immune dysregulation, characteristic of autoimmune disease, should not be disturbed by immunotherapy. Therefore, allergic diseases occurring in subjects with systemic lupus erythematosus, rheumatoid arthritis, and other collagen vascular diseases are usually not treated with immunotherapy.

IMMUNODEFICIENCY. IgE dysregulation may be associated with congenital immunodeficiency diseases, such as Wiskott-Aldrich syndrome, and noncongenital immunodeficiency syndromes, such as AIDS (Wright et al, 1990). There are no studies of immunotherapy in the setting of immunodeficiency, but as with autoimmune disease states, immunotherapy is usually not practical.

UNSTABLE ASTHMA. The majority of fatalities associated with immunotherapy have occurred in asthmatics, many with asthma symptoms immediately preceding or coincident with allergen administration (Committee on Safety of Medicine, 1989; Reid et al, 1993; Stewart and Lockey, 1992). Extreme caution should be exercised in this situation, with initiation and continuation of immunotherapy relatively contraindicated when significant asthma symptoms are present or the treated subject has a significant increase in airway obstruction compared to baseline values. Some investigators do not recommend the administration of immunotherapy if pulmonary function is not greater than 70% of predicted values (Bousquet et al, 1994).

ADMINISTRATION OF IMMUNOTHERAPY

Inhalant Extracts

The usual route of immunotherapy is subcutaneous, with the deltoid region of the arm as the most commonly utilized site. If a single injection is given, the usual practice is to alternate arms with each injection. A 0.5- or 1.0-ml syringe should be used to facilitate accurate measurement of the volume of extract administered. A ⅜- to ½-inch needle of

25 gauge or greater is preferable. Care should be exercised to withdraw the plunger of the syringe after insertion of the needle through the skin to be certain that the injection is not given intravenously. The needle should never be removed after the injection to permit reuse of the syringe since aspiration of blood and body fluids into the syringe occurs during removal (Koepke et al, 1985). The treated subject should be observed for 20 to 30 minutes following the injection since the overwhelming majority of systemic reactions occur within this time period (Committee on Safety of Medicine, 1989; Lockey et al, 1987; Reid et al, 1993; Stewart and Lockey, 1992). Individuals at higher risk should be observed for 30 minutes or longer. These include subjects with asthma who are suffering a flare or seasonal exacerbation, patients with higher degrees of sensitivity, and individuals receiving beta blockers (Anderson et al, 1990; Bukantz and Lockey, 1991). Allergen extracts should be stored at 4°C for maximum potency, and if the temperature of an extract warms to greater than 40°C, the vial should be discarded.

The number of injections administered at any given time is ideally one, although two or more may be required if there is clinical sensitivity to more than six to eight allergens. Increasing the number of allergens in a given vial of extract dilutes the amount of any single allergen given with each injection. This could jeopardize a beneficial response to treatment, since improvement is associated with larger amounts of each selected allergen administered (Bruce et al, 1988; Franklin and Lowell, 1967; Van Metre et al, 1982). Allergen extracts are generally mixed in variable combinations dictated by the pattern of sensitivity of the treated subject. The protease activity contained in dust mite extracts leads some clinicians to avoid mixing dust mite extract with pollen extracts (Edwards et al, 1992). The concern is that the protease may accelerate the loss of potency of pollen allergens in the extract. This point has not been validated.

DOSAGE SCHEDULE. Immunotherapy may be given intermittently during the year (a preseasonal or co-seasonal schedule) or throughout the year (a perennial schedule) (Van Metre et al, 1991). The perennial schedule has been best studied and is the generally recommended regimen. Variations of the perennial schedule include rush immunotherapy or cluster immunotherapy. The latter two give several injections on a given day and usually on more than one day a week (Bousquet et al, 1986; Bush et al, 1991; Stevens et al, 1985; Van Metre and Adkinson, 1991). The rationale is to provide benefits rapidly or to facilitate administration for a treated subject who must travel long distances. Total dose of a given allergen administered is the primary factor governing beneficial effects, so that any of these schedules is effective. There are higher rates of adverse reactions with rush and cluster immunotherapy (Stevens et al, 1985; Van Metre et al, 1982).

Traditional, perennial immunotherapy is administered on a weekly or twice-weekly schedule (Table 17–2). The starting dose is chosen to be well tolerated by most sensitive subjects, although this dose may be adjusted on the basis of clinical criteria and test results. The dose is increased with each injection until a maintenance dose is reached. The optimal maintenance dose is determined by the tolerance and sensitivity of the treated subject, but the dose should be large enough to be effective and low enough to be safe. For most well-studied allergens, the maintenance dose contains approximately 4 to 12 μg of each major allergen being administered (Golden et al, 1981; Taylor et al, 1974; Van Metre et al, 1982). The dose may be cautiously increased two- to threefold higher than the standard maintenance dose if clinical improvement does not occur. This increase in dose does augment the potential for adverse reactions and does not guarantee symptom relief.

The maintenance dose is usually administered at a 2- to 4-week interval, provided the injections are well tolerated and symptoms improve. If systemic reactions or anaphylaxis occurs, the dose of immunotherapy is reduced to the previously tolerated dose or, more conservatively, to one tenth the previous dose. Subsequently, the dose is increased as tolerated at weekly or twice-weekly intervals. The maintenance vial is replaced with a newly prepared vial every 6 to 12 months, and the dose is reduced by one third to one half with the first injection of the new vial. The dose is subsequently increased weekly or twice weekly to the routine maintenance dose. Typical large local reactions—erythema and induration of ≤2 cm—may be treated symptomatically or may necessitate dose modification to facilitate tolerance. The latter is particularly true for reactions greater than 2 cm in

TABLE 17–2. EXAMPLE OF AN IMMUNOTHERAPY TREATMENT SCHEDULE FOR INHALANT ALLERGY

Date	Extract Concentration (wt/vol)	Extract Concentration (PNU/mL)	Volume	Remarks
	1:10,000	100 PNU/mL	0.05	
			0.10	
			0.15	
			0.20	
			0.30	
			0.40	
			0.50	
	1:1000	1000 PNU/mL	0.05	
			0.10	
			0.20	
			0.30	
			0.40	
			0.50	
	1:100	10,000 PNU/mL	0.05	
			0.10	
			0.15	
			0.20	
			0.25	
			0.30	
			0.35	
			0.40	
			0.45	
			0.50	

From Grammer LC and Shaughnessy MA. Principles of immunologic management of allergic diseases due to extrinsic antigens. *In* Patterson R, Grammer LC, Greenberger PA, Zeiss CR (eds). Allergic Diseases: Diagnosis and Management. 4th ed. Philadelphia, J.B. Lippincott, 1993, p 264.

diameter. Topical application of ice to reduce local blood flow, oral antihistamine therapy, topical corticosteroid or even systemic corticosteroid therapy may occasionally be necessary to treat these reactions. There are no data to indicate that large local reactions are harbingers of systemic, anaphylactic reactions (Lockey et al, 1987). Some physicians discourage vigorous exercise 2 to 4 hours following immunotherapy administration, although there are no studies to document this concern. The dose of maintenance immunotherapy during the major pollen season may be reduced if the recipient is sensitive to the pollen and receiving the allergen in the treatment extract (Bukantz and Lockey, 1991).

Duration of Aeroallergen Immunotherapy. There are no data to identify the optimal duration of inhalant immunotherapy. General recommendations are that maintenance immunotherapy be administered until symptoms have improved to a satisfactory level for one year; until symptom improvement is noted in three consecutive annual seasons; or until 3 to 5 years of maintenance immunotherapy have been completed (Grammer et al, 1991; Bousquet et al, 1994). Relapse is possible after discontinuation. If no improvement is noted after a trial of 12 to 24 months, it is unlikely that additional therapy will be of value.

Venom and Ant Immunotherapy

Subjects treated with pure venoms are usually given each venom to which sensitivity has been documented, regardless of the insect suspected to have caused the reaction (Yunginger, 1991). White-faced hornet, yellow hornet, and yellow jacket venoms, which cross-react immunologically, are available commercially in a mixed vespid preparation to facilitate administration. Some investigators have recommended sole administration of the venom of the insect causing the original reaction (Reisman, 1990). The techniques of administration are the same as that for inhalant extracts. Testing for imported fire ant sensitivity is indicated in a clinical situation that usually differs from that of the other Hymenoptera. The clinical identification of imported fire ant stings (they leave a tell-tale pustule) is usually sufficient to exclude the possibility of other Hymenoptera stings. Therefore, it is not advisable to test for imported fire ant sensitivity when evaluating for venom sensitivity unless there is a historical reason to suspect sensitivity to the imported fire ant. Likewise, testing for venom sensitivity is not recommended when evaluating imported fire ant sensitivity unless historically indicated. Hypersensitivity to harvester ant bites also occurs, and immunotherapy to the whole-body extract of this ant is probably effective, although this requires confirmation (Lockey, 1974, 1990).

DOSAGE SCHEDULE. Various schedules have been suggested for the administration of venom immunotherapy. An examplary regimen is provided in Table 17–3 (Yunginger, 1991). The unpredictability of life-threatening reactions to insect stings frequently results in a high level of anxiety. Using an accelerated immunotherapy schedule, with several injections given on each day, expedites reaching a maintenance dose of 100 μg of each venom utilized. This dose provides the equivalent of two or more natural stings. Some investigators have reported that 50 μg of each venom may be adequate, but successful treatment is probably more likely with the higher dose. The maintenance dose is administered at 4- to 6-week intervals, with some investigators recommending 12-week intervals (Goldberg and Reisman, 1988; Golden, 1988; Reisman, 1990; Yunginger, 1991). Imported fire ant and harvester ant whole-body extract is usually administered following a schedule similar to that of inhalant immunotherapy (Stafford et al, 1989). The maintenance or protective dose has not been as well characterized for the imported fire ant as it has been for the other Hymenoptera. Maintenance dosage usually employs 0.3 to 0.5 cc of a 1:100 or 1:10 weight/volume extract, whichever is tolerated. Maintenance therapy is usually given at 2- to 4-week intervals.

DURATION OF VENOM OR IMPORTED FIRE ANT IMMUNOTHERAPY. There is no consensus to define guidelines concerning the optimal duration of immunotherapy for Hymenoptera hypersensitivity. Various investigators have proposed and/or presented data supporting three approaches: (1) measure specific IgG to the venom used and discontinue immunotherapy when a concentration of 5 μg/ml or more is reached (Golden et al, 1989; Graft et al, 1987); (2) repeat the measurement of specific IgE, either *in vitro* or by skin testing, and discontinue when the level decreases from the initial value or disappears (Randolph and Reisman, 1986); (3) discontinue without testing after immunotherapy has been given for a time period of 3 to 5 years (Reisman and Latner, 1989). It is possible that all of these approaches have clinical utility. Application of clinical judgment with utilization of some of the aforementioned guidelines is generally the course of action. Therapy can be discontinued when the skin or *in vitro* specific IgE test becomes negative. More data are necessary to determine when therapy can be safely discontinued in patients whose level of specific IgE remains elevated (Lockey, 1990).

Other Forms of Immunotherapy

LOCAL NASAL IMMUNOTHERAPY. Local nasal aeroallergen immunotherapy is an alternative form of immunotherapy using an aqueous solution of allergen to spray on the nasal mucosa at specified time intervals (Van Metre and Adkinson, 1991; Welsh et al, 1983). This form of treatment has been shown to be clinically effective, with some studies demonstrating systemic immunologic changes with treatment (Georgitis et al, 1985). The risk of anaphylactic reactions is less than with traditional immunotherapy, and administration is facilitated since the patient self-administers the extract. The primary side effects—nasal pruritus, congestion, and sneezing—are of sufficient severity in some subjects to result in discontinuation. Sufficient long-term trials are not yet available to permit recommending this form of therapy.

ORAL AEROALLERGEN IMMUNOTHERAPY. Oral immunotherapy with birch pollen extract has been shown to be efficacious utilizing various dosage schedules (Björkstin et al, 1986; Möller et al, 1986; Tari et al, 1990; Van Niekerk and Delvet, 1987). Trials with sublingual administration of allergen extracts have suggested that low-dose therapy with dust mite or grass-maize extract is efficacious in allergic rhinitis and asthma (Tari et al, 1990; Van Niekerk and Delvet, 1987). No adverse effects were described. A double-blind, placebo-controlled trial of sublingual standardized cat immunotherapy for the treatment of asthma demonstrated no benefit with this form of treatment (Nelson et al, 1987). Oral immunotherapy is of uncertain efficacy, and additional studies are needed.

TABLE 17-3. SELECTED DOSAGE REGIMENS FOR VENOM

Day	Week	Venom Immunotherapy Regimen (μg)				
		Slow	Step	Modified Rush	Rush	Rapid
1	0	0.01	1	1	0.001	0.05
			5	5	0.01	0.10
			10	10	0.1	0.20
						0.40
						0.80
						2
						5
						10
						20
						20
2		—	—	—	1	—
					5	
3		—	—	—	10	60
					20	
7		—	—	—	—	70
8	1	0.03	25	—	20	—
					30	
9		—	—	—	50	—
					50	
15	2	0.1	—	30	100	—
21	3	0.25	25	—	—	80
28	4	0.5	—	60	100	—
35	5	1.0	25	—	200*	100*
42	6	2.5	50	100		
49	7	5	—	—		
56	8	10	50	100		
63	9	20	—	—		
70	10	30	50	—		
77	11	40	100	100		
84	12	60	—	—		
91	13	80	100	—		
98	14	100	—	—		
105	15	100	100	100*		
112	16	—	—			
119	17	100	—			
126	18	—	100*			
133	19	—				
140	20	100*				

*From Golden DK, Valentine MD, Kagey-Sobotoka A, Lichtenstein LM: Regimens of Hymenoptera venom immunotherapy. Ann Intern Med 92:621, 1980; Bousquet J, Knani J, Velasquez G, et al: Evolution of sensitivity to Hymenoptera venom in 200 allergic patients followed for up to 3 years. J Allergy Clin Immunol 84:94, 1989; Bernstein DI, Mittman RJ, Kagen SL, et al. Clinical and immunologic studies of rapid venom immunotherapy in Hymenoptera-sensitive patients. J Allergy Clin Immunol 84:952, 1989.

ALUM-PRECIPITATED ALLERGEN EXTRACTS. Modification of aqueous extracts, by precipitation of proteins with aluminum hydroxide, results in a product that produces less systemic reaction than aqueous allergen extracts (Hedlin et al, 1986; Report of FDA Panel, 1985; Sundin et al, 1986). This modification permits a more rapid increase in the dosage of the treatment, and fewer total injections are required before benefits are realized (McAllen, 1969). Equivalent clinical and immunologic changes with ragweed alum–precipitated extracts required half as many injections as did aqueous ragweed extracts. Cat and grass have also been studied, and other alum-precipitated extracts would presumably be of equivalent efficacy. Although systemic reactions are decreased, some treated subjects experience prolonged local reactions following administration of alum–precipitated extracts (Van Metre and Adkinson, 1991). Alum–precipitated products are currently limited in diversity and should not be mixed with aqueous extracts.

Prior to alum precipitation, allergens can be extracted with pyridine to further reduce the potential for systemic reactions following administration. Alum–precipitated pyridine grass extracts have been shown to be efficacious, but other allergens, such as ragweed, are denatured by the pyridine treatment and rendered ineffective (Van Metre and Adkinson, 1991). The utility of alum–precipitated pyridine extracts is limited and largely unproven (Report of FDA Panel, 1985).

MODIFIED AEROALLERGEN EXTRACTS. Polymerization or aggregation of the proteins of an aqueous extract reduces the allergenicity while preserving the immunogenicity of the product. Two methods of such modification have accomplished this goal—formalin-treated allergens (allergoids) and glutaraldehyde-treated allergens (polymerized allergen extracts) (Marsh et al, 1970; Patterson et al, 1973). Regimens utilizing these extracts permit completion of an immunotherapy program with 10 to 15 weekly injections, with less than 1 percent occurrence of systemic reactions (Grammer et al, 1991; Norman et al, 1979; Van Metre and Adkinson, 1991). One trial of immunotherapy with polymerized extracts demonstrated clinical improvement lasting for at least 4 years following a course of treatment (Grammer et al, 1984). The possibility of long-term side effects, though none have been documented, has hindered commercial development of this effective modification of immunotherapy. These products offer the potential for a major advance in the treatment of inhalant allergic disorders.

ADVERSE EFFECTS OF IMMUNOTHERAPY

Immunotherapy has an inherent risk since a substance is administered to an individual with proven sensitivity to that substance. The risk of significant adverse reactions is low, ranging from 0.05 to 3.5 percent per injection using retrospective data (Van Arsdel and Sherman, 1957; Stewart and Lockey, 1992). Most of these adverse events are systemic manifestations of hypersensitivity—asthma, urticaria, laryngospasm, hypotension, angioedema. Additional immunologic adverse effects, such as vasculitis or immune complex disease, and neuropathy have been reported (Bukantz and Lockey, 1991; Phanuphak and Kohler, 1980). The limited number of such reports and other negative studies not confirming an association suggest that these latter adverse events probably are not causally related to the immunotherapy. However, the anaphylactic reactions are a definite risk from immunotherapy and remain a major concern (Bukantz and Lockey, 1991; Hejjaoui et al, 1990; Lockey et al, 1987, 1990).

In 1986 a report of fatalities from immunotherapy in the United Kingdom focused additional concern on the risk of immunotherapy (Committee on Safety of Medicine, 1986). The report summarized 26 deaths following immunotherapy from 1957 to 1985. Eleven of the deaths occurred after 1980, and five occurred in the 18 months preceding the report. The apparent increase in the occurrence of fatalities from immunotherapy is not completely explained but may be due to the increased potency of allergen extracts available in the last 10 to 15 years. All of these deaths were secondary to bronchial airway obstruction and/or anaphylaxis, and the clinical indication for immunotherapy had been asthma in 16 of 26 subjects. All but two of the reactions began within 30 minutes of administration of the immunotherapy injection. An apparent increase of anaphylactic deaths related to immunotherapy in Sweden was related to the introduction of high-potency allergen extracts. Immunotherapy in Sweden has subsequently been restricted to designated medical facilities specializing in this treatment (Norman, 1987).

Deaths from immunotherapy in the United States have been collected retrospectively by the American Academy of Allergy and Immunology, with the data published in 1987 and 1993 (Lockey et al, 1987; Reid et al, 1993). Valid data were obtained for 24 fatalities following immunotherapy between 1945 and 1984, 17 between 1985 and 1989, and 10 from 1990 through most of 1991. The majority of these cases were "highly sensitive" and most had asthma. The cause of death in almost all of the subjects with asthma was respiratory with or without anaphylactic shock. Neither the initial signs and symptoms of the systemic reaction nor the history of previous reactions to immunotherapy was predictive of fatality. Three of the fatal reactions reported began more than 30 minutes after the injection.

The risks of immunotherapy are significant and warrant strict adherence to measures to minimize the risk of fatality (Stewart and Lockey, 1992). Discussions concerning the risk benefit ratio of immunotherapy should be conducted prior to initiating treatment. Documentation of this information exchange with the treated subject is essential. Some physicians require that a consent form be completed by the patient (Fig. 17–3). Immunotherapy given to subjects at increased risk of adverse events should only be administered in medical facilities having personnel who are carefully trained to assess and treat anaphylaxis (Executive Committee Position Statement, 1990; Executive Committee Position Statement, 1994). Adequate resources should be available for treatment of hypotension, bronchospasm, laryngeal edema, and shock. If allergen extracts are administered in a facility outside the specialist's control, instructions should be provided to the treating physician defining the potential risks, signs and symptoms to be monitored, and appropriate therapeutic procedures. Emphasis should be placed on the immediate use of epinephrine if a reaction occurs or is suspected, with repeated administration to an adult of 0.1- to 0.2-cc doses of 1:1000 epinephrine rather than larger, single-dose injections. The repetition of doses of epinephrine facilitates monitoring and minimizes adverse effects of the treatment. Antihistamines should also be given and systemic glucocorticoid therapy considered. The latter two forms of treatment may be effective for minimizing the delayed anaphylaxis that may occur several hours after the initial reaction. The treated subject should be observed for 20 to 30 minutes following immunotherapy and for 60 minutes or longer if a systemic reaction occurs (Anderson et al, 1990; Executive Committee Position Statement, 1994; Stewart and Lockey, 1992).

SUMMARY

Immunotherapy has stood the test of time and remains an important treatment modality

---

IMMUNOTHERAPY PATIENT CONSENT FORM

Immunotherapy, hyposensitization, or allergy injections should be administered at a medical facility with a medical physician present since occasional reactions may require immediate therapy. These reactions may consist of any or all the following symptoms: itchy eyes, nose, or throat; nasal congestion; runny nose; tightness in the throat or chest; coughing; increased wheezing; lightheadedness; faintness; nausea and vomiting; hives; and shock, the last under extreme conditions. Reactions, even though unusual, can be serious but rarely fatal. You are required to wait in the medical facility in which you receive the injections for at least 30 minutes after each injection.

I have read (if new patient) or re-read (if established patient) the patient information sheet on immunotherapy and understand it. The opportunity has been provided for me to ask questions regarding the potential side effects of immunotherapy and these questions have been answered to my satisfaction. I understand that every precaution consistent with the best medical practice will be carried out to protect me against such reactions.

Patient (or parent if patient a minor) _____

_____ Date _____

Witness _____ Date _____

INJECTIONS ADMINISTERED AT AN OUTSIDE MEDICAL FACILITY

Please complete the following if the allergy extract will be administered at an outside medical facility.

I have read (if new patient) or re-read (if established patient) all the information about allergy injections, and I agree that I will not attempt to administer my extract to myself nor will I permit anyone who is not a licensed physician or under the supervision of a licensed physician to administer these extracts.

Patient (or parent if patient a minor) _____ Date _____

Witness _____ Date _____

FACILITY WHERE INJECTIONS WILL BE ADMINISTERED:
_____
_____

FIGURE 17–3. An example of a consent form that can be used to document the exchange of information between the treating physician and the patient concerning the potential risks of immunotherapy. (From Bukantz SC, Lockey RF. Adverse effects and fatalities associated with allergen immunotherapy. *In* Lockey RF, Bukantz SC (eds). Allergen Immunotherapy. New York, Marcel Dekker, 1991, p 253.)

for subjects suffering from inhalant allergic diseases as well as Hymenoptera sting hypersensitivity. In contrast to pharmacologic therapies, allergen avoidance and immunotherapy offer the possibility of addressing the fundamental pathophysiologic process of allergy—the release of mast cell and basophil mediators on contact with specific allergens.

REFERENCES

Alum R, Kuna P, Rozanieck J, et al. The magnitude of the spontaneous production of histamaine-releasing factor by lymphocytes in vitro. Correlation with the state of bronchial hyperreactivity in patients with asthma. J Allergy Clin Immunol 79:103, 1987.

Anderson JA, Kaliner M, Kaplan AP, et al. Position statement: The waiting period after allergen skin testing and immunotherapy. J Allergy Clin Immunol 85:526, 1990.

Björkstin B, Möller C, Broberger U, et al. Clinical and immunologic effects of oral immunotherapy with a standardized birch pollen extract. Allergy 41:290, 1986.

Bousquet J, Braquemond P, Feinberg J, et al. Specific IgE response before and after rush immunotherapy with a standardized allergen or allergoid in grass pollen allergy. Ann Allergy 56:456, 1986.

Bousquet J, Hejjaoui A, Soussana M, et al. Double-blind, placebo-controlled immunotherapy with mixed grass-pollen allergoids IV. Comparison of the safety and efficacy. J Allergy Clin Immunol 85:490, 1990.

Bousquet J, Knani J, Velasquez G, et al. Evolution of sensitivity to Hymenoptera venom in 200 allergic patients followed for up to 3 years. J Allergy Clin Immunol 84:944, 1989.

Bousquet J, Michel FB. Specific immunotherapy in asthma: Is it effective? J Allergy Clin Immunol 94:1, 1994.

Bruce CA, Norman PS, Rosenthal RR, et al. The role of ragweed pollen in autumnal asthma. J Allergy Clin Immunol 18:351, 1988.

Brunet C, Bedard P-M, Lavoie A, et al. Allergic rhinitis to ragweed pollen. I. Reassessment of the effects of immunotherapy on cellular and humoral responses. J Allergy Clin Immunol 89:76, 1992.

Bukantz SC, Lockey RF. Adverse effects and fatalities associated with allergen immunotherapy. In Lockey RF, Bukantz S (eds). Allergen Immunotherapy. New York, Marcel Dekker, 1991, pp 233–263.

Burge HA, Soloman WR. Outdoor allergens. In Lockey RF, Bukantz S (eds). Allergen Immunotherapy. New York, Marcel Dekker, 1991, pp 51–67.

Bush RK, Huftel MA, Busse WW. Patient selection. In Lockey RF, Bukantz S (eds). Allergen Immunotherapy. New York, Marcel Dekker, 1991, pp 25–50.

Committee on Safety of Medicine. CSM Update: Desensitising vaccines. Br Med J 293:948, 1986.

Creticos MD, Reed CE, Norman PS, et al. The NIAID cooperative study of the role of immunotherapy in seasonal ragweed-induced adult asthma. J Allergy Clin Immunol 91:226, 1993. (Abstract)

Creticos MD, Reed CE, Norman PS, et al. The NIAID cooperative study of the role of immunotherapy in ragweed-induced adult asthma: 3rd year clinical endpoints; cost effectiveness. J Allergy Clin Immunol 91:226, 1993. (Abstract)

Creticos PS, Marsh DG, Adkinson NF, et al. Evaluation by nasal pollen challenge of immunotherapy with rapidly released ragweed allergen. J Allergy Clin Immunol 73:141, 1984.

Creticos PS, Van Metre TE, Mardiney MR, et al. Dose of response of IgE and IgG antibodies during ragweed immunotherapy. J Allergy Clin Immunol 73:94, 1984.

D'Souza MF, Pepys J, Wells ID, et al. Hyposensitization with Dermatophagoides pteronyssinus in house dust allergy: A controlled study of clinical and immunologic effects. Clin Allergy 3:177, 1973.

Djurup DBK, Malling H, Sondergaard I, et al. The IgE and IgG subclass antibody response in patients allergic to yellow jacket venom undergoing different regimens of venom immunotherapy. J Allergy Clin Immunol 76:46, 1985.

Dominiguez MA, Sanz, ML, Lobera T, et al. T helper and T suppressor subpopulations in pollinosis. Effect of specific immunotherapy. Allergol-Immunopathol (Madr) 11:415, 1983.

Dreborg S, Agress B, Foucard T, et al. A double-blind, multicenter immunotherapy trial in children, using a purified and standardized Cladosporium herbarum preparation. I. Clinical results. Allergy 41:131–140, 1986.

Edwards TB, Trudeau WL, Fernandez-Caldas E, et al. Cysteine and serine proteinases in extracts of the storage mite, Aleuroglyphus ovatus. J Allergy Clin Immunol 90:129, 1992.

Ewan PW, Alexander MM, Snape C, et al. Effective hyposensitization in allergic rhinitis using a potent partially purified extract of house dust mite. Clin Allergy 18:501, 1988.

Executive Committee, American Academy of Allergy and Immunology. Position statement, Personnel and equipment to treat systemic reactions caused by immunotherapy with allergenic extracts. J Allergy Clin Immunol 86:775, 1990.

Executive Committee, American Academy of Allergy and Immunology. Position statement, Beta-adrenergic blockers, immunotherapy and skin testing. J Allergy Clin Immunol 84:129, 1989.

Executive Committee, American Academy of Allergy and Immunology. Position statement, Guidelines to minimize the risk from systemic reactions caused by immunotherapy with allergenic extracts. J Allergy Clin Immunol 93:811, 1994.

Fennerty AG, Jones KP, Davies BH. Immunological changes associated with a successful outcome of pollen immunotherapy. Allergy 43:415, 1988.

Frankland AW, Hughes WH, Garrill RH. Autogenous bacterial vaccines in the treatment of asthma. Br Med J 2:941, 1955.

Franklin W, Lowell FC. Comparison of two dosages of ragweed extract in the treatment of pollinosis. JAMA 201:95, 1967.

Freeman TM, Nylander R, Ortiz A, et al. Imported fire ant immunotherapy. J Allergy Clin Immunol 90:210, 1992.

Georgitis JW, Nickelsen JA, Wypych JI, et al. Local nasal immunotherapy: Efficacy of low-dose aqueous ragweed extract. J Allergy Clin Immunol 75:496, 1985.

Goldberg A, Reisman RE: Prolonged interval maintenance venom immunotherapy. Ann Allergy 61:177, 1988.

Golden DBK: Guidelines for venom immunotherapy. Ann Allergy 61:159, 1988.

Golden DBK, Addison BI, Gadde J, et al. Prospective observations on stopping prolonged venom immunotherapy. J Allergy Clin Immunol 84:162, 1989.

Golden DBK, Kagey-Sobotka A, Valentine MD, et al. Dose dependence of Hymenoptera venom immunotherapy. J Allergy Clin Immunol 67:370, 1981.

Graft DF, Schuberth KC, Kagey-Sobotka A, et al. Assessment of prolonged venom immunotherapy in children. J Allergy Clin Immunol 30:162, 1987.

Grammer LC, Shaughnessy MA, Patterson R. Administration of allergen extracts. In Lockey RF, Bukantz SC (eds). Allergen Immunotherapy. New York, Marcel Dekker, 1991, pp 191–207.

Grammer LC, Shaughnessy MA, Suszko IM, et al. Persistence of efficacy after a brief course of polymerized ragweed allergens: A controlled study. J Allergy Clin Immunol 73:484, 1984.

Haugaard L, Dahl R. Immunotherapy in patients allergic to cat and dog dander: I. Clinical results. Allergy 47:249, 1992.

Haugaard L, Dahl R, Jacobsen L. A controlled dose-response study of immunotherapy with standardized, partially purified extract of house dust mite: Clinical efficacy and side effects. J Allergy Clin Immunol 91:709, 1993.

Hedlin G, Graff-Lonnevig V, Heiborn H, et al. Immunotherapy with cat- and dog-dander extracts. II. In vivo and in vitro effects observed in a one-year double-blind placebo study. J Allergy Clin Immunol 77:488, 1986.

Hejjaoui A, Dhivert H, Michel FB, et al. Immunotherapy with a standardized Dermatophagoides pteronyssinus extract. IV. Systemic reactions according to the immunotherapy schedule. J Allergy Clin Immunol 85:473, 1990.

Hirsch SR, Kalbfleisch, JH, Golbert TM, et al. Rinkel injection therapy. A multi-center controlled study. J Allergy Clin Immunol 68:133, 1981.

Hoffman DR, Jacobson RS, Schmidt M, et al. Allergens in Hymenoptera venom. XXIII. Venom content of imported fire ant whole body extract. Ann Allergy 66:29, 1991.

Horst M, Hejjaoui A, Horst V, et al. Double-blind, placebo controlled rush immunotherapy with a standardized Alternaria extract. J Allergy Clin Immunol 85:460, 1990.

Hseih KH. Decreased production of CD8 (T8) antigen after immunotherapy. J Allergy Clin Immunol 91:111, 1989.

Hunt KJ, Valentine MD, Sobotka AK, et al. A controlled trial of immunotherapy in insect hypersensitivity. N Engl J Med 229:157, 1978.

Johansson SGO, Nordvall S, Ledford D, et al. Specific IgE and IgG responses in immunotherapy with imported fire ant and whole body extract in imported fire ant hypersensitivity. J Allergy Clin Immunol 75:208, 1985.

Johnstone DE. Study of the value of bacterial vaccines in the treatment of bronchial asthma associated with respiratory infections. Am J Dis Child 94:1, 1974.

Kaplan AP, Anderson JA, Valentine MD, et al. Position statement: Beta-adrenergic blockers, immunotherapy and skin testing. J Allergy Clin Immunol 84:129, 1989.

Katelaris CH, Walls RS. A study of possible ill effects from prolonged immunotherapy in treatment of allergic diseases. Ann Allergy 53:257, 1984.

Koepke JW, Reller LB, Masters HA, et al. Viral contamination of intradermal skin test syringes. Ann Allergy 55:776, 1985.

Kuna P, et al. The effect of preseasonal immunotherapy on the production of histamine-releasing factor (HRF) by mononuclear cells from patients with seasonal asthma: Results of a double-blind placebo-controlled randomized study. J Allergy Clin Immunol 83:816, 1989.

Lockey RF. Systemic reactions to stinging ants. J Allergy Clin Immunol 54:132, 1974.

Lockey RF. Immunotherapy for allergy to insect stings. N Engl J Med 323:1627, 1990. (Editorial)

Lockey RF, Benedict LM, Turkeltaub PC, et al. Fatalities from immunotherapy and skin testing. J Allergy Clin Immunol 79:660, 1987.

Lockey RF, Turkeltaub PC, Olive CA, et al. The Hymenoptera venom study. III: Safety of venom immunotherapy. J Allergy Clin Immunol 86:775, 1990.

Løwenstein H, Graff-Lonnevig V, Hedlin G, et al. Immunotherapy with cat- and dog-dander extracts. J Allergy Clin Immunol 77:497, 1986.

Løwenstein H, Matthiesen F, Ipsen H. Preparation and standardization of allergen extracts (pollens, mites, molds, dander, and venoms). In Lockey RF, Bukantz S (eds). Allergen Immunotherapy. New York, Marcel Dekker, 1991, pp 161–170.

Malling HJ, Dreborg J, Week B. Diagnosis and immunotherapy of mould allergy: V. Clinical efficacy and side effects of immunotherapy with Cladosporium herbarum. Allergy 41:507, 1986.

Marsh DG, Lichtenstein LM, Campbell DN. Studies on allergoids prepared from naturally occurring allergens. I. Assay of allergenicity and antigenicity of formalinized rye Group I component. Immunology 18:705, 1970.

McAllen MK. Hyposensitization in grass pollen hay fever. A double-blind trial of alum precipitated pollen extract. Acta Allergol 24:421, 1969.

Mendoza GR, Minagawa K. Subthreshold and suboptimal desensitization of human basophils. I. Kinetics of decay of releasability. Int Arch Allergy Appl Immunol 61:101, 1982.

Meriney DK, Kothari H, Chinoy P, et al. The clinical and immunologic efficacy of immunotherapy with modified ragweed extract (allergoid) for ragweed hay fever. Ann Allergy 56:34, 1986.

Metzger WJ, Turner E, Patterson R. The safety of immunotherapy during pregnancy. J Allergy Clin Immunol 61:268, 1978.

Möller C, Dreborg S, Lanner A, et al. Oral immunotherapy of children with rhinoconjunctivitis due to birch pollen allergy. Allergy 41:271, 1986.

Morrey CB: Vaccination with mixed cultures from the nose in hay fever. JAMA 61:1806, 1913.

Muller UR, Morris T, Bischof M, et al. Combined active and passive immunotherapy in honeybee-sting allergy. J Allergy Clin Immunol 78:115, 1986.

Nelson HS, Oppenheimer J, Vatsia GA, et al. A double-blind, placebo-controlled evaluation of sublingual immunotherapy with standardized cat extract. J Allergy Clin Immunol 92:229, 1993.

Norman PS. Fatal misadventures. J Allergy Clin Immunol 59:572, 1987.

Norman PS, Lichtenstein LM. The clinical and immunologic specificity of immunotherapy. J Allergy Clin Immunol 61:370, 1978.

Norman PS, Marsh DG, Lichtenstein LM. A long-term immunotherapy with ragweed allergen and allergoid. J Allergy Clin Immunol 63:167, 1979.

Ohman JL, Findlay SR, Leiterman KM. Immunotherapy in cat-induced asthma. Double-blind trial with evalua-

tion of *in vivo* and *in vitro* responses. J Allergy Clin Immunol 74:230, 1984.
Oppenheimer JJ, Nelson HS, Bock SA. Treatment of peanut allergy with rush immunotherapy. J Allergy Clin Immunol 90:256, 1992.
Ortolani C, Pastorello E, Moss RB. Grass pollen immunotherapy: A single year double-blind, placebo-controlled study in patients with grass pollen-induced asthma and rhinitis. J Allergy Clin Immunol 73:283, 1984.
Patterson R, Suszko IM, Pruzansky JJ, et al. Polymerized ragweed antigen E. II. *In vivo* elimination studies and reactivity with IgE antibody systems. J Immunol 110:1413, 1973.
Paull BR, Coghlan TH. Fire ant allergy: Whole body extract treatment failures. J Allergy Clin Immunol 78:141, 1986.
Phanuphak P, Kohler PF. Onset of polyarteritis nodosa during allergic hyposensitization treatment. Am J Med 68:479, 1980.
Pienkowski MD, Norman PS, Lichtenstein LM. Suppression of late-phase skin reactions by immunotherapy with ragweed extract. J Allergy Clin Immunol 76:729, 1985.
Price JF, Warner JO, Hey EN, et al. A controlled trial of hyposensitization with tyrosine adsorbed *Dermatophagoides pteronyssinus* antigen in childhood asthma: In vivo aspects. Clin Allergy 14:209, 1988.
Randolph CC, Reisman RE. Evaluation of decline in serum venom-specific IgE as a criterion for stopping venom immunotherapy. J Allergy Clin Immunol 77:823, 1986.
Reed CE, Yuninger JW, Evans R. Quality assurance and standardization of allergy extracts in practice. J Allergy Clin Immunol 84:4, 1989.
Reed MA, deShazo RD, Ortiz AA, et al. Comparison between RAST with imported fire ant whole body extracts and venom. J Allergy Clin Immunol 79:217, 1987.
Reid MJ, Lockey RF, Turkeltaub PC, et al. Survey of fatalities from skin testing and immunotherapy 1985–1989. J Allergy Clin Immunol 92:6, 1993.
Reid MJ, Moss RB, Yoa-Pi H, et al. Seasonal asthma in northern California: Allergic causes and efficacy of immunotherapy. J Allergy Clin Immunol 78:590, 1986.
Reisman RE. Insect Hypersensitivity. *In* Current Views in Allergy and Immunology, Volume XVIII. Atlanta, School of Medicine of the Medical College of Georgia and the American Academy of Allergy and Immunology, 1990.
Reisman RE, Latner R. Further observations of stopping venom immunotherapy: Comparison of patients stopped because of a fall in serum venom-specific IgE to insignificant levels with patients stopped prematurely by self-choice. J Allergy Clin Immunol 83:1049, 1989.
Report of FDA panel on review of allergenic extracts. Fed Register 50:382, 1985.
Rinkel HJ. The management of clinical allergy. Part III. Inhalant allergy therapy. Arch Otolaryngol 77:215, 1963.
Rocklin RE, Sheffer AL, Greineder DK, et al. Generation of antigen-specific suppressor cells during allergy desensitization. N Engl J Med 302:1213, 1980.
Sadan N, Rhyne MB, Mellits ED, et al. Immunotherapy of pollinosis in children. Investigation of immunologic basis of clinical improvement. N Engl J Med 280:624, 1969.
Salvaggio JE, Burge HA, Chapman JA. Emerging concepts in mold allergy: What is the role of immunotherapy? J Allergy Clin Immunol 92:217, 1993.
Schatz M, Hoffman CP, Zeiger RS, et al. The course and management of asthma and allergic disease during pregnancy. *In* Middleton E, Reed CE, Ellis EF, Adkinson NF, Yunginger JW (eds). Allergy: Principles and Practice. 4th ed. St Louis, Mosby–Year Book, 1993, vol II, pp 1301–1342.
Stafford CT, Rhoades RB, Bunker-Soler AL, et al. Survey of whole-body extract immunotherapy for imported fire ants and other Hymenoptera-sting allergy. Report of the Fire Ant Subcommittee of the American Academy of Allergy and Immunology. J Allergy Clin Immunol 83:1107, 1989.
Stevens WJ, Verhelst JA, van den Bogaert W, et al. Clinical and biological evaluation of a semi-rush and ordinary immunotherapy schemes in type I allergic respiratory diseases. Allergy 40:447, 1985.
Stewart GA, Thompson PJ, McWilliam AS: Biochemical properties of alloallergens: Contributory factors in allergic sensitization. Pediatr Allergy Immunol 4:163, 1993.
Stewart GE, Lockey RF. Systemic reactions from allergen immunotherapy. J Allergy Clin Immunol 90:567, 1992. (Editorial)
Strom GB, Boswell RN, Jacobs RI. *In vivo* and *in vitro* comparison of fire ant venom and fire ant whole body extract. J Allergy Clin Immunol 72:46, 1983.
Sundin B, Lilja G, Graff-Lonnevig V, et al. Immunotherapy with partially purified and standardized animal dander extracts. J Allergy Clin Immunol 77:497, 1986.
Tamir R, Castracane JM, Rocklin RE. Generation of suppressor cells in atopic patients during immunotherapy that modulate IgE synthesis. J Allergy Clin Immunol 79:591, 1987.
Tari MG, Maccino M, Mouni C. Efficacy of sublingual immunotherapy in patients with rhinitis and asthma due to house dust mite: A double-blind study. Allergol Immunopathol 18:277, 1990.
Taylor B, Sanders SS, Norman AP. A double-blind controlled trial of house mite-fortified house dust vaccine in childhood asthma. Clin Allergy 4:35, 1974.
Toogood JH. Risk of anaphylaxis in patient receiving beta-blocker drugs. J Allergy Clin Immunol 77:727, 1988. (Editorial)
Van Arsdel PP, Sherman W. The risk of inducing constitutional reactions in allergic patients. J Allergy 28:251, 1957.
Van Metre TE Jr, Adkinson NF Jr. Immunotherapy for allergic disease. *In* Middleton E, Reed CE, Ellis EF, Adkinson NF Jr, Yunginger JW (eds). Allergy: Principles and Practice. 4th ed. St Louis, Mosby–Year Book, 1991, vol II, pp 1489–1510.
Van Metre TE Jr, Adkinson NF Jr, Amodio FJ, et al. A comparison of immunotherapy schedules for injection treatment of ragweed pollen hay fever. J Allergy Clin Immunol 69:181, 1982.
Van Metre TE Jr, Marsh DG, Adkinson NF Jr, et al. Immunotherapy for cat asthma. J Allergy Clin Immunol 82:1055, 1988.
Van Niekerk CH, DeWet JI. Efficacy of grass-maize pollen oral immunotherapy in patients with seasonal hay fever: A double-blind study. Clin Allergy 17:507, 1987.
Watkins DJ, Reed MA, Jones T, et al. Crossed immunoelectrophoretic studies of imported fire ant whole body extracts and venom. J Allergy Clin Immunol 79:217, 1987.

Weeke B, Søndergaard I, Lind P, et al. Crossed immunoelectrophoresis for identification of allergens and determination of the antigenic specificities of patients' IgE. Scand J Immunol 17:265, 1983.

Welsh PW, Butterfield JH, Yunginger JW, et al. Allergen-controlled study of intranasal immunotherapy for ragweed hay fever. J Allergy Clin Immunol 71:454, 1983.

Wright DN, Nelson RP, Ledford DK, et al. Serum IgE and human immunodeficiency virus (HIV) infection. J Allergy Clin Immunol 85:445, 1990.

Yang Wh, Dorvla G, Osterland CK, et al. Circulating immune complexes during immunotherapy. J Allergy Clin Immunol 63:300, 1979.

Yunginger JW. Insect allergy. *In* Middleton E, Reed CE, Ellis EF, Adkinson NF, Yunginger JW (eds). Allergy: Principles and Practice. St Louis, Mosby–Year Book, 1991, 4th ed. vol II, pp 1511–1524.

ACKNOWLEDGMENTS: The authors are grateful for the review of this manuscript by Dr. Sam Bukantz.

Chapter 18

Identification and Management of Psychosocial Factors

Stephen J. Gaioni, Ph.D., Edwin B. Fisher, Jr., Ph.D., and Robert C. Strunk, M.D.

PSYCHOLOGICAL FACTORS IN ASTHMA

Successful management of a chronic illness such as asthma typically requires that the patient obtain regular medical care, adhere to a medical regimen, and make significant changes in life style. These are health management *behaviors* and hence fall within the realm of psychology. Often these behaviors must be maintained for the remainder of the individual's life. The maintenance of these behaviors usually requires good communication with the physician and other primary health care providers, education about the disease and its management, strong social support, a sense of having some control over one's life, and hope for a decent quality of life. On the negative side, chronic illness can cause psychological dysfunction that interferes with these health management behaviors. Depression and anxiety may arise from a sense of despair over one's illness; a feeling of hopelessness for the future; a fear of death; feelings of being different, inadequate, or abnormal; a diminished quality of life; or perhaps biologic factors common to both the disease and the mood disorder. Beyond the individual, the chronic illness may place a variety of strains on the family resulting in family dysfunction that reduces social support and makes medical compliance more difficult.

Emotional Triggers of Asthma

Strong emotional responses such as fear, anger, and excitement are known to be triggers of asthma. Isenberg et al (1992) reviewed the empiric literature on the effect of emotions on bronchoconstriction, and found that approximately 40 percent of asthmatic subjects tested across five studies showed significant decreases in either peak expiratory flow rate or forced expiratory volume in one second (FEV_1) after exposure to an emotional trigger. These studies did not use a common protocol to induce emotional responses. Viewing a "gory" film, visualizing an anxiety-provoking event, listening to an anger- or fear-eliciting tape recording, and receiving a hypnotic suggestion of fear or anger all appeared to be effective in inducing bronchoconstriction. Control subjects without asthma showed little or no bronchoconstriction in these studies.

In a related series of experiments, researchers have examined the response of asthmatic subjects to the suggestion of the delivery of an allergen or irritant nebulization. These studies are based on a protocol, developed by Luparello et al (1968), in which asthmatic subjects are led to believe that they are inhaling allergens or irritants when they are inhaling only nebulized physiologic saline. The subject's response is then compared to that when the subject is correctly informed of the inhaled saline or is misinformed that the saline is a bronchodilator. Luparello et al found that 19 of 40 (45 percent) of the asthmatics tested showed an increase in airway resistance of at least 20 percent, and 12 of these developed "full-blown clinical attacks of asthma with dyspnea and wheezing." None of 40 control subjects without asthma showed significant changes in airway resistance. This significant reduction in airflow as a result of suggestion in asthmatic subjects, but not nonasthmatic controls, has been frequently replicated, although other researchers have failed to observe the clinical symptoms observed by Luparello and his colleagues.

Isenberg et al (1992) propose that both emotional arousal and suggestion decrease airflow (increase airway reactivity) through increases in parasympathetic activity of the vagus nerve. A study by Janson-Bjerklie et al (1986), however, suggests that the effects of emotional arousal and suggestion on bronchoconstriction may not be based on the same underlying mechanism. These investigators correlated subjects' self-reports about whether their asthma could be emotionally triggered with their susceptibility to suggestion using the Luparello et al paradigm. Ten of 29 subjects displayed a greater than 20 percent increase in airway resistance, replicating the basic suggestion finding. However, the subjects' susceptibility to suggestion was not related to their reports of perceived emotional triggers of asthma. Further work is needed to disentangle the relationships between suggestion, emotional arousal, and bronchoconstriction.

Psychological Factors in Daily Functioning of Asthmatics

Research by Ludwick et al (1986) on the cardiopulmonary endurance of a group of children with moderately severe to severe asthma referred for rehabilitation indicated that approximately 50 percent of the children had levels of fitness in the significantly abnormal range on maximal exercise bicycle ergometer testing. However, almost all of the children (93 percent) were able to reach normal fitness levels with training within 2 to 16 weeks, suggesting that this lack of fitness was not a necessary limitation of their asthma. Subsequent research by Strunk and his colleagues indicates that psychological factors may be more important than medical factors in determining the physical fitness of these children.

Strunk et al (1989) prospectively studied the relationships between cardiopulmonary fitness, disease severity, and psychological functioning in 90 patients with moderately severe to severe asthma. Of these patients, 90 percent had a history of exercise-induced asthma, 20 percent had a history of respiratory failure or a hypoxic seizure, and 66 percent had used oral corticosteroids the previous year. Medical characteristics examined included length of disease, presence of a severe complication of asthma, steroid use in the year before evaluation, steroid dose at the time of evaluation, history of exercise-induced asthma, number of hospitalizations for asthma, and pulmonary function at the time of evaluation. Psychological functioning was assessed by a structured interview conducted by social workers and by a parent questionnaire. None of the medical characteristics of asthma was significantly correlated with cardiopulmonary functioning. Further, of the medical characteristics, only the number of hospitalizations was significantly correlated with psychological functioning. In contrast, psychological functioning, as determined by the structured interviews (but not the parent questionnaire), was significantly correlated with cardiopulmonary functioning.

Strunk and his colleagues (Gutstadt et al, 1989; Bender et al, 1987) also studied the relationships between medical characteristics of asthma, psychological functioning, and both school performance and fine and gross motor coordination in these children with moderately severe to severe asthma. In contrast to their cardiopulmonary functioning, these children were in the normal to slightly above normal range on school performance and motor coordination. Like the cardiopulmonary results, however, psychological functioning was correlated with these variables, whereas medical characteristics of asthma were not. These results indicate that attention needs to be paid to the psychological functioning of patients with asthma if we are to optimize their quality of life.

Anxiety, Asthma, and Psychosocial Development

Bowlby (1969) has argued that the roots of an individual's psychosocial development are formed in early mother-child interactions.

Anxiety plays a crucial role in Bowlby's theory. When a mother is sensitive to the needs of the young child and consistently responds to those needs, the young child develops relatively free of anxiety and confronts the world confidently, using mother as a secure base. Such a child develops an attachment style in which he or she is secure in self and in interactions with others. In contrast, when a mother is inconsistent or ineffective in meeting the young child's needs, the child is likely to become more anxious and to be more ambivalent about confronting the world. Such a child is likely to be less secure about self and about interactions with others. There is growing empiric support that young children do develop different attachment styles and that these styles carry over into adulthood, where they continue to exert an influence on an individual's interactions with others (Ainsworth et al, 1978; Hazan and Shaver, 1987).

An asthma attack must be very frightening not only to a young child but also to a parent. Often a mother feels helpless in coping with such an attack. Not only may the young child become anxious about confronting the world, but the mother may become overly protective because of her own anxiety. The anxiety of both child and mother may conspire to prevent the child from growing independent of the mother, resulting in an anxious rather than secure attachment style. This might be evidenced by abnormal separation anxiety in the young child. In an adult, this might be evidenced in a patient who is overly dependent on others for control of his asthma.

The existing empiric literature is consistent with the view that children with asthma are more likely to have problems developing secure attachment styles than children without asthma. Mrazek et al (1984) compared parent-child interactions of 26 severely asthmatic preschool children between the ages of 36 and 72 months with 22 healthy children of the same ages. The asthmatic children showed twice as much separation anxiety as the healthy children, although this difference largely disappeared in the 60- to 72-month-old children. The asthmatic children displayed much more negative affect, and their mothers were more likely to respond to this behavior in a negative manner. Maternal reports indicated that many of the asthmatic children appeared to suffer from depressed mood. Williams (1975) also demonstrated that asthmatic children had a greater reaction to separation and were judged more dependent than children who were healthy or had cystic fibrosis. McNichol and Williams (1973a,b,c) studied 315 asthmatic children in Australia. The more severely asthmatic children were more anxious during medical visits, during contacts with social workers, and in school. They were more demanding and socially immature.

There is also clear evidence that asthmatic adults suffer from greater anxiety than the population at large (see below). The extent to which this anxiety can be traced to early attachment styles is unclear; no research has addressed this interesting issue.

Social Support and Management of Asthma

In our culture, which praises independence and self-reliance, benefit from social support is sometimes viewed as a sign of weakness rather than a valuable asset (Strunk et al, 1993). When one considers the complexity of successful asthma self-management, however, it is clear that social support facilitates this management. Social norms that view asthma as a serious disease requiring regular care create a supportive milieu for appropriate management behaviors. Cooperation from family members, friends, and co-workers makes the avoidance of asthma triggers much easier. Encouragement from others increases the likelihood that learned self-management skills will be put into action. Indeed, Bowlby (1973) has written that social support and secure attachment are the basis of self-reliance rather than its opposite.

One aspect of social support known to be important is the presence of a confidant upon whom one can depend in time of need. Lowenthal and Haven (1968), in a study of the elderly, found that the presence of a confidant was highly correlated with a high degree of satisfaction with life and a low incidence of depression. Hopper and Schechtman (1985) extended this research to diabetics. They found the presence of a confidant was correlated with glucose control, as measured by fasting blood sugar. The literature suggests that the presence of even a single confidant may make a significant difference in an individual's physical and psychological well-being.

Recently, we have been examining the effects of social isolation on the asthma care that inner-city African-American mothers, or other primary caregivers, provide their children (Fisher et al, 1993). Caregivers answered questions about the number of close friends and relatives they had and the number of emergency department visits their children had made for asthma during the previous year. The quality of asthma management was assessed through interviews with the children. Social isolation was significantly associated with poorer asthma management ($r = 0.14$, $p < 0.01$) and more emergency department visits ($r = 0.36$, $p < 0.05$). Subsequent analyses suggested that social isolation leads to poor asthma management which, in turn, leads to increased emergency department visits. To help alleviate these effects of social isolation, we are involved in a project in which neighborhood residents serving as CASS workers (Change Asthma with Social Support) provide social support to the caregivers. The social support literature (House et al, 1988) suggests that these neighbors helping neighbors may produce a significant improvement in asthma management, bringing with it a significant reduction in emergency department visits.

Psychological Factors that Interfere with Asthma Management

Asthma places added psychosocial stress on afflicted individuals and their families. Thus it is not surprising that there should be a higher incidence of psychopathology among asthmatics than in the general population. In particular, one might expect to find higher than normal incidence of anxiety disorders, depression, and behavioral disturbance (see below).

The inability to breath is a frightening event. When such an event occurs repeatedly, it is not surprising that high levels of anxiety might result. To the extent that these attacks are not under the control of the asthmatic individual, the anxiety will be greater. In addition, facing a serious chronic disease can lead to feelings of hopelessness and despair characteristic of depression. These feelings can be exacerbated by feelings of isolation from being different. Further, the strain on family members trying to cope with the emotional, social, and economic strain of asthma can lead to increased family dysfunction. When family dysfunction is combined with increased anxiety and depression in the asthmatic child (and his or her parents), behavioral problems are more likely to occur. These psychological problems all make effective asthma management more difficult. As a result, the disease is likely to worsen, producing a vicious cycle. Aggressive intervention to interrupt this cycle is critical to effective asthma management. Such a cycle is common to many chronic illnesses. For example, there is a much higher incidence of anxiety disorders and depression in people with diabetes than in the general population. Depressed and anxious diabetics have worse metabolic control of their diabetes and feel more distress from this lack of control than do non-depressed and non-anxious diabetics (Lustman et al, 1986).

There is a growing body of evidence that severe asthmatics with psychological problems are at far greater risk for death from asthma attack. For example, Strunk et al (1985) examined variables that discriminated between a group of 21 asthmatic children who died during a severe asthma attack from a control group of severely asthmatic children who did not die. They identified 14 variables that discriminated between these groups, of which 10 were psychological in nature (Table 18–1).

Kravis (1987) examined 15 children's deaths from asthma in Philadelphia. Two thirds had been referred for psychiatric evaluations because psychological factors appeared to be important in the course of their asthma. Of those referred, 30 percent were found to have serious psychosocial pathology, and another 30 percent severe family dysfunction. Rea et al (1986), in a case-controlled study of

TABLE 18–1. PSYCHOLOGICAL VARIABLES PREDICTING DEATH IN CHILDREN WITH SEVERE ASTHMA

- Disregard of perceived asthma symptoms
- Self-care not appropriate for age
- Patient-staff conflict
- Parent-staff conflict
- Patient-parent conflict
- Manipulative use of asthma
- Emotional disturbance
- Depressive symptoms
- History of emotional/behavioral reactions to loss or separation
- Family dysfunction

From Strunk et al. Physiological and psychological characteristics associated with deaths from asthma in childhood: a case-controlled study. JAMA 254:1193–1198, 1985.

asthma deaths in New Zealand, found that adults with documented psychosocial problems had 3.5 times the relative risk of dying from asthma. Sears et al (1986), in a 2-year study of all deaths due to asthma in New Zealand, found that half of the 16 children less than 15 years of age who died from asthma came from dysfunctional families. Detjen et al (1992) conducted a case study of six patients with potentially fatal asthma, defined in terms of survival from major asthma events such as respiratory failure requiring mechanical ventilation, and two episodes of acute pneumothorax or pneumomediastinum. They noted that three of six patients had significant psychosocial problems and five of six had denial of the severity of their illness.

CO-MORBIDITY OF PSYCHOLOGICAL PROBLEMS WITH ASTHMA

In recent years there has been a growing appreciation of the high co-morbidity of asthma and psychological disorders. The evidence is strongest for the anxiety disorders, although there is some evidence for depressive disorders as well.

Asthma and Anxiety Disorders

Shavitt et al (1992) studied 107 consecutive asthma center outpatients, 83 women and 24 men, with a mean age of 26.8 years and a standard deviation of 8.9 years. Patients were given a screening questionnaire about phobic and anxiety symptoms. Patients who responded positively (n = 56) were given psychiatric interviews. Those who showed evidence of anxiety or phobic avoidance were given a structured psychiatric interview, the relevant sections of the Structured Clinical Interview (SCID) for the DSM III-R. Twenty one of the original 107 patients (19.6 percent) met the diagnostic criteria for either agoraphobia (14 = 13.1 percent) or panic disorder (7 = 6.5 percent). (Agoraphobia is a fear of being caught in places or situations, for example, driving in a car or being in a crowded store, where panic symptoms might occur and it would be difficult or embarrassing to escape.) These percentages are considerably higher than the estimated *lifetime* prevalence rates for agoraphobia and panic disorder in the general population, 3 to 9 percent and 1 to 3 percent, respectively. Interestingly, none of these patients had ever been diagnosed or treated for their anxiety disorder. The authors suggested that clinicians may mislabel panic attacks for crises of asthma. They note that there is a large overlap of symptoms between panic and asthma attacks and that medical tradition is biased toward looking for a single diagnosis. They, and Yellowlees and Kalucy (1990), have noted the potentially vicious circle of anxiety disorders and asthma: asthma attacks can trigger panic or phobic avoidance and anxiety symptoms can trigger asthma attacks.

Yellowlees and his colleagues (Yellowlees et al, 1988; Yellowlees and Ruffin, 1989; Yellowlees and Kalucy, 1990) have examined psychiatric morbidity in 25 patients with life-threatening asthma (near-miss asthma deaths [NMAD], defined as an episode of severe acute asthma with respiratory failure and/or an altered state of consciousness), compared to 40 patients with less severe asthma. Psychiatric diagnoses were based on two structured interviews, one specifically developed by the authors and the other the Diagnostic Interview Schedule (DIS). There were not significant differences between the proportions of NMAD patients and less severe asthmatics who suffered from anxiety disorders. Thirty-four percent of the total of 65 patients had anxiety disorders: 17 percent panic disorders, 11 percent post-traumatic stress disorders, and 6 percent phobic disorders. Although the mix of anxiety disorders differs between Yellowlees' and Shavitt's studies, both reveal that anxiety disorders are apparently much more prevalent among asthmatics than in the general population.

The research on anxiety disorders in patients with asthma is consistent with research showing an increased incidence of anxiety disorders in patients with a wide variety of chronic diseases, including other chronic lung diseases, arthritis, diabetes, heart disease, and high blood pressure (Wells et al, 1989). The recent and lifetime prevalence of anxiety disorders in patients with these chronic diseases typically is two to three times that of healthy subjects.

Asthma and Depression

The National Institute of Mental Health Epidemiological Cachement Area study indicates that the 6-month prevalence of major depressive episodes is approximately 1.5 to 2 percent for males and 4 percent for females in the general population (Meyers et al, 1984). In contrast, research on chronic diseases indicates that individuals with chronic lung disease, arthritis, heart disease, hypertension, and diabetes all have lifetime rates of major depression (14.3 to 18.6 percent) that are two to three times the lifetime prevalence rates for healthy individuals (6.9 percent; Wells et al, 1989). Data from a tertiary referral center suggest that the prevalence of depression in seriously asthmatic children may be as high as 25 percent (Miller, 1987). Mrazek et al (1984) observed that preschool children with severe asthma had significantly higher levels of depressed symptoms than nonasthmatic controls, based on a behavioral screening questionnaire completed by the mother.

PRACTICAL ISSUES FOR THE PHYSICIAN

How to Recognize Psychological Problems

Often the best screening method for psychological problems is the physician's self-questioning about the presence of such problems during routine care (Strunk et al, 1993). Table 18–2 provides some questions which, when asked in the course of caring for a patient, may give some indication of problems.

The physician should also be aware of several other issues with respect to screening for psychological problems that might interfere with asthma management. One such issue relates to childhood depression. Until recently, many psychiatrists and psychologists doubted the existence of depression in children. There is now a growing consensus recognizing that depression does occur, even in young children, although symptoms may differ somewhat from those of adults. It is particularly noteworthy that children with depressed mood often show an increased sensitivity of mood, for example, crying or throwing temper tantrums at the least provocation. Lethargy may be less pronounced than in adults; rather, agitation is commonly observed. General somatic complaints, such as headaches or stomach aches, also may be common (Carlson, 1988).

An important point of *similarity* between depressed children and adults is that suicidal ideation is not uncommon (Carlson, 1988). The physician needs to be sensitive to the issue of suicide, particularly with older children and adolescents. Signs that should make one consider the possibility of suicidal ideation include loss of interest in life, isolation from friends, comments about the meaninglessness of life, recent suicide of a peer, and the giving away of valued possessions. If suicide potential is suspected, the best approach is a direct one: the patient should be asked in a straightforward fashion, "Have you ever thought of hurting yourself or killing yourself? Have you thought about it recently?" Asking about suicide does not make a person any more likely to carry out a suicide attempt, and questioning of suicidal potential is a necessary first step in assessing suicide risk, as well as a first step in therapy. The risk of suicide grows as a function of previous suicide attempts, specificity of suicidal thoughts and plans, lethality of a plan, and accessibility to the planned means. If a patient admits to suicidal ideation, these points need to be assessed, as well as possible barriers to suicide (Table 18–3). Needless to say, if the physician is too uncomfortable making such a preliminary assessment or if such an assessment reveals any signs of potential suicide, *immediate* referral should be made to an appropriate mental health care provider.

Physicians also should be aware that the

TABLE 18–2. QUESTIONS SUGGESTING POTENTIAL PSYCHOLOGICAL PROBLEMS

Is there evidence of persistent medical noncompliance or poor self-care?
Am I aware of anger, frustration, or antagonism toward the patient and/or family?
Have there been important losses to the patient, such as death of spouse, parent, or child; divorce; loss of employment; or geographic relocation?
Am I concerned about depression or have there been references to death, self-harm, guilt, and/or expression of hopelessness?
Have there been notable personality changes, unusual behavior, emotional lability, decline in school or work function, or onset of drug or alcohol use/abuse?
Is there evidence of sexual or physical abuse?

From Strunk et al. Use of prospective disease management to minimize asthma symptoms and maximize potential. *In* Gershwin ME, Halpren GM (eds). Bronchial Asthma: Principles of Diagnosis and Practice. Totowa, NJ, Humana, 1994, pp 661–690.

TABLE 18–3. SUICIDE ASSESSMENT

For assessing suicide risk, a direct approach is preferable. There is no evidence that mentioning suicide to a patient makes the patient more likely to attempt suicide. On the contrary, the physician's open concern may help to counteract the sense of hopelessness and isolation that underlies many suicide attempts. The following points should be assessed.
1. Is the patient thinking about hurting or killing himself/herself? For example, you might ask "Have you thought of hurting or killing yourself?"

If the answer to the first question is positive, then:

2. Has the patient made a suicide attempt in the past?
3. Dose the patient have a specific plan for killing himself/herself?
   Has the patient taken any steps towards enacting this plan?
   How lethal is this plan?
   How accessible is the means of committing suicide? For example, is there a gun in the home?
4. Does the patient know anyone who has committed or attempted suicide?
5. Are there any barriers to suicide? For example, is the patient concerned over the potential effects of suicide on his or her family?

Positive answers to 1 through 4 and a negative answer to 5 indicate high suicide risk.

---

caretaker of a child with severe asthma may be more susceptible to depression. Worry and feelings of guilt over the child's health, stress over the cost of medical care, loss of sleep, and other stresses all place the parent at increased risk for the development of depression. The risk is intensified if the parent is a single mother living in the inner city with a low socioeconomic status and little social support. Further exacerbating this situation, asthma is much more common in this population (Weitzman et al, 1990). Such a parent almost certainly will not be able to consistently carry out an asthma management program involving her child.

When Should a Mental Health Care Provider Become Involved in Asthma Co-Management?

As we have seen throughout this chapter, psychological problems and concerns are inextricably interwoven with asthma (or any other serious chronic disease). Because of this, we believe that, whenever possible, a mental health care provider (e.g., psychologist, psychiatrist, social worker, psychiatric nurse) should be a part of the asthma management team. A psychological screening by the mental health staff member should be made a routine part of the initial work-up/assessment for a new patient with asthma. This would allow for the early identification and treatment of psychological problems likely to impede asthma management. It also creates in the patient the perception that psychological factors are important in the management of chronic asthma and reduces the social stigma of dealing with any psychological problems that may arise.

Whenever concerns over potential psychological problems arise, they should be addressed promptly during ongoing management of the patient's asthma. We would recommend that the physician have a low threshold for obtaining a psychological consultation if such problems are not yielding to the approach used by the physician and a mental health care provider is not part of the management team, or if the severity of these problems is beyond the expertise of that team member (e.g., possible suicides, as discussed above). In many situations, psychological evaluation may be best obtained early in the course of treatment rather than ordering a number of physiologic tests to determine that there is not a problem in other areas. This helps to avoid the implication that "It's all in your head" and conveys to the patient that the physician perceives psychological issues to be important in asthma management.

The following illustrates how a physician might broach a psychological referral with a patient:

"You appear to be anxious (depressed . . .) about your (your child's) asthma. That's not surprising given all the stress and worry you've had to go through. Many of my patients show similar reactions to their asthma. This anxiety can really interfere with our managing your asthma effectively. In these situations, I like to refer my patients to Dr. _____ who's a psychologist on our team. She has some techniques that are highly effective in helping people control their anxiety. We've been very successful working together. Let's set up an appointment for you to see her."

Such an approach directly addresses the concern over the psychological problem, normalizes the problem for the patient ("You are not abnormal; other patients with asthma often have this problem"), creates an expectation of a positive outcome, and treats a psychological referral as routine as a medical referral would be.

What to Expect Once a Psychological/Psychiatric Referral Is Made

Referral

Ideally, referral should be made to a mental health care provider with knowledge of medical and psychological aspects of asthma, or at least with experience working with patients with chronic diseases. Other criteria for selecting a referral source would include: Does the psychologist have experience working with the relevant age group and ethnic group? If the referral problem is family related, does the social worker have experience with family therapy?

After a referral is made, the issue of confidentiality needs to be addressed among the patient and the professionals involved. All parties need to understand at the outset what information will or will not be communicated back to the physician (and vice versa).

Psychological Assessment

Following referral to a psychologist, assessment typically would include a detailed interview, including information on: the problem as viewed by the patient and other relevant family members, history relevant to the problem, behavioral observations (e.g., physical appearance, pattern of speech, nonverbal communication such as eye contact), and a brief check of mental status, both cognitive and emotional. (Is the patient alert and oriented? Is there any evidence of hallucinations or delusions? Is the patient's affect normal?) During this initial assessment, the psychologist is also attempting to begin to develop a therapeutic relationship, building rapport and conveying to the patient that the psychologist cares about the patient and that his or her problems are amenable to treatment.

Depending on the nature of the problems to be addressed, the assessment may also include self-report (or parent-report) questionnaires and/or standardized psychological tests. The assessment phase typically lasts one or two sessions. At its conclusion, the psychologist should be able to provide the physician with a clear statement of the problem (other problems may, of course, be uncovered as therapy proceeds), a description of the treatment approach, and an estimate of the duration of treatment. The psychologist should be willing to "translate" any technical terms into language understandable to the physician.

Treatment Methods

The most common psychological problems likely to be encountered by a physician involve patients whose asthma care is complicated by anxiety, depression, possibly including suicidal ideation, and family dysfunction. Fortunately, these problems have proved to be amenable to therapeutic intervention. We briefly describe some to the major treatment modalities for these problems and cite, where available, relevant research literature involving the use of these treatment modalities on patients with asthma.

PHARMACOTHERAPY. Severe depression in adults generally will require pharmacotherapy and should be accompanied by psychotherapy, whereas mild or moderate depression often is treatable by psychotherapy alone. There has been little research on the use of antidepressants in children and adolescents (Carlson, 1988).

There are case studies suggesting that some tricyclic antidepressants, such as amitryptiline and imipramine, may have a beneficial effect on asthma symptoms by producing bronchodilation. This may be due to anticholinergic effects (Mrazek, 1992; Miller, 1987; Carlson, 1988). Patients sensitive to tartrazine, a dye used in certain antidepressants, should avoid imipramine, desipramine, and trazodone (Mrazek, 1992; Kanner et al, 1989).

There is evidence that the tricyclic antidepressant imipramine is also effective in the treatment of anxiety disorders. However, a study by Kanner et al (1989) suggests that caution is required in prescribing imipramine to asthmatics, especially children. These authors conducted a pilot study using imipramine to treat five children with chronic intractable asthma suffering from separation anxiety disorder (four) and major depressive disorder (one). Both psychiatrist and child ratings indicated that the treatment with imipramine improved the anxiety disorder in all four children tested, although it had no effect on the depression in the one child. Further, wheezing improved in all four anxiety disorder children. Unfortunately, serious side effects in all four anxiety patients required the termination of this study. One patient had a generalized epileptic seizure after 10 weeks of treatment. This patient had theophylline blood levels of 28 µg/ml, well above therapeutic range, and in a range known to cause seizures. However, this patient had previously had equally high theophylline levels on several occasions without seizures. A second patient developed a cardiac arrhythmia consisting of auricular premature contractions. A third patient developed diastolic hypertension, and a fourth patient displayed increased motor activity, insomnia, impulsive behavior, and transitory moderate postural hypotension.

COGNITIVE/BEHAVIORAL THERAPIES. Cognitive/behavioral techniques have been demonstrated to be highly effective in the treatment of anxiety disorders, including panic disorder, agoraphobia, and post-traumatic stress disorder (Barlow, 1988). Studies comparing behavioral therapies with pharmacotherapies in the treatment of anxiety disorders typically have shown the behavioral therapies to be at least as effective, with lower dropout rates and without potential drug complications. The common element across different behavioral therapies that have been shown to be successful in the treatment of anxiety disorders is repeated enforced exposure to the anxiety-arousing stimulus or situation so that the anxiety habituates. Typically, the amount of exposure to the anxiety-arousing stimulus is gradually increased. This gradual exposure works at least as well as more rapid exposure and reduces patient dropout rates. The exposure treatment is often combined with relaxation or deep breathing techniques and cognitive techniques to help the patient restructure his or her thinking about anxiety. Barlow (1988) describes in detail the clinical and research literature on anxiety disorders and their treatments.

Several psychotherapies have been demonstrated to be effective in the treatment of depression in adults (Elkin et al, 1989). For mild and moderate depression they are as effective as pharmacotherapy. Perhaps the most widely used is a form of cognitive therapy first developed by Beck and his associates (Beck, 1976; Beck et al, 1979). This therapy is based on the theoretic view that emotional problems are often the result of faulty thinking patterns. With respect to depression, Beck argues that there are a triad of faulty cognitions about oneself, the world, and the future. The therapist and the client work together examining and correcting these faulty cognitions. There is a major behavioral component to this process. Beck notes that depressed patients often suffer from a reduced activity level and a lack of rewards or sources of pleasure in their lives. Thus, patients are given assignments to increase their daily activities, are taught to monitor the pleasure they obtain from their actions, practice breaking tasks down into manageable components so that successes can occur, and are taught to test behaviorally their faulty cognitions. With this therapy, significant changes in mood and behavior typically occur within a relatively short time frame (e.g., a couple of months).

There has been little outcome research on the treatment of childhood depression (Matson and Carey, 1988). The few studies that have been conducted suggest that a cognitive/behavioral approach may also be effective with this population. An important component of such an approach applied to children may be the facilitation of social interactions through social skills training. With such training, children receive instruction on how to interact socially, they observe models, they practice the social interactions themselves, and they receive feedback and reinforcement for their performance.

FAMILY THERAPY. Successful management of childhood asthma requires the cooperative efforts of the entire family. Family dysfunction can easily disrupt asthma management. A rebellious adolescent may refuse parental requests to comply with his or her medical regimen, or a depressed mother may lack the energy to adequately oversee the child's care. Unfortunately, the psychological, economic, social, and practical burdens placed on a family by a serious chronic disease such as asthma increase the probability of family dysfunction. Thus, when psychological problems interfere with asthma management, they are often best dealt with at the level of the family rather than the patient alone.

Although there are a variety of types of family therapy, all share a focus on treating the family as an interactive system. An individual's psychopathology is seen as arising from this system, and it, in turn, feeds back and influences the functioning of the system. Therapy attempts to change dysfunctional patterns of family interaction (Lask and Matthew, 1979; Wells, 1988).

There have been few controlled studies examining the effect of family therapy on childhood asthma (Lask and Matthew, 1979; Gustafsson et al, 1986). These studies, however, have shown impressive positive results and deserve replication on a larger scale. Lask and Matthew randomly assigned moderate to severe asthmatic children between 4 and 14 years of age to a family therapy (17 families with 21 asthmatic children) or control group (16 families with 16 asthmatic children). Both groups received routine medical care over a 4-month period, and the family therapy group also received six 1-hour family therapy sessions (one every 3 weeks). These sessions focused on helping the whole family to develop less extreme and more realistic attitudes and feelings about different concerns involving the child's asthma. The family therapy group, in comparison to the control group, showed significantly better thoracic gas volumes and significantly less wheezing. The therapy group also showed a significant improvement in their peak expiratory flow rate over the course of the study, whereas the control group did not.

The Gustafsson et al study involved the 20 most severe chronic cases of bronchial asthma from approximately 600 patients who attended the pediatric outpatient clinic at a university hospital in Sweden. The children ranged in age from 6 to 15 years, and all had asthma grade D (McNichol and Williams, 1973a,b,c). Children were randomly assigned to a family therapy (n = 9) or control (n = 8) group. (Two families refused to participate in the study, and one family served as a pilot case.) Two family therapy subjects did not attend any family therapy sessions but were included in the data analyses for the family therapy group. Following an 8-month baseline, the family therapy group received family therapy over 8 months (between 2 and 21 sessions, mean of 8.8) while the control group received no treatment. Then, control group families were offered family therapy; four accepted and were treated. Thus, a total of 12 families received family therapy at some time in the study (one pilot family, seven experimental group families, and four initial control group families), and six families never received therapy (two experimental families who did not attend any therapy sessions and four control families). Finally, 18 months later, the children were reevaluated for an additional 8-month period. The children were clinically evaluated three times during each 8-month period by a pediatric allergist who was blind to the patients' experimental condition. This evaluation included: a general pediatric assessment with regard to the severity and frequency of asthma symptoms, clinical grading of daily functioning, peak expiratory flow (PEF), patient compliance to prescribed medications and treatments, emergency department visits, days of functional impairment from parents' diaries, doses of β_2 agonists, nights when β_2 agonists were used, and prescriptions of steroids for longer than 2 months.

The initial between-group comparisons revealed significant improvements in the family therapy group relative to the control group on general pediatric assessment and days of functional impairment. When within-patient changes over time were examined, patients who received family therapy showed significant improvements in general pediatric assessment, clinical grading, PEF, functionally impaired days, doses of β_2 agonist, and nights using β_2 agonists. There was also a near-significant decrease in emergency department visits from 2.67 days/year to 0.17 days/year ($p = 0.06$). In the non-family therapy cases there were no significant changes in any of these measures over time. Although these results are promising, the study has a number of important limitations. As the authors acknowledge, this study does not allow one to separate specific benefits due to family therapy from a nonspecific placebo effect. Also, comparison of within-patient changes over time between the therapy and no-therapy patients must be interpreted with great caution since this separation of patients was not random.

Overall, these initial studies suggest that relatively small amounts of family therapy (approximately eight sessions) may be effective in producing large amounts of change in the condition of asthmatic children. These results are particularly impressive when one considers that the families selected for these studies were apparently *not* chosen based on a high degree of family dysfunction. Children of such families might be expected to profit even more from family therapy.

SUMMARY

As we have seen, psychological factors are woven through asthma and its treatment. Emotional factors can trigger asthma attacks. The psychological functioning of children with asthma appears to play a larger role than in just their medical condition, with effects on their physical and social functioning. There is a high co-morbidity of asthma with anxiety, depression, and family dysfunction. These psychological problems affect immediate management of asthma, sometimes resulting in life-threatening situations. They also can have long-term effects on the psychosocial development of children with asthma.

On the positive side, psychological interventions have been shown to be highly effective in the treatment of these psychological problems, and initial results indicate that their resolution results in improved asthma management. Further, social support has been shown to facilitate the management of chronic diseases, including asthma. Thus, it is important for the physician to recognize when psychological factors are triggering asthma or interfering with its management, so that they can be aggressively treated. Consideration of psychological factors is an integral part of successful asthma management.

REFERENCES

Ainsworth MDS, Blehar MC, Waters E, Wall S. Patterns of Attachment: A Psychological Study of the Strange Situation. Hillsdale, NJ, Erlbaum, 1978.

Barlow DH. Anxiety and Its Disorders. The Nature and Treatment of Anxiety and Panic. New York, Guilford Press, 1988.

Beck A. Cognitive Therapy and Emotional Disorders. New York, International Universities Press, 1976.

Beck AT, Rush AJ, Shaw BF, Emery G. Cognitive Therapy of Depression. New York, Guilford Press, 1979.

Bender BG, Belleau L, Fukuhara JT, Mrazek DA, Strunk RC. Psychomotor adaptation in children with severe chronic asthma. Pediatrics 79(5):723–727, 1987.

Bowlby J. Attachment and Loss. Vol. 1. Attachment. New York, Basic Books, 1969.

Bowlby J. Self-reliance and some conditions that promote it. In Gosling R (ed). Support, Innovation, and Autonomy. (Tavistock Clinic Golden Jubilee Papers) London, Tavistock Publications Ltd, 1973.

Carlson GA. Depression: Pharmacotherapies. In Matson JL (ed). Handbook of Treatment Approaches in Childhood Psychopathology. New York, Plenum Press, 1988, pp 345–366.

Detjen PF, Greenberger PA, Grammer LC, Patterson R. Malignant potentially fatal asthma: A management strategy. Allergy Proc 13(1):27–33, 1992.

Elkin S, Shea MT, Watkins JT, Imber SD, Sotsky SM, Collins JF, Glass DR, Pilkonis PA, Leber WR, Docherty JP, Fiester SJ, Parloff MB. National Institute of Mental Health Treatment of Depression Collaborative Research Program: General effectiveness of treatments. Arch Gen Psychiatry 46:971–982, 1989.

Fisher EB Jr, Sylvia SC, Sussman LJ, Arfken CL, Sykes RK, Strunk RC. Social isolation of caretakers of African American children with asthma is associated with poor asthma management. Paper presented at Annual Meeting of the American Thoracic Society, San Francisco, May, 1993.

Gustafsson PA, Kjellman M, Cederblad M. Family therapy in the treatment of severe childhood asthma. J Psychosom Res 30(3):369–374, 1986.

Gutstadt LB, Gillette JW, Mrazek DA, Fukuhara JT, LaBrecque JF, Strunk RC. Determinants of school performance in children with chronic asthma. Am J Dis Child 143:471–475, 1989.

Hazan C, Shaver P. Romantic love conceptualized as an attachment process. J Pers Soc Psychol 52:511–524, 1987.

House JS, Landis KR, Umberson D. Social relationships and health. Science 241:540–544, 1988.

Hopper S, Schechtman K. Factors associated with diabetic control: Utilization patterns in a low-income, older adult population. Patient Educ Counseling 7:275–288, 1985.

Isenberg SA, Lehrer PM, Hochron S. The effects of suggestion and emotional arousal on pulmonary function in asthma: A review and a hypothesis regarding vagal mediation. Psychosom Med 54:192–216, 1992.

Janson-Bjerklie S, Boushey HA, Carrieri VK, Lindsey AM. Emotionally triggered asthma as a predictor of airway response to suggestion. Res Nurs Health 9:163–170, 1986.

Kanner AM, Klein RG, Rubinstein B, Mascia A. Use of imipramine in children with intractable asthma and psychiatric disorders: A warning. Psychother Psychosom 51:203–209, 1989.

Kravis LP. An analysis of fifteen childhood asthma fatalities. J Allergy Clin Immunol 80(3, Part 2):467–472, 1987.

Lask B, Matthew D. Childhood asthma. A controlled trial of family psychotherapy. Arch Dis Child 54:116–119, 1979.

Lowenthal MF, Haven C. Interaction and adaptation: Intimacy as a critical variable. Am Sociol Rev 33:20–30, 1968.

Ludwick SK, Jones JW, Jones TK, Fukuhara JT, Strunk RC. Normalization of cardiopulmonary endurance in severely asthmatic children after bicycle ergometry therapy. J Pediatr 109:446–451, 1986.

Luparello T, Lyons HA, Bleecker BA, McFadden ER Jr. Influences of suggestion on airway reactivity in asthmatic subjects. Psychosom Med 30(6):819–825, 1968.

Lustman PJ, Griffith LS, Clouse RE, Cryer PE. Psychiatric illness in diabetes: relationship to symptoms and glucose control. J Nerv Ment Dis 174:736–742, 1986.

Matson JL, Carey M. Depression: Psychological therapies. In Matson JL (ed). Handbook of Treatment Approaches in Childhood Psychopathology. New York, Plenum Press, 1988, pp 327–344.

McNichol KN, Williams HE. Spectrum of asthma in children—I, clinical and physiological components. Br Med J 4:7–11, 1973a.

McNichol KN, Williams HE. Spectrum of asthma in children—II, allergic components. Br Med J 4:12–16, 1973b.

McNichol KN, Williams HE, Allan J, McAndrew I. Spectrum of asthma in children—III, psychological and social components. Br Med J 4:16–20, 1973c.

Meyers JK, Weissman MM, Tischler GL, Holzer CE III, Leaf PJ, Orvaschel H, Anthony JC, Boyd JH, Burke JD, Kramer M, Stoltzman R. Six-month prevalence of psychiatric disorders in three communities. Arch Gen Psychiatry 41:959–967, 1984.

Mrazek DA, Anderson IS, Strunk RC. Disturbed emotional development of severely asthmatic preschool children. J Child Psychol Psychiatry 4(suppl):81–94, 1984.

Mrazek DA. Psychiatric complications of pediatric asthma. Ann Allergy 69:285–293, 1992.

Rea HH, Scragg R, Jackson R, Beaglehole R, Fenwick J, Sutherland DC. A case control study of deaths from asthma. Thorax 41:833–839, 1986.

Sears MR, Rea HH, Fenjwick J, et al. Deaths from asthma in New Zealand. Arch Dis Child 61:6–10, 1986.

Shavitt RG, Gentil V, Mandetta R. The association of panic/agoraphobia and asthma. Contributing factors and clinical implications. Gen Hosp Psychiatry, 14:420–423, 1992.

Strunk RC, Fisher EB Jr, Davis SG, Sussman L. Use of prospective disease management to minimize asthma symptoms and maximize potential. In Gershwin ME, Halpren GM (eds). Bronchial Asthma: Principles of Diagnosis and Practice. Totowa, NJ, Humana, 1994, pp 661–690.

Strunk RC, Mrazek DA, Fuhrmann GSW, LaBrecque J. Physiological and psychological characteristics associated with deaths from asthma in childhood: A case-controlled study. JAMA 254:1193–1198, 1985.

Strunk RC, Mrazek DA, Fukuhara JT, Masterson J, Ludwick SK, LaBrecque JF. Cardiovascular fitness in children with asthma correlates with psychological functioning of the child. Pediatrics 84:460–464, 1989.

Weitzman M, Gortmaker S, Sobol A. Racial, social, and environmental risks for childhood asthma. Am J Dis Child 144:1189–1194, 1990.

Wells KC. Family therapy. In Matson JL (ed). Handbook of Treatment Approaches in Childhood Psychopathology. New York, Plenum Press, 1988, pp 45–64.

Wells KB, Golding JM, Burnam MA. Affective, substance use, and anxiety disorders in persons with arthritis, diabetes, heart disease, high blood pressure, or chronic lung conditions. Gen Hosp Psychiatry 11:320–327, 1989.

Williams JS. Aspects of dependence. Independence conflict in children with asthma. J Child Psychol Psychiatry 16:199–218, 1975.

Yellowlees PM, Haynes S, Potts N, Ruffin RE. Psychiatric morbidity in patients with life-threatening asthma: Initial report of a controlled study. Med J Aust 149:246–249, 1988.

Yellowlees PM, Ruffin RE. Psychological defenses andcoping styles in patients following a life-threatening attack of asthma. Chest 95(6):1298–1303, 1989.

Yellowlees PM, Kalucy RS. Psychobiological aspects of asthma and the consequent research implications. Chest 97(3):628–634, 1990.

Chapter 19

Patient Education: Creating a Partnership for Effective Asthma Care

Virginia Silver Taggart, M.P.H., and Gary S. Rachelefsky, M.D.

Asthma is a common and serious chronic condition affecting between 9 and 12 million Americans. The prevalence of asthma among children—already 6 percent—is rising. Mortality rates and hospitalizations increased dramatically from 1979 to 1989 (U.S. Department of Health and Human Services, 1992). During this period, children with asthma missed twice as much school as their classmates, and one quarter of the children with asthma missed more than 11 days of school in one year (Fowler et al, 1992). Over 10 million school days a year were lost because of asthma. One third of children with asthma restricted their physical activities (Newachek and Taylor, 1992). Adults with asthma experience similar disruptions: 3 million workdays lost among persons 18 years old or older as well as restrictions on normal daily activities (Weiss et al, 1992).

The burden of asthma can be substantial—not only in terms of illness, academic problems, limited activities, disruption of family life, but also in lost productivity of adults with asthma, or even parents while caring for a sick child, a loss that equalled 1 billion dollars in 1990 (Weiss et al, 1992). The burden of asthma on a physician's practice includes unscheduled visits and the problems inherent in treating an illness that can be difficult to resolve.

CREATING A PARTNERSHIP

Fortunately, therapies now exist that enable most patients with asthma to participate fully in all activities, but statistics noted earlier have not changed proportionately. Are we getting the right therapy to our patients with asthma? Equally important, are we giving patients adequate education so that they can and will use the therapy appropriately?

Numerous studies document that patient education can improve adherence to therapy and improve health outcomes (Rachelefsky, 1987). This education is not the traditional kind that focuses almost entirely on giving information and simply tells patients what to do. Studies repeatedly show that with such traditional health provider messages only 30 to 40 percent of the patients understand or follow the physician's instructions. Giving information is necessary, but by itself it is rarely enough to effect the behavior change needed for adequate asthma management.

Behavior change depends, obviously, on one's knowing what to do, but it also depends on one's believing the recommended action is worth doing, on being able to do it, and on being reinforced for doing it (Parcel and Baronowski, 1981). Patient education that fosters behavior change is most effectively accomplished by getting patients and parents to take responsibility for specific actions, that is, by helping them to become partners in asthma care.

A partnership is a relationship involving cooperation among parties with specific and joint rights and responsibilities. The major responsibilities of the patient/parent are to learn the skills necessary to manage asthma, to adhere to the treatment plan, and to make adjustments to the plan as arranged with the clinician. When adherence to the treatment plan is difficult or produces adverse effects, the patient must let the clinician know so that a new treatment plan can be negotiated. The clinician's responsibilities are to provide the medical expertise to assess the patient's asthma and select the most appropriate treatment plan, to teach the patient the skills necessary to follow the plan and manage asthma at home, to negotiate for the best possible adherence, and to be available to the patient for education and support.

In a pediatric practice, the child must become a partner in asthma care as well as the parents. It is increasingly well documented that children have considerable access to medications and that they start taking over-the-counter medications on their own at early ages (Bush and Ianotti, 1990). Children make numerous decisions on their own that can profoundly affect their asthma. They decide, for example, whether to play with a friend's pet, report early symptoms, or cooperate with medication regimens. Thus it is important to prepare them to make appropriate decisions by actively including them in the asthma care partnership as early as possible. Children as young as 3 and 4 years of age can be the central focus of the clinician's communication with the family. Some clinicians find that directing their comments to the child—even when answering the parent's questions—has two benefits: (1) it improves the child's participation and sense of personal efficacy, and (2) it ensures that the parent will understand while avoiding the appearance of "talking down" to a parent.

THE FIVE Rs OF TEACHING

How can patient education be organized and delivered to make a partnership among the clinician, patient, and family possible? The "Five Rs of Teaching," based on social learning theory and the experience of successful asthma education programs, provide a framework: reach agreement on goals, rehearse asthma management skills, repeat messages, reinforce appropriate behavior, and review.

Reach Agreement on Goals

It is realistic, with current therapies, to expect that most patients with asthma can control their asthma. The first "R" is to *reach* agreement on goals. These goals for therapy should be as close as possible to those established by the National Asthma Education Program (National Heart, Lung, and Blood Institute, 1991):

- Maintain (near) normal pulmonary function rates.
- Maintain normal activity levels, including exercise.
- Prevent chronic and troublesome symptoms (e.g., coughing or breathlessness in the night, in the early morning, or after exertion).
- Prevent recurrent exacerbations of asthma.
- Avoid adverse effects from asthma medication.

Many patients do not realize that their quality of life could and should be normal. They have accepted sleepless nights, persistent cough, and limited activities as the nature of asthma. It is often up to the clinician to raise patient and parent expectations for asthma care. Some parents resist a diagnosis of asthma because they fear that this means their child cannot lead a normal life or that the asthma is psychological. It is important to assure parents and children that this is not the case. Although asthma is a chronic disease of the lungs (not the mind) and although there is no cure for asthma, it *is* controllable. However, the clinician's goals may not be the same as the patient's goals, or the patient may perceive the "price" of accomplishing them to be too high. For example, a clinician may want a patient to have lung function at 100 percent of that predicted and be totally free of symptoms, which would require daily medicine and removal of a beloved family pet. But these requirements may be difficult for the patient to accept. Further, the recommendation of daily therapy may run counter to the patient's belief that asthma is episodic and can be handled by just getting through the asthma episodes as quickly, and with as little medicine, as possible. Discussion with this patient is necessary to develop realistic goals for therapy and to shape appropriate beliefs about asthma and what will accomplish these goals.

To reach agreement on goals for therapy, the discussion between the clinician and patient or parent should focus on clarifying expectations for therapy, developing a treatment plan together, negotiating details for implementing the plan, and providing a written plan.

CLARIFY EXPECTATIONS. Patient education for a partnership in asthma care cannot be limited to discussing only those things the physician thinks the patient needs to know and do. It must incorporate and accommodate what the patient and parents perceive as their own needs and concerns. Patients and parents cannot attend adequately to what physicians recommend until their own expectations, needs, fears, and concerns are addressed (Korsch et al, 1968). Addressing patient needs is critical. A patient who is dissatisfied is less likely to follow recommendations, and a patient *is* dissatisfied if the clinician does not listen to concerns or meet the patient's expectations (Korsch et al, 1968).

There are several methods for eliciting the patient expectations. Some physicians send a letter to new patients (or parents) asking them to think about their asthma and their hopes for asthma care and to bring in a list for the initial visit. Others encourage patients to review a list of key questions about whether their goals for therapy have been met or whether their asthma is troublesome before each visit or phone call. In any case, the critical step is to ask the patient and parents directly. It is most effective to use open-ended questions such as:

What does asthma mean to you?
What bothers you about your asthma?
What problems has it created for you?
What have you tried? Did it help?
What do you expect from treatment?
Many people worry about asthma medications. What do you worry about?
What would you like from this visit today?

Clarifying patient (and parent) expectations helps to identify what the patient understands about asthma, what the patient is already doing, and what the patient wants. The clinician uses this opportunity to respond to specific concerns, relieve fears, correct inappropriate beliefs, and adjust teaching to the particular patient's needs—building on what the patient already knows and is doing appropriately. This leads to a discussion about the nature of asthma and key aspects of effective treatment. The key messages are brief: Asthma is a chronic inflammatory disease of the airways with acute exacerbations of airway narrowing and related symptoms. Therapy is aimed at (1) preventing these exacerbations (through environmental control and anti-inflammatory pharmacologic therapy) and (2) for exacerbations that do occur, treating exacerbations promptly at the earliest signs of worsening. Such signs are detected by symptom and peak flow monitoring.

DEVELOP A TREATMENT PLAN TOGETHER. The discussion of expectations for therapy provides the basis for developing a treatment plan together, a plan that the clinician knows is medically indicated and the patient or parent knows is practical and worthwhile.

Every treatment plan has two parts:

1. A plan for the daily management of asthma that specifies the medication (name, dose, and times of administration) and environmental measures necessary to maintain control.
2. An action plan for handling exacerbations. This plan tells patients:

- How to recognize signs of deterioration (increasing symptoms, especially at night, and declining peak flow)
- What kind, and what dose of medication to add at what times
- When and whom to call for help, day- and night-time phone numbers for the physician, the emergency department, and ambulance

Because patients often consider asthma an episodic disease, it may be difficult for them to understand why daily medications are recommended. Teaching patients about the two entirely different types of medications—"preventer" medications and "quick relief" medications—provides an essential rationale for treatment, increases the patient's confidence that there are treatments that can control asthma, and thus may improve adherence.

NEGOTIATE DETAILS. Tailoring the medication schedule to the patient's daily routine enhances adherence. It is helpful to ask the patient or parent to suggest the best time for taking medicines and what difficulties there might be taking medicine in, for example, a day care or school setting. This can make a difference in the type and timing of medication. Perhaps a child can have a nebulizer treatment at home before going to day care and use an MDI at the day care site. Perhaps the school child or employed adult should take larger doses twice a day, early in the morning and at night rather than three times a day. The patient may have clear preferences among spacer devices or inhaler techniques, and the patient should choose what is most comfortable and practical in order to increase the likelihood of adherence. For example, one teenager agreed to use a spacer device at home but only the open-mouth inhaler technique at school. Agreeing on and writing down specific times of the day to take medicines, rather than simply recommending, for example, "take this twice a day," may foster a commitment to the regimen.

Frequency of peak flow monitoring is particularly amenable to negotiation. For example, after an initial 2- to 3-week assessment period of twice-a-day measures, the clinician and patient may discover that the patient's own perception of symptoms may be sensitive enough to render unnecessary daily peak flow monitoring. Measures just once a day, once or twice a week, or less, may provide sufficient monitoring information.

Environmental control measures are especially important to negotiate. All too often a patient or parent is given a lengthy list of allergens to eradicate from the home environment without any discussion of priorities or practicality. Many patients and parents interpret this as all or nothing. Faced with a daunting behavioral change effort that affects the entire family, many opt for "nothing." Behavioral change efforts are often most successful when an easier change is identified first. The success of accomplishing that one change improves motivation to take on the next step. Thus, it is preferable to explain that the goal is to reduce exposure to identified allergens as much as possible, not necessarily eradicate all allergens. The clinician and patient together can select areas that are either most critical (i.e., will yield the most significant results) or easiest to accomplish. Some compromise will be required. For example, most but not all of the stuffed animals can be removed from a child's bed, and the remaining few can be washed periodically. A clinician may state strongly that the family cat must be removed from the house. However, the disruption this may create for the entire family may lead the family to ignore the recommendation and blame the clinician's "insensitivity" rather than the cat for problems in getting asthma under control. The clinician could state clearly that although the ideal is removal, perhaps something short of that is worth trying. Measures to clean the patient's bedroom, ban the cat entirely from the bedroom, and wash the cat once a week may help to reduce the patient's symptoms or medication requirements. Such negotiation conveys that the clinician takes the partnership seriously and is willing to work with the patient and family to develop the most appropriate, and thus more likely to be followed, treatment plan.

PROVIDE A WRITTEN PLAN. A written asthma management plan serves as the "contract" for the partnership. By writing down the plan and reviewing it with the patient, the clinician reduces confusion about the recommendations. Further, written plans can be taken home as important reminders. Some clinicians use a standardized form and fill in information particular to the patient's needs. The sample form illustrated in Figure 19–1 has an action plan based on a traffic light system and symptom. The use of green, yellow, and red lights adapted to a peak flow and symptom zone system makes it easier for patients to remember what actions to take when their peak flow measures and symptoms are at different levels (Lewis et al, 1984). Other clinicians prefer to create a plan for each patient. Some physicians have the patient (including children) write the plan down themselves to make certain that they can read the plan and to increase a sense of involvement and ownership.

For children, copies of the management plan, especially the action plan for handling exacerbations, should be made available to all of the adults responsible for caring for the child, including teachers, day care providers, and relatives. Patients of all ages find it helpful to have several copies to post at home or at work. Some clinicians encourage patients to set up a small bulletin board dedicated to information about asthma, including the treatment plan, and the physician's phone numbers.

Asthma Control Plan for _____
(Name of Patient)

Prepared by _____
(Name of Clinician)

This plan will help you control your asthma and know what to do if you have an asthma episode. Keeping your asthma under control will help you:

- **Be active without having asthma symptoms. This includes being active in exercise and sports.**
- **Sleep through the night without having asthma symptoms.**
- **Prevent asthma episodes (attacks).**
- **Have the best possible peak flow number—lungs that work well.**
- **Avoid side effects from medicines.**

Here are three ways to control your asthma:
- Follow your medicine plan (see the next page).
  — Follow your **Green Zone** plan every day to keep most asthma symptoms from starting.
  — Recognize your symptoms of an asthma episode. Act quickly to stop them.
  — Follow the **Yellow Zone** plan to stop asthma symptoms and to keep an asthma episode from getting serious.
  — Follow the **Red Zone** plan to take care of a serious episode. This is an emergency plan!
- Whenever possible, stay away from things that bring on your asthma symptoms. Follow your asthma trigger control plan to reduce the number of things in your home, workplace, or classroom that bother your asthma.
- See your doctor regularly. Talk about this plan with your doctor when you visit him/her. Your doctor will mark (check) on the plan what you should do.

Important Information:

Doctor _____

Telephone Number _____

Address _____

Hospital

Address _____

Telephone Number _____

Ambulance

Telephone Number _____

Friend/Relative To Call

Telephone Number _____

Taxi

Telephone Number _____

FIGURE 19–1. Asthma control plan. (From National Asthma Education Program. Teach Your Patients About Asthma: A Clinician's Guide. Bethesda, MD, U. S. Department of Health and Human Services, National Heart, Lung, and Blood Institute, 1992.)

Follow the symptoms and action steps in these three zones to help you control your asthma.

Green Zone: All Clear
This is where you should be every day.

Peak flow_____
(80-100%
of personal best)*

No symptoms of an asthma episode. You are able to do your usual activities and sleep without having symptoms.

☐ Take these medicines.

Name of medicine	How much to take	When to take it
_____	_____	_____
_____	_____	_____

☐ Follow your asthma trigger control plan to avoid things that bring on your asthma.

☐ Take _____ before exercise.
   (Name of medicine)

Yellow Zone: Caution
This is not where you should be every day. Take action to get your asthma under control.

Peak flow_____
(50-80%
of personal best)*

Symptoms of an asthma episode may be mild or moderate. You may be coughing, wheezing, feeling short of breath, or feeling like your chest is tight. These symptoms may keep you from your usual activities or keep you from sleeping.

☐ First, take this medicine.

Name of medicine	How much to take	When to take it
_____	_____	_____

☐ Next, if you feel better in 20 to 60 minutes and your peak flow is over _____ take the medicine listed below:
   (70% of personal best)

Name of medicine	How much to take	When to take it
_____	_____	_____

☐ Keep taking your green zone medicine(s).

But if you DO NOT feel better in 20 to 60 minutes or your peak flow is under _____, **Follow the Red Zone Plan.**
(70% of personal best)

Let the doctor know if you keep going into the Yellow Zone. Your Green Zone medicine may need to be changed to keep other episodes from starting.

Red Zone: Medical Alert
This is an emergency! Get help. Your asthma symptoms are serious.

Peak flow_____
(below 50%
of personal best)*

You may be coughing, very short of breath, and/or the skin between your ribs and your neck may be pulled in tight. You may have trouble walking or talking. You may not be wheezing because air cannot move out of your airways.

*This is a general guideline only. Some people have asthma that gets worse very fast. They may need to have a **Yellow Zone** start at 90 percent of their personal best.*

☐ First, take this medicine.

Name of medicine	How much to take	When to take it
_____	_____	_____

☐ Next, **call the doctor** to ask about what you should do next. Tell him/her this is an emergency.

But, see the doctor **RIGHT AWAY** or go to the hospital if *any* of these things are happening:
- Lips or fingernails are blue.
- You are struggling to breathe.
- You do not feel any better 20 to 30 minutes after taking the extra medicine and your peak flow is still under_____.
  (50% of personal best)
- Six hours after you take the extra medicine, if you still need inhaled beta$_2$-agonist medicine every 1 to 3 hours and your peak flow is under _____.
  (70% of personal best)

FIGURE 19–1 *Continued*

Rehearse Asthma Management Skills

After the clinician and the patient reach agreement on the treatment plan, the patient needs to learn exactly what is required to implement the plan. The second R for teaching is to *rehearse* asthma management skills. The key skills are identifying asthma triggers, recognizing early warning signs of deterioration, conducting home peak flow monitoring, taking medicine correctly (which involves administering the medicine and following a stepwise action plan), taking preventive actions, and seeking help appropriately. The emphasis is on skill development, not acquisition of knowledge.

Teaching skills effectively relies on demonstration and practice, that is, rehearsal. A technique used in school classrooms as well as adult education classes is to explain that the desired skill has several complicated tasks that will be discussed individually after the learner has a chance to see and try the whole skill. The skill is then demonstrated in slow motion without any discussion. The patient tries it. Then each task is walked through and feedback is given along the way.

A performance checklist may be helpful. One study among adults demonstrated significant improvement and retention of inhaler technique with the use of a performance checklist (Windsor et al, 1990). Written handouts with illustrations of the steps involved in using a device (inhaler, nebulizer, peak flow meter) are valuable reference points for a demonstration and for the patient to take home. Illustrated handouts help make a patient's family or a child's other caregivers aware of proper techniques. Videotape demonstrations may also be helpful and can be an efficient way to introduce a new skill. In some settings the office nurse teaches techniques first, and then the physician observes the patient and reviews the skill.

It is essential for the clinician to observe the patient's asthma management techniques and to have the patient practice until he or she can demonstrate appropriate techniques. It is not uncommon for treatment failure to be due to improper inhaler technique rather than inadequate prescriptions. Research has indicated that a majority of patients do not have appropriate inhaler technique (King et al, 1991; Manzella et al, 1989). Further, inappropriate peak flow technique yields unreliable monitoring information and discourages adherence. Unless patient technique is observed, it cannot be corrected.

Repeat Messages

Repetition is a cardinal principle of education. The third R for teaching is *repeat* messages. One study of adult patient recall of a single message from the physician showed that 5 minutes after the message was given, only 50 percent of the patients could recall the message. When the same message was repeated three times, 100 percent recalled the message. This can be done easily within an office visit; the clinician can give the message, other staff in the office can repeat it, written materials can be given, and, perhaps most importantly, the patient can repeat it to the staff in his/her own words (Doak et al, 1985).

Repeated review of patient skills is also critical. Education is a continuous process. Patients meet new circumstances that require adjustments in therapy and new skills; patients get confused by multiple medications; they forget tasks or develop inappropriate or "sloppy" habits over time. Thus, it is important to review key skills, such as inhaler technique, at every visit. This review must include the patient's demonstration of medication use, preferably using his or her own equipment. It is not uncommon to see patients put the wrong medication into a nebulizer or to hear that the patient takes the inhaled corticosteroid on an "as needed" basis. It is often helpful to spend some time alone with children, especially those over 5 years old. They may be embarrassed to discuss problems or defensive when their skills need to be corrected in front of their parents.

Reinforce Appropriate Behavior

Reinforcement is important to shape and maintain new behaviors. The fourth R for teaching is *reinforce* appropriate behavior. Diaries are helpful because they provide both a repetitive drill for monitoring asthma and a feedback mechanism at home that can reinforce the medication regimen. Diaries do not have to be elaborate, but can be kept on a standard form, on school or work paper, or on calendars. Some patients enjoy creating their own diaries on the computer. Figure 19–2 illustrates diaries, including the diary used by a clinician with a young girl that helped reinforce the need to act promptly when peak flow measures declined. Diaries can also provide documentation and justification for daily therapy when a patient can observe improvements in peak flow and daily symptom scores over time. Reviewing diaries can improve adherence and can be done quickly during the return visits. An efficient and well-received method consists of having patients fax their diary to the clinician, who can then write comments on the diary and return it by fax. Children also benefit from this technique. This can also be done through the mail, and all children enjoy receiving mail. Daily diaries can be cumbersome for some patients; keeping a 1- to 2-week diary when therapy is adjusted, or for the week prior to a follow-up visit, can still provide valuable information.

Praise is a powerful reinforcer; success does breed success. Praising appropriate behavior and fostering in the patient a confidence that he or she can perform well increases the patient's efforts. The time demands of a patient visit may lead to focusing on what is going wrong and needs to be corrected. It is helpful at each visit to find at least one thing the patient is doing right and to praise it.

Prizes or rewards for completing tasks offer incentive and praise for a job well done. In one practice, children work for "Asthma Achievement Dollars" by taking their medication, taking peak flow measures, and reporting problems promptly. These dollars can be earned at the office and can be turned in for a prize from a basket of inexpensive toys or coupons. Alternatively, the child can select a prize that has personal meaning and value and earn the dollars at home. Adults also respond favorably to reward systems. In one practice, tokens were turned in for lottery or raffle tickets, cassette tapes, books, or rewards the patient bought himself.

Habit and routine are also reinforcers. The more asthma management tasks are linked with the patient's existing routines, the more likely they are to be performed. For example, the patient could take a morning peak flow right after turning off the alarm and take medication right before brushing teeth.

The telephone is an effective way to provide reinforcement and reassurance. Having a set call-in time assures patients that they can reach the clinician to go over concerns that are not urgent but are nonetheless too bothersome to wait for the next visit. "Calling out" is also important—by either the nurse or physician. Reminder calls can improve appointment keeping 20 to 30 percent (Becker, 1985). Calling a patient within several days of starting new therapy or within a day of an urgent care visit or phone call from the patient demonstrates concern and may contribute substantially to the patient's satisfaction with his or her care. Being available goes a long way. Extending hours or having Saturday hours can be helpful, especially for avoiding conflict with after-school activities or work schedules.

The asthma care partnership should be expanded to include other people who have significant relationships with the patient. Spouses, siblings, caretakers, and school personnel can help to encourage a patient's efforts to follow his or her asthma management plan, help reduce identified allergens or irritants in the patient's environment, and provide an additional source of reinforcement and support. The clinician has an important role in recruiting these people into the partnership. For example, providing a written management plan for students to take to school will facilitate communication between the family and school; direct discussion with the school nurse or teacher may be necessary for some children. See Chapter 56, Allergies in the School, for samples of school forms. Nurses in the physician's office can help to link patients with other patients. For example, one office finds it useful to have a teenager or young adult in the practice who has successfully managed his or her asthma (especially one who is also a successful student and athlete) talk to a younger, new patient and family. Such a technique provides an effective role model for the patient and family as well as effective reinforcement. A recent study among adults with asthma indicated that small group education was as effective as individual education. Patients appeared to benefit from peer support and education, and educators perceived the group interaction especially valuable in eliciting fears and concerns of patients and addressing them in a way that promoted appropriate self-management (Wilson et al, 1993).

Support groups, either longstanding groups that meet regularly or short-term groups formed for an asthma management education class, give patients and parents an opportunity to learn in a group setting, have peer role models, exchange practical tips and coping strategies, and expand patient and parent networks for support. This is vital because research indicates that many asthma patients feel a sense of isolation as they try to cope with asthma. A pilot study showed that social isolation explained 70 percent of the variability in asthma management and 16 percent of the variability in emergency department visits (Fisher, 1992). Clinical trials have demonstrated that patients with social support enlisted to help with managing chronic illnesses have greater compliance and disease control than those who do not. Clinicians have a role in making support groups happen and work well, for both children and parents. The number of groups available for teens is increasing.

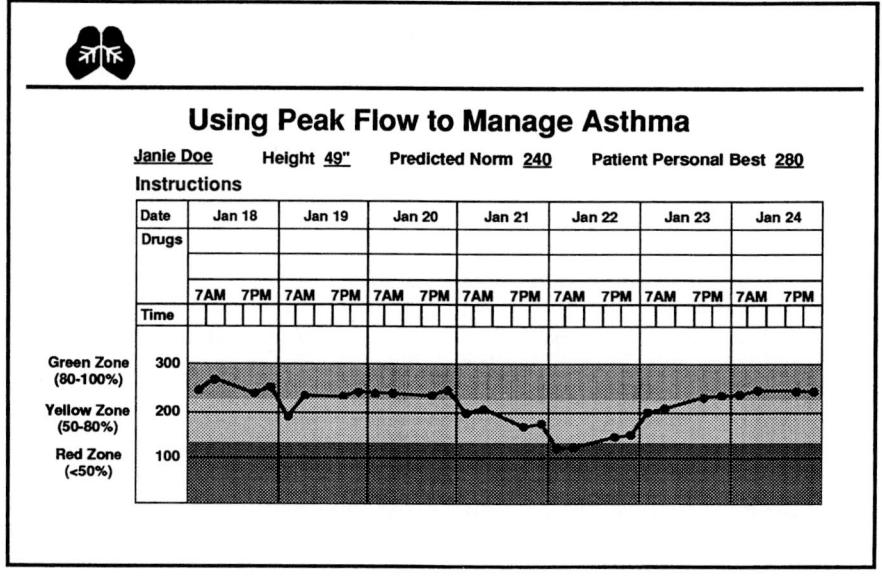

This figure describes how peak flow readings are used to manage asthma. In this case, a child's predicted/personal best PEFR is 280--her Green Zone. Following antigen exposure when she visited her friend who had a cat, there was a significant reduction in her PEFR that she noticed when she took her PEFR. She was not experiencing significant symptoms. She took her "Yellow Zone" medicine--a $beta_2$-agonist metered dose inhaler and quickly returned to normal. She continued to do well until she developed a respiratory infection and essentially ignored her declining PEFR and symptoms--which may have been confused with symptoms of the infection. Her PEFR continued to deteriorate until she dipped into her Red Zone and was facing a full blown exacerbation that required more aggressive therapy--oral corticosteroids--and took more time to return to normal. Thus, this illustrates how PEFR monitoring and appropriate response to declining PEFR results in more effective asthma management.

FIGURE 19–2. Sample diaries. (From National Asthma Education Program. Guidelines for the Diagnosis and Management of Asthma. Bethesda, MD, U.S. Department of Health and Human Services, National Heart, Lung, and Blood Institute, 1991, and from Pedipress, 1993.)

Clinicians can help patients to meet each other, start support groups or asthma education classes in the practice, or give referrals to existing groups. Each of these roles provides a group experience that can be a valuable supplement and positive reinforcement to the care a patient receives in the medical office.

Review

The fifth R for teaching and the final phase of the patient education process is *review*. The review serves as a source of feedback on the entire process and often directs the patient and clinician to a renewed educational cycle. For example, review may indicate a deficiency in skills, which requires another round of rehearsal. In this sense, the five Rs for teaching represent a continuous effort.

At each visit, the patient and clinician should review whether the goals for therapy have been met, identify barriers to meeting the goals, and explore ways to overcome the barriers. The clinician can quickly assess whether goals have been met by asking whether the patient has had night-time

ASTHMA DIARY

Name: Carla Freed
See back for instructions.
Please bring to each visit.

○ – Before bronchodilator
X – After bronchodilator

		12/8	12/9	12/10	12/11	12/12	12/13	12/14	12/15	12/16	12/17	12/18
Date →	Triggers, Comments			Has cold	Feels better	More active	Cough-cold air	Stomach ache	Stomach ache	Very tired		

Peak Flow Rate
- Green Zone — 100% 200
- High Yellow Zone — 80% 160
- Low Yellow Zone — 65% 130
- Red Zone — 50% 100

Medicines*
- Cromolyn — Intal – 4 amps
- Inhaled steroid
- Albuterol — Ventolin – 0.5 cc
- Oral steroid — Prelone – 1½ t.
- Theophylline

Medicine	12/8	12/9	12/10	12/11	12/12	12/13	12/14	12/15	12/16	12/17	12/18
Cromolyn		√√	√√	√√	√√	√√	√√	√√	√√	√√	√√
Inhaled steroid											
Albuterol		√	√	√	√	√	√	√	√√	√√	√√
Oral steroid							√	√	√	√	√
Theophylline											

Signs

	12/8	12/9	12/10	12/11	12/12	12/13	12/14	12/15	12/16	12/17	12/18
Wheeze	1	0	0	0	0	0	0	0	0	0	0
Cough	1	1	1	0	0	0	0	0	0	0	0
Activity	0	0	0	0	0	0	0	0	0	0	0
Sleep	1	0	0	0	0	0	0	0	0	0	0

Signs

◆ **Wheeze:**
- None 0
- Exhale only 1
- Throughout entire exhale 2
- Both inhale and exhale. 3

◆ **Cough:**
- None 0
- Less than one per minute 1
- One to four per minute. 2
- More than four per minute 3

◆ **Activity:**
- Fully active 0
- Can run short distance. 1
- Can walk only 2
- Missed school or stayed indoors 3

◆ **Sleep:**
- Fine 0
- Slight wheeze or cough 1
- Awake 2-3 times, wheeze or cough 2
- Awake most of the time 3

Books available from Pedipress (800-344-5864)
- *Children with Asthma: A Manual for Parents*
- *One Minute Asthma: What You Need to Know*
- *El asma en un minuto*
- *Winning Over Asthma*

*Medicines: • Cromolyn (Intal) • Inhaled steroid (AeroBid, Azmacort, Beclovent, Vanceril) • Albuterol (Proventil, Ventolin) • Oral steroid (prednisone, Prelone, Pediapred) • Theophylline (Slo-bid capsules, Theo-Dur tablets.) Your doctor may prescribe others.

© 1993 Pedipress, Inc. All rights reserved. Adapted from *Asthma Charts and Forms* by Thomas F. Plaut, M.D. and Carla Brennan.

FIGURE 19-2 *Continued*

symptoms, how often the patient has used the inhaled beta$_2$-agonist therapy, and in what way the patient's asthma has interfered with his or her normal activities. A review of a peak flow diary provides valuable information. Most importantly, open-ended questions should be asked about how well the patient thinks the management plan is working and about what problems the patient has had with asthma or with the management plan since the previous visit.

Physicians often doubt the reliability of a patient's reports of adherence. The question, "Are you taking the medication as we planned?" only invites the patient to please the physician. Carefully framed questions can elicit accurate information, such as "Many people have difficulty following a medication plan like yours; what problems have you had?" "Describe for me how and when you take your medicines and if this works out well for you." "I know it's hard to always follow our plan all the time. How often have you had to change it?"

Review also includes observation of the patient's asthma management techniques and corrective education as appropriate, as discussed earlier.

Through the review process, the clinician can identify patient barriers to adherence or performance of adequate skills. Common barriers to adherence are either a lack of conviction that the treatment can help or fears about treatment. Fear of toxicity, fear of loss of effect, fear of addiction, and fear that inhaled corticosteroids are the same as anabolic steroids have been reported to be key concerns (Clark et al, 1980). These fears can be alleviated through careful discussion and additional reading materials for the patient to take home. Inconvenient schedules or multiple medications are also barriers to adherence. As discussed earlier, it helps to keep the regimen as simple as possible, to establish priorities for environmental control, and to tailor the plan to the patient's or parent's life style. Costs of medications and environmental control measures can be a significant burden, which can be eased somewhat if patients are referred to support services or support groups that can secure discounts for medical devices.

Questioning the patient about the efficacy and acceptability of the treatment plan reminds both the clinician and the patient or parents that asthma care is a partnership effort. The patient and parents are recruited into the problem-solving effort and become part of removing the barriers, renegotiating, and recommitting to the treatment plan.

INTEGRATING PATIENT EDUCATION INTO MEDICAL PRACTICE

Various methods are available for including the five Rs of patient teaching in the medical practice setting. All require some investment of time. Each asthma management skill may take 5 to 10 minutes to teach and 3 to 5 minutes to review. This may necessitate scheduling patients for longer than the standard brief office visit. There are several methods for organizing the patient education effort. Some clinicians prefer to have a 1-hour initial visit to review all aspects of asthma management. For children under 4, this may mean a brief visit with the child and a return visit only with the parents. Some clinicians schedule these educational visits at the end of the day or on Saturdays when the practice is not as busy and working parents are available. Follow-up visits may use 10 to 15 minutes for education.

Many offices cannot schedule 1-hour visits; many patients (adults as well as children) cannot absorb an intensive 1-hour educational session with a variety of skills taught all at once. An alternative is to offer either a series of evening or Saturday asthma management group sessions or refer the patient to a local Lung Association or Asthma and Allergy Foundation chapter for organized classes. The classes can provide basic information and training about asthma. Research involving controlled designs has documented the benefits of group classes in improving health outcomes (Rachelefsky, 1987; Wilson-Pessano and McNabb, 1985; Wilson et al, 1993), and the group format has the additional advantages of being able to include several members of the family directly in the educational effort and of being less costly. However, many patients and families prefer not to attend classes or find them difficult to schedule. Further, the classes are meant to be a supplement to, not a replacement for, a clinician's personal education and advice tailored to the specific needs of the patient.

An important method is to integrate education into the medical care routine (Taggart et al, 1991) and to identify separate topics for education to cover briefly in a series of office visits, with the order of topics determined by the patient's or parent's needs. Typically, the first visit may focus on reaching agreement on goals, developing a treatment plan, teaching medication use, and identifying key elements of environmental control. Subsequent visits can include more on peak flow monitoring, extensive discussion of environmental control, and how to deal with special situations at school, work, and social events that involve exposure to allergens or irritants, and during exercise programs or sports. Of course, review of the patient's medication techniques and diaries occurs at every visit. An educational record in the patient's chart can help track progress (Fig. 19–3) and to highlight areas most in need of the clinician's attention.

Most importantly, education takes place at each clinical visit. Clinicians must take advantage of teachable moments at every visit. This can be done in the following ways:

- Before the visit starts, by having the patient and/or parent write down key expectations for the visit. The clinician can ask: "What questions do you want to ask the doctor today?" "What problems have you had with your asthma since the last visit?" "What problems do you have with your medication?"
- In the waiting room or laboratory testing area, by having the patient read or watch educational videos
- In the examining room, by having the nurse teach and/or review inhaler techniques while the patient waits to see the physician
- While taking the history, by reviewing the diary and asking questions about adherence to the treatment plan
- During the physical examination by taking a peak flow reading as part of the physical examination and giving instant feedback on technique
- During the exit interview, by reviewing the medication technique and agreeing upon adjustments in the medication plan before prescribing any refills or additional medication.

All these techniques are designed to use the clinician's time with the patient as effectively as possible. Many clinicians fear that patient education will take too much time. It is important to remember that in clinical practices that rely on traditional information-giving, up to half the patients do not adhere to the clinician's recommendations. In essence, half the clinician's time might be wasted (Mellins and Evans, 1992). The five Rs of teaching promote more efficient use of time with the patient through an effective and satisfying partnership in asthma care.

RESOURCES FOR PATIENT MATERIALS

National Asthma Education and Prevention Program
Information Center
P.O. Box 30105
Bethesda, MD 20824-0105
(301) 251-1222

Allergy and Asthma Network
Mothers of Asthmatics, Inc.
3554 Chain Bridge Road, Suite 200
Fairfax, VA 22030-2709
1-800-878-4403

American Academy of Allergy and Immunology
611 East Wells Street
Milwaukee, WI 53202
1-800-822-2762

American College of Allergy and Immunology
85 W. Algonquin Road, Suite 550
Arlington Heights, IL 60005
1-800-842-7777

American Lung Association
American Thoracic Society
Check for local chapter or contact:
1740 Broadway
New York, NY 10019-4374

Asthma and Allergy Foundation of America (AAFA)
1125 15th Street, N.W. #502
Washington, DC 20005
1-800-7-ASTHMA

National Jewish Center of Immunology and Respiratory Medicine
1400 Jackson Street
Denver, CO 80206
1-800-222-LUNG

Pedipress, Inc.
125 Redgate Lane
Amherst, MA 01002
1-800-344-5864

PROGRAM PARTICIPATION:	Date/Initial	Comments
Slide Show/Video/etc. Demonstration Pamphlet and Discussion		

Score Patient's Progress:	Visit 1	Visit 2	Visit 3	Visit 4	Visit 5
Triggers: (circle patient's triggers: exercise, pollens, animal, dust mites, smoke, weather) o Uses avoidance measures list recommendations:) _____ _____					
Correct use of medicine: o Agrees to medicine plan and schedule o Knows difference between prevention and prn med. o Takes medicine correctly					
Peak flow meter: o Uses PF meter correctly o Knows when to use PF o Completes diary					
Warning signs: o Knows early signs and symptoms o Knows PF green, yellow, red zones					
Manages attacks: o Agrees to action plan o Moves away from trigger o Takes medicine correctly o Relaxes o Monitors response with PF o Knows when to get help					

SCORING KEY:
- 0: Patient has no understanding
- 1: Patient can list items
- 2: Patient can demonstrate skills and illustrate how they fit his/her own situation

COMMENTS ON PROGRESS	
Date	Comments

FIGURE 19-3. Sample asthma education patient record.

REFERENCES

Becker MH. Patient adherence to prescribed therapies. Med Care 23:539–555, 1985.

Bush PJ, Iannotti RJ. A children's health belief model. Med Care 28:69–86, 1990.

Clark N, Feldman CH, Freudenberg N, et al. Developing education for children with asthma through study of self-management behavior. Health Educ Q 7:278–296, 1980.

Doak C, Doak L, Root J. Teaching patients with low literacy skills, Philadelphia, JB Lippincott, 1985.

Fisher E. Patient education with adults. Conference proceedings: First National Conference on Asthma Management, 1992. National Asthma Education Program, Crystal City, Virginia.

Fowler M, Davenport M, Gary R. School Functioning of U.S. children with asthma. Pediatrics 90:939–944, 1992.

King D, Earnshaw SM, Delaney JC. Pressurized aerosol inhalers: The cost of misuse. Br J Clin Pract 42:48–49, 1991.

Korsch BM, Gozzi EF, Francis V. Gaps in doctor-patient communications. Doctor-patient interaction and patient satisfaction. Pediatrics 42:855–871, 1968.

Lewis CE, Rachelefsky G, Lewis MA, et al. A randomized trial of ACT (asthma care training) for kids. Pediatrics 74:478–486, 1984.

Manzella B, Brooks C, Richard J, et al. Assessing the use of metered dose inhalers by adults with asthma. J Asthma 26(4):223–230, 1989.

Mellins, RB, Evans, D. Patient compliance: Are we wasting our time and don't know it? Am Rev Respir Dis 146:1376–1377, 1992.

National Heart, Lung, and Blood Institute. National Asthma Education Program Expert Panel Report: Guidelines for the Diagnosis and Management of Asthma. Washington, DC, National Institutes of Health, 1991. NIH Pub. No. 91-3042.

Newacheck P, Taylor W. Childhood chronic illness: Prevalence, severity and impact. Am J Public Health 82:364–369, 1992.

Parcel GS, Baronowski T. Social learning theory and health education. Health Educ Monogr 12:14–18, 1981.

Rachelefsky G. Review of asthma self-management programs. J Allergy Clin Immunol 80:506–511, 1987.

Taggart V, Zuckerman A, Sly R, et al. You can control asthma: Evaluation of an asthma education program for hospitalized inner-city children. Patient Educ Couns 17:35–47, 1991.

U.S. Department of Health and Human Services. Morbidity and Mortality 1992: Chartbook on Cardiovascular, Lung, and Blood Diseases. Washington, DC, National Heart, Lung, and Blood Institute, May 1992.

Weiss K, Gergen P, Hodgson T. An economic evaluation of asthma in the United States. N Engl J Med 326:862–866, 1992.

Wilson-Pessano SR, McNabb WL. The role of patient education in the management of childhood asthma. Prev Med 14:670–687, 1985.

Wilson SR, Scamagas P, German DF, et al. A controlled trial of two forms of self-management education for adults with asthma. Am J Med 94:564–576, 1993.

Windsor RA, Bailey WC, Richard JM, et al. Evaluation of the efficacy and cost effectiveness of health education methods to increase medication adherence among adults with asthma. Am J Public Health 80(12):1519–1521, 1990.

Chapter 20

Risk Factors and Prevention of Allergy

Noah J. Friedman, M.D., and Robert S. Zeiger, M.D., Ph.D.

The ability to prevent disease before it occurs has been a desire of physicians in various disciplines for many years. Techniques of preventing allergy could be aimed at: (1) *primary prevention*: inhibition of IgE sensitization; (2) *secondary prevention*: deterrence of disease expression despite prior IgE sensitization; or (3) *tertiary prevention*: suppression of symptoms despite occurrence of IgE-mediated disorder.

This chapter will focus on primary prevention of allergy in infants, a goal that has become elusive because of both scientific and societal limitations. With the revolutionary breakthroughs in molecular genetics and our ever-increasing knowledge of immunomodulatory mechanisms, the direct ability to modulate IgE synthesis, mediator release, and end-organ sensitivity may be within our grasp in the near future. For now, however, practical efforts at primary allergy prevention in infants are limited to environmental manipulation or restricting infants' allergen exposure by ingestion or inhalation.

In order to determine practical guidelines for such environmental and dietary manipulation, some basic questions need to be answered: Which infants would warrant such manipulation? What is the crucial period of time needed to carry out effective prevention? What type of environmental and dietary manipulation would be most effective?

RISK FACTORS AND PREDICTION OF ATOPY IN INFANTS

Like so many conditions, the development of allergy appears to be influenced by both genetic and environmental factors. Efforts at prevention at this point must, of course, be focused on the latter, but the genetic inheritance of allergy is critical for determining which patients would warrant environmental manipulation. Numerous physiologic and sociologic factors have been employed with varying degrees of success to determine which infants are likely to develop atopy (Table 20–1). Several of these determinants warrant further discussion here.

Role of Family History

The pattern of inheritance of the predisposition toward allergy seems to be explained best by a multifactorial or polygenic mode. Maimonides was the first to note the familial inheritance pattern of asthma as noted in his *Treatise on Asthma* in the twelfth century. However, not until over 700 years later, in 1923, did the studies of Coca and Cooke first indicate this mode of inheritance.

A variety of retrospective studies in the United States and Sweden (Zeiger et al, 1992) have estimated the risk of developing allergic disease ranging from about 13 percent without a parental history of allergic disease to approximately 30 percent with a single parent history and nearly 50 percent with a bilateral history. These data are limited because of the methodologic problems encountered in retrospective questionnaires. Prospective studies over the past 30 years (Zeiger et al, 1992), with varying degrees of methodologic limitations, have estimated the risk of allergy with a positive family history to be even greater: from 38 to 58 percent with a unilateral his-

TABLE 20–1. PROPOSED RISK FACTORS AND MARKERS FOR ALLERGIC DISEASE IN INFANCY

General	Specific
Genetic/Immunologic	Family atopic history
	Increased cord blood IgE
	Increased specific IgE
	Increased blood eosinophilia in infancy
	Increased nasal eosinophilia in infancy
	Increased cord blood IgE binding factors
	Decreased CD8 + T cells in infancy
	Increased cord blood phosphodiesterase activity
	Cord blood thrombocytopenia
	Increased cord blood linoleic acid
Environmental	Feeding practices:
	Brief feeding
	Food allergens in breast milk
	Early solid foods
	Magnitude of inhalant allergen exposure
	Early inhalant allergen exposure
	Intrauterine exposure to drugs
	Infections
	Exposure to passive tobacco smoke and pollutants

Modified from Zeiger RS. Prevention of food allergy in infancy. Ann Allergy 65:430, 1990.

tory and 60 to 80 percent with a bilateral history. Furthermore, offspring of atopic parents not only have a higher risk of developing allergic disease, but are likely to manifest allergies earlier in life. For example, studies by Kjellman and Johansson (1979) estimated the risk for children of two atopic parents of developing allergic disease within the first 18 months of life to be 42 percent.

Role of Cord Blood IgE as a Predictor of Atopy

Studies during the early 1980s suggested that IgE levels in cord blood were highly predictive of early development of allergic disease. For example, a retrospective study by Bousquet et al in 1983 determined by a physician-directed questionnaire that a cord blood IgE > or = 1.0 IU/ml was 85 percent sensitive at predicting allergy by age 2 while maintaining a specificity of 58 percent. A contemporary Swedish study by Kjellman and Croner (1984), using a parent-directed questionnaire, suggested that a cord blood IgE > or = 0.9 IU/ml was more specific than, nearly as sensitive as, and significantly more efficient than a positive family history in predicting atopy by age 7.

More recent studies and longer prospective follow-up by the initial investigators, however, have tempered this initial enthusiasm for cord blood IgE as a highly sensitive and specific marker for early allergic disease. In 1990, Croner and Kjellman published an 11-year follow-up of their initial patient cohort and concluded that while cord blood IgE had a higher screening efficiency than family history and that an immediate family history in addition to elevated cord blood IgE has a very high predictive value for atopic disease by age 11, the sensitivity of either of the factors taken alone was disappointingly low. This would preclude the use of either of these tests as a sensitive enough marker for the routine detection of candidates for allergy prevention.

Effect of Ingestants on Allergic Sensitization

Since Grulee and Sanford suggested in 1936 that feeding infants breast milk instead of cow's milk (CM) might decrease the risk for developing eczema, research has focused on what dietary manipulation might modulate the expression of a preprogrammed allergic genotype. Though later studies have both supported and refuted these findings, there has been substantial evidence that early introduction of highly allergenic food in an infant's diet will generally have an adverse effect on the subsequent development of atopy.

Savilahti et al (1987) noted that prolonged exclusive breast-feeding can significantly lower serum levels of IgG, IgA, and IgM in infants without increasing the risk of infection. While increases in these immunoglobulin classes generally represent normal, nonpathologic responses to foreign proteins, this would suggest that the infant's immune system does indeed respond to ingested food as foreign.

Eastham et al (1978) reported that five infants given casein hydrolysate (Nutramigen) for 3 months developed significantly lower levels of whey hemagglutinins than five infants fed CM formula. Similarly, Zeiger et al noted in 1992 that infants "at risk for atopy" (with positive family histories) who were either exclusively breast-fed or supplemented with casein hydrolysate formula for 1 year had significantly lower levels of IgG to beta-lactoglobulin (BLG) than did similar infants who were fed or supplemented with standard CM formula. This blunted immunologic response was noted at 4 and 12 months and remained suppressed even at 24 months, after CM was introduced in both groups. These studies lend credence to the notion that breast milk and protein hydrolysate formulas are less immunogenic than CM in infants at risk for atopy.

Moreover, May et al (1982) compared the immunologic response of infants fed either CM formula or soy formula for 4 months. Both groups responded with increased serum IgG and IgA to their respective formula protein; early ingestion of soy did not significantly blunt an immunologic response to milk protein when it was introduced after 4 months, suggesting that soy does not offer any protection against an eventual immunologic response to milk. Of course, it must be noted that these data only address the question of *immunogenicity* rather than *allergenicity* of these foodstuffs when introduced early in infancy.

Hattevig et al (1984) studied prospectively the IgE immunologic responses of 86 healthy newborns (~50 percent from atopic families) to such foods as egg, milk, and soy. No IgE directed against milk or egg was noted in the cord blood despite ingestion of these foodstuffs by the mothers during pregnancy. This supports lack of prenatal sensitization to foods. There was a peak incidence of IgE antibodies to these ingestants by 8 months of age. A greater incidence of higher antibody levels to egg (22 percent of infants at 8 months) occurred than to milk (9 percent) or soy (6 percent). Finally, healthy, nonatopic children tended to have lower food-specific IgE as noted by radioallergosorbent testing (RAST) than atopic children who manifested symptoms of food allergy. Research has shown that while high levels of food-specific IgE correlate well with clinical atopy, lower levels of IgE to certain foods may represent transient, clinically insignificant sensitization.

The early introduction of solid food into an infant's diet has also been raised as a possible risk factor for the development of atopy. Numerous studies have been performed to examine this relationship with varying results. A large cohort study from New Zealand noted a significant relationship between the number of solid foods introduced during the first 4 months of life and the development of one episode of eczema by 2 (Fergusson et al, 1981) and 3 (Fergusson et al, 1982) years of age and the development of chronic eczema by age 10 (Fergusson et al, 1990). This study, however, depended on chart review for the diagnosis of eczema and lacked immunologic investigation into the cause of eczema. Other studies have suggested that postponing the introduction of solid foods will only delay, but not prevent, the development of food allergy.

No relationship has been found between early feeding practices and the development of asthma (Fergusson et al, 1983). This is most likely due to the fact that infections, rather than food allergy, are generally considered the leading cause of asthma in early childhood.

Effect of Breast-Feeding on the Prediction of Atopy

Many studies have suggested that breast-feeding reduces atopy. However, this should not imply that there are no adverse immunologic effects to this practice. By studies early in this century employing the method of transfer of passive cutaneous anaphylaxis (Shannon, 1921) and more recent studies using more sensitive assays, small quantities of maternally ingested foods have been shown to pass into the breast milk. For example, three common milk antigens—beta-lactoglobulin (BLG), casein, and bovine IgG (Stuart et al, 1984)—as well as egg (Cant et al, 1985) and wheat (Troncone et al, 1987) proteins have been measured in nanogram concentrations in a majority of lactating women who are not avoiding milk, eggs, or wheat. These substances have been detected in human breast milk by 2 to 6 hours after maternal ingestion and can persist for as long as 1 to 4 days.

Well-controlled studies have determined that the amount of these antigens found in human breast milk is not a predictor of the development of atopic disease in the infant (Cant et al, 1985; Machtinger and Moss, 1986). However, there have been numerous studies that suggest, though not conclusively, that early sensitization (as early as 1 week) to highly allergenic foods can occur in "exclusively breast-fed infants" through maternal ingestion of these foods (Van Asperen et al, 1983). Though many of these studies were sound—symptoms were tested clinically by maternal elimination or food challenges in the infants and confirmed by sensitive immunologic tests such as prick skin tests or RAST—the studies failed to control for the possibility that the infants were sensitized to these foodstuffs inadvertently via caretakers or even via the environment or anti-idiotypic antibodies. Although the true frequency of sensitization of infants to highly allergenic food such as milk, egg, and peanut through breast milk cannot be accurately ascertained, numerous reports have documented the ability of maternally ingested foodstuffs to *exacerbate* allergic symptoms in *already sensitized* breast-fed infants.

Thus, although breast-feeding, with or without maternal elimination diets, cannot be a true predictor of the development of atopic disease, proper control of the early ingestion of highly allergenic foodstuffs continues to be investigated as a means of preventing allergic disease in the first few years of life, as will be discussed later in this chapter.

Inhalants as a Risk Factor for Atopy

Although it is somewhat harder to quantitate exposure to inhalant allergens than to foods, investigations have been ongoing to determine the risk of early exposure to inhalant allergens and irritants with regard to the subsequent development of allergic disease. Studies have approached this question from several directions.

Several studies have tried to relate month of birth to the development of allergy (Bjorksten et al, 1980; Zeiger et al, 1992), assuming that a critical time might exist during the first year of life when large exposure to pollen might put an infant at greater risk of subsequent IgE sensitization. Results have been varied and inconclusive, but many researchers have presented data that clearly suggest a relationship.

Dust mites, molds, and animal danders are all important indoor allergens and may be measured more directly within homes of infants to correlate early exposure with subsequent IgE sensitization. In a recent study by Sporik et al (1990), it was determined that high levels of the dust mite antigen *Der p1* in bedding and carpets during infancy led to (1) an increased risk of becoming sensitized to this antigen, as determined by RAST and puncture test, (2) an earlier age of onset of asthma, and (3) an increased risk of developing asthma by age 11. The relative risk of the latter was noted to be 4.8 with *Der p1* levels in household dust of 10 µg/ml during infancy. Warner et al (1990) studied the influence of early exposure to a variety of airborne allergens (e.g., dust mite, cat, pollen, and molds) in 68 atopic asthma patients at ages 2 to 14. The conclusions drawn included the following: (1) a high risk of developing IgE sensitization to dust mite and cat with high levels of *Der p1* or the cat allergen *Fel d1* in the household environment, (2) a higher risk of developing cat allergy if cats were present in the home at birth, (3) *Fel d1* detected in homes without cats present, suggesting that cat allergen may be brought into homes indirectly, and (4) tree but not grass or mold exposure increased the risk for ultimately developing positive skin tests. Several retrospective studies have led to similar conclusions.

The mechanism of this relationship between early sensitization and the subsequent development of atopy remains unknown. As noted above, the lion's share of asthma in infants and toddlers is not allergy related but rather exacerbated by respiratory infections. As it has been postulated that IgE regulation occurs, to at least some degree, at the T cell level, one might surmise that early exposure to allergen might prime T cells to become allergen-specific memory T cells, which must await some later event to become triggered to stimulate IgE production.

In addition to the inhalation of allergens, irritants such as cigarette smoke and air pollution have been suspected as risk factors in the development of allergic disease, through either local mucosal damage or immunomodulation. Second-hand cigarette smoke has been shown to increase the risk of an infant to develop persistent wheezing (Fergusson et al, 1980; Cogswell et al, 1987), a reduced level of growth and pulmonary function (Tager, 1986), earlier onset of wheezing and allergic rhinitis (Suoniemi et al, 1981), and an increased risk of serous otitis media (Kraemer et al, 1984). Several studies have confirmed higher serum IgE levels in children from households with smoking parents (Kjellman, 1981; Zeiger et al, 1992).

Similarly, a variety of international studies have determined an increased risk, as high as twofold, of developing respiratory allergy from living in more polluted areas, such as near roadsides or factories (Ishizaki et al,

1987; Aberg, 1989). This risk was further increased in children whose exposure to pollution from factories or highways was coupled with exposure to cigarette exposure in the household (Andrae et al, 1988).

PREVENTION OF ALLERGY

In 1936, Grulee and Sanford followed 20,000 infants and concluded that breast-feeding significantly decreased the prevalence of eczema when compared to ingestion of CM. Recent studies have also suggested that avoidance of common inhaled allergens during early infancy may have an effect on the subsequent development of respiratory allergy. However, the results of numerous studies aimed at pinpointing whether or not environmental or dietary manipulation can indeed alter the expression of a predetermined allergic phenotype have been conflicting.

Though it is simpler to monitor what allergens an infant ingests than to determine what potential allergens he or she is inhaling, neither determination is, by any means, a clear-cut process. For example, besides observing what foods an infant directly ingests through formula and solid food feedings, one must also take into account what antigens have potentially led to sensitization via the placenta (by maternal ingestion during gestation), through the breast milk (because of the mother's diet during lactation), and inadvertently via airborne droplets, house dust, and the like. These potential exposures have, to a certain degree, confounded efforts to determine what steps need be taken to prevent the development of atopic disease by dietary manipulation during infancy.

This section will attempt to summarize various studies that have dealt with this issue and point out some of the pitfalls encountered.

Breast-Feeding versus Cow's Milk Formula Feeding

Much has been written in recent years, in both the medical and lay press, concerning the documented benefit of breast-feeding compared with bottle feeding with regard to nutritional content, immunologic protection, and maternal-infant bonding. However, whether or not breast-feeding can actually decrease or delay the development of atopic disease remains controversial.

Table 20–2 summarizes numerous prospective infant feeding studies that compare breast-feeding to CM formula feeding. Many retrospective studies have also been undertaken but will not be reviewed here; the reader is referred to numerous recent review articles for a more thorough summary (Zeiger, 1993).

The major design flaw in the studies summarized herein is the lack of randomization between the CM- and formula-fed groups. Self-selection of the study groups invites bias, as parents self-selecting breast-feeding tend to be more educated, less likely to smoke, and have a greater level of home care, which might lead to an increased tendency toward atopy in the formula-fed group irrespective of feeding practice. In contrast, some of the studies suggest that there is an increased frequency of a bilateral allergic family history in the patient groups electing to breast-feed, biasing the results in the opposite direction. Nevertheless, many valuable observations have been made and some bear review here.

Over the past two decades several prospective studies have supported the original findings of Grulee and Sanford. For example, in 1979, Saarinen et al showed that serum IgE was lower at ages 1, 2, and 4 months in infants who were exclusively breast-fed and whose parents practiced allergy prevention as compared with those infants who were fed whole CM and did not have allergen avoidance practiced in the home. Infants who were fed CM formula had intermediate levels of serum IgE. At 1 year of age, however, after weaning and the introduction of solid foods, IgE levels were statistically similar in all three groups. Similarly, in a Canadian study, Chandra et al (1985) demonstrated a significant decrease in the prevalence of allergic disease (defined as eczema and/or three or more episodes of asthma) by 2 years of age in infants from allergic families who were exclusively breast-fed as compared to similar infants who were fed CM formula. Though infants with high IgE concentrations in cord blood were more likely to develop atopy than those with normal cord blood IgE, the lower prevalence of allergy in breast-fed infants than in formula-fed infants was noted irrespective of this difference. Furthermore, although the groups were not prospectively randomized, factors such as family income, household pets, pa-

TABLE 20-2. PROSPECTIVE NONRANDOMIZED STUDIES COMPARING THE EFFECTIVENESS OF BREAST-FEEDING WITH THAT OF COW'S MILK FEEDING ON THE DEVELOPMENT OF ALLERGIC DISEASE

Study (Reference)	Year	B (n)/CM (n)	Interval (yr)	Eczema (E)/Allergy (A)/ Asthma (As) Outcomes	Design Weaknesses†
A. Supportive of allergy preventive effect from breast-feeding					
Grulee	1936	9749/1707	0.75	E: 0.6% B vs 4% CM**	2, 3, 4, 5, 6
Matthew	1977	23/19	1	E: 13% B vs 47% CM*	1, 2, 3, 5, 7, 8, 9
Saarinen	1979	25/19	3	E: 12% B vs 26% CM*	2, 3, 5, 9
Chandra	1979	37/37	3	E: 11% B vs 59% CM**	2, 3, 5, 9, 10
Ziering	1979	25/25	2	A: 32% B vs 65% CM*	2, 3, 5, 9
Gruskay	1982	48/201	15	A: 28% B vs 53% CM*	2, 3, 5, 6
Businco	1983	34/41	2	A: 18% B vs 37% CM*	1, 2, 3, 5, 9
Pratt	1984	19/58	5	E: 16% B vs 38% CM*	2, 5, 6, 9
Chandra	1985	72/48	2	A: 17% B vs 52% CM**	2, 3, 5, 9
B. Nonsupportive of allergy preventive effect from breast-feeding (p>0.1)					
Kaufman	1972	38/54	2	E: ~50% B and CM	1, 2, 3, 5, 8, 9
Halpern	1973	193/349	0.5–7	A: ~16% B and CM	1, 2, 3, 4, 5, 6
Kaufman	1976	38/56	2	E: 32% B vs 23% CM	1, 2, 3, 5, 8, 9
Hide	1981	204/62	1	A: 45% B vs 53% CM	1, 2, 3, 5, 6, 7
Gordon	1982	112/85	2	A: 22% B vs 13% CM	1, 2, 3, 5
Van Asperen	1984	54/25	1.3	E: 52% B vs 40% CM	2, 3, 5, 8, 9
Van Asperen	1984	19/60	1.3	E: 58% B vs 45% CM	2, 3, 5, 8, 9
Hide	1985	35/132	4	E: 17% B vs 15% CM As: 9% B vs 11% CM	2, 6, 8

Modified from Zeiger RS. Prevention of food allergy in infancy. Ann Allergy 65:430, 1990.
Abbreviations: B = breast-feeding; CM = cow's milk feeding.
†Design weaknesses: 1 = late solids in B; 2 = not randomized; 3 = unmasked; 4 = unselected sample; 5 = compliance not documented; 6 = no immunologic documentation; 7 = differential environmental control in B; 8 = dropout high; 9 = inadequate sample size; 10 = B < 4 months.
#p = 0.08; * p<0.05; **p<0.01

rental smoking, family history of atopy, and age at introduction of solid foods were similar among the groups, lending more credence to the findings.

Duchateau and Casimir (1983) determined that 10 percent of 660 unselected infants had IgE levels greater than 1.0 IU/ml at 5 days of age. Among these infants with elevated IgE, 10 of 19 (53 percent) fed CM developed atopic dermatitis by 1 month of age, as compared to only 2 of 18 (11 percent) of solely breast-fed infants. This clinical observation was supported by significantly higher serum IgE levels at 1 month of age in the CM-fed infants than in the breast-fed babies. No difference in either the development of atopic dermatitis or 1-month serum IgE levels was noted between breast-fed infants and CM-fed infants among those patients with serum IgE levels less than 1.0 IU/ml at 5 days of age.

As noted above, the studies that have shown a beneficial effect of breast-feeding with regard to the development of atopic disease need to be interpreted with caution because of poor randomization of the study groups. Other design flaws encountered in many of these studies include lack of control of when solid foods were introduced to the different groups, lack of blinding, and poor monitoring of compliance.

Unfortunately, investigations that have failed to document a reduction in the amount of allergic disease by breast-feeding have similar weaknesses of design.

In 1982, Gordon et al noted that 22 percent of infants who were exclusively breast-fed for 3 months developed atopic disease by age 2, as compared to only 15 percent of bottle-fed infants. Some immunologic confirmation was provided in that both groups had a similar incidence of elevated serum IgE. Similarly, Van Asperen et al (1984) determined that 4 months of exclusive breast-feeding did not protect infants of atopic parents from developing either atopic disease or specific IgE to foods when compared to infants who were either bottle-fed or had solid foods introduced early. In 1985, Hide and Guyer noted similar clinical findings comparing infants who were exclusively breast-fed for 6 months versus those who were breast-fed only briefly followed by early introduction of solid food. This third study was not supported by any immunologic data.

Rowntree et al (1985) noted that breast feeding for 3 months did not protect infants against the development of eczema or food allergy within the first year of life or respiratory allergy by age 5. Immunologic confirmation was provided by an increased prevalence of skin test positivity to milk and egg in the breast-fed group and no increased sensitization to dust mite or ryegrass by age 5.

The only prospective, randomized study comparing the effects of breast-feeding versus those of CM feeding in the development of atopic disease was performed in 1990 by Lucas et al. They studied 446 unselected preterm neonates, 227 of whom were randomly assigned to receive banked human milk while 219 received preterm CM formula. One would theoretically expect preterm infants to be at a higher risk for allergic sensitization because of decreased gut maturity and enhanced exposure to dietary antigens. Within the entire cohort, the incidence of allergic reactions by 18 months was the same between the two groups. However, within the subgroup with a family history of allergy, the infants fed CM formula had a 41 percent chance of developing one or more allergic reactions compared to 16 percent of the breast-fed infants, with eczema most responsible for the difference. Objective immunologic support was lacking. Nonetheless, these data strongly support the protective effect of breast-feeding on the development of allergic disease.

Maternal Avoidance Diets During Pregnancy

Although initial studies reported specific IgE sensitization to foods (Michel et al, 1980), more recent reports suggest that such an occurrence probably occurs in less than 0.3 percent of monitored pregnancies (Zeiger, 1990). Moreover, studies that have examined the effect of maternal diets devoid of either milk and egg (Lilja et al, 1989) or milk, egg, and peanut (Falth-Magnusson and Kjellman, 1987) have failed to demonstrate a prophylactic effect on the development of atopy in high-risk infants who were otherwise maintained on a hypoallergenic diet postnatally. Because of this evidence, it would be inappropriate and potentially harmful to recommend maternal avoidance diets during pregnancy in order to prevent allergic disease in their children.

Maternal Avoidance Diets During Lactation

A major factor in all of the studies reviewed in the previous section that could explain, at least in part, the tremendous discrepancies is that maternal diet was not controlled. As noted earlier, there is evidence to suggest that infants can be sensitized to various foodstuffs through the breast milk if these foods were ingested by the mother. One might therefore suspect that while breast-feeding by mothers who have a diet high in allergenic foods such as milk, egg, or peanut might lead to an increase in food allergy in the recipient of that breast milk, breast-feeding by mothers whose diet restricts these foods might offer a protective effect (Table 20–3).

In 1989, Hattevig et al compared two groups of infants of atopic mothers selected and divided according to the site of hospital affiliation, both of whom were given breast milk, casein hydrolysate formula, and hypoallergenic diets during the first 6 months of life. The mothers of the infants in the study group were on diets devoid of egg, CM, and fish during the first 3 months of breast-feeding, while the mothers of the infants in the control group were on normal diets. The infants in the study group had less atopic dermatitis than the controls at both 3 months and 6 months and a lower detectable level of serum IgE to milk and/or egg at 3 months of age. Levels of specific IgE to egg or milk were similar in both groups after 6 months, most likely due to the introduction of these foods into the diet after this time. There was no suppression in the development of specific IgE or IgG antibodies to ovalbumin or BLG in the study group. It also appeared that the infants who developed IgG antibodies to ovalbumin did not have a decreased incidence of IgE antibodies to this egg-white protein, suggesting that IgG antibodies to food do not offer protection against allergic sensitization.

These findings were similar to those of Chandra et al (1989) who, in a prospective, randomized, controlled study, determined the incidence of atopic dermatitis by 18 months in two groups of infants of atopic families who were exclusively breast-fed for 6 months. The mothers of the infants in the study group maintained a lactation diet

TABLE 20–3. PROSPECTIVE RANDOMIZED CONTROLLED STUDIES OF FOOD ALLERGEN AVOIDANCE ON THE DEVELOPMENT OF ATOPIC DISEASE IN INFANTS OF ATOPIC PARENTS

Study (Reference)	Subjects (n)	Mom Pregnancy Diet	Mom Lactation Diet	Infant Diet	Follow-up	SPT/RAST	DBPCFC	Atopic Disease	Comments
Magnusson et al (1987) (1988) (1992)	197	3rd trimester (No egg, CM) vs No restriction	None	Breast +/or casein hydrolysate (3 Mo); Solids (>4 Mo); CM (>6 Mo); egg/fish (>9 Mo)	5 Yr	Not significant	No	Not significant	Pregnancy diet had no effect on infant atopy, SPT, or IgE
Lilja et al (1989) (1991)	162	3rd trimester (No egg, CM) vs No restrictions	None	Exclusive breast (5–6 Mo) vs No restrictions	1.5 Yr	Not significant	No	Not significant	Pregnancy diet had no effect on infant atopy, SPT, or IgE
Chandra et al (1986)	71	Entire pregnancy (No egg, CM, fish, peanut, beef) vs No restrictions	Entire lactation (same as pregnancy) vs No restrictions	Exclusive breast (5–6 Mo) vs No restrictions	1 Yr	Not determined	No	Reduced AD severity by 1 Yr*	No immunologic or food challenge confirmation. Benefit probably derives from infant diet and/or maternal lactation diet and not pregnancy diet
Zeiger et al (1989) (1992) (1993)	288	3rd trimester (No egg, CM, peanut) vs No restrictions	Entire lactation (same as pregnancy) vs No restrictions	Breast +/or casein hydrolysate (12 Mo); Solids (>6 Mo); CM, soy, corn (>12 Mo); egg, fish, peanut (>24 Mo) vs AAP guidelines	4 Yr	Reduced CM-IgE prevalence at 1* and 2 Yr**	Yes; half consented, 80% positive challenges	Reduced current prevalence of AD* and food allergy** at 1 Yr. Asthma, AR unaffected	Benefits probably derive from infant diet and/or maternal lactation diet and not pregnancy diet (see Magnusson and Lilja above)
Hattevig et al (1989) (1990) Sigurs et al (1992)	115	None	1st 3 Mo of lactation (No egg, CM, fish) vs No restrictions	Breast +/or casein hydrolysate (6 Mo); CM/solids (>6 Mo); egg/fish (>9 Mo)	4 Yr	Reduced # of CM +/or egg-IgE tests at 3 Mo**	No	Reduced AD at 3**, 6*, and 48** Mo	Groups assigned by hospital rather than by true randomization
Chandra et al (1989)	97	None	Entire lactation (No egg, CM, peanuts, soy, fish) vs No restrictions	Exclusive breast (~6 Mo), Solids (~6 Mo)	1.5 Yr	Not determined	No	Reduced AD by 1.5 Yr*	No immunologic or food challenge confirmation
Chandra et al (1989)	124 (3 groups)	None	None	Exclusive casein hydrolysate vs CM or soy. No breast feeding	1.5 Yr	Not determined	No	Reduced AD* by 1.5 Yr with casein hydrolysate	AD prevalence exceptionally high; no immunologic or food challenge confirmation
Chandra et al (1989) Chandra and Hamed (1991)	288 (4 groups)	None	None	Exclusive partial whey hydrolysate (6 Mo) vs CM, soy, or breast feeding (6 Mo)	1.5 Yr	No difference in CM-IgE at 2 and 6 Mo	No	Reduced 6 and 12 Mo AD cumulative prevalence*	No immunologic or food challenge confirmation; Cord blood + CM/Soy-IgE unexplainably high incidence

Table continued on following page

TABLE 20–3. PROSPECTIVE RANDOMIZED CONTROLLED STUDIES OF FOOD ALLERGEN AVOIDANCE ON THE DEVELOPMENT OF ATOPIC DISEASE IN INFANTS OF ATOPIC PARENTS (Continued)

Study (Reference)	Subjects (n)	Mom Pregnancy Diet	Mom Lactation Diet	Infant Diet	Follow-up	SPT/RAST	DBPCFC	Atopic Disease	Comments
Lucas et al (1990)	75 (Preterm)	None	None	Human milk vs preterm formula for 1.5 mo	1.5 Yr	Not determined	No	Reduced AD by 1.5 Yr*	No immunologic or food challenge confirmation. Only randomized study of human milk compared to CM feedings
Vandenplas, et al (1992)	67	None	None	Partial whey hydrolysate (6 Mo) vs CM formula	1 Yr	No difference in CM-IgE at 2 and 6 Mo	Blinded but not DBPCFC	Reduced CMA/CMPI prevalences at 6** and 12* Mo	Exceptionally high 6 Mo prevalence of AD (77%) and CMA/CMPI (34%) in controls; CMA/CMPI during (n = 1) and after (n = 3) hydrolysate
Arshad et al (1992)	120	None	Entire lactation (No egg, CM, fish, nuts) vs No restrictions	Breast +/or soy hydrolysate (9 Mo); CM/soy (9 Mo); egg (11 Mo); all others (12 Mo) plus mite avoidance (acaricide and encasings) vs No restrictions	1 Yr	Not significant	No	Reduced AD* and asthma* by 1 Yr	Control group with more smoking mothers (p = 0.11) and dual family atopy (p <0.05), but multivariate analyses confirmed benefit. Protective effect seen after exclusion of smokers

Modified from Zeiger RS. Pediatr Allergy Immunol 1994, in press.
Abbreviations: CM = cow's milk; AD = atopic dermatitis; CMA = CM allergy; CMPI = CM protein intolerance; AR = allergic rhinitis; DBPCFC = double-blind, placebo-controlled food challenge; Mo = month; Yr = year.
*p <0.05; **p <0.01

avoiding milk products, egg, fish, peanut, and soy, while the control group maintained a normal diet. The cumulative incidence of eczema in the study group was 22 percent (11 of 49), while in the control group it was 48 percent (21 of 48). Although these clinical results are impressive, no immunologic confirmation was provided, thereby weakening the cause and effect relationship.

Soy Formula in the Prevention of Allergy

In the early 1950s, it was suggested, based on data obtained in a retrospective study, that genetically allergy-prone children fed CM from birth were four times more likely to develop atopic disease—including eczema, asthma, and allergic rhinitis—than children in whom CM was largely replaced by soybean-based formula. This study led, in part, to the development of the large soy formula industry. Numerous prospective studies, aimed at confirming these results, have been performed since that time with varying degrees of methodologic loopholes that weaken their conclusions. One study in particular (Johnstone and Dutton, 1966), which found no evidence of protection against atopic dermatitis with the use of soy formula, did find a decreased incidence of respiratory allergy in children who were fed soy (a conclusion that would be counterintuitive to our current knowledge of allergic disease in infancy and early childhood). This study did not control for the ingestion of solid food nor the degree of environmental control carried out by the study and control groups.

Kjellman and Johansson (1979), on the other hand, performed a particularly well-controlled, randomized, immunologically supported prospective study in which infants with bilateral atopic family histories were fed either milk or soy formula. Their findings demonstrated a similar occurrence of atopy in the two groups, greater than 60 percent in each, a strikingly high proportion. These conclusions are not unexpected, inasmuch as infant sensitization to soy protein has been documented on numerous occasions. It has even been estimated that as many as 10 to 15 percent of children with CM allergy may also have soy allergy and IgE antibodies to soy.

Therefore, routine use of soy-based formulas cannot be routinely recommended as a choice for a "hypoallergenic" formula in the prevention of allergic disease. However, it may be an appropriate choice as a formula for selected infants with CM allergy.

Protein Hydrolysate Formula in the Prevention of Allergy

Protein hydrolysate formulas (Table 20–4) were first developed in the early 1940s for use in feeding infants with food intolerances, food allergies, and malabsorption. In more recent years several other attempts have been made at developing such formulas, with an attempt at minimal allergenicity, via the use of small peptides, while maintaining palatability and acceptable cost (Knights, 1985). Ideally, these formulas should contain <1 percent peptides >1.5 kilodaltons in size, contain no intact proteins, show no evidence of anaphylaxis in animals, reveal protein determinant equivalents less than 1 millionth of the original protein, determinant equivalents less than 1 millionth of the original protein, and be shown safe in milk-allergic infants by both double-blind placebo-controlled food challenge and by open challenge.

The extensively hydrolyzed casein hydrolysate formulas, Nutramigen and Alimentum, have been documented to fulfill these immunologic and clinical criteria and can be termed hypoallergenic (Sampson et al, 1991), while the recently developed partially hydrolyzed whey hydrolysate, Good Start, has numerous peptides >4 kilodaltons in size and has been shown to frequently cause allergic reactions in patients with documented IgE to CM (Businco et al, 1989; Ellis et al, 1991). Because of this, only fully hydrolyzed formulas should be considered truly hypoallergenic, whereas partially hydrolyzed formulas should be avoided in patients with IgE-mediated milk allergy. Even so, it must be realized that even the fully hydrolyzed formulas, on rare occasions, have caused allergic reactions in milk-allergic patients (Lifschitz et al, 1988; Bock, 1989). Thus prudence dictates that any formula prescribed for milk-allergic patients first be administered under medical supervision with preparation to treat possible anaphylaxis. For patients who cannot tolerate protein hydrolysate formulas, the elemental formula Neocate (Scientific Hospital Supplies, Gaithersburg, MD), which is not yet commercially available in the United States, would be a safe alternative if it can be obtained from the manufacturer (Sampson et al, 1992).

Logic would suggest that the use of a protein hydrolysate formula might prevent or delay the development of atopic disease in infants. In contrast to soy and other formulas,

TABLE 20–4. CHARACTERISTICS OF SEVERAL COMMERCIAL PROTEIN HYDROLYSATES (PH) AND AN ELEMENTAL AMINO ACID–DERIVED FORMULA

Characteristic	Nutramigen	Alimentum	Good Start	Neocate
Introduced in USA	1942	1989	1989	Pending approval
Formula	CM Casein PH	CM Casein PH	CM Whey PH	Elemental amino acid
Oil	Corn	Safflower	Coconut/palm	Safflower/soy/coconut
Carbohydrate	Corn syrup solids	Sucrose/tapioca	Lactose	Maltodextrin
Peptides >1500 Daltons	Rare	Rare	Frequent	None
Residual CM antigen <10^{-6} of original CM	Yes	Yes	No	No CM antigen determinants
+ DBPCFC in IgE-CMA patients	Rare	Rare	Frequent	None reported
Hypoallergenic	Yes	Yes	No	Yes
Recommended in CMA	Yes	Yes	No	Yes

Modified from Zeiger RS. Prevention of food allergy in infancy. Ann Allergy 65:430, 1990.
CM = cow's milk; CMA = cow's milk allergy; DBPCFC = double-blind placebo-controlled food challenge.

extensive casein hydrolysates have been documented to lack sensitizing capacity in animals (McLaughlan et al, 1981). For this reason, several prospective randomized studies have been recently performed to evaluate a possible role for protein hydrolysate formulas in the prevention of allergic disease in infants.

In 1989, Zeiger et al reported the results of a study of infants from allergy-prone families given either CM formula (n = 161) or Nutramigen (n = 89) as supplements during weaning from or in lieu of breast-feeding. After 1 year, 4.3 percent of the CM formula-fed infants developed skin and/or gastrointestinal manifestations of allergic disease with demonstration of milk-specific IgE as compared to none in the Nutramigen-fed group. Additionally, Nutramigen was shown to suppress the IgG BLG response after milk was introduced at 1 year, suggesting significant hypoallergenicity.

Chandra et al (1989) noted that the cumulative incidence of eczema by 18 months was only 21 percent in infants fed Nutramigen versus 70 percent in CM-fed and 63 percent in soy-fed infants. This group has also documented a decreased 6-month cumulative prevalence of eczema in infants fed Good Start. Unfortunately, no immunologic data were presented to support these findings.

In summary, these data suggest but do not prove that protein hydrolysate formulas may be able to play a role in the prevention of food allergy in selected infants. Though it has been suggested that partial hydrolysates may decrease the prevalence of food allergy, these formulas have also been shown to cause anaphylaxis in children who have already been sensitized to CM protein. As the infants in whom one may attempt to prevent sensitization may accidentally ingest CM protein from a variety of sources, caution would probably dictate the use of the most hydrolyzed type of formula available, such as the casein hydrolysates, as a safe way to potentially prevent or delay milk sensitization in infancy. Definitive, prospective, randomized double-blind studies using double-blind, placebo-controlled food challenges to define adverse outcomes must demonstrate a protective effect of these formulas before any can be universally recommended for the prevention of food allergy, particularly CM allergy.

Delayed Introduction of Solid Foods

Infants directly exposed to a variety of solid foods early in infancy appear to have higher rates of eczema (Fergusson et al, 1990). A genetically prone infant with an immature gut is likely to have difficulty excluding a variety of proteins from its blood stream, thereby potentially priming the IgE system and hence increasing its risk of developing allergic disease later in infancy or childhood.

In 1983, Kajosaari and Saarinen reported the results of a prospective, nonrandomized study in which 115 infants with atopic family histories either were exclusively breast-fed for 6 months or had solid foods introduced at 3 months as a supplement to breast-feeding. In the exclusively breast-fed group, 14 percent developed atopic dermatitis and food allergy by 1 year of age compared to 35 percent of the group supplemented with solid food. While the results of this study may seem intuitively pleasing, the nonrandomized nature of the study weakens its conclusions. Therefore, although the withholding of solid foods during early infancy may be beneficial, additional studies would strengthen this notion and lead to more clear recommendations.

Combined Maternal and Infant Avoidance of Allergenic Foods

Two recent studies have attempted to determine whether an attempt at restricting the consumption of allergenic foods by infants could decrease the incidence of allergic disease, realizing that there are numerous sources from which an infant can become sensitized. In 1986, Chandra et al reported the results of a prospective, randomized, unblinded study of 71 infants with atopic siblings, which concluded that maternal avoidance of milk, egg, peanut, fish, and beef during the entire pregnancy and lactation period, coupled with exclusive breast-feeding and delayed introduction of solid foods for 6 months, led to a decreased severity of eczema. Although compliance with the maternal avoidance diet was well documented, no immunologic confirmation, such as skin test or food challenge data, was provided.

More recently, Zeiger et al (1989 and 1992) evaluated the role of combined infant and maternal avoidance diets, compared to standard feeding practices, in the prevention of allergic disease in infants born to documented atopic parents. In a prenatally randomized, physician-blinded, controlled study, 103 mother/infant pairs were placed on a regimen that included (1) maternal avoidance of milk, egg, and peanut during the third trimester of pregnancy and during lactation, (2) either exclusive breast or Nutramigen feedings for 6 months in the infants, and (3) the child's avoidance of milk, corn, soy, citrus, and wheat for 1 year and avoidance of egg, peanut, and fish for 2 years. The 185 children in the control group followed standard maternal and infant feeding practices recommended by the American Academies of Obstetrics and Gynecology and Pediatrics. The results showed that the children in the restricted diet group had: (1) decreased periods (current) and cumulative prevalences of atopic diseases at 1 year, (2) decrease in milk-specific IgE at 1 year, (3) marginally lower serum IgE at 4 months, but (4) no decrease in the prevalence of allergic rhinitis, asthma, or IgE to inhalant allergens at 4 years, when compared to the control group.

In contrast, Lilja et al (1991) observed no reduction in food allergy when combined maternal and infant food avoidance was carried out for less than 6 months, suggesting that a time period of dietary restriction of somewhere between 6 and 12 months may be necessary for some effective prophylaxis of food allergy.

The Role of Avoidance of Both Ingested and Inhaled Allergens in the Prevention of Atopic Disease

One might imagine that if one would minimize infant exposure to both allergenic foodstuffs and highly allergenic inhalants such as dust mite and cat dander, it might be possible to protect against atopic dermatitis as well as allergic rhinitis and asthma. Recently, Arshad et al (1992) reported that maternal and infant avoidance diets during infancy, combined with the use of acaricide, an anti–dust mite spray, significantly reduced the development of asthma and atopic dermatitis by 1 year. Further studies with longer follow-up periods would be indicated.

CONCLUSIONS

The studies cited in this review suggest that one may indeed be able to prevent or delay the development of atopic disease by first predicting which patients are at risk for developing allergy and then recommending a program of environmental and dietary manipulation aimed at minimizing exposure to likely allergens. Based on past research, the emerging consensus is that the greater degree of avoidance measures carried out (i.e., maternal restriction diets during lactation, delayed introduction of solid foods to infants, breast milk supplementation only with hypoallergenic formulas, as well as dust mite and animal avoidance from early infancy), the greater are the chances of delaying or preventing the development of allergy.

Three caveats must therefore be presented before recommending such control measures to large numbers of patients. First, as the majority of studies conducted have had varying degrees of design flaws, *the* definitive study has yet to be performed regarding what environmental and dietary manipulation is clearly the most effective. Second, it is not clear through long-term follow-up whether or not the development of allergic disease is prevented or merely delayed by carrying out allergen avoidance measures during infancy, a fact that must be made clear to patients before such manipulation is recommended. Third, stringent environmental and dietary manipulation requires a tremendous amount of motivation on the part of the families and caretakers of the infants involved. The effort involved in markedly restricting the diet of both infant and mother, as well as carrying out dust mite avoidance measures and removing household pets in some instances, makes a prophylactic regimen practical for only the most motivated of families, particularly until more definitive studies are performed. Clearly, smoking should be discouraged in the homes of all children, not just in the households of those children at risk for atopy.

In the meantime, a provisional strategy for potentially preventing or delaying the development of atopic disease in those at most risk for developing allergy is outlined in Table 20-5.

With the rapid advances made in genetics and molecular biology, one would expect that in the near future our emphasis will shift from hypoallergenic diets and allergy avoidance to more direct methods to alter the phenotypic expression of a predetermined allergic genotype. It is not hard to foresee a future in which we might be able, through direct genetic engineering, to alter the genes responsible for IgE synthesis, or via immunomodulation, to alter the effect of cytokines or end-

TABLE 20–5. PROVISIONAL RECOMMENDATIONS FOR THE PREVENTION OF FOOD AND OTHER ALLERGIC DISORDERS IN NEWBORNS/INFANTS AT HIGH-RISK FOR ATOPY

STRATEGY	METHOD OR MEASURE
1. Identify high-risk infant prenatally or early postnatally	Atopic family (biparental, parent and sibling) or elevated cord blood IgE
2. Avoid infant exposure to:	
a. Food allergens	
In utero	Dietary intervention not indicated and potentially harmful
In breast milk	Maternal lactation diet with no egg, CM, peanut (consider?)
	Supplement maternal diet with 1500 mg calcium daily
In infant diet	Breast-feed for at least 4–6 mo, preferably the latter
	Supplement or wean with nutritious and hypoallergenic extensively hydrolyzed protein hydrolysate formula
	No solid foods for 6 mo, then add least allergenic first
	After 1 yr, add biweekly or monthly, if tolerated, CM, wheat, soy, citrus, egg, peanut, fish. Delay egg, peanut, and fish longer in food atopic infants
b. Aeroallergens	Reduce household mite, mold, pet concentrations
	Use air conditioners/air purifiers, acaricides, denaturants, mite-proof bedding encasings
3. Avoid nonspecific environmental adjuvants	No smoking prenatally or postnatally by caretakers
	Reduce pollution
	Minimize infections (breast-feed, avoid early day care)

Modified from Zeiger RS. Prevention of food allergy in infancy. Ann Allergy 65:430, 1990.

organ receptors necessary to express allergic disease. Such breakthroughs would revolutionize the way in which we would approach the prevention of atopy well into the next millennium.

REFERENCES

Aberg N. Asthma and allergic rhinitis in Swedish conscripts. Clin Allergy 19:59, 1989.

Andrae S, Axelson O, Bjorksten B, et al. Symptoms of bronchial hyperreactivity and asthma in relation to environmental factors. Arch Dis Child 63:473, 1988.

Arshad SH, Matthews S, Gant C, et al. Effect of allergen avoidance on development of allergic disorders in infancy. Lancet 339:1493, 1992.

Bjorksten F, Suoniemi I, Koski V. Neonatal birch pollen contact and subsequent allergy to birch pollen. Clin Allergy 10:585, 1980.

Bock SA. Probable allergic reaction to casein hydrolysate formula. J Allergy Clin Immunol 84:272, 1989. (Correspondence)

Bousquet J, Menardo JL, Viala JL, et al. Predictive value of cord serum IgE determination and the development of "early onset atopy." Ann Allergy 51:291, 1983.

Businco L, Marchetti F, Pellegrini G, et al. Predictive value of cord blood IgE levels in "at-risk" newborn babies and influence of type of feeding. Clin Allergy 13:503, 1983.

Businco L, Cantani A. Longhi AL, et al. Anaphylactic reactions to a cow's milk whey protein hydrolysate (Alfa-Re, Nestle) in infants with cow's milk allergy. Ann Allergy 62:333, 1989.

Cant A, Narsden RA, Kilshaw PJ. Egg and cow's milk hypersensitivity in exclusively breast-fed infants with eczema, and detection of egg protein in breast milk. Br Med J 291:932, 1985.

Chandra RK. Prospective studies on the effect of breast feeding on incidence of infection and allergy. Acta Paediatr Scand 68:691, 1979.

Chandra RK, Puri S, Cheema PS. Predictive value of cord blood IgE in the development of atopic disease and role of breast feeding in its prevention. Clin Allergy 15:517, 1985.

Chandra RK, Puri S, Suraiya C, et al. Influence of maternal food antigen avoidance during pregnancy and lactation on incidence of atopic eczema in infants. Clin Allergy 16:563, 1986.

Chandra RK, Shakuntla P, Hamed A. Influence of maternal diet during lactation and use of formula feeds on development of atopic eczema in high-risk infants. Br Med J 299:228, 1989.

Chandra RK, Hamed A. Cumulative incidence of atopic disorders in high risk infants fed whey hydrolysate, soy and conventional cow milk formulas. Ann Allergy 67:129, 1991.

Coca AF, Cooke RA. On the classification of the phenomena of hypersensitization. J Immunol 8:163, 1923.

Cogswell JJ, Mitchell EB, Alexander J. Parental smoking, breast feeding, and respiratory infection in development of allergic diseases. Arch Dis Child 62:338, 1987.

Croner S, Kjellman NIH. Development of atopic disease in relation to family history and cord blood IgE levels. Eleven year follow-up in 1654 children. Pediatr Allergy Immunol 1:14, 1990.

Duchateau J, Casimir G. Neonatal serum IgE concentrations as predictor of atopy. Lancet 1:413, 1983.

Eastham EJ, Lichauco T, Grady MI. Antigenicity of infant formulas: Role of immature intestine on protein permeability. J Pediatr 93:561, 1978.

Ellis MH, Short JA, Heiner DC. Anaphylaxis after ingestion of a recently introduced hydrolyzed whey protein formula. J Pediatr 118:74, 1991.

Falth-Magnusson K, Kjellman NIM. Development of atopic disease in babies whose mothers were receiving exclusion diets during pregnancy—a randomized study. J Allergy Clin Immunol 80:868, 1987.

Falth-Magnusson K, Kjellman NIM, Magnusson KE. Antibodies IgG, IgA and IgM to food antigens during the first 18 months of life in relation to feeding and development of atopic disease. J Allergy Clin Immunol 81:743, 1988.

Falth-Magnusson K, Kjellman NIM. Allergy prevention by maternal elimination diet during pregnancy—a 5-year follow-up of a randomized study. J Allergy Clin Immunol 89:709, 1992.

Fergusson DM, Horwood LJ, Shannon FT. Parental smoking and respiratory illness in infancy. Arch Dis Child 55:358, 1980.

Fergusson DM, Horwood LJ, Beautrias AL, et al. Eczema and infant diet. Clin Allergy 11:325, 1981.

Fergusson DM, Horwood LJ, Shannon FT. Risk factors in childhood eczema. J Epidemiol Community Health 36:118, 1982.

Fergusson DM, Horwood LJ, Shannon FT. Asthma and infant diet. Arch Dis Child 58:48, 1983.

Fergusson DM, Horwood LJ, Shannon FT. Early solid feeding and recurrent childhood eczema: A 10-year longitudinal study. Pediatrics 86:541, 1990.

Gordon RR, Ward AM, Noble DA, et al. Immunoglobulin E and the eczema-asthma syndrome syndrome in early childhood. Lancet 1:72, 1982.

Grulee CG, Sanford HN. The influence of breast and artificial feeding on infantile eczema. J Pediatr 9:223, 1936.

Gruskay FL. Comparison of breast, cow and soy feedings in the prevention of onset of allergic disease: A 15-year prospective study. Clin Pediatr 21:486, 1982.

Halpern SR, Sellars WA, Johnson RB, et al. Development of childhood allergy in infants fed breast soy or cow milk. J Allergy Clin Immunol 51:139, 1973.

Hattevig G, Kjellman B, Johansson SGO, et al. Clinical symptoms and IgE responses to common food problems in atopic and healthy children. Clin Allergy 14:551, 1984.

Hattevig G, Kjellman B, Siqurs N, et al. Effect of maternal avoidance of eggs, cow's milk and fish during lactation upon allergic manifestations in infants. Clin Exp Allergy 19:27, 1989.

Hattevig G, Kjellman B, Siqurs N, et al. The effect of maternal avoidance of eggs, cow's milk and fish during lactation on the development of IgE, IgG and IgA antibodies in infants. J Allergy Clin Immunol 85:108, 1990.

Hide DW, Guyer BM. Clinical manifestations of allergy related to breast and cow's milk feeding. Arch Dis Child 56:172, 1981.

Hide DW, Guyer BM. Clinical manifestations of allergy related to breast and cow's milk feeding. Pediatrics 76:973, 1985.

Ishizaki T, Koizumi K, Ikemore R, et al. Studies of prevalence of Japanese cedar pollenosis among the residents in a densely cultivated area. Ann Allergy 58:265, 1987.

Johnstone DE, Dutton Am. Dietary prophylaxis of allergic diseases in children. N Engl J Med 274:715, 1966.

Kajosaari M, Saarinen UM. Prophylaxis of atopic disease by six months' total solid food elimination. Arch Paediatr Scand 72:411, 1983.

Kaufman HS. Diet and heredity in infantile atopic dermatitis. Arch Dermatol 105:400, 1972.

Kaufman HS, Frick OL. The development of allergy in infants of allergic parents: A prospective study concerning the role of heredity. Ann Allergy 37:410, 1976.

Kjellman MN, Croner S. Cord blood IgE determination for allergy prediction—a follow-up to seven years of age in 1,651 children. Ann Allergy 53:167, 1984.

Kjellman NIM. Effect of parental smoking on IgE levels in children. Lancet 1:993, 1981.

Kjellman NIM, Johansson SGO. Soy versus cow's milk in infants with a biparental history of atopic disease: development of atopic disease and immunoglobulins from birth to 4 years of age. Clin Allergy 9:347, 1979.

Knights RJ. Processing and evaluation of the antigenicity of protein hydrolysates. In Lifshitz F (ed). Nutrition for Special Needs in Infancy: Protein Hydrolysis. New York, Marcel Dekker, 1985.

Kraemer MJ, Marshall SG, Richardson MA. Etiologic factors in the development of chronic middle ear effusions. Clin Rev Allergy 2:319, 1984.

Lifschitz CH, Hawkins HK, Guerra C, et al. Anaphylactic shock due to cow's milk protein hypersensitivity in a breast-fed infant. J Pediatr Gastroenterol Nutr 7:141, 1988.

Lilja G, Dannaeus A, Foucard T, et al. Effects of maternal diet during late pregnancy and lactation on the development of atopic disease in infants up to 18 months of age—in vivo results. Clin Exp Allergy 19:473, 1989.

Lilja G, Dannaeus A, Foucard T, et al. Effects of maternal diet during late pregnancy and lactation on the development of IgE and egg- and milk-specific IgE and IgG antibodies in infants. Clin Exp Allergy 21:195, 1991.

Lucas A, Brooke OG, Morely R, et al. Early diet of preterm infants and development of allergic or atopic disease: randomized prospective study. Br Med J 300:837, 1990.

Machtinger S, Moss R. Cow's milk allergy in breast-fed infants. The role of allergen and maternal secretory IgA antibody. J Allergy Clin Immunol 77:341, 1986.

Maimonides M. Treatises on asthma. In Muntner S (ed). The Medical Writings of Moses Maimonides. Vol. I. Philadelphia, JB Lippincott, 1963.

Matthew DJ, Taylor B, Norman AP. Prevention of eczema. Lancet 1:321, 1977.

May CD, Fomon SJ, Remigio L. Immunologic consequences of feeding infants with cow's milk and soy products. Acta Paediatr Scand 71:43, 1982.

McLaughlan P, Anderson KJ, Widdowson EM, et al. Effect of heat treatment on the anaphylactic sensitizing capacity of cow's milk, goat's milk and various infant formulae fed to guinea pigs. Arch Dis Child 56:165, 1981.

Michel FB, Bousquet J, Greillier P, et al. Comparison of cord blood immunoglobulin E and maternal allergy for the prediction of atopic disease in infancy. J Allergy Clin Immunol 65:422, 1980.

Pratt HF. Breast-feeding and eczema. Early Human Dev 9:283, 1984.

Rowntree S, Cogswell JJ, Platts-Mills TAE, et al. Development of IgE and IgG antibodies to food and inhalant allergens in children at risk of allergic disease. Arch Dis Child 60:727, 1985.

Saarinen UM, Backman A, Kajosaari M, et al. Prolonged breast-feeding as prophylaxis for atopic disease. Lancet 2:163, 1979.

Sampson HA, Bernhisel-Broadbent J, Yang E, et al. Safety of casein hydrolysate formula in children with cow milk allergy. J Pediatr 118:520, 1991.

Sampson HA, James JM, Bernhisel-Broadbent J. Safety

of amino acid-derived infant formula in children allergic to cow milk. Pediatrics 90:463, 1992.

Savilahti E, Salmenpera L, Tainio VM, et al. Prolonged exclusive breast-feeding results in low serum concentrations of immunoglobulin G, A and M. Acta Paediatr Scand 76:1, 1987.

Shannon WR. Demonstration of food proteins in human breast milk by anaphylactic experiments on guinea pigs. Am J Dis Child 22:223, 1921.

Sigurs N, Hattevig G, Kjellman B. Maternal avoidance of eggs, cow's milk and fish during lactation: Effect on allergic manifestations, skin prick tests and specific IgE antibodies in children at age 4 years. Pediatrics 89:735, 1992.

Sporik R, Holgate ST, Platts-Mills TAE, et al. Exposure to house-dust mite allergen (Der p I) and the development of asthma in childhood. A prospective study. N Engl J Med 323:502, 1990.

Stuart CA, Twiseton R, Nicholas MF, et al. Passage of cow's milk protein in breast milk. Clin Allergy 14:533, 1984.

Suoniemi I, Bjorksten F, Haahtela T. Dependence of immediate hypersensitivity in the adolescent period on factors encountered in infancy. Allergy 36:263, 1981.

Tager IB. "Passive smoking" and respiratory health in children—sophistry or cause for concern? Am Rev Respir Dis 133:959, 1986.

Troncone R, Scarcella A, Donatiello A, et al. Passage of gliadin into human breast milk. Acta Paediatr Scand 76:453, 1987.

Van Asperen PP, Kemp AS, Mellis CM. Immediate food hypersensitivity reactions on the first known exposure to the food. Arch Dis Child 58:253, 1983.

Van Asperen PP, Kemp AS, Mellis CM. Relationship of diet in the development of atopy in infancy. Clin Allergy 14:525, 1984.

Vandenplas Y, Hauser B, Van den Bore C, et al. Effect of a whey hydrolysate prophylaxis of atopic disease. Ann Allergy 68:419, 1992.

Warner JA, Little SA, Pollock I, et al. The influence of exposure to house dust mite, cat, pollen and fungal allergens in the home on primary sensitization in asthma. Pediatr Allergy Immunol 1:79, 1990.

Zeiger RS, Heller S, Mellon MH, et al. Effect of combined maternal and infant food allergen avoidance on development of atopy in early infancy: A randomized study. J Allergy Clin Immunol 84:72, 1989.

Zeiger RS. Prevention of food allergy in infancy. Ann Allergy 65:430, 1990.

Zeiger RS, Heller S, Mellon MH, et al. Genetic and environmental factors affecting the development of atopy through age 4 in children of atopic parents: a prospective randomized study of food allergen avoidance. Pediatr Allergy Immunol 3:110, 1992.

Zeiger RS. Development and prevention of allergic disease in childhood. In Middleton E Jr, Reed CE, Ellis EF, et al (eds). Allergy: Principles and Practice. 4th ed. vol II. St. Louis, Mosby-Year Book, 1993.

Ziering R, O'Connor R, Mellon M, et al. University of California in San Diego prophylaxis of allergy in infancy study: An interim report. J Allergy Clin Immunol 63:199, 1979.

Section Four
SYSTEMIC REACTIONS AND ANAPHYLAXIS

Chapter 21
Specific and Idiopathic Anaphylaxis: Pathophysiology and Treatment

Phillip L. Lieberman, M.D.

The term "anaphylaxis" refers to a systemic, immediate hypersensitivity reaction due to IgE-mediated immunologic release of mediators from mast cells and basophils. The term "anaphylactoid reaction" refers to a clinically similar event not mediated by IgE.

Portier and Richet coined the term "anaphylaxis" in 1902 (Portier and Richet, 1902). It literally means "without or against protection." Portier and Richet were trying to establish immunity to the sting of the sea anemone. During the immunization process they sensitized dogs (the animal used in the experiment) to the venom. These dogs thus unexpectedly reacted fatally to a previously nonlethal dose of venom. This phenomenon was the opposite of their desired goal of prophylaxis. They therefore coined the term "anaphylaxis" to identify this event.

INCIDENCE AND CAUSATIVE AGENTS

Overall Incidence

The exact incidence of anaphylaxis is unknown. A review of the literature between

1895 and 1923 revealed 41 cases of fatal anaphylaxis (Lamson, 1924). A subsequent review from 1923 to 1935 recorded 68 fatal cases (Vaughn and Pipes, 1936). In great Britain 140 cases, 41 of which were fatal, were reported to the Committee on Safety of Medicines between 1966 and 1975 (Davies, 1977).

The Boston Collaborative Drug Surveillance Program, in 1973, reported six anaphylactic reactions and 0.87 deaths per 10,000 patients monitored (Boston Collaborative Drug Surveillance Program, 1973). In 1977 this collaborative study recorded a series of 32,812 continuously monitored patients in selected medical wards. Drug-induced anaphylaxis occurred in 12 (0.04 percent), and there were two deaths (Porter and Jick, 1977). In a review of patients admitted to a university hospital during 1990 there were nine cases of anaphylaxis out of a total of 20,064 admissions (0.04 percent) (Amornmarn et al, 1992). In the province of Ontario, the overall documented incidence was reported as four cases per 10 million population (Orange and Donsky, 1978).

Of course, these studies permit only an approximation of the true incidence of anaphylaxis. Many do not take into consideration reactions to foods, Hymenoptera stings, and other causes. In addition, they are subject to error because of the well-recognized tendency for many drug reactions to go unreported (Barclay, 1979).

Factors Affecting Incidence

Age, race, geographic location, sex, route of administration of antigen, constancy of administration of antigen, and atopy have been evaluated for their effects on the incidence of anaphylaxis. Race and geographic location exert no effect on incidence (Lieberman, 1981). In most instances sex is not a significant factor. However, there are possible exceptions to this observation. Anaphylactic reactions to intravenous muscle relaxants have been reported to occur more frequently in women (Vervloet et al, 1979). This may be related to the fact that the quaternary ammonium ion found in muscle relaxants is also found in some cosmetics, and thus females may be sensitized by previous exposure. A similar increased incidence in females has been reported for reactions to aspirin (Harnett et al, 1978) and latex (Hamann, 1993). The increased incidence of anaphylaxis to latex is probably due to an increased exposure to latex gloves in women. In addition, insect sting anaphylaxis has been reported to occur more frequently in men (Reisman, 1978). This also is probably a function of exposure.

The incidence and/or severity of anaphylaxis and anaphylactoid reactions to radiocontrast media (Lieberman, 1992), Hymenoptera (Parrish, 1963), plasma expanders (Watkins and Clarke, 1978), and anesthetics (Watkins and Clarke, 1978) has been reported to be greater in adults than in children. However, fatal reactions can occur in children. Whether this apparent effect of age is due to an increased frequency of exposure, heightened level of hypersensitivity, or both is conjectural.

The route of administration of the provocative agent is important in regard to both frequency of occurrence and severity. Anaphylaxis has occurred in association with all routes of administration including oral, subcutaneous, intramuscular, intravenous, intranasal, intraocular, cutaneous, intravaginal, intrarectal, and endotracheal. Attacks seem to be more frequent and more severe when the agent is injected versus ingested. This is a point of clinical relevance when prevention of anaphylactic episodes is considered.

The constancy of administration of antigen is of note. For example, in most patients with insulin allergy the anaphylactic reaction does not occur as long as there is uninterrupted administration of the drug. Sensitivity is enhanced when administration of the drug is resumed after cessation of therapy (Lieberman, 1991b).

In addition, the time elapsing between an original episode of anaphylaxis and the readministration of antigen is an important variable. The likelihood of a second episode decreases as the time interval between the original attack and readministration increases. This is probably due to the catabolism and decreased synthesis of IgE after cessation of antigen administration.

The role of atopy as a predisposing factor varies. The significance of the atopic state appears to be dependent on several factors including the antigen involved and the route of administration. Early investigations found that anaphylaxis to penicillin was more common in atopic individuals (Levine, 1966; Kern and Wimberley, 1953), but more recent reviews have not confirmed this observation. In a multi-center cooperative study of penicillin allergy by the American Academy of Allergy there was no correlation between penicillin reactivity and a personal or family history of atopy (Green and Rosenblum, 1971). In 1973, in a study involving 1433 subjects, there was no difference in the incidence of positive skin tests to penicillin between atopic and non-atopic individuals (Stember and Levine, 1973). In one review of 1030 penicillin allergic subjects and 1344 patients with pollen allergy, it was found that atopics had a *lower* than normal risk for immediate hypersensitivity to penicillin (Filip, 1988). Similar observations have been made regarding anaphylactic reactions to insulin (Lieberman et al, 1971) and Hymenoptera stings (Settipane et al, 1978). On the other hand, the incidence of anaphylaxis to latex is clearly increased in atopic individuals (Slater, 1993; Fernandez de Corres et al, 1993). This probably relates to the nature of the antigen and its cross-reactivity with foods (bananas, avocado, chestnuts) to which atopic individuals have been sensitized (Fernandez de Corres et al, 1993). Indeed, reactions to food in general, an antigen to which exposure is mucosal, are more frequent in atopics. This is in keeping with experimental data showing that atopic individuals appear to be more prone to develop IgE antibody when antigen is administered topically but show little preference to do so when it is administered by injection (Salvaggio et al, 1964). Atopics appear to be predisposed to anaphylaxis and anaphylactoid reactions in general, since they account for an inordinate percentage of cases in random series (Kemp et al, 1993) and in series of cases of idiopathic anaphylaxis (Orfan et al, 1992), exercise-induced anaphylaxis (Horan and Sheffer, 1992), and anaphylactoid reactions to radiocontrast material (Katayama et al, 1990). This predisposition may well be related to the phenomenon of basophil "hyperreleasability" seen in atopics. In patients with food allergy (Frieri et al, 1992; May, 1976), atopic dermatitis (Sampson and Broadbent, 1987), and asthma and bronchopulmonary aspergillosis (Ricketti et al, 1983; Patterson et al, 1988), spontaneous basophil histamine release is enhanced compared to controls. This *in vitro* phenomenon could be responsible for increased *in vivo* sensitivity to agents capable of causing mast cell and basophil degranulation (Patterson et al, 1988).

In atopics the time of year the antigen is administered may also play a role, as evidenced by the increase in frequency of anaphylactic reactions to allergen immunotherapy during pollen season (Van Metre and Adkinson, 1988).

Of course, frequency of exposure is an important factor in terms of the incidence of anaphylactic reactions. This is self-evident in most instances but can be cryptic in others. For example, diabetics treated with protamine-containing insulin are 40 to 50 times more likely to have reactions to protamine when this agent is administered to reverse heparin anticoagulation (Gottschlich et al, 1988). Also, previous administration of protamine for heparin neutralization can sensitize a patient to insulin preparations containing protamine. Reactions to these preparations can be confused with anaphylactic reactions to insulin per se, and the previous sensitization experience to protamine can be missed. This can result in delayed recognition of protamine as the responsible agent (Kim et al, 1991; Dykewicz and Orfan, 1991).

Table 21–1 summarizes the effect of these factors on the incidence and severity of anaphylactic and anaphylactoid reactions.

PATHOLOGY

Death from anaphylaxis is usually due to respiratory obstruction and/or cardiovascular collapse (Delage and Irey, 1972; James and Austen, 1964; Hunt, 1993; Lamson, 1929; Sheppe, 1980; Delage et al, 1973).

In patients dying from respiratory obstruction there is edema of the airway and pulmonary hyperinflation. Upper airway edema can be found in about 60 percent of deaths (Delage and Irey, 1972; James and Austen, 1964). Bronchial obstruction with hyperinflation of the lungs occurs in about half the cases (Delage and Irey, 1972; James and Austen, 1964; Hunt, 1993; Lamson, 1929). Bronchial obstruction is due to a combination of spasm, submucosal edema, and secretions (Delage and Irey, 1972; James and Austen, 1964). Upper airway edema is secondary to the accumulation of transudate in the submucosal tissue (James and Austen, 1964).

In deaths due to cardiovascular collapse there may be no pathologic finding. However, myocardial damage can be detected in the majority of cases (Delage et al, 1973). Dilatation of the right ventricle may also be found (James and Austen, 1964).

TABLE 21–1. FACTORS AFFECTING THE INCIDENCE AND/OR SEVERITY OF ANAPHYLAXIS AND ANAPHYLACTOID REACTIONS

Factor	Effect	Reference
Age	More frequent in adults than children for some agents—radiocontrast plasma expanders, anesthetics; may be function of exposure frequency	Reisman, 1978; Lieberman, 1992; Parrish, 1963
Sex	Reportedly more frequent in females for latex, aspirin, and muscle relaxants; more frequent in males for Hymenoptera; may be function of exposure frequency	Lieberman; 1981; Vervloet et al, 1979; Hamann and Curtis, 1993
Route of administration	Oral less likely to produce reaction and reaction usually less severe	Lieberman, 1981
Constancy of administration	Gaps in administration may predispose to reactions	Lieberman et al, 1971
Time since last reaction	The longer the interval the less likely the recurrence for many allergens	Lieberman, 1981; Erffmeyer, 1992
Atopy	Higher incidence in anaphylaxis due to ingested antigens, exercise anaphylaxis, idiopathic anaphylaxis, radiocontrast reactions, latex reactions; probably equal incidence for insulin, penicillin, and Hymenoptera reactions	Kern and Wimberley, 1953; Green and Rosenblum, 1971; Stember and Levine, 1973; Lieberman et al, 1971; Settipane et al, 1978; Slater, 1993; Orfan et al, 1992; Horan and Sheffer, 1992
Geographic location	No known effect	
Race	No known effect	

Other findings include diffuse eosinophilic infiltration of the pulmonary vessels, laminae propria of the gastrointestinal tract, and sinusoids of the spleen. There is also congestion of the abdominal viscera (Delage and Irey, 1972; James and Austen, 1964).

Of more recent interest is the observation that postmortem determination of specific IgE and serum tryptase may be useful in establishing anaphylaxis as the cause of death in patients experiencing sudden death of unknown cause (Yunginger et al, 1991; Schwartz et al, 1988; Ansari et al, 1993; Schwartz et al, 1993).

In one study, IgE antivenom (RAST) was assayed in postmortem blood samples taken from patients dying unexpectedly from spring through autumn; 23.2 percent of sera showed significant levels of IgE anti-Hymenoptera venom (Schwartz et al, 1988). In a follow-up of that study (Schwartz et al, 1993), 68 remaining sera previously examined for the prevalence of IgE antivenom were analyzed for tryptase. Nine of these cases (13 percent) demonstrated elevation of serum tryptase (greater than 10 ng/ml). There was some degree of correlation between elevated tryptase levels and the previously assayed antivenom IgE levels. In three samples with markedly elevated antivenom IgE levels, one showed elevation of serum tryptase. In 17 samples with moderate elevations of antivenom IgE, three (18 percent) demonstrated elevated tryptase levels. In the 47 samples with no increase in venom-specific IgE, five (11 percent) demonstrated elevated tryptase levels.

The specificity and sensitivity of specific IgE and tryptase levels have been demonstrated by their assay in patients who have died from documented anaphylactic episodes (Yunginger et al, 1991). Mast cell-derived tryptase and specific IgE antibody levels were measured in sera obtained prior to or within 24 hours after death from anaphylaxis in 19 subjects. Serum tryptase levels were elevated in nine of nine Hymenoptera sting fatalities, six of eight food-induced fatalities, and two of two deaths due to diagnostic/therapeutic agents. This contrasted with normal serum tryptase levels in 57 postmortem control patients. Serum IgE antibodies were elevated in five of the nine Hymenoptera fatalities and eight of the eight fatal food reactions.

An interesting observation of this evaluation was that serum tryptase levels were higher in those to whom the allergen was administered parenterally (Hymenoptera venoms and injections) than in those in whom the allergen was encountered orally (foods). The authors postulated that this was due to the fact that connective tissue mast cells were preferentially degranulated when the antigen was injected, and that mucosal mast cells were preferentially degranulated when the antigen was ingested. Connective tissue mast cells contain more tryptase than mucosal mast cells (Schwartz et al, 1987).

The implications of these findings are important for two reasons. First, they imply that the incidence of anaphylactic death may be underestimated, and that a significant proportion of unexplained sudden deaths may be due to anaphylaxis. Second, they are of clinical importance since they offer a diagnostic modality with the potential of determining the cause of unexpected death. The authors recommended that sera should be obtained antemortem (if possible) and postmortem for the analysis of tryptase and allergen-specific IgE (Yunginger et al, 1991). Sera should be frozen and stored at $-20°$ C until assay. Of note is the fact that pleural and pericardial fluids were not satisfactory for tryptase quantitation. The authors also suggested that unconsumed portions of foods eaten by the victim before the episode should be saved to construct "custom" RAST reagents (Yunginger et al, 1991).

A summary of the pathologic findings in anaphylaxis and anaphylactoid reactions is seen in Table 21–2.

PATHOPHYSIOLOGY

Anaphylaxis and anaphylactoid events are the result of the activation of several pathways of inflammation. A classification of the role of these pathways is seen in Table 21–3.

Anaphylactic reactions are defined as those mediated through antigen-induced IgE mast cell and basophil degranulation. The most common causes of these reactions are foods, drugs and biologicals, and insect stings and bites. In addition, some cases of exercise-induced anaphylaxis (food-dependent) are also mediated through this mechanism (Okazaki et al, 1992).

Anaphylactoid reactions are those reactions that are clinically similar to anaphylactic episodes but have a different underlying pathophysiology. One of the most common mechanisms of production of anaphylactoid reactions involves the direct (non-IgE) release of mediators from mast cells and basophils. This occurs in anaphylactoid reactions to drugs and biologicals, most cases of idiopathic anaphylaxis, probably the majority of cases of exercise-induced anaphylaxis, and anaphylaxis to other physical factors such as cold and sunlight. For example, numerous drugs including radiocontrast media (2pc), opioids (Marone et al, 1991), and several other agents (Lieberman, 1981) are capable of producing anaphylactoid events through this mechanism.

Aspirin and NSAID probably produce some anaphylactoid reactions via the aberrant me-

TABLE 21–3. PATHOPHYSIOLOGIC CLASSIFICATION OF ANAPHYLAXIS AND ANAPHYLACTOID REACTIONS

I. Anaphylaxis—IgE-mediated reaction
  A. Food
  B. Drugs
  C. Insect bites and stings
  D. Perhaps some cases of exercise
II. Anaphylactoid
  A. Direct release of mediators from mast cells and basophils
    1. Drugs
    2. Idiopathic
    3. Exercise
    4. Physical factors such as cold, sunlight
  B. Disturbances in arachidonic acid metabolism
    1. Aspirin
    2. Nonsteroidal anti-inflammatory drugs
  C. Immune aggregates
    1. Gamma globulin
    2. IgG anti-IgA
    3. Possibly dextran and albumin
  D. Cytotoxic
    Transfusion reactions to cellular elements
  E. Miscellaneous and multimediator activity
    1. Non–antigen-antibody-mediated complement activation
      a. Radiocontrast material
      b. Possibly some cases of protamine reactions
      c. Dialysis membranes
    2. Activation of contact system
      a. Dialysis membranes
      b. Radiocontrast material

TABLE 21–2. MAJOR PATHOLOGIC FINDINGS IN ANAPHYLACTIC DEATHS

Commonly no findings are noted	Dilatation of right ventricle
Pulmonary hyperinflation	Congestion of abdominal viscera
Airway edema	Eosinophilic infiltrate
Laryngeal	Lungs
Tracheal	Sinusoids of spleen
Epiglottal	Abdominal viscera
Hypopharyngeal	Serum tryptase elevation
Bronchial	Elevation of specific IgG
Myocardial ischemia	

tabolism of arachidonic acid (Manning et al, 1992). However, some reactions to these agents may be due to the direct degranulation of mast cells since elevations of histamine and tryptase occur (Lee et al, 1991; Bosso et al, 1991).

Immune aggregate anaphylaxis can occur when the complement system is activated by antigen-antibody complexes or other protein aggregates. This type of anaphylactoid reaction has been reported to occur after administration of protamine (Westaby et al, 1985; 5pc), dextran (Hedin and Richter, 1982), albumin (Ring, 1991), and after transfusions or gamma globulin given to patients with IgA deficiency (Vyas and Fudenberg, 1969).

In cytotoxic anaphylactoid reactions the antigen is cell-fixed. Such reactions occur during incompatible transfusions when there are complement-fixing antibodies to formed elements of the blood such as red cells, white cells, and platelets. Complement activation is thought to play a role in the production of these events.

Finally, several agents such as radiocontrast material (Lieberman, 1992) and protamine (Weiss and Adkinson, 1991) produce anaphylactoid reactions through activation of multiple inflammatory pathways. These include complement as well as the contact (kallikrein) system.

Basophil and Mast Cell Degranulation Syndromes

It is likely that the majority of anaphylaxis and anaphylactoid events involve basophil and mast cell degranulation. It is therefore important to be familiar with the contents of these cells. The mediators released from basophils and mast cells and their possible role in the production of anaphylaxis and anaphylactoid reactions are seen in Table 21–4. The major pathophysiologic events due to the release of these mediators include smooth muscle spasm (especially of the bronchus, coronary arteries, and gastrointestinal tract), an increase in vascular permeability, vasodilatation, stimulation of sensory nerve endings with reflex activation of vagal effector pathways and antidromic pathways, and myocardial depression. These effects result in the classic symptoms of flush, urticaria and angioedema, wheeze, fall in blood pressure with potential shock, gastrointestinal smooth muscle contraction with nausea, vomiting and diarrhea, and myocardial ischemia.

In addition, many of these mediators are capable of activating other inflammatory pathways. Mast cell kininogenase (Proud et al, 1985) and basophil kallikrein (Newball et al, 1979) can activate the kinin system. Tryptase also has kallikrein activity and can activate the complement cascade as well as cleave fibrinogen (Holgate et al, 1993). In addition, chemotactic agents, by calling forth eosinophils and other cells, have the capacity to prolong and intensify reactions. Other agents perhaps modify the pathophysiologic events. Heparin can inhibit clotting, plasmin, and kallikrein. It also modulates the effects of tryptase and has anticomplementary activity. Chymase is capable of converting angiotensin I to angiotensin II and therefore theoretically could enhance the compensatory response to hypotension.

It can be seen, by visualizing the summation effect of these mediators, that late-phase and protracted anaphylactic and anaphylactoid events could occur due to their release. Case reports of such events have been described (Popa and Lerner, 1984).

Since histamine infusion has been shown to produce the majority of the symptoms of anaphylaxis (Kaliner et al, 1982), and since it has been the most intensively studied mediator, the effects of this agent will be reviewed in more detail.

Histamine

The vast majority of the body's store of histamine is found in mast cells and basophils. Histamine formation and storage also occur in the central nervous system, gastric mucosa, and epidermal cells.

The actions of histamine are mediated through three receptor types (H_1, H_2, H_3). There are other, less well-defined receptors (non-H_1, non-H_2, non-H_3) that exist as well. Table 21–5 lists the activities, salient to anaphylaxis, mediated through H_1 and H_2 receptors.

The overall effect of histamine on the vascular bed is dilatation. This produces flushing and a lowering of peripheral resistance with a subsequent fall in systolic pressure. There is also an increase in vascular permeability due to a separation of endothelial cells at the postcapillary venule level. This exposes the permeable basement membrane. Vasodilatation

TABLE 21-4. MAST CELL AND BASOPHIL MEDIATORS THAT MAY PLAY A ROLE IN ANAPHYLAXIS AND ANAPHYLACTOID REACTIONS

Mediator	Pathophysiologic Event	Possible Clinical Manifestations
Histamine	Acts through H_1, H_2 receptors Increased vascular permeability Vasodilatation Contraction of smooth muscle Exocrine gland secretion Irritation sensory nerves	Flush, urticaria, angioedema, wheeze, hypotension, abdominal cramps, diarrhea

Arachidonic acid metabolites
  Lipoxygenase pathway
    LTB4
    LTC4
    LTD4
	
	Chemotaxis
	Contraction airway smooth muscle
	Increased vascular permeability
	Goblet and mucosal gland secretion
		
		Possible role in late phase response
		Possible production of wheeze and hypotension

Cyclooxygenase pathway
    PG D_2
    PG $F_{2\alpha}$
    Thromboxane A_2
	
	Peripheral vasodilatation
	Contraction airway smooth muscle
	Coronary vasoconstriction
	Goblet, submucosal gland secretion
		
		Flush, hypotension
		Possible production of wheeze, myocardial ischemia

Prostaglandin-generating factor of anaphylaxis	Formation of arachidonic acid metabolites of both cyclooxygenase and lipoxygenase pathways	Same as arachidonic acid metabolites above
Platelet-activating factor	Contraction airway smooth muscle Vascular permeability	Wheeze, hypotension
Eosinophil and neutrophil chemotactic factors	Infiltration of and activation of eosinophils and neutrophils	Unclear; theoretically could prolong and intensify reaction, producing late phase reaction
Tryptase	May activate complement by cleavage C_3 to C_{3a} Cleaves fibrinogen Possibly has kallikrein activity	Unclear; may recruit other pathways of inflammation
Mast cell kininogenase and basophil kallikrein	Activate contact system with formation kinins	Unclear
Chymase	Cleaves neuropeptides Converts angiotensin I to angiotensin II	May play role in response to hypotension with conversion of angiotensin; could have salutary effect by inactivation neuropeptides
Heparin	Inhibits clotting, plasmin, and kallikrein Also anticomplementary	May have salutary (anti-inflammatory) effect

is mediated by both H_1 and H_2 receptors. H_2 receptors exert their effect by a direct action on the vascular smooth muscle. H_1 receptors exert their effect directly but also indirectly by stimulation of endothelial cells. Endothelial cell stimulation causes the production of a smooth muscle relaxing factor, nitric oxide (Moncada and Martin, 1993; Palmer et al, 1987). This indirect vasodilatory reaction plays an important role in the cumulative vasodilatory response.

The effects of histamine on the heart are mediated primarily through the H_2 receptor, but the H_1 receptor also plays a role. H_2 receptor stimulation increases both the rate and force of atrial and ventricular contraction, probably by enhancing calcium influx. This increases cardiac oxygen need. H_1 receptor activity increases the heart rate by hastening diastolic depolarization at the SA node. The H_1 receptor also produces coronary artery vasospasm (Lieberman, 1990).

Histamine produces varying effects on extravascular smooth muscle. It causes smooth muscle contraction in the bronchial tree. This is mediated entirely via the H_1 receptor. H_1 receptor stimulation also causes modest contraction of the human uterus, and H_2 receptor stimulation can produce uterine relaxation. The predominant effect of histamine on the gastrointestinal smooth muscle is contraction mediated via the H_1 receptor.

Glandular secretion is mediated by both H_1 and H_2 receptors. Glycoprotein secretion from

TABLE 21–5. ACTIONS OF HISTAMINE PERTINENT TO ANAPHYLAXIS MEDIATED THROUGH H_1 AND H_2 RECEPTORS

H_1	H_2	REQUIRES H_1 AND H_2 FOR MAXIMUM EFFECT
Smooth muscle contraction	Cardiac effects	Vasodilatation
Stimulation of nerve endings	Positive inotropic	Flush
Vagal irritant receptors	Positive chronotropic	Headache
Pruritus	Decreased fibrillation threshold	Hypotension
Neuropeptide release	Vasodilatation	Increased amount mucous gland secretion
Vascular permeability	Mucous glycoprotein secretion from goblet cells and bronchial glands	
Vasodilatation		
Endothelial cell relaxing factor (nitric oxide)		
Direct effect		
Cardiac effects		
Increased rate of depolarization of SA node		
Coronary artery vasospasm		
Increased viscosity mucous gland secretion		

goblet cells and bronchial glands is produced by stimulation of the H_2 receptor, whereas stimulation of the H_1 receptor increases mucus viscosity.

Infusion of histamine into man produces symptoms similar to those observed during anaphylaxis, including flushing, headaches, tachycardia, and hypotension. For maximal inhibition of flushing, headaches, and hypotension, a combination of H_1 and H_2 receptor blockade is required. Increases in heart rate could be effectively blocked by an H_1 receptor antagonist, but for optimal protective effects, both an H_1 and H_2 antagonist were required (Kaliner et al, 1982).

The role of other basophil and mast cell mediators has not been as clearly defined. However, as noted above, these agents are potentially strong candidates for the production of the pathophysiologic events responsible for anaphylaxis and anaphylactoid events.

Recruitment of Other Inflammatory Pathways

From the discussion above, it is clear that mast cell and basophil contents have the capability of activating a number of inflammatory pathways including the kinin system, complement system, clotting, and clot lysis (disseminated intravascular coagulation). There is strong *in vivo* evidence to indicate that these recruitment pathways play an important role in clinical events (Smith et al, 1980; van der Linden et al, 1993a; Kaplan et al, 1977; van der Linden et al, 1990; Hermann and Ring, 1990; Pavek et al, 1982).

One of the first demonstrations of the activation of other inflammatory pathways in human anaphylaxis occurred during controlled studies of immunotherapy for insect hypersensitivity (Smith et al, 1980; Kaplan et al, 1977). In subjects experiencing only generalized urticaria to insect sting challenge there were no changes in blood histamine levels or recruitment of other mediator pathways. However, in three patients who experienced shock, peak histamine levels rose dramatically and correlated with the severity of hypotension. In addition, two of the three patients with the more severe episodes had diminutions in factor V, factor VIII, fibrinogen, and high-molecular-weight kininogen. In one of these patients there were diminished levels of C_4 and C_3.

A later evaluation of eight patients with previous reactions to wasp stings who were rechallenged with a sting demonstrated a relationship between levels of the anaphylatoxin C_{3a} and the severity of the anaphylactic event. There was no change in C_{3a} in one patient who showed no reaction and only a slight rise in three patients with mild reactions. In contrast, C_{3a} rose substantially in four patients with severe reactions. The presence of this cleavage product of C_3 indicated activation of the complement cascade (van der Linden et al, 1990).

Other investigations have demonstrated activation of the kallikrein-kinin system (van der Linden et al, 1993a; Pavek et al, 1982).

Kallikrein-C_1-inhibitor complexes, factor XIIa-C_1-inhibitor complexes, antigenic prekallikrein, and antigenic factor XII were measured in serial blood samples obtained from 16 subjects with a history of insect sting anaphylaxis immediately after insect sting challenge (van der Linden et al, 1993b). Peak levels of kallikrein-C_1-inhibitor complexes and factor XIIa-C_1-inhibitor complexes were found 5 minutes after the onset of symptoms. By 15 minutes, antigenic prekallikrein levels had decreased in patients with angioedema as a component of the anaphylactic event. These findings only occurred in subjects experiencing reactions. Thus, activation of the contact system (kallikrein-kinin) was strongly related to the development of angioedema after sting challenge.

As previously noted, recruitment of other inflammatory pathways could be due to tryptase, mast cell kininogenase, and basophil kallikrein. In addition, the cellular and biochemical events (e.g., hypoxia, endothelial damage) occurring during shock could activate the contact system, clotting system, and complement system. Activation of these systems has been noted in severe hypotensive shock of other etiologies (cardiovascular shock, endotoxic shock). Table 21–6 summarizes the multiple inflammatory pathways involved.

Abnormal Physiologic Events

Many of the pathophysiologic events that occur during anaphylactic shock are easily explained by the action of the mediators cited above. For example, wheeze, increase in airway resistance, and fall in Po_2 (Smith et al, 1980) can be attributed to the direct contractile activity of histamine and other mediators on the smooth muscle of the lung. Similar explanations are evident for flush, urticaria, angioedema, and gastrointestinal symptoms. However, the mechanism of production of hypotension and shock is more complicated and deserves mention.

Much of the data regarding the mechanism of production of shock in human beings has been obtained from the evaluation of patients experiencing anaphylaxis or anaphylactoid reactions during anesthesia or cardiac catheterization (Nordström et al, 1978; Fisher, 1977; Obeid et al, 1975). This has allowed for hemodynamic measurements during the event. Although the hemodynamic changes occurring during anaphylaxis and anaphylactoid reactions can vary (van der Linden, 1993a; Hanashiro and Weil, 1967; Silverman et al, 1984), the major factors causing cardiovascular abnormalities are universal and are due to an initial loss of intravascular fluid and vasodilatation, which may be followed shortly thereafter by vasoconstriction and then myocardial depression.

Increased vascular permeability can produce a rapid and dramatic loss of intravascular volume. Fluid shifted to the extravascular space can result in a loss of 50 percent of vascular volume within 10 minutes (Fisher, 1989; Fisher, 1986). This loss of blood volume results in compensatory mechanisms that involve both the secretion of catecholamines, such as norepinephrine and epinephrine (Fahmy, 1981; Moss et al, 1981; van der Linden, 1993a), and activation of the angiotensin system with conversion of angiotensin I to angiotensin II and increased production of these agents (van der Linden, 1993a; Hermann et al, 1980; von Tschirschnitz et al, 1993; Hermann et al, 1992a; Hermann et al, 1992b). On the other hand, attempts to correlate elevations of vasopressin and oxytocin with anaphylactic episodes have shown inconsistent results (Hermann et al, 1980; Hermann et al, 1992a).

These internal compensatory vasopressor responses can produce variable results. In some patients with anaphylactic and anaphylactoid episodes, the peripheral resistance can be abnormally elevated (indicating maximal vasoconstriction) owing to this response (Ha-

TABLE 21–6. MULTIMEDIATOR RECRUITMENT OCCURRING DURING ANAPHYLAXIS AND ANAPHYLACTIC EVENTS

Pathway Activated	Reference
Coagulation pathway	Smith et al, 1980;
Decreased factor V	Kaplan et al, 1977
Decreased factor VIII	
Decreased fibrinogen	
Complement cascade	
Decreased C_4	Smith et al, 1980
Decreased C_3	Smith et al, 1980
Formation C_{3a}	Van der Linden et al, 1990
Contact system (kinin formation)	
Decreased high-molecular-weight kininogen	Kaplan et al, 1977
Formation of kallikrein-C_1-inhibitor complexes, factor XIIa-C_1-inhibitor complexes	Van der Linden et al, 1993a

nashiro and Weil, 1967). Whereas in other subjects, despite elevation of catecholamines, systemic vascular resistance falls (Fahmy, 1981).

It has been suggested that failure to mobilize these compensatory mechanisms may predispose patients to anaphylaxis (Hermann and Ring, 1992). In a study comparing baseline plasma angiotensin I and angiotensin II levels in Hymenoptera-sensitive patients and normal controls, the former group had significantly lower amounts. An inverse correlation between angiotensin levels and the severity of the anaphylactic episodes was noted; the lower the levels, the more severe the symptoms.

Further hemodynamic changes contributing to, or occurring as a result of, the fall in arterial pressure include a decrease in cardiac output, decrease in pulmonary wedge pressure and pulmonary artery pressure, and increases in pulmonary vascular resistance. These latter changes can result in "shock lung" or adult respiratory distress syndrome with pulmonary edema (Edde and Burtis, 1973).

Falls in blood pressure can be correlated with elevations of histamine, tryptase (van der Linden et al, 1992; Smith et al, 1980) and C_{3a} (van der Linden et al, 1990). However, levels of these mediators do not correlate with the presence of urticaria, flush, or wheeze (Smith et al, 1980; van der Linden et al, 1992). Angioedema may be related to the appearance of activation products of the contact (kinin-kallikrein) system (van der Linden et al, 1993a).

These changes are highly important from a therapeutic standpoint. It is obvious that the one consistent and most important finding in regard to the production of hypotension is the loss of effective intravascular volume due to fluid extravasation into the extravascular space. In addition, because of internal compensatory mechanisms (secretion of epinephrine and norepinephrine, and production of angiotensin II), such patients with shock may be maximally vasoconstricted and therefore unresponsive to pressor agents. Thus fluid replacement and volume expanders, not vasoconstrictor agents, are the treatments of choice in such cases.

SIGNS AND SYMPTOMS

The clinical manifestations of anaphylaxis can be ascertained best by a review of several series of patients experiencing anaphylactic episodes. An analysis of four such series consisting of a total of 743 patients is summarized in Table 21–7. These series include patients suffering exclusively from exercise-induced anaphylaxis (Wade et al, 1989), patients with idiopathic anaphylaxis (Orfan et al, 1992), and two series of patients with anaphylaxis due to a variety of etiologies (Kemp et al, 1993; Wiggins, 1991).

The signs and symptoms of anaphylaxis as reported in these articles are remarkably similar. In all instances urticaria and angioedema were the most commonly occurring manifestations. In fact, in the series on idiopathic anaphylaxis (Orfan et al, 1992), involving 225 patients, all subjects experienced urticaria and angioedema. In both series involving patients with multiple causes (Wiggins, 1991; Kemp et al, 1993), 90 percent of patients experienced this complaint, and in exercise-induced anaphylaxis (Wade et al, 1989), 83 percent of cases had urticaria and angioedema. In most studies, the next most common complaint was lower respiratory in nature with shortness of breath, dyspnea, or wheeze. Flush was reported in a significant number of cases in patients suffering from exercise-induced anaphylaxis but was only

TABLE 21–7. FREQUENCY OF OCCURRENCE OF SIGNS AND SYMPTOMS OF ANAPHYLAXIS

SIGNS/SYMPTOMS	NUMBER	PERCENT
Urticaria and angioedema	657	88
Dyspnea, wheeze	354	47
Dizziness, syncope, hypotension	246	33
Nausea, vomiting, diarrhea, cramping abdominal pain	227	30
Flush*	225	46
Upper airway edema*	237	56
Headache*	73	15
Rhinitis*	44	16
Substernal pain*	16	6
Itch without rash*	12	4.5
Seizure*	4	1.5

Based on a compilation of data from the following references: Kemp et al. A review of 267 cases of anaphylaxis in clinical practice. J Allergy Clin Immunol 91(suppl):153, 1993. (Abstract); Wade et al. Exercise-induced anaphylaxis: Epidemiological observations. Proc Clin Biol Res 297:175, 1989; Wiggins CA. Characteristics and etiology of 30 patients with anaphylaxis. Immunol Allergy Pract 13:313–316, 1991; Orfan et al. Idiopathic anaphylaxis: Total experience in 225 patients. Allergy Proc 13:35–43, 1992.

*Symptom or sign not reported in all four series; therefore, total number may be underrepresented and percent of subjects may be a more accurate representation.

reported as a symptom in one other series (Kemp et al, 1993). In this series it occurred in 28 percent. Dizziness, syncope, and hypotension constituted the next most common symptom complex. Overall these symptoms occurred in approximately 33 percent of subjects when all series were totaled. Gastrointestinal symptoms including nausea, vomiting, diarrhea, and cramping abdominal pain occurred in 30 percent of subjects when all series were totaled. Upper airway edema was reported as a symptom in only three of the four studies but did involve 56 percent of subjects in those three. Headache was a somewhat unique complaint, occurring in a significant percentage of subjects with exercise-induced anaphylaxis (30 percent), but not reported in two of the other series and occurring in only 5 percent of a series of patients with anaphylaxis due to various causes (Kemp et al, 1993). Several symptoms—including rhinitis, substernal pain, itch without rash, and seizures—were reported only in one study in a small minority of patients (Kemp et al, 1993).

In sum, urticaria and angioedema are by far the most frequent manifestations of anaphylaxis and anaphylactoid reactions, the next most common being lower respiratory tract symptoms followed by dizziness, syncope, and gastrointestinal manifestations.

It should be noted that cardiovascular collapse with shock can occur immediately without any cutaneous or respiratory symptoms (Viner and Rhamy, 1975). In fact, in a series of 27 severely affected patients treated by anesthesiologist-staffed ambulance and helicopter crews (Soreide and Harboe, 1988), only 70 percent of patients with circulatory and/or respiratory failure had cutaneous symptoms; 30 percent of these had gastrointestinal symptoms and 85 percent had neurologic symptoms (seizures, impaired consciousness, muscle spasms). However, the relative paucity of cutaneous symptoms in these patients may have been due to the fact that data were recorded only from signs observed after arrival to the scene. Another possible explanation is the difference in severity between these cases and those in the series included in Table 21–8. Of the 27 patients reported in this series, there were two deaths and 23 hospitalizations (Soreide and Harboe, 1988).

Symptoms usually begin within 5 to 30 minutes when antigen has been administered by injection. However, there can be a delay of an hour or more. After oral administration of antigen, symptoms usually occur within the first 2 hours after ingestion but can be delayed in onset for several hours. It is believed that there is a direct correlation between the immediacy of onset of symptoms and the severity of a given attack. The more rapid the onset, the more severe the episode.

An episode can abate and then exhibit a recrudescence several hours after symptoms have disappeared. This has been termed "biphasic anaphylaxis" (Popa and Lerner, 1984).

TABLE 21–8. DIFFERENTIAL DIAGNOSIS OF ANAPHYLAXIS AND ANAPHYLACTOID REACTIONS

I. Anaphylaxis and anaphylactoid reactions
   A. Anaphylaxis and anaphylactoid reactions to exogenously administered agents
   B. Physical factors
      Exercise
      Cold, heat, sunlight
   C. Idiopathic
II. Vasodepressor reactions
III. Flush syndromes
   A. Carcinoid
   B. Postmenopausal
   C. Chlorpropamide-alcohol
   D. Medullary carcinoma thyroid
   E. Autonomic epilepsy
IV. "Restaurant syndromes"
   A. MSG
   B. Sulfites
   C. Scombroidosis
V. Other forms of shock
   A. Hemorrhagic
   B. Cardiogenic
   C. Endotoxic
VI. Excess endogenous production of histamine syndromes
   A. Systemic mastocytosis
   B. Urticaria pigmentosa
   C. Basophilic leukemia
   D. Acute promyelocytic leukemia (tretinoin treatment)
   E. Hydatid cyst
VII. Nonorganic disease
   A. Panic attacks
   B. Munchausen's stridor
   C. Vocal cord dysfunction syndrome
   D. Globus hystericus
VIII. Miscellaneous
   A. Hereditary angioedema
   B. "Progesterone" anaphylaxis
   C. Urticarial vasculitis
   D. Pheochromocytoma
   E. Hyperimmunoglobulin E, urticaria syndrome
   F. Neurologic (seizure, stroke)
   G. Pseudoanaphylaxis
   H. Red man syndrome (vancomycin)

In addition, attacks can be protracted, persisting for over 24 hours. This is especially true for cardiovascular symptoms. Protracted shock and adult respiratory tract distress symptoms can occur in spite of appropriate therapy (Edde and Burtis, 1973). Death can occur at any time during the course of protracted anaphylaxis.

The cardiac manifestations of anaphylaxis can be varied and profound (Criep and Woehler, 1971; Sullivan, 1982; Brasher and Sanchez, 1974). Characteristically, anaphylaxis is associated with a compensatory tachycardia that occurs in response to a decreased effective vascular volume. This has often been used as a sign to differentiate an anaphylactic episode from a vasodepressor reaction. However, bradycardia, presumably due to increased vagal reactivity, can also occur in anaphylaxis (Simon, 1989; Jacobsen and Secher, 1988). This is probably due to the Bezold-Jarisch reflex. This cardioinhibitory reflex has its origin in sensory receptors in the inferoposterior wall of the left ventricle. Unmyelinated vagal C fibers carry the reflex, which is activated by ischemia.

Myocardial depression with decreased cardiac output due to contractile depression can occur and can persist for several days. This is thought to be due to hypoxemia (Raper and Fisher, 1988). Coronary artery vasospasm has been documented with coronary angiography (Austin et al, 1984). Vasospasm can result in myocardial infarction (Cisteró et al, 1992). Electrocardiographic abnormalities include ST segment elevation, flattening of T waves, inversion of T waves, and arrhythmias (Booth and Patterson, 1970; Antonelli et al, 1984). Cardiac enzyme elevations also occur.

Arterial blood gas abnormalities usually consist of a fall in Po_2 and Pco_2 early in the course. If severe respiratory difficulty supervenes, the hypoxia worsens, and an elevation of Pco_2 may occur along with a fall in pH that is probably due to a combination of CO_2 retention and metabolic acidosis (van der Linden et al, 1993b).

Anaphylactoid reactions can be indistinguishable from those due to anaphylaxis. However some anaphylactoid reactions have singular characteristics that bear mention. Reactions to gamma globulin administration can produce nausea, vomiting, chills, fever, low back pain, and a sensation of chest tightness and constriction. These symptoms can be somewhat delayed in onset.

DIFFERENTIAL DIAGNOSIS

The differential diagnosis of anaphylaxis and anaphylactoid events is seen in Table 21-8. This classification includes conditions that should be considered by the physician seeing the patient during the acute event as well as conditions that should be considered when the patient is seen after the episode for the purpose of determining the cause of the event.

Perhaps the most common condition mimicking anaphylaxis is the vasodepressor reaction. Vasodepressor reactions are characterized by hypotension, pallor, weakness, nausea, vomiting, and profuse diaphoresis. They are usually the result of a threatening event or emotional trauma. Bradycardia occurs in vasodepressor reactions. This can be used as a differential diagnostic factor to distinguish an anaphylactic event from a vasodepressor reaction, but cannot be trusted as the sole differential determinant since the pulse may be slow or normal in anaphylaxis (Simon, 1989; Smith et al, 1980). An important distinguishing feature is the fact that vasodepressor reactions are not accompanied by cutaneous manifestations (e.g., urticaria, angioedema, flush).

Entities that produce flush should be considered in the differential diagnosis. These include carcinoid syndrome, postmenopausal flush, chlorpropamide-alcohol–induced flush, flush associated with medullary carcinoma of thyroid, and autonomic epilepsy.

It is not surprising that carcinoid syndrome can produce symptoms similar to anaphylaxis since carcinoid tumors secrete histamine, kallikrein, neuropeptides, and prostaglandins in addition to 5-hydroxytryptamine (serotonin) (Aldrich et al, 1988). Patients with carcinoid syndrome have flushing, diarrhea, abdominal pain, cardiovascular disease, and wheezing.

Approximately 50 percent of patients with postmenopausal flush present with flushing of the face, neck, upper chest, and breasts. This flush lasts 3 to 5 minutes and can occur several times a day. It can be aggravated by alcohol and stress. There is no fall in blood pressure.

Alcohol, ingested while taking a sulfonylurea agent, especially chlorpropamide, can produce a flush that is associated with hypoglycemia and all of its accompanying symptoms. The flush usually begins about 3 to 5 minutes after the ingestion of alcohol and peaks in about 15 minutes. There is no fall in blood pressure or syncope, and gastrointestinal symptoms are not noted.

Medullary carcinoma of the thyroid can cause a protracted flush of the face and upper extremities. Patients usually have telangiectasia, a positive family history for the disease, and sometimes mucosal neuromas. This tumor can secrete prostaglandins, histamine, substance P, and 5-hydroxytryptamine.

Autonomic epilepsy is a rare disease thought to be due to paroxysmal autonomic discharges. The blood pressure may fall or rise, and tachycardia, flush, and syncope occur.

In many patients the cause of flushing cannot be determined. These patients are said to have idiopathic flush reactions. This occurs more frequently in women. It can be associated with palpitations, diarrhea, syncope, and hypotension. There is no wheezing or abdominal pain (Aldrich et al, 1988).

Certain postprandial syndromes resemble anaphylaxis. These have been attributed to the ingestion of monosodium glutamate, sulfites, and saurine (Settipane, 1986). They are referred to as "the restaurant syndromes."

High concentrations of sulfites can be found in pickles, gelatin, dried fruits, wine, fruit juices, sausages, and shellfish. After ingestion of these agents some patients experience flushing, bronchospasm, and hypotension.

Monosodium glutamate (MSG) ingestion can produce chest pain, facial burning, flushing, paresthesias, sweating, dizziness, headaches, palpitations, nausea, and vomiting. Children can experience shivering and chills, irritability, screaming, and delirium. The occurrence of these symptoms has been referred to as the "Chinese restaurant syndrome." The mechanism of production of this condition is unknown, but it is thought that MSG causes a "transient acetylcholinosis." Fifteen to 20 percent of the general population appears to be sensitive to small doses of MSG, but reactions can occur in any individual should the dose be large enough. Symptoms usually begin no later than 1 hour after ingestion, but can be delayed in onset up to 14 hours. There may be a familial tendency to develop these reactions (Settipane, 1986).

Scombroidosis occurs after the ingestion of spoiled fish (Hughes and Merson, 1976). Symptoms consist of flushing, urticaria and itching, headache, and nausea and vomiting. *Klebsiella pneumoniae* and *Proteus morgani* have been incriminated. These bacteria decarboxylate histidine, resulting in the production of saurine, a chemical with histamine-like activity. Everyone eating sufficient quantities of the fish experiences the reaction. Patients taking isoniazid appear to be especially susceptible (Settipane, 1986).

There are several syndromes characterized by excessive endogenous production of histamine. These include systemic mastocytosis, leukemias associated with an overproduction of histamine-containing cells (acute promyelocytic leukemia, basophilic leukemia), and hydatid cysts. Anaphylaxis can occur in such patients after appropriate stimuli. For example, episodes can be precipitated in patients with systemic mastocytosis upon the ingestion of opiates, and in patients with promyelocytic leukemia when treated with tretinoin (Koike et al, 1992).

Nonorganic disease can mimic anaphylaxis. Such episodes can be involuntary, as in panic attacks or the vocal cord dysfunction syndrome (Goodman et al, 1991), or can be consciously self-induced, as in Munchausen's stridor (Patterson and Schatz, 1975).

Panic attacks are accompanied by tachycardia, flushing, gastrointestinal symptoms, and shortness of breath.

Vocal cord dysfunction syndrome and Munchausen's stridor have similar presentations. The former is due to an involuntary adduction of the vocal cords occluding the glottal opening. There is a bunching together of the false vocal cords. This produces obstruction in both inspiration and expiration. The patient is unaware of the process. The term Munchausen's stridor was coined to describe patients who intentionally adduct their vocal cords and present to emergency rooms with self-induced manifestations of laryngeal edema. This entity occurs in psychologically disturbed individuals (Patterson and Schatz, 1975). It can be distinguished from vocal cord dysfunction syndrome (Goodman et al, 1991) by laryngoscopy during the acute episode and by the fact that patients with Munchausen's stridor can be distracted from their vocal cord adduction if they are asked to perform maneuvers such as coughing (Patterson and Schatz, 1975).

Other entities traditionally listed in the differential diagnosis of anaphylaxis include hereditary angioedema, progesterone anaphylaxis, anaphylaxis associated with recurrent and chronic urticaria, pheochromocytoma, neurologic disorders, tracheal foreign body, the pseudoanaphylactic syndrome occurring after the administration of procaine penicillin, and the "red man syndrome" that can occur after the administration of vancomycin.

Hereditary angioedema can present with laryngeal edema, abdominal pain, and an erythematous rash that could be confused with urticaria. Thus, it should be included in the differential diagnosis. In most instances, however, it is not difficult to distinguish between these two entities.

Patients previously thought to have idiopathic anaphylaxis have been found to have progesterone-related anaphylactic episodes (Alater et al, 1987; Meggs et al, 1984). Patients with this disorder experience anaphylactoid reactions to the infusion of luteinizing hormone-releasing hormone (LHRH) and after the intradermal injection of medroxyprogesterone. LHRH analog therapy is beneficial. The mechanism of production of this disorder is unknown, but it has been postulated that the increased level of progesterone associated with menses predisposes subjects to their anaphylactic events. This entity should be considered in women, usually over age 35, who present with recurrent episodes of anaphylaxis exhibiting a temporal relationship with the menstrual cycle (Burstein et al, 1991).

The vast majority of patients with chronic idiopathic urticaria or recurrent episodes of urticaria are not considered at risk for the development of anaphylaxis or anaphylactoid episodes. In rare instances, however, anaphylaxis can occur in patients who previously had only recurrent episodes of acute urticaria (Greenberger, 1984) or chronic urticaria (Guillet and Jeune, 1983). The subject with recurrent episodes of acute urticaria that culminated in an episode of anaphylaxis also had hyperimmunoglobulinemia E (Greenberger, 1984). The subject with chronic episodes of urticaria had urticarial vasculitis, which was associated with an episode of shock, leukopenia, and thrombocytopenia. In this instance the reaction was thought to be due to activation of the complement cascade (Guillet and Jeune, 1983).

It would be unusual to confuse a pheochromocytoma with anaphylaxis, but occasionally such patients can have symptoms suggestive of an anaphylactic reaction.

Pseudoanaphylaxis is a term used to describe patients who develop syncope and neurologic symptoms after the administration of procaine penicillin. These reactions are due to the procaine and not to the penicillin (Kraus and Green, 1976). Similar episodes have been reported after the administration of lidocaine (Kraus and Green, 1976).

The laboratory might be helpful, in some instances, in making a diagnosis of anaphylaxis or ruling out other causes. If carcinoid syndrome or pheochromocytoma is being considered, blood levels of serotonin and urinary 5-hydroxyindole acetic acid, catecholamines, and vanillylmandelic acid are indicated. If a patient is seen shortly after an anaphylactic episode, plasma and urinary histamine (or histamine metabolites) and serum tryptase determinations may be helpful. Plasma histamine levels begin to rise within 5 to 10 minutes and remain elevated for 30 to 60 minutes (Schwartz et al, 1989; LaRoche et al, 1991). Thus, they are of little help if the patient is seen as long as an hour after the onset of the event (Schwartz et al, 1989). However, urinary histamine and its metabolites are elevated for a longer duration and therefore might be useful (Kaliner et al, 1984). Serum tryptase levels peak 1 to 1½ hours after the onset of anaphylaxis and persist longer than plasma histamine levels. Elevated tryptase levels may be found as long as 5 hours after the onset of symptoms (LaRoche et al, 1991). Therefore, serum tryptase levels may be useful in establishing the diagnosis (Schwartz et al, 1989; Schwartz et al, 1987). The best time to measure serum tryptase is between 1 to 2 hours but no longer than 6 hours after the onset of symptoms (LaRoche et al, 1991). The best time to measure plasma histamine is between 10 minutes and 1 hour after the onset of symptoms (LaRoche et al, 1991). It is interesting to note that there may be a dysjunction between histamine and tryptase levels, with some patients exhibiting elevations of only one of these mediators (LaRoche et al, 1991). It might also be beneficial to obtain serum for the analysis of specific IgE against suspected antigens and, if vomiting occurs, to obtain unconsumed portions of food because extracts of these might be useful for the creation of "custom" RAST reagents to test for food-specific IgE antibodies in search of an etiologic agent (Yunginger et al, 1991).

Once the diagnosis of anaphylaxis has been established, it should be recognized that the specific agent may not be identifiable in the majority of instances (Kemp et al, 1993). The search for such an agent should include, when appropriate, tests for foods. Such tests have been reported to determine the offending agent in some cases previously designated idiopathic (Stricker et al, 1986). Tests should include not only foods but also spices and vegetable gum productions (Yeates and Jenson, 1991). Of course, a detailed and intense history is the most important of "tests." This history should be repeated after each episode. Occasionally serial histories will reveal a previously undetermined cause (Seligman and Witkin, 1993).

PREVENTION AND MANAGEMENT

Prevention: General Measures

Anaphylactic reactions are an unavoidable aspect of the practice of medicine. However, the incidence and severity of such reactions can be decreased by general and specific preventive measures (Table 21–9).

A thorough history for drug allergy should be taken in every patient. Proper interpretation of this history requires a knowledge of the immunologic and biochemical cross-reactivity between drugs. When the history of an allergic reaction to a drug is present, a substitute, noncross-reactive drug should be administered whenever possible. Parenteral administration of medication usually produces more severe reactions than oral administration. Therefore, drugs should be administered orally whenever possible. When parenteral administration is required, the patient should remain in the office for 20 to 30 minutes after the drug is given. Instances of anaphylaxis due to drug mislabeling are rare but do occur. Therefore, proper labeling of drugs is essential, and whenever a drug is suspected as the cause of an episode, the contents of the container should be checked against the label.

Patients subject to anaphylaxis should wear a MedicAlert bracelet or necklace and should carry an identification card in a wallet or purse. Such patients should be supplied with kits for the self-injection of epinephrine and should be told to keep the kit nearby at all times. β-blockers and angiotensin-converting enzyme inhibitors (ACE inhibitors) should not be taken by patients at risk for anaphylaxis or anaphylactoid episodes if any other agents will suffice.

Management of the Acute Event

This discussion of the treatment of anaphylaxis and anaphylactoid episodes will emphasize office management. However, the therapy of prolonged attacks requiring hospitalization will also be mentioned.

The drugs used to treat anaphylaxis and suggested dosage regimens are seen in Table 21–10. Therapy may be divided into those procedures that should be performed immediately and those that may be initiated after further evaluation. These steps are listed in Table 21–11.

Rapid recognition and treatment are essential. It is believed that prompt initiation of therapy prevents fatalities. It is important to stress that the steps seen in Table 21–11 are subject to the discretion of the physician managing the care of the patient, and variations in their sequence and performance depend on the physician's judgment. In addition, when a patient should be transferred to a tertiary care center is also dependent on the skill, experience, and assessment of the individual physician.

Obviously, in order to initiate therapy, the medication and apparatus must be available. There is disagreement as to what constitutes the preferred office inventory of drugs and equipment needed to treat anaphylaxis.

TABLE 21–9. MEASURES TO REDUCE THE INCIDENCE OF ANAPHYLAXIS AND ANAPHYLACTIC DEATHS

General measures
  Obtain thorough history for drug allergy.
  Avoid drugs with immunologic or biochemical cross-reactivity with any agents to which the patient is sensitive.
  Administer drugs orally rather than parenterally when possible.
  Check all drugs for proper labeling.
  Keep patients in office 20 to 30 minutes after injections.
Measures for patients at risk
  Have patient wear and carry warning identification.
  Teach self-injection of epinephrine and caution patients to keep epinephrine kit with them.
  Discontinue β-adrenergic blocking agents and ACE inhibitors.
  Use preventive techniques when patient is required to undergo a procedure or take an agent that places him at risk. Such techniques include:
    Pretreatment
    Provocative challenge
    Desensitization

TABLE 21-10. DRUGS AND OTHER AGENTS USED IN THE TREATMENT OF ANAPHYLAXIS AND ANAPHYLACTOID REACTIONS

Drug	Dose and Route of Administration	Comment
Epinephrine	1:1000 0.3–0.5 ml SC or IM (adult); 1:1000 0.01 mg/kg or 0.1–0.3 ml SC or IM (child)	Initial drug of choice for all episodes Should be given immediately; may repeat q 10–15 min
	0.1 to 1.0 ml of 1:1000 aqueous epinephrine diluted in 10 ml normal saline IV (see text for details)	If no response to SC or IM administration and patient in shock with cardiovascular collapse
Antihistamines		
Diphenhydramine	25 to 50 mg IM or IV (adult) 12.5 to 25 mg PO, IM, or IV (child)	Route of administration depends on severity of episode
Ranitidine or cimetidine	300 mg IV (adult)	Cimetidine should be administered slowly since rapid administration has been associated with hypotension; dose in children not established (possibly 150 mg)
Corticosteroids		
Hydrocortisone	100 mg to 1 gram IV or IM (adult) 10 mg to 100 mg IV (child)	Exact dose not established; other preparations such as methylprednisolone can be used as well; for milder episodes, prednisone 30 to 60 mg may be given (see text)
Drugs for Resistant Bronchospasm		
Aerosolized β-agonist (albuterol, metaproterenol)	Dose as for asthma (0.25 to 0.5 cc in 1½ to 2 cc saline q4h, prn)	Useful for bronchospasm not responding to epinephrine
Aminophylline	Dose as for asthma	Rarely indicated for recalcitrant bronchospasm; β-agonist is drug of choice
Volume Expanders		
Crystalloids (normal saline on Ringer's lactate)	1000 to 2000 cc rapidly in adults; 30 ml/kg in first hour in children	Rate of administration titrated against blood pressure response for IV volume expander; after initial infusion further administration requires tertiary care monitoring; in patients who are β-blocked, larger amounts may be needed
Colloids (hydroxyethyl starch)	500 ml rapidly followed by slow infusion in adults	
Vasopressors		
Dopamine	400 mg in 500 cc dextrose (5%) in water as IV infusion; 2 to 20 μg/kg/min	Dopamine probably the drug of choice; the rate of infusion should be titered against the blood pressure response; continued infusion requires tertiary care monitoring
Levarterenol	4 mg in 500 cc dextrose (5%) in water as IV infusion; initial dose is 4 to 8 μg/min in adults	
Drugs Employed in Patients Who Are β-blocked		
Atropine sulfate	0.3 to 0.5 mg IV; may repeat every 10 min to a maximum of 2 mg in adults	Glucagon is probably the drug of choice, with atropine useful only for treatment of bradycardia
Glucagon	Initial dose of 1 to 5 mg IV followed by infusion of 5 to 15 μ/min titrated against blood pressure	

Abbreviations: SC = subcutaneous; IM = intramuscular; IV = intravenous; PO = by mouth.

Therefore any attempt to formalize a list of such material should be one of consensus. Unfortunately, at present, there is no recently published consensus. The last two consensus lists found by the author were published in 1973 by the American Academy of Pediatrics Committee on Drugs (American Academy of Pediatrics Committee on Drugs, 1973) and in 1986 by the American Academy of Allergy and Immunology (Journal of Allergy and

TABLE 21-11. THERAPY OF ANAPHYLAXIS

Immediate action
  Assessment
    Check airway and secure if needed
    Rapid assessement of level of consciousness
    Vital signs
  Treatment
    Epinephrine
    Supine position, legs elevated
    Oxygen
    Tourniquet proximal to injection site
Dependent on evaluation
  Start peripheral intravenous fluids
  H_1 and H_2 antagonist
  Vasopressors
  Corticosteroids
  Aminophylline
  Glucagon
  Atropine
  Electrocardiographic monitoring
  Transfer to hospital
Hospital management
  Military anti-shock trousers
  Continued therapy with above-noted agents and management of complications

Clinical Immunology Position Statement, 1986). These lists, with revisions, have been used to compile the suggested inventory seen in Table 21–12. It should be emphasized that the materials noted in this table are simply suggestions. Any such inventory is subject to the judgment of the individual physician. The suggestions noted here are reasonably extensive and may not be needed in every situation.

The initial step in the management of anaphylaxis is a rapid assessment of the patient's status with emphasis on evaluation of the airway and the state of consciousness. If the airway is compromised, it should be secured at that time. Blood pressure and pulse should be obtained. The patient should be placed in the supine position with feet elevated. However, modification of this Trendelenburg position may be necessary if the patient is wheezing. In addition, the increase in intrathoracic pressure produced by this position can reduce the pressure gradient between the right atrium and the inferior vena cava and thus limit the benefit of the increased venous return (Eon et al, 1991). If the antigen has been injected, a tourniquet should be placed proximal to the injection site. This tourniquet should be released every 5 minutes (for a minimum of 3 minutes) during therapy. It should be left on no longer than a total of 30 minutes. Oxygen should be started. During this time an estimate of the patient's weight should be made to help guide dosage decisions.

Epinephrine should be administered almost simultaneously with the above measures. The dose and route of administration of epinephrine depends on the severity of the reaction. In almost all instances of office management, the intramuscular or subcutaneous route can be utilized. The dose in adults is 0.3 ml to 0.5 ml (0.3 to 0.5 mg) and in children is 0.01 mg/kg. The initial dose can be repeated two or three times as needed at 10- to 15-minute intervals.

If severe hypotension is present, epinephrine can be given intravenously. There is no established dose (Barach et al, 1984), and numerous regimens have been suggested (Eon et al, 1991; Barach et al, 1984; Levy and Levi, 1992; Fath and Cerra, 1984; Saryan and O'Loughlin, 1992). Regardless of the dose and regimen used, care should be taken and the patient monitored for arrhythmias. The amount administered will depend on the severity of the episode and should be titered

TABLE 21-12. EQUIPMENT AND MEDICATION FOR THERAPY OF ANAPHYLAXIS IN OFFICE

Primary
  A. Tourniquet
  B. 1-ml and 5-ml disposable syringes
  C. Oxygen tank and mask/nasal prongs
  D. Epinephrine solution (aqueous) 1:1000
  E. Diphenhydramine injectable
  F. Ranitidine or cimetidine injectable
  G. Injectable corticosteroids
  H. Ambu bag, oral airway, laryngoscope, endotracheal tube, No. 12 needle
  I. Intravenous setup with large-bore catheter
  J. IV fluids: 2000 cc crystalloid, 1000 cc hydroxyethyl starch
  K. Aerosol β_2 bronchodilator and compressor nebulizer
  L. Glucagon
  M. Electrocardiograph
  N. Normal saline 10 cc vial for epinephrine dilution
Supporting
  A. Suction apparatus
  B. Dopamine
  C. Sodium bicarbonate
  D. Aminophylline
  E. Atropine
Optional
  A. Defibrillator
  B. Calcium gluconate
  C. Neuroleptics for seizures
  D. Lidocaine

against the response. A suggested protocol is as follows: The intravenous preparation can be prepared by diluting 0.1 ml (0.1 mg) of a 1:1000 aqueous epinephrine solution in 10 ml of normal saline. This 10-ml dose can be infused over 5 to 10 minutes (resulting in a total dose of 100 µg at a rate of 10 to 20 µg/minute) and repeated, depending on the response (Barach et al, 1984). The dose can be increased in more critical situations; 1 ml (1.0 mg) of a 1:1000 solution of epinephrine can be diluted in 10 cc normal saline (for a concentration of 0.1 mg/ml) and a dose of 1 to 2 ml (1.0 to 2.0 mg) administered every 5 to 20 minutes as indicated (Levy and Levi, 1992). A constant intravenous infusion can be started if needed.

If intravenous access cannot be obtained, sublingual injection (rather than subcutaneous or intramuscular) has been suggested as an alternate route because of the rich vascularity of this area. The intramuscular dose should be injected in the posterior third of the sublingual area.

If the patient has an endotracheal tube in place, the intravenous dose can be administered via long catheter through the endotracheal tube into the area near the carina. It is absorbed rapidly and dispersed in 5 to 10 breaths (Powers and Donowitz, 1984).

If the antigen responsible for the episode was injected, 0.3 cc (0.1 to 0.3 ml in children) of 1:1000 aqueous epinephrine can be injected into the original site in order to slow antigen absorption.

After the above procedures, further therapy is dictated by the clinical course and findings.

Antihistamine therapy can be useful as adjunctive treatment with epinephrine. Although antihistamine therapy is not considered lifesaving, it can at times offer dramatic relief of symptoms (Vidovich et al, 1992; Kambam et al, 1989; Mayumi et al, 1987; De Soto and Turk, 1989; Yarbrough et al, 1989). Based upon clinical trials (Runge et al, 1992) and the known effects of histamine as previously discussed, a combination of an H_1 and H_2 antagonist appears to be superior to an H_1 antagonist alone (Vidovich et al, 1992; Kambam et al, 1989; Mayumi et al, 1987; De Soto and Turk, 1989; Yarbrough et al, 1989). Thus, therapy should be instituted with diphenhydramine and ranitidine or cimetidine in the dosages noted in Table 21–10. The rapid infusion of cimetidine has been associated with falls in blood pressure, and therefore this drug should be administered slowly. The route of administration, as with epinephrine, depends on the severity of the episode. The intramuscular or intravenous route can be used for diphenhydramine and the intravenous route for the H_2 antagonist.

The exact role of corticosteroids in the management of anaphylaxis and anaphylactoid reactions has not been established. However, based on an extrapolation of their effect in other allergic diseases, their administration is indicated. Patients with severe anaphylactic episodes or patients who had previously been on systemic glucocorticoid therapy within the previous several months should receive corticosteroids. Perhaps the most salient theoretical rationale for their use relates to their effects on the late-phase reaction. Since anaphylaxis can be biphasic, a role for steroids in preventing such a recurrence can be postulated. There is no established dose or drug of choice. Suggested intravenous doses for severe episodes are seen in Table 21–10. In addition, it is probably wise to give oral prednisone (30 to 60 mg) to patients who have experienced mild anaphylactic symptoms and been discharged from therapy.

If wheezing unresponsive to epinephrine occurs, aerosolized β-adrenergic agents and, if necessary, intravenous aminophylline can be employed. The doses are the same as those used in asthma. Aerosolized β-adrenergics are the drug of choice. Aminophylline should be reserved for recalcitrant bronchospasm not responding to epinephrine and aerosolized β-adrenergic agents.

Perhaps the manifestation of anaphylaxis that is the most difficult to treat and the most threatening, except for acute upper airway obstruction, is profound, protracted hypotension. Hypotension can be severe and resistant to therapy. This was evident in a study of insect sting reactions whereby patients were deliberately stung in an intensive care unit. Severe, persistent hypotension occurred that was unresponsive to fluid therapy and large doses of intravenous epinephrine (Smith et al, 1980).

As previously discussed, hypotension is due to a shift of fluid from the intravascular to the extravascular space. The mainstay of treatment should be the restoration of intravascular volume. This is best accomplished by the rapid administration of large volumes of fluid. There is debate as to whether colloids or crystalloids should be used, and there are arguments to support both forms of therapy (Shine et al, 1980). However, the most important component of fluid therapy initially is not the composition of the fluid itself but rather the rate of administration (Mueller and Noxon, 1990). Large volumes of crystalloid are often required; 1000 to 2000 cc of lactated Ringer's or normal saline should be given rapidly, depending on the blood pressure, at a rate of 5 to 10 ml/kg in an adult in the first 5 minutes (Eon et al, 1991). Children should receive up to 30 ml/kg of crystalloid solution in the first hour (Saryan and O'Loughlin, 1992). An alternative to crystalloid therapy would be the colloid, hydroxyethyl starch. Adults should receive rapid infusion of 500 ml followed by slow infusion thereafter. In patients who have β-adrenergic blockade due to the administration of a β-adrenergic blocking agent, the volume of fluid required may be much greater (5 to 7 liters) before stabilization occurs (Eon et al, 1991). Of course, should fluid therapy of this magnitude be indicated, the patient should be transferred to a tertiary care facility. Further administration of fluid will depend on cardiovascular monitoring including central venous pressure, pulmonary artery wedge pressure, cardiac output, oxygen consumption, urinary output, and electrocardiographic monitoring.

Although fluids are clearly the most important element, along with epinephrine, in the therapy of hypotension, the use of other vasopressors may also be indicated. However, their effectiveness can be diminished since hypotension often occurs in patients who have increased peripheral resistance due to endogenous compensatory mechanisms (Fisher, 1977; Hanashiro and Weil, 1967). In such patients the hypotension is, as noted, due to fluid shift and perhaps decreased cardiac output. However, vasopressors have been employed for many years and can be helpful. The drug of choice is dopamine administered at a rate of 2 to 20 μg/kg per minute. The rate should be titrated using the blood pressure. Any patient requiring dopamine, of course, should be transferred to a tertiary care unit.

The patient who has β-adrenergic blockade presents a special problem in the therapy of anaphylaxis (Toogood, 1987). Such patients can be resistant to standard therapeutic regimens (Hart and Sue, 1988; Kivity and Yarchovsky, 1990; Newman and Schultz, 1981). They can experience refractory hypotension (Zaloga et al, 1986), bradycardia, and relapsing manifestations (Kivity and Yarchovsky, 1990). In such patients both inotropic and chronotropic functions of the heart are suppressed, resulting in marked hypotension with bradycardia. Two drugs, atropine and glucagon, have been recommended for therapy in patients with β-adrenergic blockade. Atropine is useful only for bradycardia but does not exert a beneficial effect on the inotropic function of the heart. The dose of atropine sulfate is 0.3 to 0.5 mg every 10 minutes to a maximum of 2 mg. Glucagon, a polypeptide hormone produced by the α cells of the pancreas, has both a positive inotropic and chronotropic effect on the heart. This inotropic effect is not dependent on catecholamines or their receptors and is therefore unaltered by β-adrenergic blockade (Glick et al, 1968). Thus glucagon is probably the drug of choice in the therapy of patients who are β-blocked. The dose of glucagon is 1 to 5 mg intravenously as a bolus followed by an infusion of 5 to 15 μg per minute titrated against the clinical response. The cardiotonic effects of glucagon are not associated with increased myocardial irritability (Lvoff and Wilcken, 1972). Cardiotonic effects are seen in 1 to 5 minutes and are maximal at 5 to 15 minutes following a single 5-mg bolus. Nausea and vomiting are the major limiting factors of therapy.

In addition to the above medications, MAST (Military Anti-Shock Trousers, David Clark Incorporated, Worcester, Massachusetts) will provide rapid redistribution of intravascular fluid. Inflation of the MAST suit redirects fluid from the venous circulation of the legs and abdomen to the upper circulation. This redistribution of the intravascular volume can cause an immediate rise in blood pressure in the upper extremities (Shine et al, 1980).

Because of the possibility of the occurrence of a biphasic episode, the patient should be observed, after the symptoms have subsided, before discharge. There is no established period of observation. It would appear that a 2-hour observation period would be reasonable for mild episodes and perhaps as long as 24 hours for severe episodes.

REFERENCES

Alater JE, Raphael G, Cutler BG, Loriaux DL, Meggs WJ, Kaliner M. Recurrent anaphylaxis in menstruating women: Treatment with a luteinizing hormone-releasing hormone agonist—a preliminary report. Obstet Gynecol 70:542–546, 1987.

Aldrich LB, Moattari R, Vinik AI. Distinguishing features of idiopathic flushing and carcinoid syndrome. Arch Intern Med 148:2614–2618, 1988.

American Academy of Pediatrics Committee on Drugs. Anaphylaxis. Pediatrics 51:136–140, 1973.

Amornmarn L, Bernard L, Kumar N, Bielory L. Anaphylaxis admissions to a university hospital. J Allergy Clin Immunol 89(suppl):349, 1992. (Abstract)

Ansari M, Zamora J, Lipscomb M. Postmortem diagnosis of acute anaphylaxis by serum tryptase analysis: A case report. Am J Clin Pathol 99:101–103, 1993.

Antonelli D, Koltun B, Barzilay J. Transient ST segment elevation during anaphylactic shock. Am Heart J 108:1052–1054, 1984.

Austin SM, Barooah B, Kim CS. Reversible acute cardiac injury during cefoxitin-induced anaphylaxis in a patient with normal coronary arteries. Am J Med 77:729–732, 1984.

Barach EM, Nowak BM, Lee TG, Tomlanovich MC. Epinephrine for treatment of anaphylactic shock. JAMA 251:2118–2122, 1984.

Barclay WR. Adverse drug reactions. JAMA 242:656, 1979.

Booth BH, Patterson R. Electrocardiographic changes during human anaphylaxis. JAMA 211:627–631, 1970.

Bosso JV, Schwartz LB, Stevenson DD. Tryptase and histamine release during aspirin-induced respiratory reactions. J Allergy Clin Immunol 88:830–837, 1991.

Boston Collaborative Drug Surveillance Program. Brief reports: Drug-induced anaphylaxis. JAMA 224:613, 1973.

Brasher GW, Sanchez SA. Reversible electrocardiographic changes associated with wasp sting anaphylaxis. JAMA 229:1210–1211, 1974.

Burstein M, Rubinow A, Shalit M. Cyclic anaphylaxis associated with menstruation. Ann Allergy 66:36–38, 1991.

Cisteró A, Urías S, Guindo J, Lleonart R, Garcia-Moll M, Geli A, Bayés deLuna A. Coronary artery spasm and acute myocardial infarction in naproxen-associated anaphylactic reaction. Allergy 47:576–578, 1992.

Criep LH, Woehler TR. The heart in human anaphylaxis. Ann Allergy 29:399–409, 1971.

Davies DM (ed). Anaphylaxis and the community nurse. In Adverse Drug Reaction Bulletin. Newcastle Upon Tyne: Regional Postgraduate Institute of Medicine & Dentistry, 1977, vol 65, p 228.

Delage C, Irey NS. Anaphylactic deaths: A clinical pathologic study of 43 cases. J Forensic Sci 17:525, 1972.

Delage C, Mullick FG, Irey NS. Myocardial lesions in anaphylaxis. Arch Pathol Lab Med 95:1985, 1973.

De Soto H, Turk M. Cimetidine in anaphylactic shock refractory to standard therapy. Anesth Analg 69:260–269, 1989.

Dykewicz MS, Orfan N. Anaphylaxis to protamine component in NPH human insulin. J Allergy Clin Immunol 87(suppl):276, 1991. (Abstract)

Edde R, Burtis B. Lung injury in anaphylactoid shock. Chest 63:636–637, 1973.

Eon B, Papazian L, Gouin F. Management of anaphylactic and anaphylactoid reactions during anesthesia. In Clinical Reviews in Allergy. The Humana Press, Inc. 9:415–429, 1991.

Erffmeyer J. Reactions to antibiotics. Immunol Allergy Clin North Am 12:633–648, 1992.

Fahmy NR. Hemodynamics, plasma histamine and catecholamine concentrations during an anaphylactoid reaction to morphine. Anesthesiology 55:329–331, 1981.

Fath JJ, Cerra FB. The therapy of anaphylactic shock. Drug Intell Clin Pharm 18:14–21, 1984.

Fernandez de Corres L, Moneo I, Munoz D, Bernaola G, Fernandez E, Audicana M, Errutia I. Sensitization from chestnuts and bananas in patients with urticaria and anaphylaxis from contact with latex. Ann Allergy 7:35–39, 1993.

Filip V. Anaphylactic reactions incidence in allergic and atopic patients: Allergol et Immunopathol 16:73–75, 1988.

Fisher M. Blood volume replacement in acute anaphylactic cardiovascular collapse related to anesthesia. Br J Anaesthesiol 49:1023, 1977.

Fisher M. Clinical observations on the pathophysiology and implications for treatment. In Vincent JL (ed). Update in Intensive Care and Emergency Medicine. New York, Springer-Verlag, 1989, pp 309–316.

Fisher MM. Clinical observations on the pathophysiology and treatment of anaphylactic cardiovascular collapse. Anaesth Intensive Care 14:17–21, 1986.

Frieri M, Madden J, Nolte H. Spontaneous basophil histamine release (BHR) in atopic patients with food hypersensitivity. J Allergy Clin Immunol 89:195, 1992. (Abstract)

Glick G, Parmley WW, Wechsler AS. Glucagon: Its enhancement of cardiac performance in the cat and dog and persistence of its inotropic action despite β-receptor blockade with propranolol. Circ Res 22:789–792, 1968.

Goodman DL, O'Connell MA, Sklarew PR. Vocal cord dysfunction (VCD) presenting as anaphylaxis. J Allergy Clin Immunol 87:278, 1991. (Abstract)

Gottschlich GM, Gravlee GP, Georgitis JW. Adverse reactions to protamine sulfate during cardiac surgery in diabetic and non-diabetic patients. Ann Allergy 61:277–281, 1988.

Green GR, Rosenblum A. Report of the penicillin study group, American Academy of Allergy. J Allergy Clin Immunol 48:331, 1971.

Greenberger PA. Life-threatening idiopathic anaphylaxis associated with hyperimmunoglobulinemia E. Am J Med 76:553–556, 1984.

Guillet G, Jeune R. Urticarial vasculitis with shock, leukopenia, and thrombocytopenia, possible due to anaphylatoxin release. Br J Derm 108:605–608, 1983.

Hamann, Curtis P. Natural rubber latex protein sensitivity. Am J Contact Derm IV: 4–21, 1993. (Review)

Hanashiro PK, Weil MH. Anaphylactic shock in man: Report of two cases with detailed hemodynamic and metabolic studies. Arch Intern Med 119:129, 1967.

Harnett JC, Spector SL, Farr RS. Aspirin idiosyncrasy: Asthma and urticaria. In Middeton Jr E, Reed CE, Ellis EF (eds). Allergy Principles and Practice. St. Louis, Mosby–Year Book, 1978, p 1004.

Hart LL, Sue D. Potentiated anaphylaxis during chronic beta-blocker therapy. Drug Intell Clin Pharm 22:720–721, 1984.

Hedin H, Richter W. Pathomechanisms of dextran-induced anaphylactoid/anaphylactic reactions in man. Int Arch Allergy Appl Immunol 68:122–126, 1982.

Hermann K, Hertenberger B, Rittweger R, Jakob T, Ring J. Urine levels of methylhistamine, angiotensin I and II, vasopressin and oxytocin in patients with anaphylactoid reactions. J Allergy Clin Immunol 85:228, 1980. (Abstract)

Hermann K, Ring J. Hymenoptera venom anaphylaxis: May decreased levels of angiotensin peptides play a role? Clin Exper Allergy 20:569–570, 1990.

Hermann K, Rittweger, Ring J. Urinary excretion of angiotensin I, II, arginine vasopressin and oxytocin in patients with anaphylactoid reactions. Clin Exper Allergy 22:845–853, 1992a.

Hermann K, Rittweger M, Phillips MI, Ring J. Presence of angiotensin peptides in human urine. Clin Chem 38:1768–1772, 1992b.

Hermann K, Ring J. Changes in angiotensin peptides in plasma and urine in patients with anaphylaxis. Int Arch Allergy Appl Immunol 99:446–448, 1992.

Holgate ST, Robinson C, Church M. Mediators of immediate hypersensitivity. In Middleton E Jr, et al. Allergy Principles and Practice. 4th ed. Mosby–Year Book, St. Louis, 1993, pp 267–301.

Horan RF, Sheffer AL. Exercise-induced anaphylaxis. Immunol Allergy Clin North Am 12:559–570, 1992.

Hughes JM, Merson MH. Fish and shellfish poisoning. N Engl J Med 295:1117–1120, 1976.

Hunt EL. Death from allergic shock. N Engl J Med 228:502, 1993.

Jacobsen J, Secher NH. Slowing of the heart during anaphylactic shock: A report of five cases. Acta Anaesthesiol Scand 32:401–403, 1988.

James Jr LP, Austen KF. Fatal and systemic anaphylaxis in man. N Engl J Med 270:597, 1964.

Journal of Allergy and Clinical Immunology. Position Statement. J Allergy Clin Immunol 77:271–273, 1986.

Kaliner M, Shelhamer JH, Ottesen EA. Effects of infused histamine: Correlation of plasma histamine levels and symptoms. J Allergy Clin Immunol 69:283–289, 1982.

Kaliner M, Dyer J, Merlin S, et al. Increased urine histamine and in contrast media reactions. Invest Radiol 19:116, 1984.

Kambam JR, Merrill WH, Smith BE. Histamine$_2$ receptor blocker in the treatment of protamine-related anaphylactoid reactions: Two case reports. An J Anaesth 36:463–465, 1989.

Kaplan AP, Hunt KJ, Sobotka AK, Smith P, Horakova Z, Gralnick H, Lichtenstein LM. Human anaphylaxis: A study of mediator systems. Clin Research 25:361A, 1977.

Katayama H, Yamaguchi K, Kozuka T, et al. Adverse reactions to ionic and nonionic contrast media: A report from the Japanese committee on the safety of contrast media. Radiology 175:621, 1990.

Kemp S, Lieberman P, Wolf B. A review of 267 cases of anaphylaxis in clinical practice. J Allergy Clin Immunol 91(suppl):153, 1993. (Abstract)

Kern RA, Wimberley NA, Jr. Penicillin reactions: Their nature, growing importance, recognition, management and prevention. Am J Med Sci 226:357, 1953.

Kim HW, Lieberman P, Yoo TJ. Protamine hypersensitivity reaction presenting as an insulin reaction. J Allergy Clin Immunol 87(suppl):286, 1991. (Abstract)

Kivity S Yarchovsky J. Relapsing anaphylaxis to bee sting in a patient treated with β-blocker and Ca blocker. J Allergy Clin Immunol 85:669–670, 1990.

Koike T, Tatewaki W, Aoki A, Yoshimoto H, Yagisawa K, Hashimoto S, Furukawa T, Saitoh H, Takahashi M, Li-Bo Y, Ying W, Shibata A. Brief report: Severe symptoms of hyperhistaminemia after the treatment of acute promyelocytic leukemia with tretinoin (all-transretinoic acid). N Engl J Med 327:385–387, 1992.

Kraus SJ, Green RL. Pseudoanaphylactic reactions with procaine penicillin. Cutis 17:765, 1976.

Lamson RW. Sudden death associated with the injection of foreign substances. JAMA 82:1091, 1924.

Lamson RW. So-called fatal anaphylaxis in man with a special reference to diagnosis and treatment of clinical allergies. JAMA 93:1775, 1929.

LaRoche D, Vergnaud M, Sillard B, Soufarapis H, Brickard H. Biochemical markers of anaphylactoid reactions to drugs. Comparison of plasma histamine and tryptase. Anesthesiology 75:945–949, 1991.

Lee TH, Smith CM, Arm JP, Christie PE. Mediator release in aspirin-induced reactions. J Allergy Clin Immunol 88:827–829, 1991.

Levine BB. Immunologic mechanisms of penicillin allergy: A haptenic model system for the study of allergic disease of man. N Engl J Med 275:1115, 1966.

Levy JH, Levi R. Diagnosis and treatment of anaphylactic/anaphylactoid reactions. In Assem E-SK (ed). Allergic reactions to anaesthetics. Clinical and basic aspects. Monogr Allergy 30:130–144, 1992.

Lieberman P, Patterson P, Metz R, Lucena G. Allergic reactions to insulin. JAMA 215:1106, 1971.

Lieberman P. Anaphylaxis and anaphylactoid reactions. In Spittel JA (ed). Clinical Medicine. Philadelphia, Harper & Row, 1981, pp 1–16.

Lieberman P. The use of antihistamines in the prevention and treatment of anaphylaxis and anaphylactoid reactions. J Allergy Clin Immunol 86:684–797, 1990.

Lieberman P. Anaphylactoid reactions to radiocontrast material. Clin Rev Anesthesiol Allergy 9:319–338, 1991a.

Lieberman P. Difficult allergic drug reactions. Immunol Allergy Clin North Am 11(1):213, 1991b.

Lieberman P. Anaphylactoid reactions to radiocontrast material. Immunol Allergy Clin North Am 12:649–670, 1992.

Lvoff R, Wilcken DEL. Glucagon in heart failure and in cardiogenic shock. Circulation 45:534–539, 1972.

Manning M, Stevenson D, Mathison D. Reactions to aspirin and other nonsteroidal antiinflammatory drugs. Immunol Allergy Clin North Am 12:611–631, 1992.

Marone G, Stellato C, Mastronardi P, Mazzarella B. Nonspecific histamine-releasing properties of general anesthetic drugs. Anesth Allergy: Clin Rev Allergy 9:269–280, 1991.

May CD. High spontaneous release of histamine in vitro from leukocytes of persons hypersensitive to food. J Allergy Clin Immunol 58:432–437, 1976.

Mayumi H, Kimura S, Asano M, Shimokawa T, Au-Yong TF, Yayama T. Intravenous cimetidine as an effective treatment for systemic anaphylaxis and acute allergic skin reactions. Ann Allergy 58:447–450, 1987.

Meggs WJ, Pescovitz OR, Metcalfe D, Loriaux DL, Cutler G, Kaliner M. Progesterone sensitivity as a cause of recurrent anaphylaxis. N Engl J Med 311:1236–1238, 1984.

Moncada S, Martin J. Vasodilatation–evolution of nitric oxide. Lancet 341:1511, 1993.

Moss J, Fahmy NR, Sunder N, Beaven MA. Hormonal and hemodynamic profile of an anaphylactic reaction in man. Circulation 63:210–213, 1981.

Mueller DL, Noxon JO. Anaphylaxis: Pathophysiology and treatment. The Compendium 12:157–171, 1990.

Newball HH, Berninger RW, Talamo RC, Lichtenstein LM. Anaphylactic release of a basophil kallikrein-like activity. I. Purification and characterization. J Clin Invest 64:457–465, 1979.

Newman BR, Schultz LK. Epinephrine-resistant anaphylaxis in a patient taking propranolol hydrochloride. Ann Allergy 47:35–37, 1981.

Nordström L, Fletcher R, Pavek K. Shock of anaphylactoid type induced by protamine: A continuous cardiorespiratory record. Acta Anaesthesiol Scand 22:195, 1978.

Obeid AI, Johnson L, Potts J, Mookherjee S, Eich RH. Fluid therapy in severe systemic reaction to radiopaque dye. Ann Intern Med 83:317, 1975.

Okazaki M, Kitani H, Mifune T, Mitsunobu FM, Saito S, Asaumi N, Tanizaki Y. Food-dependent exercise-induced anaphylaxis. Intern Med 31:1052–1055, 1992.

Orange RP, Donsky GJ. Anaphylaxis. In Middleton E Jr, Reed CE, Ellis EF (eds). Allergy Principles and Practice. St. Louis, Mosby–Year Book, 1978, p 564.

Orfan NA, Stoloff RS, Harris KE, Patterson R. Idiopathic anaphylaxis: Total experience with 225 patients. Allergy Proc 13:35–43, 1992.

Palmer RMJ, Ferrige AG, Moncada S. Nitric oxide release accounts for the biological activity of endothelium derived relaxing factor. Nature 327:524–526, 1987.

Parrish HM. Analysis of 460 fatalities from venomous animals in the U.S. Am J Med Sci 245:129–141, 1963.

Patterson R, Schatz M. Factitious allergic emergencies: Anaphylaxis and laryngeal "edema." J Allergy Clin Immunol 56:152–159, 1975.

Patterson R, Pruzansky JJ, Dykewicz MS, Lawrence ID. Basophil-mast cell response syndromes: A unified clinical approach. Allergy Proc 9:611–620, 1988.

Pavek K, Wegmann A, Nordström L, Schwander D. Cardiovascular and respiratory mechanisms in anaphylactic and anaphylactoid shock reactions. Klin Wocheschr 60:941–947, 1982.

Popa VT, Lerner SA. Biphasic systemic anaphylactic reaction: Three illustrative cases. Ann Allergy 53:151–155, 1984.

Porter J, Jick H. Boston Collaborative Drug Surveillance Programs: Drug-induced anaphylaxis, convulsions, deafness, and extrapyramidal symptoms. Lancet 1:587, 1977.

Portier P, Richet C. De l'action anaphylactique de certains venins. C R Soc Biol (Paris) 54:170, 1902.

Powers RD, Donowitz LG. Endotracheal administration of emergency medications. South Med J 77:340–341, 1984.

Proud D, Macglashan DW, Newball HH, Schulman ES, Lichtenstein LM. Immunoglobulin E-mediated release of a kininogenase from purified human lung mast cells. Am Rev Respir Dis 132:405–408, 1985.

Raper RF, Fisher M McD. Profound reversible myocardial depression after anaphylaxis. Lancet I:386–388, 1988.

Reisman RE. Insect allergy. In Middleton E Jr, Reed CE, Ellis EF (eds). Allergy Principles and Practice. St. Louis, Mosby–Year Book, 1978, p 1100.

Ricketti AJ, Greenberger PA, Pruzansky JJ, Patterson R. Hyperreactivity of mediator-releasing cells from patients with allergic bronchopulmonary aspergillosis as evidenced by basophil histamine release. J Allergy Clin Immunol 72:386–392, 1983.

Ring J. Anaphylactoid reactions to intravenous solutions used for volume substitution. Clin Rev Allergy 9:397–414, 1991.

Runge JW, Martinez JC, Caravati EM, Williamson SG, Hartsell SC. Histamine antagonists in the treatment of acute allergic reactions. Ann Emerg Med 21:237–242, 1992.

Salvaggio JE, Cavanaugh JJA, Lowell FC, Leskowitz S. A comparison of the immunologic responses of normal and atopic individuals to intranasally administered antigens. J Allergy 35:62, 1964.

Sampson HA, Broadbent K. "Spontaneous" histamine release and histamine releasing factor in patients with atopic dermatitis and food hypersensitivity. J Allergy Clin Immunol 79:249, 1987. (Abstract)

Saryan JA, O'Loughlin JM. Anaphylaxis in children. Pediatr Ann 21:590–598, 1992.

Schwartz LB, Irani AMA, Roller K, Castells MC, Schechter NM. Quantitation of histamine, tryptase, and chymase in dispersed human T and TC mast cells. J Immunol 138:2611–2615, 1987.

Schwartz LB, Yunginger JW, Miller J, et al. The time course of appearance and disappearance of human mast cell tryptase in the circulation after anaphylaxis. J Clin Invest 83:1551–1555, 1989.

Schwartz LB, Metcalfe DD, Miller JS, Earl H, Sullivan T. Tryptase levels as an indicator of mast cell activation in systemic anaphylaxis and mastocytosis. N Engl J Med 316:1622–1626, 1987.

Schwartz HJ, Sutheimer C, Gauerke M, Yunginger JW. Hymenoptera venom-specific IgE antibodies in post-mortem sera from victims of sudden, unexpected death. Clin Allergy 18:461–468, 1988.

Schwartz HJ, Yunginger J, Schwartz LB. Unrecognized anaphylaxis may be a cause of sudden unexpected death. J Allergy Clin Immunol 91(suppl):154, 1993. (Abstract)

Seligman MJ, Witkin S. Not so idiopathic anaphylaxis. J Allergy Clin Immunol 91:155, 1993.

Settipane GA, Klein DE, Boyd GK. Relationship of atopy and anaphylactic sensitisation: A bee sting allergy model. Clin Allergy 8:259, 1978.

Settipane GA. The restaurant syndromes. Arch Intern Med 146:2129–2130, 1986.

Sheppe WM. Fatal anaphylaxis in man. J Lab Clin Med 16:372, 1980.

Shine K, Kuhn M, Young L, Tillisch J. Aspects of the management of shock. Ann Intern Med 93:723–734, 1980.

Silverman HJ, Van Hook C, Haponik EF. Hemodynamic changes in human anaphylaxis. Am J Med 77:341–344, 1984.

Simon MR. Anaphylaxis associated with relative bradycardia. Ann Allergy 62:495–497, 1989.

Slater J. Latex allergies. Ann Allergy 70(1):1–2, 1993. (Editorial)

Smith PL, Kagey-Sobotka A, Bleecker ER, Traystman R, Kaplan AP, Gralnick H, Valentine MD, Permutt S, Lichtenstein LM. Physiologic manifestations of human anaphylaxis. J Clin Invest 66:1072–1080, 1980.

Soreide E, Harboe S. Severe anaphylactic reactions outside hospital: Etiology, symptoms, and treatment. Acta Anaesthesiol Scand 32:339–342, 1988.

Stember RH, Levine BB. Prevalence of allergic diseases, penicillin hypersensitivity, and aeroallergen hypersensitivity in various populations. J Allergy Clin Immunol 51:100, 1973. (Abstract)

Stricker WE, Anorve-Lopez E, Reed CE. Food skin testing in patients with idiopathic anaphylaxis. J Allergy Clin Immunol 77:516–519, 1986.

Sullivan TJ. Cardiac disorders in penicillin-induced anaphylaxis: Association with intravenous epinephrine therapy. JAMA 248:2161–2162, 1982.

Toogood JH. Beta-blocker therapy and the risk of anaphylaxis. Can Med Assoc J 136:929–933, 1987.

Van der Linden PW, Hack CE, Kerckhaert J, Struyvenverg A, van der Zwan JC. Preliminary report: Complement activation in wasp-sting anaphylaxis. Lancet 336:904–906, 1990.

Van der Linden PWG, Hack CE, Poortman J, Vivie-Kipp

YC, van der Zwan JK. Insect-sting challenge in 138 patients: Relationship between clinical severity of anaphylaxis and mast cell activation. J Allergy Clin Immunol 90:110–118, 1992.

Van der Linden PWG, Hack CE, Eerenberg AJM, Struyvenberg A, van der Zwan JK. Contact-system activation and angioedema in insect-sting anaphylaxis. J Allergy Clin Immunol 91:282, 1993a. (Abstract)

Van der Linden PWG, Struyevenberg A, Kraaijenhagen RJ, Hack CE, van der Zwan JK. Anaphylactic shock after insect-sting challenge in 138 persons with a previous insect-sting reaction. Ann Intern Med 118:161–168, 1993b.

Van Metre TE Jr, Adkinson NF. Immunotherapy for allergic disease. In Middleton E Jr, et al. Allergy Principles and Practice. 3rd ed. St. Louis, Mosby–Year Book, 1988, p 1338.

Vaughn WT, Pipes DM. On the probable frequency of allergic shock. Am J Dig Dis 3:558, 1936.

Vervloet D, Arnaud A, Vellieux P, Keplanski S, Charpin J. Anaphylactic reactions to muscle relaxants under general anesthesia. J Allergy Clin Immunol 63:348, 1979.

Vidovich RR, Heiselman DE, Hudock D. Treatment of urokinase-related anaphylactic reaction with intravenous famotidine. Ann Pharmacother 26:782–783, 1992.

Viner NA, Rhamy RK. Anaphylaxis manifested by hypotension alone. J Urol 113:108, 1975.

Von Tschirschnitz M, von Eschenback CE, Hermann K, Ring J. Plasma angiotensin II in patients with Hymenoptera venom allergy during hyposensitization. J Allergy Clin Immunol 91:283, 1993. (Abstract)

Vyas GN, Fudenberg HH. Isoimmune anti-IgA causing anaphylactoid transfusion reactions. N Engl J Med 280:1073–1074, 1969.

Wade JP, Liang MH, Sheffer AL. Exercise-induced anaphylaxis: Epidemiological observations. Prog Clin Biol Res 297:175, 1989.

Watkins J, Clarke RSJ. Report of a symposium: Adverse responses to intravenous agents. Br J Anesthesiol 50:1159, 1978.

Weiss ME, Adkinson NF Jr. Allergy to protamine. Anesth Allergy: Clin Rev Allergy 9:339–356, 1991.

Westaby S, Turner MW, Stark J. Complement activation and anaphylactoid response to protamine in a child after cardiopulmonary bypass. Br Heart J 53:574–576, 1985.

Wiggins CA. Characteristics and etiology of 30 patients with anaphylaxis. Immunol Allergy Pract 13:313–316, 1991.

Yarbrough JA, Moffitt JE, Brown DA, Stafford CT. Cimetidine in the treatment of refractory anaphylaxis. Ann Allergy 63:235–238, 1989.

Yeates HM, Jenson KK. Chronic anaphylaxis caused by ingestion of vegetable gum products. J Allergy Clin Immunol 87:274, 1991. (Abstract)

Yunginger JW, Nelson DR, Squillace DL, Jones RT, Holley KE, Hyma BA, Biedrzycki L, Sweeney K, Sturner W, Schwartz L. Laboratory investigation of deaths due to anaphylaxis. J Forensic Sci 36:857–865, 1991.

Zaloga GP, Delacey W, Holmboe E, Chernow B. Glucagon reversal of hypotension in a case of anaphylactoid shock. Ann Intern Med 105:65–66, 1986.

Chapter 22

Drug Hypersensitivity

Paul P. VanArsdel, Jr., M.D.

An adverse reaction may occur when any therapeutic agent is used. Furthermore, as more drugs are introduced for the cure or control of life-threatening diseases, the spectrum of adverse reactions will continue to expand. Although allergic reactions constitute only a small proportion of adverse reactions, their heterogeneity, unpredictability, and potential severe—including fatal—consequences require continuing reassessment in the context of the proliferation of knowledge regarding immunologic mechanisms.

CLASSIFICATION OF ADVERSE REACTIONS

Most adverse reactions are toxic rather than allergic. They occur because of overdosage, impaired metabolism (or excretion), or drug interaction. Since allergic reactions can be understood and diagnosed most reliably within the context of all adverse reactions, a general classification of drug reactions is presented here (Table 22–1). The following brief discussion is based on this classification. Toxic reactions that mimic allergic reactions are of particular importance to this discussion and are reviewed subsequently. Some disease-associated reactions also may be triggered by drugs, particularly by antimicrobials. The classic reaction of this group was first described at the turn of the century by Jarisch and Herxheimer, who observed it during the treatment of syphilis with mercury (Bryceson, 1976). When penicillin was introduced, treatment was associated with more severe reactions. Symptoms and signs included chills, fever, localized edema, skin rash, adenopathy, headache, and, most typically, a flare-up of the syphilitic skin lesions. When such a reaction develops, the knowledgeable physician will continue necessary antimicrobial treatment while the reaction subsides. Other drugs may produce similar reactions during treatment of spirochetal, enteric, parasitic, and fungal infections (VanArsdel, 1983).

Ampicillin is associated with a high frequency of skin rashes when given to patients with infectious mononucleosis or lymphocytic leukemia and patients with gout treated also with allopurinol. The mechanisms involved remain speculative. In children particularly, the occurrence of skin eruptions during treatment with any antimicrobial drug may be entirely coincidental. Most eruptions, including urticaria, are manifestations of the illnesses being treated.

TABLE 22–1. CLASSIFICATION OF ADVERSE DRUG REACTIONS

Predictable risks
  Toxic: overdose or side effect, delayed expression
    (e.g., teratogenicity, malignancy)
  Allergy-like side effects
  Superinfection
  Drug interactions
Disease-associated risks
  Impaired degradation, excretion of drugs, or both due
    to organ system failure (increased toxicity)
  Conditions mimicking allergic reactions
    Jarisch-Herxheimer reaction
    Ampicillin reactions with infectious mononucleosis
      and other diseases
Coincidental risks
  Exanthematous infectious diseases
  Controversial: Stevens-Johnson syndrome and other
    disorders with many suspected causes
  Psychogenic
Risks to a susceptible subpopulation
  Intolerance
  Idiosyncrasy
  Allergy

Psychophysiologic reactions can take many forms. Anxiety, lassitude, drowsiness, nausea, and headache are fairly obvious. Most physicians and other medical professionals are less aware of the possibility that allergy-like symptoms also can be psychogenic. Perhaps this is best known to those who conduct placebo-controlled clinical drug trials. Subjects not infrequently complain of nasal congestion, urticaria, angioedema, and even anaphylactoid reactions while receiving only placebos.

DEFINITIONS. The last section of Table 22–1 lists three categories, which are defined here along with a few other terms:

- *Intolerance:* That condition in which a drug produces its expected toxic side effects at an unusually low dose.
- *Idiosyncrasy:* That condition in which the adverse reaction is strange and pharmacologically unexpected (i.e., different from the usual toxic reactions). Reactions of intolerance and idiosyncrasy may be related to the presence of enzyme defects in some patients.
- *Allergy:* An acquired potential for developing an adverse reaction that is immunologically mediated. *Allergy and hypersensitivity* will be used interchangeably in this chapter. In practice, of course, many reactions that are generally considered to be allergic could in fact be idiosyncratic, since no immune mechanism has been identified.
- *Anaphylactoid:* An adverse reaction that mimics an allergic reaction but is produced by toxic rather than immune release of potent vasoactive and smooth muscle reactive mediators.
- *Carrier:* A substance with immunogenic potential that, when coupled with a low-molecular-weight drug or metabolite, renders that chemical (the *hapten*) immunogenic.
- *Cross-reaction:* The reaction of an antibody or antigen-specific lymphocyte with an antigen other than one that induced its formation.
- *Hapten:* A substance that can react with specific antibody but is of a molecular weight too low for it to be immunogenic by itself.

GENERAL ASPECTS OF HYPERSENSITIVITY REACTIONS

By strict definition, hypersensitivity reactions should be associated with specific and reproducible abnormal immune findings. In fact, such proof is not often available. Furthermore, there is good evidence that some allergy-like reactions are not immunologically mediated. These so-called *pseudoallergic reactions* are discussed separately from allergic reactions in the sections to follow.

Allergic Drug Reactions

BACKGROUND. Human hypersensitivity reactions to therapeutic agents were first recognized after the introduction of horse serum antitoxins. Serum sickness was the most common major manifestation of iatrogenic allergic reactions until the 1930s. Little is known about reactions to the few specific drugs that were in general use before 1900 other than the obvious toxicity of these natural poisons. New synthetic drugs then began to appear. By 1930, adverse reactions that were presumably allergic were beginning to be reported, for example, 3 percent of patients given phenobarbital developed reactions that were probably allergic in nature. Ironically, aspirin, one of the first synthetic drugs reported after the turn of the century to produce angioedema and asthma, probably does so on a nonimmune basis (*vide infra*). Allergy to synthetic small-molecular-weight drugs did not become a prominent problem until the first sulfonamides were introduced in the late 1930s.

CHARACTERISTICS. The features that characterize an allergic drug reaction are listed in Table 22–2. Perhaps the most reliable clinical feature is the latent period between the start

TABLE 22–2. FEATURES OF AN ALLERGIC DRUG REACTION

Previous treatment without adverse effects.
Reaction usually appears only after several days of treatment, especially if no previous exposure to the drug.
Risk of reaction exists at doses far below therapeutic range.
Clinical manifestations do not resemble the general pharmacologic effects of the drug and cannot be predicted from animal testing.
Reaction occurs in a small proportion of the population.
Reaction usually is restricted to a limited number of syndromes generally accepted as allergic in nature.
Antibodies or T lymphocytes have been identified that react specifically with the drug or a metabolite, in a few instances.
A similar reaction can be reproduced on administration of a small amount of the suspected drug or drugs of similar chemical structure.

of treatment and the onset of the adverse reaction. Even this is not absolute, because the patient may have forgotten about previous treatment or may have had some non-therapeutic exposure (e.g., penicillin in cow's milk). Ideally, hypersensitivity testing should prove or exclude the diagnosis of drug allergy. In practice, however, objective sensitivity tests are reliable for only a few categories of drugs. These are as follows:

- Proteins and large polypeptides (xenogenic sera, hormones, enzymes).
- Drugs responsible for hematologic reactions.
- Small-molecular-weight drugs in which immunologically reactive intermediates have been identified (penicillin is the best example).
- Drugs responsible for allergic contact dermatitis.

The provocative challenge test is the most reliable test to confirm or exclude the diagnosis of allergy to most drugs. The suspected drug is readministered and the patient observed for a reaction similar to the previous one. Usually the risk of such a challenge is greater than any benefit one can hope to gain by such proof. One general exception is the patch test for determining the cause of allergic contact dermatitis. This test, when properly done by experienced personnel, will provide the necessary proof safely and reliably (VanArsdel and Larson, 1989).

INCIDENCE. Although adverse allergic reactions to xenogenic sera and the first sulfonamides were common a few decades ago (10 percent or more of those treated reacted), recent data, based primarily on hospital populations, indicate that the incidence of drug allergy is relatively low. For most drugs, it is less than 2 percent. In a well-known study of hospitalized patients reported by the Boston Collaborative Drug Surveillance Program, the overall incidence of skin eruptions associated with all drugs, per course of drug therapy, was only 0.2 percent. Among the commonly used drugs, only the semisynthetic penicillins, trimethoprim-sulfamethoxazole, cephalosporins, and transfusions were associated with reaction rates over 2 percent: trimethoprim-sulfamethoxazole headed the list at 56/1000 patients treated (Bigby et al, 1986).

RISK FACTORS FOR ALLERGIC REACTIVITY. In *children* the incidence of all adverse drug reactions has been reported for both outpatients and inpatients by several groups. In one study, drug reactions were responsible for 2 percent of hospital admissions (McKenzie et al, 1976). Very few of these (11 of 3556) were classified as allergic. Allergic reactions are thought to be less common in children than in adults, and this appears to be so at least for penicillin (Bierman and VanArsdel, 1969; Graff-Lonnevig et al, 1988) and drug fever (Whyte and Greenan, 1977). However, in the Bigby study cited previously, there was no significant age association in the occurrence of skin rashes in hospitalized patients, although the reactions did occur more often in female than in male patients, independent of age. Once the patient is sensitized, there is no known age difference in the nature or severity of a reaction if the drug is readministered.

A history of a previous allergic reaction to the same drug (or one that is chemically similar) is by far the most reliable evidence that giving the drug would be risky. Perhaps multiple drug exposure (so common in hospitalized patients!) increases the risk of a reaction to a newly introduced medication. Some patients are more prone to develop allergic reactions to several unrelated drugs, especially antibiotics, than are others (Kamada et al, 1991). Whether this is a general risk from multiple drug treatment or represents a unique susceptibility of a subset of patients has yet to be determined.

At one time, a history of atopic disease was generally considered to be an important risk factor. However, this assumption may not be correct. For example, the prevalence of penicillin allergy among patients with ragweed hay fever does not differ significantly from that among normal control subjects, nor is there reliable evidence for an association of atopy with allergy to any other drug. However, atopic patients who do have a systemic reaction to a drug tend to react more severely than non-atopic patients (VanArsdel, 1991a).

Genetic factors that control drug metabolism may influence the risk of drug hypersensitivity. Patients who are slow acetylators are more likely than those with fast acetylator phenotypes to develop adverse reactions. Examples are drug-induced systemic lupus erythematosus (Gilliland, 1991) and certain severe sulfonamide reactions (Rieder et al, 1989). A few associations between histocompatibility types and certain adverse reactions have been reported, but none of any major significance (VanArsdel 1991a).

Immunosuppression may enhance the sensitizing potential of some drugs. The principle is interesting. An immunosuppressed patient may become deficient in those suppressor T cells that regulate IgE antibody synthesis. A bone marrow transplant recipient developed an allergic reaction to polymyxin B (an extremely unusual occurrence) and was found to have an IgE anti-polymyxin B antibody (Lakin et al, 1975).

In recent years, immunosuppression associated with human immunodeficiency virus infections has become a major risk factor for adverse drug reactions. Over half the patients with AIDS develop adverse reactions when treated with trimethoprim-sulfamethoxazole. The incidence of reactions to amoxicillin-clavulanate is inversely proportional to CD4+ cell counts (Kovacs et al, 1984; Battegay et al, 1989). Several other drugs have been found to have a higher than expected tendency to produce adverse reactions in HIV-infected patients. Most are mild-to-moderate skin eruptions, but the risk of anaphylaxis and even toxic epidermal necrolysis may also be enhanced with HIV infection (Bayard et al, 1992; Coopman et al, 1993; VanArsdel, 1991a).

Topical medication to the skin (apparently not to the mucous membranes) is the most likely to sensitize, and oral administration the least likely. Intravenous administration of a drug is less likely to sensitize than are other parenteral approaches.

Finally, the risk of drug allergy is related to the chemical nature of the drug and to the route of administration. As will be discussed later, the allergenicity of a drug is related to its potential to form stable conjugates with carrier proteins either directly or via a reactive metabolite.

Pseudoallergic Reactions

Allergy-like side effects can be produced directly by certain drugs in the absence of any evidence of hypersensitivity. In contrast to true allergic reactions, these occur promptly the first time the drug is given, if the dose is sufficiently high, appear only when the dose is increased, or, with an intravenous drug, when the rate of administration is increased. Table 22–3 is a classification of these reactions. The *histamine releasers* produce reactions that are similar to anaphylaxis. Since they are not immunologically mediated, they are referred to as *anaphylactoid* reactions. The mechanism of the anaphylactoid reaction is similar to the antigen-induced one; the drug induces a calcium-dependent noncytotoxic and energy-dependent reaction in mast cells and basophils that results in granule exocytosis and release or activation of potent vasoactive and smooth muscle–reactive mediators. The reaction occurs most frequently when the offending substance is given rapidly and intravenously, producing a diffuse flush, pruritus, urticaria, and transient hypotension followed by headache. Phytonadione (colloidal vitamin K) also can produce such a reaction if given intravenously, and a few fatalities have been reported. The reaction may be caused by a dispersing or emulsifying agent rather than by the vitamin itself (Gilman et al, 1990). Among the opiates, codeine, morphine and meperidine are histamine releasers, whereas fentanyl, sufentanyl, methadone, and naloxone are not.

TABLE 22–3. PSEUDOALLERGIC REACTIONS

Histamine-releasing drugs
   Deferoxamine
   Atracurium and tubocurarine
   Opiates
   Pentamidine
   Phytonadione
   Polymyxins
   Radiographic contrast media
   Vancomycin
Complement activities
   Endotoxins
   Foreign proteins
   Human gamma globulin (aggregated)
   Protamine
   Radiographic contrast media
Autonomic drugs
   Beta-adrenergic blocking agents
   Reserpine and other antihypertensive agents
   Parasympathetic agonists and anticholinesterases
Enzyme inhibitors
   Angiotensin-converting enzyme inhibitors
   Anticholinesterases
   Nonsteroidal anti-inflammatory drugs

Complement activation has been an important but often unrecognized cause of systemic reactions during most of this century. Reactions could be induced by peptones, aggregated proteins, bacterial endotoxins, and various impurities. When complement is activated, anaphylatoxins are generated. These polypeptide cleavage products of complement components, C3a, C4a, and C5a, act by releasing histamine. Furthermore, C5a is a strong chemotactic agent (VanArsdel, 1991b). The most commonly used agents that activate complement are the radiographic contrast media (Lasser, 1991). Protamine is also causing an increasing number of systemic reactions with its expanded use in relatively high doses to terminate heparin autocoagulation after cardiopulmonary bypass surgery. It may produce reactions either by the direct activation of complement or by reactions involving IgE and IgG antibodies (Weiss et al, 1989).

Angiotensin-converting enzyme (ACE) inhibitors, commonly used to treat hypertension, are also kininases. A dose-related pruritic, maculopapular skin eruption that occurs with one ACE inhibitor, captopril, is probably caused in part by the inhibition of kinin degradation. A more important side effect is cough, which can occur in as many as 10 percent of patients treated with any ACE inhibitor. Angioedema, another side effect, is much less common (Israeli and Hall, 1992; VanArsdel, 1991b).

Antihypertensive drugs may produce or aggravate respiratory symptoms. The best known is reserpine, which produces predictable dose-related nasal stuffiness, discharge, or both. Others are hydralazine and alpha-adrenergic blockers. Anticholinesterase and histamine-releasing drugs also may produce nasal symptoms. Asthma can be made worse by beta-adrenergic blocking agents and by anticholinesterases. Rhinitis and asthma in some patients are aggravated by aspirin and other nonsteroidal anti-inflammatory drugs, possibly via their enzyme-inhibitory actions. These topics are discussed further in Chapter 38, Drug-Induced Asthma.

IMMUNE PATHOGENESIS

Immunochemical Principles

Only a few therapeutic agents are complete antigens. Foreign proteins, such as horse serum antitoxins and antithymocyte globulins, are antigenic and induce IgG antibody formation in all individuals who are capable of normal immune responses. If the titer of such antibodies is high enough, immune complexes may activate a sufficient amount of complement-derived mediators (anaphylatoxins, chemotactic factors) to produce allergic symptoms. Some individuals (not necessarily those with atopic diatheses) will produce specific IgE antibodies and develop typical anaphylactic manifestations. Larger polypeptide hormones are similarly immunogenic. Immunogenicity is weak when the molecular weight is less than 5000 daltons, and as a rule molecules containing fewer than seven amino acids are not immunogenic.

Most drugs in common use are simple organic chemicals with molecular weights under 1000 daltons. For such chemicals to produce specific immune responses, they must be conjugated to some macromolecule, usually a protein or large polypeptide, termed a *carrier*. This phenomenon was first established by Landsteiner's pioneering work over a half-century ago (Landsteiner and Jacobs, 1935). Such conjugation must be firm; the usual serum binding of drugs is not sufficient. Conjugation of virtually any drug to a carrier can be achieved artificially in the laboratory by use of such activating chemicals as the carbodiimides and diisocyanates. The drug is proved to be immunogenic by injecting the conjugate into appropriate experimental animals and demonstrating the appearance of antibodies that bind specifically to the drug (the *hapten*) rather than to the carrier protein. The role of the carrier in producing immunogenicity is not clear; it may stimulate the activation of helper T cells. Highly selective monoclonal antidrug antibodies that are induced by these conjugates are now used widely for the immunoassay of drug concentrations in biologic fluids.

Beginning with Landsteiner's findings, practically all effective conjugates prepared in the laboratory have covalent hapten-carrier bonds. Such conjugation does not occur readily *in vivo*. A few organic compounds can form covalent bonds with carriers without synthetic manipulation. These compounds are as follows: acid anhydrides, acid chlorides, aromatic halides, isocyanates, isothiocyanates, mercaptans, quinones, and diazonium salts (Levine, 1966). Few of these are known to play a role in the pathogenesis of drug hypersensitivity.

The beta-lactam antimicrobial drugs have in common an oxazolone group (a type of anhydride) in the beta-lactam ring. The oxazolones of the penicillins, monobactams, and carbapenems form stable covalent bonds with proteins and polypeptides, thus forming conjugates that are potentially allergenic. This reaction was identified over 20 years ago and is used to prepare the skin-testing conjugate, benzylpenicilloyl polylysine. The comparable metabolites of the other class of beta-lactam drugs—the cephalosporins—are unstable and do not form any recognizable allergenic conjugates. Other penicillin metabolites have free-SH groups and have the potential to form stable mixed disulfides with cysteine in carrier proteins.

The experience derived from research on penicillin hypersensitivity over 20 years ago led to considerable optimism that allergic reactions to many other drugs would prove to be mediated by metabolites rather than by the drugs themselves, and thus reliable diagnostic tests could be developed. So far, though, immunogenic metabolites have been identified as responsible for clinical adverse reactions caused by only a handful of drugs; the methods used have not yet emerged from research laboratories and have not been confirmed as useful for clinical testing (see VanArsdel, 1991a, for reviews).

Mechanisms

The four Coombs and Gell types of human hypersensitivity, as originally described, are useful in classifying drug reactions and are reviewed briefly.

CONDITIONS ASSOCIATED WITH IgE ANTIBODIES. A diverse number of macromolecules (allergens) are responsible for the production of anaphylaxis and urticaria and for the production or aggravation of asthma, rhinitis, and some adverse reactions to foods. In a sensitive person, an allergen reacts with specific IgE antibody on the surface of mast cells and basophils, resulting in the release or activation of histamine, leukotrienes, and other potent mediators. Macromolecular therapeutic agents can produce similar types of sensitivity. Allergenic extracts used in immunotherapy fall into this category, as do xenogenic sera, large polypeptide hormones, and macromolecular contaminants in various biologic products. Small-molecular-weight drugs also can produce such reactions by conversion to immunogenic haptens (the penicillins, for example). Quaternary ammonium muscle-relaxing drugs such as succinylcholine are small molecules that may sensitize without forming hapten-carrier conjugates. They have reactive determinants that are spaced far enough apart so that they act as bivalent antigens, bridging specific IgE antibodies on mast cells, and thus inducing mediator release (Birnbaum and Vervloet, 1991).

CYTOTOXIC ANTIBODY REACTIONS. Essentially all cytotoxic antibody-mediated reactions to therapeutic agents involve injury to formed elements of the blood. The most obvious ones occur when mismatched erythrocytes, leukocytes, or platelets are administered. These are injured by IgG and IgM antibodies in the presence of complement and subsequently destroyed. Drug-induced reactions fall into the three following general categories:

The Hapten-Cell Reaction. The offending drug reacts with cell surfaces to form a stable immunogenic complex, which stimulates antibody that is drug-specific. The main example is penicillin-induced hemolytic anemia, confirmed by demonstrating that the patient's serum agglutinates erythrocytes that have been preincubated with penicillin. The agglutinin is an IgG antibody that does not fix complement; presumably the red blood cell destruction occurs entirely in the reticuloendothelial system.

The Immune Complex Reaction. Although this reaction belongs in the next category, it is included here for contrast. It is thought to be responsible for most allergic drug reactions involving blood cells. A drug or metabolite reacts with antibody in the circulation. The soluble immune complex that is formed, along with complement, affixes to the cell surface, and injury is produced by the membrane attack complex of complement. The drug-antibody complex may remain on the cell only transiently after activating complement, which remains behind.

Drug-Induced Autoimmune Reaction. This is a hemolytic anemia thought to be caused when the offending drug induces autoantibody production against apparently normal red blood cell determinants by an unknown mechanism. In the case of methyldopa, at least, the IgG antibody that develops reacts against Rh determinants.

OTHER IMMUNE COMPLEX REACTIONS. Nonhematologic reactions thought to be caused by drug-IgG antibody complexes can be systemic or local in their manifestations. The classic systemic reaction, produced by xenogenic serum, is serum sickness. Much of the information about immune complex disease has been generated by the production of experimental serum sickness in animals; this is a standard model for studying immune complex nephritis. Human serum sickness differs in that renal manifestations are minor in most patients, and it almost always coexists with IgE-mediated phenomena. Serum sickness-like reactions are produced by several drugs, including penicillin. In the case of penicillin sensitivity, in which specific serum antibodies can be measured, IgG antibody is found usually in fairly high titer. However, there is no evidence that this antibody is responsible for any allergic manifestations. It does not fix complement and appears to cause no harm to the fetus after crossing the placenta. Infiltrative lung disease associated with inhaled drug allergens also is associated with the presence of IgG antibody. In the past, it developed occasionally from the inhalation of a biologic product, such as posterior pituitary powder, but rarely is seen nowadays. In any event, a T cell–mediated mechanism may play a more important role than the humoral one.

CELL-MEDIATED CONDITIONS. These are mediated by specifically sensitized T lymphocytes. The great majority of the reactions occur after cutaneous contact and are characterized by infiltration of lymphocytes and other mononuclear cells. There is little reason to doubt that various lymphocyte mediators (lymphokines) are responsible for tissue injury, but little proof of this has come from *in vitro* studies on lymphocyte reactivity. Studies that measure responses, such as mitogenic transformation, tritiated thymidine uptake, and migration inhibition factor (MIF) generation from cells cultured in the presence of the suspected drug, have not led to any consistently reliable laboratory indicator for allergic contact dermatitis, let alone other drug reactions (mostly cutaneous) of uncertain pathogenesis. Although some evidence exists that cell-mediated mechanisms do play some role in special circumstances (Rocklin, 1974; Knutsen et al, 1984), the tests are not sufficiently reliable for general use in the diagnosis of drug allergy.

The best confirmed of the systemic cell-mediated reactions are not those suspected from *in vitro* tests, but those that occur in a person with preexisting contact allergy who is given the offending agent parenterally. Such reactions from theophylline-ethylenediamine (aminophylline) given to patients with contact allergies to ethylenediamine have been reported so often in recent years that the phenomena have become model examples of systemic T cell–mediated reactions.

TYPES OF CLINICAL REACTIONS

Clinical reactions that are generally accepted as allergic or possibly allergic are outlined in Table 22–4. This outline is used in the following discussion. The listing of drugs that are possible causes of the various kinds of reactions is derived from several sources. The most comprehensive are standard references in pharmacology (Gilman et al, 1990 and AMA Drug Evaluation subscriptions, through spring, 1993). These were supplemented by textbooks on adverse drug reactions (Cluff et al, 1975; Davies, 1991), the reports of the Boston Collaborative Drug Surveillance Program (Bigby et al, 1986), selected reviews and reports in various journals, and The Physicians' Desk Reference (PDR), 1995.

Mast Cell–Mediated Reactions

SYSTEMIC ANAPHYLAXIS. (See also Chapter 21.) The patient who suffers this reaction develops one or more of the following symptoms, usually within a few minutes after the drug is given: generalized flush, palpitations, weakness, dizziness, tingling of the extremities or tongue, urticaria, angioedema, and ap-

TABLE 22–4. CLASSIFICATION OF ALLERGIC DRUG REACTIONS

Mast cell–mediated
  Systemic anaphylaxis
  Urticaria and angioedema
  Some pruritic maculopapular eruptions
  Serum sickness (in part)
  Anaphylactoid (nonimmune)
T lymphocyte–mediated
  Allergic eczematous contact dermatitis
Photodermatitis
Other cutaneous reactions (mechanism uncertain)
  Maculopapular or exanthematous
  Fixed eruptions
  Toxic epidermal necrolysis
Drug fever
Systemic lupus erythematous and other autoimmune
  reactions
Organ systems
  Blood
    Eosinophilia, hemolytic anemia, thrombocytopenia,
      granulocytopenia
  Lung
  Liver
  Kidney
  Heart
Reactions with inconsistent drug associations
  Erythema multiforme
  Exfoliative dermatitis
  Vasculitis

prehension. Angioedema may obstruct the upper airway. If the reaction is not treated, it may progress to difficulty breathing, shock, seizures, incontinence, coma, and death. Fortunately, anaphylaxis is rare. The most reliable information on incidence comes from the experience with penicillin treatment in venereal disease clinics. Anaphylaxis occurred in 1 of every 1820 patients treated (Rudolph and Price, 1973). One fatality from penicillin occurred in approximately 50,000. The incidence of fatal reactions to macromolecular drugs or agents is undoubtedly higher, and an important recent example is the antitumor agent, asparaginase.

Some drugs produce mast cell–mediated reactions that are not immune. As mentioned previously, mast cell release of mediators is a predictable toxic side effect of such drugs. Because their mechanism is different from the immunologically mediated one, these are called anaphylactoid reactions. Drugs that are known to produce anaphylactic or anaphylactoid reactions are listed in Table 22–5. The most common offenders are foreign sera, allergenic extracts, dextrans, injected enzymes, polypeptide hormones, penicillins, and radiographic contrast media. Gold sodium thiomalate, but not aurothioglucose, can produce an anaphylactoid reaction with nitritoid features; the vehicle rather than the gold is thought to be responsible. Aspirin and nonsteroidal antiinflammatory agents (NSAIDs) are not included in the table because their reactions, which may be anaphylactoid when severe, are complex and are discussed elsewhere. Other drugs not listed in the table are those in which reactions are reported in the medical literature because of their rarity and not because of significant risk of anaphylaxis. Examples are glucocorticoids, H_2 antagonists, and tetracyclines.

CUTANEOUS REACTIONS. Most reactions are urticarial; occasionally, they can be morbilliform. Often they are accompanied by angioedema of extremities, mucous membranes, or genitalia. A reaction may appear explosively (e.g., in a previously sensitized patient) after the first dose of the drug (alone or as part of systemic anaphylaxis) or may not appear for several days. The clinical characteristics of urticaria and angioedema are described in Chapter 46. There is nothing distinctive about the appearance of drug-induced reactions. Drugs responsible for these reactions include those listed in Table 22–5 as well as additional drugs listed in Table 22–6. Most cases of urticaria clear up in a few days after treatment with the suspected drug is stopped. One should look for an alternative explanation if the reaction lasts more than a week and should realize that many cases of chronic urticaria of unknown cause have started during some drug-treated illness.

SERUM SICKNESS. Patients with reactions to foreign sera develop urticaria, angioedema, arthralgias with adjacent edema, and low-grade fever from a few hours (the accelerated form) to 3 weeks after receiving the sera. The more severe reactions may include temporomandibular arthritis, adenopathy, and mononeuritis multiplex. A few reactions have been associated with glomerulitis. The reactions seen with small-molecule drugs usually are limited to urticaria and arthralgias. The most common causes of serum sickness today are hydralazine, penicillins, sulfonamides, and thiazide diuretics. Although reactions to animal sera products are not as common as they

TABLE 22–5. DRUGS RESPONSIBLE FOR ANAPHYLACTIC OR ANAPHYLACTOID REACTIONS

Macromolecules	Clindamycin
Allergic extracts*	Ethambutol
Dextrans	Fluoroquinolones
(including iron dextran)*	Lincomycin
Enzymes	Ondansetron
Asparaginase*	Polymyxin B†
Chymotrypsin	Spectinomycin
Trypsin	Sulfonamides
Chymopapain*	Tetracyclines
Gelatin	Vancomycin†
(in some vaccines)	Other drugs
Heparin	Bleomycin†
Hormones	Cisplatin
(e.g., ACTH, insulin)	Colchicine
Human gamma globulin	Cytarabine
Organ extracts	Dimethylsulfoxide†
Protamine	Ethylene oxide
Vaccines	Gold sodium thiomalate
Xenogenic sera*	Latex
Diagnostic agents	Meprobamate
Dyes	Muscle relaxants
Iodinated contrast media†	Opiates†
Antimicrobials	Suramin
Aminoglycosides	Thiobarbiturates
Amphotericin B	Tolmetin
Beta-lactams*	Triamterene

*These agents either are frequent causes of anaphylaxis because of extensive use or are responsible for a relatively high incidence of reactions. They also are the most commonly implicated in urticaria and angioedema.

†These agents produce anaphylactoid (nonimmune) reactions in most instances.

TABLE 22–6. URTICARIA-PRODUCING DRUGS

Antimicrobials	Ergotamine
Isoniazid	Ethchlorvynol
Metronidazole	Ethosuximide
Miconazole	Lipid-lowering
Nalidixic acid	agents
Quinine	Meprobamate
Rifampin	Metoclopramide
Tetracyclines*	Nafarelin
Other drugs	NSAIDs
Acetaminophen/phenacetin*	Penicillamine
Allopurinol*	Pentazocine*
Anticoagulants (oral)*	Phenothiazines
Calcitonin	Procainamide
Chloral hydrate	Quinidine
Clonidine	Sulfonylureas
Cyclophosphamide	Ticlopidine
Dantrolene	
Digitalis*	
Doxorubicin	

*Reactions of urticaria and angioedema are rarely associated with these agents.

once were, xenogenic antiserum is still needed for treatment of botulism and poisonous bites. Furthermore, it is being used with increasing frequency for the immunomodulation of organ transplant patients and those with certain malignancies. An interesting pattern has been observed in patients who react to antithymocyte globulin (ATG) (Bielory et al, 1985); a majority of the cutaneous reactions were morbilliform rather than urticarial, and more than half the patients developed distinctive serpiginous bands of erythema on their hands and feet at the margin of palmar or plantar skin. The lesions were frequently purpuric, as might be anticipated in thrombocytopenic patients. The treatment program in this group of patients included methylprednisolone as well as ATG; this probably is the reason for the low incidence of urticaria.

A few other drugs produce reactions that are not really similar to serum sickness but do not fit easily in any other classification. Aminosalicylic acid, for example, causes a syndrome similar to infectious mononucleosis, and phenytoin not uncommonly produces adenopathy without other stigmata of serum sickness.

One should not forget that a serum-sickness syndrome thought to be caused by a drug may actually be caused by the illness that the drug is being used to treat. Infectious diseases, in particular, may have serum sickness–like features. These diseases include hepatitis B, rubella, and infectious mononucleosis. The symptoms are likely to be mediated by immune complexes, but there is no evidence for such complexes playing any role in the production of reactions produced by small-molecular-weight drugs. For the same reason, laboratory tests are of little value in the diagnosis of this class of drug allergy.

T Lymphocyte–Mediated Reactions

Most of these reactions result from the use of topical medications on the skin. The offending drug produces a pruritic, erythematous, papulovesicular, and even bullous eruption that is called *allergic eczematous contact dermatitis*. The general clinical, pathologic, and immune features of this condition are presented in Chapter 45. Most commonly, the reaction develops during topical therapy of a preexisting dermatosis.

Allergic contact dermatitis in general is uncommon in children; the prevalence of sensitivity increases with age. This would be true for drug sensitivity as well except that topical medications are used so frequently in treating skin rashes in young children that the development of contact sensitivity is a common event. In one study, 24 percent of 2000 patients with eczema had developed contact allergy to one or more drugs (Cronin et al, 1970).

Some drugs, notably antihistamines, penicillin, and sulfonamides, were such common sensitizers that they are now rarely used on the skin. However, these drugs and others still can sensitize the medical or manufacturing personnel who handle them. Table 22–7 lists these drugs separately from the therapeutic (topical) agents. Drugs that are fairly common sensitizers are bacitracin, benzocaine, idoxuridine, and neomycin. Other potential sensitizers are added to numerous medications as stabilizers and preservatives and include ethylenediamine, thimerosal, and parabens. The patient who develops contact allergy to one of these agents runs some risk of developing a generalized reaction if treated with a systemic drug containing that agent (Storrs, 1991). Local or systemic symptoms from prosthetic implants could, theoretically, develop on the basis of T cell sensitization to metals (especially nickel) in stainless steel devices. Such sensitization is exceedingly rare, however. Recently, certain practitioners have claimed that hypersensitivity to mercury amalgam in tooth fill-

TABLE 22–7. DRUGS THAT CAN PRODUCE ALLERGIC ECZEMATOUS CONTACT DERMATITIS

Occupational
  Ampicillin
  Benzalkonium chloride
  Chlorpromazine
  Formaldehyde
  Glutaraldehyde
  Hexachlorophene
  Local anesthetics
  Opiates
  Penicillin
  Phenothiazines
  Streptomycin
  Thimerosal
Therapeutic
  Antihistamine (H$_1$)
  Bacitracin
  Benzocaine
  Ethylenediamine
  Fluorouracil
  Formaldehyde
  Glucocorticoids
  Hydroxyquinolines
  Idoxuridine
  Lanolin
  Neomycin
  Parabens
  Para-aminobenzoic acid
  Propylene glycol
  Sulfonamides
  Therapeutic dyes
  Thimerosal

ings could be responsible for ailments such as acne, depression, fatigue, and multiple sclerosis. In fact, such sensitivity occurs rarely, and the resulting reaction is a local one; *there is no evidence that it is ever responsible for other symptoms* (Mackert and Fisher, 1985).

Other Cutaneous Reactions

PHOTODERMATITIS. Photosensitivity reactions occur when skin is exposed to ultraviolet light during a time when a patient is taking the offending drug, either topically or internally. There are two types, *toxic* and *allergic*. The two are differentiated as are other toxic and allergic reactions. Toxic reactions develop immediately after drug treatment is started, assuming a sufficient amount of ultraviolet light exposure occurs. The reaction is provoked by "sunburn" wavelengths (285 to 310 nm). Photoallergic reactions are activated by longer wavelengths (320 to 450 nm) and appear only after the drug has been taken for a period of time sufficient for sensitization to develop (5 to 21 days). Whereas the toxic reaction has the characteristics of a typical sunburn, the allergic reaction may be erythematous, urticarial, edematous, eczematous, or exudative. Phototoxic drugs absorb and concentrate ultraviolet energy in the skin. Those drugs or metabolites responsible for allergic reactions may conjugate to dermal proteins and serve as haptens to a significant degree only in the presence of ultraviolet energy.

Table 22–8 lists some systemic drugs that are responsible for photodermatitis. The most common phototoxic drugs are chlorpromazine, demeclocycline, and doxycycline. The most common systemic drugs responsible for photoallergy are griseofulvin, nalidixic acid, psoralens, and sulfonamides. With the exception of coal-tar derivatives and psoralens, the reactions to topically applied agents are photoallergic. Most topical sensitizers have been removed from the market in the United States. The halogenated salicylanilides, used as antiseptics in soaps and cosmetics, are the best known sensitizers still in common use. Others are hexachlorophene and para-aminobenzoic acid (PABA) esters.

The diagnosis of photodermatitis usually is obvious because of eruption during drug therapy and its appearance on exposed skin only. If further proof is needed, the photopatch test can be used. This is done by applying the suspected agents to skin sites in duplicate for at least 24 hours, then exposing one of the sites to natural sunlight or an artificial source of ultraviolet light for 20 minutes. The next day the sites are inspected and interpreted in the same manner as in conventional patch tests (see subsequent section on testing).

There is no way to predict who is at risk of a reaction, but it is prudent to warn the patient to avoid sunlight exposure during treatment with a known offender, such as doxycycline. Sunscreen agents may protect from unavoidable exposure, but some of them may be photoallergenic because they contain PABA esters.

FIXED DRUG ERUPTIONS. Fixed drug eruptions consist of one or more macular, erythematous, edematous, round, or oval plaques that are sharply demarcated. The more severe reactions may be eczematous or even bullous. The lesions heal with scaling after treatment with the offending drug is

TABLE 22–8. SYSTEMIC PHOTOSENSITIZING DRUGS

Amiodarone	Naproxen
Azithromycin	Oxaprozin
Carbamazepine	Phenothiazines
Demeclocycline*	Psoralens*
Doxycycline*	Quinethazone
Gold salts	Sulfonamides*
Griseofulvin*	Sulfonylureas
Imipramine	Thiazide diuretics
Lincomycin	Triamterene
Nalidixic acid	

*Reactions to these drugs are relatively common.

stopped, leaving a sharply demarcated area of dark red, violet, or brown-pink pigmentation. Lesions may occur anywhere, including mucous membranes. Occasionally they are pruritic, but there are no systemic symptoms. Evidence for an allergic etiology is historically convincing. First, the drug may be given several times, even over the course of years, before the reaction develops. Second, the fixed eruption can be reproduced without significant risk by readministering the drug. Despite the convincing clinical evidence, the immune mechanism remains in doubt. The most likely is a localized T cell sensitivity, but numerous experimental studies using patch testing and skin grafting have produced conflicting or inconsistent results (Ackroyd, 1985). Over 50 drugs and food additives have been reported to cause fixed drug eruptions (Derbes, 1964), but most of these are rare. Drugs that have been implicated are barbiturates, gold salts, iodides, metronidazole, NSAIDs, penicillins, phenolphthalein, sulfonamides, and tetracyclines.

GENERALIZED SKIN RASHES. Other drug-induced skin rashes that are thought to be allergic are characterized generally by pruritus, erythema, and maculopapular eruptions. Some are described as scarlatiniform or exanthematous. To emphasize the connection, the otherwise unenlightening term *dermatitis medicamentosa* may be used. These are the most common allergic drug reactions, amounting to 46 percent of the total in one study from a dermatology service (Kuokkanen, 1972). The onset of these eruptions usually is late in treatment, and there is nothing unique to differentiate them from infectious disease exanthemata. The reactions are thought to be allergic, possibly on a T cell–mediated basis, but definitive proof is lacking. Sometimes, as in the case of most ampicillin-induced rashes, the evidence is to the contrary; usually, the eruption is not reproduced when the patient is rechallenged with the drug. There are no helpful laboratory features to support or exclude the possibility of drug allergy.

Most drugs have produced skin eruptions at one time or another. The most common offenders are ampicillin, aminoglycoside antibiotics, barbiturates, benzodiazepines, gold salts, phenytoin, and sulfonamides. Listing all drugs that have been implicated would serve no useful purpose. Instead, Table 22–9 is a list of commonly used drugs that rarely are responsible for skin eruptions.

TABLE 22–9. COMMONLY USED DRUGS THAT RARELY OR NEVER CAUSE SKIN ERUPTIONS

Acetaminophen	Lithium
Adrenergic agents	Local anesthetics
Androgens	Meperidine
Antacids	Morphine
Antihistamines	Nystatin
Aspirin	Paraldehyde
Atropine	Pentazocine
Bromocriptine	Prednisone
Cascara	Progesterone
Clomiphene	Spironolactone
Codeine	Tetracycline
Digoxin-digitoxin	Theophylline
Emollient laxatives	Thyroid hormones
Estrogens	Tubocurarine
Ganglionic-blocking agents	Vitamins
Glucocorticoids	Warfarin
Hydrochlorothiazide	
Levodopa	

If a maculopapular eruption develops, and for some reason treatment with the responsible drug is continued, the outcome is unpredictable. Sometimes the rash will resolve, suggesting either that it was not drug induced or that continuing the treatment has produced tolerance. The risk, of course, is that the eruption will evolve into something more severe and potentially fatal. The possibilities are *exfoliative dermatitis* and severe bullous reactions. The former is thought to be the more likely, but the evidence is scanty. Furthermore, the causal relationship is often uncertain because exfoliative dermatitis and bullous reactions are not necessarily caused by drugs. For this reason, exfoliative dermatitis is discussed in a subsequent section. However, a severe form of bullous reaction, *toxic epidermal necrolysis (TEN)*, will be considered next because of an increasing consensus in recent years that this type of reaction more often than not is drug induced.

TOXIC EPIDERMAL NECROLYSIS (TEN). This reaction, also called Lyell's syndrome, begins with the development of an erythematous rash, which soon is followed by the appearance of large, confluent bullae. Occasionally, the reaction may be difficult to distinguish from severe *erythema multiforme* (Stevens-Johnson syndrome, discussed in a subsequent section). TEN may be associated with, or preceded by, malaise and fever. Rarely, the reaction may be associated with eosinophilia, renal failure, or both. In the more severe reactions, bullae become widespread and confluent, and the epidermis sloughs off in large sheets, leaving large areas of raw dermis. The reaction is similar to a severe thermal injury with attendant fluid, electrolyte, and infection problems. Drugs that have been implicated as causes of TEN include allopurinol, barbiturates, carbamazepine, chloramphenicol, ethambutol, ibuprofen, ketorolac, lovastatin, penicillin, phenolphthalein, phenylbutazone, phenytoin, sulfonamides, and sulindac. In rare instances, the offending drug has been given again inadvertently, and the ensuing maculopapular eruption (fortunately, self-limited) has confirmed the relationship (Pegram et al, 1981).

The staphylococcal scalded skin syndrome (SSSS), usually seen in children, was classified with TEN until recently. Since it is not drug induced, the general impression developed that TEN also was not often drug induced. Skin biopsy findings, however, have proved that the two conditions are not the same. In TEN, the whole epidermis separates; in the more benign SSSS, the tissue that separates is intraepidermal.

Fever

Body temperature is regulated in the preoptic region of the anterior hypothalamus. This thermoregulatory center maintains body temperature under normal circumstances within a narrow range by controlling heat production and conservation via both autonomic and skeletal motor neural pathways. Fever can occur when macrophages are stimulated to produce endogenous pyrogens. These include interleukin-1 (IL-1), tumor necrosis factor, and interferon alpha (VanArsdel, 1991a). It is believed that they act by generating E prostaglandins from arachidonic acid. This increase has an important temperature-raising influence on the hypothalamic center. Several factors are known to stimulate generation of these cytokines. These include bacteria or bacterial products (gram-negative endotoxins and exotoxins), viruses, fungi, and antigen-antibody complexes. Since body temperature can be raised also by other mechanisms, such as inadequate heat dissipation, excessive heat production, and direct hypothalamic effect, it should not be surprising that different therapeutic agents might produce fever in different ways. Some well-recognized febrile reactions to drugs are not immunologically mediated. These are listed in Table 22–10. The first four categories in this table are self-explanatory. Increased tissue metabolism often is associated with autonomic dysfunction, leading to severe and potentially fatal reactions, as in malignant hyperthermia induced during inhalation anesthesia by succinylcholine and perhaps other agents. Reactions of comparable severity, associated with hyperpyrexia and rigidity, have been reported with the use of haloperidol and similar drugs (i.e., "neuroleptic malignant syndrome") (Szabadi, 1984). Hyperpyrexia in children caused by certain psychotropic drugs has been recognized as an occasional problem for several years (Feigin and Shearer, 1976).

Prostaglandins are now used therapeutically and are frequently pyrogenic via a direct central effect. Alprostadil (PGE_1) should be of particular interest to pediatricians. It is used to help maintain patent ductus arteriosus in infants with congenital heart disease, and 14

TABLE 22–10. NONALLERGIC CAUSES OF DRUG FEVER

Mechanism	Examples
Endogenous release of bacterial pyrogen	Jarisch-Herxheimer reaction
Administration of exogenous pyrogen	Contaminated fluids or drugs
	Fever therapy; injection of endotoxin or typhoid vaccine
Release of endogenous pyrogen	Sterile inflammation after intramuscular drug injection
Secondary to another type of adverse reaction producing tissue injury	Hemolysis, hepatitis
Increased tissue metabolism	General anesthetics, succinylcholine (malignant hyperthermia)
	Neuroleptic malignant syndrome
Peripheral vasoconstriction and reduced heat loss	Norepinephrine effect
Central effect	Amphetamine intoxication
	Prostaglandins and prostaglandin-generating agents
Hormonal	Etiocholanolone fever

percent of these infants so treated develop hyperpyrexia.

Recombinant interferon alpha is also pyrogenic. It is an immunomodulating cytokine used for treatment of some virus infections and hairy cell leukemia. It produces fever by generating PGE_2 production in the hypothalamus (Dinarello et al, 1988).

Some other drugs probably are direct pyrogens, being commonly associated with fever, but the mechanisms are not known. Amphotericin B is the best known example; others are bleomycin, cimetidine, iron dextran, calcium disodium edetate, and dimercaprol. In children, *epinephrine as well as norepinephrine can cause fevers.* Atropine (even eye drops) and phenothiazine may inhibit sweating sufficiently to raise the body temperature above normal.

Perhaps the earliest description of allergic fever produced by a drug was reported by Jadassohn in 1896 (see Samter, 1969). He described a patient with contact dermatitis who subsequently swallowed a small amount of the offending chemical; several hours later, the patient developed fever and generalized erythroderma. Allergic fever can be part of drug-induced vasculitis, which may include manifestations similar to those of serum sickness. It may be the first sign of drug-induced hepatitis, or it may be the only physical manifestation. When allergic fever occurs alone, the patient may lack other symptoms associated with a febrile illness. This is a noteworthy feature to recognize when a fever due to an antimicrobial drug allergy appears after resolution of a fever caused by an infection. When treatment with the offending drug is stopped, the temperature almost always drops to normal within 48 hours. One exception is phenytoin. This drug has a high tissue affinity, and the temperature may not return to normal for several days after treatment is stopped.

Table 22–11 lists drugs that have been reported to cause allergic fevers without other allergic manifestations. The most commonly implicated are blood products, carbamazepine, cephalosporins, hydroxyurea, iodides, methyldopa, penicillamine, penicillins, phenytoin, procainamide, quinidine, and vancomycin. Fever is relatively uncommon among all forms of adverse drug reactions in hospitalized patients but may make up as much as 25 percent of the total number of allergic reactions. In one study of 146 children with fevers of unknown origin, three had drug fevers (Feigin and Shearer, 1976).

The mechanism of allergic drug fever has not been established. Because the clinical features are consistent with allergy and because the fever has been produced in sensitized rabbits by a penicilloyl conjugate (Chusid and Atkins, 1972), there is general consensus that allergic drug fever is caused by the release of IL-1 and other cytokines during phagocytosis of complexes of antibody with drug-carrier conjugates.

TABLE 22–11. DRUGS THAT CAN CAUSE FEVER WITHOUT OTHER SIGNS OF ALLERGY

ANTIMICROBIALS	OTHER DRUGS
Cephalosporins	Allopurinol
Chloramphenicol	Antithymocyte globulin
Erythromycin	Blood products
Griseofulvin	Carbamazepine
Isoniazid	Heparin
Kanamycin	Hydralazine
Nitrofurantoin	Hydroxyurea
Penicillins	Iodides
Pyrazinamide	Methyldopa
Quinine	Penicillamine
Streptomycin	Phenobarbital
Sulfonamides	Phenytoin
Tetracyclines	Pneumococcal vaccine
Trimethoprim	Procainamide
Vancomycin	Quinidine

Autoimmune Reactions

SYSTEMIC LUPUS ERYTHEMATOSUS (SLE). First reported in patients receiving hydralazine treatment over 30 years ago, a syndrome similar to SLE has subsequently been associated with treatment with many other drugs. However, most cases have been caused by hydralazine or procainamide. The most frequent symptoms are malaise, fever, arthralgias, and pleuritic pain. A few patients also develop pericarditis, adenopathy, skin rash, and hepatosplenomegaly. Most develop mild anemia and leukopenia and demonstrate an elevated erythrocyte sedimentation rate. The lupus cell preparation and antinuclear antibody (ANA) titer become positive. In contrast to true SLE, central nervous system or renal involvement is unusual, serum complement remains normal, and antibodies to double-stranded DNA are absent. Over 90 percent of patients with symptomatic procainamide-induced SLE have antihistone antibodies. By contrast, patients with true SLE have nuclear antibodies. The prevalence of positive ANA titers increases with the duration of treatment and the incidence of clinical manifestations may be dose related. The prevalence is so high (over 50 percent with positive ANAs from procainamide treatment and up to 12 percent with symptoms from hydralazine treatment) that the SLE syndrome is often considered toxic rather than allergic. Indeed, the reaction may be the outcome of a pharmacologic effect. Procainamide and hydralazine inhibit DNA methylation. Experimentally, DNA hypomethylation tends to generate autoreactivity. There is no evidence that the drugs unmask latent SLE, and symptoms and ANA titers gradually diminish after drug treatment is stopped.

Other drugs that are documented causes of the SLE syndrome are chlorpromazine, isoniazid, methyldopa, penicillamine, and quinidine. At least a dozen more drugs have been implicated, but the evidence for a causal association is weak (Gilliland, 1991).

OTHER AUTOIMMUNE DISORDERS. Penicillamine has been implicated in several immune complex disorders in addition to SLE. These include dermatomyositis, polymyositis, Goodpasture's syndrome, hypersensitivity pneumonitis, immunocytopenias, membranous glomerulonephritis, myasthenia gravis, and pemphigus/bullous pemphigoid. The last disorder is noteworthy because antiacetylcholine receptor antibodies and antistriated muscle antibodies have been identified in the sera of some patients being treated with D-penicillamine (Vincent et al, 1978). A syndrome similar to myasthenia gravis also has been reported during treatment with trimethadione and with quinidine.

Lovastatin, pravastatin, and simvastatin are cholesterol-lowering agents that act by inhibiting 3-hydroxy-3-methylglutaryl, coenzyme A (HMG-CoA) reductase. This class of enzyme inhibitors has been associated with the development of a complex hypersensitivity syndrome that may include SLE, vasculitis, polymyalgia rheumatica, cytopenias, anaphylaxis, urticaria, and erythema multiforme.

Organ System Reactions

Hematologic Reactions

EOSINOPHILIA. Eosinophilia usually accompanies other allergic manifestations of drug allergy, or it may be the first sign to appear. Although its appearance may serve as a warning of worse manifestations to come, this rarely is appreciated at the time. Furthermore, the appearance of eosinophilia alone is not a reason to terminate important therapy. Drugs that are commonly associated with eosinophilia are listed in Table 22–12. Only occasionally is eosinophilia the only manifestation of drug allergy. It is curious that eosinophilia alone is common during treatment with streptomycin (50 percent), kanamycin (10 percent), and digitalis, even though clinical allergy to the last is extremely rare.

The association between a drug and eosinophilia may not indicate cause and effect, particularly with antibiotic therapy. Eosinophilia is not an uncommon part of convalescence from infections, such as pneumococcal pneumonia.

HEMOLYTIC ANEMIA. As indicated previously, it is useful to categorize drug-related cell destruction according to three types of mechanisms.

Hapten-Cell Type. In this type of reaction, the offending drug or its reactive intermediate binds to some portion of the red blood cell membrane. The immunogenicity of the drug may relate more to its serum protein binding than to its binding to that membrane. Accordingly, the effect of the reaction of antibody with the drug is more analogous to passive hemagglutination than to that of a reaction with a drug-membrane-protein carrier. Thus, the mechanism may be more appropriately termed "drug-adsorption" than "hapten-cell" (Petz, 1985). This reaction was first described with high-dose benzylpenicillin treatment in association with high-titered IgG antibody. The diagnosis is supported if the direct Coombs

TABLE 22–12. DRUGS ASSOCIATED WITH EOSINOPHILIA

ANTIMICROBIALS	OTHER DRUGS
Cephalosporins	Allopurinol
Erythromycin	Carbamazepine
Isoniazid	Chloral hydrate
Kanamycin	Clonazepam
Nalidixic acid	Digitalis
Nitrofurantoin	Ethosuximide
Penicillins	Papaverine
Rifampin	Penicillamine
Streptomycin	Phenothiazines
Sulfonamides	Probucol
Tetracyclines	Tricyclics

antiglobulin reaction is positive; the diagnosis is confirmed if the indirect test results, using normal drug-treated cells, also are positive (VanArsdel, 1970). A similar mechanism is responsible for the reaction to the antitumor drug, cisplatin. Cephalothin, commonly responsible for a positive Coombs test result, rarely causes hemolytic anemia. This positive test result is an artifact caused by nonspecific protein adsorption.

Immune Complex Type. When IgG or IgM antibody develops with specificity for an epitope on a drug or drug metabolite, the antibody forms a complex with the antigen (most likely bound to a macromolecular carrier) in the circulation. In susceptible individuals, this complex, after reacting with complement, develops a high affinity for red blood cells and attaches to them nonspecifically. After such an attachment, the antigen-antibody complex may remain on the cells only transiently, while the membrane attack complex of complement remains on the cell to produce injury. For this reason, the direct Coombs test result in drug-induced immune anemia may be positive only if a complement antiserum is used. For many years the binding to red cells or other formed elements was thought to be nonspecific, and Shulman (1964) applied the term, "innocent bystanders" to these cells. However, it is now known that drug-induced antibody binding to red cells occurs only if the cells contain certain specific blood group systems (Gilliland, 1991). This indicates that binding is an active immunologic process. Drugs in common use that can cause this kind of anemia are acetaminophen, chlorpropamide, isoniazid, quinidine, rifampin, sulindac, and tolmetin.

The more severe reactions have been associated with evidence of intravascular hemolysis. An antidepressant drug, nomifensine, has been observed recently to produce these reactions in several patients. Although the drug is not used in the United States, investigation of patients receiving it in Germany has provided further insight into the immune mechanism of drug hypersensitivity. Some complement-fixing IgG and IgM antibodies were found with drug specificity, but most antibodies were reactive with drug metabolites. The most consistent reactions were found using, as an antigen source, the urine from a normal person who had been given the drug. Most of the *"ex vivo"* reactive metabolites so obtained have not yet been identified (Salama and Mueller-Eckhardt, 1985).

Autoimmune Reaction. In this type of reaction, drug administration may lead to the production of IgG autoantibodies directed against red cell antigens with Rh specificity. The direct Coombs antiglobulin test is strongly reactive, but the anticomplement test is not. The most commonly implicated drug, methyldopa, inhibits suppressor lymphocyte function, including those cells that prevent the unrestrained production of autoimmune antibodies (Kirtland et al, 1980). Levodopa, mefenamic acid, and procainamide are others that may be responsible for this type of reaction.

THROMBOCYTOPENIA. An immune complex mechanism probably is responsible for most cases of drug-induced immune thrombocytopenia, although, as with anemia, the binding may be more active than previously thought. The sensitized patient will react within 30 minutes of receiving even a minute dose of the offending drug (e.g., quinine in tonic water) with chills, fever, petechiae, and mucous membrane bleeding as the platelet count drops precipitously. The antibody involved usually is an IgG immunoglobulin, which may have specificity for a platelet membrane glycoprotein. In the laboratory, the suspected drug is incubated with the patient's serum and normal platelet-rich plasma. A positive reaction may be detected by complement fixation, platelet factor release, or serotonin uptake inhibition. Drugs now in common use that have been associated with immune thrombocytopenia are listed in Table 22–13. The most frequent offenders are gold salts, heparin, hydantoins, interferon alpha, isonia-

TABLE 22–13. DRUGS CAUSING IMMUNE THROMBOCYTOPENIA

Acetaminophen	Mefenamic acid
Acetazolamide	Meprobamate
Acetylsalicylic acid	Methyldopa
Amrinone	Penicillamine
Carbamazepine	Phenacetin
Chloramphenicol	Phenylbutazone
Chlorpheniramine	Procainamide
Danazol	Quinidine
Desipramine	Quinine
Digitoxin	Ranitidine
Ethchlorvynol	Rifampin
Gold salts	Stibophen
Heparin	Sulfonamides
Hydantoins	Sulfonylureas
Interferon-alpha	Thiazide diuretics
Isoniazid	Valproic acid
Levodopa	

zid, NSAIDs, procainamide, quinidine, quinine, rifampin, sulfonamides, and thiazide diuretics. In the case of acetaminophen, the responsible antigen was a sulfate metabolite.

GRANULOCYTOPENIA. Immune granulocytopenia is associated with the appearance of acute chills, fever, and arthralgias, accompanied by a rapid fall in the leukocyte count. By contrast, toxic or idiosyncratic leukopenia caused by bone marrow depression develops insidiously and becomes apparent if the patient is monitored with periodic blood counts or if an infection, such as stomatitis or pharyngitis, develops. Drugs causing immune granulocytopenia are few in number compared with those causing predictable suppressive effects on bone marrow. Aminopyrine was the first drug reported to produce immune granulocytopenia; sensitivity was confirmed by demonstrating leukoagglutinating antibodies that transferred the sensitivity passively to normal recipients. Leukoagglutinins to other drugs have been identified inconsistently. The results may be inconsistent because granulocytes altered by drug-antibody complexes have short half-lives and remove the complexes when they are cleared from the circulation. Thus, any leukoagglutinin is present only transiently. A test based on the opsonization of normal neutrophils by sera of neutropenic patients receiving various drugs appears to be more reliable than leukoagglutination (Weitzman et al, 1978). Immune granulocytopenia from any drug is rare. The more familiar drugs that have been associated with drug-dependent antibodies against mature neutrophils are beta-lactam antimicrobials, flecainide, gold salts, phenytoin, procainamide, and quinidine. Evidence of drug-dependent immune reactivity against granulocyte precursors has been identified in patients with neutropenia induced by ibuprofen, phenytoin, and quinidine (Gilliland, 1991).

Hepatic Reaction

The liver, being a major site for drug metabolism, should be particularly susceptible to drug injury. Perhaps because the liver is such a vulnerable target, few drugs that are primarily hepatotoxic remain in use today. Occasionally, toxic dose-related reactions occur from acetaminophen or intravenous tetracycline; necrosis and fibrosis are calculated risks in treatment with methotrexate or mercaptopurine. In children, idiosyncratic hepatotoxic reactions to aspirin may occur during the treatment of juvenile rheumatoid arthritis and allied diseases (Anderson, 1980). Most hepatic reactions have characteristics more consistent with allergy, although the evidence is based primarily on clinical clues such as the delay in the onset of symptoms or signs and the association with other signs of allergy. To the degree that the risk of sensitization correlates with the generation of reactive metabolites by hepatic enzymes such as those in the cytochrome P450 system, it should not be surprising that the liver is a prime target for drug injury, immune and otherwise (Willson, 1991).

The two main subclasses of hypersensitivity are *cholestatic* and *hepatocellular*. Drugs that may produce hepatic reactions are listed according to these two subclasses in Table 22–14. Jaundice usually is the first sign of a cholestatic reaction but may be preceded by the appearance of eosinophilia. Phenothiazines and erythromycin estolate have been more often responsible for the cholestatic reaction, although the latter is rarely used now because of this side effect. The clinical picture of hepatocellular reaction may be similar to that of viral hepatitis. Fever may be the first manifestation, or signs of obstructive jaundice may develop. The liver becomes enlarged and tender. A skin rash and arthralgias, eosinophilia, or both may develop. The reaction oc-

TABLE 22–14. DRUGS CAUSING HYPERSENSITIVE HEPATIC REACTIONS

Primarily cholestatic	Griseofulvin
Chlorzoxazone	Halothane
Erythromycin estolate	Hydantoins
Ethchlorvynol	Isoniazid
Haloperidol	Ketoconazole
Imipramine	Methyldopa
Nalidixic acid	Monoamine oxidase
Nitrofurantoin	inhibitors
Papaverine	Nitrofurantoin
Phenothiazines	Oxyphenisatin
Sulindac	Phenylbutazone
Sulfamethoxazole	Propylthiouracil
Sulfonylureas	Pyrazinamide
Troleandomycin	Quinidine
Primarily hepatocellular	Rifampin
Aminosalicylic acid	Sulfonamides
Amphotericin B	Sulindac
Ethacrynic acid	Trimethadione
Furosemide	Valproic acid
Gold salts	

curs frequently with pyrazinamide, rifampin, and aminosalicylic acid, and is the most frequent reaction in children treated with valproic acid. Rarely, the anesthetic agent halothane can produce an allergic hepatitis after repeated exposure, and some deaths have been reported. Recent evidence supports the concept that, in susceptible individuals, a reactive metabolite of halothane generates neoantigens that are responsible for the allergic reaction (Pohl et al, 1989). Patients with cholestatic hepatitis always recover completely when drug treatment is stopped. Most with hepatocellular injury also recover, but in rare instances the reaction may lead to postnecrotic cirrhosis and can be fatal.

Granulomatous hepatitis has been associated with several drugs, but these associations may be coincidental. It has developed during allopurinol treatment along with other signs of vasculitis (see subsequent discussion), and a few cases of *chronic active hepatitis* have been reported following treatment with methyldopa, nitrofurantoin, and oxyphenisatin.

Pulmonary Reaction

ASTHMA. Asthma most often is a part of a generalized systemic reaction to an injected allergenic extract. It may occur occasionally as part of an anaphylactic drug reaction in a patient with an asthmatic diathesis. It rarely is the only manifestation of a systemic allergic reaction but has been reported in a few patients treated with ondansetron, a new selective serotonin (5HT$_3$) receptor antagonist that is used for treatment of nausea. Indeed, if asthma alone follows administration of some drug, it probably is a pharmacologic side effect of that drug. Such reactions are discussed elsewhere in this chapter. Inhaled agents such as antimicrobials and enzymes may provoke asthmatic reactions in sensitive individuals but are reported much more commonly from occupational exposure than from therapeutic use. (See also Chapter 38.)

INFILTRATIVE REACTIONS. These are acute reactions that usually develop 2 to 10 days after onset of treatment, with cough and dyspnea that are often associated with chills, fever, and malaise. A maculopapular rash may develop. The physical findings usually are limited to a few focal or basilar coarse rales. In contrast, the chest radiograph usually shows the following impressive changes: diffuse alveolar, reticulonodular, and focal migratory fluffy infiltrates. The reaction has been reported from inhaled drugs, even cromolyn, but is exceedingly rare. Reactions reported to be caused by systemic drug administration are listed in Table 22–15. *Eosinophilic pneumonitis* usually is associated with few symptoms or physical signs, but marked eosinophilia develops, followed by the radiographic appearance of nodular or fluffy infiltrates in the chest. In the *"other"* category are drugs that produce a diffuse interstitial infiltrate. Sometimes, patients develop symptoms and signs suggesting pulmonary edema, particularly with nitrofurantoin. This drug is the most common cause of acute reactions. Evidence that the acute reactions are allergic is mostly circumstantial. Sometimes a reaction occurs that has features of both toxicity and hypersensitivity. The most striking example is amiodarone pneumonitis (Obermiller and Lakshminarayan, 1991). There are scattered reports of drug-induced stimulation of a patient's lymphocytes in tissue culture, suggesting a cell-mediated hypersensitivity mechanism, but no consistent immune pattern has emerged.

FIBROTIC REACTIONS. These are slowly developing reactions that are probably toxic-idiosyncratic. They are characterized by the gradual development of cough and dyspnea without any associated systemic symptoms. Responsible drugs are also listed in Table 22–15. Pulmonary toxicity of certain antineoplastic agents, particularly bleomycin, is a predict-

TABLE 22–15. DRUGS CAUSING INFILTRATIVE PULMONARY REACTIONS

Probably allergic	Fibrotic
Eosinophilic	Bleomycin
pneumonitis	Busulfan
Carbamazepine	Methysergide
Chlorpropamide	Mitomycin
Gold salts	Nitrofurantoin
Naproxen	Nitrogen mustards
Penicillamine	Nitrosoureas
Penicillin	
Phenytoin	
Sulfonamides	
Other	
Amiodarone	
Gold salts	
Melphalan	
Methotrexate	
Nitrofurantoin	
Procarbazine	
Sulfonamides	
Thiazide diuretics	

able, dose-related side effect. Fibrosis may continue to progress after drug treatment is terminated.

Renal Reaction

Interstitial nephritis is the most common drug-induced hypersensitivity reaction. It is characterized by hematuria, proteinuria, pyuria, and varying degrees of azotemia. The reaction tends to be milder and of shorter duration in children than in adults. Most patients have other findings that suggest an allergic reaction, such as fever, skin rash, and eosinophilia of blood and urine. The renal biopsy specimen shows tubular degeneration and necrosis with infiltrates containing mononuclear cells, plasma cells, and eosinophils. The results of immunofluorescent studies have been variable and inconsistent. Methicillin has been the most common identified cause of interstitial nephritis. Other probable causes among drugs in common use are other beta-lactam drugs, captopril, cimetidine, diuretics (furosemide and thiazides), rifampin, and sulfonamides. Nonsteroidal anti-inflammatory drugs (NSAIDs) also can produce interstitial nephritis, but the symptoms and signs are those of nephrotic syndrome, and associated allergic features are rare. The predominant cells in the interstitial infiltrate are T lymphocytes. Allopurinol and phenytoin may produce interstitial nephritis, but usually reactions from these drugs are heterogeneous with vasculitis and variable glomerular involvement (Adler et al, 1985).

A patient with a drug-induced immune *glomerular injury* usually presents with nephrotic syndrome. Commonly, renal function is only mildly impaired. The biopsy findings are typical of membranous glomerulopathy, including the immunofluorescence findings of finely granular IgG and C3 deposits (Adler et al, 1985). Drugs that are most often implicated are captopril, gold salts, NSAIDs, and penicillamine.

Cardiac Reaction

Drug-induced eosinophilic myocarditis is a rare condition that is usually recognized postmortem. The possibility should be suspected if the patient develops unexplained tachyarrhythmias and other ECG changes, along with signs of hypersensitivity such as skin rash and eosinophilia. The reaction has been attributed to methyldopa, penicillins, and sulfonamides. Interleukin-2 (IL-2) treatment has been associated with a dose-related biopsy-proven eosinophilic myocarditis (Schuchter et al, 1990).

Reactions with Inconsistent Drug Associations

ERYTHEMA MULTIFORME. This is an eruption characterized by concentric or "target"-shaped skin eruptions along with various combinations of macular, papular, urticarial, vesicular, and purpuric lesions. A severe form, called the *Stevens-Johnson syndrome,* is characterized by bullous skin lesions with mucous membrane and conjunctival involvement. It generally is preceded by fever, malaise, or other constitutional symptoms. Some authorities consider TEN (discussed earlier) to be a severe form of this syndrome. Establishing or excluding a drug association usually is difficult, because the reaction can be associated with mycoplasma and other infections, neoplasms, connective tissue diseases, and even radiation therapy. As mentioned previously, a drug being used for treatment of a disease may be mistakenly blamed for a reaction that is actually a result of the disease itself. Nevertheless, hypersensitivity to the suspected drug has been proved in a few instances; the drug was inadvertently given again, and the skin eruption reappeared. Drugs so implicated in published cases are minoxidil, phenolphthalein, rifampin, sulfapyridine, and trimethoprim-sulfamethoxazole (VanArsdel, 1983). Commonly used drugs that have been implicated on circumstantial evidence alone are carbamazepine, gold salts, hydralazine, NSAIDs, penicillins, phenylbutazone, phenytoin, and sulfonylureas.

EXFOLIATIVE DERMATITIS. This is a potentially fatal reaction that may begin as an apparently benign maculopapular eruption but progresses to a diffuse, highly pruritic desquamative erythroderma. If uncontrolled, it may become edematous and exudative and lead to severe fluid loss and secondary infection. About 10 percent of cases are thought to be drug induced; the remainder are associated with underlying diseases such as psoriasis, atopic dermatitis, and lymphocytic malignancies. There is only scanty evidence for an immune pathogenesis. The best evidence is clinical. Patients with known contact allergy to ethylenediamine may develop exfoliative erythroderma if treated with parenteral aminophylline (Petrozzi and Shore, 1976). Exfoliative dermatitis has been implicated as an unusual or rare adverse effect from treatment with the drugs listed in Table 22–16. Carbamazepine may be the most frequent offender (Kuokkanen, 1972). In children, exfoliative dermatitis may be a toxic reaction; it is one of several symptoms and signs of vitamin A poisoning.

VASCULITIS. This reaction has other names, e.g., *allergic angiitis, hypersensitivity angiitis, and allergic purpura.* The patient presents with erythematous and maculopapular lesions that usually appear first on dependent areas. Frequently, purpuric lesions then appear. These are raised ("palpable purpura") and may become bullous and necrotic. Occasionally, urticaria and target lesions also are present. There may be systemic symptoms, such as fever, malaise, arthralgias, headache, and abdominal pain. A biopsy specimen of a typical skin lesion shows fibrinoid necrosis in walls of small venules and arterioles, endothelial swelling, hemorrhage, platelet thrombi, and disintegrating nuclei in the leukocyte infiltrate (*leukocytoclastic vasculitis*). Vasculitis is probably an immune complex disease, but most of the convincing laboratory evidence for this is found in patients with vasculitis that is not drug induced, i.e., vasculitis related to hepatitis B. In fact, most cases are not drug induced; only 4 of 39 cases reported in one survey were considered to be drug induced (Mackel and Jordon, 1982). Drugs in common use that have been implicated are allopurinol, cimetidine, furosemide, hydantoins, penicillins, phenylbutazone, and sulfonamides. There is at least one report of vasculitis that reappeared when the offending drug (cimetidine) was taken again. The biopsy findings were positive both times (Mitchell et al, 1983).

TABLE 22–16. DRUGS IMPLICATED IN EXFOLIATIVE DERMATITIS

Allopurinol	Penicillin
Aminophylline (ethylenediamine)	Phenobarbital
Carbamazepine	Phenothiazines
Captopril	Phenytoin
Dapsone	Sulfonamides
Glutethimide	Trimethadione
Gold salts	Trimethoprim
Iodides	

OTHER. There is no evidence other than a small number of anecdotal reports that any drug causes either *erythema nodosum* or *Henoch-Schönlein purpura.*

Pseudoallergic Reactions

These reactions have been outlined previously (see Table 22–3) and discussed briefly. Three groups of drugs (NSAIDs, radiographic contrast media, and various additives) merit further discussion.

NSAIDs. One year after aspirin was first approved in 1909 by the Council on Pharmacy and Chemistry of the American Medical Association, a 40-year-old woman with a history of asthma developed acute difficulty in breathing after ingesting 5 grains of aspirin for a headache. Within a few years, aspirin reactions were thought to be among the most common examples of drug allergy. However, when similar reactions began to appear from anti-inflammatory drugs of significantly different chemical structure, it became clear that the commonality among these drugs was not immunochemical cross-reactivity, but pharmacologic similarity. Starting with aspirin and indomethacin, this commonality now encompasses a substantial number of drugs—the NSAIDs—that share the property of inhibiting the enzyme cyclooxygenase and, thus, the generation of prostaglandins from arachidonic acid. The first reported patient is typical of patients who develop intolerance to aspirin and other NSAIDs. All such patients have a history of asthma, chronic rhinosinusitis, or both. Many have nasal polyps, and most have blood and tissue eosinophilia. Many do not have an atopic background, and most developed their first respiratory symptoms as adults. About 4 percent of unselected adult asthmatic patients give histories of symptoms provoked by NSAIDs, and as many more will show drops in ventilatory function after drug challenge. Up to 40 percent of patients with asthma, rhinosinusitis, and nasal polyps are intolerant or will become so. Some have the symptoms for several years before intolerance develops, although it is not uncommon for one with a history of rhinosinusitis to have the first asthma attack provoked by aspirin.

The NSAIDs produce or provoke both asthma and symptoms of rhinosinusitis in most intolerant patients; about 10 percent develop one or the other only. The degree of intolerance varies widely. Some patients may show nothing more than a 15 percent reduction in the forced expiratory volume in 1 second (FEV_1) and no symptoms when challenged with a full therapeutic dose; others may develop symptoms when challenged with a tenth that amount. Severe reactions can be anaphylactoid, leading to shock and death. Although most intolerant patients are adults, intolerance can develop in adolescents and in older children. Young atopic patients who have the misfortune to have asthma or allergic rhinitis complicated by chronic sinusitis and nasal polyps are at risk.

The mechanism of intolerance to NSAIDs is probably related in some way to their pharmacologic action. The most obvious explanation is that the inhibition of cyclooxygenase by these drugs increases arachidonic metabolism via the lipoxygenase pathway, thus increasing leukotriene generation. However, if the mechanism were this simple, NSAIDs should have an adverse effect on all asthmatic patients. There is no doubt that sensitive patients are hyperreactive physiologically and biochemically. Their mast cells are more labile, they generate more leukotrienes, and their airways are much more responsive to LTE_4 inhalation challenge than is the case with nonsensitive subjects (Manning and Stevenson, 1991). (See also Chapter 38, Drug-Induced Asthma.)

Aspirin also aggravates symptoms of about one fourth of patients with chronic urticaria. The mechanism might be immune, but proof is lacking. Urticaria and other skin eruptions initiated by aspirin are rare.

RADIOGRAPHIC CONTRAST MEDIA. Flushing, urticaria, wheezing, angioedema, and syncope with hypotension are occasional adverse reactions to the injection of iodine-containing radiopaque substances. Contrary to some assertions, the risk of reaction is completely independent of any sensitivity to iodine, to iodides in the diet, or to shellfish. Reactions are much less frequent following arterial injections than intravenous ones. Even though the symptoms may seem to be allergic, most reactions in fact are the results of the direct release or activation of mast cell–derived and complement-derived vasoactive mediators. (See Chapter 24 for further discussion of reactions to radiocontrast media.)

SULFITES AND OTHER FOOD AND DRUG ADDITIVES. Sulfiting agents have been used for centuries to aid in food preservation. Sulfur dioxide, sodium sulfite, sodium and potassium bisulfite, and sodium and potassium metabisulfite are antioxidants and sanitary agents. They delay bacterial spoilage; minimize discoloration of various foodstuffs during processing, storage, and distribution; and inhibit undesirable microorganisms during wine making and other fermentation processes. Although the presence of metabisulfites in "salad bar" lettuce, processed potatoes, and shrimp has received the most publicity, sulfiting agents are found in a variety of other foods as well and are used in numerous drugs, including some bronchodilator solutions (see Settipane, 1984, for detailed tables listing foods and drugs that contain sulfites). Symptoms produced by sulfiting agents in susceptible individuals are flushing, urticaria and angioedema, laryngeal edema, asthmatic wheezing, and potentially fatal anaphylactoid shock. Some develop various gastrointestinal symptoms alone or in addition to the anaphylactoid symptoms. The reactions are potentially fatal. The prevalence of sulfite reactivity may be as high as 10 percent among asthmatic patients, and asthma has been provoked even by the small amount of sodium metabisulfite in the ophthalmic solution dipivefrin (Schwartz and Sher, 1985). There is no increase in the risk of sulfite sensitivity in patients who are sensitive to aspirin and NSAIDs. Sulfite reactions probably are mediated via irritant receptors in the upper airways through neural reflexes and vagal efferent pathways. In the recent past, about 80 percent of the sulfite reactions have occurred in restaurants. Through the efforts of the FDA, state regulatory agencies, and the National Restaurant Association, the use of sulfites in restaurants has been drastically curtailed.

Compared with sulfites, other additives produce rare or inadequately documented adverse reactions. Tartrazine (FD&C Yellow No. 5) has received the most attention because of reported reactions in some aspirin-sensitive asthmatic patients. However, such sensitivity rarely has been confirmed by proper placebo-controlled challenge testing. The evidence for intolerance to other food and drug coloring agents and to substances, such as sodium benzoate, is even less convincing. The role of food additives in the genesis of hyperactivity in children remains controversial; in general, the association has not been confirmed in properly controlled clinical studies (Lipton and Mayo, 1983).

MANAGEMENT

Prevention

REDUCING DRUG EXPOSURE. The most effective way to prevent an adverse reaction to a drug is—don't use it! Hospital surveys have shown repeatedly that the number of adverse reactions is proportional to the number of drugs prescribed. The use of important drugs should be restricted to important conditions. For example, potentially lifesaving antimicrobial drugs should not be prescribed for minor illnesses or for questionable indications. One or more earlier courses of treatment given for questionable indications may sensitize a patient to an important drug, making it difficult to use the drug safely later when it is really necessary.

PRODUCT REFINEMENTS. Improvements in the manufacturing methods and in the components of biologic products have reduced, but not eliminated, the sensitizing potential of many therapeutic agents. Examples are as follows:

- Reduction in the use of sensitizing preservatives, such as parabens and thimerosal.
- Elimination of impurities, including immunogenic polymers, from penicillin and its homologues.
- Development of purified insulin and manufacture of inexpensive human insulin by recombinant DNA technology.
- Substitution with synthetic polypeptides for pituitary polypeptide hormones of animal origin.
- Replacement of equine antitoxins with human antitoxins.
- Employment of purified gamma globulin instead of whole serum when an animal product must be used (e.g., antithymocyte serum).
- Development of vaccines free of egg and other animal proteins.

IMPORTANCE OF THE HISTORY. Taking a careful history is the best possible action to minimize allergic drug reactions. However, a positive history must be interpreted carefully. For example, one that elicits a background of mild atopic disease should not exert a significant influence on therapeutic decision making. It is of paramount importance, though, to document any previous drug reaction. The patient, or whoever is best informed about the patient's previous medical problems, should be asked not only the name of the drug, but also the kinds of symptoms, the severity of the adverse reaction, and the nature of the illness being treated at the time. The physician should be able to determine whether any previous reaction was caused by a drug that is immunochemically or pharmacologically similar to the drug being considered for treatment. However, it is important to be careful in selecting and prescribing *any* drug for someone who gives a history of allergy to several different drugs.

Inevitably, some patients will be labeled as allergic who actually are not. By careful questioning alone, one may be able to correct the record. Symptoms of the previous reaction could be nonallergic (e.g., nausea, vomiting, diarrhea, and/or headache). The patient who gives a history of penicillin allergy may have been given ampicillin (or some other homologues with an unfamiliar name) some time after the alleged penicillin reaction with no problem. As mentioned previously, ampicillin treatment may be associated with the development of a skin rash, but the patient may not be allergic to the drug. In a child, cutaneous and serum sickness-like reactions commonly accompany acute viral infections, and it is likely that a sick child will be given drugs of some sort, including antimicrobials. It is worth remembering that allergic drug reactions are uncommon in children, except for those who require repeated treatment, e.g., patients with cystic fibrosis.

As the promotion and distribution of nonorthodox medicines increase, so do adverse reactions to their various ingredients. In taking a thorough history, one should not forget to ask tactfully about the use of aberrant remedies. Herbal products may be "fortified" with glucocorticoids, NSAIDs, psychotropic agents, or thiazide diuretics. The herbal products themselves may contain a wide variety of plant allergens capable of aggravating asthma or even provoking anaphylaxis. Chamomile tea is prepared from flower heads that cross-react with ragweed. Ginseng can produce skin eruptions as well as toxic side effects. Alfalfa seeds may induce a reaction similar to systemic lupus erythematosus. "Bee pollen" causes severe anaphylactic reactions. The eosinophilia-myalgia syndrome, induced by L-tryptophan ingestion, reached epidemic proportions a few years ago and was associated with some fatalities (Obermiller and Lakshminarayan, 1991). "Cellular therapy," consisting of injections of various animal tissues, has obvious and potentially severe risks. The many adverse effects of nonorthodox treatment schemes have been reviewed in detail recently by Vulto and de Smet (1988).

ROUTINE TESTING OR PREMEDICATION. All patients should undergo skin tests for possible anaphylactic sensitivity before receiving any xenogenic protein or large polypeptide agent. A prick test is done with a 1:10 dilution of serum. If the reaction is negative in 10 minutes, this dilution is used again for an intradermal test reaction which, if negative, is followed by an intradermal test with the undiluted substance. A negative test reaction is one with a wheal diameter less than 5 mm 15 minutes after the test is placed. Skin testing for penicillin allergy is discussed subsequently. Suffice it to say that a recent multicenter study found that when all hospitalized patients about to receive penicillin were tested, allergy was identified in such a small number with no history of penicillin allergy that the potential benefit was not worth the effort expended!

Premedication of all patients about to be treated has not proved to be practicable. For example, premedication is no longer used routinely before administering a radiographic contrast agent unless there is a history of a previous reaction.

The Patient with a Positive History

Frequently, a patient develops a problem in which it would be desirable to use a particular drug or diagnostic agent, but gives a history of suspected allergy or idiosyncrasy to that substance or a similar one. The decision pathways to use for such a patient are depicted in Figure 22–1 and are discussed next.

ALTERNATIVE DRUGS. If possible, a drug that is not known to cross-react with the suspect drug, but is equally effective, should be used. The risk of toxicity from the alternative drug, however, should not be overlooked. For example, vancomycin and aminoglycosides are alternatives to penicillins but are substantially more toxic. It might be a better choice to prescribe one of the cephalosporins, even

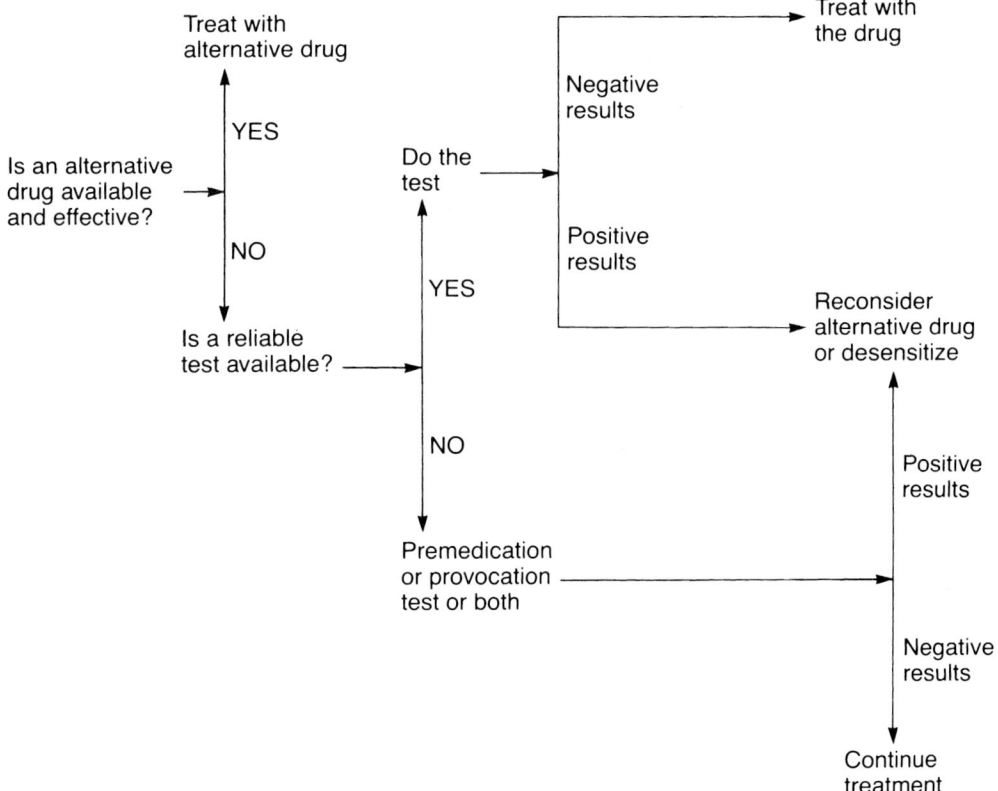

FIGURE 22–1. Decision pathway for assessing patients with positive histories of drug allergies.

though there is some statistical probability of cross-reactivity; fewer than 5 percent of patients with histories of penicillin allergy will react also to a cephalosporin. This is an acceptable risk unless the patient had an anaphylactic reaction to penicillin. Anaphylactically reactive patients should be tested for penicillin allergy (see subsequent discussion) or treated cautiously, beginning with small test doses. There is also significant cross-reactivity between penicillin allergy and skin test sensitivity to imipenem, a relatively new beta-lactam drug of the carbapenem group. However, no cross-reactivity has been demonstrated with aztreonam, a monobactam (Shepherd, 1991).

IMMUNOLOGIC TESTING. As discussed in the previous section, prick and intradermal skin testing are reliable for identifying IgE-mediated allergy to macromolecules, such as xenogenic sera and large polypeptides or polysaccharides. For most purposes, the skin test is sufficient to establish whether sensitivity is present. Serologic methods for measuring IgE antibodies, namely, the radioallergosorbent test (RAST) and the enzyme-linked immunosorbent assays (ELISAs), are available for testing to some agents but are more expensive, less sensitive, take longer, and add no further information than skin testing. Whereas routine skin testing to macromolecular agents can begin with a 1:10 dilution, it is prudent to start with a dilution of 1:1000, if the patient gives a history of a prior allergic reaction or is about to receive an agent about which little clinical experience has been accumulated. If severe anaphylaxis was the previous reaction, the first test should be a prick test using a 10^{-5} dilution.

Before testing can be done for allergy to drugs of small molecular weight, the immunogenic metabolites and, ideally, the mode of their conjugation to macromolecular carriers should be identified. With the exception of penicillin, this goal has been achieved only rarely; a few isolated examples of metabolites responsible for hematologic reactions were previously cited. Testing for penicillin allergy has become a well-established procedure for screening patients who give histories of suspected previous reactions to one of the penicillins. One principal and immunogenic penicillin metabolite that forms a stable conjugate *in vitro* with protein or polypeptide carriers has been identified. It is commercially available as penicilloyl polylysine (PPL). Skin test reactions using this so-called *major determinant* reagent will be positive in most patients who are truly allergic. However, it will not detect sensitivity in some patients in whom reliable testing is needed the most: those at risk for anaphylactic reactions. Fortunately, almost all such individuals have positive skin reactions to penicillin G (PG) itself; a very small number have been found to react only to other metabolites, e.g., benzylpenicilloate, benzylpenilloate, and penicilloyl-n-propylamine. Collectively, PG and these metabolites are called *minor determinants*. A standardized mixture called the minor determinant mixture (MDM) has been tested extensively on hospitalized patients in eight medical centers around the United States and should be released for general use soon. In the meantime, the closest approximation to MDM that is generally available for testing is a fresh solution of PG. The standard procedure at the University of Washington Hospitals uses PPL, 6×10^{-5} M, and PG, 1000 μ/ml. Any patient with a history of a severe, rapid-onset reaction should be tested first with 1:100 dilutions of these reagents. Prick tests are done first; if these reactions are negative after 10 minutes, intracutaneous tests are then done, delivering not more than 0.02 ml into the skin. If the resulting wheal is less than 5 mm in diameter after 15 minutes, treatment probably is safe. Because of the rare allergic patient who is sensitive neither to PPL nor to PG, it is prudent to give the patients whose reactions are negative a small dose (1000 units or the equivalent) 30 minutes before the full therapeutic dose. Some consultants will perform skin tests also to the specific beta-lactam drug that is to be used. This seems reasonable, especially if new evidence regarding the role of side-chain specificity on the immunogenicity of drugs such as ampicillin can be confirmed.

In our study of hospitalized patients who underwent skin testing with PPL and MDM, approximately 85 percent of those who gave histories of penicillin allergy were no longer allergic by skin testing, and these findings were confirmed by subsequent uneventful treatment (VanArsdel et al, 1986). This study was part of a nationwide project involving 726 hospitalized patients in eight medical centers. Overall, 81 percent of these had negative tests, and only seven (1.2 percent) had mild or moderate skin reactions to subsequent treatment (Sogn et al, 1992). We did not attempt to treat any patients with positive test reactions with a penicillin because effective alternative drugs were available. In earlier studies, approximately two thirds of patients with positive skin test reactions had systemic allergic reactions when penicillin treatment was attempted (Levine and Zolov, 1969).

Despite the demonstrated safety of re-treating patients with a history of penicillin allergy who have negative skin tests, these patients may become sensitized once again following an uneventful course of penicillin treatment (Parker et al, 1991). Accordingly, it is prudent to test all such patients once again before beginning any subsequent courses of treatment. The risk of a recurrence of sensitivity is even greater after treatment of history-positive test-positive patients who have been desensitized (see below).

Systemic allergy to local anesthetics, whatever the chemical structure, is extremely rare. Skin testing is an effective way to rule out allergy. Each drug to be tested is obtained epinephrine free and is diluted 1:10 and 1:100. The patient first undergoes prick testing with the 1:100 dilution. This is followed by intradermal tests to the 1:100, 1:10, and undiluted drug 15 minutes apart. A test dose of 0.5 ml can then be given subcutaneously or into the area to be anesthetized as a final precaution. In over 100 patients tested at the University of Washington Hospital, we have yet to identify a patient who was allergic to a local anesthetic. Furthermore, we have not observed any reactions that were caused by sensitivity to parabens or any other additives.

Skin testing for allergy to other drugs of low molecular weight is in general not reliable, although recent observations on the predictive value of skin tests for certain muscle-relaxing drugs and non-beta-lactam antimicrobials are encouraging (Birnbaum and Vervloet, 1991; Brandt et al, 1993). Serologic tests are only useful to confirm drug-induced hematologic reactions, and most of these are done reliably only in research laboratories. Since T cell–mediated allergy is suspected in a large proportion of drug reactions, several laboratories over the last two decades have tested suspected drugs for their possible blastogenic and lymphokine-producing effects on lymphocytes in tissue culture. Reports continue to appear of positive responses to a few drugs by lymphocytes from patients who have had recent allergic reactions. The most reliable reports have come from research laboratories interested in the immune mechanisms of the reactions (Knutsen et al, 1984). The *in vitro* lymphocyte response is a valuable research procedure, but its usefulness for diagnosing drug allergy, either prospectively or retrospectively, has yet to be established.

PROVOCATIVE TESTING. The only definitive test for drug sensitivity is to give the drug again under controlled conditions. The best example of a provocative test is the *patch test*. This is used to identify the cause of drug-induced allergic eczematous contact dermatitis. The drug or drugs in question are applied to the skin, in an appropriate vehicle, under an occlusive adhesive patch. Any positive reaction will develop within 48 (occasionally 72) hours as a pruritic, erythematous, and vesicular eruption similar to the original reaction but limited in severity and in scale. Other situations in which a provocation test may be advisable (i.e., when the offending drug is in doubt) are those in which the anticipated reaction is benign. Two common examples are the fixed-drug eruption and uncomplicated fever.

Whenever a drug is the probable cause of a reaction that is potentially serious, challenge rarely is justified. When the relationship is in doubt, the prior reaction was not a life-threatening one, and the suspected agent is clearly the best available one to use, then careful challenge testing will be necessary. This is done by giving a small dose at first, orally if possible. The starting dose can be 1 percent of the therapeutic dose unless the prior reaction was a severe one, in which case, the starting amount should be 100- or 1000-fold lower. Doses should be repeated in tenfold increments every 15 to 60 minutes (depending on the route of administration). If any symptoms appear, the test either should be terminated or, if the need for the drug is sufficiently great, should evolve into a desensitization attempt. Properly maintained emergency resuscitative equipment must always be kept at hand whenever provocation testing, desensitization, or both are carried out.

PREMEDICATION. Various drugs have been used for several decades to suppress possible reactions from antituberculous drugs, transfusions of blood products, and allergen immunotherapy injections. Premedication usually includes some combination of glucocorticoids, NSAIDs, antihistamines, and adrenergic drugs. Such therapy may be applied routinely or initiated if and when allergic symptoms develop during provocation testing or desensitization. Premedication is a necessary part of the preparation of patients who have had previous reactions to radiographic contrast media. At one center, patients are given oral prednisone, 50 mg every 6 hours for three doses before the procedure; diphenhydramine, 50 mg intramuscularly, and sometimes ephedrine, 25 mg subcutaneously, are given 1 hour before. This pretreatment reduced the reaction rate to below 10 percent when conventional contrast media were used, and below 1 percent when a low-osmolality agent was used (Greenberger and Patterson, 1991).

DESENSITIZATION. The strategies used in provocation testing and in premedication can be applied to desensitization as well. These strategies were used for many years to overcome sensitivity to antituberculosis drugs when alternative, first-line drugs were not available. Recent published reports have described the successful slow desensitization of patients to drugs such as allopurinol, carbamazepine, metronidazole, sulfasalazine, and trimethoprim-sulfamethoxazole. *Desensitization to sulfasalazine* has become fairly common because no comparable alternative drug is available for treatment of inflammatory bowel disease (Purdy et al, 1984). The usual starting dose is 1 mg, doubled daily until the 2-gm therapeutic dose is achieved. The dose is reduced temporarily if a reaction occurs; medication for the reaction usually is not needed. Desensitization schemes for the other drugs are similar in principle.

Desensitization to other agents is done more rapidly. The patient who is sensitive to *xenogenic serum* is given 0.1 ml subcutaneously of the smallest tenfold dilution that gives a positive skin test reaction (see previous section, Premedication). The dose is doubled every 15 minutes until 1 ml of the undiluted serum has been given. This dose is then given intramuscularly, followed by the full therapeutic dose. Because the procedure is required only when there is an immediate and urgent need for the drug, *penicillin desensitization* also is done rapidly. The patient with a positive skin test reaction to one or more of the penicillin determinants can usually be desensitized in a few hours, and the skin test reaction becomes negative (for the duration of treatment, at least). Desensitization can be carried out successfully through oral or parenteral routes. The oral program begins with 100 units as a rule; it is safe and takes up to 5 hours to complete (Sullivan et al, 1982). The intravenous route should be used if the patient cannot take oral medication or if absorption from the gut is uncertain. Intravenous administration has an advantage over other routes because one can control both the concentration and the rate of administration. Furthermore, a reaction can be identified at the first hint of symptoms, and corrective action can be taken promptly. With emergency equipment and drugs at hand, a dilute solution of benzylpenicillin or a homologue is delivered intravenously according to the method given in Table 22–17. Each infusion is given slowly at first, then gradually more rapidly until warning symptoms such as pruritus and flush develop. If any symptoms develop, the flow rate is reduced and the patient is given an antihistamine and a glucocorticoid drug. The flow rate is increased again when the symptoms are gone. Thirty minutes should be sufficient to administer each dilution. A report of children and young adults with cystic fibrosis, who were allergic to penicillin, described the successful use of intravenous desensitization in preparation for treatment with semisynthetic penicillins (Moss et al, 1984).

It also is customary to use *rapid desensitization for insulin allergy*, whether or not a sense of urgency exists. Insulin is a complete antigen, but systemic reactions to insulin are extremely rare unless there has been a lapse in treatment. Before desensitization is considered, one of the several alternative products

TABLE 22–17. INTRAVENOUS METHOD FOR PENICILLIN DESENSITIZATION*

BAG NO.	CONCENTRATION† μ/ml or μg/ml	TOTAL DOSE† μ or μg
1‡	0.01	0.5
2	0.1	5
3	1	50
4	10	500
5§	100	5000
6	1,000	50,000
7	10,000	500,000
8	Full dose	

*All solutions prepared in dextrose and water. 50-ml plastic bags for "piggyback" delivery.
†For simplicity of preparation, a unit of benzylpenicillin is equated with 1 μg rather than with the actual value of 0.6 μg.
‡Starting point if prick test reaction is strongly positive.
§Starting point if only the intradermal test reaction is positive.

should be tried, e.g., pork insulin, sulfated insulin, single peak insulin (partially purified), single component insulin (highly purified), and human insulin. The possibility of sensitivity to protamine or even zinc should not be overlooked. Patients who react even to human insulin are rare, but do exist (Grammer et al, 1985). Experience with human insulin desensitization is still limited. Conventional desensitization (using pork insulin) starts with the lowest concentration that gives a positive skin test reaction, proceeding with tenfold increments given subcutaneously as often as every 15 minutes until a local reaction occurs. The next dose is lower, and the following doses are increased at smaller increments. For a review of insulin allergy in children see Ross (1984).

A few patients with rheumatoid arthritis and allied conditions who are intolerant to *aspirin* and other NSAIDs would benefit greatly if these drugs could be used. Desensitization is possible (Manning and Stevenson, 1991). Tolerance usually can be achieved (albeit with some risk of severe asthmatic reactions) by giving gradually increasing doses every 3 hours, beginning with an amount previously determined to be the threshold for a reaction; it may be as little as 10 mg. Tolerance is maintained by taking the drug every day; it may lapse if the drug is not taken for more than 2 days.

TREATMENT

Stopping the drug treatment may be sufficient to terminate relatively benign reactions, such as fever and nonpruritic fixed and generalized eruptions. Indeed, the presence of such reactions does not necessarily require that effective drug treatment be discontinued.

Urticaria and other pruritic skin eruptions can be treated with antihistaminic drugs with sedative or tranquilization properties. Hydroxyzine (25 to 100 mg, or 1 mg/kg two to three times daily) or diphenhydramine (25 to 100 mg, or 1 mg/kg four times daily) usually is effective. Urticaria that develops rapidly after a drug is given should be treated in addition with epinephrine, 0.01 mg/kg or 0.3 to 0.5 mg subcutaneously, in anticipation of a possible anaphylactic reaction. Anaphylaxis is discussed in detail in Chapter 21. Briefly, epinephrine is effective for most of the features of anaphylaxis. Any patient taking a beta-adrenergic blocking drug may not respond to epinephrine and should be treated with glucagon (Zaloga et al, 1986). Other essentials of treatment are as follows:

- Prevent the absorption of the offending agent (if injected) with local infiltration of epinephrine and application of a tourniquet.
- Maintain plasma volume with ample amounts of intravenous fluids.
- Give drugs, including epinephrine intravenously (by slow drip), if the patient is hypotensive.
- Give oxygen and maintain patency of the upper airway; an intravenous antihistaminic may help.
- Watch for bronchospasm, and treat it.
- Monitor for cardiac dysrhythmias and cardiogenic shock.
- Consider glucocorticoid therapy to suppress a late reaction after the aforementioned have been done.

Pain of serum sickness, SLE syndrome, vasculitis, and some cases of urticaria may require analgesic therapy with a NSAID. Systemic glucocorticoid therapy should be started without hesitation for treatment of severe urticaria, contact dermatitis, exfoliative dermatitis, and erythema multiforme. It may hasten recovery from pulmonary, hematologic, and hepatic reactions as well. The usual dosage range is 40 to 80 mg/day of prednisone or its equivalent, and the dose can be tapered rapidly as soon as the lesions begin to subside, usually within 3 days. Toxic epidermal necrolysis, vasculitis, and interstitial nephritis do not usually respond to glucocorticoid treatment, but a short trial may be appropriate. Topical glucocorticoids are ineffective in the treatment of urticaria and other pruritic dermatoses. Although they may be of some benefit in contact dermatitis, their systemic use is much more effective and just as safe over the usual short treatment period.

REFERENCES

Ackroyd JF. Fixed drug eruptions. Br Med J 290:1533, 1985.

Adler SG, Cohen AH, Border WA. Hypersensitivity phenomena and the kidney: Role of drugs and environmental agents. Am J Kidney Dis 5:75, 1985.

Anderson JA. Drug allergies. *In* Bierman CW, Pearlman DS (eds). Allergic Diseases of Infancy, Childhood and Adolescence. Philadelphia, WB Saunders, 1980.

Battegay M, Opravil M, Wuthrich B, et al. Rash with

amoxycillin-clavulanate therapy in HIV-infected patients. Lancet 2:1100, 1989.
Bayard PJ, Berger TG, Jacobson MA. Drug hypersensitivity reactions and human immunodeficiency virus disease. J Acquired Immune Deficiency Syndromes 5:1237, 1992.
Bielory L, Yancey KB, Young NS, et al. Cutaneous manifestations of serum sickness in patients receiving antithymocyte globulin. J Am Acad Dermatol 13:411, 1985.
Bierman CW, VanArsdel PP, Jr. Penicillin allergy in children. J Allergy 43:267, 1969.
Bigby M, Jick S, Jick H, Arndt K. Drug-induced cutaneous reactions: A report from the Boston collaborative drug surveillance program on 15,438 consecutive inpatients, 1975 to 1982. JAMA 256:3358, 1986.
Birnbaum J, Vervloet D. Allergy to muscle relaxants. Clin Rev Allergy 9:281, 1991.
Brandt MA, Gruchalla RS, Sullivan TJ. Skin testing and *in vitro* testing to detect IgE to antimicrobial drugs. J Allergy Clin Immunol 91:263, 1993.
Bryceson ADM. Clinical pathology of the Jarisch-Herxheimer reaction. J Infect Dis 133:696, 1976.
Chusid MJ, Atkins E. Studies on the mechanism of penicillin-induced fever. J Exp Med 136:227, 1972.
Cluff LE, Caranasos GJ, Stewart RB. Clinical Problems with Drugs. Philadelphia, WB Saunders, 1975.
Coopman SA, Johnson RA, Platt R, et al. Cutaneous disease and drug reactions in HIV infection. N Engl J Med 328:1670, 1993.
Cronin E, Bandmann HJ, Calnan CD, et al. Contact dermatitis in the atopic. Acta Dermvenereol 50:183, 1970.
Davies DM (ed). Textbook of Adverse Drug Reactions. 4th ed. New York, Oxford University Press, 1991.
Derbes VJ. The fixed eruption. JAMA 190:765, 1964.
Dinarello C, Cannon JG, Wolff SM. New concepts on the pathogenesis of fever. Rev Infect Dis 10:168, 1988.
Feigin RD, Shearer WT. Fever of unknown origin in children. Curr Prob Pediatr vol. 6, no. 10, 1976.
Gilliland BC. Drug-induced autoimmune and hematologic disorders. Immunol Allergy Clin North Am 11:525, 1991.
Gilman AG, Rall TW, Nies AS, Taylor P (eds). Goodman and Gilman's The Pharmacological Basis of Therapeutics, 8th ed. New York, Macmillan, 1990.
Graff-Lonnevig V, Hedlin G, Lindfors A. Penicillin allergy—a rare paediatric condition? Arch Dis Child 63:1342, 1988.
Grammer LC, Roberts M, Patterson R. IgE and IgG antibody against human (recombinant DNA) insulin in patients with systemic insulin allergy. J Lab Clin Med 105:108, 1985.
Greenberger PA, Patterson R. The prevention of immediate generalized reactions to radiocontrast media in high-risk patients. J Allergy Clin Immunol 87:867, 1991.
Israeli ZH, Hall WD. Cough and angioneurotic edema associated with angiotensin-converting enzyme inhibitor therapy. Ann Intern Med 117:234, 1992.
Kamada MM, Twarog F, Leung DYM. Multiple antibiotic sensitivity in a pediatric population. Allergy Proc 12:347, 1991.
Kirtland HH, III, Mohler DN, Horwitz DA. Methyldopa inhibition of suppressor-lymphocyte function. A proposed cause of autoimmune hemolytic anemia. N Engl J Med 302:825, 1980.
Knutsen AP, Anderson J, Satayaviboon S, et al. Immunologic aspects of phenobarbital hypersensitivity. J Pediatr 105:558, 1984.
Kovacs JA, Hiemenz JW, Macher AM, et al. *Pneumocystis carinii* pneumonia: A comparison between patients with the acquired immunodeficiency syndrome and patients with other immunodeficiencies. Ann Intern Med 100:663, 1984.
Kuokkanen L. Drug eruptions: a series of 464 cases in the Department of Dermatology, University of Turku, Finland, during 1966–1970. Acta Allergol 27:407, 1972.
Lakin JD, Grace WR, Sell KW. IgE antipolymyxin B antibody formation in a T cell-depleted bone marrow transplant patient. J Allergy Clin Immunol 56:94, 1975.
Landsteiner K, Jacobs J. Studies on the sensitization of animals with simple chemical compounds. J Exp Med 61:643, 1935.
Lasser EC. Pseudoallergic drug reactions: Radiographic contrast media. Immunol Allergy Clin North Am 11:645, 1991.
Levine BB. Immunochemical mechanisms of drug allergy. Ann Rev Med 17:23, 1966.
Levine BB, Zolov DM. Prediction of penicillin allergy by immunological tests. J Allergy 43:231, 1969.
Lipton MA, Mayo JP. Diet and hyperkinesis—an update. J Am Diet Assoc 83:132, 1983.
Mackel SE, Jordon RE. Leukocytoclastic vasculitis: A cutaneous expression of immune complex disease. Arch Dermatol 118:296, 1982.
Mackert JR, Fisher AA. Hypersensitivity to mercury from dental amalgams. J Am Acad Dermatol 12:877, 1985.
Manning ME, Stevenson DD. Pseudoallergic drug reactions: Aspirin, nonsteroidal anti-inflammatory drugs, dyes, additives, and preservatives. Immunol Allergy Clin North Am 11:659, 1991.
McKenzie MW, Marchall GL, Netzloff ML, et al. Adverse drug reactions leading to hospitalization. J Pediatr 89:487, 1976.
Mitchell GG, Magnusson AR, Weiler JM. Cimetidine-induced cutaneous vasculitis. Am J Med 75:875, 1983.
Moss RB, Babin S, Hsu YP, et al. Allergy to semisynthetic penicillins in cystic fibrosis. J Pediatr 104:460, 1984.
Obermiller T, Lakshminarayan S. Drug-induced hypersensitivity reactions in the lung. Immunol Allergy Clin North Am 11:575, 1991.
Parker PJ, Parrinello JT, Condemi JJ, et al. Penicillin resensitization among hospitalized patients. J Allergy Clin Immunol 88:213, 1991.
Pegram PS, Mountz JD, O'Bar PR. Ethambutol-induced toxic epidermal necrolysis. Arch Intern Med 141:1677, 1981.
Petrozzi JW, Shore RN. Generalized exfoliative dermatitis from ethylenediamine. Arch Dermatol 112:525, 1976.
Petz LD. Drug-induced immune hemolysis. N Engl J Med 313:510, 1985.
Pohl LB, Saton H, Christ DD, et al. Neoantigens associated with halothane hepatitis. Drug Metab Rev 20:203, 1989.
Purdy BH, Philips DM, Summers RW. Desensitization for sulfasalazine skin rash. Ann Intern Med 100:512, 1984.
Rieder MJ, Uetrecht J, Shear NH, et al. Diagnosis of sulfonamide hypersensitivity reactions by *in-vitro* "rechallenge" with hydroxylamine metabolites. Ann Intern Med 110:286, 1989.
Rocklin RE. Clinical applications of *in vitro* lymphocyte tests. In Schwartz RS (ed). Progress in Clinical Immunology. Vol. 2. New York, Grune and Stratton, 1974.
Ross JM. Allergy to insulin. Pediatr Clin North Am 31:675, 1984.

Rudolph AH, Price EV. Penicillin reactions among patients in venereal disease clinics: a national survey. JAMA 223:499, 1973.

Salama A, Mueller-Eckhardt C. The role of metabolite-specific antibodies in nomifesine-dependent immune hemolytic anemia. N Engl J Med 313:469, 1985.

Samter M (ed). Excerpts from Classics in Allergy (see Jadassohn J, page 27). Columbus, Ohio, Ross Laboratories, 1969.

Schuchter LM, Hendricks CB, Holland KH, et al. Eosinophilic myocarditis associated with high-dose interleukin-2 therapy. Am J Med 88:439, 1990.

Schwartz HJ, Sher TH. Bisulfite intolerance manifests as bronchospasm following topical dipivefrin hydrochloride therapy for glaucoma. Arch Ophthalmol 103:14, 1985.

Settipane GA. Adverse reactions to sulfites in drugs and foods. J Am Acad Dermatol 10:1077, 1984.

Shepherd GM. Allergy to β-lactam antibiotics. Immunol Allergy Clin North Am 11:611, 1991.

Shulman NR. A mechanism of cell destruction in individuals sensitized to foreign antigens and its implications in autoimmunity: combined clinical staff conference at the National Institutes of Health. Ann Intern Med 60:506, 1964.

Sogn DD, Evans R, Shepherd GM, et al. Results of the National Institute of Allergy and Infectious Diseases collaborative clinical trial to test the predictive value of skin testing with major and minor penicillin derivatives in hospitalized adults. Arch Intern Med 152:1025, 1992.

Storrs FJ. Contact dermatitis caused by drugs. Immunol Allergy Clin North Am 11:509, 1991.

Sullivan TJ, Yecies LD, Schatz GS, et al. Desensitization of patients allergic to penicillin using orally administered beta-lactam antibiotics. J Allergy Clin Immunol 69:275, 1982.

Szabadi E. Neuroleptic malignant syndrome. Br Med J 288:1399, 1984.

VanArsdel PP Jr. Serum antibodies to red cell conjugates in penicillin allergy. In Stewart GT, McGovern JP (eds). Penicillin Allergy. Springfield, Charles C Thomas, 1970.

VanArsdel PP Jr. Adverse drug reactions. In Middleton E, Reed CE, Ellis EF (eds). Allergy: Principles and Practice. 2nd ed. St. Louis, CV Mosby, 1983.

VanArsdel PP. Classification and risk factors for drug allergy. Immunol Allergy Clin North Am 11:475, 1991a.

VanArsdel PP. Pseudoallergic drug reactions: Introduction and general review. Immunol Allergy Clin North Am 11:635, 1991b.

VanArsdel PP, Larson EB. Diagnostic tests for patients with suspected allergic disease: Utility and limitations. Ann Intern Med 110:304, 1989.

VanArsdel PP Jr, Martonick GJ, Johnson LE, et al. The value of skin testing for penicillin allergy diagnosis. West J Med 144:311, 1986.

Vincent A, Newsom-Davis J, Martin V. Anti-acetylcholine receptor antibodies in D-penicillamine-associated myasthenia gravis. Lancet 1:1254, 1978.

Vulto AG, de Smet PAGM. Drugs used in non-orthodox medicine. In Dukes MNG (ed). Meyler's Side Effects of Drugs. 11th ed. Amsterdam, Elsevier Science Publishing, 1988.

Weiss ME, Nyhan D, Peng Z, et al. Association of protamine IgE and IgG antibodies with life-threatening reactions to intravenous protamine. N Engl J Med 320:866, 1989.

Weitzman SA, Stossel TP, Desmond M. Drug-induced immunological neutropenia. Lancet 1:1068, 1978.

Whyte J, Greenan E. Drug usage and adverse drug reactions in paediatric patients. Acta Paediatr Scand 66:767, 1977.

Willson RA. The liver: Its role in drug biotransformation and as a target of immunologic injury. Immunol Allergy Clin North Am 11:555, 1991.

Zaloga GP, Delacey W, Holmboe E, et al. Glucagon reversal of hypotension in a case of anaphylactoid shock. Ann Intern Med 105:65, 1986.

Chapter 23
Allergic Reactions to Insect Stings

David B.K. Golden, M.D.

The globe is covered almost in its entirety with insects, many of which have plagued mankind since antiquity. Insect bites and stings cause a wide range of reactions in humans; most are toxic but some are allergic. At their worst, insect stings have long been recognized as a potential cause of severe and often life-threatening reactions in susceptible individuals. Attempts at treatment have had limited success, and only in the past 15 years has medical research established effective modes of therapy and acquired sufficient understanding of the disease to guide therapy intelligently.

Insect bites and stings usually cause transient local inflammation, and some can cause toxic symptoms (especially when they are multiple). Allergic reactions can cause more severe local or generalized reactions. Large local reactions often represent late-phase allergic reactions which evolve over 24 to 48 hours to a maximal induration of 8 cm or more and resolve in 2 to 7 days. Systemic (generalized) reactions may include any of the signs and symptoms of anaphylaxis. Unusual patterns of reaction have been reported including nephropathy, central and peripheral neurologic syndromes, idiopathic thrombocytopenic purpura, and rhabdomyolysis; most of these are not IgE mediated. The danger from the notorious africanized honeybee ("killer bee") stems from the numbers of stings because of the swarm-and-attack behavior of this strain of honeybee rather than any greater allergenicity or toxicity of their venom, which is in fact similar to that of other honeybees.

EPIDEMIOLOGY AND NATURAL HISTORY

Surveys of children and adults have shown that insect sting allergy is more common than previously thought. In published surveys, systemic allergic reactions were reported by approximately 3 percent of adults, whereas less than 1 percent of children had severe sting reactions. The frequency of large local reactions is uncertain but is estimated at 10 percent in adults. There are at least 50 fatal sting reactions each year in the United States, and it is believed that many other sting fatalities are unrecognized. It has recently proved possible to document the presence of venom-specific IgE antibodies as well as elevated serum tryptase in postmortem blood samples, demonstrating the pathophysiology of the fatal reaction in cases of unexplained sudden death. However, the presence of IgE antibodies to Hymenoptera venom is not at all unusual. Recent surveys suggest that allergic sensitization is common: over 30 percent of adults stung in the previous 3 months showed venom-specific IgE by skin test or RAST, and over 20 percent of all adults tested positive (Golden et al, 1989c). The majority of subjects have no history of allergic sting reactions and constitute a previously unrecognized group with asymptomatic sensitization and a potential risk of future anaphylaxis. Sensitivity is often transient, disappearing more rapidly than it does in patients with a history of anaphylaxis. Although the venom-specific IgE became negative in 50 percent after 3 to 5 years in one study, those who remained positive showed a significant 15 to 20 percent risk of a systemic reaction to a sting (Golden et al, 1992).

The natural history of Hymenoptera venom sensitivity has only recently come under study, but it is crucial in clinical decision making. It was the lack of this information that led to the mistaken conclusion that whole-body extract therapy was effective in the prevention of anaphylaxis. The apparent efficacy ("success") of whole-body extracts was overestimated because many low-risk patients were studied along with the patients who had recent sting anaphylaxis. We now know that the maximum risk of reaction is 50 percent, as shown in the placebo-controlled trial of venom immunotherapy (Hunt et al, 1978). Furthermore, low-risk patients include the majority of children (because most have had strictly cutaneous sting reactions and have less than 10 percent risk) (Valentine et al, 1990) and patients with large local reactions (<10 percent risk). In addition, the allergy is self-limited in many cases, but this was not reliably reflected by the whole-body extract skin tests used at that time for diagnostic identification. When these various factors are added together, our current knowledge would predict a "success" rate of over 80 percent even for placebo in the collections of patients studied. The actual risk of reaction in "high-risk" patients falls from 50 percent initially to 35 percent after 3 to 5 years, and perhaps 20 percent risk with a remote history of reaction more than 10 years earlier (Reisman, 1992). However, there remain individuals in whom the risk of anaphylaxis persists for decades even with no intervening stings.

Allergy to insect sting can occur at any age, often following a number of uneventful stings. Sensitization requires at least one previous sting, but this may be remote and forgotten. Allergic reactions to insect stings occur more frequently in cases of frequent exposure and intermittent stings, as in individuals engaged in agriculture, landscaping, or beekeeping and in children and other people who spend a great deal of time outdoors. Although often familial, this condition is not statistically more likely in those with a family history of sting reactions, and there is only a weak correlation with other allergic conditions.

The common symptoms and signs of allergic reactions to insect stings in adults and children are shown in Table 23–1. Children have a higher frequency of isolated cutaneous reactions and a lower frequency of vascular symptoms and anaphylactic shock compared to adults. Systemic reactions can become progressively more severe with each sting in some cases but usually follow a more predictable and reproducible pattern for each individual patient. It is important to note that any single manifestation can occur alone, making a diagnosis more difficult. Objective evidence of hypotension, wheezing, stridor, airflow reduction, or typical urticaria/angioedema facilitates the diagnosis. There are no specific laboratory measurements that diagnose anaphylaxis; however, serum tryptase levels can be measured hours or days after the event. Skin or serologic tests for IgE antibodies to the suspected insect venoms should be performed days or weeks later to confirm the diagnosis.

TABLE 23–1. SYMPTOMS AND SIGNS OF INSECT STING ANAPHYLAXIS IN ADULTS AND CHILDREN

	FREQUENCY	
SYMPTOM OR SIGN	Adults	Children
Cutaneous only	15	60
Urticaria/angioedema	80	95
Dizziness/hypotension	60	10
Dyspnea/wheezing	50	40
Throat tightness/hoarseness	40	40
Loss of consciousness	30	5

From Golden DBK, Lichtenstein LM. Insect sting allergy. *In* Kaplan AP (ed). Allergy. New York, Churchill Livingstone, 1985, pp 507–524.

ETIOLOGY

Anaphylaxis, although reported to occur from bed bugs and kissing bugs (*Triatoma* spp), is exceedingly rare from biting insects. Allergic reaction due to inhalation of insect-derived proteins is not within the scope of this review. Only stinging insects cause significant problems with anaphylaxis, and the only insects that possess true stingers are those of the order Hymenoptera. There are three families of importance; bees (honeybees, bumblebees) and vespids (yellow jackets, hornets, wasps) are best known. In recent years, fire ants (*Solenopsis* spp) have become a rapidly increasing public health hazard in the southeast and south central states, especially on the Gulf Coast of the United States (DeShazo et al, 1990). Early attempts to prevent sting anaphylaxis by immunotherapy were directed by a misconception that the sensitivity was related to an "intrinsic bee protein" thought to be present in the whole body and in venom. Ultimately, the application of immunologic and epidemiologic methods demonstrated that whole-body extract therapy was no more effective than placebo, and that venom immunotherapy is 98 percent effective in the prevention of anaphylaxis (Golden et al, 1981; Hunt et al, 1978).

The immunochemical characteristics of Hymenoptera venoms have been thoroughly studied and their immunogenetic relationships elucidated through protein sequencing (Hoffman, 1993). The three important allergenic proteins in honeybee venom are phospholipase A_2, hyaluronidase, and acid phosphatase, although the quantitatively greatest component is mellitin. The allergens are immunochemically distinct from the three major allergens in vespid venoms: phospholipase, hyaluronidase, and the primary allergen, antigen 5. The vespid venoms have a high degree of cross-reactivity and contain essentially the same allergens. The yellow jacket and hornet venoms are so closely related that 95 percent of vespid-allergic patients have positive skin tests to all three of the common vespid skin test preparations: yellow jacket, yellow hornet, white-faced hornet. *Polistes* wasps are more distantly related to the other vespids, and only 50 percent of patients allergic to yellow jacket have positive tests to wasp venom. Fire ant venoms are quite different in that they contain very little protein in an unusual suspension of alkaloid toxins, which cause the characteristic painful vesicular eruption, often in a circle where the insect has pivoted on its mandible while stinging repeatedly. The allergenic proteins are unique except for one, which shows limited cross-reactivity with vespid allergen 5.

DIAGNOSIS

The diagnosis of insect sting allergy rests primarily on the history since venom-specific IgE antibodies are also present in many clinically nonreactive individuals. A positive skin test to insect venom is confirmatory evidence of the allergic sting reaction and helps to define the allergenic specificity of the reaction. The history is of paramount importance and should be reviewed in detail with respect to the nature and timing of stings in the past, the time course of the reaction, and all associated symptoms and treatments. Symptoms are sometimes exaggerated by fear, panic, exercise, heat, alcohol, or underlying cardiorespiratory disease (arrhythmia, heart failure, angina, COPD, asthma). However, symptoms can also be subtle, leading some patients to underestimate their significance. The identity of the insect is a notoriously unreliable part of the history, but the location and timing of the sting or the location of the nest may suggest the type of insect. Honeybee stings are much more common in children and others who run barefoot; in the United States, the large majority of stings in adults is due to yellow jackets.

The standard method of testing is with the intradermal skin test technique using the five Hymenoptera venom protein extracts. Whole-body extracts, still commercially available despite an FDA advisory against their use, contain little or no venom, and do not distinguish allergic from nonallergic individuals. An important exception is the case of fire ant sensitivity, which can be tested with reasonable diagnostic sensitivity and specificity utilizing whole-body extracts of imported fire ants. Preliminary studies suggest the superiority of fire ant venom extract, but commercial preparations are still under development. For Hymenoptera venom testing, prick tests at 0.001 µg/ml may be used initially for patients with a history of severe reactions. Intradermal tests are performed with venom concentrations beginning with 0.001 µg/ml and increasing to to 1.0 µg/ml to find the minimum concentration giving a positive (5/20 mm) result. Even when there has only been a single reaction to a sting, sensitization may have occurred to multiple venoms, and skin testing should be performed with a complete set of Hymenoptera venoms, as well as the usual negative diluent (HSA-saline) control and a positive histamine control.

Skin test results are easily interpreted in most cases because the vast majority of those with a convincing history are clearly positive and a few are clearly negative. Negative skin tests in a history-positive patient are usually associated with lack of contact with the insect for many years and may represent the loss of sensitivity (see Epidemiology and Natural History). In patients with more recent sting anaphylaxis, negative skin tests are rare but occur during the refractory period of "anergy" for several weeks after a sting reaction. Skin tests may be repeated after 1 to 6 months, when they may become positive. Some cases of apparent sting anaphylaxis are thought to be non-IgE-mediated. It is unclear whether they represent subclinical mastocytosis or simply mast cell hyperreleasability with nonimmune release of mast cell mediators. There are many different patterns of venom skin test sensitivity. Most importantly, the degree of skin test sensitivity does not correlate reliably with the degree of clinical sting reaction. The strongest skin tests often occur in patients who have had only large local reactions and have a very low risk of anaphylaxis, whereas some patients who have had abrupt and near-fatal anaphylactic shock show only weak skin test or serologic sensitivity. In fact, almost 25 percent of patients presenting for systemic allergic reactions to stings have been skin test positive only at the 1.0 µg/ml concentration, demonstrating the importance of skin testing with the full diagnostic range of concentrations. These cases emphasize that it is the history that is primarily responsible for the diagnosis.

The diagnosis of insect allergy by detection of allergen-specific IgE antibodies in serum (typically by RAST or similar serologic tests) is a method of high potential but variable performance. The test is often qualitative, poorly standardized, and negative in at least 15 to 20 percent of patients skin testing positive for sting allergy. When it is clearly elevated, a high level of venom-specific IgE is diagnostic, and the level has been used as a marker for the effectiveness of therapy in diminishing sensitivity.

TREATMENT

Acute reactions to insect stings are treated symptomatically with ice, rest, and antihistamines for local reactions. Massive local reactions, especially involving the head and neck, are best treated with a brief burst of prednisone (30 to 40 mg, tapering to zero in 4 days). Hives may respond to antihistamines alone, but any sign of hypotension or respiratory obstruction should be treated promptly with aqueous epinephrine 1:1000, 0.3 to 0.5 cc subcutaneously, and should have full emergency medical attention and observation for 6 hours or more (see also Chapter 21). Some individuals are resistant to epinephrine, especially those on beta blockers. Anaphylaxis is often prolonged or recurrent for 6 to 24 hours and may require intensive medical care. Emergency medical care of anaphylaxis is generally efficient, but there are two major problems. Patients themselves usually do not seek medical attention since the reaction subsides spontaneously after 1 to 2 hours in most cases and is misjudged to be a chance occurrence. Even in medical history taking, patients often fail to admit sting reactions without specific inquiry. A second problem is the follow-up information given (or not given) to the patient on discharge from emergency care. Many patients are not specifically instructed in the need for an epinephrine kit, an allergy consultation, and preventive treatment. Pediatric-dose epinephrine injection kits are also available. All patients should understand that using the kit is not a substitute for emergency medical attention. The best treatment is prevention, and the best prevention is education.

VENOM IMMUNOTHERAPY

Venom immunotherapy is the preventive treatment of choice but requires the careful selection of patients, a period of initial treatment to induce a protective immune state, regular monitoring during maintenance therapy, and long-term decisions about when to stop. Current indications for venom immunotherapy require a history of previous systemic allergic reaction to a sting and evidence of a positive venom skin test. Patients with a negative skin test are not eligible regardless of history: they may have lost sensitivity but a few seem to have non-IgE-mediated reactions. Some patients with positive skin tests do not need venom immunotherapy because they are judged to be at low risk for anaphylaxis. Epidemiologic studies have helped to estimate the risk of reaction. The highest risk, in those with a recent history of anaphylaxis and a positive skin test, is 50 percent since only half of these individuals react to a challenge sting. A low risk (<10 percent) has been found in children and adults with a history of large local reactions, and in children with reactions limited to cutaneous signs and symptoms but with no respiratory or vascular manifestations (Reisman, 1992). In these cases, venom immunotherapy is not required, but some patients will still request treatment because of their fear of reaction and the impact on their life style. There are insufficient data on the risk of anaphylaxis in adults with strictly cutaneous reactions, especially since this presentation is unusual in adults but is the predominant form in children (see Table 23–1). Since there are cases of progression in adults from cutaneous reactions to life-threatening anaphylaxis on subsequent stings, adults with cutaneous systemic reactions are still advised to undergo venom immunotherapy. Unfortunately, both for large local and cutaneous reactors, there is no test that predicts which patients will progress to more severe reactions. In some cases the decision regarding immunotherapy is complicated by factors that would seem to reduce the risk but are of unknown significance. When the sting reaction was in the remote past, especially when intervening stings have caused little or no reaction, even a positive skin test is not always convincing enough to require venom immunotherapy. Some patients report reactions only with multiple or sequential stings, but not from isolated single stings.

Initial venom immunotherapy follows a schedule, which may vary according to the recommendations of the source laboratory that has prepared the allergen extract. The common "modified rush" regimen is more rapid than traditional regimens, achieving maintenance dose in eight weekly injections, instead of the 4- to 6-month regimens that are more commonly utilized for inhalant allergen immunotherapy. With this regimen, adverse reactions are no more common than in traditional regimens of inhalant allergen therapy, and the mean venom-specific IgG antibody response is greater and more rapidly achieved, although both regimens are equally effective. The recommended maintenance dose is 100 µg of each venom giving a positive skin test. Lower doses may not give an adequate immune response in 15 to 20 percent of patients, whereas standard therapy is at least 98 percent effective in completely preventing the systemic allergic reaction. The same recommendations have been made for children age 3 and over; there are few reports of half-dose therapy in children, although their immune response to venom immunotherapy is double that of adults (Fig. 23–1).

The selection of venom extracts to be used for immunotherapy is dependent on the venom skin test reaction to those venoms. Therapy should include all that are positive,

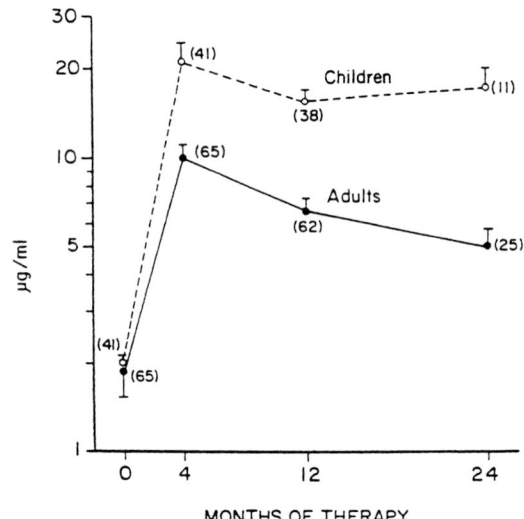

FIGURE 23–1. Anti–yellow jacket venom IgG concentration (µg/ml; mean + SEM) during venom immunotherapy in children and adults (n for each point shown in parentheses). (From Golden DBK, Valentine MD. Allergen-specific IgG antibody measurements in the management of immediate hypersensitivity to Hymenoptera venoms. J Clin Immunoassay 6:172–176, 1983.)

since a guarantee of not reacting to the next sting is not possible without therapy if the skin test is positive. For this reason, the most common therapy when vespids are involved is with the mixed vespid venoms preparation (equal parts yellow jacket, yellow hornet, and white-faced hornet venoms). Although therapy with yellow jacket venom alone has been shown to protect against hornet stings because of the marked cross-reactivity of the *Vespula* venoms, there are also reports that therapy with any single venom gives 15 to 20 percent less immune response and less reliable clinical protection than mixed vespid venoms. The three component venoms in mixed vespid venom effectively present double the yellow jacket allergen load as that of any single venom. The skin test is also positive to *Polistes* wasp venoms in at least 50 percent of vespid-allergic patients; when positive it is usually included in therapy as a separate injection. Therapy with yellow jacket or mixed vespid venoms can protect against wasp stings, but this has only been established for patients whose wasp-specific IgE showed complete cross-reactivity with yellow jacket venom as assessed by RAST inhibition (Hamilton et al, 1993).

Fire ant immunotherapy is still at an early

stage of development since the natural history of fire ant allergy is still unclear (DeShazo et al, 1990). However, there is a clear and increasing need for effective immunotherapy. Ongoing trials suggest that fire ant whole-body extract immunotherapy is reasonably safe and effective and should be employed in cases of significant systemic reaction. More reliable clinical protection with improved safety is the goal of current studies to develop the fire ant venoms for clinical diagnostic and therapeutic use.

Adverse reactions to venom immunotherapy are no more common than reactions during inhalant allergen immunotherapy. Systemic symptoms occur in 5 to 15 percent of patients during the initial weeks of treatment, regardless of the regimen used. Most reactions are mild, and fewer than 5 percent require epinephrine. In the unusual case of recurrent systemic reactions to injections, therapy may be streamlined to a single venom and given in divided doses, 30 minutes apart. Rarely, therapy has to be suspended for 6 to 12 months in order to be able to advance toward protective maintenance doses. Large local reactions are common, occurring in up to 50 percent of patients, especially in the dose range of 20 to 50 μg. Unlike standard inhalant immunotherapy, there is a uniform target dose in venom immunotherapy, and so it is occasionally necessary to advance the dose in the face of moderately severe local reactions (8 to 10 cm), beyond what might otherwise be considered the "maximum tolerated dose."

Maintenance therapy is administered every 4 weeks for at least a year, and then may be given at lengthening intervals of every 6 to 8 weeks over several years in most cases. For those patients and physicians who seek confirmation of the immune protection, only some assays for venom-specific IgG have correlated strongly with clinical protection (see Fig. 23–1). The test is used to confirm protective levels after initial therapy and then to determine whether the venom-specific IgG level is adequately maintained at longer maintenance intervals. In the most extensively validated assay, the IgG level was considered protective when >3 μg/ml during 1 to 4 years of maintenance therapy, but when the monthly maintenance dose is first reached (4 to 6 months), the IgG should preferably achieve levels >5 μg/ml. Repeat skin tests or RASTs are performed to determine when there has been a significant decline in venom-specific IgE, usually every 2 to 3 years. Skin tests generally remain unchanged in the first 2 to 3 years, but show a significant decline after 4 to 6 years. Less than 20 percent of patients are skin test negative after 5 years, but 50 to 60 percent become negative after 7 to 10 years (Golden et al, 1989b). Venom-specific IgE antibody levels before immunotherapy average 10 ng/ml in adults and 20 ng/ml in children; the level rises in the first months of therapy, returns to baseline after 12 months, and then declines steadily during maintenance treatment (even after therapy is stopped and even after a sting) (Golden et al, 1989a).

The duration of venom immunotherapy is still not uniformly defined. The question is no longer whether venom immunotherapy can be discontinued, but when and with what risk factors. The original recommendations approved for the product insert in the United States were that therapy should be continued until the skin tests (or RASTs) become negative. This has been successful in the small number of patients who do become negative. Skin test positive patients who prematurely discontinue therapy after 1 to 2 years still have a substantially increased risk of systemic reaction to a sting. However, study of over 100 adults and children has shown that even when there is persistent venom-specific IgE, venom immunotherapy may be stopped after 5 years with a 5 to 10 percent risk of systemic symptoms after a sting, but only a 2 percent risk of a reaction requiring epinephrine treatment (Golden et al, 1989a). In the patients who did relapse, there was an association with a lack of skin test suppression during immunotherapy and with a history of a systemic reaction to a sting or an injection during the period of venom immunotherapy. In this study, there was no greater reaction rate in patients with a history of near-fatal pretreatment sting reactions than in the patients who had milder reactions. Further studies will have to examine whether therapy may be stopped sooner in patients with a history of milder reactions or in children (Reisman, 1992). Reassuring, too, is the observation that even after stopping venom treatment, the venom-specific IgE declines steadily with time and shows no sign of persistent increase after challenge stings. Venom-specific IgG levels fall to subtherapeutic levels within months of discontinuing therapy and are unrelated to the apparent loss of reactivity to the sting. Current immunologic evidence supports the hypothesis that a cellular suppression is induced by high-dose immunotherapy but only after 4 or 5 years. Some patients will prefer the security of continuing treatment even though the apparent risk of stopping therapy is in the 5 percent range judged acceptable for other "low-risk" patients (large local reactors and children with cutaneous systemic reactions).

CONCLUSION

Insect sting allergy is common but should be preventable. Public education is needed to encourage people to tell their physicians about allergic reactions to insect stings (or foods, drugs, or latex for that matter), to encourage emergency room staff to provide information to patients who have had anaphylaxis about the need for allergy consultation, preventive immunotherapy, and how to use an epinephrine self-treatment kit. These kits should be more readily available to affected individuals in schools and in public recreation and transportation areas. Venom immunotherapy has been a model not only for public education in allergy, but also of the clinical use of highly purified and standardized allergenic extracts to virtually cure a life-threatening anaphylactic sensitivity.

REFERENCES

DeShazo RD, Butcher BT, Banks WA. Reactions to the stings of the imported fire ant. N Engl J Med 323:462–466, 1990.

Golden DBK, Langlois J, Valentine MD. Treatment failures with whole body extract therapy of insect sting allergy. JAMA 246:2460–2463, 1981.

Golden DBK, Addison BI, Gadde J, Kagey-Sobotka A, Valentine MD, Lichtenstein LM. Prospective observations on patients who discontinue venom immunotherapy. J Allergy Clin Immunol 84:162–167, 1989a.

Golden DBK, Kwiterovich KA, Kagey-Sobotka A, Valentine MD, Lichtenstein LM. Discontinuing venom immunotherapy: Determinants of clinical reactivity. J Allergy Clin Immunol 83:273, 1989b.

Golden DBK, Marsh DG, Kagey-Sobotka A, et al. Epidemiology of insect sting allergy. JAMA 262:240–244, 1989c.

Golden DBK, Addison BI, Kwiterovich KA, et al. Natural history of Hymenoptera venom allergy in adults. J Allergy Clin Immunol 89:291, 1992.

Hamilton RH, Wisenauer JA, Golden DBK, Valentine MD, Adkinson NF Jr. Selection of Hymenoptera venoms for immunotherapy based on patients' IgE antibody cross-reactivity. J Allergy Clin Immunol 92:651–659, 1993.

Hoffman DR. Allergens in Hymenoptera venom. XXV. The amino acid sequence of Antigen 5 molecules. The structural basis of antigenic crossreactivity. J Allergy Clin Immunol 92:707–716, 1993.

Hunt KJ, Valentine MD, Sobotka AK, et al. A controlled trial of immunotherapy in insect hypersensitivity. N Engl J Med 299:157–161, 1978.

Reisman RE. Natural history of insect sting allergy: Relationship of severity of symptoms of initial sting anaphylaxis to re-sting reactions. J Allergy Clin Immunol 90:335–339, 1992.

Valentine MD, Schuberth KC, Kagey-Sobotka A, et al. The value of immunotherapy with venom in children with allergy to insect stings. N Engl J Med 323:1601–1603, 1990.

Chapter 24

Radiocontrast, Local Anesthetic, and Latex Reactions

Frank S. Virant, M.D.

RADIOCONTRAST

Intravascular radiocontrast is used in over 10 million radiologic examinations annually in the United States. The overall frequency of adverse reactions is 5 to 8 percent, and life-threatening reactions occur with a frequency of 0.05 to 0.1 percent (Bush and Swanson, 1991). Over the last decade, with the increased usage of lower osmolality media, the overall risk of adverse reaction has been reduced by 70 to 80 percent. Nonetheless, reactions still occur, and as a practical point, the conventional agents still tend to be used more frequently because they are significantly less expensive.

Appropriate intervention in response to adverse radiocontrast reactions should be based on an understanding of the mechanism of such events. With this knowledge, the clinician can promptly institute corrective therapy when adverse reactions occur. Also, many adverse reactions to intravascular contrast can be prevented by the use of pre-treatment protocols and recognition of the high-risk patient (see also Chapter 21).

Adverse Reactions

Classification

Intravascular radiocontrast reactions are either anaphylactoid or chemotoxic. Although anaphylactoid reactions are more common, the chemotoxic effects of radiocontrast may account for more severe events, particularly in the debilitated patient. Since many adverse reaction events are vascular in nature, it is important to differentiate clinical signs of the reaction from aspects of the patient's underlying disease.

Anaphylactoid (anaphylaxis-like) reactions to radiocontrast are independent of the dosage or concentration of the offending agent. Clinically, these reactions may resemble allergic hypersensitivity events, and yet they do not appear to result from antigen-antibody interactions (Thrall, 1990). There is evidence that radiocontrast can directly release histamine from mast cells, and yet there does not appear to be a correlation between the amount of histamine release and the severity of adverse effects. Activation of other systems, including complement, kinin, and coagulation also may occur after the administration of radiocontrast, leading to the release of a variety of vascular mediators. However, the degree of system activation by radiocontrast does not correlate with the production of observable adverse events. On the other hand, if these systems are pre-activated, the patient may be more susceptible to an adverse reaction to radiocontrast.

Chemotoxic reactions to radiocontrast are directly related to a physicochemical effect of the medium, and such reactions are dose and concentration dependent. Chemotoxic events are largely due to the hyperosmolar character of radiocontrast, but are also affected by calcium-binding properties and ionic strength (Table 24–1). Clinically, chemotoxic reactions

TABLE 24-1. CHEMOTOXIC EFFECTS OF RADIOCONTRAST MEDIA*

Vascular
  Increased osmolality → Hypervolemia, ↑ Cardiac output
  Altered permeability → Inflammation, Pain, Microthrombi
  Dilated vessels → Altered blood flow/pressure, pain
Cerebral
  Dilated external carotid artery
  Stimulate chemoreceptors → Altered blood pressure, Heart rate†
  Altered blood-brain barrier permeability
  Altered neuro-electrical activity
Cardiac
  Dilated coronary artery
  Altered EKG → Bradycardia, Conduction delays
  Ventricular fibrillation‡
  Decreased myocardial contractility‡
Renal
  Renovascular constriction → Decreased renal blood flow
  Altered glomerular permeability
  Proteinuria
  Osmotic diuresis

Adapted from Bush WH, Swanson DP. Acute reactions to intravascular contrast media: Types, risk factors, recognition, and specific treatment. Am J Roentgenol 157:1154, 1991.
*Reactions due to hyperosmolality except as noted.
†Also due to sodium ion concentration.
‡Secondary to calcium binding effects.

appear as local or systemic vascular irritant effects: pain, altered blood flow, altered blood pressure, abnormal cardiac conduction, and decreased renal function.

Prevalence

Among the 5 to 8 percent of patients who experience an adverse reaction to conventional radiocontrast, most have minor reactions that require no specific treatment (Shehadi and Toniolo, 1980). About 1 percent of patients will have a moderate reaction such as severe vomiting, diffuse urticaria, or angioedema, which requires therapy. Life-threatening reactions occur in one of every 1000 to 2000 examinations in which conventional radiocontrast is used. Although studies quote a wide spectrum of mortality, a reasonable estimate is one in every 75,000 patients (Katayama et al, 1990).

With the recent development of lower osmolality radiocontrast media, it would appear that the overall risk of anaphylactoid reactions is decreased to about one fifth that of conventional media (Bettman, 1990). On the other hand, the relative risk of adverse renal effects in patients receiving radiocontrast does not seem to be significantly different between conventional and lower osmolality contrast media (Schwab et al, 1989).

Risk Factors

The prevalence of adverse radiocontrast reactions appears to be greatest for 20- to 50-year-old patients. This prevalence rate is lowest for patients under 20 years of age. When adverse reactions to radiocontrast occur, however, they are frequently most severe in elderly persons. This is probably because older patients often have preexisting vascular disease and thus have less "reserve" when blood flow is compromised.

The patient group at highest risk for adverse radiocontrast reactions are those who have experienced a prior adverse event. This group is, in fact, three to eight times more likely to react than the general population (Witten, 1975). Other patient groups with relative increased risk include asthmatic (Bush and Swanson, 1991) and atopic patients in general (Enright et al, 1989) (Table 24-2).

Treatment of Acute Reactions

Although acute reactions may occur in many clinical combinations, it is useful to categorize adverse events as follows: nausea/vomiting; urticaria; bronchospasm; hypotension; anaphylactoid reaction; vasovagal reaction; cardiovascular collapse; and seizures. Table 24-3 and the following paragraphs reflect

TABLE 24-2. RISK FACTORS FOR ADVERSE RADIOCONTRAST REACTION

Factor	Relative Risk*
Prior radiocontrast reaction	3–8×
Asthma	5×
Allergy (atopy)	2×

*Compared to unexposed general population.

TABLE 24-3. TREATMENT OF ACUTE RADIOCONTRAST REACTIONS

Symptom	Treatment	Dosage	Max. Dose
Nausea/vomiting	Prochlorperazine	0.13 mg/kg IM, IV q3–4h	10 mg
Urticaria	Diphenhydramine	1.25 mg/kg IM, IV q2–3h	50 mg
	Cimetidine	5 mg/kg IV, q6–8h	300 mg
Bronchospasm	Epinephrine (1:1000)	0.01 mg/kg SC, q15min	0.3 mg
	Albuterol	0.1 mg/kg NEB q15min	5 mg
Hypotension	Normal Saline	10–20 ml/kg IV PRN	2 L
Anaphylactoid	Epinephrine (1:10,000)	0.01 mg/kg IV q2–3min	0.1 mg
Vagal	Atropine	0.02 mg/kg IV PRN	1 mg
Seizures	Diazepam	0.2–0.5 mg/kg IV q20min	10 mg

Adapted from Bush WH, Swanson DP. Acute reactions to intravascular contrast media: Types, risk factors, recognition, and specific treatment. Am J Roentgenol 157:1158, 1991.

treatment recommendations for these clinical events (Bush, 1990) (see also Chapter 21 for other treatment recommendations). In almost all instances, the infusion of radiocontrast media should be discontinued once symptoms begin.

NAUSEA/VOMITING. Normally nausea and vomiting are minor, self-limited reactions. Since these can represent symptoms of a more severe ensuing event, the first approach should be to slow the rate of infusion of the radiocontrast. At the same time, it is appropriate to reassure the patient that such reactions are common, usually mild, and not progressive. If nausea and vomiting do not subside with conservative treatment, prochlorperazine or other antinauseant medication can be administered.

URTICARIA. When scattered urticaria with pruritus occurs, the administration of an H_1 antihistamine such as diphenhydramine often is sufficient treatment. Diffuse urticaria may require the addition of an H_2 blocker such as cimetidine (Mayumi et al, 1987) and should also heighten suspicion of a more severe systemic adverse event.

BRONCHOSPASM. Mild-to-moderate bronchospasm can generally be managed by the administration of subcutaneous epinephrine or nebulized albuterol with oxygen at 3 liters/min. The use of subcutaneous epinephrine at 0.01 mg/kg (up to 0.3 mg) may offer some advantage if the patient is experiencing other anaphylactoid side effects (Barach et al, 1984). Otherwise, the use of nebulized albuterol at 0.1 mg/kg (5 mg maximum) should be considered first because such therapy is less invasive and has less systemic cardiovascular side effect.

HYPOTENSION. Profound hypotension without respiratory symptoms may occur after the administration of radiocontrast. Typically, such hypotension is associated with compensatory tachycardia unless the patient is on concomitant beta-adrenergic blocking agents. When hypotension is associated with bradycardia, this should be considered a vagal reaction, and usual treatment should be accompanied by the administration of atropine. The standard treatment for hypotension is the rapid infusion of large volumes of intravenous fluid, such as normal saline or Ringer's solution.

ANAPHYLACTOID REACTIONS. Anaphylactoid reactions typically are clinically apparent as hypotension, bronchospasm, laryngospasm, and angioedema. When this occurs, epinephrine, administered intravenously, is the treatment of choice since its effect is rapid and systemic. It is suggested that a low-dose epinephrine infusion be used to maximize beta-adrenergic effects and minimize alpha-adrenergic activity. Intravenous epinephrine is contraindicated in patients on noncardioselective beta blockers because the beneficial beta-adrenergic effects of the drug will be blocked, and the unopposed alpha-adrenergic effects of epinephrine may actually increase the release of histamine and leukotrienes and enhance the adverse reaction. Other important supportive therapies include those noted earlier for urticaria, bronchospasm, and hypotension. Specifically, the early administration of intravenous diphenhydramine and cimetidine can be useful in blocking an anaphylactoid reaction. Similarly, nebulized albuterol and intravenous normal saline can be helpful supportive adjuncts. Finally, intravenous corticosteroids should be considered in patients with a severe or protracted anaphylactoid event. Although corticosteroids are of little immediate value, there is evidence that they may prevent delayed generation and release of mediators (Lasser et al, 1977).

VASOVAGAL REACTIONS. Vasovagal reactions may be caused by severe anxiety and/or possibly a toxic effect of intravascular administration of radiocontrast media. Clinical manifestations of a vagal reaction are due to depression of the cardiac conductive system and simultaneous peripheral vasodilation. This combination creates sinus bradycardia with pulse less than 50 beats per minute and hypotension with systolic blood pressure less than 80 mm Hg. Untreated, this reaction can progress over 10 to 20 minutes to unresponsiveness and cardiac arrest. Appropriate therapy includes normal saline and atropine as noted previously for hypotension. If significant bradycardia persists, intravenous doses of atropine can be given every 3 to 5 minutes up to a total maximal dose of 3 mg in adults.

CARDIOVASCULAR COLLAPSE. When an anaphylactoid or severe vagal reaction progresses to cardiovascular collapse, appropriate cardiopulmonary resuscitative measures must be employed. As with any cardiopulmonary resuscitation, an airway must be established, ventilation begun, and cardiac massage employed. It is essential that intravenous access be established and cardiac monitoring be started.

SEIZURES. Seizures typically only occur after a severe anaphylactoid or hypotensive episode. In addition to routine management of the primary reaction, intravenous diazepam should be given at 0.2 to 0.5 mg/kg every 20 minutes until the seizures are controlled, using a maximum dose of 10 mg. Since repeated dosages of diazepam may cause respiratory depression, the clinician must be prepared to establish an adequate airway.

Prevention of Reactions

Anaphylactoid Reactions

Ideally, patients with previous reactions to radiocontrast or with a prior history of allergies or asthma should be pretreated with diphenhydramine and prednisone (Kelly et al, 1978). Standard protocols for this procedure include the administration of 50 mg of each drug at 13, 7, and 1 hour(s) before the procedure. Greenberger et al have noted that the addition of ephedrine, 25 mg, one hour before the procedure appeared to offer further reduction in the risk for adverse reactions, and the use of cimetidine appeared to increase the overall reaction rate (Greenberger et al, 1985). Other authors have not confirmed the observations regarding cimetidine (Ring and Messmer, 1977; Marshall and Lieberman, 1991). Greenberger et al pointed out that ephedrine should not be used in patients with a history of hypertension or prior cardiovascular disease. In addition to the pretreatment protocol, a lower-osmolality contrast medium should be used (Greenberger and Patterson, 1991).

Chemotoxic Reactions

The likelihood of chemotoxic events is much greater in patients who are debilitated or those that have underlying vascular conditions such as renal dysfunction, cardiovascular disease, and cerebrovascular disease. In such high-risk patients an alternative diagnostic procedure should be considered in which intravascular contrast is not needed. If this is not practical, a low-osmolality nonionic agent should be employed.

In addition to avoidance of "high-risk" patients, adequate hydration is the best preventive of chemotoxic reactions. Patients with pheochromocytoma should be additionally pretreated with 2 to 5 mg phentolamine intravenously prior to radiocontrast exposure (Thrall, 1990).

LOCAL ANESTHETICS

For centuries the useful properties of local anesthetics have been appreciated. Synthetic changes in the side chain of benzocaine in the early 1900s led to the first injectable agent, procaine, which remained the standard local anesthetic for nearly half a century. Nearly 50 years ago, a second class of local anesthetic was introduced in the form of lidocaine. In general, all of these drugs are well tolerated, and when adverse reactions occur, they tend to be primarily chemotoxic or not related to the local anesthetic itself. With this in mind, it is critical to understand the classes of local anesthetics, the composition of local anesthetic solutions, and a practical approach to skin testing and challenge (Sindel and deShazo, 1991).

TABLE 24-4. LOCAL ANESTHETIC CLASSIFICATION

Type	Examples
Group 1	
Benzoic acid esters	Cocaine, meprylcaine, tetracaine
p-Aminobenzoic acid esters	Procaine, chlorprocaine, butethamine
m-Aminobenzoic acid esters	Metabutethamine, isobucaine
Group 2	
Amides	Lidocaine, mepivacaine, prilocaine
	Bupivacaine, dibucaine, etidocaine
Ethers	Pramoxine
Ketones	Dyclonine
Phenetidin-type	Phenacaine
Antihistamines	Chlorpheniramine

Adapted from Sindel LJ, deShazo RD. Accidents resulting from local anesthetics: True or false allergy? Clin Rev Allergy 9:379–395, 1991.

Classification of Local Anesthetics

Local anesthetics can be divided into two major groups: group 1 includes esters of benzoic acid; group 2 includes a more diverse group containing amides, ethers, ketones, phenetidine derivatives, and antihistamines (Table 24-4). There does not appear to be significant cross-reactivity between group 1 and group 2 drugs in patients who demonstrate hypersensitivity. Further studies are in progress to determine whether significant cross-reactivity exists among the group 2 constituents.

Historically, group 1 anesthetics are more likely to cause allergic or pseudoallergic reactions, possibly because they are metabolized almost completely by pseudocholinesterases in the plasma. Accordingly, potentially reactive metabolites of the ester type agents are rapidly produced after injection. Group 2 agents, in contrast, are metabolized in the liver, where degradation is much slower so that relatively fewer reactive metabolites are available (Savarese and Covino, 1986).

Local Anesthetic Solutions

The typical local anesthetic consists of three chemical portions: a hydrophilic amino terminus, an intermediate connecting group, and a lipid-soluble aromatic residue. The classification of the local anesthetic is determined by the linkage between the intermediate and aromatic groups (e.g., an ester linkage as in procaine or an amide linkage as in lidocaine). Interestingly, the chemical structure of benzoic acid esters is very similar to that of methylparaben—a compound historically used as a preservative in local anesthetics and now more commonly used in topical products. Not only is methylparaben a contact sensitizer, but there are at least two convincing case reports to suggest that it may cause anaphylaxis when given intravenously (Nagel et al, 1977).

Local anesthetics often contain vasoconstrictors such as epinephrine and preservatives such as sodium bisulfite. In other research, sulfites, in the form of stable salts or sulfur dioxide gas, have been implicated as a cause of anaphylactoid symptoms including bronchospasm in susceptible individuals (Stevenson and Simon, 1981). Affected patients appear to be uniformly deficient in sulfite oxidase, an enzyme that is important for metabolism of sulfite to sulfate. Despite such data, the role of sulfite sensitivity in alleged local anesthetic reactions is unclear.

Adverse Reactions

Classification

Adverse reactions to local anesthetics can be divided into four types: allergic/pseudoallergic, chemotoxic, non-drug-related, and idiosyncratic (Table 24-5).

ALLERGIC/PSEUDOALLERGIC REACTIONS. Although anaphylaxis-like reactions have been reported after local anesthetics, including urticaria, angioedema, bronchospasm, and hypotension, it would seem unlikely that such reactions occur on an IgE-mediated basis. Since local anesthetics have a typical weight of 200 to 300 daltons, an IgE-mediated response would depend on the ability of these molecules to conjugate with carrier proteins.

TABLE 24-5. ADVERSE REACTIONS TO LOCAL ANESTHETICS

Allergic/pseudoallergic	Non-drug-related
Anaphylaxis/anaphylactoid	Psychomotor
Urticaria/angioedema	Sympathetic stimulation
Contact dermatitis	Operative "trauma"
Chemotoxic	Idiosyncratic
Central nervous system stimulation/depression	Methemoglobulinemia
Cardiovascular	

Such an event of conjugation has not been demonstrated with either local anesthetics or their metabolites (Parker, 1975). Furthermore, local anesthetics appear to be monovalent antigens, not the polyvalent type generally required for mast cell activation. If systemic reactions are in fact drug related, it would appear that an anaphylactoid mechanism is more likely, similar to that which occurs after radiocontrast in some patients. In fact, some ester-type local anesthetics at high dosages cause wheal and flare reactions in the skin, suggesting that they may be nonspecific mast cell mediator releasers.

CHEMOTOXIC REACTIONS. Virtually all local anesthetics can stimulate the central nervous system, manifest clinically as excitement, anxiety, agitation, or even seizures (deJong, 1978). At higher doses, local anesthetics can induce central suppression leading to hypotension, apnea, and stupor. Another attribute of some local anesthetics is the quinidine-like effect, which can, in fact, be therapeutically useful in certain patients by decreasing cardiac irritability. At toxic levels, these agents can induce dangerous new cardiac rhythms (Covino, 1972a, 1972b).

NON-DRUG-RELATED REACTIONS. Ironically, the most common type of adverse reaction to local anesthetics does not appear to be directly related to the agent itself. Anxiety reactions including hyperventilation and vasovagal events are common, particularly in dental situations, in which fainting occurs in 2 to 3 percent of patients. Similarly, sympathetic stimulation may often occur independent of the drug and is probably due to anxiety associated with procedures. It is unlikely that epinephrine administered with a local anesthetic is an important factor in such reactions since the maximum acceptable dose of local anesthetic will be reached far before the maximal epinephrine dose (given the small amount contained in some local anesthetic preparations). Finally, many cases of large, local swelling are more probably due to operative "trauma" than to any effects of the agents contained in local anesthetic solutions.

IDIOSYNCRATIC REACTIONS. In general, such reactions are rare, although methemoglobinemia has been reported with prilocaine.

Diagnostic Tests

A composite view of research studies provides many useful points to consider in evaluating patients with alleged local anesthetic reactions (Sindel and deShazo, 1991; Schatz and Fung, 1986; Chandler et al, 1987). First, most patients labeled allergic are in fact not allergic to local anesthetics, and this can often be determined based on the history of the reaction alone. Second, positive skin tests with dilute local anesthetics are rare and may suggest immunologic sensitivity; this is true even for full-strength prick and 1:100 intradermal tests. Finally, skin test reactions to full-strength intradermal local anesthetics are uniformly falsely positive. Accordingly, any testing with full-strength local anesthetics should be considered part of a systemic challenge rather than a meaningful local reaction. As a practical point, the presence of paraben in testing solutions makes no difference in skin test results. Based on the above cumulative data, Sindel and deShazo have suggested a protocol for skin testing and incremental challenge in patients with a history of adverse reactions to local anesthetics (Table 24–6) (Sindel and deShazo, 1991).

Management of Reactions

The initial approach to patients with alleged local anesthetic reactions is to thoroughly review the history. Often it will be readily ap-

TABLE 24–6. SKIN TESTING AND CHALLENGE PROTOCOL FOR LOCAL ANESTHETIC AGENTS*

	SKIN TESTS		
Step	Vol (ml)	Dilution	Route
1†	—	1:100	PP
2	—	FS	PP
3†	0.02	1:100	ID
	CHALLENGE		
Step	Vol (ml)	Dilution	Route
4†	0.1	FS	SC
5	0.5	FS	SC
6	1.0	FS	SC

Adapted from Sindel LJ, deShazo RD. Accidents resulting from local anesthetics: True or false allergy? Clin Rev Allergy 9:379–395, 1991.

FS = full strength; PP = prick-puncture; ID = intradermal; SC = subcutaneous.

*Agent = 1% local anesthetic without epinephrine or paraben. Steps performed at 15–20 minute intervals unless history suggests delayed reaction. Protocol stopped with positive skin test or anaphylactoid symptoms (generalized urticaria, laryngeal edema, hypotension).

†Placebo tests may be added at these steps with phosphate-buffered saline (same route).

parent that the nature of the reaction was due to a chemotoxic property of one of the agents or that the adverse event was psychosomatic in nature. With such a history, reassurance alone may be adequate. An alternative approach, if the offending agent is known, is to choose an agent from a different group. The rationale for this comes from two studies demonstrating cross-reactivity between ester local anesthetics, but lack of such cross-reactivity between the ester and nonester compounds (Rothman et al, 1945). Although appropriate skin testing and challenge protocols have not proved this cross-reactivity phenomenon, clinical experience seems to demonstrate that this approach is useful.

For other patients who have a history suggestive of an allergic reaction, or in whom the nature of the apparent reaction is vague, it is appropriate to proceed with testing either to establish whether sensitivity to a suspected anesthetic exists or to demonstrate safety for future administration of a specific agent. This is particularly prudent if the offending initial agent is unknown. Testing may reasonably include a local anesthetic from each of the two major groups (Sindel and deShazo, 1991; Ruzicka et al, 1987). Simultaneous skin testing with phosphate-buffered saline can also be valuable in patients who have a history that is more suggestive of an anxiety-based reaction to the prior agent. When the inciting agent is known, a practical approach, even with an allergic history, is simply to choose an agent from another chemical group or an antihistamine for local anesthesia. In such patients, antihistamines do not typically provide adequate pain relief for dental procedures (Smith, 1961).

LATEX

Adverse reactions to natural rubber latex gloves, principally in the form of local dermatitis, were first reported 60 years ago (Downing, 1933). Clinically, it was believed that reactions were due to delayed hypersensitivity and that the responsible antigens were not latex, but rather thiurams, mercaptobenzothiazoles, and carbamates (Heese et al, 1991). Evidence for IgE-mediated reactions to latex proteins has only been firmly demonstrated over the last 14 years (Förström, 1980). Reports of allergic reactions to latex have increased exponentially with the advent of AIDS-related universal precaution requirements, as has the rate of production of latex gloves (FDA, 1991). This has raised speculation that some manufacturers may have altered their production process in an effort to produce more product, and that an alteration in the production may be increasing the degree of antigenicity in latex products.

Antigens

Natural latex is harvested, principally in Southeast Asia and West Africa, from the rubber tree *Hevea brasiliensis*. Raw liquid is obtained by placing a special chisel into the phloem of the tree. Subsequently, ammonia and sulfites are typically added as preservatives. Following centrifugation to increase the concentration of latex, a variety of "compounding" agents are added to enhance processing or to achieve various physical properties in the ultimate product. These compounding agents include carbamates, mercaptobenzothiazoles, thiurams, dithiodimorpholine, aldehydeamines, thioureas, and xanthines. Other potential antigens that may be added at this stage include emulsifiers, colorants, stiffeners, biocides, ultraviolet light absorbers, and fragrances. Latex gloves, for example, are then formed by dipping porcelain molds into the compounding slurry. Subsequent steps include heating, water baths, and a vulcanization process to enhance strength, which includes the addition of sulfur and prolonged heating at 100°C. A final production step includes the application of cornstarch powder prior to removal of the gloves from the molds. To produce a powder-free glove, a chlorination wash is required, which has the additional benefit of reducing water-soluble antigen (although it may also decrease the life span and physical properties of the glove). Several groups have used immunoblot, HPLC, or filtration techniques to search for IgE affinity proteins in latex. Sources of antigen in these studies have included natural latex, gloves, condoms, and balloons. Despite multiple antigen sources and variable techniques of isolation, these studies collectively suggest two likely major antigens with molecular weights of 14.5 kd and 30 kd (Makinen-Kiljunen et al, 1992; Alenius et al, 1991; Turjanmaa et al, 1988a; Jaeger et al, 1992; Slater and Chhabra, 1992).

Although cornstarch powder has also been

implicated as a potential antigen in finished products, no maize-specific IgE has been identified in alleged cases (Seggev et al, 1990; Fisher, 1987). At the same time, there is good evidence that cornstarch powder absorbs natural rubber latex protein and thus increases the antigenicity, particularly when absorbed as an aerosol by the conjunctival or airway mucosa (Swanson et al, 1992; Seaton, 1990).

Adverse Reactions

Clinical Presentation

The clinical presentation of latex allergy is variable and depends on the amount of available antigen and the type of exposure. Aerosolized latex powder may create rhinoconjunctivitis, asthma, or even full-blown anaphylaxis. Adverse reactions to latex gloves may be minimal, such as exacerbation of chronic eczema or localized vesicular dermatitis, or the response can be systemic disseminated urticaria or anaphylaxis (Losada et al, 1992).

In general, most severe or life-threatening reactions to natural rubber latex protein are associated with parenteral or mucosal exposure. Examples include exposure to natural rubber latex cuffs during barium enema procedures (Ownby et al, 1991), intraoperative patient exposure to latex surgical gloves, oral or sexual organ exposure to latex gloves during examination, lip exposure to balloons, and sexual organ exposure to condoms (Fisher, 1991).

Risk Factors

There is no accurate information on the risk of latex sensitivity in various populations. At the same time, it is clear that the prevalence of latex allergy is significantly increased in patients with frequent exposure, including patients with meningomyelocele (Slater et al, 1991), workers in latex factories (Tarlo et al, 1990), operating room doctors and nurses (Turjanmaa, 1987), hospital employees (Turjanmaa, 1987), and atopic patients (Kelly et al, 1991; Shield et al, 1992) (Table 24–7). It is likely that the most significant factors that contribute to latex sensitivity include the frequency and duration of exposure as well as the specific amount of available protein content of the product. Accordingly, both the incidence of latex sensitivity and the

TABLE 24–7. LATEX ALLERGY RISK FACTORS

Factor	Prevalence	References
Meningomyelocele patients	18–50%	Slater et al, 1991
Latex glove plant workers	11%	Tarlo et al, 1990
Operating room doctors	7.4–10%	Turjanmaa, 1987
Operating room nurses	5.6–10%	Turjanmaa, 1987
Hospital employees	4.5%	Turjanmaa, 1987
Allergic children	3.8%	Shield et al, 1992
Non-health-care employees	0.8%	Turjanmaa, 1987

Adapted from Hamann CP. Natural rubber latex protein sensitivity in review. Am J Contact Dermatitis 4:4–21, 1993.

degree of clinical manifestation of allergy can be greatly influenced by the latex protein source. Assays of natural rubber latex gloves have demonstrated great ranges in relative concentrations of total protein, ranging from 1 to 2960 latex allergy units/m^2 (Jones et al, 1992). It appears the most important factors in lowering potential allergen exposure are leaching and steam sterilization of the latex product (Leynadier, 1991).

In addition to degree of chronic latex protein exposure, other factors that appear to increase the likelihood of sensitization include chronic eczema (Kleinhans, 1984) and possibly cross-reactivity with banana, avocado, passion fruit, and chestnut proteins (Ceuppen et al, 1992; M'Raihi et al, 1991; Fernández-deCorres et al, 1990; Young et al, 1992). In fact other plants, including poinsettias (Santucci et al, 1985) and *Ficus benjamina* (Axelsson et al, 1990), have also been demonstrated to contain proteins which bind to latex-specific IgE. Possibly, this could increase the likelihood of sensitization in nursery or florist workers.

Diagnostic Tests

A suggestive clinical history of latex hypersensitivity should prompt further diagnostic evaluation. This includes patients who experience rhinoconjunctivitis, asthma, urticaria, pruritus, or angioedema in association with relevant exposures including latex gloves, condoms, balloons, and catheters. In addition, preoperative patients from high-risk groups—including allergic patients with hand eczema, patients with a history of contact urticaria to latex, and patients with a previous history of idiopathic intraoperative anaphylaxis—should be evaluated (Hamann, 1993).

Serologic tests for latex allergy have limited utility. A total IgE is generally increased with latex hypersensitivity but is neither sensitive nor specific (Jaeger et al, 1992). A latex-specific radioallergosorbent test (RAST) is available (Pharmacia, Piscataway, New Jersey) which is highly specific but ranges in sensitivity from 40 to 70 percent (Fuchs and Wahl, 1992). Accordingly, negative latex-specific RAST results do not rule out latex sensitivity.

In an effort to improve sensitivity, another common test is the use test (Turjanmaa et al, 1988b). In this test, the patient's wet hands are exposed to rubber latex gloves versus tactylon or vinyl gloves as controls. Initially, one finger is exposed for 15 minutes, and if there is no reaction, the whole hand is exposed for an additional 15 minutes. A positive test is manifested as clinical urticaria.

Although a standardized natural latex antigen reagent is not yet available, the preferred and most sensitive diagnostic method is the prick test (Turjanmaa et al, 1988b; Seaton, 1990). Testing material is prepared by extracting latex protein from twenty 1 cm × 1 cm latex glove squares for 30 minutes in 5 ml phosphate-buffered saline. Positive reactions are evident if the wheal induced by latex extract is at least equal to one half the histamine control after 15 minutes. Although this method appears to be highly sensitive, there is also some concern about the potential risk of anaphylaxis with such testing (Sussman et al, 1992). Accordingly, it would seem prudent in a patient with a history of previous possible systemic reaction to latex to consider serial dilutions of the prick test material prior to advancing to full-strength testing (Sussman et al, 1992). The diagnostic specificity of a positive prick test result is not well defined, and accordingly, the presence of IgE antibody to latex should be interpreted only in the context of a clinically suggestive history. It is also reassuring to demonstrate prick test negativity in several low-risk, history-negative controls.

Management

The treatment for latex rubber allergy is complete avoidance. "Hypo-allergenic" latex gloves are available, including dry rubber or powder-free preparations, but these gloves may still contain enough protein to cause anaphylaxis (Warpinski et al, 1991). Safer, appropriate alternatives to latex include polyvinyl chloride, polychloroprene, polynitriles,

TABLE 24–8. COMMON LATEX SOURCES

General medical	Anesthesia	Surgical
Blood pressure cuff	Breathing circuit	Implant
Burn bandage	Endotracheal tube	Instrument mat
Elastic bandage	Epidural catheter adapter	Surgical glove
Electrode pad	Induction mask	Texas catheter
Enema retention cuff	Nasal/oral airway	Urine bag/strap
Esophageal dilator	Reservoir breathing circuit	Vascular catheter
Esophageal protector	Teeth protector	Wound drain
Examination glove	Ventilator bellows	
Eye dropper	Ventilator tubing	Other
Face mask elastic		Adhesive
Feeding tube	Dental	Baby bottle nipple
Finger cot	Bite block	Baby pacifier
Foley catheter	Dental dam	Balloon
Hemodialyzer	Orthodontic elastic	Carpet backing
Hot water bottle	Prophy cup	Elastic in underwear
Latex injection port		Household glove
Rubber sheet/pillow	Gynecologic	Paint
Rubber stopper	Cervical cap	Raincoat
Syringe stopper	Cervical dilator	Rubber band
Tourniquet	Condom	Rubber toy
Ultrasound cover	Diaphragm	Shoe
Warming blanket	Douche bulb	
Wheelchair tire		

Adapted from Hamann CP. Natural rubber latex protein sensitivity in review. Am J Contact Dermatitis 4:4–21, 1993.

or substituted polystyrene derivatives (e.g., tactylon). Although some studies suggest that latex-sensitive patients can be successfully premedicated with antihistamines and hydrocortisone to allow safe intraoperative exposure to latex (Swartz et al, 1990), others have shown the failure of this approach (Kwittken et al, 1992). It is emphasized, therefore, that the only safe approach would appear to be complete avoidance of any source of latex (Table 24–8).

Until FDA standards are developed which ensure low latex protein content of latex-related materials, and hence, lower likelihood of sensitization, it is important from a clinical perspective to minimize latex exposure in high-risk groups so that sensitization will not occur, especially patients with meningomyelocele, latex plant workers, and allergic health care personnel (Hamann, 1993).

REFERENCES

Alenius H, Turjanmaa K, Palosuo T. Surgical latex glove allergy: Characterization of rubber protein allergens by immunoblotting. Int Arch Allergy Appl Immunol 96:376–380, 1991.

Axelsson IG, Johansson SG, Larsson PH, Zetterstrom O. Characterization of allergenic components in sap extract from weeping fig. Int Arch Allergy Appl Immunol 91:130–135, 1990.

Barach EM, Nowak RM, Tennyson GL, Tomlanovich MC. Epinephrine for treatment of anaphylactic shock. JAMA 251:2118–2122, 1984.

Bettman MA. Ionic versus nonionic contrast agents for intravenous use: Are all the answers in? Radiology 175:616–618, 1990.

Bush WH. Treatment of systemic reactions to contrast media. Urology 35:145–150, 1990.

Bush WH, Swanson DP. Acute reactions to intravascular contrast media: Types, risk factors, recognition, and specific treatment. Am J Roentgenol 157:1153–1161, 1991.

Ceuppen JL, Van Durme P, Dooms-Goossens A. Latex allergy in patient with allergy to fruit. Lancet 339:493, 1992. (Letter)

Chandler MJ, Grammer LC, Patterson R. Provocative challenge with local anesthetics in patients with a prior history of reaction. J Allergy Clin Immunol 79:883–886, 1987.

Covino BG. Local anesthesia 1. N Engl J Med 286:975–983, 1972a.

Covino BG. Local anesthesia 2. N Engl J Med 286:1035–1042, 1972b.

DeJong RH. Toxic effects of local anesthetics. JAMA 239:1166–1168, 1978.

Downing JG. Dermatitis from rubber gloves. N Engl J Med 208:196–198, 1933.

Enright T, Chua-Lim A, Duda E, Lim DT. The role of a documented allergic profile as a risk factor for radiographic contrast media reaction. Ann Allergy 62:302–305, 1989.

Fernández-deCorres L, Moneo I, Munoz D, Bernaola G, Fernández E, Audicana M, Urrutia I. Contact urticaria. Sensitization to chestnuts and bananas in patient with contact urticaria from latex. Contact Dermatitis 23:277, 1990.

Fisher AA. Condom conundrums: Part II. Cutis 48:433–434, 1991.

Fisher AA. Contact urticaria and anaphylactoid reaction due to cornstarch surgical glove powder. Contact Dermatitis 16:224–225, 1987.

Food and Drug Administration. Allergic reactions to latex-containing medical devices. FDA Medical Bulletin July, 1991.

Förström L. Contact urticaria from latex surgical gloves. Contact Dermatitis 6:33–34, 1980.

Fuchs T, Wahl R. Immediate reactions to rubber products. Allergy Proc 13:61–66, 1992.

Greenberger PA, Patterson R. The prevention of immediate generalized reactions to radiocontrast media in high-risk patients. J Allergy Clin Immunol 87:867–872, 1991.

Greenberger PA, Patterson R, Tapio CM. Prophylaxis against repeated radiocontrast media reactions in 857 cases. Arch Intern Med 145:2197–2200, 1985.

Hamann CP. Natural rubber latex protein sensitivity in review. Am J Contact Dermatitis 4:4–21, 1993.

Heese A, Hintzenstern JV, Peters KP, Koch HU, Hornstein OP. Allergic and irritant reactions to rubber gloves in medical health services. J Am Acad Dermatol 25:831–839, 1991.

Jaeger D, Kleinhans D, Czuppon AB, Baur X. Latex specific proteins causing immediate-type cutaneous, nasal, bronchial, and systemic reactions. J Allergy Clin Immunol 89:759–768, 1992.

Jones RT, Bubak ME, Grosselin VA, Yunginger JW. Relative latex allergen contents of several commercial latex gloves. J Allergy Clin Immunol 89:225, 1992. (Abstract)

Katayama H, Yamaguchi K, Kozuka T, Takashima T, Seez P, Matsuura K. Adverse reactions to ionic and nonionic contrast media: A report from the Japanese Committee on the Safety of Contrast Media. Radiology 175:621–628, 1990.

Kelly JF, Patterson R, Lieberman P, Mathison DA, Stevenson DD. Radiographic contrast media studies in high-risk patients. J Allergy Clin Immunol 62:181–184, 1978.

Kelly K, Setlock M, Davis JP. Anaphylactic reactions during general anesthesia among pediatric patients—United States Jan 1990-Jan 1991. MMWR Morb Mortal Wkly Rep 40:437, 443, 1991.

Kleinhans D. Contact urticaria to rubber gloves. Contact Dermatitis 10:124–125, 1984.

Kwittken PL, Becker J, Oyefara B, Danziger R, Pawlowski NA, Sweinberg S. Latex hypersensitivity reactions despite prophylaxis. Allergy Proc 13:123–127, 1992.

Lasser EC, Lang J, Sovak M, Kolb W, Lyon S, Hamlin AE. Steroids: theoretical and experimental basis for utilization in prevention of contrast media reactions. Radiology 125:1–9, 1977.

Leynadier F. Shared reaction of prick test positivity from both increased leaching and steam sterilization. Allergy 46:619–625, 1991.

Losada E, Lázaro M, Marcos C, Quirce S, Fraj J, Dávila I, Igea JM, Sánchez-Cano M. Immediate allergy to natural rubber latex: Clinical and immunological studies. Allergy Proc 13:115–120, 1992.

Makinen-Kiljunen S, Turjanmaa K, Palosuo T, Reunala

T. Characterization of latex antigens and allergens in surgical gloves and natural rubber by immunoelectrophoretic methods. J Allergy Clin Immunol 90:230–235, 1992.

Marshall G, Lieberman P. Comparison of three pretreatment protocols to prevent anaphylactoid reactions to radiocontrast media. Ann Allergy 67:70–74, 1991.

Mayumi H, Kimura S, Asano M. Intravenous cimetidine as an effective treatment for systemic anaphylaxis and acute allergic skin reactions. Ann Allergy 50:447–451, 1987.

M'Raihi L, Charpin D, Pons A, Bongrand P, Vervloet D. Cross-reactivity between latex and banana. J Allergy Clin Immunol 87:129–130, 1991.

Nagel J, Fuscaldo J, Fireman P. Paraben allergy. JAMA 237:1594–1595, 1977.

Ownby DR, Tomlanovich M, Sammons N, McCullough J. Anaphylaxis associated with latex allergy during barium enema examinations. J Allergy Clin Immunol 156:903–908, 1991

Parker CW. Drug Allergy. N Engl J Med 292:511–514, 1975.

Ring J, Messmer K. Incidence and severity of anaphylactoid reactions to colloid volume substitutes. Lancet 1:466, 1977.

Rothman S, Orland FJ, Flesch P. Group specificity of epidermal allergy to procaine in man. J Invest Dermatol 6:191–199, 1945.

Ruzicka T, Gerstmeier M, Przybilla B, Ring J. Allergy to local anesthetics: Comparison of patch test with prick and intradermal test results. J Am Acad Dermatol 16:1202–1208, 1987.

Santucci B, Picardo M, Cristaudo A. Contact dermatitis from *Euphorbia pulcherrima*. Contact Dermatitis 12:285–286, 1985.

Savarese JJ, Covino BG. Basic and clinical pharmacology of local anesthetic drugs. *In* Miller RD (ed). Anesthesia. New York, Churchill Livingstone, 1986.

Schatz M, Fung DL. Anaphylactic and anaphylactoid reactions due to anesthetic agents. Clin Rev Allergy 4:215–227, 1986.

Schwab SJ, Hlatky MA, Peiper KS, Davidson CJ, Morris KG, Skelton TN, Bashore TM. Contrast nephrotoxicity: A randomized controlled trial of a nonionic and an ionic radiographic contrast agent. N Engl J Med 320:149–153, 1989.

Seaton A. Latex as aeroallergen. Lancet 336:808–809, 1990.

Seggev JS, Mawhinney TP, Yuninger JW, Braun SR. Anaphylaxis due to cornstarch surgical glove powder. Ann Allergy 65:152–155, 1990.

Shehadi WH, Toniolo G. Adverse reactions to contrast media. Radiology 137:299–302, 1980.

Shield S, Blaiss MS, Gross S. Prevalence of latex sensitivity in children evaluated for inhalant allergy. J Allergy Clin Immunol 89:224, 1992. (Abstract)

Sindel LJ, deShazo RD. Accidents resulting from local anesthetics: True or false allergy? Clin Rev Allergy 9:379–395, 1991.

Slater JE, Chhabra SK. Latex antigens. J Allergy Clin Immunol 89:673–678, 1992.

Slater JE, Mostello LA, Shaer C. Rubber-specific IgE in children with spina bifida. J Urol 146:578–579, 1991.

Smith J. Diphenhydramine hydrochloride used as a local anesthetic for tooth removal: Report of case. J Oral Surg 19:418–419, 1961.

Stevenson DD, Simon RA. Sensitivity to ingested metabisulfites in asthmatic subjects. J Allergy Clin Immunol 68:26–32, 1981.

Sussman GL, Bonnekoh B, Merk HF. Safety of latex prick skin testing in allergic patients. JAMA 267:2603, 1992. (Letter)

Swanson MC, Bubak ME, Hunt LW, Reed CW. Occupational respiratory allergic disease from latex. J Allergy Clin Immunol 89:225, 1992. (Abstract)

Swartz J, Braude BM, Gilmour RF, Shandling B, Gold M. Intraoperative anaphylaxis to latex. Can J Anaesth 37:589–592, 1990.

Tarlo SM, Wong L, Roos J, Booth N. Occupational asthma caused by latex in a surgical glove manufacturing plant. J Allergy Clin Immunol 85:626–631, 1990.

Thrall JH. Adverse reactions to contrast media. *In* Swanson DP, Chilton HM, Thrall JH (eds). Pharmaceuticals in Medical Imaging. New York, Macmillian, 1990.

Turjanmaa K. Incidence of immediate allergy to latex gloves in hospital personnel. Contact Dermatitis 17:270–275, 1987.

Turjanmaa K, Laurita K, Makinen-Kiljunen S, Reunala T. Rubber contact urticaria: Allergenic properties of 19 brands of gloves. Contact Dermatitis 19:362–367, 1988a.

Turjanmaa K, Reunala T, Rasanen L. Comparison of diagnostic methods in latex and surgical glove contact urticaria. Contact Dermatitis 19:241–247, 1988b.

Warpinski JR, Folgert J, Cohen M, Bush RK. Allergic reaction to latex: An unsuspected risk factor for anaphylaxis. Allergy Proc 12:95–102, 1991.

Witten DM. Reactions to urographic contrast media. JAMA 231:974–977, 1975.

Young MC, Osleeb C, Slater J. Latex and banana anaphylaxis. J Allergy Clin Immunol 89:226, 1992. (Abstract)

Chapter 25
Food-Induced Systemic Reactions and Anaphylaxis

John A. Anderson, M.D.

Food anaphylaxis is a manifestation of food allergy characterized by a systemic reaction to food protein exposure in susceptible individuals as the result of IgE sensitization to a food allergen, subsequent re-exposure to the allergen, followed by cutaneous and systemic respiratory, gastrointestinal, and cardiovascular symptoms. Historically, anaphylaxis was described as an outcome during pioneering research involving animals (see Chapter 21). Charles Richet and Paul Portier, in 1902, introduced the theory behind this reaction and coined the term "anaphylaxis" (a lifting up or removal of protection), as opposed to "prophylaxis" (favoring of protection).

The tissue mast cell and, to some degree, the blood basophil are the effector cells in the pathogenesis of anaphylactic reactions (see Chapter 21). The signs and symptoms of anaphylaxis are the result of mast cell or basophil chemical mediators—either preformed and released upon degranulation or generated in the surrounding tissue.

Anaphylactoid reactions to foods or food additives occur on the basis of direct exposure of these substances to effector mast cells (or basophil) followed by mediator release without involving immune processes. The symptoms of anaphylaxis and anaphylactoid reactions look the same and are sometimes called "allergic-like." In the case of food anaphylaxis, prior exposure to the food protein, usually intermittently, is necessary in order for IgE sensitization to take place; once sensitization has occurred, exposure to the food allergen is necessary before anaphylaxis. In the case of food or food additive anaphylactoid reactions, prior exposure to offending substances is not necessary. Typically in anaphylaxis, following allergy sensitization, a small quantity of food protein re-exposure can result in a maximum systemic reaction. In the case of anaphylactoid food reactions, however, the amount of substance involved in stimulating the reaction is more important, with the degree of systemic symptoms more closely following a classic dose-response immune curve.

CLINICAL MANIFESTATIONS OF ANAPHYLAXIS AND ANAPHYLACTOID FOOD REACTIONS

The initial symptoms of systemic anaphylaxis or anaphylactoid reaction usually begin within 30 minutes and almost always before 2 hours after exposure (Yunginger, 1992). The signs and symptoms of anaphylaxis or anaphylactoid reactions may be divided into cutaneous (usually mild) and systemic (which are more serious). Regardless of the cause of anaphylaxis or anaphylactoid reaction, the clinical manifestations are similar. A description of these clinical manifestations can be found in Chapter 21. A major risk factor for death in systemic anaphylaxis is the presence of concurrent asthma. In a group of 13 children and adolescents who either died of food anaphylaxis or nearly died, all had asthma as well as food allergy (Sampson et al, 1992b). In 12 of the 13 situations, the asthma was under good control immediately before the food anaphylaxis event occurred.

Three defined clinical patterns of anaphylaxis have been described: uniphasic, biphasic, and protracted (Stark and Sullivan, 1986). It has been reported that 52 percent of individuals with systemic anaphylaxis experience a short-lived uniphasic clinical pattern. Another 20 percent develop a biphasic reaction, with early and late phase separated by an interval of 1 to 8 hours. Finally, 28 percent of patients were found to have severe protracted and persistent symptoms that lasted 5 to 32 hours. Anaphylaxis due to oral agents, including foods, were more likely to result in biphasic or protracted symptoms rather than a uniphasic pattern.

Two relatively new anaphylactic syndromes related to food allergy have been described. The first is food-dependent exercise-induced anaphylaxis (EIA). EIA, a form of physical allergy, was first described in 1969 and relates to urticaria, angioedema, or hypotension associated with physical exertion (see Chapter 26). This condition may occur with any vigorous exercise, but jogging is a frequent cause in the United States. A recent epidemiologic survey of 199 individuals with EIA showed that food ingestion within 2 hours of exercise was a factor in the development of attacks in 54 percent of cases (Horan and Sheffer, 1991). The precise pathophysiology of EIA, or the way the process of eating affects the development of attacks, is unknown although it is clear that histamine release occurs. The specific food ingestions that have been reported to be associated with EIA include: celery, shrimp, oysters, chicken, peaches, and wheat.

Another syndrome of food-related anaphylaxis is the oral allergy syndrome (OAS) (Amlot et al, 1987). In this syndrome, adults and children who are allergic to inhaled pollens and who usually have seasonal allergic rhinitis may also develop concurrent allergies to a series of fresh fruits and raw vegetables. Allergens in these fruits and vegetables specifically cross-react with certain pollen allergens (Moller, 1989). The clinical manifestations of OAS usually are confined to the mouth parts and involve pruritus and angioedema of the lips, tongue, and palate as a result of the direct contact of the fresh fruit or raw vegetable. Uncommonly, reactions to these fruits and vegetables can progress to systemic anaphylaxis reactions (Amlot et al, 1987).

Specific cross-reactivity has been identified between ragweed pollen and watermelon, other melons, and members of the gourd family including cucumber and squash (Enberg et al, 1987). Specific cross-reactivity between birch pollen and celery, mugwort, apples, and hazelnut has also been found (Calkhoven et al, 1987; Ebner et al, 1991). Other fresh fruit and vegetable allergen cross-reactivities with grass and tree pollen are also probably important in the development of OAS symptoms (Ortolani et al, 1989).

Vasovagal reactions are probably the most common clinical reaction confused with anaphylaxis or anaphylactoid reactions. This reaction is usually characterized by prompt onset of pallor, diaphoresis, weakness, and possibly fainting. Although the patient becomes hypotensive to some degree, the pulse rate is low or bradycardic (not tachycardic as would be expected with histamine release of anaphylaxis). Characteristics of an allergic reaction such as urticaria or angioedema or other signs of systemic anaphylaxis are not present. Other syndromes or conditions that have to be considered in the differential diagnosis of systemic anaphylaxis or anaphylactoid reaction include cardiac arrhythmia, seizure disorder, aspiration, and drug overdose. Although systemic mastocytosis occurs in children, symptoms are usually limited to urticaria. Individuals with either hereditary angioedema (HANE) or the acquired form of C_1 esterase inhibitor deficiency develop edema without urticaria. Cold urticaria, which is the most common form of physical urticaria in children, in rare instances may be associated with systemic symptoms due to a massive chemical mediator release such as sudden or prolonged chilling after swimming in cold water.

PREVALENCE OF SYSTEMIC REACTIONS TO FOOD AND FOOD ADDITIVES

The incidence of systemic reactions to food is unknown (Bock, 1992). The prevalence of adverse reactions to foods, confirmed by a double-blind, placebo-controlled food challenge (DBPCFC), was found to be 8 percent among 480 consecutively born infants in Denver, Colorado (Bock, 1987). Of these infants, 25 (5.2 percent) were probably allergic to milk, but only 11 (2.3 percent) were confirmed by DBPCFC to be allergic to milk (Bock, 1987). In a well-controlled prospective study of a cohort of 1749 newborns born in 1985, in a single hospital in a municipality in Denmark, 39 or 2.2 percent were found to have systemic adverse reactions after cow's milk protein challenge (Horst and Halken, 1990). The generally accepted estimate of the incidence of food allergy in older children or adults is 1 to 2 percent of the population.

Bock, in an attempt to obtain an estimate of the prevalence of anaphylaxis and other serious systemic reactions to food, performed a prospective survey involving 73 Colorado emergency departments over a 2-year period in which all severe allergic-like reactions that may have involved diet were tabulated (Bock, 1992). Twenty-five individuals, ages 2 to 71 years, who had anaphylaxis or anaphylactoid reactions were identified. Nine individuals (36 percent) were below the age of 18. Twenty of the 25 individuals required epinephrine injections. Two required cardiopulmonary resuscitation and one patient died. On the basis of this study, it was estimated that 950 severe reactions to food, requiring emergency intervention, could be expected to occur in the United States yearly (Bock, 1992).

The incidence of intolerance to food additives is unknown, especially in children. A study involving reactions to common food additives among 4274 Danish school children, ages 5 to 16 years, was reported recently (Fuglsang et al, 1993). Following screening by a questionnaire and selection by a 2-week elimination diet, both children with no complaints and those with allergic-like symptoms were challenged with a mixture of food preservatives, colors, and flavors using an open method. None of the 98 healthy control children reacted on food additive challenge, but 17 of 173 children reporting symptoms to these agents had positive open food additive challenges. Of individuals who reacted, one had gastrointestinal symptoms, 13 had aggravation of their atopic dermatitis, and three developed urticaria. Twelve of the 17 individuals underwent DBPCFC with food additives and six were positive (one with urticaria and five with exacerbation of atopic dermatitis). Five of the six reacted to colors, and one patient reacted to citric acid (Fuglsang et al, 1993). On the basis of these studies, the authors estimated that the prevalence of food additive intolerance in Danish school children to be 1 to 2 percent. It should be noted that in none of these cases could the reaction be described as systemic in nature. All previous reactions were cutaneous, either as exacerbation of atopic dermatitis rash or acute urticaria (one case).

FOODS AND ADDITIVES INVOLVED IN DIETARY ANAPHYLAXIS AND ANAPHYLACTOID REACTIONS

A wide variety of individual foods, processed foods, and food additives have been reported to be associated with anaphylaxis or anaphylactoid events (Stricker et al, 1986) (Table 25–1). Absolute proof (using DBPCFC) of an association with a specific food exposure and the anaphylactic event is often lacking in the reports of these reactions (Bock et al, 1988). In many clinical situations, the presence of a good history and evidence of *in vitro* IgE allergen-specific antibody or a positive IgE-mediated reacting food-specific skin test is enough to make a presumptive diagnosis of food anaphylaxis for reporting purposes (Bock, 1992). This is also true of reports of reactions to processed foods. As an example, an 18-year-old who was reported to have a sudden reaction to chicken soup was found to have a positive wheal and flare skin test reaction to packaged chicken soup mix as well as to peanuts, parsley, carrots, celery, cucumber, and grapefruit, but not to chicken (Staff and Fink, 1992). Although challenge testing to each allergen was considered, it was not done because of the fear of precipitating another episode of anaphylaxis.

On the other hand, a good example of detective work can be found in the case of a 14-year-old who developed systemic reactions on two occasions while eating marinated chicken. It was later found that he was reactive (on DBPCFC) to coriander spice in the teriyaki sauce used in the preparation of the chicken (Bock, 1993). Occasionally, individuals may react to known allergens in finished processed foods which inadvertently got there through the manufacturing process. Such is the case of individuals reported to react to cow's milk protein in "non-dairy products" (Gern et al, 1992; Jones et al, 1992). In some

TABLE 25–1. DIETARY AND OTHER SUBSTANCES REPORTED TO BE ASSOCIATED WITH ANAPHYLAXIS OR ANAPHYLACTOID REACTIONS

Foods*				Processed Foods and Other Substances	Food Additives
Abalone[1]	Chili pepper	Honey[8]	Psyllium seed	Breakfast cereal (psyllium)[15]	*Antioxidants*
Allspice	Chocolate	Hops	Raspberry	Bee pollen[9]	Butylated hydroxyanisole (BHA)
Almond	Cinnamon	Horseradish	Red snapper[1]	Beignet (mite)[16]	
Anise seed	Clam	Juniper berry	Rye[7]	Burrito[9]	
Apple	Clove	Kiwi[9]	Sage	Cake[10]	Butylated hydroxytoluene (BHT)
Artichoke	Coconut	Lentil	Salmon	Candy[10]	
Avocado[2]	Cod fish[1]	Lima bean	Scallop[9]	Catsup[9]	
Baker's yeast	Coriander[4]	Lobster	Sesame seed[11]	Chicken soup[17]	*Aspartame* (sweetening agent)
Banana	Corn	Mango	Shrimp[12]	Cookie[10]	
Bay leaf	Cotton seed	Mahi mahi[1]	Sole[1]	Cupcake[10]	*Food coloring*
Bean	Crab[5]	Milk	Soy	Diaper rash ointment (milk-contact)[18]	Yellow (FD&C 5,6)
Beet	Cumin seed	Millet	Squash[13]		Red (FD&C 3, 4, 5)
Black pepper	Cuttlefish	Mushroom	Squid[1]	Hamburger roll[17]	Blue (FD&C 1 & 2)
Brazil nut	Dill seed	Nutmeg	Strawberry	Immunoglobulin (oral)[19]	
Brewer's yeast	Egg	Orange	Sunflower[8]	Measles vaccine (egg)[20]	*Nitrates/Nitrites*
Buckwheat	Fennel seed	Oyster	Sweet potato	M&M plain chocolate (peanuts)[21]	*Monosodium glutamate (MSG)*
Cantaloupe	Filbert nut	Pea	Tangerine		
Caraway seed	Flax seed	Peach	Tapioca	MMR vaccine (egg) (gelatin-inj)[11, 22]	
Cashew nut	Flounder[3]	Peanut	Thyme		
Castor bean	Garbanzo bean[1]	Pecan[10]	Trout[1]	Muffin[9]	
Celery	Garlic	Perch[1]	Tumeric	Pastry[23]	
Chamomile	Gelatin[6]	Pine nut	Tuna[11]	Potato salad[9]	
Chestnut[3]	Ginger	Pistachio	Vanilla	Sandwich[23]	
Chicken	Grape[7]	Poppy seed	Walnut	Spice[4, 9]	
Chicory	Halibut	Potato	Wheat[7, 14]	Sesame seed oil[24]	
				Sunflower honey (pollen)[8]	
				Teriyaki sauce[4]	
				Vinegar[9]	

*Modified from Stricker WE, Anorne-Lopez E, Reed CE. Food skin testing in patients with idiopathic anaphylaxis. J Allergy Clin Immunol 77:519, 1986.

References indicated by superscript numerals: 1, de Martino et al, 1990; 2, Moneret-Vantrin et al, 1993; 3, de Martino et al, 1992; 4, Bock, 1993; 5, Cartier et al, 1986; 6, Ebner et al, 1992; 7, Bock et al, 1988; 8, Birnbaum et al, 1989; 9, Bock, 1992; 10, Sampson et al, 1992; 11, Fasano et al, 1991; 12, Daul et al, 1990; 13, Enberg et al, 1987; 14, Dohi et al, 1991; 15, James et al, 1991; 16, Erben et al, 1993; 17, Staff and Fink, 1992; 18, Jarmoc and Primack, 1987; 19, Bernhisel-Broadbent et al, 1991; 20, Herman et al, 1983; 21, Keating et al, 1990; 22, Kelso et al, 1993; 23, Perkin, 1990; 24, Chin and Haydik, 1991.

cases, the manufacturers are aware of the fact that minimum amounts of allergen may contaminate a finished product and warn consumers, e.g., by peanut labeling of plain chocolate candies (Keating et al, 1990).

Allergic individuals may develop anaphylaxis when ingesting a food product containing non-food protein. Fortunately, foods containing significant amounts of antibiotics are uncommon in the United States today, but penicillin anaphylaxis because of penicillin-containing foods, particularly milk, has been reported (Yunginger, 1992). Recently, there was a report of an adult allergic to house dust mite who ate a beignet made from a commercial mix contaminated with house dust mite (Erben et al, 1993). Several individuals have been reported to react to psyllium seed contained in a breakfast cereal (James et al, 1991).

Individuals, including children, may be exposed to food products by routes other than oral consumption. An example of a contact exposure is contained in a report of an infant exposed to cow's milk protein contained in a diaper rash ointment (containing 5 percent "calcium caseinate") (Jarmoc and Primack, 1987). Ten minutes after the ointment was applied to a severely excoriated diaper area, a 12-month-old infant developed generalized urticaria and wheezing, which responded to epinephrine injections and antihistamines. Children and adults who are allergic to fish or seafood are warned not to handle these foods and to avoid areas where there is a strong odor of these foods, particularly during the cooking process. Initial IgE allergen-specific sensitization, as well as IgE-mediated reactions, may occur through exposure to the aerosolized fish or seafood protein. The importance of this method of exposure to food allergens was validated in studies involving snow crab processors (Cartier et al, 1986).

Biologic therapeutics containing food protein may be a problem for allergic infants and children. Hypersensitivity to measles-mumps-rubella (MMR) vaccine has been described in chicken egg–allergic infants (Aukrust et al, 1980; Herman et al, 1983). There is a small but detectable amount of chicken egg protein in measles and MMR vaccine. Most children proven to be egg-allergic (by DBPCFC), however, can tolerate routine MMR vaccine (Fasano et al, 1991; Beck et al, 1991). Those allergic individuals potentially at risk for MMR vaccine reaction can be identified by the use of an epicutaneous (prick) immediate-reacting IgE skin test using MMR vaccine (Beck et al, 1991).

Of the 28 reports of anaphylactic reactions to measles or MMR vaccine, only a small percentage are due to egg allergy (Kelso et al, 1993). An allergic reaction to neomycin contained in MMR vaccine has been reported in a single patient (Rietschel and Bernier, 1981). Recently, a 17-year-old, who was not allergic to eggs and had no reaction to her first MMR vaccine at 15 months of age, developed diffuse itching, hives/angioedema, rhinitis, choking, and hypotension 10 minutes after MMR vaccine injection (Kelso et al, 1993). This individual was found, subsequently, to be allergic to the gelatin used in the vaccine as a stabilizer. Gelatin is a protein prepared by hydrolysis of collagen from bovine and porcine hides and bones. Passive immunization using orally administered immunoglobulin preparations derived from various sources, including bovine products or chicken egg, has been proposed as a treatment for enteric diseases. Children proven to be allergic to cow's milk and chicken egg protein are at risk with exposure to these preparations (Bernhisel-Broadbent et al, 1991).

A newly recognized cause of life-threatening systemic anaphylaxis has been identified in reactions to natural rubber latex (Ownby et al, 1991). Some patients who have documented latex sensitivity also have been found to react clinically to a variety of fresh fruits and vegetables such as banana, chestnuts, avocado, and kiwi fruit (Moneret-Vautrin et al, 1993; Miraihi et al, 1991; Fernández de Corres et al, 1993). A partial cross-reactivity between natural rubber latex and banana food allergens has been identified (Ross et al, 1992). New preliminary information points to the existence of cross-reacting proteins (IgE reactive) between natural rubber latex, ragweed, and blue grass pollens (Appleyard et al, 1994). Clinical cross-reactions have been described between fruit and vegetable exposure and pollen sensitivities in the oral allergy syndrome (OAS) (Enberg et al, 1987; Calkhoven et al, 1987; Ortolani et al, 1989).

FOOD ADDITIVES

Thousands of different agents are added to processed foods eaten by humans (Simon and Stevenson, 1993). Most of these agents are added to preserve the food against bacterial or other contamination, to stabilize the content, or to increase the appeal of processed food through color or flavor. The food additives listed in Table 25–1 are those that are usually reported to be involved in an allergic or an allergic-like reaction (Simon and Stevenson, 1993). They include the antioxidants butylated hydroxyanisole (BHA) and butylated hydroxytoluene (BHT); aspartame sweetener; the yellow, red, and blue colors; nitrates and nitrites; monosodium glutamate (MSG); sodium benzoate; and the sulfiting agents plus SO_2 (as preservatives).

In 1985 the USA Food and Drug Administration (FDA) established a self-reporting mechanism called the adverse reaction monitoring system (ARMS). Of the common food additives listed above, aspartame and sulfites account for 95 percent of the complaints (Perkin, 1990). Only some of the adverse reactions reported to be related to food additives are allergic-like in nature. They include: (1) urticaria, angioedema, and anaphylaxis and (2) asthma (Fuglsang et al, 1993; Simon and Stevenson, 1993; Perkin, 1990; deMartino et al, 1992).

Urticaria, Angioedema, and Anaphylaxis

There are reports that children with recurrent or persistent urticaria or angioedema react up to 36 to 64 percent of the time when challenged to colors, sodium benzoate, and aspartame (deMartino et al, 1992). On the other hand, in a well-done study, the prevalence of intolerance reactions among 4952 unselected 5- to 16-year-old school children in Denmark was shown to be only 1 to 2 percent (Fuglsang et al, 1993).

The relationship between tartrazine ingestion and urticaria goes back to a report by Lockey who described three adults who developed hives after ingestion of a medication containing tartrazine (Lockey, 1959). This was substantiated in one patient by open challenge. Other studies have been reported which link urticaria with tartrazine ingestion. Unfortunately, the majority of these studies were not controlled (Simon and Stevenson, 1993). Using the strict criteria of DBPCFC, only occasional patients have been identified who develop urticaria when exposed to tartrazine (Stevenson et al, 1986). As far as the other colors are concerned, urticaria reactions have been proved only in rare individuals (Perkin, 1990). For instance, there is a single report in the English literature involving three adults who reacted on open challenge to a color mix (Murdock et al, 1987). When rechallenged, using DBPCFC techniques with individual colors, two of these three individuals developed urticaria when challenged with sunset yellow (FD&C #6). These positive challenge results were correlated with increased urine histamine and prostaglandin increases.

According to Simon and Stevenson (1993), there are only two reports (a total of two adult patients) in the English literature that documented sulfite-induced urticaria, angioedema, or anaphylaxis. In both situations, positive immediate-reacting IgE skin tests and passive transfer tests (Prausnitz-Küstner [PK]) demonstrated the rare presence of IgE sulfite-specific antibodies (Prenner and Stevens, 1976; Yang et al, 1986).

The incidence of urticarial reactions to sodium benzoate has been reported to be as high as 57 percent in a group of Italian children with recurrent urticaria (deMartino et al, 1992). Investigators in the United States have been unable to document a case (Simon and Stevenson, 1993). Urticarial reactions to BHA and BHT are rare. Two adults with chronic urticaria, who improved on a color- and preservative-free diet, were found to be challenge-positive to BHA and BHT during a DBPCFC technique (Goodman et al, 1990).

The most commonly reported adverse reaction associated with MSG flavor enhancer is the Chinese restaurant syndrome (Warner, 1993). This syndrome includes the following symptoms: nausea, headache, sweating, facial flushing, "tightness" and burning sensation of the face and chest, abdominal pain, and a "crawling" sensation of the skin. MSG-induced angioedema has been reported in rare instances (Simon and Stevenson, 1993).

Aspartame, an artificial sweetener, is a common source of complaints related to food additives (Perkin, 1990). The major complaint appears to be headache. Of 570 complaints reported to the FDA which were investigated by the US Center for Disease Control (CDC), 15 percent were allergic-like in nature (Geha et al, 1993). Two cases of aspartame-proved urticaria/angioedema confirmed by DBPCFC have been reported in the United States (Kulczycki, 1986). Claims have been made that 48 percent of children with chronic urticaria reacted to aspartame (deMartino et al, 1992). In spite of these reports, a recent, well-done and controlled, multi-center United States and Canadian study was unable to substantiate any relationship between urticaria or angioedema and aspartame (Geha et al, 1993).

Asthma

The principal food additive agents responsible for asthma exacerbation are the sulfite preservatives or SO_2. In 1973, an asthmatic child was reported who developed an acute attack after opening a cellophane package and ingesting part of the dried fruit content which had been treated with SO_2 (Kochen, 1973). Studies have shown that asthmatics may wheeze when exposed to less than 1.0 part per million (ppm) of SO_2 (Simon and Stevenson, 1993). Although sulfiting agents have been used in foods, beverages, and the restaurant industry world-wide for many years, it was not realized until the early 1980s that asthmatics might wheeze while ingesting these foods. Of particular concern have been fruits and vegetables ingested in restaurant salad bars where fruits and vegetables had been sprayed or dipped with sulfiting solutions (Taylor et al, 1988). The principal mechanism behind acute asthma exacerbation with sulfite exposure is the inhalation of the gas SO_2, released when foods containing sulfite are chewed and ingested. Other mechanisms that may be important in selected individuals include a rare IgE-mediated response and sulfite oxidase deficiency (Simon and Stevenson, 1993).

It is estimated that 3.9 percent of asthmatics are at risk for sulfite/SO_2-induced acute asthma (Bush et al, 1986). Of these, the risk is approximately 8.4 percent in serious or "steroid-dependent" asthmatics and 0.8 percent in mild-to-moderate asthmatics. Recently, federal legislation has been introduced to better regulate the use of sulfites in the United States, and consequently, reports of acute asthmatic exacerbations due to these agents have decreased. Sulfite content now must be noted in the labeling of foods, and less sulfite residues are allowed in foods and wines. The FDA has largely banned the use of sulfites on fresh fruits and vegetables.

A few individuals have been reported to have developed acute asthma attacks after ingesting foods containing monosodium glutamate (Allen et al, 1987). Using control studies, however, other investigators have been unable to substantiate these claims upon open oral challenge with up to 7.5 mg of MSG (Germano et al, 1991).

The other food additive most frequently implicated in provoking asthma reactions, according to the medical literature, has been tartrazine (yellow FD&C #5) (Simon and Stevenson, 1993). In the 1950s, artificial colorings were identified as a cause of asthma in children (Speer, 1958). Although numerous studies over the years claim to link tartrazine ingestion with asthma exacerbation, most well-done DBPCFC studies have failed to confirm this association. In one study of seven of 44 asthmatics who first reacted to tartrazine on single-blind challenge, none reacted on DBPCFC (Weber et al, 1979). Furthermore, in studies at Scripps Clinic in La Jolla, California, involving 150 proven aspirin-sensitive adult asthmatics, six individuals were found on single-blind screening to have a decrease in pulmonary function with oral tartrazine challenge, but none were found to react when challenged by means of double-blind methods (Stevenson et al, 1986).

TREATMENT OF ACUTE DIETARY SYSTEMIC REACTIONS

The treatment of systemic anaphylaxis and anaphylactoid reactions is outlined in Chapter 21. Management is based on (1) the initial treatment, (2) the approach if significant blood pressure decrease occurs (hypotension or shock), and (3) the approach if complications such as laryngeal edema or asthma occur.

The most important aspect of the initial treatment of anaphylaxis or anaphylactoid systemic reaction is the prompt use of subcutaneous aqueous epinephrine (American Academy of Allergy and Immunology, 1993). Although there are misconceptions that the patient or the caretaker of the patient can "wait and see" whether the condition gets worse before using epinephrine, the reaction may progress rapidly to a life-threatening situation. In a study of children and adolescents who either died or almost died of food anaphylaxis, one of the most important risk factors distinguishing death from near-death is how quickly epinephrine was administered (within one hour) after the first symptoms of anaphylaxis began (Sampson et al, 1992). For situations in which the individual is aware of the risk of reaction to a food, it is important that epinephrine be available to be used by patients, caretakers, and other responsible individuals should anaphylaxis occur (American Academy of Allergy and Immunology, 1993; American Academy of Pediatrics, 1990). Epinephrine is available for patient use in an autoinjector (Epi-Pen, 0.3 cc 1:1000 aqueous epinephrine, or Epi-Pen Jr, 0.15 cc 1:2000 aqueous epinephrine) or in a preloaded plastic syringe (AnaKit, two doses, 0.3 cc each of 1:1000 aqueous epinephrine) (see Chapter 21). All individuals who develop anaphylaxis or anaphylactoid reactions should go promptly to an emergency department for medical attention, whether or not epinephrine is administered immediately.

LABORATORY STUDIES

Mast cell tryptase has been shown to remain elevated in the serum for 1 to 4 hours following the onset of anaphylaxis or anaphylactoid reactions (Schwartz et al, 1989). Unfortunately, finding an increase of mast cell tryptase in the serum does not identify the cause. Also unfortunately, elevations in serum tryptase levels cannot always be found in milder anaphylactic reactions (including those to foods) and are not found in every case of severe systemic anaphylaxis.

In indeterminate cases of systemic reactions due to food ingestion, samples of the meal consumed by the patient can be frozen and saved for possible allergen-specific immunoassay studies (Keating et al, 1990; Yunginger et al, 1991). An IgE food allergen–specific *in vitro* assay may confirm the immunologic sensitivity of the patient. In most cases of serious systemic reactions, this test is sensitive enough to be positive if the proper allergen is tested. Food allergen IgE immediate-reacting epicutaneous (prick/puncture) skin testing can also be done, but in severe reactions, it is more risky than the identification of *in vitro* allergen-specific antibody (Yunginger, 1992). Not infrequently, when dealing with processed foods, the exact food allergen that was actually important in precipitating symptoms requires considerable detective work for the physician (Bock, 1993). Although provocative oral challenge feeding, preferably using DBPCFC methods, is an ideal way to confirm the involvement of a specific food or food additive in these reactions, these types of challenge tests are frequently avoided because of the risk involved (Yunginger, 1992).

In the case of other types of systemic reactions to dietary items such as suspected reactions to food additives, IgE *in vitro* or IgE epicutaneous immediate-reacting skin testing is not helpful since allergy is not involved. Only dietary challenge can confirm association with the suspected agent, preferably by the DBPCFC method. When asthma is suspected of being a symptom of dietary exposure, serial pulmonary function tests can be effectively used as end point (Stevenson et al, 1986; Taylor et al, 1988; Weber et al, 1979).

PREVENTION OF SYSTEMIC REACTIONS TO FOOD AND FOOD ADDITIVES

The best method of preventing repeated systemic reaction to foods or food additives is to identify the specific agent and then avoid future contact with that food or food additive (Yunginger, 1992). Although recently introduced federal regulations have improved product labeling in the United States, the public still has difficulty relying strictly on "label reading" as an absolute method by which one can obtain a processed food product free of ingredients that are offensive. Very often the food protein is called by different names, which are misleading (e.g., "caseinate" or "whey" for cow's milk protein). Incidences of falsely labeled food products have also surfaced, often because of food protein contamination during the manufacturing process (Gern et al, 1992; Jones et al, 1992). The food-allergic individual, especially the one who develops anaphylaxis, is particularly vulnerable when away from home, as in restaurants, school cafeterias, or social affairs. Often the offensive food protein is disguised in processed foods such as bakery products, candy, sauces, soups, sandwiches, or salads/dressings (Sampson et al, 1992; Yunginger et al, 1988). Although the anaphylactically sensitive individual must be cautious when eating away from home, this is often not enough. The sensitive person should carry a syringe of epinephrine (see Chapter 21), such as an Epi-Pen or Epi-Pen Jr. autoinjector or an AnaKit. Epinephrine should be used immediately at the first sign of a reaction, and then the patient should go, or be taken, for further medical treatment in a emergency department. Physicians are advised to prescribe three (e.g., home, car, person) or more epinephrine devices. Use of Medic Alert jewelry should be encouraged (Medic Alert Foundation, Turlock, California). Patient support for food-allergic individuals can be obtained through the Food Allergy Network, 4744 Holly Avenue, Fairfax, VA 22030—telephone number (703) 691-3179; or through local chapters of the Asthma and Allergy Foundation of America, 1125 15th Street NW, Suite 502, Washington DC 20005—telephone number (800) 727-8462.

Most medical authorities do not recommend food allergen immunotherapy as a method of food allergy prevention. Studies involving pollen allergen immunotherapy have failed to show protection of children with the OAS to exposure to fruits and vegetables. However, allergen immunotherapy for protection from generalized anaphylaxis from food has come under recent reappraisal (Sampson, 1992). Research into this form of immune modulation and protection for the anaphylactically sensitive individual has been advanced (Oppenheimer et al, 1992; Sampson, 1992). Peanut allergy was picked as the subject of the initial studies because of the high potential of peanut to cause sensitization, at an early age, as well as the high relative risk of re-exposure to a small but significant amount of peanut protein disguised in prepared or processed foods. In controlled studies, it has been shown that most infants of atopic parents are exposed to peanuts by the age of 2 years (Zeiger et al, 1989). Once peanut sensitization occurs, that sensitization lasts for at least 14 years and is presumed to be "life-long" (Bock and Atkins,

1989). Generally, individuals allergic to peanuts are able to tolerate other foods in the same family (e.g., soy, peas, beans). In deaths or near-deaths from food allergens in the United States, peanuts lead the list of agents involved (Yunginger et al, 1988; Sampson et al, 1992). Only carefully controlled future research studies will determine whether food allergen immunotherapy is a worthwhile, safe, and efficacious mode of food anaphylaxis prevention.

REFERENCES

Allen DH, Deloheny J, Baker G. Monosodium L-glutamate induced asthma. J Allergy Clin Immunol 80:503, 1987.

American Academy of Allergy and Immunology (AAAI). Position Statement. Use of epinephrine in the treatment of anaphylaxis. AAAI News & Notes. AAAI, Milwaukee WI, Oct, 1993, pp 6–7.

American Academy of Pediatrics. Committee on School Health. Guidelines for urgent care in schools. Pediatrics 86:999, 1990.

Amlot PL, Kemeny DM, Zachary C, et al. Oral allergy syndrome (OAS). Symptoms of IgE-mediated hypersensitivity to foods. Clin Allergy 17:33, 1987.

Appleyard JK, McCullough JA, Ownby DR. Cross-reactivity between latex, ragweed, and blue grass allergens. J Allergy Clin Immunol 93:182, 1994.

Aukrust L, Almend TL, Refsum D, Aas K. Severe hypersensitivity or intolerance to measles vaccine in six children. Allergy 35:581, 1980.

Beck S, Williams L, Shirrell A, Burks AW. Egg hypersensitivity in measles–mumps–rubella vaccine administration. Pediatrics 88:913, 1991.

Bernhisel-Broadbent J, Yolken RH, Sampson HA. Allergenicity of orally administered immunoglobulin preparations in food-allergic children. Pediatrics 87:208, 1991.

Birnbaum J, Tafforeau M, Vervloet D, et al. Allergy to sunflower honey associated with allergy to celery. Clin Exp Allergy 19:229, 1989.

Bock SA. Anaphylaxis to coriander; a sleuthing story. J Allergy Clin Immunol 91:1232, 1993.

Bock SA. The incidence of severe adverse reactions to foods in Colorado. J Allergy Clin Immunol 90:683, 1992.

Bock SA. Prospective appraisal of complaints of adverse reactions to foods in children during the first three years of life. Pediatrics 79:683, 1987.

Bock SA, Atkins FM. The natural history of peanut allergy. J Allergy Clin Immunol 83:900, 1989.

Bock SA, Sampson HA, Atkins FM, et al. Double-blind, placebo-controlled food challenge (DBPCFC) as an office procedure: A manual. J Allergy Clin Immunol 82:986, 1988.

Bush RK, Taylor SL, Holden K, et al. Prevalence of sensitivity to sulfiting agents in asthmatic patients. Am J Medicine 81:816, 1986.

Calkhoven PG, Aalbense M, Koshte V, et al. Cross-reactivity among birch pollen, vegetable and fruit as detected by IgE antibodies is due to at least three distinct cross-reactive structures. Allergy 42:382, 1987.

Cartier A, Malod L, Ghezzo H, McCants M, Lehrer SA. IgE sensitization in snow crab-processing workers. J Allergy Clin Immunol 78:244, 1986.

Chin JT, Haydik IB. Sesame seed oil anaphylaxis. J Allergy Clin Immunol 88:414, 1991.

Daul C, Morgan J, Lehrer S. The natural history of shrimp hypersensitivity. J Allergy Clin Immunol 86:88, 1990.

DeMartino M, Novembre E, Galli L, et al. Allergy to different fish species in cod-allergic children: *In vitro* and *in vivo* studies. J Allergy Clin Immunol 86:909, 1990.

DeMartino M, Peruzzi M, Galli L, et al. Food-additive intolerance and its correlation with atopy in children with recurrent or intermittent urticaria-angioedema. Pediatr Allergy Immunol 3:33, 1992.

Dohi M, Suko M, Sugiyama H, et al. Food-dependent, exercise-induced anaphylaxis: A study of 11 Japanese cases. J Allergy Clin Immunol 87:34, 1991.

Ebner C, Birkner T, Valenta R, et al. Common epitopes of birch pollen and apples—studies by western and northern blot. J Allergy Clin Immunol 88:588, 1991.

Enberg R, Leickly F, McCullough J, et al. Watermelon and ragweed share allergens. J Allergy Clin Immunol 79:867, 1987.

Erben A, Rodriguez JL, McCullough J, Ownby DR. Anaphylaxis after ingestion of beignets contaminated with *Dermatophygoidies farinae*. J Allergy Clin Immunol 92:846, 1993.

Fasano MB, Wood RA, Sampson HA. Egg allergy and adverse reaction to measles, mumps, rubella (MMR) vaccine. J Allergy Clin Immunol 87:175, 1991.

Fernández de Corres L, Moneo I, Munoz D, et al. Sensitization from chestnuts and bananas in patients with urticaria and anaphylaxis from contact with latex. Ann Allergy 70:35, 1993.

Fuglsang G, Madsen C, Saval P, Osterballe O. Prevalence of intolerance to food additives among Danish school children. Pediatr Allergy Immunol 14:123, 1993.

Geha R, Buckley CE, Greenberger P, et al. Aspartame is no more likely than placebo to cause urticaria/angioedema: Results of a multicenter, randomized, double-blind, placebo-controlled, cross-over study. J Allergy Clin Immunol 92:513, 1993.

Germano P, Cohen SG, Hahn B, Metcalfe DD. An evaluation of clinical reactions to monosodium glutamate (MSG) in asthmatics using a blinded, placebo-controlled challenge. J Allergy Clin Immunol 87:177, 1991.

Gern JE, Yange E, Eurand HM, Sampson HA. Allergic reactions to milk containing "non-dairy products." N Engl J Med 324:976, 1992.

Goodman DL, McDonnell JT, Nelson HS, Vaugh TR, Weber RW. Chronic urticaria exacerbated by the antioxidant food preservatives, butylated hydroxysole (BHA) and butylated hydroxytoluene (BHT). J Allergy Clin Immunol 86:570, 1990.

Herman JJ, Radin R, Schneider R. Allergic reactions to measles (rubella) vaccine in patients hypersensitive to egg protein. J Pediatrics 102:196, 1983.

Horan RF, Sheffer AL. Food-dependent exercise-induced anaphylaxis. Immunol Allergy Clin North Am 11:757, 1991.

Horst A, Halken S. A prospective study of cow's milk allergy in Danish infants during the first 3 years of life. Allergy 45:587, 1990.

James J, Cooke S, Barnett A. Anaphylactic reactions to a psyllium containing cereal. J Allergy Clin Immunol 88:402, 1991.

Jarmoc L, Primack W. Anaphylaxis to cutaneous exposure to milk protein in a diaper rash ointment. Clin Pediatrics 26:154, 1987.

Jones RT, Squillocs DL, Yunginger JW. Anaphylaxis in a milk allergic child after ingestion of milk-contaminated kosher "pareve-labeled" dairy-free dessert. Ann Allergy 68:273, 1992.

Keating MU, Jones RT, Worley NJ, et al. Immunoassay of peanut allergens in food-processing materials and finished foods. J Allergy Clin Immunol 86:41, 1990.

Kelso JM, Jones RT, Yunginger JW. Anaphylaxis to measles, mumps, and rubella vaccine mediated by IgE to gelatin. J Allergy Clin Immunol 91:867, 1993.

Kochen J. Sulfur dioxide, a respiratory irritant, even if ingested. Pediatrics 52:145, 1973.

Kulczycki A. Aspartane-induced urticaria. Ann Intern Med 104:207, 1986.

Lockey SD. Allergic reactions due to FD&C yellow #5, tartrazine, an aniline dye used as a coloring and identifying agent in various steroids. Ann Allergy 17:719, 1959.

Miraihi L, Charpin D, Pon A, Bongrand P, Vervloet D. Cross-reacting between latex and banana. J Allergy Clin Immunol 87:129, 1991.

Moller C. The effect of immunotherapy on food hypersensitivity on children with birch pollinosis. Ann Allergy 62:343, 1989.

Moneret-Vautrin DA, Beaudouin E, Widmer S, et al. Prospective study of risk factors in natural rubber latex hypersensitivity. J Allergy Clin Immunol 92:668, 1993.

Murdock D, Pollock I, Young E, Lessof MH. Food additive-induced urticaria: Studies of mediator release during provocative tests. J Royal College Physicians London 4:262, 1987.

Oppenheimer JJ, Nelson HS, Bock SA, et al. Treatment of peanut allergy with rush immunotherapy. J Allergy Clin Immunol 90:256, 1992.

Ortolani C, Ispnao M, Pastorello EA, et al. Comparison of results of skin prick tests (with fresh foods and commercial food extracts) and RAST in 100 patients with oral allergy syndrome. J Allergy Clin Immunol 83:683, 1989.

Ownby D, Tomlanovich M, Sammons N, McCullough J. Fatal anaphylaxis during a barium enema examination associated with latex allergy. Am J Radiol 156:903, 1991.

Perkin JE. Adverse reactions to food additives and other food constituents in food allergies and adverse reactions. In Perkin JE (ed). Food Allergies and Adverse Reactions. Gaithersburg, MD, Aspen, 1990, pp 129–170.

Prenner BM, Stevens JJ. Anaphylaxis after ingestion of sodium bisulfite. Ann Allergy 37:180, 1976.

Rietschel RL, Bernier R. Neomycin sensitivity and MMR vaccine. JAMA 13:245, 1981.

Ross BD, McCullough J, Ownby DR. Partial cross-reactivity between latex and banana allergens. J Allergy Clin Immunol 90:409, 1992.

Sampson HA. Food allergy and the role of immunotherapy (Editorial). J Allergy Clin Immunol 90:151, 1992.

Sampson HA, Mendelson L, Rosen J. Fatal and near-fatal anaphylactic reactions to foods in children and adolescents. N Engl J Med 327:380, 1992.

Schwartz LB, Yunginger JW, Miller J, et al. The time course of the appearance and disappearance of human mast cell tryptase in circulation after anaphylaxis. J Clin Invest 83:1551, 1989.

Simon RA, Stevenson DD. Adverse reactions to food and drug additives. In Middleton E Jr, Yunginger JW, Busse WW (eds). Allergy: Principles and Practice. 4th ed. St. Louis, Mosby–Year Book, 1993, pp 1687–1704.

Speer K (ed). The Management of Childhood Asthma. Springfield, IL, Charles C Thomas, 1958, p 23.

Staff RH, Fink JN. Anaphylaxis to chicken soup: A case report and a brief history of chicken in medicine. J Allergy Clin Immunol 89:1061, 1992.

Stark BJ, Sullivan TJ. Biphasic and protracted anaphylaxis. J Allergy Clin Immunol 78:76, 1986.

Stevenson DD, Simon RA, Lumrey WR, et al. Adverse reactions to tartrazine. J Allergy Clin Immunol 78:182, 1986.

Stricker WE, Anorne-Lopez E, Reed C. Food skin testing in patients with idiopathic anaphylaxis. J Allergy Clin Immunol 77:516, 1986.

Taylor SL, Bush RK, Selner JC, et al. Sensitivity to sulfated foods among sulfite-sensitive subjects with asthma. J Allergy Clin Immunol 81:1159, 1988.

Warner JO. Food and behavior. Pediatr Allergy Immunol 4:112, 1993.

Weber RW, Hoffman M, Raine DA, Nelson HS. Incidence of bronchoconstriction due to aspirin, azo dyes, nonazo dyes, and preservatives in a population of perennial asthmatics. J Allergy Clin Immunol 64:32, 1979.

Yang WH, Purchase ECR, Rivington RN. Positive skin tests and Prausnitz-Kutsner reactions in metabisulfite sensitive subjects. J Allergy Clin Immunol 78:443, 1986.

Yunginger JW. Anaphylaxis to foods. Immunol Allergy Clin North Am 12:543, 1992.

Yunginger JW, Nelson DR, Squillace DL, et al. Laboratory investigation of deaths due to anaphylaxis. J Forensic Sci 36:857, 1991.

Yunginger JW, Sweeney KG, Sturner WQ, et al. Fatal food-induced anaphylaxis. JAMA 260:1450, 1988.

Zeiger RS, Heller S, Mellon MH, et al. Effect of combined maternal and infant food-allergen avoidance on development of atopy in early infancy: A randomized study. J Allergy Clin Immunol 84:72, 1989.

Chapter 26

Exercise-Induced Anaphylaxis

Richard F. Horan, M.D., and Albert L. Sheffer, M.D.

Anaphylaxis is the most urgent manifestation of allergic disease. The clinical features of this syndrome result, at least in part, from the release of potent biologically active substances by activated mast cells and basophils, with subsequent elicitation of characteristic responses in target organs. Clinical manifestations of anaphylaxis may involve skin and subcutaneous tissue (suffusion and flushing, pruritus, urticaria, and angioedema), upper respiratory tract (laryngeal edema and rhinitis), lower respiratory tract (bronchospasm), gastrointestinal tract (abdominal colic, nausea, diarrhea, and gastrointestinal bleeding), cardiovascular system (vascular collapse with hypotension), and other tissues. Thus, symptoms and signs may range from merely disquieting to immediately life-threatening. Mortality or end-organ damage caused by shock may ensue.

Exercise-induced anaphylaxis (EIA) is a syndrome that has been recognized for about a quarter century. In EIA, symptoms similar to those of anaphylactic reactions due to classic type I hypersensitivity occur in association with exercise. This syndrome, which is classified among the physical allergies, may present with initial findings of pruritus, cutaneous suffusion and warmth, urticaria, and angioedema, and may in some instances progress to upper respiratory obstruction, vascular collapse, or both (Sheffer and Austen, 1980; Sheffer and Austen, 1984; Sheffer et al, 1983). The exact pathogenesis of this syndrome is not understood. Participation of the mast cell appears important in the pathophysiology of at least some cases (Sheffer et al, 1985). On clinical grounds, EIA has been differentiated from a number of other exercise-associated adverse reactions. Recognition of EIA is increasing, in association with increased popular interest in physical fitness through exercise. However, the incidence, pathophysiology, and natural history of this condition remain poorly understood.

CLINICAL FEATURES OF EIA

Recognition of a clinical syndrome of exercise-induced anaphylaxis dates back more than a quarter century, but it was not until 1980 that a group of patients with this condition was described. Prior to this, the earliest report in the literature is probably that of Mathews and Pan, in 1970 (Mathews and Pan, 1970). Over the past decade, clinical experience with EIA has increased, and multiple case reports, small series, and controlled clinical studies have documented the existence of this entity, which is now well recognized by the practicing allergist (Sheffer and Austen, 1980; Sheffer and Austen, 1984; Sheffer et al, 1983; Sheffer et al, 1985; Casale et al, 1986; Lewis et al, 1981; Wade et al, 1989; Sonsiridej and Busse, 1983).

The initial series of 16 patients with EIA reported in 1980 consisted of 11 male and 5 female patients, ranging in age from 12 to 54 years (mean age 24 years) (Sheffer and Austen, 1980). In most of these patients, symptoms of EIA had been noted for several years prior to the initial assessment. The frequency of occurrence of episodes of EIA varied from a single occurrence to several attacks annually for a period of 16 years. All patients in this series were accomplished athletes. EIA had occurred in association with such activities as jogging, running, sprinting, performing tennis warmups, playing tennis, or playing soccer. Most patients in this series exercised daily, two exercised three times per week, and two exercised once per week. Early on, it was noted that, in contrast to other forms of physical allergy in which application of the physical stimulus is reproducibly and invariably associated with the development of symptoms, attacks of EIA were not consistently noted in a given patient, even when the patient was undergoing apparently identical degrees of exertion. The inconsistent development of EIA after apparently similar degrees of exertion suggests the possible importance of other factors in the development of clinically overt EIA. The nature of such factors and their precise role in the pathogenesis of EIA remain speculative. In the initial series, exercise in the postprandial state, exercise after ingestion of aspirin or of caffeine, and exercise in higher ambient temperatures appeared to be associated with an increased likelihood of development of symptoms. In one patient in this series, exercise in the rain was associated with prolonged collapse on two occasions.

Episodes of EIA have been noted to have a characteristic evolution, and this was described in the initial series of patients reported and has subsequently been validated by further clinical experience. Premonitory symptoms include fatigue, diffuse warmth and pruritus, and development of cutaneous erythema. An urticarial eruption generally ensues, with the development of areas of confluence, often with angioedema. Angioedema of the face, palms, and soles has been a prominent feature in many individuals afflicted with EIA. Cutaneous findings of urticaria and angioedema tend to persist throughout the attack, which generally lasts from 30 minutes to 4 hours. Vascular collapse with transient loss of consciousness is common, and in the initial series, 12 of 16 patients collapsed after the interruption of exercise. Choking and stridor, gastrointestinal colic, nausea, and vomiting are common. Headache, often disabling, has been a late sequela of episodes of EIA and can persist for as long as 72 hours.

A recent epidemiologic survey of EIA provided detailed information that had been obtained by questionnaire from 199 individuals believed on clinical grounds to be afflicted with this disorder. Of these, 134 were female and 65 were male. The mean age at the time of assessment was 32.8 years (range 9 to 80 years); the mean age at the onset of symptoms was 24.7 years (range 4 to 74 years). The most common pattern clinically was that of twice-weekly episodes, with the frequency of attacks ranging from a single episode to innumerable attacks. Jogging was the most common activity reported to precipitate attacks, but a variety of other activities including walking, bicycling, racquet sports, skiing, and aerobic exercise were noted to have been associated with the development of episodes. The clinical features of the attacks were similar to those that had been described in earlier reports, with pruritus the most frequent and earliest symptom in most individuals. Urticaria, angioedema, and flushing were also common, and upper respiratory symptoms were described by 59 percent of respondents. Thirty-two percent of individuals surveyed had experienced loss of consciousness, and gastrointestinal symptoms had been present in 30 percent. Gastrointestinal colic was described by 30 percent of patients. Most episodes resolved within 2 hours, but persistent symptoms for 12 or more hours were noted by a minority of respondents, and headache was the most typical prolonged manifestation of the disorder.

Most respondents in this survey described additional factors that they believed to precipitate an attack eventuating in conjunction with exercise. These factors included antecedent ingestion of alcohol (5 percent of respondents), aspirin ingestion before exercise (6 percent of respondents), use of other medications before exercise, and environmental factors. Exercise in a warm environment was cited by 127 of 199 respondents as tending to increase the likelihood of an attack, whereas cold weather was believed to increase the probability of an attack by 46 respondents to this survey. Humidity was believed by 63 respondents to increase the likelihood of an attack. Twenty-five of 134 female respondents thought that the phase of the menstrual cycle affected the probability of development of EIA. Numerous additional reports have suggested an association between exercise in the postprandial state and the development of EIA. The antecedent use of aspirin has also been cited elsewhere as a factor tending to increase the likelihood of a clinical attack (Dohi et al, 1990).

Numerous patients have been described in whom the antecedent ingestion of a specific food (varying from patient to patient, and generally reflected by positive prick test sensitivity or elevated RAST test titers to the food in question) was a prerequisite for an attack of EIA. Other patients have been described in whom exercise in the postprandial state either was requisite to the occurrence of an attack (without requirement for ingestion of a specific food), or increased the probability of development of a clinical episode.

EIA requiring the ingestion of a specific food antecedent to exercise was first reported by Maulitz et al (Maulitz et al, 1979). The authors reported the development of anaphylaxis associated with running after ingestion of shrimp or oysters in a 31-year-old atopic man. Long distance running without prior ingestion of shellfish, and ingestion of shellfish without subsequent exertion, provoked no reaction. Prick testing showed positive tests to oysters and shrimp as well as to clams, crabs, peanuts, and several aero-allergens. Subsequently, additional patients have been described in whom the antecedent ingestion of shellfish, celery, peach, wheat or other grains, or chicken is essential for the development of a reaction (Akutsu et al, 1989; Armentia et al, 1990; Buchbinder et al, 1983; Dohi et al, 1990; Dohi et al, 1991; El-Dieb, 1984; Kidd et al, 1983; Kivity et al, 1988; Kushimoto and Aoki, 1985; Laufer, 1987; Lin and Barnard, 1993; McNeil and Strauss, 1988; Silverstein et al, 1986; Watanabe et al, 1990). Specific foods noted by a variety of responders to an epidemiologic survey as important in the genesis of their attacks have included shellfish (8 percent of respondents), celery (6 percent), or cabbage (6 percent) (Wade et al, 1989).

EIA occurring only in the postprandial state (without requirement for ingestion of a specific food) was first described by Novey et al in a 1983 case report (Novey et al, 1983). Subsequently, additional patients have been described in whom the development of clinically overt EIA appears only when exercise is undertaken postprandially (Dohi et al, 1991). Of the 16 patients described by Sheffer and Austen in 1980, three believed that symptoms were worse when exercise was conducted in the postprandial state (Sheffer and Austen, 1980). The epidemiologic survey conducted by Wade et al indicated that food ingestion within 3 to 4 hours prior to exercise was believed to be an important factor in increasing the likelihood of attacks by more than half of respondents (Wade et al, 1989). Antecedent ingestion of alcohol was believed to be important by 5 percent of respondents. Patients with postprandial EIA whose attacks are exacerbated by the use of aspirin have also been described.

Personal and family histories of atopy are more common in individuals with EIA, both in patients assessed first-hand and on the basis of epidemiologic survey information. At least one study has suggested that the incidence of atopy is particularly increased in individuals with onset of EIA at an earlier age (Dohi et al, 1991). Familial EIA has been reported occasionally (Grant et al, 1985; Longley and Panush, 1987).

EXERCISE CHALLENGE IN EIA

Exercise challenge involving running on a treadmill while wearing a plastic occlusive suit has been described in seven patients with a history of EIA seen at our center (Sheffer et al, 1983). Clinical responses to exercise challenge were noted in only four of these subjects and were characterized by the development of pruritus and flushing without urticaria. Angioedema developed in four instances in two subjects. On one of these occasions, a subject had symptoms of upper respiratory obstruction with coughing, which required administration of epinephrine for symptomatic relief. With rechallenge, this subject developed severe headache in addition to the aforementioned symptoms in attenuated form. None of the subjects assessed in this report or subsequently participating in experimental exercise challenge at our center experienced vascular collapse or loss of consciousness. Wheezing has not been noted in any individual so challenged. Pruritus and erythema generally resolve within 30 minutes after cessation of exercise challenge, thus representing a somewhat shorter duration than in the naturally occurring attack. No changes in pulmonary function testing have been noted in patients undergoing exercise challenge. In those subjects participating in the foregoing series who experienced a clinical response to exercise challenge, significant increase in serum histamine levels was noted, whereas in individuals not experiencing clinical symptoms, significant increase in serum histamine could not be documented. Elevations in serum histamine level during symptomatic episodes returned to normal in approximately 20 minutes, slightly before the resolution of clinical signs and symptoms. Other routine laboratory studies and assessment of the complement system have been unremarkable in patients with EIA evaluated at our center. In one other series, the use of exercise challenge was augmented by passive elevation of body temperature, with patients with true EIA not demonstrating a reaction with passive temperature elevation, in contrast to patients with cholinergic urticaria.

DIFFERENTIAL DIAGNOSIS OF EIA

This syndrome of exercise-associated development of pruritus, cutaneous warmth and erythema, urticaria, vascular collapse, upper respiratory distress, gastrointestinal colic, and other associated findings has been designated EIA because of its similarity to the naturally occurring attack of anaphylaxis caused by IgE-dependent mechanisms after ingestion or injection of a foreign antigenic substance. EIA appears to be clinically distinct from other exercise-associated syndromes (Table 26–1). Arrhythmias or other isolated cardiovascular events are not associated with pruritus, cutaneous erythema, urticaria, and angioedema, or true upper respiratory obstruction and gastrointestinal symptoms, as seen in EIA, do not form a part of the presentation of the patient with an arrhythmia. Exercise-induced asthma is characterized by prominent wheezing, in contrast to the occasional development of evanescent wheezing occurring in EIA. In experimental exercise challenges of patients with EIA, pulmonary function testing has been normal (although exercise challenges have not been noted to produce full-blown attacks of the syndrome and, indeed, are intended to produce an attenuated form of the naturally occurring attack, with discontinuation at the initial manifestations of anaphylaxis, so that the experimental challenge may not be entirely adequate to assess pulmonary function changes that might be seen with more advanced, naturally occurring episodes). Cutaneous warmth and erythema, pruritus, urticaria, and angioedema are not seen in exercise-induced asthma, nor does upper respiratory obstruction or vascular collapse characterize that condition.

Cholinergic urticaria is a physical allergy characterized by the development of punctate (1 to 3 mm diameter), intensely pruritic wheals with surrounding erythematous flares, occurring after elevation of core body temperature (e.g., with exertion, fever, or hot baths or showers), as well as in association with stress (thus possibly implicating a neurogenic mechanism). Although most patients with EIA develop urticarial lesions greater than several millimeters in diameter (that is to say, develop "common hives"), a minority of individuals experiencing the clinical syndrome of cutaneous pruritus, warmth, vascular collapse, upper respiratory obstruction, and gastrointestinal symptoms has been noted to present with cutaneous lesions more consistent with cholinergic urticaria (Sheffer and Austen, 1980; Sheffer and Austen, 1984; Casale et al, 1986). The differentiation of EIA from generalized symptoms consequent to severe cholinergic urticaria has thus at times been difficult. However, the clinical syndrome of EIA has a sufficient degree of uniformity of presentation to suggest that EIA represents a discrete clinical entity distinct from cholinergic urticaria. Pulmonary function test abnormalities are common in cholinergic urticaria (Soter et al, 1980), but have not been noted in controlled clinical exercise challenges in EIA. Conversely, vascular collapse

TABLE 26–1. CLASSIFICATION OF EXERCISE-INDUCED PHYSICAL ALLERGY

Type	Precipitating Event	Urticaria: Morphology	Associated Collapse	Bronchospasm		Elevated Serum Histamine
				Clinical	Functional	
Cholinergic	Heat, stress, exercise	Punctate (2–5 mm)	−	±	+	+
Variant	Exercise	Punctate	+	−	−	+
Anaphylactic	Exercise	Conventional (10–15 mm)	+	−	−	+

− = absent; + = present; ± = equivocal.
From Sheffer AL, et al. Exercise-induced anaphylaxis: A distinct form of physical allergy. J Allergy Clin Immunol 71:311, 1983.

and upper respiratory obstruction, although common in patients with EIA, are rare in individuals afflicted with cholinergic urticaria. Patients with EIA, moreover, do not develop symptoms after a hot bath or shower, with febrile episodes, or with anxiety or stress (see Table 26–1). A passive heat challenge has been described as useful in differentiating the two entities (Casale et al, 1986). The development of cholinergic urticaria appears more consistent and reproducible than is the case with EIA, which alone among the described physical urticarias does not invariably occur following application of the defined physical stimulus. Although elevation of serum histamine levels has been described in experimental challenge of individuals with cholinergic urticaria (Soter et al, 1980), and although involvement of the mast cell appears to be important in both of these forms of physical allergy, ultrastructural changes during experimental challenge in EIA and in cholinergic urticaria appear to be distinct. In exercise challenge in individuals with EIA, mast cell ultrastructural changes are similar to those seen in IgE-Fc-dependent activation-secretion response of dispersed human pulmonary mastocytes (anaphylactic granulation) (Maulitz et al, 1979). In contrast, cholinergic urticaria has preliminarily been associated with a novel ultrastructural appearance termed zonal degranulation. Although passive transfer experiments have suggested an IgE-mediated mechanism in at least some individuals with cholinergic urticaria, no such studies have as yet been performed in EIA. Nonetheless, the causes of each of these forms of physical urticaria remain unknown, and it may well be that factors affecting mast cell lability are common to the pathophysiology of each of these disorders.

PATHOPHYSIOLOGY OF EIA

The sequence of biochemical events in the development of an attack of EIA is unknown. The similarity of clinical presentations of the findings seen in IgE-mediated anaphylaxis caused by ingestion or injection of an antigenic substance has suggested the possibility of a significant role for mast cells, basophils, or both types of cells. Experimental challenges have been associated with an increase in serum histamine levels in EIA in several studies (Sheffer et al, 1983; Casale et al, 1986; Dohi et al, 1991), and elevated tryptase level has been described in one patient. Morphologic evidence of mast cell involvement has been adduced with evidence of anaphylactoid degranulation following exercise challenge in patients with EIA (Sheffer et al, 1985). Before exercise challenge, ultrastructural evaluation of cutaneous mast cells showed no abnormality in patients with EIA compared with normal controls. After exercise challenge, however, the development of clinical response was associated with a number of ultrastructural changes in dermal mast cells, including a loss of electron density and internal substructure of mast cell granules; fusion of granule membranes with membranes of adjacent granules and mast cell membrane; and a decrease in the number of intact granules per mast cell. These changes, as above, are similar to those seen in the IgE-Fc-dependent activation-secretion response of dispersed human pulmonary mast cells and to alterations seen in mast cells after *in vivo* challenge by intradermal injection of ragweed extract into an allergic individual.

Aside from the demonstration of elevation of serum histamine levels in association with development of clinical symptoms, studies assessing other mast cell–derived mediators of inflammation and other inflammatory mediators in general have not been undertaken. Although several reports describe complement abnormalities in individual patients with EIA (Obata et al, 1989), no abnormalities of the complement system have been appreciated in most patients reported in the literature (Sheffer and Austen, 1980; Sheffer and Austen, 1984; Lewis et al, 1981).

The pathogenesis of EIA thus remains obscure. However, it is clear that a variety of physiologic inputs can induce mast cell degranulation or alter the threshold for degranulation (Holgate et al, 1989; White et al, 1989). Such inputs include neuropeptides, endogenous opiates, inflammatory cell-derived histamine-releasing factors, and other cytokines. The importance of neural inputs on the mast cell, particularly the input of the nonadrenergic, noncholinergic autonomic nervous system, is increasingly being appreciated. Also possibly significant in connection with the importance of neurohumoral input on the mast cell is the finding that, although both norepinephrine and epinephrine levels increase in response to exercise, the response is significantly more marked for norepinephrine, and thus an alpha adrenergic influence on mast cell tone could conceivably be important in the pathophysiology of EIA (Dimsdale et al, 1984). Transient fluctuations in extracellular fluid electrolyte concentrations, respiratory water, and heat loss during exercise, or conceivably even alterations in cutaneous blood flow during exercise, could also be relevant. Patients in whom the postprandial state is either requisite or conducive to the development of EIA might have abnormal responses to autonomic efferents in the postprandial state, or to neuropeptide elaboration. In this regard, it is interesting that, at physiologic concentrations, gastrin has been shown to stimulate mediator release from cutaneous mast cells *in vitro* and *in vivo* (Tharp et al, 1984).

Kivity and coworkers have speculated that the development of clinical episodes of EIA in individuals with specific food allergies might be a consequence of an antigen-IgE interaction, which would in itself represent a subthreshold exposure, potentiated by a nonspecific effect of physical stimulus causing decreased mast cell threshold, with consequent mediator release (Maulitz et al, 1979). This concept seems more plausible given the clinical observation of dermatographism occurring during penicillin therapy in individuals allergic to that drug. To further assess this hypothesis, five atopic individuals with histories of exercise-induced urticaria and angioedema who had specific food allergen sensitivity on prick skin testing were evaluated. Cutaneous whealing caused by intradermal injection of compound 48/80 and of histamine was measured after exercise challenge was performed in individuals who had ingested a meal free of foods to which they reacted. Cutaneous whealing was also measured in patients after ingestion of a meal containing foods to which prick tests had been positive and, in a further study, after exercise following ingestion of a meal containing food to which patients had positive prick tests. Symptoms could be reproduced in only four of the five patients tested. In these individuals, the development of symptoms after a combination of ingestion of skin test positive foods plus exercise challenge was associated with marked increase in the cutaneous wheal response to compound 48/80, but not to histamine, whereas ingestion of skin test positive foods alone or exercise challenge without prior ingestion of skin test positive foods did not produce any significant change in cutaneous reactivity to either compound 48/80 or histamine. These findings are consistent with increased mast cell releasability to specific food allergens after exercise, thus lending credibility to the hypothesis that at least some cases of food-dependent EIA might represent food-dependent, IgE-mediated immediate hypersensitivity reactions, which would be subthreshold in the absence of exercise, but which, because of a synergistic influence of exercise on mast cell lability, become clinically overt.

The development of the clinical phenomenon of EIA in a sensitive individual thus might be the result of an abnormal post-exercise concentration of a mast cell secretagogue normally present at a lower concentration in unafflicted individuals; the exercise-associated elaboration of a mast cell secretagogue not present in unafflicted individuals; aberrations in neural tone; or an abnormal sensitivity of mast cells, or a subpopulation thereof, or some other cell type to an exercise-associated secretagogue or to exercise-associated neural efferents. In some individuals, such a mechanism or mechanisms might potentiate an IgE-mediated reaction to the requisite food coupled with nonspecific humoral or neural abnormalities operative in other patients with EIA. Alternatively, the exertion in question could possibly have been associated with augmented distribution of the specific food allergen at appropriate concentrations to peripheral sites with subsequent IgE-mediated reaction and tissue response. (Further support for the role of IgE-mediated mechanisms may be lent by reports of individuals who experience their EIA symptoms during their allergic rhinitis seasons.)

MANAGEMENT OF EIA

The emergency management of EIA is identical to that of anaphylaxis of any cause and includes the subcutaneous administration of epinephrine, intravenous volume repletion, oxygen therapy, and vigilance for upper airway compromise, with endotracheal intubation or tracheotomy should this be required. Antihistamines may be helpful in blunting the severity of the acute attack, but prompt treatment of acute manifestations with administration of epinephrine, volume repletion, and airway management is crucial.

Bronchospasm may be addressed with inhalational bronchodilators, subcutaneous epinephrine, or aminophylline, as in other forms of anaphylaxis. The occurrence of a late-phase reaction in human anaphylaxis has not been definitely established, but continued observation of an individual presenting with EIA for an appropriately prolonged period (e.g., 6 hours) seems prudent. The utility of administration of glucocorticoids in anaphylaxis in the human has not been definitely established, although it is frequently undertaken on an empiric basis in the emergency room setting, and glucocorticoids have been useful in chronic management of many patients with idiopathic anaphylaxis.

PREVENTION

Recognition of the exercise-associated nature of the event is critical if the afflicted individual is to avoid recurrent attacks. A close historical review of the events surrounding the presenting episode, as well as any prior episodes, should be conducted, and the history should include information concerning ingestants and any other factors that might conceivably bear on precipitation of the episode, including antecedent use of aspirin or nonsteroidal anti-inflammatory drugs (as is common among athletes). The importance of environmental factors, particularly ambient temperature and humidity at the time of the attack, should be considered. In atopic patients with EIA, the seasonal occurrence of EIA should be considered.

The prophylactic use of antihistamines before exercise has been noted by some individuals with EIA to be associated with some amelioration or blunting of the naturally occurring attack. However, antihistamines do not appear to fully prevent attacks of EIA, and their prophylactic use should therefore not be relied upon. More important is recognition of the prodromal manifestations of the EIA attack, so that exercise can be discontinued at the earliest warning signs. Modification of the individual's exercise program by reduction in intensity or duration of exertion may be required to avoid early manifestations of EIA. Avoidance of exercise on warm or humid days is prudent, and given that the postprandial state seems important as a conducive factor in many afflicted individuals and that our knowledge of the pathophysiology of EIA in a given patient is limited, it also seems appropriate that as a general rule individuals with EIA defer significant exercise for 4 to 6 hours postprandially. Given the association of antecedent aspirin ingestion with EIA in some patients, avoidance of salicylates, nonsteroidal anti-inflammatory drugs, and cyclooxygenase inhibitors in conjunction with exercise also seems prudent. Individuals in whom ingestion of aspirin or nonsteroidal anti-inflammatory drugs has clearly been associated with the development of EIA should certainly avoid exertion with the use of these medications.

Individuals with EIA should be aware of the need to discontinue exercise at the earliest symptoms of pruritus or cutaneous warmth. Ideally, such individuals should be accompanied during exercise by a companion aware of their condition and capable of rendering emergency assistance. Patients with EIA should have materials for self-administration of subcutaneous epinephrine on their person during exercise and should wear a medical identification bracelet.

The degree of risk of mortality or significant morbidity associated with EIA is currently unknown. Nonetheless, the similarity of the EIA attack to anaphylaxis occurring as IgE-mediated mechanisms, and the known risk of death or significant organ damage associated with anaphylaxis of the latter cause, mandate a prudent approach to the management of patients with EIA.

REFERENCES

Akutsu I, Motojima S, Ikeda Y, et al. Three cases of food-dependent exercise-induced anaphylaxis. Arerugi 38:277, 1989.

Armentia A, Martin-Santos JM, Blanco M, et al. Exercise-induced anaphylactic reaction to grain flours. Ann Allergy 65:149, 1990.

Buchbinder EM, Bloch KJ, Moss J, et al. Food-dependent, exercise-induced anaphylaxis. JAMA 250:2973, 1983.

Casale TB, Keahey TM, Kaliner M. Exercise-induced anaphylactic syndromes: Insights into diagnostic and pathophysiologic features. JAMA 255:2049, 1986.

Dimsdale JE, Hartley LH, Guiney T, et al. Postexercise peril: Plasma catecholamines and exercise. JAMA 251:630, 1984.

Dohi M, Suko M, Sugiyama H, et al. Food-dependent exercise-induced anaphylaxis: A study on 11 Japanese cases. J Allergy Clin Immunol 87:34, 1991.

Dohi M, Suko M, Sugiyama H, et al. Three cases of food-dependent exercise-induced anaphylaxis in which aspirin exacerbated anaphylactic symptoms. Arerugi 39:1598, 1990.

El-Dieb MR. Food-dependent, exercise-induced anaphylaxis. JAMA 251:3224, 1984. (Letter)

Grant JA, Farnam J, Lord RA, et al. Familial exercise-induced anaphylaxis. Ann Allergy 54:35, 1985.

Holgate S, Benyon RC, Lowman MA, et al. Activation of human mast cells after immunoglobulin E-dependent and neuropeptide stimulation. Prog Clin Biol Res 297:103, 1989.

Kidd JM III, Cohen SH, Sosman AJ, et al. Food-dependent exercise-induced anaphylaxis. J Allergy Clin Immunol 71:407, 1983.

Kivity S, Sneh E, Greif J, et al. The effect of food and exercise on the skin response to compound 48/80 in patients with food-associated exercise-induced urticaria-angioedema. J Allergy Clin Immunol 81:1155, 1988.

Kushimoto H, Aoki T. Masked type I wheat allergy. Relation to exercise-induced anaphylaxis. Arch Dermatol 121:355, 1985.

Laufer P. Exercise-induced anaphylactic reaction to chicken dependent on the quantity ingested. Immunol Allergy Pract 9:213, 1987.

Lewis J, Lieberman P, Treadwell G, et al. Exercise-induced urticaria, angioedema, and anaphylactoid episodes. J Allergy Clin Immunol 68:432, 1981.

Lin RY, Barnard M. Skin testing with food, codeine and histamine in exercise-induced anaphylaxis. Ann Allergy 70:475, 1993.

Longley S, Panush RS. Familial exercise-induced anaphylaxis. Ann Allergy 58:257, 1987.

Mathews KP, Pan P. Post-exercise hyperhistaminemia, dermographia, and wheezing. Ann Intern Med 72:241, 1970.

Maulitz RM, Pratt DS, Schocket AL. Exercise-induced anaphylactic reaction to shellfish. J Allergy Clin Immunol 63:433, 1979.

McNeil D, Strauss RH. Exercise-induced anaphylaxis related to food intake. Ann Allergy 61:440, 1988.

Novey HS, Fairshter RD, Salness K, et al. Postprandial exercise-induced anaphylaxis. J Allergy Clin Immunol 71:498, 1983.

Obata T, Kishida M, Okuma M, et al. A case of exercise-induced anaphylaxis: Evidence of an association with the complement system. Acta Paediatr Jpn Overseas Ed 31:340, 1989.

Sheffer AL, Austen KF. Exercise-induced anaphylaxis. J Allergy Clin Immunol 66:106, 1980.

Sheffer AL, Austen KF. Exercise-induced anaphylaxis. J Allergy Clin Immunol 73:699, 1984.

Sheffer AL, Soter NA, McFadden ER Jr, et al. Exercise-induced anaphylaxis: A distinct form of physical allergy. J Allergy Clin Immunol 71:311, 1983.

Sheffer AL, Tong AK, Murphy GF, et al. Exercise-induced anaphylaxis: A serious form of physical allergy associated with mast cell degranulation. J Allergy Clin Immunol 75:479, 1985.

Silverstein SR, Frommer DA, Dobozin B, et al. Celery-dependent exercise-induced anaphylaxis. J Emerg Med 4:195, 1986.

Sonsiridej V, Busse WW. Exercise-induced anaphylaxis. Clin Allergy 13:317, 1983.

Soter NA, Wasserman SI, Austen KF, et al. Release of mast cell mediators and alterations in lung function in patients with cholinergic urticaria. N Engl J Med 302:604, 1980.

Tharp MD, Thirlby R, Sullivan TJ. Gastrin induces histamine release from human cutaneous mast cells. J Allergy Clin Immunol 75:159, 1984.

Wade JP, Liang MH, Sheffer AL. Exercise-induced anaphylaxis: Epidemiologic observations. Prog Clin Biol Res 297:175, 1989.

Watanabe T, Sakamoto Y, Tomonaga H, et al. A case of food-dependent exercise-induced anaphylaxis. Arerugi 39:1523, 1990.

White MV, Kowalski ML, Kaliner MA. Mast cell secretagogues. Prog Clin Biol Res 297:83, 1989.

Chapter 27

Adverse Reactions to Vaccines: The Complexity of Vaccine Safety

Vincent A. Fulginiti, M.D.

"Vaccines are safe and effective, but not perfectly safe and effective." This statement has been used for decades to describe the expectations from the use of vaccines. This chapter deals with the "safe . . . (but) . . . not perfectly safe" aspect of immunization.

Use of vaccines has altered life for millions of the world's citizens. Smallpox has been eradicated—a disease that killed hundreds of thousands and maimed and disabled millions (World Health Organization 1980). Poliomyelitis is on the way to potential eradication, and other childhood diseases have been drastically reduced (Patriarca et al, 1993). The benefits of immunization cannot be overstated, and the focus in this chapter on allergic and other adverse reactions should not detract from the enormously positive benefit-to-risk ratio for all vaccines.

QUESTIONS PERTAINING TO ADVERSE REACTIONS

There is nothing that we do in health care interventions that is without risk: some with high risk and others with minimal risk to the patient. Vaccines are no exception. Whether they are manipulated natural infectious agents, detoxified products of natural agents, or manufactured by modern genetic recombinant techniques, they all have some side effects. Virtually any substance foreign to the human host when injected, inhaled, ingested, or placed in contact with skin or mucous membrane will evoke a defensive reaction—as slight as local vasodilation and mild inflammation or as severe as central nervous system disturbance or death. When considering adverse reactions to vaccine products, one must take into account a variety of questions:

1. Did the vaccine actually cause the observed effect?
2. If so, by what mechanism?
3. What is the frequency of such reactions among those vaccinated?
4. What is the severity of the individual reaction—the range of severity among all recipients of the vaccine?
5. What is the duration and long-term consequence of the reaction?
6. What effect does the occurrence of the reaction have on subsequent use of that vaccine, related vaccines, any other vaccine, or any other product?
7. How are such reactions diagnosed?
8. What can be done to treat such reactions?
9. How can we prevent the reaction?
10. How can we design new vaccine products with the least potential for adverse reactions?

Some of these questions are not germane

to this text, but all are of concern to medicine and to the individuals responsible for vaccine development, testing, manufacture, and delivery to the individual patient. For the purposes of this chapter, it is pertinent to explore some of these in depth and others in more generic fashion.

Did the Vaccine Actually Cause the Observed Effect?

Unfortunately, vaccines are administered to individuals who have risks and vulnerabilities independent of the vaccine's effect. For example, we administer a variety of vaccines to 2- to 6-month-old infants, in a period of life during which predictable central nervous system disorders occur unrelated to vaccine. This is especially true for infantile myoclonic seizures, a disorder that has been attributed to pertussis vaccine, although considerable evidence indicates there is a temporal but not causal connection (Lombroso, 1983; Bellman et al, 1983). Thus, if a given child receives a vaccine and then comes down with such an independent disorder, the tendency of parents and some physicians is to immediately identify a causal association. On the other hand, if a vaccine truly causes an effect such as urticaria, but urticaria also occurs among the vaccinees as a result of other influences, it may be difficult to correctly discern the connection. This dilemma has hampered efforts to accurately identify adverse effects of vaccines. Only carefully conducted clinical trials with adequate numbers and appropriate controls analyzed statistically can yield even a first approximation of cause and effect. For an extensive discussion of these issues, refer to the Institute of Medicine reports on adverse events associated with vaccine (Institute of Medicine, 1991, 1994).

Some have suggested criteria for establishing such an association, but these are not perfect instruments. Among the issues suggested are the questions that follow.

Is the Observed Reaction Biologically Plausible, Given the Nature of the Vaccine?

For some products (e.g., recombinant hepatitis B surface antigen) the precise chemical constitution of the vaccine is known and plausibility can be inferred from known characteristics or experience with that chemical configuration. For others, such as the whole-cell form of pertussis vaccine, the composition is complex and varies from lot to lot; it may be impossible to infer effect, and worse, to rule out the possibility of association. Biologic plausibility in itself cannot establish causality, however. Also, current knowledge may not permit us to assume biologic plausibility, but it may be a correct explanation only to be verified later as more information is uncovered.

Is the Time Interval Observed Between Vaccine Receipt and Occurrence Appropriate to the Pathogenesis of the Adverse Event?

This is also a difficult parameter in that the vaccine must be absorbed, a process that may take time, and could be metabolized to a harmful by-product. Hence, the observed interval may be more prolonged than projected by knowledge of the nature of the reaction. Nevertheless, long intervals between vaccine receipt and putative reaction, longer than is plausible, suggest a lack of relationship. If the interval is appropriate for the known pathogenesis of the reaction, the other factors loom larger in the determination of causation.

Is the Sample Size Adequate to Detect Rare Events?

This is critical. If an event occurs once in every 100,000 vaccine administrations, or less frequently, then the usual FDA-approved trials are unlikely to detect it. They are sensitive at the 1:10,000 level (Hopps et al, 1988). Hence, only when a vaccine has "passed" the phase II and III clinical trials may it be deployed among hundreds of thousands to millions of recipients. Rare events may then come to light but go unrecognized as causally related because the event was not detected during trials. This factor requires that we have adequate post-licensing surveillance, and at this writing, there is no such mandatory, effective system. Rather, there is dependence on voluntary, random reporting (CDC, 1994). Only aggregation of rare adverse events over time permits association to be confirmed, or at least to be the subject of further scrutiny.

Is There an Inherent Susceptibility in the Host That is Consistent with the Observed Reaction?

If the recipient is allergic to mercury and a mercury compound is used in preservatives in the vaccine, this condition has been met provided also that the reaction is biologically consistent with mercury sensitivity (Murphy and Strunk, 1985; Herman et al, 1983). To generalize, the person receiving the vaccine must have a condition or disease that permits susceptibility to a potential untoward effect of one or more constituents of the vaccine. Apart from the allergic example, an individual immunodeficient in response to viruses might suffer from a generalized, even severe, infection from an attenuated vaccine virus that produces an adequate immune response in normal individuals, without manifest disease.

Can One Identify the Putative Factor in a Complex Vaccine or in Situations When Multiple Vaccines are Given Simultaneously?

For example, if a child has an urticarial reaction within hours of receipt of DTP, and the other factors are satisfied, is it diphtheria toxoid, tetanus toxoid, or some component in the complex pertussis vaccine that is responsible? Or, if a reaction occurs in a child who has received MMR, is it the measles, rubella, or mumps virus that is responsible, or some other constituent of the specific vaccine formulation? Consider the implications of this question when some children today are simultaneously receiving DTP, OPV (three viruses), MMR (three viruses), and *Haemophilus influenzae,* type B conjugate vaccine. This involves 10 different viral and bacterial agents and products, and a variety of other substances used in the suspension (e.g., preservatives) or mixed in with the desired antigens. A reaction after receipt of such a combination may defy logical analysis.

MECHANISMS PRODUCING ADVERSE EVENTS AFTER IMMUNIZATION

Adverse events following immunization usually can be classified into one of the following pathophysiologic mechanisms: *mechanical or toxic, immunologic, or infectious.*

Mechanical or Toxic Events

Mechanical or toxic pathogenesis will not be considered further, except to note that they occur and can be confused with immunologic reactions.

One generic issue, irrespective of etiology, is management of the large local reaction to a single dose of vaccine. Many individual physicians have "split" subsequent doses of vaccine in an effort to reduce the local reaction. This is not recommended for the following reasons:

1. Reactions may not be prevented if they are nonmechanical (e.g., due to an immunologic reaction to some component of the vaccine).

2. All immunologic effectiveness data are based on experience with full doses; hence, reduction of the dose does not guarantee that satisfactory response has been elicited, leading to false expectations of the efficacy of the vaccine. (Report of Committee on Infectious Diseases, American Academy of Pediatrics, 1994).

Immunologic Events (Gell and Coombs Classification)

Type I: Immediate Hypersensitivity; Anaphylaxis

Most commonly these reactions are a response to noninfectious components of various vaccines, e.g., egg sensitivity in influenza virus vaccine recipients, antibiotic sensitivity in various vaccine recipients (trace amounts of antibiotics remaining in the final product). On occasion, they may occur in response to a component of the infectious agent, but often this is difficult to separate from reactions to noninfectious components (e.g., urticaria following DTP). One additional factor in many vaccine preparations is the inclusion of adjuvants, which can enhance the potentiality of a type I response to an antigen. Reactions vary from minimal urticarial reactions to life-threatening anaphylaxis. Symptoms may include hives, swelling of the mucous membranes, laryngospasm, hypotension, and shock. Usually, such reactions are seen soon after administration of the vaccine, upon absorption of the inciting antigen and tissue exposure to specific IgE antibody.

Anaphylactic reactions have been attributed to influenza vaccine (egg antigen related); to live measles virus vaccine (chick embryo antigens related to egg sensitivity—disputed); to yellow fever vaccine (egg); to a variety of vaccines containing neomycin or other antibiotics; and to adjuvant vaccines (influenza, inactivated poliovirus vaccine). Links are often based solely on the occurrence of the reaction, without establishing proof of causality. Exceptions are the documented IgE reactivity in egg/chick antigen-related reactions to both influenza vaccine and live measles virus vaccine (Murphy and Strunk, 1985; Herman et al, 1983).

Type II Reactions

Cytotoxic reactions engendered by vaccines are not common and usually involve the hematopoietic system. Certain vaccines have been associated with immune thrombocytopenia, but the association is often difficult to prove conclusively (Institute of Medicine, 1994).

Type III Reactions

Autoimmune disorders have occurred after immunization. Again, the major difficulty is in tying the reaction to the vaccine in causal fashion. Most frequently the temporal relationship and the multiple occurrences of the disorder are suggestive but not conclusive proof of a causal link. The enhanced susceptibility of infants who received either inactivated respiratory syncytial virus vaccine or inactivated measles virus vaccine was believed by some to be an autoimmune disorder attendant on an inordinately high IgG antibody produced against the viral antigens, which then attacked normal tissues infected with the wild measles virus (Buser, 1967). This hypothesis implied that inactivation led to alteration of the virus to eliminate critical antigens to which an antibody response would have been protective. Instead, the antibody response was transient and to antigens other than the critical one(s) on the viral particle. When confronted with natural wild virus, the individual overreacted with high antibody production and tissue tropism associated with the distribution of the viral antigens. The resultant disease was manifest by such disorders as polyserositis, characteristic of an autoimmune process. Some investigators disagreed with this hypothesis and felt that the patients were experiencing a type IV reaction because of a dissociation between antibody production and cell-mediated immunity upon exposure to the viral vaccine (Fulginiti et al, 1967). The vaccines have been removed from the market, and no other instances of this type of reaction have been recorded for other vaccines.

Type III reactions meet the test of biologic plausibility because the matching natural virus infections have been associated with such effects. Both animal experimental data and human disease models have been linked with autoimmune disorders.

Type IV Reactions

These lymphocyte-mediated delayed reactions may be the most difficult to link to vaccine because of the timing and lack of definitive testing. These reactions have been suspected in a variety of vaccine administrations, but rarely have been proved (Fulginiti et al, 1967).

Management of Hypersensitivity Reactions: Reactions to Egg or Egg-Related Antigens

Measles and influenza vaccines are the most common vaccines linked to egg-related allergic reactions. Less frequently, mumps and yellow fever vaccines have been implicated. Skin testing with the vaccine product to be administered has been recommended in the past, but other experts have questioned the predictive value of this technique on the basis that components other than egg-related antigens may be responsible for the reaction. (Report of Committee on Infectious Diseases, American Academy of Pediatrics, 1994). However, in most expert's view, skin testing should continue to be performed until this issue is clarified. Additionally, package inserts accompanying vials of these vaccines recommend skin testing in appropriate individuals. Candidates for skin testing include those who experience systemic anaphylactic symptoms (generalized urticaria, shock, upper or lower airway obstruction) after ingesting eggs.

TESTING TECHNIQUE. The technique recommended by the Academy of Pediatrics Redbook Committee is as follows:

Scratch, Prick, or Puncture Test. A drop of 1:10 dilution of the vaccine in physiologic saline is applied at the site of a superficial scratch, prick, or puncture on the volar surface of the forearm. Positive (histamine) and negative (saline) control tests should also be used. The test is read after 15 to 20 minutes. A positive test is a wheal 3 mm in size or larger than that of the saline control, usually with surrounding erythema. The histamine control must be positive for valid interpretation. If the result of this test is negative, an interdermal test should be performed.

Intradermal Test. A dose of 0.02 ml of a 1:100 dilution of the vaccine in physiologic saline is injected intradermally; positive and negative control skin tests are performed concurrently. A wheal 5 mm in size or larger than the negative control with surrounding erythema is considered a positive reaction.

Cautions. Some have recommended the use of a puncture test using undiluted vaccine or an intradermal test using a 1:100 dilution as the only skin test necessary for vaccines containing measles virus antigen. Scratch, prick, or puncture tests with some allergens have resulted in fatal reactions in highly sensitized individuals; such reactions have not been reported for vaccine product testing, but all such procedures should be performed in settings in which emergency treatment can be carried out with experienced personnel, necessary equipment and drugs for counteracting anaphylaxis readily available (see Chapter 21).

DESENSITIZATION. If an individual is found to be hypersensitive to the vaccine in question as a result of skin testing, the following desensitization procedure is recommended. (American Academy of Pediatrics Redbook Committee, 1994):

Subcutaneous Method. Administer the following doses at 15- to 20-minute intervals, provided no reaction has occurred after each dose:

1. 0.05 ml of 1:10 dilution
2. 0.05 ml of full-strength vaccine
3. 0.10 ml of full-strength vaccine
4. 0.15 ml of full-strength vaccine
5. 0.20 ml of full-strength vaccine.

Desensitization should be performed in a setting in which experienced personnel, equipment, and drugs to counteract anaphylaxis are readily available.

NOTE: Many primary care health professionals may prefer to refer patients to a knowledgeable allergist or immunologist for testing and for desensitization procedures.

Infection

Any live agent in a vaccine administered to humans has the potential to produce a serious infectious disease. All such vaccines rely on some degree of infection to produce the desired immune response, but the adverse events are beyond this limited replication and represent a potential for any live agent administered as a vaccine. This potential is tempered by the genetic susceptibility of the "normal" host; by established, congenital, or acquired immune deficiency in the host; and by the capacity of the vaccine live agent to either produce disease or to revert to a more virulent form upon replication in a given host.

Examples of infection after live-agent immunization are multiple. BCG vaccine, a live, attenuated tubercle-like bacillus, can produce local infection and inflammation in regional lymph nodes and systemic infection in unusually susceptible hosts (Mande, 1968). Live poliovirus vaccine can result in poliomyelitis either in the infant recipient, or in an adult contact exposed to the virus excreted in the primary vaccinee's stool (CDC MMWR, 1986). Live measles virus in the vaccine has been capable of resulting in a lethal infection in children with leukemia or other severe immune deficits, particularly of the cell-mediated immune type (Granoff and Osterholm, 1987).

ADVERSE REACTIONS ASSOCIATED WITH SPECIFIC VACCINES

Diphtheria and Tetanus Toxoids

Given the long history of these toxoids, it is surprising that there are virtually no data to confirm with scientific certainty the reactions that have been "attributed" to these products. Reactions included anaphylaxis, a variety of peripheral and central neurologic disorders, arthritis, and a variety of skin disorders. Associations have been based on case reports, uncontrolled observations, even some "series" of patient reactions. A select committee of the Institute of Medicine, in reviewing all of the available information, concluded that there was a causal relationship between some instances of anaphylaxis and DT, Td, and tetanus toxoid vaccines (Institute of Medicine, 1994). They indicated that there were no controlled studies that substantiate these observations in individual patients, and that the events occur at an "extraordinarily low" rate.

The committee also concludes that the evidence reviewed favored a causal relationship for the Guillain-Barré syndrome in association with DT/Td/T vaccines. There appears to be substantial evidence favoring a direct causal relationship between tetanus toxoid administration and anaphylaxis, although the frequency of such occurrences is low.

Poliovirus Vaccines

INACTIVATED POLIOVIRUS VACCINE (IPV, KILLED, SALK). Virtually no significant reactions have been attributed to properly manufactured killed poliovirus vaccine. Some have claimed that IPV can be associated with the Guillain-Barré syndrome, but there is no precise evidence for this as a causal relationship (Institute of Medicine, 1994).

ORAL POLIOVIRUS VACCINE (OPV, ATTENUATED, LIVE, SABIN). Many case reports with appropriate viral isolation linking the virus recovered to the vaccine strains have associated nonparalytic and paralytic disease in both recipients and in contacts of vaccinees. Biologic plausibility and the impossibility of controlled studies combined with contrast with IPV experience and the virologic studies alluded to above have convinced most scientists that OPV produces paralytic infection, albeit rarely, in susceptible recipients. The accepted rates for recipients of OPV at present are one case per 520,000 first doses of OPV and 1 case per 12.3 million subsequent doses administered (Institute of Medicine, 1994). The data do not provide a frequency in contacts of vaccinees, although such instances are well documented. In some of these infections, death may ensue from the infection, particularly in the immunocompromised individual. There is enough suggestive information for the special IOM committee to state that the evidence favors acceptance of a causal relationship between OPV and the Guillain-Barré syndrome, estimated to be a relative risk of 3.5 for adults and the risk difference is approximately 2.5 per 100,000 people.

Haemophilus Influenzae, Type B Vaccines (HIB)

Two types of vaccine have been used: one is the simple polyribophosphate product (PRP) and the other PRP linked with a variety of protein moieties. The PRP vaccines appeared to enhance susceptibility to invasive infection with the organism soon after immunization in some areas of the Unites States (Granoff and Osterholm, 1987). The conjugated PRP vaccines have not had this phenomenon associated with their use (American Academy of Pediatrics, 1991; 1994). Neither vaccine has been associated with other significant, proven adverse reactions.

Hepatitis B Virus Vaccine (HBVV)

No data exist for proven reactions of any type. However, case reports of anaphylactic reactions have occurred with sufficient frequency to suggest a relationship (Hudson et al, 1991).

Live Measles Virus Vaccine (LMV)

Apart from the expected 5 to 15 percent frequency of fever and rash that may occur within a week or so of immunization, LMV does not appear to have any significant side effects in normal individuals that can be proved, except for anaphylaxis due to egg sensitivity and some instances of thrombocytopenia. In individual instances, causation may be difficult to prove since most recipients receive MMR, and any of the components may be responsible. Case reports of central nervous system disorders have appeared from time to time, but no definitive link with vaccine has been provided, given the background incidence of these disorders in the general population.

As has been noted, fatal infections have occurred in the immunocompromised individual (Monofo et al, 1994).

Live Mumps Virus Vaccine (LMuV)

This vaccine has been reported to be associated with parotitis, but the fact that other viruses can produce parotitis and the lack of consistent evidence to link this disorder with the vaccine has cast doubt on its causal relationship. Few other adverse reactions have been attributed or noted, and none proved, for LMuV.

Live Rubella Virus Vaccine (LRuV)

Although the evidence is disputable, many experts accept chronic arthritis as a complication of LRV (Institute of Medicine, 1991). This is based on the known occurrence of arthralgia and arthritis after LRV immunization, particularly among adolescent and adult females, and on some case reports (Mitchell et al, 1993). Also supportive of this hypothesis is the natural occurrence of arthritis in wild rubella virus infection, which lends biologic credibility to that observed after vaccine virus. Less frequently, a peripheral neuropathy syndrome may be seen after rubella immunization. The potential for thrombocytopenia with rubella viruses, either the wild or vaccine type, has been mentioned previously.

Despite the occurrence of congenital rubella in natural disease, inadvertent administration of rubella virus during pregnancy has not resulted in fetal disease, although a low rate of infection has been noted in either the placenta or the fetus.

Pertussis Vaccine

Killed whole bacterial pertussis vaccine has been the center of much controversy as to its efficacy and the adverse reactions associated with it. An exhaustive analysis of all reported information was provided by the Institute of Medicine (Institute of Medicine, 1991). The modern view is that the vaccine is effective but not 100 percent protective, and that it does produce a number of toxic, local, and systemic reactions that are temporary, but rarely produces lingering effects or lethal complications. Reactions at the site of injection are common, and fever occurs with significant frequency, but more serious problems are uncommon to rare. Seizures occur once in every 1750 administrations and are probably related to fever and/or familial tendency to seizures. The so-called hypotonic-hyporesponsive (collapse syndrome) episodes in which respiratory and/or cardiac collapse are observed occur once in every 1750 doses. These episodes are transient, and neither the seizure nor the collapse syndrome produces permanent sequelae. In rare instances, death has been recorded in children experiencing the collapse syndrome. The cause of this adverse event is unknown, but some suspect an endotoxin-type reaction.

Central nervous system complications, especially encephalopathies, were once thought to be a consequence of pertussis immunization. The best evidence today militates against this relationship; at worst, if these complications do occur, they must do so rarely, and in an individual case cause and effect are impossible to judge. Complicating this analysis is the fact that certain neurologic disorders (e.g., infantile myoclonic seizures), occur in the same age group as that receiving DTP, irrespective of whether DTP has been received. When a child destined to develop infantile myoclonic seizures receives pertussis vaccine, the temptation is to assign a cause and effect relationship, solely on the basis of temporal association.

SUMMARY

Vaccines currently used for "routine" preventive care in children are extraordinarily safe and effective. There are known side effects and adverse reactions, as detailed in this chapter and covered exhaustively in the two committee reports of the Institute of Medicine. Physicians and other health professionals should become familiar with these possibilities and, to the extent possible, avoid immunization of individuals in whom such reactions are likely to occur. For authoritative and complete information on all aspects of childhood immunizations, the reader is referred to the Redbook, official publication of the American Academy of Pediatrics Committee on Infectious Diseases.

REFERENCES

American Academy of Pediatrics, Committee on Infectious Diseases. *Haemophilus influenzae* vaccines: Recommendations for immunization of infants and children 2 months of age or older. Update. Pediatrics 88:169–171, 1991.

Bellman MH, Ross EM, Miller DL. Infantile spasms and pertussis immunization. Lancet 1:1031–1034, 1983.

Buser F. Side reaction to measles vaccine suggesting the Arthus phenomenon. N Engl J Med 277:250–251, 1967.

CDC. Poliomyelitis—United States 1975–1984. MMWR 35:180–182, 1986.

CDC. Reporting of adverse events following vaccination. MMWR (General Recommendations on Immunization) 43:27, 1994.

Fulginiti VA, Eller JJ, Downie AW, Kempe CH. Atypical measles in children previously immunized with inactivated measles virus vaccine. Altered reactivity to measles virus. JAMA 202:1075–1078, 1967.

Granoff DM, Osterholm MT. Safety and efficacy of *Haemophilus influenzae*, type B polysaccharide vaccine. Pediatrics 80:590–592, 1987.

Herman JJ, Radin R, Schneiderman R. Allergic reactions to measles (rubeola) vaccine in patients hypersensitive to egg proteins. J Pediatr 102:196–199, 1983.

Hopps HE, Meyer BC, Parkman PD. Regulation and testing of vaccines. In Plotkin S, Mortimer E (eds). Vaccines. Philadelphia, WB Saunders, 1988.

Hudson TJ, Newkirk M, Gervais F, Shuster J. Adverse response to acute hepatitis B vaccine. J Allergy Clin Immunol 85:821–822, 1991.

Institute of Medicine. Adverse Effects of Pertussis and Rubella Vaccines. Washington, DC, National Academy of Sciences, 1991.

Institute of Medicine. Adverse Events Associated with Childhood Vaccines: Evidence Bearing on Causality. Washington, DC, National Academy of Sciences, 1994.

Lombroso CT. A prospective study of infantile spasms: Clinical and therapeutic correlations. Epilepsia 24:135–158, 1983.

Mande R. Cases of fatal generalized BCG disease. In Mande R (ed). BCG Vaccination. London, Dawsons, 1968.

Mitchell LA, Tingle AJ, Shukin R, Sangeorzan JA, McCune J, Braun DK. Chronic rubella vaccine-associated arthropathy. Arch Intern Med 153:2268–2274, 1993.

Monofo WJ, Haslam DB, Roberts RL, Zaki SR, Bellini WJ, Coffin CM. Disseminated measles infection after vaccination in a child with a congenital immunodeficiency. J Pediatr 124:273–276, 1994.

Murphy KR, Strunk RC. Safe administration of influenza vaccine in asthmatic children hypersensitive to egg proteins. J Pediatr 106:931–933, 1985.

Patriarca PA, Foege WH, Swartz TA. Progress in polio eradication. Lancet 342:1461–1464, 1993.

Report of the Committee on Infectious Diseases (Redbook), Elk Grove Village, Illinois, American Academy of Pediatrics, 1994.

World Health Organization. The global eradication of smallpox. History of International Public Health. No. 4, Geneva, WHO, 1980.

Section Five

UPPER RESPIRATORY TRACT DISEASES

Chapter 28

Physiology and Diseases of the Nose

George Philip, M.D., and Robert M. Naclerio, M.D.

The nose is the major portal for air between the external and internal environments. However, the nose is much more than a passive conduit: it conditions air for the lower airways, samples the content of air through olfaction, and serves as a first defense system against inhaled potential pathogens through nasal reflexes and local immune function. Though a wide variety of pathologic processes can affect the nose, by virtue of its structure and functions, the nose has a relatively limited palette of clinical manifestations of disease, i.e., mostly obstruction, drainage, and irritation.

This chapter begins with an overview of the embryology, anatomy, and physiology of the nose because a basic understanding of the nose helps to provide insight into disease processes and directions in treatment. Next, a general approach to nasal disease is given with attention to classification of nasal disease and to some diagnostic methods. Finally, more detailed discussion is provided for two common diseases of the nose—allergic rhinitis and nonallergic rhinitis.

STRUCTURE OF THE NOSE

Development

By the fifth week of human development, the nose begins to develop as two nasal pits separated by a large frontal process with no connection to the oral cavity. As the nasal pits deepen and approach the ectoderm of the oral cavity, the bucconasal membrane is formed. During the seventh week the bucconasal membrane ruptures, yielding two openings into the anterior part of the oral cavity, the primitive choanae. As the tongue descends during the seventh week, lateral palatine processes fuse with each other in the midline and with the medial palatine process anteriorly. Simultaneously, the nasal septum grows posteriorly. By the end of the eleventh week, the separation of the right and left nasal chambers from each other and from the oral cavity is complete (Jaffe, 1981).

In the pediatric patient with nasal symptoms, a few disorders of development should be considered (Table 28–1). Choanal atresia results from failure of the bucconasal membrane to disintegrate and may be unilateral or bilateral. In the obligate nose-breathing neonate, complete bilateral choanal atresia presents as a relative respiratory emergency at birth, which resolves with crying. Unilateral choanal atresia, the more common form, may remain asymptomatic beyond the neonatal period (Flowers and Naclerio, 1990). The patient usually presents with persistent unilateral nasal discharge; however, obstruction of the contralateral nasal cavity from an upper respiratory infection may cause respiratory distress. Less common causes of congenital nasal obstruction include dermoid cysts, encephaloceles, and gliomas. Malformations of the nasal structure include nasal agenesis, clefts, and facial dysostosis. The cleft lip-nose deformity, characterized by the triad of nasal tip deformity, dorsal displacement of the nasal dome, and buckling of the alar cartilage, is the most common problem.

External Nose

The external nose protrudes from the anterior aspect of the skull in the form of a pyramid, which is shaped by a combination of bone and cartilage. The apex of the pyramid, called the nasion, is where the paired nasal bones meet the frontal bone in the midsagittal plane. Inferiorly, the nasal bones lead to the piriform aperture, which is the bony opening for the external nose. The cartilaginous framework of the external nose consists of two pairs of nasal cartilages. The upper lateral cartilages provide shape to the middle third of the external nose. They are attached to the undersurface of the nasal bones and frontal processes of the maxilla, and they join to the cartilaginous septum medially. The lower lateral cartilages each have a horseshoe shape; medially, they extend along the cartilaginous septum and laterally they provide shape to the alae of the nose. A group of alar muscles are present to dilate the anterior nares; they are innervated by buccal branches of the facial nerve.

Nasal Cavity

The anterior nares are separated by the columella—that portion of the membranous septum which is covered with skin—and open into the nasal vestibules. Posterior to the vestibule, the floor of the nasal cavity is generally flat and consists of the maxillary and palatine bones, while the superior aspect of the nasal cavity arches upward to the cribriform plate. The lateral nasal wall is composed of the ethmoid bone, from which the superior and middle turbinates extend, and the separate bone of the inferior turbinate, which joins the maxilla and palate. The nasal cavity is continuous with the nasopharynx through the posterior choanae, which are two oval-shaped openings posterior and perpendicular to the palate.

NASAL VALVE. The nasal vestibules funnel toward the inferior turbinates, forming the nasal valve. The airway in this region is slit-shaped, having a cross-sectional area of only 30 to 40 mm^2 on each side. The funnel shape creates air turbulence that assists in warming and humidifying inspired air. The nasal valve accounts for approximately half the total airway resistance from atmosphere to alveoli (Swift and Proctor, 1977). An increase in the tone of the dilator naris muscle, as occurs during labored breathing, increases the cross-sectional area and flow across the nasal valve. With greater airflows, as during sniffing, relative negative pressure in the nose causes collapse of the lower lateral cartilages and contraction of the nasal valve. The limit to nasal inspiratory airflow placed by the nasal valve is overcome by switching to oronasal breathing.

TABLE 28–1. CONGENITAL NASAL ABNORMALITIES

Choanal atresia: unilateral or bilateral
Dermoid cysts
Encephaloceles
Gliomas
Nasal agenesis
Clefts (e.g., cleft lip-nose deformity)
Facial dysostosis

THE SEPTUM. The nasal septum divides the nasal cavity into two separate compartments. The septum is approximately 10 to 14 cm in length and is composed of cartilage anteriorly and bone posteriorly. Deviations of the septum from midline are relatively common. Severe deviations or deviations located in critical areas will impede airflow and/or predispose to sinus infection.

TURBINATES. Two main turbinates, inferior and middle, are shelves of bone that project from the lateral nasal wall. They curve inferiorly then laterally to present a convex surface toward the nasal septum (Fig. 28–1). Their main roles are to increase surface area of the nasal airway to about 100 to 200 cm^2 and to control airflow characteristics in the nasal airway by means of vascular congestion. Based on animal studies, the turbinates may play a role in body thermoregulation. A third or even fourth turbinate may be seen, but they are of little functional significance.

MEATUSES. The two main turbinates divide each side of the nasal cavity into three horizontal passages or meatuses: inferior, middle, and superior (Figs. 28–1 and 28–2). The inferior meatus is the largest of the three and lies between the inferior turbinate and the floor of the nose. The opening of the nasolacrimal duct lies under the inferior turbinate to drain tears into the inferior meatus. The middle meatus, lateral to the middle turbinate, is the most important meatus as it drains the ostia of the frontal, maxillary, and anterior ethmoid sinuses. Mucosal disease or anatomic abnormalities in this area, termed the ostiomeatal complex, can predispose to sinus obstruction and possible infection. The superior meatus, also called the ethmoid fissure, is slit-like and lies between the septum and the ethmoid bone above the middle turbinate. The sphenoethmoid recess, located above and behind the superior meatus, receives the ostia of the sphenoid sinus and the posterior ethmoid sinuses.

Vasculature

The nose receives blood from both the internal and external carotid arteries. The anterior and posterior ethmoidal arteries branch from the ophthalmic artery passing through the orbit to enter the nose. The sphenopalatine artery branches from the external carotid artery to enter the nose through the posterior lateral wall. These vessels anastomose with branches of the facial artery in the cartilaginous septum of the vestibule to form Kiesselbach's plexus (Fig. 28–3). This area is the most common site of epistaxis. Veins draining the nasal cavity run adjacent to the arteries into the pterygoid and ophthalmic venous plexuses and partially into the cavernous sinus.

The arterioles that supply the subepithelial and glandular zones travel toward the mucosal surface and give off arteriovenous anastomoses to venous sinusoids before forming a subepithelial network of fenestrated capillaries. The fenestrations face the respiratory surface and probably are the major source of fluid for humidification (Cauna, 1982). The

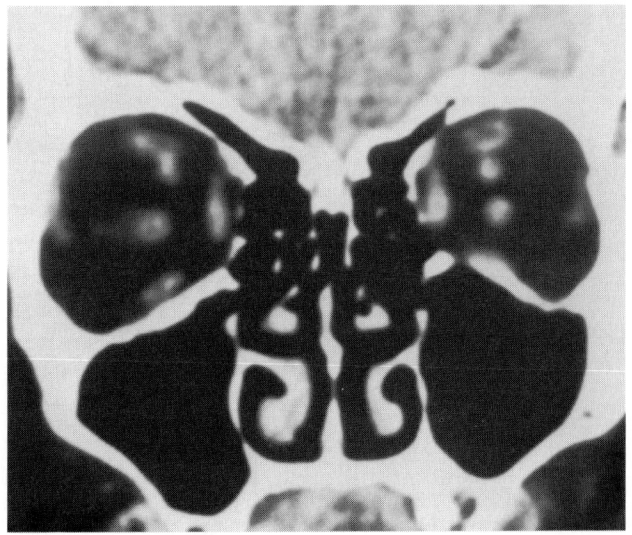

FIGURE 28–1. Normal anatomy of the nasal airway viewed by a coronal CT scan. (From Naclerio RM. The embryology, anatomy and physiology of the upper airway. *In* Middleton E, Reed CE, Ellis EF, Adkinson NF Jr, Yunginger JW [eds]. Allergy: Principles and Practice. 4th ed. St. Louis, Mosby–Year Book, 1993, Vol 1.)

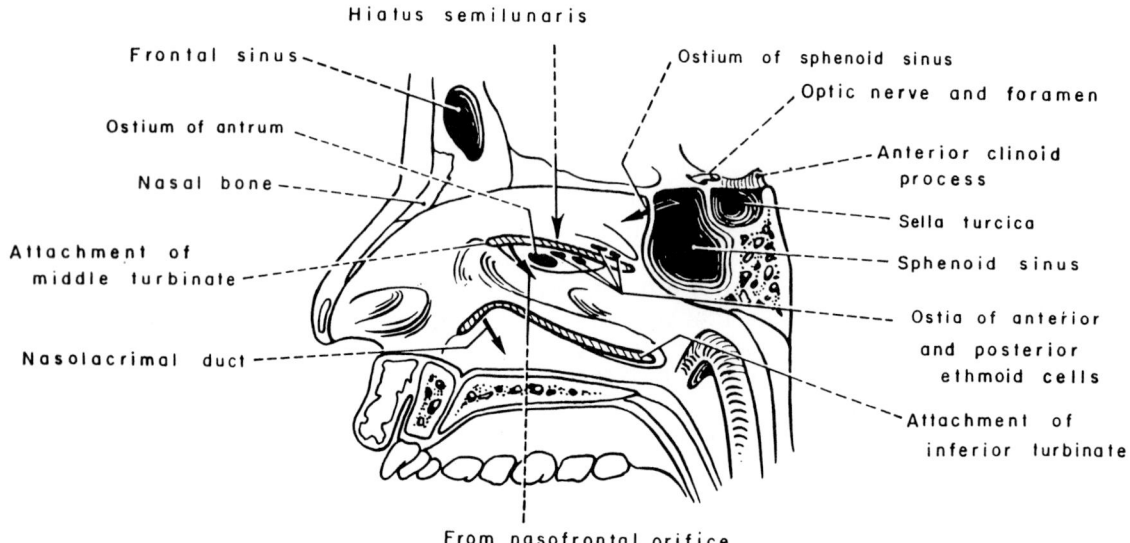

FIGURE 28–2. Lateral nasal wall with middle and inferior turbinates cut away to display openings of sinuses into the meatuses. (From Montgomery WW. Surgery of the Upper Respiratory System. Philadelphia, Lea & Febiger, 1971, Vol I, p 43.)

capillaries from this subepithelial network form venules, which drain into superficial veins and then into the venous sinusoids.

The venous sinusoids, or cavernous plexus, consist of networks of large, valveless, anastomosing veins found mostly over the inferior and middle turbinates and the mid-level of the septum. When the arteriovenous anastomoses open, the sinusoids fill rapidly with blood to function as capacitance vessels. This cavernous plexus changes volume in response to neural, mechanical, thermal, psychological, or chemical stimuli. When vascular engorgement occurs in these vessels, which lie in and around the nasal valve, symptoms of nasal congestion ensue.

Lymphatics from the nasal vestibules drain toward the external nose, while those of the

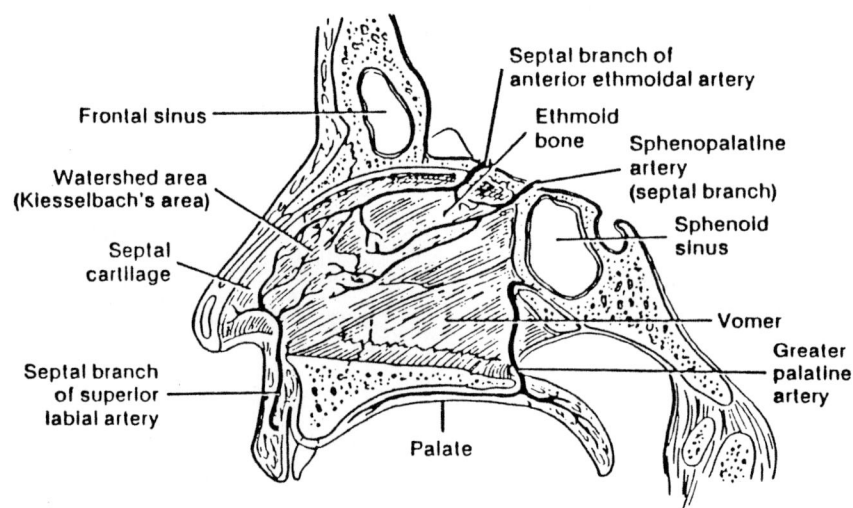

FIGURE 28–3. Arterial supply to the nasal septum. Kiesselbach's plexus is the most common site of epistaxis. (From Maceri DR. Epistaxis and nasal trauma. *In* Cummings CW, et al [eds]. Otolaryngology—Head and Neck Surgery. 2nd ed. St. Louis, Mosby–Year Book, 1993, p 728.)

main nasal cavity drain toward the nasopharynx. Two main collecting trunks flow above and below the eustachian tube orifice. Their first-order lymph nodes are the lateral retropharyngeal nodes, which cannot be palpated. This pattern explains the rare observation of lymphadenopathy with isolated rhinitis and sinusitis.

Innervation

OLFACTION. The roof of the nasal cavity and the area extending inferiorly for 8 to 10 mm along the septum and lateral nasal wall constitute the olfactory area. The olfactory mucosa located in this area has a surface area in man of about 200 to 400 mm^2. The olfactory epithelium contains bipolar neurons from the first cranial nerve, the most peripheral portion of the central nervous system. Odorant-binding proteins have been identified in animals, and these proteins chaperone lipophilic odorant molecules through hydrophilic mucus to reach the olfactory epithelium.

SENSORY INNERVATION. Sensory innervation to the nose is provided by branches of the trigeminal nerve. The ophthalmic division of the trigeminal supplies the upper and anterior areas of the septum and lateral nasal wall via the ethmoidal nerve, while the maxillary division supplies the lower and posterior areas via the posterior nasal nerve. Only mechanical and pain receptors have been clearly identified in the nasal mucosa. Thermoreceptors have not been identified but are presumably concentrated in the skin of the nasal vestibule, where they sample the temperature of inhaled air. Thin unmyelinated fibers from the trigeminal nerve have endings that penetrate into the nasal epithelium. These fibers may be activated by inhalation of irritants or by mediators of inflammation such as histamine.

PARASYMPATHETIC INNERVATION. The parasympathetic fibers originate in the midbrain and then travel with the fibers of the seventh cranial nerve. At the geniculate ganglion in the temporal bone, these fibers separate to form the greater superficial petrosal nerve, which traverses the floor of the anterior cranial fossa to synapse in the sphenopalatine ganglion. From this point, parasympathetic fibers distribute to mucosal and submucosal appendages via the vidian nerve. Stimulation of the parasympathetic nerves induces both glandular secretions and vasodilation, effects that also occur following nasal challenge with cholinergic agents.

SYMPATHETIC INNERVATION. Sympathetic fibers originate in the hypothalamus, synapse in the superior cervical ganglion, and then travel with the carotid plexus until joining with parasympathetic fibers to form the vidian nerve. The sympathetic fibers, in contrast to the parasympathetic, do not synapse in the sphenopalatine ganglion. Stimulation of the sympathetic system causes vasoconstriction, with a concomitant decrease in nasal airway resistance. Exercise stimulates the sympathetic system causing nasal decongestion, which can be blocked by anesthesia of the superior cervical ganglion.

NONADRENERGIC, NONCHOLINERGIC INNERVATION. In addition to classic cholinergic and adrenergic autonomic innervation, the nose also possesses a nonadrenergic, noncholinergic (NANC) system. This autonomic system functions via release of small peptides from sensory, parasympathetic, or sympathetic nerves upon stimulation (Barnes et al, 1991). Many of these so-called neuropeptides have been identified in the human nasal mucosa and may be important in nasal function, both in health and in disease.

Neuropeptides of the NANC system include substance P, calcitonin gene-related peptide (CGRP), vasoactive intestinal peptide (VIP), and neuropeptide Y. Substance P and CGRP are both released from peripheral endings of sensory nerves upon stimulation of these nerves. These peptides function to increase vascular permeability and cause vasodilation. Thus, release of these peptides may mediate a local inflammatory response to sensory nerve activation at the site of an irritant stimulus. VIP is co-released with acetylcholine on stimulation of parasympathetic nerves, and has vasodilatory and secretagogue actions. An increase in VIP-immunoreactive nerves has been reported in the nasal mucosa of patients with nonallergic rhinitis. Neuropeptide Y is co-released with norepinephrine on stimulation of sympathetic nerves and is one of the most potent vasoconstrictors known. Although the pathophysiologic role of the NANC system is still not clear, further understanding may lead to therapeutic advances.

Mucosa

A thin, moderately keratinized, stratified squamous epithelium lines the nasal vestibule, while the majority of the nasal cavity is lined by pseudostratified columnar epithelium. The transition between these epithelial types is under the influence of airflow and begins in the region of the anterior tip of the turbinates. Epithelial cells do more than provide a protective barrier in that they produce inflammatory mediators and the secretory portion of IgA. All cells of the pseudostratified columnar ciliated epithelium contact the basement membrane, but not all reach the epithelial surface. Within the epithelium, three types of cells are identified: basal, goblet, and columnar, which are either ciliated or nonciliated (Mygind et al, 1982).

Basal cells lie on the basement membrane and do not reach the airway lumen. Currently, basal cells are believed to help in the adhesion of columnar cells to the basement membrane. The *goblet* cells produce apocrine-type secretions, which contribute to the mucous blanket. The mucous granules give the mature cell its characteristic goblet shape, in which only a narrow part of the tapering basal cytoplasm touches the basement membrane. The lumenal surface, covered by microvilli, has a small opening, or stoma, through which the granules secrete their content. All *columnar* cells, ciliated and nonciliated, are covered by 300 to 400 microvilli, uniformly distributed over the entire apical surface. These are not precursors of cilia but are short and slender fingerlike cytoplasmic expansions, which increase the surface area of the epithelial cells to promote exchange processes across the epithelium. The microvilli also prevent drying of the surface by retaining moisture essential for ciliary function. The nonciliated columnar cell population is probably the progenitor of airway epithelium.

In man, ciliated epithelium lines the majority of the airway from the nose to the respiratory bronchioles, as well as the paranasal sinuses, the eustachian tube, and parts of the middle ear. Cilia are cellular projections that show intrinsic motility, resulting in propulsion of surface fluid. In the human nose, they are 5 μm long and consist of a shaft covered by cell membrane. The number of cilia per cell are reported to be 250 in the human trachea and 50 to 100 in the anterior part of the human nose. The shaft consists primarily of microtubules made of the globular protein, tubulin. Microtubules are found in the core of each shaft and also arranged peripherally around the core. Half of the peripheral microtubules possess dynein arms. These proteins contain ATPase activity that provides the energy for active sliding of the microtubules against each other and consequent ciliary motion.

The submucosa, or lamina propria, is separated from the epithelial layer by a basement membrane and contains primarily nerves, blood vessels, and tubuloalveolar glands. During inflammatory reactions, circulating cells enter the interstitium of the submucosa. However, unlike the gut and bronchial mucosa, the nasal mucosa does not routinely contain lymphoid aggregates. B and T cells found in the nasal mucosa arrive from the blood stream after maturation in the palatine, lingual, and nasopalatine (adenoidal) tonsils. The function of tonsils is thus similar to that of the lymphoid aggregates in the bronchi and gut.

Glands

There are two main types of nasal glands, which are located in the submucosa. The *anterior nasal glands*, serous glands 2 to 20 mm in length, have ducts that open into small crypts located in the nasal vestibule. The contribution of these glands to the total production of secretions is minimal, and they probably represent a phylogenetic rudiment. The orifices of the *seromucous glands* measure from 50 to 75 μm in diameter. The main duct is lined with simple cuboidal epithelium. This duct divides into two side ducts, which collect secretions from several tubules lined either with serous or mucous cells. At the ends of the tubules are acini, which may similarly be serous or mucous. Serous glands predominate over mucinous by a ratio of about 8:1. The total number of glands on the septum in newborns and adults is in the same range, implying that the glands are already formed at birth with no postnatal increase in number. The total number of glands is approximately 40,000.

Mucus

A mucous blanket, 10 to 15 μm deep, covers the entire nasal cavity. It consists of a sol and a gel phase. The sol phase is of low viscosity and envelops the shafts of the cilia; the gel phase, more viscous, rides over the periciliary layer and thus on the distal tips of the cilia.

Water-soluble gases, such as formaldehyde and carbon dioxide, dissolve in the mucus. Insoluble particles caught in the gel phase move as a consequence of ciliary beating. The mucus effectively filters and removes nearly 100 percent of particles greater than 5 μm in diameter. Besides filtration, the mucous layer provides water for humidification.

Estimates of daily nasal mucus production range from 0.1 to 0.3 mg/kg/day, and this is composed of 2 to 3 percent glycoproteins, 1 to 2 percent salts, and 95 percent water. One of the glandular products is mucin, a unique glycoprotein that has an extremely large molecular weight (2.3×10^6 Daltons) but comprises only a small portion of the total protein content. Mucin gives mucus its unique attributes of protection and lubrication. In contrast to serum, immunoglobulins make up the largest portion of the protein in mucus, especially secretory IgA. Other substances in nasal secretions include lysozyme, lactoferrin, albumin, alpha-antitrypsin, transferrin, lipids, histamine, urea, cells, and bacteria.

Mucociliary Action

Mucus and the ciliated epithelial cells function together in mucociliary transport. Mucociliary transport moves mucus and its contents toward the nasopharynx, with the exception of the anterior portion of the inferior turbinates, where transport is anterior. This anterior current prevents many of the particles deposited in this area from progressing further into the nasal cavity. The particles transported posteriorly toward the nasopharynx are periodically swallowed. Clearance of mucus can be aided by sniffing, sneezing, and nose blowing.

Cilia move in a characteristic manner. During the recovery phase they bend and move in the sol layer. During the effector stroke they straighten, contacting the gel phase, thus moving the mucus in only one direction. Cilia beat frequency is approximately 1000 beats per minute, which translates to surface material motion of 3 to 25 mm per minute, or about 10 to 20 minutes to clear inhaled particles from the anterior nasal cavity. In patients with Kartagener's syndrome, dynein arms are not present and the cilia are motionless. The addition of the dynein protein and magnesium induces reappearance of the arms and ciliary motion. Besides congenital structural abnormalities, mucociliary transport can be altered by a variety of factors, including viral infection, transient or permanent injury to the mucociliary system by physical trauma, dehydration, or excessively viscid secretions, as in cystic fibrosis. Disorders of ciliary movement present clinically with pooled secretions on the floor of the nasal cavity (Rossmann et al, 1984).

The composition of mucus may affect the rate of mucociliary transport. Pharmacologic agents can alter the composition of mucus and affect clearance. Guaifenesin decreases the viscosity of respiratory secretions, thus conceptually providing more effective clearing of secretions by mucociliary transport. The efficacy in humans of guaifenesin has not been proved in controlled studies. Anticholinergic agents increase the viscosity of secretions and may decrease clearance.

FUNCTION OF THE NOSE

OLFACTION. The olfactory airway, high in the nasal vault, is only 1 to 2 mm wide and is relatively poorly ventilated, as most of the inhaled air passes through the lower portion of the nasal cavity. Sniffing brings air into this part of the nasal cavity to raise the proportion of air reaching the olfactory epithelium by 5 to 20 percent. If obstruction impedes airflow to this area, hyposmia or anosmia may result. Septal deformities may alter the airflow path in the nose, directing air away from the olfactory area. Two other regions important in preserving olfactory function are the area 10 to 15 mm below the cribriform plate and medial to the middle turbinate, and the area high in the nasal cavity anterior to the cribriform plate (Leopold, 1988). If these regions are obstructed by mucosal inflammation, polyps, or other structural abnormalities, olfactory ability may decrease. Although less important to humans than to lower animals, olfaction aids the perception of taste, including identification of spoiled foods, and warns of environmental hazards, such as the mercaptans placed in natural gas to warn of a gas leak.

NASAL AIRFLOW. The nose provides the main pathway through which air reaches and leaves the lower airways. The preference for nasal breathing begins in newborns, who are obligate nose-breathers till the age of 5 to 6 months, and persists in adult life, with about 85 percent of adults breathing by nose. The shift to oronasal or oral breathing is seen only under demanding conditions, such as exercise, voice use, or nasal obstruction.

Changes in direction of airflow, as well as the irregularities of the nasal walls, disrupt laminar flow and promote turbulence. These factors allow the nose to perform its primary functions of heat and moisture exchange and of filtering inspired air. On inspiration, air first passes upward into the vestibules, then changes its direction from vertical to horizontal just prior to the nasal valve. As mentioned previously, the cross-sectional area of the airway decreases dramatically at the nasal valve, which separates the vestibules from the remainder of the nasal cavity; consequently, air velocity increases as it traverses the valve. Because of this airflow, the bulk of large particles that enter the nose impact just beyond the nasal valve onto the anterior portion of the inferior turbinate. After traversing the nasal valve, inspired air flows into the main nasal airway, which has a width of 1 to 3 mm. Here, the cross-sectional area increases, and air velocity decreases. The nature of flow also changes from laminar, before and at the nasal valve, to more turbulent posteriorly. This turbulence causes smaller particles to impact more posteriorly in the nasal cavity, and it also allows mixing of air for efficient heat and moisture exchange.

Spontaneous changes in the blood content of the nasal mucosa cause changes in mucosal volume, which alternate between the two nasal cavities. This phenomenon, termed the "nasal cycle," leads to alternating congestion and decongestion of the right and left nasal cavities. Because of reciprocity in the resistance changes between the two sides of the nose, total nasal resistance remains unchanged throughout the nasal cycle. The duration of one cycle varies between 50 minutes and 4 hours and is controlled by autonomic innervation. The nasal cycle is interrupted by the vasoconstrictive effects of medications or exercise.

Conditioning of Air. Inspired air is warmed and humidified in an extremely efficient process, which is facilitated by the turbulent characteristics of nasal airflow. During normal breathing, air that may be at 20°C in ambient air is warmed to 31°C in the pharynx and 35°C in the trachea. As the air is warmed, it also is fully humidified from relative humidities as low as 9 percent to a relative humidity of nearly 100 percent. Because rewarming of the nasal mucosa is a relatively slow process, the temperature of the nasal mucosa at expiration remains lower than that of expired air. As expiratory air passes through the nose, it therefore gives up heat to the cooler nasal mucosa, which also causes condensation of water vapor. In this way, roughly 35 percent of the heat and moisture content of expired air is retained by the nasal mucosa. Blood flow changes in the nasal mucosa markedly affect mucosal rewarming and thus modify respiratory air conditioning. Glandular secretion is a major source of water for humidification of inspired air. Other sources include transudation of fluid from the blood vessels of the nose, secretions from goblet cells, and lacrimation via the nasolacrimal duct.

Filtration of inspired air begins at the vibrissae, the hairs that grow in the nasal vestibule, which are able to filter airborne particles larger than 15 μm in diameter. Thereafter, turbulent airflow causes smaller particles to impact the mucus layer. The mucus effectively filters and removes almost all particles greater than 5 μm in diameter. Only a small percentage of particles smaller than this are permitted by the nose to enter the lower airway. The nose even partially filters some gases, such as ozone, which dissolve in mucus and are eliminated by mucociliary clearance.

Nasal Protective Reflexes. The most familiar reflex originating in the nose is the sneeze. After irritation of a sensory nerve, the sneeze begins as one or more spasmodic inspirations. The glottis and velopharyngeal aperture close, allowing an increase in lower airway pressure. These structures suddenly open, allowing a blast of air to push through the nose and mouth in an attempt to clear the nasal passage (Baroody and Naclerio, 1990). This reflex occurs with viral infection, irritants, exposure to allergens, and in some individuals, exposure to bright light.

Reflex stimulation may also cause nasal secretion, which then helps the nose respond to environmental insults. Challenge of one nostril with allergen or cold dry air can induce secretion on both sides of the nose, illustrating a nasonasal secretory reflex. Nasal secretion also occurs on eating hot or spicy foods, so-called gustatory rhinitis. Cholinergic reflex stimulation is involved in these responses because they are inhibitable by parasympathetic blockade (Raphael et al, 1991). Finally, neuronal stimulation originating within the nose can affect function elsewhere. Mucosal irritation can initiate the diving reflex, consisting of apnea, glottic closure, bradycardia, and vasoconstriction, in an attempt to protect the heart and brain by redistributing blood flow to these vital organs. Other nasopulmonary reflexes have occasionally been documented but are of unclear significance.

MUCOSAL IMMUNITY. Immunoglobulins comprise about 70 percent of the protein content of mucus. IgA constitutes the majority, with the rest distributed among the IgG, IgE, IgM, and IgD classes. The transport of IgA into mucosal secretions has been well studied (Strober and James, 1991). IgA is synthesized locally by plasma cells in the submucosa. Monomeric IgA combines with the J chain, also synthesized by IgA plasma cells, to form $(IgA)_2$–J dimers. The J chain of the dimers then binds noncovalently with secretory component, which is synthesized by epithelial cells. This complex is endocytosed by the epithelial cell for transport to the apical surface of the cell. En route, dimeric IgA becomes covalently linked to secretory component in order to form secretory IgA, which is released by the epithelial cell into nasal secretions. A similar mechanism involving J chain and secretory component results in translocation of smaller amounts of pentameric IgM through secretory epithelial cells into nasal secretions.

Other immunoglobulins contribute to humoral immunity of the nasal mucosa. Serum-derived IgG is present in large concentrations in the extravascular space and can thus reach nasal secretions by passive diffusion between epithelial cells or through minor breaks in the mucosa. Monomeric IgA and some IgE reach secretions by the same method. This mode of immunoglobulin transfer through the surface epithelium is accelerated in the presence of mucosal inflammation. Any stimulus that enhances vascular leakage in the nasal mucosa increases extravascular concentrations and thus the amount of these immunoglobulins in nasal secretions.

In the upper airway, the tonsils and adenoids are favorably located to mediate immunologic protection of the upper airway, as they are exposed to airborne antigens. The tonsils and adenoids are covered by stratified squamous epithelium, which extends into deep branched crypts well suited for trapping foreign material. Antigen transporting cells, HLA-DR–positive mononuclear cells, and T and B lymphocytes are found in tonsillar crypt epithelium. Tonsillar B cell blasts probably contribute to the IgA dimer-producing plasma cells of the upper airway, including the nasal mucosa (Brandtzaeg, 1984). The tonsils may likewise be a major source of the relatively high number of IgG plasma cells normally found in this region. Thus the tonsils seem to support the nasal mucosal immune response in a comparable fashion to gut and bronchus associated lymphoid tissues.

CLINICAL APPROACH TO NASAL DISEASE

History

A careful history is essential. The history begins with the onset of disease and the duration of symptoms, giving particular emphasis to temporal relationships with seasons and with life events (e.g., acquiring a pet, trauma). The history should define current symptoms as to the amount and characteristics of secretions (clear versus purulent), degree of airflow obstruction, itching/sneezing (very characteristic of atopic disease), and the presence or absence of pressure and pain over the sinus areas. Exacerbating factors must be identified; these may be allergens (e.g., pollens, dust, animals) or nonspecific irritants (e.g., cigarette smoke, chemical fumes, cold air). Such factors are part of a complete environmental history. Inquiry into the sense of smell aids in determining the degree of airflow obstruction. Severe nasal obstruction decreases the sense of smell, which is usually perceived as a loss of taste. Ocular symptoms associated with allergic rhinitis include conjunctival itching, tearing, injection, and edema of the eyelids and periorbital area. Pharyngeal symptoms or cough may be related to postnasal drainage. Questions should be directed at disturbances of sleep. Snoring frequently is seen with nasal obstruction, but apneic episodes may occur which signify sleep apnea with sequelae including daytime fatigue and pulmonary complications. Mouth breathing due to nasal obstruction leads to morning complaints of sore throat. Patients may be noted to have paroxysmal nocturnal coughing spells. Halitosis as a complaint by the parent or spouse may indicate infection. The history should detail previous treatments. Patients easily discuss prescription medications used but infrequently mention over-the-counter preparations, including aspirin or topical medications. Evidence of other allergic diseases, such as asthma or atopic dermatitis, as well as a family history of allergic diathesis are important components of the initial history.

Physical Examination

A complete ear, nose, and throat examination is essential for all patients complaining of nasal symptoms. Tenderness over the sinuses may reflect an underlying infection, whereas numbness raises suspicion of a tumor. The nasal examination begins with the external face. Perennial nasal obstruction, whether mechanical or functional in origin, presents with an open mouth. Black or blue discoloration beneath the lower eyelids ("allergic shiners") is secondary to chronic periorbital edema and venous stasis; these changes may occur in conjunction with adenoidal hypertrophy. Chronic nasal obstruction originating in childhood is thought to cause underdevelopment of the zygoma, nasal processes, and maxillary sinuses, resulting in the flattened "adenoid facies." Structural deviations or asymmetry should raise suspicion of trauma or congenital deformities.

After examining the external nares, a nasal speculum should be used to examine the anterior third of the nasal cavity. Color and amount of nasal secretion are recorded as well as color and size of the turbinates. Although classic descriptions of the nasal mucosa exist in textbooks, no consistent physical finding definitively rules in allergic rhinitis. Rather, the examination rules out other potential causes of similar nasal symptoms. Unilateral signs, particularly purulent drainage, should raise suspicion about foreign bodies. Pooling of secretions under the inferior turbinate is seen with immotile cilia syndrome or with total nasal obstruction.

Applying a topical decongestant permits better visualization of the deeper portions of the nasal cavity. The position and surface of the nasal septum should be noted. Lateral to the anterior portion of the middle turbinates lie the openings for the frontal, maxillary, and anterior ethmoidal sinuses where nasal polyps usually originate. A slow or absent response to a decongestant indicates a hyperplastic nasal mucosa or may be consistent with rhinitis medicamentosa. Examination of the oral cavity may reveal a high arched, V-shaped palate with poor dental occlusion related to chronic mouth breathing during facial development. Posterior cervical lymphadenopathy may signal adenoiditis, whereas tonsillar infections drain to jugular digastric lymph nodes.

Classification

A simple approach to the evaluation of rhinitis is shown in Table 28–2.

ACUTE VERSUS CHRONIC RHINITIS. Acute rhinitis is usually associated with an upper respiratory infection. Symptoms include rhinorrhea, nasal obstruction, and sometimes fever. The most common acute rhinitis is viral. It is manifest by nasal mucosal edema and clear nasal drainage, which may become cloudy due to cellular debris. Foreign body rhinitis must be considered, especially in children; suggestive findings include unilateral drainage that is blood-stained or malodorous. Infectious rhinitis may be confused with allergic rhinitis when patients complain of a "constant cold." If such symptoms persist beyond 2 or 3 weeks, evaluation should include causes other than viral infection.

CHRONIC RHINITIS. Chronic nasal symptoms frequently have an allergic basis. How-

TABLE 28–2. BRIEF DIFFERENTIAL DIAGNOSIS OF RHINITIS BASED ON A SIMPLIFIED APPROACH TO THE EVALUATION OF NASAL DISEASE (FRAMEWORK FOR EVALUATION OF NASAL DISEASE)

BASED ON TIME COURSE OF SYMPTOMS	
Acute	*Chronic*
Upper respiratory infection	Allergic disease
Viral	Persistent/recurrent
Bacterial	infections
Foreign body	Anatomic disease
Trauma	Congenital
	Septal deviation
	Other nonallergic disease

BASED ON USE OF ADDITIONAL TESTING	
Allergy Tests: Positive	*Allergy Tests: Negative*
Allergic Rhinitis	Nonallergic Rhinitis
Seasonal	Unknown etiology
Perennial	Known etiologies
Perennial with seasonal	(see Table 28–3)
exacerbations	
Episodic	

ever, it is incumbent on the physician to keep in mind other diseases that manifest chronic nasal symptoms. In particular, chronic sinusitis commonly produces nasal complaints. Although frequently associated with allergic rhinitis, chronic sinusitis often occurs in the absence of allergic disease.

Anatomic bases for chronic rhinitis must be considered. Congenital choanal atresia can be a cause of nasal obstruction with discharge in infants. Enlarged adenoids are a frequent cause of nasal obstruction and mouth breathing in children. Septal deviation may follow trauma, including passage through the birth canal. Mucosal swelling of rhinitis may make such a septal deviation clinically significant, leading to nasal obstruction and predisposing to unilateral chronic sinusitis.

Other conditions also lead to chronic nasal symptoms. Rhinitis medicamentosa is a condition of chronic nasal congestion with roughened, erythematous mucosa, which develops after prolonged use of topical vasoconstrictors. Pregnancy can be associated with persistent nasal blockage which disappears after delivery. Malignancies and Wegener's granulomatosis may first present with "perennial rhinitic" symptoms; hemorrhagic secretions, unilateral symptoms, or pain may raise the suspicion of such conditions, which must be pursued by endoscopic and/or radiographic imaging.

ALLERGIC VERSUS NONALLERGIC RHINITIS. The diagnosis of an inhalant nasal allergy can usually be made when history, physical examination, and allergy testing are combined. However, the decision of allergic versus nonallergic disease is not always simple. Mild false-positive allergy tests may point toward allergic rhinitis, which is not actually significant. Negative allergy testing may reflect the lack of complete knowledge of inhalant allergens to be tested or the use of poor-quality preparations for testing. Perennial rhinitis, especially, is seldom completely allergic or nonallergic as nonspecific irritants tend to trigger symptoms in allergic as well as nonallergic disease. Nonetheless, differentiation of allergic versus nonallergic rhinitis is useful because it can direct therapy between allergen-specific treatments (avoidance, antihistamines, immunotherapy) and relatively nonspecific pharmacologic treatments. This differentiation also affects the likelihood of a satisfactory response to therapy, as allergic rhinitis tends to respond more completely to currently available treatments.

Diagnosis

ALLERGY TESTING. The diagnosis of allergic rhinitis is based on history and physical findings as supplemented by *in vivo* or *in vitro* allergy tests (see Chapter 11). Allergy testing should be considered in all patients with a suspected diagnosis of allergic rhinitis. Such diagnostic tests can support the history but do not replace it; on the other hand, a history without supporting tests can be questioned. Positive tests without a plausibly positive clinical history are consistent with sensitization but do not necessarily indicate clinical disease. Only when historical findings and diagnostic testing coincide should allergen-specific treatment be recommended.

NASAL CYTOLOGY. Samples of superficial nasal mucosal cells can be obtained by blowing the nose into plastic wrap or by use of a cotton swab. More consistent specimens can be obtained by scraping the surface of the middle portion of the inferior turbinate with a plastic curette (Rhinoprobe) (Meltzer et al, 1993). The clinical utility of nasal cytology is to rapidly differentiate infectious from noninfectious rhinitis and to subclassify perennial rhinitis. Predominance of neutrophils suggests an infectious etiology. Increased numbers of eosinophils are found in active allergic disease. On the other hand, a subcategory of perennial rhinitis can be identified, which is not associated with positive allergy tests but nonetheless shows significant eosinophilia. Presence of eosinophilia in nasal cytology portends a greater likelihood of good clinical response to topical intranasal steroids. Unfortunately, the variability in nasal smears is so great that a single examination often does not give a conclusive result.

FIBEROPTIC RHINOSCOPY. Endoscopic evaluation provides a far superior examination of the nasal cavity in comparison to anterior rhinoscopy with a speculum. On the whole, however, the allergic nose shows little other than watery secretion and a swollen mucosa. The real utility of endoscopy is to rule out other structural abnormalities that may present as rhinitis or may help predispose to sinus disease. Most children over 5 years of age will permit an endoscopic examination to view the nasopharynx. In children, the contribution of the adenoids to nasal obstruction must be appreciated; rarely, a unilateral choanal atresia may be noted. Dermoid cysts, encephaloceles, and gliomas may also be noted intranasally. Other abnormalities that may be seen in adults include posterior septal deviation, concha bullosa (a bulbous enlargement of the middle turbinate because it contains an ectopic air cell), and various bony abnormalities of the lateral nasal wall. In addition, tumors (e.g., squamous cell carcinoma, nasopharyngeal carcinoma) and other conditions such as Wegener's granulomatosis may be first appreciated by nasal endoscopy.

ALLERGIC RHINITIS

Pathophysiology

Many insights have been gained into allergic disease in the nose by means of *in vitro* and *in vivo* studies. Individuals with a genetic predisposition for allergic disease become sensitized on exposure to allergens. The specificity of this response is presumably provided by $CD4^+$ T_{H2} phenotype T cells, which possess both the correct antigen specificity and the ability to produce appropriate cytokines. The cytokines produced on activation of these cells, especially IL-4, then stimulate B cell differentiation into IgE-producing plasma cells.

Allergen-specific IgE antibodies bind to high-affinity receptors on mast cells and basophils and to low-affinity receptors on certain other cells, which may include monocytes, eosinophils, lymphocytes, and platelets. On re-exposure to antigen via surface IgE, mast cells degranulate, releasing multiple inflammatory mediators such as histamine and leukotrienes. These mediators can be detected in nasal lavage fluid after allergen challenge (Naclerio et al, 1983). The released mediators stimulate the nasal end organs to produce itching, sneezing, rhinorrhea, and congestion. However, the immediate anaphylactic release of mediators from nasal mast cells does not entirely explain the clinical disease. This is supported by the fact that systemic corticosteroids, which have no direct inhibitory effect on mast cell degranulation, nonetheless are extremely effective in treating the clinical disease.

Following the early reaction, symptoms and the levels of mediators detected in nasal lavage fluid subside, and the patients enter a clinically quiescent phase. In some individuals, symptoms spontaneously recur 3 to 11 hours after the initial challenge. Accompanying these symptoms is a concomitant release of some mediators and an influx of cells into nasal secretions. This late phase response may provide insight into the pathophysiology of more prolonged clinical disease, such as during the weeks, months, or years of allergic manifestations associated with seasonal or perennial allergic rhinitis.

The cellular influx includes eosinophils, neutrophils, basophils, and mononuclear cells. There is preliminary evidence to support the recruitment of T_{H2} phenotype T cells into the nasal mucosa of allergic rhinitics after allergen challenge to the nasal mucosa. Not only are cytokines produced by T_{H2} cells able to induce IgE production, but they also may selectively attract and activate basophils and eosinophils. In addition, mast cells may also produce cytokines able to stimulate basophil and eosinophil influx. Strong correlations exist between the number of basophils and the level of histamine in the late reaction and between the number of eosinophils and the amount of major basic protein in the late reaction (Naclerio, 1991). These observations suggest that hours after nasal provocation these cells enter the nose and degranulate. Thus, while mast cell degranulation underlies the release of histamine in the early response, basophil influx appears to explain histamine release (and perhaps the associated symptoms) in the late response. The neutrophil represents the cell entering the nose in greatest number, but whether the neutrophil actually participates in the late reaction is still undetermined.

The existence of a priming response, an augmented response to a second allergen challenge given hours after an initial allergen challenge, may effectively model the repetitive challenges that occur during the allergy season. This increased responsiveness is not allergen specific, is a transient phenomenon, and does occur with environmental exposure during the natural pollen season. Associated with increased clinical sensitivity are increased levels of mediators such as histamine and kinins. This increase in mediator release could result, at least in part, from the stimulation of additional cells that have arrived as part of an inflammatory cell influx. Another potential, and not mutually exclusive, explanation of priming is hyperreactivity of end organs, i.e., an equivalent amount of mediator release induces greater responses and symptoms. This could explain the increase in nonspecific reactivity often seen during seasonal exposure. Chronic allergen exposure, such as during a pollen season, leads to other changes including migration of mast cells within the nasal mucosa. Our understanding of more prolonged allergen exposure needs to be investigated, including the mechanisms for the resolution of inflammation.

In conclusion, allergen inhalation induces the rapid release of inflammatory mediators from nasal mucosal mast cells in allergic individuals. Antagonism of these mediators, by agents such as antihistamines, can significantly ameliorate the clinical manifestations during the early response. However, the nasal reaction to allergen challenge is not limited to this early response. Some more prolonged manifestations of allergic rhinitis, including the late-phase reaction and the priming response, are probably related to the influx of lymphocytes, basophils, eosinophils, and other cells into the nasal mucosa. These findings are consistent with the efficacy in allergic rhinitis of corticosteroids, which prevent the influx and activation of these cells.

Epidemiology

Allergic rhinitis is the most common chronic disease suffered by humans. Estimates of prevalence in the American population range from 9 to 21 percent, although some of these studies are based on patients' self-reported histories only. The onset of allergic rhinitis occurs most commonly during childhood or young adulthood, although up to 30 percent of patients have their onset after age 30. The single most important risk factor for allergic rhinitis is a positive family history of allergic disease, especially in those patients whose onset is during childhood. Interestingly, there apparently has been an increase in the occurrence of allergic rhinitis in many if not all industrialized countries, especially over the past two decades (Smith, 1993). In light of these findings, further research is clearly of importance to understand the interplay between genetic predisposition, allergen exposure, immunologic response, and disease manifestation in this large population of patients who suffer allergic rhinitis.

Seasonal Versus Perennial Allergic Rhinitis

A fairly simple differentiation exists within allergic rhinitis with regard to the time frame of allergen exposure and thus the temporal pattern of associated symptoms. Seasonal allergic rhinitis occurs in temperate climates in which allergenic pollens (and fungal spores) are airborne during circumscribed times of the year. In many areas of the United States, pollen is released from trees in the early spring, grasses in the late spring, and ragweed in the early fall. Certain allergenic fungi also have seasonal patterns of spore release. Seasonal allergic rhinitics classically have symptoms that they note only during the spring or fall. Their complaints are often characterized by frequent paroxysms of sneezing, itching, profuse rhinorrhea, and conjunctival symptoms. In some parts of the United States, the pollen and mold seasons are long enough to overlap for much of the year. Allergic patients in these areas may thus have "seasonal" symptoms that occur for much of the year.

Perennial allergic rhinitis is classically associated with exposure to indoor allergens such as dust mites. Interestingly, these patients tend to complain less of sneezing and conjunctival symptoms and more of chronic nasal obstruction. The nature of these allergens makes it possible to reduce allergen exposure, especially in the bedroom. Thus, measures to reduce exposure to dust mites or animals can make a real difference in the severity of disease. Although perennial rhinitics are responsive to antihistamines, the chronic nature of their exposure often requires chronic anti-inflammatory therapy such as topical nasal steroids. For those patients who have allergies to outdoor as well as indoor allergens, their disease, which is characterized by perennial rhinitis with seasonal exacerbations, is often responsive to all of these measures.

A final category of allergic rhinitis is episodic disease. An example is a cat-sensitive patient who suffers an almost immediate onset of acute allergic rhinitis upon visiting a home with a cat. While avoidance is important, social and other commitments may require exposure to allergens; thus, prophylactic strategies must be devised.

Treatment

A general approach to the management of allergic rhinitis is presented in Figure 28–4. This section will discuss options in the treatment of allergic rhinitis.

AVOIDANCE. The elimination of offending

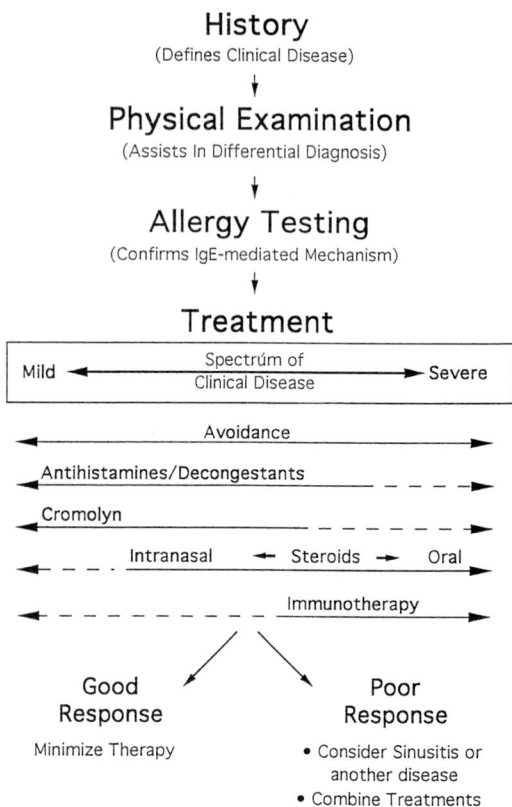

FIGURE 28–4. Flow chart depicting an approach to the management of allergic rhinitis.

agents from the patient's environment theoretically provides the potential for cure. As mentioned above, most perennial allergens are encountered in the home. Dust mites, a major component of dust, feed on human epithelial scales and organic debris. Washing bedding in hot water kills them, although the inanimate allergen may remain. Mattresses and pillows should be encased in protective linings. Fungi can be reduced in the home by cleaning and dehumidifying the basement. Pets may be the direct etiology of the problem or may act indirectly by carrying pollens into the home on their coats. Seasonal allergies can be problematic both inside the home and outdoors. Air conditioners in cars and homes reduce pollen exposure. Outdoor activities such as grass cutting, picnics, and camping trips are best avoided during appropriate seasons.

ANTIHISTAMINES. Antihistamines are the most utilized agents in the treatment of allergic rhinitis (see Chapter 16). They show greatest efficacy in the relief of sneezing, itching, and rhinorrhea. Symptoms of seasonal allergic rhinitis are thus more likely to respond to antihistamines than are symptoms of perennial rhinitis. In general, the long clinical experience with these medications makes them a safe choice for prolonged treatment.

DECONGESTANTS. Since antihistamines have limited efficacy in the treatment of nasal congestion, they are frequently combined with systemic and topical decongestants. Topical decongestant sprays or drops are more effective in achieving nasal decongestion than their oral counterparts and lack the side effects associated with oral administration. The main disadvantage of these medications, however, is the development of rhinitis medicamentosa with prolonged usage. Consequently, use of a topical decongestant is recommended only for a few days. In the young child, nasal drops should be instilled with the patient supine and the head turned to one side. The drops are then placed into the dependent nostril and the position maintained for one minute. Nasal sprays are administered with the head tilted forward, and the patient is instructed to sniff during insufflation of the medicine.

CROMOLYN. Cromolyn sodium, administered topically, has been shown to be clinically efficacious in the treatment of seasonal and perennial allergic rhinitis. To be effective, the drug should be used prior to the onset of symptoms and continued through the period of allergen exposure. Its major disadvantage is the relatively short duration of action, often requiring administration four times a day. It also appears relatively less effective than topical nasal steroids in seasonal allergic rhinitis.

CORTICOSTEROIDS. Systemic steroids have long been known to be efficacious in the treatment of allergic disease, but the risk of complications from systemic administration outweighs their benefit for the prolonged management of allergic rhinitis. Nonetheless, short courses of oral steroids may be indicated for intractable allergic rhinitis or for rhinitis medicamentosa. In both these situations, disease severity renders antihistamine/decongestants and topical corticosteroids ineffective. A 1- to 2-week course of prednisone, starting at 30 mg per day, generally provides a rapid clinical response. Once disease severity has been reduced sufficiently by a course of systemic steroids, a topical nasal steroid can be started and then continued with effective disease control.

Topical nasal corticosteroids avoid the risks

of systemic steroids while achieving site-specific efficacy. Many patients expect nasal steroid sprays to work, like topical decongestants, within minutes. However, the topical steroid effect reaches its maximum benefit after several days to weeks of use (although some effect may be noted sooner); the patient must be so informed. Patients should also be cautioned to aim the medication straight back into the nasal cavity and not toward the septum. Any local irritation noted on physical examination should be followed closely to prevent the rarely reported complication of a septal perforation.

Other problems relate to the delivery mechanism. One method delivers topical steroid as a dry powder propelled into the nose by pressurized freon. Alternatively, a topical steroid may be made aqueous as a microsuspension with polyethylene glycol or methylcellulose for delivery by metered dose spray. Because of these vehicles, which must be used for delivery, local irritation has been a side effect of intranasal steroids. The choice between aqueous or freon-delivered forms often come down to patient preference. Many patients find the blast of medication from a pressurized canister uncomfortable and opt for an aqueous form. Others, especially those with profuse rhinorrhea and postnasal discharge, do not like the additional fluid volume of the aqueous forms and prefer a freon-delivered form. As only a subset of patients with associated eye symptoms find relief with topical nasal steroid treatment, many will require additional medications. In patients with olfactory complaints, a method designed to optimize delivery of medications toward the roof of the nasal cavity may be helpful. One way to achieve this goal is to have the patient spray an aqueous steroid while lying supine on a bed with his head extended off the bed.

IMMUNOTHERAPY. As this topic is covered in Chapter 17, only a few comments will be made. The decision to choose immunotherapy is best made by patient and physician preference, depending on the duration and severity of symptoms, as well as the degree of symptom control attained with other forms of therapy. The decision to treat with immunotherapy commits the patient to an extended period of therapy. Frequent injections are time consuming, costly, and may be associated with adverse systemic allergic reactions. Daily medications themselves, however, may cause problems with compliance and adverse effects. Both types of therapy are not mutually exclusive. A patient receiving immunotherapy with a symptomatic exacerbation during the pollen season may benefit from the addition of antihistamines or topical nasal steroids during the time of peak symptoms.

SURGERY. Surgery is not a treatment for allergic rhinitis, but it may play an adjuvant role. Surgery can cure nasal airflow obstruction secondary to mechanical factors. Correcting a septal deviation can provide better access for topical therapy and may eliminate a predisposing factor for recurrent sinusitis. The role of enlarged adenoids in children should also be considered. Consultation from an otolaryngologist can aid in the management of patients with allergic rhinitis who are not responding to therapy. Patients who have undergone surgical intervention previously should have an otolaryngology consultation.

NONALLERGIC RHINITIS

A number of patients with chronic nasal complaints undergo allergy evaluation, including allergy tests, only to find no identifiable allergic etiology. In addition, obvious mechanical and other identifiable causes from the differential diagnosis are able to be eliminated. By exclusion, these patients are categorized as having nonallergic rhinitis. In patients with chronic rhinitis who were studied in allergy and otolaryngology clinics, the prevalence of nonallergic disease ranged from 28 to 60 percent (Togias, 1993). This large variation probably stems in part from differences in definitions of disease and in diagnostic testing. The lack of wide agreement on the parameters of disease makes the study and understanding of nonallergic rhinitis difficult. Even available terminology is confusing: "vasomotor rhinitis" has been used to describe this entity despite the fact that no "vasomotor" dysfunction of the nasal mucosa has been clearly identified. This rather misleading term is therefore best avoided.

The initial approach to nonallergic rhinitis is to rule out a number of conditions with nasal manifestations and specific etiologies (Table 28–3). Drugs can often be implicated in nasal complaints. Rhinitis medicamentosa is due to overuse of topical α-adrenergic ago-

TABLE 28–3. NONALLERGIC RHINITIS: DIFFERENTIAL DIAGNOSIS OF KNOWN ETIOLOGIES

Associated drugs
   α-Adrenergic agonists (i.e., rhinitis medicamentosa)
   Vasodilator antihypertensives
   Oral estrogens
   Ophthalmic β-adrenergic blockers
   Aspirin and other NSAIDs
Infections
   Chronic sinusitis
   Granulomatous infections
      Tuberculosis
      Syphilis
   Fungal infections
Systemic conditions
   Cystic fibrosis
   Immunodeficiencies
   Immotile cilia syndrome
   Rhinitis of pregnancy
   Hypothyroidism
Granulomatous diseases
   Wegener's granulomatosis
   Sarcoidosis
   Midline granuloma
Primary atrophic rhinitis
Relapsing polychondritis
Neoplasms
   Squamous cell carcinoma
   Nasopharyngeal carcinoma
Structural abnormalities
   Congenital
   Septal deviation
   Concha bullosa
   Other bony abnormalities of the lateral nasal wall

nists. Vasodilator antihypertensives, oral estrogens, and ophthalmic β-adrenergic blockers are all associated with nasal congestion. Aspirin and other nonsteroidal anti-inflammatory agents (NSAIDs) may cause rhinorrhea, especially as part of the syndrome of aspirin-sensitivity with nasal polyps and asthma. Systemic conditions that have been associated with nasal complaints include cystic fibrosis, immunodeficiencies, immotile cilia syndrome, rhinitis of pregnancy, and hypothyroidism. Primary atrophic rhinitis is associated with nasal congestion, mucosal atrophy, dry crusts, and a constant bad smell (ozena) in the nose; the prevalence of this condition has decreased in developed countries. Other diseases with nasal manifestations include granulomatous diseases (e.g., Wegener's granulomatosis, sarcoidosis, midline granuloma) and infections (e.g., tuberculosis, syphilis) as well as nasal neoplasms.

Once these relatively unusual conditions have been ruled out, most patients with non-allergic rhinitis are left with symptoms that are of unclear etiology and difficult to treat. As with perennial allergic rhinitis, patients generally complain of nasal obstruction, anterior rhinorrhea, postnasal discharge, sinus pressure or pain, and occasional sneezing and pruritus. But when compared to patients with perennial allergic rhinitis, these patients complain less of sneezing and conjunctival symptoms and more of sinus pressure and pain. In fact, one diagnosis that may have important clinical overlap with nonallergic rhinitis is chronic sinusitis. It may be difficult to separate these two entities in some patients, as nonallergic rhinitis may predispose to sinusitis, and symptoms of chronic sinusitis may mimic those of chronic nonallergic rhinitis. Especially in those patients who complain of sinus pressure or pain, and postnasal discharge, an aggressive search for sinusitis may be indicated, including a coronal sinus CT scan. If suggestive evidence is found, an extended course of antibiotics may resolve the problem (see Chapter 30).

A frequent finding in nonallergic rhinitis is nasal sensitivity to nonspecific factors. These patients note nasal secretion and/or obstruction on exposure to irritants, such as cigarette smoke, perfumes, hair sprays, chemical fumes, or pollutants; to changes in environment, such as sudden changes in temperature (e.g., leaving or entering an air-conditioned room), humidity, or barometric pressure; or to exposure to cold weather or hot spicy foods. Patients with perennial allergic rhinitis also complain of such sensitivities, but generally find them less troublesome than exposure to their clearly identifiable allergens. Some nonallergic rhinitics complain of predominant obstructive symptoms, and others of predominant secretory symptoms; as yet, this contrast has not yielded insights into the pathogenesis of nonallergic rhinitis, but it may help to direct the use of symptomatic therapeutic agents.

Attempts to understand the pathophysiology of nonallergic rhinitis have pursued models of nasal reactions that can be studied in the laboratory. Two nonallergic stimuli that have been studied are nasal inhalation of cold dry air and ingestion of hot spicy food. Both of these models have in common an apparent neural component as both apparently induce reflex-mediated nasal secretion, which can be blocked by anticholinergic agents. What makes certain patients susceptible to such stimuli remains an open question; there is evidence that subjects who are sensitive to nasal inhalation of cold dry air have a defect in efficient humidification of inspired air (Togias, 1993). There is also evidence that sensory nerves may be hyperresponsive in at least a subpopulation of nonallergic rhinitics. Capsaicin, the pungent principle of hot peppers, specifically activates certain sensory nerves in the mucosa; this agent caused greater nasal secretion in subjects with nonallergic rhinitis who complain predominantly of rhinorrhea than in normal subjects (Stjärne et al, 1989).

MANAGEMENT. Patients with nonallergic rhinitis tend to be less responsive to treatment than those with allergic rhinitis. Although mechanisms of disease are not known, many agents used for treatment of allergic rhinitis also have efficacy in nonallergic disease. Antihistamines do have some benefit; it may be the anticholinergic effects of first-generation antihistamines that play a role in control of rhinorrhea. Decongestants are also of use; unfortunately, topical treatment is unsuitable for long-term use, and these patients with chronic disease are left with the relatively less effective oral agents. Perhaps because of their efficacy in allergic rhinitis, topical nasal steroids have become "first-line" therapy. Although some clinical efficacy has been demonstrated, these agents often do not provide the same relief as they do in allergic rhinitis. For those patients who complain of rhinorrhea, anticholinergic agents have clinical benefit. Atropine and ipratropium bromide both have been shown to be effective in treating the rhinorrhea of nonallergic rhinitis. Topical anticholinergic preparations for the nose are not yet available in the United States. Some uncontrolled trials have suggested a role for capsaicin desensitization in the treatment of nonallergic rhinitis, but this method needs more study before it can be generally recommended. Surgical approaches have been used in the past, including vidian neurectomy (Mackay, 1993). Cutting this nerve, which carries the parasympathetic fibers as well as some sympathetic fibers to the nose, is an attempt to reduce nasal secretion; however, any improvement has proved to be short-lived, probably due to reinnervation. Other than surgical treatment of impaired sinus drainage, which may contribute to an associated chronic sinusitis, surgery is of little benefit in the management of nonallergic rhinitis.

NASAL POLYPS

Nasal polyps are non-neoplastic collections of inflammatory mucosal tissue that generally originate from sinus mucosa. These simple mucous polyps become symptomatic when they enlarge to cause obstruction of sinuses and the nasal cavity. Histologically, polyps consist of grossly edematous submucosa covered by respiratory epithelium. Within the sparsely vascularized submucosa, there is a cellular infiltrate composed of plasma cells, lymphocytes, and an often striking eosinophilia.

Nasal polyps generally present by causing nasal obstruction that is usually bilateral, though not necessarily equal in severity. Hyposmia, due to obstruction adjacent to the olfactory epithelium, is a frequent and frustrating accompanying complaint; it is usually the most difficult symptom to treat. Sinus obstruction may lead to sinusitis causing sinus pressure or pain and purulent discharge.

Polyps are usually seen in the nares, appearing as whitish to pale yellow, glistening, semitranslucent masses. A nasal decongestant will often allow more of the polyp to be seen by shrinking the adjacent turbinate mucosa. CT scans invariably show mucosal disease: polyps contained within a maxillary sinus will appear sessile and rounded; polyps that have extended into the nasal cavity, frequently from ethmoid sinuses, will be polypoid and may have a long stalk. Nasal polyps are usually multiple and bilateral. A unilateral mass suggests a tumor or other noninflammatory lesion. A "polyp" noted before 2 years of age may be a defect of the anterior cranial fossa or a dermoid cyst.

Pathogenesis of nasal polyposis remains unclear. Despite occasional use of the term "allergic polyp," studies have shown no greater incidence of allergic disease in polyp patients than in the general population (Settipane and Chafee, 1977). On the other hand, nasal polyps can be associated with other airway diseases. Late-onset asthma, usually nonallergic, occurs in 20 to 40 percent of patients with polyps. A further subset of these patients have (or will develop) sensitivity to aspirin and other nonsteroidal anti-inflammatory drugs; they suffer naso-ocular reactions and/or acute exacerbations of asthma on ingestion of these agents. This presentation (nasal polyposis, nonallergic asthma, and aspirin sensitivity) has been termed Samter's triad (see Chapter

28) and occurs in about 8 percent of patients with nasal polyps (Samter and Lederer, 1958). Polyps occur in some patients with cystic fibrosis, especially those with respiratory manifestations of the disease. In fact, because benign simple nasal polyps occur so rarely before 20 years of age, any child with nasal polyps should undergo a sweat test.

MANAGEMENT. The initial approach to nasal polyps generally is medical. Many cases respond to corticosteroid treatment, though the degree of response varies. Topical nasal corticosteroids, delivered at the same doses used to treat allergic rhinitis, often produce a clinical response (i.e., decreased nasal obstruction) within 1 to 3 months. If so, this treatment may be continued as maintenance therapy. Oral steroids are also effective, but cannot be generally recommended for the long courses required to cause regression of polyps.

If the polyps do not regress sufficiently with steroid treatment, they may be removed surgically. Often, surgery is combined with perioperative and short-term use of oral steroids. Because recurrence of polyps is so frequent after surgery, these patients should be maintained on intranasal steroid treatment to prevent or slow this regrowth.

REFERENCES

Barnes PJ, Baraniuk JN, Belvisi MG. Neuropeptides in the respiratory tract. Am Rev Respir Dis 144:1391–1399, 1991.

Baroody FM, Naclerio RM. A Review of Anatomy and Physiology of the Nose. Self-instructional Package from the Committee on Continuing Medical Education, Alexandria, Va, American Academy of Otolaryngology–Head and Neck Surgery, 1990.

Brandtzaeg P. Immune function of human nasal mucosa and tonsils in health and disease. *In* Bienenstock J (ed). Immunology of the Lung and Upper Respiratory Tract. New York, McGraw-Hill, 1984.

Cauna N. Blood and nerve supply of the nasal lining. *In* Proctor DF, Anderson IB (eds). The Nose: Upper Airway Physiology and the Atmospheric Environment. Amsterdam, Elsevier Biomedical Press, 1982, pp 45–70.

Flowers BK, Naclerio RM. The Nose. *In* Naspitz CK, Tinkelman DG (eds). Childhood Rhinitis and Sinusitis: Pathophysiology and Treatment. New York, Marcel Dekker, 1990, pp 147–192.

Jaffe BF. Classification and management of anomalies of the nose. Otolaryngol Clin North Am 14:989–1004, 1981.

Leopold DA. The relationship between nasal anatomy and human olfaction. Laryngoscope 98:1232–1238, 1988.

Mackay IS. Surgical treatment. *In* Mygind N, Naclerio RM (eds). Allergic and Nonallergic Rhinitis: Clinical Aspects. Copenhagen, Munksgaard, 1993, pp 149–152.

Meltzer EO, Orgel HA, Jalowaiski AA. Cytology. *In* Mygind N, Naclerio RM (eds). Allergic and Nonallergic Rhinitis: Clinical Aspects. Copenhagen, Munksgaard, 1993, pp 66–81.

Mygind N, Pederson M, Nielsen M. Morphology of the upper airway epithelium. *In* Proctor DF, Anderson IB (eds). The Nose: Upper Airway Physiology and the Atmospheric Environment. Amsterdam, Elsevier Biomedical Press, 1982.

Naclerio RM. Allergic rhinitis. N Engl J Med 325:860–869, 1991.

Naclerio RM, Meier HL, Kagey-Sobotka A, Adkinson NF Jr, Meyers DA, Norman PS, Lichtenstein LM. Mediator release after nasal airway challenge with allergen. Am Rev Respir Dis 128:597–602, 1983.

Raphael GD, Baraniuk JN, Kaliner MA. How and why the nose runs. J Allergy Clin Immunol 87(2):457–467, 1991.

Rossmann CM, Lee R, Forrest JB, Newhouse MT. Nasal ciliary ultrastructure and function in patients with primary ciliary dyskinesia compared with that in normal subjects and in subjects with various respiratory diseases. Am Rev Resp Dis 129:161–167, 1984.

Samter M, Lederer F. Nasal polyps: Their relationship to allergy, particularly bronchial asthma. Med Clin North Am 42:175–197, 1958.

Settipane G, Chafee F. Nasal polyps in asthma and rhinitis. J Allergy Clin Immunol 58:17–21, 1977.

Smith JM. Epidemiology. *In* Mygind N, Naclerio RM (eds). Allergic and Nonallergic Rhinitis: Clinical Aspects. Copenhagen, Munksgaard, 1993, pp 15–22.

Stjärne P, Lundblad L, Lundberg JM, Änggård A. Capsaicin and nicotine-sensitive afferent neurones and nasal secretion in healthy human volunteers and in patients with vasomotor rhinitis. Br J Pharmacol 96:693–701, 1989.

Strober W, James SP. The mucosal immune system. *In* Terr AI, Stites DP (eds). Basic and Clinical Immunology. Norwalk CT, Appleton & Lange, 1991, pp 175–186.

Swift DL, Proctor DF. Access of air to the respiratory tract. *In* Brain DJ, Proctor DF, Reid LM (eds). Respiratory defense mechanisms. New York, Marcel Dekker, 1977.

Togias AG. Nonallergic rhinitis. *In* Mygind N, Naclerio RM (eds). Allergic and Nonallergic Rhinitis: Clinical Aspects. Copenhagen, Munksgaard, 1993, pp 159–166.

Chapter 29
Diseases of the Ear

David P. Skoner, M.D., and
Margaretha L. Casselbrant, M.D., Ph.D.

Diseases of the ear encompass a variety of disorders, affecting the externally visible structures of the ear (congenital anomalies), the external auditory canal (otitis externa or "swimmer's ear"), the middle ear, and the inner ear. However, most commonly, the middle ear is affected by inflammatory disease processes, which are collectively termed "otitis media." This chapter will therefore be heavily focused on middle ear disease, and will address diseases of the external ear and inner ear to a lesser extent. Excellent reviews of these latter topics have been presented elsewhere (Paparella et al, 1991).

EXTERNAL EAR

Cerumen Impaction

Cerumen impaction obstructs the view of the tympanic membrane and can cause a conductive hearing loss if it completely obstructs the ear canal. The cerumen is usually removed by use of a curet under direct vision. Irrigation with a syringe or a Water Pik can be performed if it is known that the tympanic membrane is intact. The water should be at body temperature because a caloric reaction can occur if the water is too cold or too warm.

Foreign Bodies

Foreign bodies in the external ear canal, such as erasers, raisins, and pieces of crayons, are often found in children. They can be difficult to remove, especially if they are medial to the isthmus of the external ear canal. The skin in the canal can easily be macerated by minimal trauma, causing bleeding, and care must be taken to avoid injuries to the tympanic membrane and ossicles. An operating microscope usually facilitates the removal of the foreign bodies by means of different curets, hooks, and loops. Irrigation can also be used for removal of small foreign bodies if the tympanic membrane is intact. General anesthesia may sometimes be necessary in younger children.

Otitis Externa

Otitis externa, or inflammation of the external auditory canal, is very common and there are many local contributory factors. The use of bobby pins, Q-tips, or the tip of a pencil to clean the canal may cause abrasion of the skin, as can trauma during removal of cerumen. Swimming and washing with soap may also interfere with the local defense against infection in the external ear canal. Systemic disorders, such as anemia, vitamin deficiency, and various dermatoses, may predispose to infection by lowering the host defense. Patients usually present with ear pain that can be severe, swelling and discharge from the ear canal, tenderness on palpation of the tragus, and sometimes fever and cellulitis with displacement of the auricle. In more chronic cases, the symptoms may be itching of the ear, with or without discharge, and hearing loss. The most common organism isolated is *P. aeruginosa*. Other organisms include *Proteus* species, *S. aureus, S. epidermidis, E. coli,* streptococci, and diphtheroids. Fungi can also be isolated.

Treatment should initially be directed toward relief of pain, cleaning of the external ear canal, and application of topical acidifying drops or antibiotic/steroid drops. An ear wick may be used during the first few days to facilitate contact between the drops and the ear canal. The elimination of predisposing factors is important. In severe or persistent cases, culture of the external ear canal should be done. Sometimes systemic antimicrobials are necessary.

Malignant Otitis Externa

Malignant otitis externa is a progressive, sometimes fatal infection of the external ear canal, surrounding tissue, and base of the skull caused by *P. aeruginosa*. The infection occurs most often in elderly patients with diabetes mellitus. The treatment consists of control of the diabetes and the use of antimicrobial agents effective against *P. aeruginosa*, including topical and systemic antipseudomonal agents. Local wound care may require aggressive debridement of the infected tissue in attempting to reduce associated morbidity and mortality.

Furuncle

Furuncles (otitis externa circumscribed) may form in the outer third of the external ear canal. They are usually staphylococcal infections of the pilosebaceous glands and present with the same symptoms as otitis externa. Although they are usually treated with analgesics, other forms of therapy may be necessary. These can include systemic and topical antimicrobial agents, and incision and drainage.

Tumors

There are many different lesions and abnormalities that can arise in the ear canal, as there are two embryologic germ layers (ectodermal and mesodermal) that constitute the various components of the external canal (Table 29-1). These lesions are more common in adults than in children (Paparella et al, 1991).

MIDDLE EAR

Middle Ear Inflammation

One of the signs of otitis media is the accumulation of a purulent, serous, or mucoid middle ear effusion. Microscopically, otitis

TABLE 29-1. BENIGN LESIONS AND MALIGNANT TUMORS OF THE EXTERNAL EAR

Benign lesions
    Skin and soft tissue cysts and tumors
    Vascular tumors
    Cartilaginous lesions
    Osseous tumors
Malignant tumors
    Auricle
        Squamous cell carcinoma
        Basal cell carcinoma
        Malignant melanoma
    External ear canal
        Basal cell carcinoma
        Adenocarcinoma
        Sarcoma

media is characterized by a middle ear mucosa that is thickened and edematous, with glandular hypertrophy. There is also engorgement of capillaries and small venules, and a cellular infiltrate of lymphocytes, neutrophils, and rarely eosinophils.

Otitis media is usually classified into several types, including acute otitis media (rapid onset of symptoms and signs of acute inflammation such as fever, pain, irritability), otitis media with effusion (fluid in the middle ear without symptoms and signs of acute inflammation, often accompanied by hearing loss), and chronic suppurative otitis media (prolonged or intermittent drainage through a perforation of the tympanic membrane). Based on epidemiologic studies, the pathogenesis of otitis media is best viewed as a disease continuum in both children and adults (Giebink, 1992). These studies showed that chronic otitis media with effusion often followed acute otitis media, and that intractable chronic otitis media (with granulation tissue and ossicle damage) frequently followed recurrent acute otitis media and chronic otitis media with effusion. This suggests that each of the currently employed classifications of otitis media represents a stage in the continuum of a single middle ear disease process.

Acute otitis media is common. Indeed, of 877 children who were followed prospectively soon after birth, 62 percent had an episode of acute otitis media by their first birthday, and 17 percent had ≥3 episodes. By age 3 years, 83 percent had ≥1 episode and 46 percent had ≥3 episodes (Teele et al, 1989). Although less common than in young children, acute otitis media persists as a health care problem in older children, adolescents, and adults (Bernstein et al, 1984).

The incidence and prevalence of otitis media with effusion is also high in children. Of 103 children 2 to 6 years of age who were evaluated monthly over a 2-year period with otoscopy and tympanometry in a Pittsburgh day-care center, 53 percent had at least one episode of otitis media with effusion during the first year of the study, and 61 percent during the second year. Thirty percent had recurrent bouts, but 80 percent of episodes cleared within 2 months (Casselbrant et al, 1985). In a similar study of 126 Pittsburgh school children 5 to 12 years of age, the incidence of otitis media with effusion was found to be much lower in children 6 years of age and older than in those younger than 6 years (Casselbrant et al, 1986).

The social impact of otitis media is tremendous. It is considered the most common diagnosis in children less than 15 years of age, with health care expenditures estimated at 2.5 billion dollars per year (Stool and Field, 1989). However, adults are also affected, since approximately 3 to 15 percent of otitis media patients referred to otolaryngology clinics are adults (Sade, 1979; Oppenheimer, 1975). In most children, the fluid resolves in 1 to 2 months (Casselbrant et al, 1985), but in 10 percent of children, the fluid persists for 3 months or longer after the onset of the first episode of acute otitis media (Teele et al, 1989). Moreover, the sequelae of otitis media in children, including hearing loss, can persist into the adult years. Therefore, much of this chapter is focused on the pediatric age group, with reference to the adult population when indicated.

Pathophysiology

The pathophysiology of otitis media is complex and multifactorial. Epidemiologic relationships have been established between otitis media in children and such diverse factors as nutrition (lack of breast-feeding), environment (allergy, exposure to second-hand tobacco smoke), infection (common cold viruses, bacteria), and host immunology (role for the immune system in protection from otitis media) (Giebink, 1992; Paparella et al, 1991; Bluestone and Klein, 1995). Both epidemiologic evidence and clinical experience would strongly suggest that otitis media is frequently a complication of the common cold. However, middle ear fluid may also be triggered by traumatic forces, including barotrauma, blunt physical injury to the temporal region and ear, or destruction by cholesteatoma and surgery. Less commonly, middle ear fluid can represent leakage of cerebrospinal fluid or perilymph from the inner ear, resulting in a salty taste and rhinorrhea in the head-down position.

Although it is possible that primary middle ear inflammation is at least partially responsible for the development of otitis media, much of the research into pathophysiology has suggested a pivotal role for dysfunction of the eustachian tube (ET) in the pathogenesis of this disease. Under normal conditions, the ET is closed, but opens transiently during swallowing owing to contraction of the tensor veli palatini muscle. This feature has been exploited in tests that have been designed to evaluate ET function (Skoner et al, 1987; Skoner et al, 1988b).

The ET has a number of roles in maintaining normal function of the middle ear, including protection from potentially harmful nasopharyngeal contents, drainage of any potential middle ear fluid, and ventilation to equilibrate any abnormal pressures within the middle ear cavity.

It is hypothesized that factors that generate nasopharyngeal inflammation (e.g., infection, allergy) may also cause direct ET inflammation or may merely obstruct the orifice of the ET due to edema. Obstruction of the ET could also be the result of tumors, enlarged adenoids, or an abnormally patent or primarily dysfunctional ET. When inflamed or obstructed, the ET may no longer be able to perform its functional role optimally. Dysfunction of such a critical protective mechanism may provide a final common pathway through which a number of the factors outlined above could exert their effects.

The use of animal models has documented that experimental ET obstruction results in middle ear underpressures and the accumulation of fluid within the middle ear cavity, which are hallmark features of otitis media (Doyle, 1984; Casselbrant et al, 1988). These generally occur within 2 to 7 days of the onset of obstruction. This suggests that prolonged obstruction of the ET may be necessary for the development of otitis media, and that ET dysfunction of relatively short duration may not be sufficient.

Human experimental models have been developed to test hypotheses derived from epidemiologic studies, especially those linking allergy and viral infection with otitis media. Collectively, the term "nasal provocation challenge" has been applied to these studies, since the design involves placing allergen or virus in the nose and measuring various airway responses objectively. Distinct advantages that these models offer are control of (1) the state of health of the subject prior to challenge with virus or allergen, (2) the dose and nature of the challenge agent (e.g., ragweed, rhinovirus 39), and (3) the precise timing of the nasal challenge. Potential limitations of this methodology include the virtual restriction of their application to adult volunteers.

Nonetheless, these nasal provocation studies have provided a great deal of insight into the pathogenesis of otitis media. Experimental allergen inhalation by allergic subjects has been shown to result in both early (within 30 minutes) and late (2 to 12 hours) ET dysfunction (Friedman et al, 1983; Skoner et al, 1988a). Effective allergens included both seasonal (ragweed) and perennial (dust mite) allergens (Skoner et al, 1986). ET dysfunction was relatively short in duration, generally resolving within several hours. The results of this laboratory model were subsequently confirmed in a natural history model, whereby untreated grass allergic subjects followed during grass pollen season also developed ET dysfunction (Skoner et al, 1990). Despite the confirmed phenomenon of allergen-induced ET dysfunction, conclusive evidence of allergen-induced middle ear negative pressure and fluid has not been forthcoming in either human or animal models.

Other studies using nasal provocation with rhinovirus 39 (common cold virus) and influenza A virus have revealed more extensive, yet virus-specific, airway pathophysiologic effects. Both rhinovirus 39 and influenza A produce nasal symptoms (sneezing, rhinorrhea, and congestion), which have an onset 1 day after inoculation, peak at 2 to 4 days post inoculation, and resolve by 6 to 8 days post inoculation (Doyle et al, 1992; 1994). ET dysfunction follows a similar temporal pattern during infection with both viruses. In contrast to the allergen model, ET dysfunction has been accompanied by middle ear underpressures during these infections. Indeed, otitis media with effusion was detected in 24 percent of subjects infected with influenza A, but was documented in <5 percent of subjects infected with rhinovirus 39 (Buchman et al, 1994). Painful, typical acute otitis media with effusion requiring myringotomy was identified in one subject in the influenza virus trials. Cultures of the purulent fluid by conventional methods were negative for both virus and bacteria. However, polymerase chain reaction (PCR) for influenza virus genomic sequences was positive, potentially indicating a role for the virus in pathogenesis (Buchman et al, 1995).

The precise mechanism by which allergens and viruses cause obstruction of the ET and/or induce ear disease is not known. However, one possible, and even likely, common pathway is via the release of histamine-like inflammatory mediators, which are known to have allergen-like effects on the function of both the nose and the ET (Skoner et al, 1987; Walker et al, 1985; Doyle et al, 1990). Indeed, the local nasal release of various inflammatory mediators, including histamine, leukotrienes, prostglandins, and kinins, has been described after allergen and/or viral nasal provocation (Skoner et al, 1990; Igarashi et al, 1993; Naclerio et al, 1988). Moreover, many of these inflammatory mediators are present in high concentrations in the middle ear fluid of children with otitis media with effusion (Skoner et al, 1988b).

As shown in Figure 29–1, bacteria are frequently isolated from middle ear fluids of children with acute otitis media, and less frequently from children with chronic otitis media (Bluestone et al, 1992). The bacteriology of acute otitis media in adults is similar to that in children, with the same three bacteria predominating in middle ear aspirates (Celin et al, 1991).

A number of the bacteria cultured from middle ear aspirates have developed mechanisms of resistance against commonly employed antimicrobial agents. In children, certain strains of *H. influenzae* and *M. catarrhalis* produce the beta-lactamase enzyme, capable of degrading the beta-lactam ring of penicillin-like antibiotics and rendering them ineffective. Percentages of beta-lactamase–producing bacteria in middle ear aspirates of Pittsburgh children in 1989 ranged from 36 to 39 percent for *H. influenzae* and 88 to 100 percent for *M. catarrhalis,* with strong evidence for a recent, steady increase in number (Bluestone et al, 1992). Similar studies in adults have also revealed a high percentage of

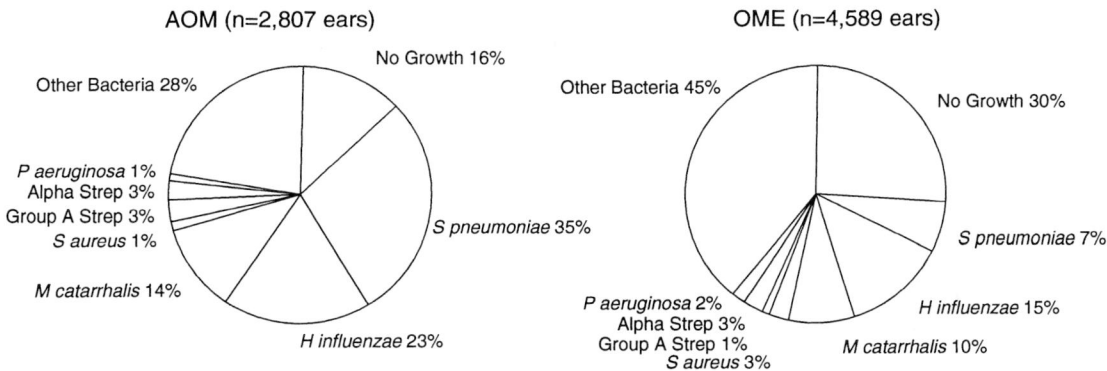

FIGURE 29-1. Results of bacterial cultures of middle ear fluids in patients with acute otitis media (AOM) and otitis media with effusion (OME). (Redrawn from Bluestone CD, Stephenson JS, Martin LM. Ten-year review of otitis media pathogens. Pediatr Infect Dis J 11:S7–S11, 1992.)

beta-lactamase–producing bacteria in middle ear aspirates (Celin et al, 1991).

Penicillin-resistant *S. pneumoniae* is also being increasingly recognized as a significant problem, even in children with otitis media. The importance of this observation is highlighted by the recent finding that the prevalence of *S. pneumoniae* isolated from acute otitis media significantly increased in Pittsburgh, from 28 percent in 1980 to 44 percent in 1989 (Bluestone et al, 1992). One recent study reported that the incidence of penicillin-resistant isolates increased from 1.7 percent in 1988 to 12.8 percent in 1989 (Ford et al, 1991). At the same institution (Texas Children's Hospital), penicillin-resistant isolates were obtained from 11 percent of middle ear cultures (Jackson et al, 1984). Indeed, isolates from the middle ear were more likely to be resistant to penicillin than were those from any other site.

As with other implicated factors in the development of otitis media, the role of bacteria in the pathogenesis of otitis media is likely to be complex and multifaceted. Whether the bacteria primarily infect the middle ear in these patients, or whether the stage for bacterial infection is set by a preceding viral infection or other exposure, is not known. However, the latter is the more likely of the two possibilities. Mechanisms by which this could develop include a permissive effect of viruses on immune parameters governing the development of bacterial infection (see below). It is more likely, however, that the virus-induced ET dysfunction and middle ear underpressure could permit the aspiration of bacteria-laden secretions into the normally sterile middle ear cavity, thus initiating the infection.

The functional capacity of the immune system is also a factor whose role in the pathogenesis of otitis media is definite, but unclear. A recent study at Children's Hospital of Pittsburgh showed that hospitalized children with primary immunodeficiencies often had otitis media, with most effusions culture positive for the same bacteria as identified in non-immunodeficient children (Haddad et al, 1992). Even though otitis media affected children with deficiencies of each of the components of the immune system (B lymphocyte, T lymphocyte, phagocytic, and complement), the majority of those affected were children with antibody deficiency syndromes (B lymphocyte). This serves to highlight the importance of a functioning humoral immune system in preventing otitis media. The role of the cell-mediated (T lymphocyte) immune system in otitis media is less clear, although variable effects on this parameter have been noted during experimental infection with rhinovirus 39 and influenza A virus (Skoner et al, 1993; Gentile et al, 1994). Immunosuppression was the dominant feature of the latter infection, where, as mentioned above, otitis media was also a frequent complication of the illness. The roles of deficiencies in the other branches of the immune system (neutrophils, complement) in predisposing to otitis media are not well delineated. However, influenza virus has also been shown to depress granulocytic function (Abramson et al, 1982), potentially playing a role in secondary bacterial infections.

Diagnosis

The history and physical examination using the pneumatic otoscope are in most instances sufficient to establish the diagnosis of otitis media. However, the use of tympanometry has become a valuable tool in determining the presence or absence of middle ear effusion. Audiometry is important in assessing the effect of the middle ear effusion on the hearing.

HISTORY

Obtaining a thorough history is essential in reaching the proper diagnosis. Information should be obtained regarding the patient's general condition, but specifically about previous history and treatment of ear disease. A thorough environmental history is also necessary to identify allergenic or irritant factors in the home, day-care center, school, or workplace that may predispose the patient to ear disease. A history of exposure to irritants, such as cigarette smoke, infections, or allergens such as house dust mite, or pets, will aid in the selection of allergy tests as well as provide information necessary to modify the patient's environment. Information regarding duration of symptoms as well as time of occurrence of symptoms, such as during pollen season, is valuable in identifying risk factors. Symptoms such as snoring, mouth-breathing, and nasal obstruction may suggest adenoidal obstruction or a severely deviated septum. Information regarding risk factors for otitis media, such as lack of breast-feeding, day-care attendance, or older siblings, should also be obtained.

PHYSICAL EXAMINATION

The physical examination should include an evaluation of the head and neck to rule out any condition that can be associated with otitis media, such as Down's syndrome or any other craniofacial abnormality. The evaluation of the oropharynx may reveal a cleft palate or large obstructing tonsils. Nasal examination may show obstruction due to large adenoids, pale boggy turbinates suggestive of allergy, or septal deviation causing mouth-breathing and hyponasal speech.

Pneumatic Otoscopy. The evaluation of the ear starts with an examination of the outer ear and external ear canal. Cerumen and debris must be cleaned from the canal so that the tympanic membrane can be inspected. The color, translucency, position, and mobility are evaluated by use of the pneumatic otoscope. The mobility of the tympanic membrane is assessed by application of positive and negative pressure (Fig. 29–2; Table 29–2). A normal tympanic membrane is thin, grayish, and translucent and moves easily when positive and negative pressure are applied. A red tympanic membrane per se does not indicate acute otitis media, as the blood vessels may engorge when a child is crying. Redness or white opacification of the tympanic membrane, fullness or bulging, and poor or no mobility due to effusion in the middle ear are signs of acute otitis media. Occasionally, this condition presents with otorrhea. A retracted tympanic membrane with poor or no mobility, on the other hand, signifies otitis media with effusion. The tympanic membrane can be pink or white and opacified, or if the middle ear effusion has been longstanding, a yellow or bluish color may be noted. Sometimes fluid levels and bubbles can be seen behind the ear drum. The mobility of the tympanic membrane is usually not affected by a small area of tympanosclerosis. However, if the tympanosclerosis is extensive, the mobil-

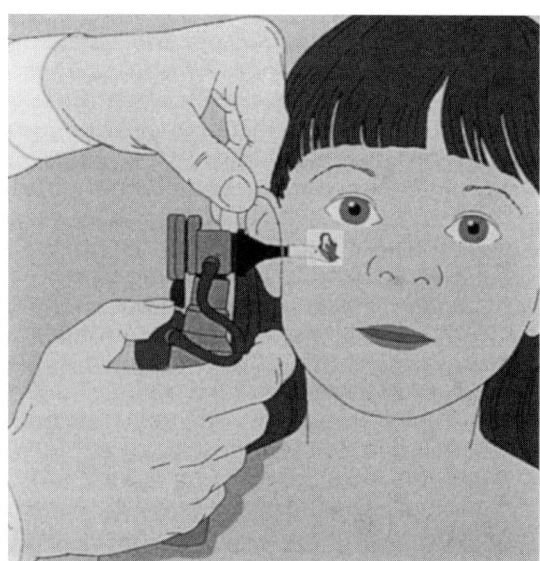

FIGURE 29–2. Two-handed positioning of diagnostic-head otoscope to minimize head movement and enhance visualization. (Adapted from Bluestone CD, Klein JO. Otitis Media in Infants and Children, 2nd ed. Philadelphia, WB Saunders, 1995.)

TABLE 29–2. CLINICAL SIGNIFICANCE OF FINDINGS IN PNEUMATIC OTOSCOPY

		Tympanic Membrane Moves to Applied Positive Pressure	
		Yes	*No*
Tympanic membrane moves to applied negative pressure	Yes	Normal middle ear pressure	Negative middle ear pressure
	No	Positive middle ear pressure	Middle ear effusion or very high negative pressure

ity of the tympanic membrane will be poor even without effusion. The tympanic membrane will be immobile if there is a perforation or patent tympanostomy tube.

Tympanometry. Acoustic immittance has been used for the identification of middle ear disease for many years. It has been used in the physician's office as well as for mass screening of children in pre-school and early elementary grade classes. Tympanometry is easy to perform and is highly sensitive to middle ear dysfunction. However, it has a low specificity, i.e., there is a high false-positive rate. Recent new ANSI standards for aural acoustic immittance testing require that absolute physical quantities are used (ANSI, 1987). Algorithms to determine the presence or absence of middle ear effusion, which were validated on old tympanometers that do not fulfill the ANSI 1987 criteria, cannot be used with the new tympanometers. Immittance variables such as peak compensated (static) admittance, tympanometric peak pressure, acoustic reflex, tympanometric shape (gradient), and tympanometric width have been studied to evaluate which of these variables have the highest sensitivity and specificity in detecting middle ear effusion. Studies by Nozza et al (1994) have shown that the tympanometric width has a high sensitivity and specificity in identifying middle ear effusions.

Audiometry. Audiometry is performed to assess the effect of middle ear effusion on the patient's hearing. In behavioral audiometry testing, methods vary with the child's age and cooperation. If hearing cannot be assessed by behavioral testing, auditory brain stem response audiometry (ABR) can be done. This test is relatively independent of the child's behavioral response and is not affected by sedation. Otoacoustic emissions testing is another objective measure to assess hearing. This method offers several advantages in hearing evaluation, as it is noninvasive and fast. Thus, it is highly suitable for testing infants and difficult-to-test children. However, even though otoacoustic emissions testing can determine the presence or absence of a hearing loss, it cannot determine hearing levels. Middle ear disease, as well as abnormal cochlear function, can affect the emission levels (Lonsbury-Martin et al, 1994). Otoacoustic emissions testing cannot differentiate between a cochlear and/or middle ear impairment. For a further review of audiologic testing, excellent references on this topic are available (Bluestone, 1990).

OTHER LABORATORY STUDIES

Aside from the laboratory studies recommended above for the diagnosis of otitis media, several other tests may be considered depending on the frequency and/or severity of ear disease, along with the presence of other characteristics. One of the main considerations is whether or not a disorder of the immune system exists (allergy, immune deficiency). In general, cases with a high degree of frequency, chronicity, or severity warrant evaluation. Coincident symptoms and signs of children with otitis media that should alert the clinician to the need for such an evaluation and the type of evaluation are summarized in Table 29–3.

Once a decision to evaluate for allergy has been made, the patient should be tested for allergy to a panel of geographically appropriate inhalant substances. There is no well-documented role for food allergy in triggering otitis media. To test for the presence of allergen-specific IgE antibodies to inhalant substances, several methods are available, including *in vivo* skin testing and *in vitro* serum testing. The advantages and disadvantages of each are summarized in Table 29–4. Generally, skin tests are preferable, since they are more sensitive and less costly, and they provide a vivid teaching example to the allergic patient about their tissue inflammatory process. However, expertise in interpretation,

TABLE 29-3. CLUES ELICITED IN THE EXAMINATION OF THE OTITIS-PRONE CHILD THAT SUGGEST THE NEED FOR EVALUATION OF THE IMMUNE SYSTEM

ALLERGY EVALUATION WARRANTED IF:

Family history	Positive for allergy and/or asthma
Sneeze, rhinorrhea, congestion	Prominent and present year-round or seasonally; interfere with normal activity
Symptom triggers	Pets, indoor allergens; or symptoms coincident with pollination
Nasal mucosa	Pale and boggy in appearance
Response to anti-allergy medical therapy	Relief with antihistamines or intranasal cromolyn or corticosteroids

IMMUNE DEFICIENCY EVALUATION WARRANTED IF:

Family history	Positive for early unexplained death or specific immune deficiency diagnosis
Frequency of infection	Elevated (>8 respiratory infections/year)
Chronicity of infection	Present
Severity of infection	High level (meningitis, sepsis)
Complication of infection	Present (e.g., mastoiditis complicating otitis media)
Site of infection	Multiple, not single, sites
Infecting organism	Opportunistic
Response to therapy	Poor, or recurring after discontinuation
Other signs	Failure to thrive, dermatitis, diarrhea

such as that provided by a board-certified allergist/clinical immunologist, is desirable. Exceptions to the general recommendation for skin testing include patients who have extensive skin disease, which precludes use of the skin for testing, who are unable to discontinue invalidating antihistamine or other therapies, or who are using beta blocker therapy, which increases the risk of skin testing. Serum testing should be used in these patients. The allergy evaluation should include the following allergens, which may vary geographically: pollens (grasses, trees, weeds), molds, dust mite, cats, and dogs. Skin tests must be interpreted in the context of reactions to both a positive (histamine) and negative (saline) control skin test. Both puncture and intradermal testing may be warranted in the evaluation. If the presence of allergy is documented, the patient is then eligible for anti-allergy therapy, including environmental control measures to reduce exposure to the allergen; anti-inflammatory medications including antihistamines, cromolyn, and corticosteroids; and allergy immunotherapy.

If immunodeficiency is suspected, the pa-

TABLE 29-4. RELATIVE ADVANTAGES OF *IN VIVO* AND *IN VITRO* TESTS IN THE DIAGNOSIS OF ALLERGIC DISEASES

IN VIVO Skin Test*	IN VITRO Serum RAST, FAST, ELISA†
Less expensive	No patient risk
Greater sensitivity	Specific and quantitative
Greater antigen availability	Not affected by drugs
Yields prompt results	Antigen stability
Technically easier	Patient convenience
Visible result useful for teaching	Useful in patients with skin conditions (e.g., dermatographism)
Good correlation with history and RAST tests	Good correlation with history and skin tests

*Puncture or intradermal.
†RAST = radioallergosorbent test; FAST = fluorescent allergosorbent test; ELISA = enzyme-linked immunosorbent assay.

tient can be screened for function of the four major branches of the immune system, including B lymphocyte, T lymphocyte, complement, and phagocytic systems, depending on the presence of other symptoms/signs of these diseases, which have been reviewed elsewhere (Buckley, 1983). Children with many of the primary immune deficiency disorders will present within the first year of life. Recurrent respiratory infections, such as otitis media, sinusitis, bronchitis, and pneumonia, are the most common presenting manifestations of the primary immune deficiencies. Often, many of these sites are involved in the same patient. Similarly, acquired immunodeficiency syndrome (AIDS) can also present with recurrent infections of the upper respiratory tract, including the middle ear.

A simple office screen for immunodeficiency, which would be capable of detecting the majority of such disorders, is presented in Table 29–5. The recurrent theme inherent in this panel of screening tests is the evaluation of both number and function for each of the individual components of the immune system. If the screening tests identify an immune deficiency, the patient should be referred to a clinical immunologist for further evaluation and therapy. As indicated in the section on pathophysiology, a disorder of the humoral antibody system would be most likely in patients with otitis media. The therapy for immune deficiency, if identified, would depend on the nature of the disorder. In humoral antibody deficiencies, the therapy may include intravenous gamma globulin and prophylactic antibiotics. Other disorders, such as those involving the T lymphocyte system, may be treatable with bone marrow transplantation.

In addition to considering abnormalities of the immune system, the clinician must also consider other possible conditions that could mimic those presentations, such as non-allergic rhinitis with eosinophilia (NARES), enlarged adenoids, submucous cleft palate, cystic fibrosis, immotile cilia syndrome, malnutrition, neoplasm, and treatment with immunosuppressive drugs. Specific diagnostic tests for these disorders may also be warranted in selected otitis-prone children. For example, cytologic examination of nasal secretions may help one distinguish between allergic, eosinophilic non-allergic, and infectious processes affecting the upper airways.

In selected cases, computerized axial tomography (CAT) may be useful to evaluate the temporal bone structure and identify cholesteatoma. Magnetic resonance imaging (MRI) can also be used, particularly in identifying acoustic neurinomas and other tumors of the middle ear and mastoid. For example, aggressive diagnostic tests for neoplasia are warranted in adults with persistent or recurrent unilateral otitis media, including computerized axial tomography, and direct nasopharyngoscopy with biopsy under local or general anesthesia. Otologic involvement has also been reported in patients with connective tissue diseases, including those with Wegener's granulomatosis, polyarteritis nodosa, allergic granulomatosis (Churg-Strauss syndrome), Sjögren's syndrome, and sarcoidosis. Depending on the presentation, an evaluation for these disorders may also be warranted, especially in the adult population.

TABLE 29–5. SUGGESTED LABORATORY SCREENING TESTS FOR OTITIS-PRONE CHILD WITH SUSPECTED IMMUNODEFICIENCY

IMMUNE SYSTEM COMPONENT	EXAMPLE OF IMMUNE DEFICIENCY	SCREENING TESTS
B lymphocyte	Bruton's agammaglobulinemia	Total lymphocyte count Quantitative immunoglobulin serum levels (IgG, IgA, IgM) Serum antibody titers to tetanus, polio, *Haemophilus influenzae*, other vaccines
T lymphocyte	Di George anomaly	Total lymphocyte count Delayed hypersensitivity skin tests (*Candida*, tetanus)
Phagocyte	Chronic granulomatous disease	Total neutrophil count Nitroblue tetrazolium reduction test
Complement	C3 deficiency	C3 and C4 complement serum levels CH_{50} (hemolytic complement)

Treatment

ACUTE OTITIS MEDIA

At present, antimicrobial therapy is recommended by the majority of physicians to treat children with acute otitis media, based on the fact that the rate of suppurative complications has been reduced in the antibiotic era (Sorenson, 1977). Also, antimicrobial agents are superior in sterilizing the middle ear compared to placebo (Howie and Ploussard, 1972). Kaleida et al (1991) showed that amoxicillin was significantly better than placebo for episodes of non-severe acute otitis media in resolving middle ear effusions. There were also significantly fewer episodes of initial treatment failures in the amoxicillin group. This effect of antimicrobial therapy was confirmed in a meta-analysis (Rosenfeld et al, 1994). Effective antimicrobial treatment should be based on the age of the patient, recent history of otitis media and antimicrobial treatment, and knowledge of the bacteriology and susceptibility patterns in the community.

Amoxicillin is the currently preferred drug for initial treatment of acute otitis media, since it is active both *in vitro* and *in vivo* against most strains of *S. pneumoniae* and *H. influenzae*. However, this may change as a result of the recent development of penicillin-resistant strains of *S. pneumoniae*. The incidence of penicillin-resistant *S. pneumoniae* strains in the community may become the determining factor in the choice of the initial antimicrobial agent, as *S. pneumoniae* is the most common organism isolated in acute otitis media. If the patient is allergic to penicillin/amoxicillin, but not to cephalosporins, then these agents may be prescribed. Erythromycin-sulfisoxazole is recommended for those patients who are allergic to both penicillins/amoxicillin and cephalosporins. Trimethoprim-sulfamethoxazole would also be an appropriate alternative, but it is not effective against *S. pyogenes*.

If the patient has not shown any clinical improvement within 48 to 72 hours of initiating antibiotic therapy, a resistant organism should be suspected, and treatment should be changed to a broad-spectrum antimicrobial agent. There is a multitude of different agents available, including amoxicillin-clavulanate, erythromycin-sulfisoxazole, trimethoprim-sulfamethoxazole, cefuroxime axetil, cefixime, loracarbef, and cefpodoxime. Cefaclor is probably effective against some of the beta-lactamase–producing organisms, but not as effective as the newer third-generation cephalosporins, which in general are more effective against gram-negative organisms. Cefixime is not effective against *S. aureus*.

Diarrhea, vomiting, diaper rashes, maculopapular rashes, and allergic reactions occur with all of these antimicrobial agents. Except for these reactions, amoxicillin has shown a remarkable record of safety. Erythromycin-sulfisoxazole and trimethoprim-sulfamethoxazole contain a sulfonamid, which has a high rate of adverse side effects that can, on rare occasions, be serious. These antibiotics, along with others, can cause fatal Stevens-Johnson syndrome. Moreover, cefaclor has been associated with a serum-sickness–like reaction.

Trimethoprim-sulfamethoxazole and the newer cephalosporins are approved for twice-a-day dosing, which may improve compliance in giving the drug. Cefixime can be given once or twice a day. The taste of the drug is important for compliance when treating children. Cefixime, followed by cefaclor, were considered to be the best tasting drugs by pre-schoolers in one study (Ruff et al, 1991). Cefuroxime axetil is not yet available in liquid form. When there is a concern that the child will not be given the medication or the child will not take the drug, ceftriaxone administered intramuscularly as a single dose could be an alternative (Green and Rothrock, 1993).

Tympanocentesis to obtain fluid from the middle ear for culture and sensitivity testing is usually not feasible in the routine clinical setting, and usually antimicrobial agents are administered without the benefit of a culture. However, a tympanocentesis should be performed for acute otitis media in a patient who (1) is seriously ill or appears toxic, (2) responds unsatisfactorily to antimicrobial therapy, (3) is already receiving antimicrobial therapy, (4) presents with suppurative complications, or (5) is immunocompromised or is a newborn (unusual organisms may be present in both).

Decongestants (systemic or local) are of value for children with nasal congestion, as are antihistamines for children with allergic rhinitis. However, there are no data available to document that they affect the course of an episode of acute otitis media.

Recurrent Acute Otitis Media

Many children have repeated episodes of acute otitis media, and if the child has three or more episodes in 6 months or four episodes in 12 months, with one episode in the last 3 months, prevention should be considered. A search for underlying factors such as respiratory allergy, immune defects, hypertrophic adenoids, and sinusitis should be done because treatment of these underlying conditions may decrease the recurrence rate of episodes of acute otitis media. If none of these conditions is present, prevention aimed primarily at the ear disease may be attempted.

Several clinical trials (Maynard et al, 1972; Gonzalez et al, 1986; Casselbrant et al, 1992) as well as a recent meta-analysis (Williams et al, 1993) have shown that antimicrobial prophylaxis is effective in preventing recurrent acute otitis media. Amoxicillin (20 mg/kg/day at bedtime) has been recommended, and sulfisoxazole (50 mg/kg/day at bedtime) should be used if the child is allergic to penicillin/amoxicillin. The incidence of side effects from amoxicillin has been low and there has not been any change in the resistance of upper respiratory tract flora (Casselbrant et al, 1992). The prophylactic regimen should be continued through the respiratory season and discontinued when the weather becomes warm. The children should be examined at regular intervals (2 to 3 months) for the development of asymptomatic middle ear effusion. If longstanding middle ear effusion develops, tympanostomy tube insertion should be considered.

Some children do not experience any relief from the prophylactic regimen, but continue to have episodes of acute otitis media. For children who are prophylactic failures and children with recurrent episodes of acute otitis media and persistent middle ear effusion between the acute episodes, tympanostomy tube insertion should be considered, as it has been shown to be effective in preventing episodes of recurrent acute otitis media (Gonzalez et al, 1986; Casselbrant et al, 1992).

Immunization against the most common organisms causing acute otitis media would be the best way to prevent otitis media. The currently available *S. pneumoniae* polysaccharide vaccine is poorly immunogenic in young children, which is the age group of children with the highest incidence of otitis media. A conjugate heptavalent *S. pneumoniae* vaccine, developed on the same principles as PedWax-HIB (*H. Influenzae* type b), is being evaluated at the present time. Also, work is in progress to develop a vaccine for nontypable *H. influenzae*, one of the major bacterial isolates in otitis media.

Otitis Media with Effusion

Treatment for this condition should be considered because of the possible impact on hearing, language, speech, and cognition. As part of the treatment plan, the child should be examined for underlying factors that may predispose to otitis media, such as respiratory allergy, immune defects, hypertrophic adenoids, and sinusitis. Treatment of these condition may improve the ear disease.

Antihistamine and decongestant preparations have been shown to be ineffective in resolving the middle ear effusion compared to placebo (Cantekin et al, 1983; Mandel et al, 1987). On the other hand, several studies, including a meta-analysis, have demonstrated some effect of systemic steroids compared to placebo in resolving the middle ear effusions (Berman et al, 1990; Persico et al, 1978; Rosenfeld et al, 1991).

As bacteria have been isolated in about one third of ears with asymptomatic middle ear effusion (see Fig. 29–1), a trial of an antimicrobial agent should be considered in a child who has not previously received such treatment, or before surgery is considered. Several studies, including a meta-analysis, have shown that antimicrobial treatment increases to some extent the likelihood of resolution (Mandel et al, 1987; Thomsen et al, 1989; Rosenfeld and Post, 1992). However, a broad-spectrum antimicrobial agent has no more favorable effect than amoxicillin in resolving the middle ear effusion (Chan et al, 1988; Mandel et al, 1991).

In children with persistent middle ear effusion, tympanostomy tube insertion has been shown to be effective (Mandel et al, 1992). Tympanostomy tube insertion is usually recommended if the fluid has persisted for 3 months or longer. Adenoidectomy with and without tympanostomy tubes has also been shown to be effective (Gates et al, 1987; Paradise et al, 1990; Maw and Bawden, 1993). Guidelines on the treatment of otitis media with effusion in children 1 to 3 years of age have recently been published (Stool and Berg, 1994).

The diagnosis of unilateral middle ear effusion in an older child or adult should make the physician suspicious of a tumor in the nasopharynx.

Complications

Complications and sequelae of otitis media can be divided into those that are intracranial and those that are intratemporal. Intracranial complications, such as meningitis or epidural, subdural, and brain abscesses, are uncommon today. Prior to the introduction of antimicrobial therapy for acute otitis media, intracranial complications were common, often resulting in severe neurologic sequelae and death (Sorenson, 1977). Intratemporal complications occur within the aural cavity and adjacent structures and are more common.

Fluctuating and persistent hearing loss is the most prevalent intratemporal complication. In most cases the hearing loss is conductive owing to the effusion in the middle ear. Sensorineural hearing loss may result from acute otitis media and is then presumed to be due to spread of the infection through the oval or round window. The sensorineural hearing loss is usually permanent, whereas the conductive hearing usually returns to normal when the fluid has resolved.

The conductive hearing loss ranges from 15 to 30 dB (Fria et al, 1985). The decreased perception of sound may cause impaired development of speech and language and learning disabilities and thus may have significant developmental consequences (Teele et al, 1984; Menyuk, 1986; Feagans et al, 1987; Teele et al, 1990). Moreover, recent studies have shown that fluid in the middle ear may affect balance (Casselbrant et al, 1983; Jones et al, 1990). This may affect motor development and may also cause the child to be more accident-prone.

A persistent perforation of the tympanic membrane may be secondary to an episode of acute otitis media or can persist after tympanostomy tubes have extruded. A large perforation may interfere with hearing. Also, an opening in the tympanic membrane (perforation or tube) may allow water to enter the middle ear during bathing and swimming, and this could cause infection with discharge from the ear.

Tympanosclerosis (calcium deposition) of the tympanic membrane is seen in children with a history of otitis media or tympanostomy tube placement. It appears as white plaques on the tympanic membrane and, if large, may cause a mild conductive hearing loss.

A cholesteatoma is an accumulation of desquamated epithelium or keratin. It may be congenital or acquired. The acquired type is commonly caused by middle ear disease, but can also be iatrogenic (following tympanostomy tube placement or other procedures). Congenital cholesteatomas are found behind an intact tympanic membrane and are not sequelae of otitis media. Cholesteatomas can enlarge and erode the bone, including the ossicular chain, causing hearing loss. They can also become infected, leading to a foul-smelling discharge from the ear. A cholesteatoma needs to be removed surgically. The recurrence rate is high, a fact that necessitates long-term follow-up.

In most instances of acute otitis media, the mastoid air cell system is involved. If treatment is not given, the infection can spread, causing acute mastoiditis with periosteitis. Clinically, the child experiences otalgia and fever, and postauricular erythema, tenderness, and swelling are noted. The pinna may be displaced with loss of the postauricular crease. Mastoiditis with periosteitis may be treated with parenteral antimicrobial therapy and myringotomy or tympanostomy tube insertion. However, if there is no improvement in 24 to 48 hours, or a coalescent mastoiditis with or without a subperiosteal abscess has developed, surgical drainage must be performed (complete mastoidectomy) to avoid further spread and complications (Bluestone and Stool, 1990).

Facial nerve paralysis or paresis may occur during an episode of acute otitis media owing to congenital bony dehiscence of the facial nerve. Treatment consists of parenteral antimicrobial therapy and drainage of the ear by myringotomy with or without tympanostomy tube insertion to decompress the middle ear.

Meningitis is the most common of the intracranial complications. The infection can spread to the meninges either directly through preformed passages or through blood. The symptoms are headache, fever, neck stiffness, and altered consciousness. The most common bacteria involved are *S. pneumoniae* and *H. influenzae* type b. Management consists of parenteral antimicrobial therapy and drainage of the middle ear. Other intracranial complications are epidural abscess, subdural empyema, and brain abscess. All of these are uncommon and require immediate attention by an otolaryngologist and a neurosurgeon.

Tumors of the Middle Ear and Mastoid

The middle ear, mastoid, and temporal bone may be affected by tumors primarily, metastatically, or by extension. The most common primary benign tumors are glomus jugulare tumors, acoustic neurinomas, meningiomas, and osteomas. Primary malignant tumors are squamous carcinoma, adenocarcinoma, and sarcomas. Tumors that may metastasize to the middle ear, mastoid, and temporal bone include adenocarcinoma of the prostate, mammary carcinoma, hypernephroma, and renal carcinoma. Systemic diseases such as leukemia, myeloma, and lymphoma may also invade the temporal bone. Tumors from adjacent structures, such as meningioma, glioma, cylindroma of the parotid gland, epidermoid carcinoma, and melanoma of the skin of the external ear canal or auricle, may invade the middle ear, mastoid, and temporal bone.

The most common symptoms are tinnitus, conductive or sensorineural hearing loss, dizziness, facial nerve paralysis, and, if the tumor extends into the skull base, other cranial nerve abnormalities. The type and degree of symptoms depend on the degree of extension of the tumor and the structures involved. The treatment is surgery, radiation chemotherapy, or a combination, depending on the type and extension of the tumor.

Otosclerosis

Otosclerosis is a disease of the otic capsule (bony labyrinth) and the ossicles, manifested by localized areas of abnormal bone. The etiology is not clear but several factors have been suggested such as hereditary, endocrine, metabolic, and vascular factors. The most classic symptom is conductive hearing loss due to otosclerotic changes in the oval window causing fixation of the stapes. The most common area of involvement is in front of the oval window. Tinnitus occurs frequently and can be a disturbing symptom in some patients. Sensorineural hearing loss can also occur, but the mechanism is not clear. Some patients may also complain about vestibular disturbance. Clinical otosclerosis is more frequent between the ages of 20 and 30 years. It is more common in women and in Caucasians.

Today, stapedectomy is the treatment of choice for the conductive component of otosclerosis. Medical treatment with sodium fluoride is recommended for patients who are poor surgical candidates owing to age, pure sensorineural hearing loss, degree of hearing loss, poor speech discrimination, or other medical problems. Sometimes this treatment is used prophylactically after surgery.

INNER EAR

Meniere's Disease

Meniere's disease is characterized by the classic triad of symptoms: episodic vertigo, fluctuating flat or low-frequency sensorineural hearing loss, and tinnitus. The patient often complains about a feeling of fullness in the affected ear. Symptoms may occur suddenly, and vertigo may be severe. Hearing usually returns to normal between the attacks in the early course of the disease, but later the hearing loss may be permanent. The disease is more common in adults but is not unlikely to occur in children 10 years or older. The etiology of Meniere's disease is endolymphatic hydrops, or distention of the endolymphatic space, which is probably due to inadequate absorption of endolymph by the endolymphatic sac.

Medical therapy consists of diuretics, salt restriction, and elimination of stress. The surgical therapy varies with the severity of the disease and the degree of hearing loss. The endolymphatic shunt operation is the most common procedure. If the hearing is poor on the affected ear and the vertigo severe, more invasive procedures may be performed.

Perilymphatic Fistula

Perilymphatic fistula is a spontaneous leakage of fluid from the perilymphatic space of the inner ear into the middle ear. Perilymphatic fistulas may occur spontaneously through a congenital weakness or defect in the temporal bone, or following head trauma with or without a fracture of the temporal bone, or from barotrauma. There are no symptoms pathognomonic of a fistula, but the following features of the history are suggestive: head injury, physical strain or stress; exposure to sudden alterations in environmental pressure (flying or diving), or sudden alterations in middle ear pressure (violent sneezing, or laughing); a sensorineural hearing loss that fluctuates, is progressive, or both; sudden hearing loss; vertigo that increases with postural changes; or a sensation of a "pop" in the ear. The diagnosis of a perilymphatic fistula may be difficult, as a noninvasive, specific test to identify the fistula is not available. An abnormality of the temporal bone such as a Mondini malformation on CT scan has been shown to be a highly reliable clue in the detection of a fistula on exploration of the ear (Supance and Bluestone, 1983).

Recently, testing of the fluid in the middle ear for beta-2-transferrin at the time of exploration has shown high sensitivity and specificity (Weber et al, 1994). The final diagnosis and treatment of perilymphatic fistulas consist of exploration of the middle ear and repair of the fistula by packing with a muscle or fascia graft.

Sudden Deafness

Sudden deafness may be defined as a sensorineural hearing loss that develops over a period of hours or a few days. It is usually unilateral but can involve both ears. The severity of the disease may vary from mild to total loss of hearing. The hearing loss may be permanent or return spontaneously to normal or near-normal. Approximately one third of patients recover completely, and one third have no recovery. An initial total loss of hearing, which is associated with severe vertigo, has a poor prognosis.

The etiology of sudden hearing loss is multifactorial: viral infections (measles, mumps, influenza, and adenovirus); acoustic neurinoma; noise; pressure changes causing breaks in Reissner's membrane or a perilymphatic fistula in the round or oval window; vascular causes (vasospasm, thrombosis, embolism, hemorrhage into the inner ear, hypercoagulation); and autoimmunity. The diagnostic work-up is complex and includes comprehensive audiologic assessment, vestibular testing, imaging of temporal bone, lumbar puncture, and laboratory tests (FTA-Abs, fasting blood glucose, total protein and albumin-globulin ratio, cholesterol and lipids, and coagulation studies).

Owing to the multitude of etiologic agents, difficulties in making a definitive diagnosis, and the high spontaneous recovery rate, there is no specific treatment available for sudden hearing loss. The treatment currently recommended includes vasodilation, anticoagulation, reduction of viscosity of the blood, vitamins, sedation, tranquilization, bed rest, and the surgical repair of the oval or round window fistulas.

Labyrinthitis

The diagnosis of labyrinthitis is often used to cover a wide range of balance disturbances. Serous or toxic labyrinthitis is a sterile inflammation of the inner ear, caused by irritation of the labyrinth by bacterial toxins or other biochemical substances from an infection in the middle ear. The symptoms consist of mild-to-moderate vertigo, with nystagmus toward the affected side and some degree of hearing loss. The treatment consists of antimicrobial therapy of the underlying cause.

Bacterial or suppurative labyrinthitis indicates a destructive process secondary to a fulminant bacterial invasion from an infection of the middle ear, such as an acute otitis media, suppurative otitis media, or meningitis. The port of entry of the infection may be through a congenital defect in the temporal bone or a defect caused by a fracture or a cholesteatoma. The patient is violently ill with severe vertigo, nystagmus toward the unaffected side, nausea and vomiting, and hearing loss. Labyrinthine infections may also be caused by viral agents such as measles, mumps, influenza, or adenovirus. The symptoms are less pronounced, but deafness may persist.

Treatment consists of maintaining fluid and electrolyte balance, and suppressing the vestibular symptoms. In suppurative labyrinthitis, the addition of appropriate antimicrobial therapy and surgery to create adequate drainage is necessary to resolve the infection and prevent intracranial complications.

Benign Paroxysmal Positional Vertigo

Benign paroxysmal positional vertigo is one of the more common vertiginous disorders. It can follow head trauma or accompany other vestibular disorders, such as endolymphatic hydrops or the post-stapedectomy condition. However, a clear etiology is usually not identifiable. Temporal bone studies have implicated degeneration of the utricle as a potential mechanism (Schuknecht, 1974). The diagnosis is usually based on the history, consisting of brief attacks of positional vertigo without any auditory symptoms. On physical examination, vertigo and nystagmus are elicited by change in head position (Hallpike maneuver). There is a short period of latency before the nystagmus appears, and the episode usually lasts less than a minute. The condition usually resolves spontaneously, and treatment consists of reassurance and explanation of the symptoms to the patient. Physical therapy has been helpful to many patients. Vestibular suppressants should be used as little as possible and only as adjunctive therapy.

REFERENCES

Abramson JS, Giebink GS, Quie PG. Influenza A virus induced polymorphonuclear leucocyte dysfunction in the pathogenesis of experimental pneumococcal otitis media. Infect Immun 36:289–296, 1982.

American National Standards Institute. American national standard specifications for instruments to measure aural acoustic impedance and admittance (aural acoustic immittance). New York, ANSI S3.39, 1987.

Berman S, Grose K, Nuss R, Huber-Navin C, Roark R, Gabbard SA, Bagnall T. Management of chronic middle ear effusion with prednisone combined with trimethoprim-sulfamethoxazole. Pediatr Infect Dis J 9:533–538, 1990.

Bernstein JM, Schatz M, Zeiger R. Immunologic ear disease in adults. Clin Rev Allergy 2:349–375, 1984.

Bluestone CD, Klein JO. Otitis Media in Infants and Children, 2nd ed. Philadelphia, WB Saunders, 1995.

Bluestone CD, Stool SE (eds). Pediatric Otolaryngology. 2nd ed. Philadelphia, WB Saunders, 1990.

Bluestone CD, Stephenson JS, Martin LM. Ten-year review of otitis media pathogens. Pediatr Infect Dis J 11:S7–S11, 1992.

Buckley RH. Immunodeficiency. J Allergy Clin Immunol 72:627–644, 1983.

Buchman CA, Doyle WJ, Skoner D, Fireman P, Gwaltney JM. Otologic manifestations of experimental rhinovirus infection. Laryngoscope 104:1295–1299, 1994.

Buchman CA, Doyle WJ, Skoner DP, Post JC, Alper CM, Seroky JT, Anderson K, Preston RA, Hayden F, Fireman P, Ehrlich GD. Brief report: Influenza A virus-induced acute otitis media. Submitted, J Infect Dis, 1995.

Cantekin EI, Mandel EM, Bluestone CD, Rockette HE, Paradise JL, Stool SE, Fria TJ, Rogers KD. Lack of efficacy of a decongestant-antihistamine combination for otitis media with effusion ("secretory" otitis media) in children. N Engl J Med 308:297–301, 1983.

Casselbrant ML, Black FO, Nashner L, Panion R. Vestibular function assessment in children with otitis media. Ann Otol Rhinol Laryngol 107:46–47, 1983.

Casselbrant ML, Brostoff LM, Cantekin EI. Otitis media with effusion in preschool children. Laryngoscope 95:428–436, 1985.

Casselbrant ML, Brostoff LM, Cantekin EI, et al. Otitis media in children in the United States. In Sade J (ed). Proceedings of the International Conference on Acute and Secretory Otitis Media. Amsterdam, Kugler Publications, 1986; pp 161–164.

Casselbrant ML, Cantekin EI, Derkmaat DC, Doyle WJ, Bluestone CD. Experimental paralysis of tensor veli palatini muscle. Acta Otolaryngol (Stockh) 106:178–185, 1988.

Casselbrant ML, Kaleida PH, Rockette HE, Paradise JL, Bluestone CD, Kurs-Lasky M, Nozza RJ, Wald ER. Efficacy of antimicrobial prophylaxis and of tympanostomy tube insertion for prevention of recurrent acute otitis media: Results of a randomized clinical trial. Pediatr Infect Dis J 11:278–286, 1992.

Celin SE, Bluestone CD, Stephenson J, Yilmaz HM, Collins JJ. Bacteriology of acute otitis media in adults. JAMA 266:2249–2252, 1991.

Chan KH, Mandel EM, Rockette HE, Bluestone CD, Bass LW, Blatter MM, Breck JM, Reisinger KS, Wolfson JH, Wucher FP, Fall P, Kim H. A comparative study of amoxicillin-clavulanate and amoxicillin (treatment of otitis media with effusion). Arch Otolaryngol Head Neck Surg 114:142–146, 1988.

Doyle WJ. Functional eustachian tube obstruction and otitis media in a primate model. Acta Otolaryngol 414:52–57, 1984.

Doyle WJ, Boehm S, Skoner DP. Physiologic responses to intranasal dose-response challenges with histamine, methacholine, bradykinin and prostaglandin in adult volunteers with and without nasal allergy. J Allergy Clin Immunol 86:924–935, 1990.

Doyle WJ, Skoner DP, Fireman P, Seroky JT, Green I, Ruben F, Kardatzke DR, Gwaltney JM. Rhinovirus 39 infection in allergic and non-allergic subjects. J Allergy Clin Immunol 89:968–978, 1992.

Doyle WJ, Skoner DP, Hayden F, Buchman CA, Seroky JT, Fireman P. Nasal and otologic effects of experimental influenza A virus infection. Ann Otol Rhinol Laryngol 103:59–69, 1994.

Feagans L, Sanyal M, Henderson F, Collier A, Appelbaum M. Relationship of middle ear disease in early childhood to later narrative and attention skills. J Pediatr Psych 12:581–594, 1987.

Ford KL, Mason EO, Kaplan SL, Lamberth LB, Tillman J. Factors associated with middle ear isolates of *Streptococcus pneumoniae* resistant to penicillin in a children's hospital. J Pediatr 119:941–944, 1991.

Fria TH, Cantekin EI, Eichler JA. Hearing acuity of children with otitis media with effusion. Arch Otolaryngol 111:10–16, 1985.

Friedman RA, Doyle WJ, Casselbrant ML, et al. Immunologic-mediated eustachian tube obstruction: A double-blind cross-over study. J Allergy Clin Immunol 71:442–447, 1983.

Gates GA, Avery CA, Prihoda TJ, Cooper JC. Effectiveness of adenoidectomy and tympanostomy tubes in the treatment of chronic otitis media with effusion. N Engl J Med 317:1444–1451, 1987.

Gentile D, Skoner D, Whiteside T, Herberman R, Wilson J, Doyle W, Fireman P. Effect of influenza A virus (FLU) infection on lymphocyte phenotype and function. J Allergy Clin Immunol 93:203, 1994.

Giebink GS. Otitis media update: Pathogenesis and treatment. Ann Otol Rhinol Laryngol 101:21–23, 1992.

Gonzalez C, Arnold JE, Woody EA, Erhardt JB, Pratt RS, et al. Prevention of recurrent acute otitis media: chemoprophylaxis versus tympanostomy tubes. Laryngoscope. 96:1330–1334, 1986.

Green SM, Rothrock SG. Single-dose intramuscular ceftriaxone for acute otitis media in children. Pediatrics 91:23–30, 1993.

Haddad J, Brager R, Bluestone CD. Infections of the ears, nose and throat in children with primary immunodeficiencies. Arch Otolaryngol 118(2):138–141, 1992.

Howie VM, Ploussard JH. Efficacy of fixed combination antibiotics versus separate components in otitis media. Clin Pediatr 11:205–211, 1972.

Igarashi Y, Skoner DP, Doyle WJ, White MV, Fireman P, Kaliner MA. Analysis of nasal secretions during experimental rhinovirus upper respiratory infections (URI). J Allergy Clin Immunol 92:722–731, 1993.

Jackson MA, Shelton S, Nelson JD, McCracken GH. Relatively penicillin-resistant pneumococcal infections in pediatric patients. Pediatr Infect Dis 3:129–184, 1984.

Jones NS, Radomskij P, Prichard AJN, Snashall SE. Imbalance and chronic secretory otitis media in children. Effect of myringotomy and insertion of ventilation tubes on body sway. Ann Otol Rhinol Laryngol 99:477–481, 1990.

Kaleida PH, Casselbrant ML, Rockette HE, Paradise JL, Bluestone CD, Blatter MM, Reisinger KS, Wald ER, Supance JS. Amoxicillin or myringotomy or both for acute otitis media: Results of a randomized clinical trial. Pediatrics 87:466–474, 1991.

Lonsbury-Martin BL, Martin GK, McCoy MJ, Whitehead ML. Otoacoustic emissions testing in young children: Middle-ear influences. Am J Otology 15:13–20, 1994.

Mandel EM, Rockette HE, Bluestone CD, Paradise JL, Nozza RJ. Efficacy of amoxicillin with and without decongestant-antihistamine for otitis media with effusion in children. N Engl J Med 316:432–437, 1987.

Mandel EM, Rockette HE, Bluestone CD, Paradise JL, Nozza RJ. Efficacy of myringotomy with and without tympanostomy tubes for chronic otitis media with effusion. Pediatr Infect Dis J 11:270–277, 1992.

Mandel EM, Rockette HE, Paradise JL, Bluestone CD, Nozza RJ. Comparative efficacy of erythromycin-sulfisoxazole, cefaclor, amoxicillin or placebo for otitis media with effusion in children. Pediatr Infect Dis J 10:899–906, 1991.

Maw R, Bawden R. Spontaneous resolution of severe chronic glue ear in children and the effect of adenoidectomy, tonsillectomy, and insertion of ventilation tubes (grommets). Br Med J 306:756, 1993.

Maynard JE, Fleshman JK, Tschopp CF. Otitis media in Alaskan Eskimo children: Prospective evaluation of chemoprophylaxis. JAMA 219:597, 1972.

Menyuk P. Predicting speech and language problems with persistent otitis media. In Davanagh JF (ed). Otitis Media and Child Development. Parkton, York Press, 1986, pp 83–96.

Naclerio RM, Proud D, Sobotka AK, Lichtenstein LM, Hendley JO, Gwaltney JM. Is histamine responsible for the symptoms of rhinovirus colds? A look at the inflammatory mediators following infection. Pediatr Infect Dis J 7:215–242, 1988.

Nozza RJ, Bluestone CD, Kardatzke D, Bachman R. Identification of middle ear effusion by aural acoustic admittance and otoscopy. Ear Hear J 15(4):310–323, 1994.

Oppenheimer RP. Serous otitis: A review of 922 cases. Eye, Ear Nose Throat Month 54:37–40, 1975.

Paradise JL, Bluestone CD, Rogers KD, Taylor F, Colborn DK, Bachman RZ, Bernard BS, Schwarzbach RH. Efficacy of adenoidectomy for recurrent otitis media in children previously treated with tympanostomy-tube placement: Results of parallel randomized and nonrandomized trials. JAMA 263:2066–2073, 1990.

Paparella MM, Shumrick DA, Gluckman JL, Meyerhoff WL. Otolaryngology. 3rd ed. Philadelphia, WB Saunders, 1991.

Persico M, Podoshin L, Fradis M. Otitis media with effusion. A steroid and antibiotic trial before surgery. Ann Otol Rhinol Laryngol 87:191–196, 1978.

Rosenfeld RM, Mandel EM, Bluestone CD. Systemic steroids for otitis media with effusion in children. Arch Otolaryngol Head Neck Surg 117:984–989, 1991.

Rosenfeld RM, Post JC. Meta-analysis of antibiotics for the treatment of otitis media with effusion. Otolaryngol Head Neck Surg 106:378–386, 1992.

Rosenfeld RM, Vetrees JE, Carr J, Cipolle RJ, Uden DL, Giebink GS, Canafax DM. Clinical efficacy of antimicrobial drugs for acute otitis media: Metaanalysis of 5400 children from thirty-three randomized trials. J Pediatr 124:355–367, 1994.

Ruff ME, Schotik DA, Bass JW, et al. Antimicrobial drug suspensions: A blind comparison of taste of fourteen common pediatric drugs. Pediatr Infect Dis J 10:30–33, 1991.

Sade J. Secretory otitis media and its sequelae. In Monographs in Clinical Otolaryngology. Vol 1. New York, Churchill Livingstone, 1979.

Schuknecht HF. Pathology of the Ear. Cambridge, MA, Harvard University Press, 1974.

Skoner DP, Doyle WJ, Chamovitz A, Fireman P. Eustachian tube obstruction (ETO) after intranasal challenge with house dust mite. Arch Otolaryngol 112:840–842, 1986.

Skoner DP, Doyle WJ, Fireman P. Eustachian tube obstruction (ETO) after histamine nasal provocation. A double-blind dose response study. J Allergy Clin Immunol 79:27–31, 1987.

Skoner DP, Doyle WJ, Boehm S, Fireman P. Late-phase eustachian tube and nasal allergic responses associated with inflammatory mediator elaboration. Am J Rhinol 2:155–161, 1988a.

Skoner DP, Stillwagon PK, Casselbrandt ML, Tanner ET, Doyle WJ, Fireman P. Inflammatory mediators in chronic otitis media with effusion (OME). Arch Otolaryngol Head Neck Surg 114:1131–1133, 1988b.

Skoner DP, Lee L, Doyle WJ, Boehm S, Fireman P. Nasal physiology and inflammatory mediators during natural pollen exposure. Ann Allergy 65:206–210, 1990.

Skoner DP, Whiteside TL, Wilson JW, Doyle WJ, Herberman RB, Fireman P. Effect of rhinovirus 39 (RV-39) infection on cellular immune parameters in allergic and non-allergic subjects. J Allergy Clin Immunol 92:732–743, 1993.

Sorenson H. Antibiotics in suppurative otitis media. Otolaryngol Clin North Am 10:45–50, 1977.

Stool SE, Berg AO. Otitis media with effusion in young children. Clinical Practice Guideline Number 12, AHCPR Publication No. 94-0622, 1994.

Stool SE, Field MJ. The impact of otitis media. Pediatr Infect Dis 8:S11–S14, 1989.

Supance JS, Bluestone CD. Perilymph fistulas in infants and children. Otolaryngol Head Neck Surg 91:663–671, 1983.

Teele DW, Klein JO, Rossner BA. Greater Boston Otitis

Media Study Group: Otitis media with effusion during the first three years of life and the development of speech and language. Pediatrics 74:282–287, 1984.

Teele DW, Klein JO, Rosner B, et al. Epidemiology of otitis media during the first seven years of life in children in greater Boston: A prospective, cohort study. J Infect Dis 160:83–99, 1989.

Teele DW, Klein JO, Chanse C, et al. Otitis media in infancy and intellectual ability, school achievement, speech, and language at age 7 years. J Infect Dis 162:685–694, 1990.

Thomsen J, Sederberg-Olsen J, Balle V, Vejlsgaard R, Stangerup SE, Bondesson G. Antibiotic treatment of children with secretory otitis media. Arch Otolaryngol Head Neck Surg 155:447–451, 1989.

Walker SB, Shapiro GG, Bierman CW, Morgan MS, Marshall SG, Furukawa CT, Pierson WE. Induction of eustachian tube dysfunction with histamine nasal provocation. J Allergy Clin Immunol 76:158–162, 1985.

Weber PC, Kelly RH, Bluestone CD, Bassiouny M. β2-transferrin confirms perilymphatic fistula in children. Otolaryngol Head Neck Surg 110:381–386, 1994.

Williams RL, Chalmers TC, Stange KC, Chalmers FT, Bowlin SJ. Use of antibiotics in preventing recurrent acute otitis media and in treating otitis media with effusion. JAMA 270:1344–1351, 1993.

Chapter 30
Sinusitis

Jonathan Corren, M.D., Gary S. Rachelefsky, M.D.,
Gail G. Shapiro, M.D., and Raymond G. Slavin, M.D.

Sinus disease is being increasingly recognized as a common and important cause of morbidity in patients of all ages. Although great advances have been made in our understanding of this disorder, many questions still remain regarding the epidemiology, pathogenesis, and optimal treatment.

EPIDEMIOLOGY

Acute sinusitis has been estimated to complicate 5 to 10 percent of viral upper respiratory infections in early childhood (Wald et al, 1991). Chronic sinus disease is also frequently reported, and was noted to be the most common chronic disease among young adults and the third most common chronic condition among older patients in the United States (National Center for Health Statistics, 1990).

DEVELOPMENT, STRUCTURE, AND FUNCTION OF THE PARANASAL SINUSES

The paranasal sinuses form as invaginations of the mucous membranes of the nasal cavity and are lined by the same mucosa as the nose. The maxillary and ethmoid sinuses begin to develop *in utero*, are present at birth, and are radiographically evident in infancy. Frontal sinuses become recognizable by the sixth to twelfth month of life and appear radiographically between the third and seventh years. The sphenoid sinuses develop by the third year of life but do not appear radiographically until the ninth year. There is great variation in the shape and size of the sinuses at all ages, particularly the frontal sinuses.

The sinuses consist of four paired structures that surround the nasal cavities and drain via ostia located in the lateral walls of the nose (Fig. 30–1). The maxillary sinuses, located in the cheekbones of the face, are bordered below by the tooth-bearing areas of the maxilla and above by the orbit of the eye. The drainage pathway of the maxillary sinus exits from a point high in the maxillary antrum and follows a circuitous path before emptying into the middle meatus.

The ethmoid sinuses are a labyrinthine network of multiple (3 to 18) small air spaces that line the medial wall of the orbit and are in close proximity to the cranial cavity. The anterior and middle ethmoids drain into the

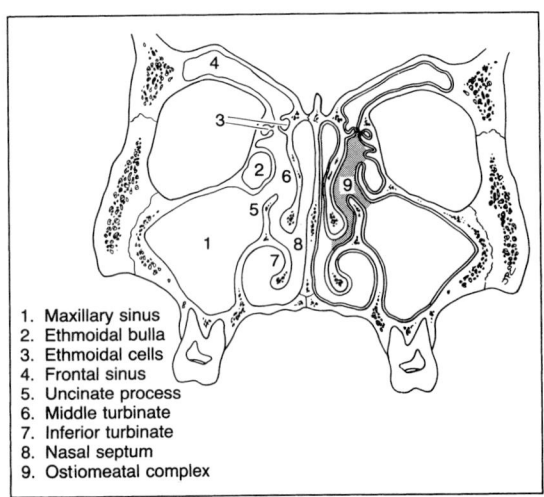

1. Maxillary sinus
2. Ethmoidal bulla
3. Ethmoidal cells
4. Frontal sinus
5. Uncinate process
6. Middle turbinate
7. Inferior turbinate
8. Nasal septum
9. Ostiomeatal complex

FIGURE 30–1. Coronal section of the nose and paranasal sinuses. The stippled area represents the ostiomeatal complex. (From Wald ER. Sinusitis in children. N Engl J Med 326:319, 1992.)

middle meatus, while the posterior ethmoids drain into the superior meatus. Drainage pathways of the maxillary and anterior ethmoid sinuses come together in a convoluted region between the middle and inferior turbinates, referred to as the ostiomeatal complex. This area is of particular importance, since even a mild degree of narrowing caused by chronic inflammation or retained secretions may result in sinus obstruction.

The frontal sinuses, which are located within the frontal bone of the skull, also drain into the middle meatus. The sphenoid sinuses, located further back in the skull beneath the pituitary, drain into the superior meatus. Isolated infection of these sinuses is unusual. However, they may become infected during an episode of pansinusitis and, importantly, may serve as foci for the spread of infection to the orbit or central nervous system.

The precise functions of the paranasal sinuses are not clear, however, some suggestions have included roles in olfaction, voice response, production of protective mucus, dampening of sudden pressure changes in the nose during respiration, and lessening of skull weight (Slavin, 1992).

PATHOGENESIS

Susceptibility to sinus infections is largely determined by four factors: patency of the ostia, ciliary function, quality of secretions, and local host immunity (Reilly, 1990).

Ostial patency appears to be the most important factor in the development of sinusitis. Obstruction of the ostium leads to the development of negative pressure within the sinus cavity, resulting in mucosal edema and serum transudation. Ostial obstruction also reduces gas exchange within the sinus, resulting in a lower Po_2. The combination of retained secretions and an anaerobic environment fosters rapid bacterial growth. The ensuing infection causes a further reduction in oxygen tension, elevation of Pco_2, and decrease in pH, all of which hinder ciliary movement and granulocyte function. If an acute episode of sinusitis (symptom duration less than one month) occurs, the sinus will usually return to normal following effective therapy. However, if therapy is incomplete or underlying etiologic factors are not treated, subacute (1 to 3 months) or chronic (greater than 3 months) sinusitis may develop. Persistent infection of the sinus mucosa may ultimately result in irreversible changes in sinus anatomy and physiology.

Causes of ostial obstruction can be divided into processes that result in direct mechanical obstruction and those that cause mucosal swelling (Table 30–1). Prominent causes of mechanical obstruction include nasal septal deviation, nasal polyps, and conchae bullosa. This latter condition is characterized by pneumatization and expansion of the middle nasal turbinate, which impinges on the middle meatus and obstructs the sinus ostia. Haller cells are aberrant ethmoid air cells that may also encroach on the ostiomeatal complex and hinder ostial drainage. Adenoid hypertrophy and/or adenoiditis probably play important adjunct roles in sinusitis in children. Although acute nasal swelling is most commonly caused by viral upper respiratory infections, persistent nasal swelling is more likely to be caused by chronic rhinitis, particularly allergic rhinitis. The role of nasal allergy in sinusitis is supported by studies showing a much higher incidence of atopy in children with sinusitis than in the general population (Shapiro et al, 1991).

Ciliary movement is critical in promoting normal drainage of the sinuses and protecting the sinuses against infection. Normal mucociliary function is particularly important to the maxillary sinuses, since the outflow tract of

TABLE 30–1. FACTORS PREDISPOSING TO SINUSITIS

Local Factors	Systemic Factors
Direct mechanical factors	Immune deficiency
Septal deviation	Cystic fibrosis
Nasal polyps	Ciliary dyskinesia
Conchae bullosa	Down's syndrome
Haller cells	Aspirin sensitivity
Enlarged adenoids	
Foreign bodies	
Choanal atresia	
Tumors	
Mucosal swelling	
Viral URI	
Chronic rhinitis (allergic and nonallergic)	
Other factors	
Trauma, barotrauma	
Dental infections	
Irritants (cigarette smoke, pollution)	
Swimming	

Modified from Shapiro GG, Virant FS. Medical management in children. Immunol Allergy Clin North Am 14:47–68, 1994.

this sinus sits high on the antral wall, making spontaneous drainage difficult. Viral infections, allergic rhinitis, and exposure to chemical irritants (such as tobacco smoke and air pollution) may result in a temporary reduction in ciliary activity. A rare cause of ciliary dysfunction is ciliary dyskinesia syndrome, a congenital group of disorders characterized by the permanent loss or derangement of the dynein arms or central core within ciliary microtubules. Patients with this syndrome invariably suffer from sinusitis, otitis, and bronchitis or bronchiectasis with or without situs inversus.

The secretory mucus blanket, consisting of deep and superficial layers, provides a medium for transporting microorganisms and particulate materials away from the nasal mucosa. Upper respiratory secretions also contain specific (e.g., immunoglobulins) and nonspecific (e.g., lactoferrin) proteins, which serve important antimicrobial functions. Viral infections and nasal allergy both result in transient abnormalities of mucus secretory activity. Patients with cystic fibrosis suffer from a permanent defect in the quality of mucus production, predisposing them to chronic infections of the upper and lower respiratory tracts.

Humoral immune mechanisms are also vital in protecting against sinus infections. Recurrent and chronic sinusitis caused by encapsulated bacteria is common in patients with humoral immune defects, including: congenital or acquired hypogammaglobulinemia, isolated IgA deficiency, and selective antibody deficiencies with or without IgG subclass deficiencies (Shapiro et al, 1991). Patients infected by HIV are also at increased risk for developing sinusitis caused by encapsulated bacteria and fungi.

MICROBIOLOGY

Although the majority of bacteriologic data have been generated by direct antral puncture of the maxillary sinuses, meaningful information has also been obtained from surgical specimens. Cultures taken directly from the nose are of limited value because of contamination by resident nasal flora.

Cultures from children with acute sinusitis have yielded predominantly aerobic bacteria, with *Streptococcus pneumoniae* accounting for 30 to 40 percent of isolates (Wald et al, 1981). *Haemophilus influenzae* and *Moraxella catarrhalis* each account for approximately 20 percent of cases and often produce beta-lactamase. Neither staphylococci nor anaerobic bacteria are commonly found in children. Respiratory viruses such as adenovirus and parainfluenzae have been cultured in less than 10 percent of cases, and the significance of these results is unclear. Pathogens identified most commonly in adults with acute sinusitis are *Streptococcus pneumoniae* and *Haemophilus influenzae*, accounting for at least 75 percent of bacterial isolates (Gwaltney et al, 1992). In some geographic regions, up to 50 percent of the *Haemophilus* species may be beta-lactamase producers. Anaerobic organisms are cultured much less commonly, with the exception of infections originating in the dental roots. As in children, respiratory viruses are cultured infrequently. Acute, hospital-acquired sinusitis is most often seen as a complication of nasogastric or nasotracheal tube placement and is typically caused by gram-negative organisms such as *Pseudomonas* and *Klebsiella*.

Bacterial isolates in children with subacute and chronic sinusitis are usually the same as those seen in acute disease. In children with more severe and protracted symptoms, however, anaerobes (such as *Bacteroides*) and staphylococci are cultured more frequently (Brook, 1981). Anaerobic organisms appear to predominate in adults with chronic sinusitis, with species of *Bacteroides* and anaerobic cocci accounting for nearly 90 percent of the isolates (Brook, 1989). Adult patients with chronic sinus disease may also develop acute exacerbations of infection, often involving the same bacterial species that cause acute sinusitis.

Fungi are a common cause of sinus disease in immunocompromised hosts, including diabetics and patients with defective cell-mediated immunity. Organisms such as *Aspergillus, Nocardia, Mucor,* and *Bipolaris* are also being increasingly identified as causes of sinusitis in patients who are otherwise healthy. Fungal sinusitis should be considered in all cases of sinusitis that has proved resistant to antibiotic therapy. Allergic fungal sinusitis is a syndrome that often occurs in young adults with asthma and has been attributed to *Aspergillus, Bipolaris, Curvularia, Helminthosporium,* and other fungal species. It is characterized by severe, hyperplastic sinusitis and associated with significant eosinophilia of sinus tissue and peripheral blood.

DIAGNOSIS

HISTORY. Acute sinusitis should be suspected if symptoms of a viral upper respiratory infection persist beyond the typical 7 to 10 days. Colored nasal discharge and cough are the most frequently reported symptoms in both children and adults, occurring in 70 to 90 percent of patients (Wald et al, 1981; Williams et al, 1992). Adults and older children often complain of headache and facial pain, which may radiate to the teeth and worsen with bending; these symptoms are unusual in children younger than age 10. Patients with subacute and chronic sinusitis generally present with indolent symptoms of nasal congestion, postnasal drip (ranging in color from mucoid to purulent), cough, facial fullness, and sore throat. If the middle ears are involved, there may also be complaints of popping or clicking in the ears and muffled hearing. Taste and smell are often reduced, and occasionally symptoms of chronic malaise and fatigue may predominate.

PHYSICAL EXAMINATION. Fever is documented in less than one-third of patients with acute sinusitis (Wald et al, 1981; Williams et al, 1992). Anterior rhinoscopy using a nasal speculum usually reveals red, swollen inferior turbinates. Although mucopus in the external nares or posterior pharynx is highly suggestive of sinusitis, its absence does not rule out infection since sinus drainage may be obstructed. Painless periorbital swelling may also be present, usually occurring early in the day. Physical findings in patients with subacute and chronic sinusitis are similar to those seen in patients with acute disease. Abnormalities predisposing to persistent or recurrent infections, such as septal deviation and nasal polyps, may also be seen. In children, middle ear effusions are often present and serve as clues to the presence of associated sinus disease.

Transillumination is an easy extension of the physical examination and can be carried out in patients older than age 10. The examination is performed in a darkened room using a special adapter attached to an otoscope handle. Transillumination of the maxillary sinuses is accomplished by placing the light over the middle of the inferior orbital rim and observing for transmission of light through the hard palate. The frontal sinuses are visualized by directing the light toward the medial border of the supraorbital ridge and assessing light transmission into the lower forehead. This technique is helpful in acute sinusitis if interpretation is confined to the extremes of transillumination, since absence of light transmission is strongly suggestive of infection, and normal transmission is good evidence that a sinus is normal (Evans et al, 1975). Transillumination is not helpful in chronic sinusitis, since many of these patients have intermediate levels of light transmission, which are unreliable in predicting whether a sinus is normal or diseased.

Flexible fiberoptic rhinoscopy is an office procedure that allows a detailed inspection of the upper nasal cavities and posterior nasopharynx and can be easily incorporated into the physical examination. It is particularly effective in visualizing the sinus drainage regions as well as lesions that may obstruct the sinus ostia, such as nasal polyps. This technique has been shown to be more sensitive than plain radiography in detecting chronic sinusitis (Castellanos and Axelrod, 1989).

LABORATORY TESTS. Nasal secretions can be easily obtained by having the patient blow into plastic wrap that is then applied to a glass slide or, alternatively, using a plastic curet or cotton-tipped applicator. The slide can be stained with Wright's or Hansel's stain to allow visualization of neutrophils, eosinophils, lymphocytes and epithelial cells. Significant neutrophilia (>5 neutrophils per high-power field) has been shown to be a sensitive but nonspecific predictor of radiographic sinus disease, whereas nasal eosinophilia (>5 to 10 percent of cells) is highly predictive of normal sinus roentgenograms (Gill and Neiburger, 1989). Nasal cytology is therefore helpful in confirming a clinical impression.

The peripheral white blood count and differential and the erythrocyte sedimentation rate are usually of no clinical value in differentiating sinusitis from other disorders. Cultures of the nasopharynx correlate poorly with cultures of antral taps and are rarely helpful.

IMAGING STUDIES. Until recently, plain films have been the principal modality in diagnosing sinusitis. Standard roentgenographic examination of the sinuses includes the following three views: the Waters (occipitomental), for visualizing the maxillary and frontal sinuses; the Caldwell (angled posteroanterior), for the frontal and ethmoid sinuses; and the lateral view, most useful for viewing the sphenoid sinuses and adenoids. Radiographic criteria indicative of acute maxillary sinusitis include the presence of air fluid levels, opacification, or mucosal thickening (greater than 50 percent opacification in children or 8 mm in adults) (Wald et al, 1981; Evans et al, 1975). Conventional films are most accurate for visualizing the maxillary and frontal sinuses but are insensitive for detecting abnormalities of the ethmoid or sphenoid sinuses or the ostiomeatal complexes. Despite its limitations, plain radiography continues to play an important diagnostic role in sinus disease, particularly acute sinusitis.

Computed tomography (CT) has become the gold standard of imaging of the paranasal sinuses and provides a detailed view of the anterior ethmoid air cells, the upper two thirds of the nasal cavity, and the ostiomeatal complex region—all of which are critical components in the pathogenesis of chronic sinusitis. CT can clarify important relationships and variations in the regional anatomy of the sinuses and provide a guide for endoscopic surgery. In some centers, a "screening" CT study (consisting of five to ten coronal or axial slices) can be obtained at the same cost as three plain film views. However, CT sinus imaging remains expensive and inaccessible for many physicians and, importantly, does require sedation for most children younger than 8 years of age. Recommendations for its use include: presurgical planning in patients who have failed medical therapy; confirmation of the diagnosis in patients with recurrent episodes of clinical sinusitis and negative plain films; and the evaluation of possible orbital extension of infection.

Magnetic resonance imaging (MRI) is extremely sensitive in detecting subtle soft-tissue abnormalities of the paranasal sinuses. For this reason, it is the technique of choice in imaging sinus neoplasms, fungal infections, and complicated infections that extend intracranially. MRI should not be used for routine diagnosis of sinusitis or for preoperative evaluation since it is very costly, requires long imaging times (necessitating sedation in children and some adults), and does not adequately display bony landmarks.

Although A-mode ultrasonography has been mentioned as a convenient radiation-free method, its value is equivocal. A study with adult patients showed >90 percent specificity for air-fluid levels or opacification, but it also showed low sensitivity (30 to 60 percent) for diagnosing maxillary or frontal sinusitis (Rohr et al, 1986). In a predominantly pediatric sample, both sensitivity and specificity were disappointing and approximated only 50 percent (Shapiro et al, 1986). It appears that ultrasonography is of limited value for diagnosing mucosal thickening, and neither the ethmoid nor sphenoid sinuses can be seen.

SINUS ASPIRATION. Indications for transnasal puncture and aspiration of the maxillary sinuses include acute sinusitis unresponsive to appropriate antibiotics, severe facial pain caused by complete ostial obstruction, or orbital or intracranial extension. Aspirates should be routinely cultured for aerobic bacteria (and if possible anaerobic organisms). Bacterial growth greater than 10^4 colony-forming units per milliliter is considered representative of true infection (Evans et al, 1975). Gram-stained secretions of the aspirate demonstrating at least one organism per high-power field correlates highly with bacterial counts of 10^5 colony-forming units per milliliter.

TREATMENT

Medical Treatment

The overall approach to the management of acute and chronic sinus disease is similar in both adults and children. Appropriate antimicrobial agents serve as the backbone of medical therapy. Adjunct therapies directed at removing secretions, reducing mucosal swelling, and improving mucociliary clearance are also important in ensuring resolution of the infectious and/or inflammatory processes.

The initial antibiotic of choice in treating acute sinusitis in both adults and children is amoxicillin or ampicillin taken for 10 to 20 days. The responsible organisms are generally sensitive, and adequate mucosal and sinus fluid concentrations of these drugs are achieved. In cases of penicillin sensitivity, trimethoprim-sulfamethoxazole may be used. Symptoms improve markedly with these antibiotics in 70 to 80 percent of patients within 2 to 3 days. If patients have not responded to the initial antibiotic within 72 hours, they should be given an alternative, beta-lactamase–resistant agent for 10 to 20 additional days. Amoxicillin-clavulanate (in children and adults), erythromycin-sulfisoxazole (in children) and cefuroxime axetil, loracarbef, and cefixime (in adults) have all proved to be effective in treating acute sinusitis. Although cefaclor has some degree of beta-lactamase resistance, in recent studies it has not proved to be any more effective than amoxicillin. Newer oral agents, including third-generation cephalosporins (cefprozil and cefpodoxime), modified erythromycins (clarithromycin), and quinolones (ciprofloxacin) appear to provide appropriate antimicrobial coverage but have not yet been formally studied in the treatment of acute sinusitis. In patients who have improved only partially after 10 days of therapy, the same antibiotic is extended for 7 to 10 additional days. Thorough eradication of residual infection theoretically reduces the possibility of developing chronic inflammatory changes. If recurrent symptoms develop 1 to 3 weeks after completion of antibiotic therapy, we assume that the original infection was incompletely treated and prescribe a different antibiotic for 21 additional days.

While there is little published data regarding antibiotic therapy for subacute or chronic sinusitis, we have found that many of our patients have failed to respond to prior repetitive courses of antibiotics given for 7 to 10 days. For this reason, a minimum of 21 days of amoxicillin or trimethoprim-sulfamethoxazole is prescribed. If the patient has not responded to this drug within 7 to 14 days, a beta-lactamase–resistant antibiotic is given for an additional 21 days. For patients with longstanding, recalcitrant disease, agents with increased anaerobic coverage such as clindamycin or metronidazole may be more effective.

Although there have been few controlled studies of ancillary therapy in treating sinusitis, several specific measures appear to be helpful in speeding resolution of symptoms and preventing recurrences in sinusitis-prone patients:

1. Removal of secretions. Steam inhalation (using a hot shower) and saline lavage effectively remove dried secretions that may block sinus ostia.

2. Reduction of swelling and inflammation. In patients with sinusitis and significant nasal obstruction, topical decongestants (oxymetolazine) given for 3 to 5 days and/or oral decongestants (pseudoephedrine or phenylpropanolamine) given for several days to weeks may be helpful in improving sinus drainage. In patients with nasal allergy or persistent sinusitis, topical nasal corticosteroids appear to play an important role in reducing nasal edema. Patients who have failed an initial course of antibiotic therapy or who suffer from concomitant nasal polyposis often appear to benefit from a 5- to 10-day tapering course of oral corticosteroids.

3. Improvement of mucociliary clearance. Mucolytic agents, such as guaifenesin, are usually given in combination with oral sympathomimetic agents and appear to thin mucus and enhance drainage in some patients.

Sinusitis should not be treated routinely with oral antihistamines, but patients with concomitant allergic rhinitis may benefit from their use. Patients with allergic nasal disease should also be counseled regarding appropriate environmental control measures and considered for possible allergy immunotherapy.

Immunologic Abnormalities and Sinusitis

Some patients with chronic sinusitis appear to have defective immunocompetence regarding the typical bacteria responsible for sinus infections. Patients who require almost continuous antibiotic therapy to avoid symptomatic disease may have structural abnormalities that require surgical intervention (see below) or may have humoral immune defects. Investigations of patients with particularly refractory sinusitis have shown low levels of immunoglobulins G and A, low levels of IgG subclasses, and poor responsiveness to polysaccharide antigens such as those presented by pneumococcal vaccine, as well as combinations of these problems (Shapiro et al, 1991).

Often these deficiencies are transient. Many patients can be managed with aggressive use of antibiotics including maintenance therapy with a prophylactic dose (one half the therapeutic dose) of an antimicrobial that appears to provide symptomatic benefit. Some recalcitrant patients have received intravenous gamma globulin therapy with benefit, but there are no controlled trials of this treatment.

Surgical Treatment

Sinusitis that persists or recurs frequently despite appropriate medical therapy may require surgical intervention. In some children with isolated maxillary sinus disease, antral lavage effectively evacuates purulent material and provides long-lasting symptom relief. In many children and most adults, however, the recently developed technique of functional endoscopic surgery has largely supplanted other surgical procedures. This method of intranasal surgery reestablishes ventilation and mucociliary clearance of the sinuses by removing chronically inflamed tissue and correcting anatomic defects in key areas, particularly the structures in and around the ostiomeatal complex. Endoscopic surgery usually results in minimal trauma to normal nasal and sinus structures and ultimately may allow nasal and sinus physiology to return to normal. Endoscopic surgery has resulted in success rates of approximately 80 percent in adults with chronic sinus disease (Mings et al, 1988), and a growing number of reports suggest that children can also be effectively and safely treated with this technique (Lusk and Muntz, 1990).

RELATIONSHIP BETWEEN SINUSITIS AND BRONCHIAL ASTHMA

Clinicians have noted for many years that sinusitis is often associated with bronchial asthma. Several series of patients have revealed that there is a high incidence of abnormal sinus radiographs (40 to 60 percent) in both adult and pediatric patients with reactive airways disease (Corren and Rachelefsky, 1994). Some investigators suggest that chronic sinusitis and asthma are manifestations of the same inflammatory disease process occurring in different parts of the respiratory tract. This viewpoint is supported by histologic studies revealing that sinus tissue from asthmatics is heavily infiltrated with eosinophils, closely resembling the pathologic picture of bronchial asthma (Harlin et al, 1988). However, multiple published observations document that patients with refractory asthma often improve when concurrent sinus disease is treated. Rachelefsky and co-workers (1984) studied 48 asthmatic children and found that 70 percent of the group were able to discontinue bronchodilators after appropriate treatment of their sinus disease. In a study of severe adult asthmatics, 60 percent of patients noted a marked improvement in their asthma symptoms following bilateral intranasal sphenoethmoidectomy for refractory sinusitis (Mings et al, 1988). Mounting experimental evidence suggests that inflammatory events in the nasal mucosa may cause alterations in airway caliber and/or bronchial responsiveness via reflex pathways.

Patients with difficult-to-control asthma should be carefully evaluated for sinus disease. It should be kept in mind that chronic sinusitis often is minimally symptomatic in asthmatics. Therefore, radiographic studies or nasal endoscopy should be appropriately utilized and sinusitis treated aggressively when it is identified.

Accurate diagnosis and appropriate treatment of sinusitis continue to be challenging tasks for all physicians. As our understanding of this complex disease improves, we hope to reduce the number of patients who develop chronic, disabling symptoms.

REFERENCES

Brook I. Bacteriologic features of chronic sinusitis in children. JAMA 246:967–969, 1981.
Brook I. Bacteriology of chronic maxillary sinusitis in adults. Ann Otol Rhinol Laryngol 98:426–428, 1989.
Castellanos J, Axelrod D. Flexible fiberoptic rhinoscopy in the diagnosis of sinusitis. J Allergy Clin Immunol 83:91–94, 1989.
Corren J, Rachelefsky GS. Interrelationship between sinusitis and bronchial asthma. Immunol Allergy Clin North Am 14:171–184. 1994.
Evans FO, Sydnor JB, Moore WEC, et al. Sinusitis of the maxillary antrum. N Engl J Med 293:735–739, 1975.
Gill FF, Neiburger JB. The role of nasal cytology in the diagnosis of chronic sinusitis. Am J Rhinol 3:13–15, 1989.
Gwaltney JM, Scheld WM, Sande MA, Syndor AS. The microbial etiology and antimicrobial therapy of adults with acute community-acquired sinusitis: A fifteen-year experience at the University of Virginia and review of other selected studies. J Allergy Clin Immunol 90(suppl):457–462, 1992.
Harlin SL, Ansel DG, Lane SR, et al. A clinical and pathologic study of chronic sinusitis: The role of the eosinophil. J Allergy Clin Immunol 81:867–875, 1988.
Lusk RP, Muntz HR. Endoscopic sinus surgery in children with chronic sinusitis: A pilot study. Laryngoscope 100:654–658, 1990.
Mings R, Friedman WH, Linford P, Slavin RG. Five-year follow-up of the effects of bilateral intranasal sphenoethmoidectomy in patients with sinusitis and asthma. Am J Rhinol 1:123–132, 1988.
National Center for Health Statistics. National Health Interview Survey, 1990.
Rachelefsky GS, Katz RM, Siegel SC. Chronic sinus dis-

ease with associated reactive airway disease in children. Pediatrics 73:526–529, 1984.

Reilly JS. The sinusitis cycle. Otolaryngol Head Neck Surg 103:856–862, 1990.

Rohr AS, Spector SL, Siegel SC, et al. Correlation between A-mode ultrasound and radiography in the diagnosis of maxillary sinusitis. J Allergy Clin Immunol 78:58–61, 1986.

Shapiro GG, Virant FS, Furukawa CT, et al. Immunologic defects in patients with refractory sinusitis. Pediatrics 87:311–316, 1991.

Shapiro GG, Furukawa CT, Pierson WE, et al. Blinded comparison of maxillary sinus radiography and ultrasound for diagnosis of sinusitis. J Allergy Clin Immunol 77:59–64, 1986.

Slavin RG. Nasal polyps and sinusitis. In Middleton E Jr, Reed CE, Ellis EF, et al (eds). Allergy: Principles and Practice. 4th ed. St. Louis, Mosby–Year Book, 1992, pp 1455–1470.

Wald ER, Milmore GJ, Bowen A, et al. Acute maxillary sinusitis in childhood. N Engl J Med 304:749–754, 1981.

Wald ER, Guerra N, Byers C. Upper respiratory tract infections in young children: Duration of and frequency of complications. Pediatrics 87:129–133, 1991.

Williams JW, Simel DI, Robers L, Samsa GP. Clinical evaluation for sinusitis: Making the diagnosis by history and physical examination. Ann Intern Med 117:705–710, 1992.

Chapter 31

Obstructive Diseases of the Larynx and Trachea

Elizabeth Rose, M.D., and Sylvan E. Stool, M.D.

Correct management of airway obstruction is possible only after a precise diagnosis has been made; the initial treatment depends on the degree of obstruction, the progression of the symptoms, and other associated problems. Nonlaryngeal and laryngeal causes of stridor are included in the differential diagnosis (Tables 31–1 and 31–2).

Compared with that of an adult, a child's larynx is relatively and absolutely of smaller diameter and is placed higher in the neck (Otherson, 1991; Bluestone and Stool, 1990). The cartilages are softer and therefore more compressible, and the submucosa is looser, allowing greater spread of edema. It is therefore possible for a foreign body in the esophagus to cause extrinsic obstruction of the trachea (Bluestone and Stool, 1990).

The site and cause of airway obstruction may be established from the history, physical examination, and appropriate radiologic examination, but in some situations there is severe respiratory distress with cyanosis and retractions, and an airway must be established immediately. If possible, a history is taken of previous intubations, laryngeal surgery, tobacco and alcohol use, and exposure to chemicals and radiation (Bailey, 1993; Becker et al, 1989). If the obstruction has been present since birth, a congenital lesion is most likely; a gradual, progressive course is typical of neoplasia; sudden onset is probably from inflammation or trauma, including foreign body aspiration.

CLINICAL ASSESSMENT

Management of airway obstruction depends on establishing an accurate diagnosis based on history, physical examination, and radiologic and endoscopic examination.

Symptoms and Signs

Symptoms associated with laryngeal obstruction are listed in Table 31–3. *Stridor* is the most common symptom and is produced by rapid, turbulent flow of air through a narrow segment of the respiratory tract. The pitch and phase of the stridor can be helpful in the localization of the lesion. With obstruction above the thoracic inlet it is inspiratory; in laryngomalacia it is low-pitched, and in bilateral vocal cord paralysis it is high-pitched. Subglottic narrowing can produce biphasic stridor and tracheomalacia involving the intrathoracic trachea produces expiratory stridor (Otherson, 1991; Bluestone and Stool, 1990).

The *cough* in subglottic narrowing has a barking sound. The *voice* or *cry* may be normal in bilateral vocal cord paralysis but weak in

TABLE 31–1. NONLARYNGEAL CAUSES OF STRIDOR

Nose and pharynx	Choanal atresia
	Tonsil and adenoid hypertrophy
Trachea	Congenital
	Vascular compression
	Webs and cysts
	Stenosis
	Inflammatory
	Tracheitis
	Trauma
	Foreign body—tracheal or esophageal
Chest	Diaphragmatic hernia
Abdomen	Large mass

TABLE 31–2. LARYNGEAL CAUSES OF STRIDOR

Congenital	Laryngomalacia (60%)
	Vocal cord paralysis (10%)
	Subglottic stenosis
	Vascular compression
	Webs and cysts
	Subglottic hemangioma
Inflammatory	Laryngotracheobronchitis
	Epiglottitis
	Angioneurotic edema
	Fungal infections
	Granulomas
	Tuberculosis
	Sarcoidosis
	Wegener's
Vocal cord paralysis	See Table 31–4
Neuromuscular	Myasthenia gravis
	Botulism
Muscles	Polymyositis
	Muscular dystrophy
Trauma	Internal
	Foreign body
	Intubation
	External
Neoplasia	Benign
	Hemangioma/lymphangioma
	Papillomas
	Chondromas
	Neurofibromas
	Malignant
	Squamous cell carcinoma (92%)
	Verrucous carcinoma
	Lymphoma

unilateral paralysis. *Feeding* is difficult if there is supraglottic obstruction but is often normal with glottic and subglottic pathology, unless there is severe respiratory compromise. In tracheoesophageal fistula, there may be complete airway obstruction when feeding is attempted. In infants with compression by a vascular ring there can be reflex apnea, with cyanosis on feeding.

On inspection, in severe obstruction there is tachycardia, tachypnea, cyanosis, flaring of the nasal alae, and retractions of the neck, intercostal spaces, and abdomen. A child with epiglottitis will sit forward with the neck extended and drool; one with acute laryngotracheobronchitis will lie down and be restless.

Palpation of the neck determines whether the larynx and trachea are in the midline and whether there is loss of prominences or subcutaneous emphysema in trauma. Masses such as a cystic hygroma or enlarged thyroid gland may also be found. In laryngeal cancer, regional lymph nodes may be involved.

Sequential auscultation over the nose, mouth, neck, and chest may localize the site of maximum stridor; this valuable method is frequently omitted but is highly cost-effective. The presence or absence of breath sounds on both sides of the chest should be noted, as should any adventitial sounds.

Altering the position of the patient may be useful; stridor is reduced when the patient is lying prone with the neck extended in conditions such as laryngomalacia, micrognathia, and innominate artery compression. In unilateral vocal cord paralysis, the airway is improved by positioning the patient on the affected side; this maneuver allows the cord to drop away and thus opens the glottis.

For cooperative patients, several methods of examination are available, but in cases of severe respiratory distress, the airway should not be further compromised. Dynamic assessment is made of the supraglottic cartilages for laryngomalacia and of the vocal cords for mobility, as well as for a structural lesion. The common examinations are: (1) *indirect laryngoscopy* using a mirror; (2) *flexible nasopharyngolaryngoscopy,* which is possible in uncooperative patients; (3) *rigid telescopic laryngoscopy,* which allows good resolution; and (4) *videolaryngoscopy* with simultaneous voice recording and videographic documentation.

Radiologic Examination

Radiologic examination may be valuable, but it should not precede the securing of an adequate airway.

Plain films of the neck demonstrate the steeple sign of narrowing of the glottis and subglottis in laryngotracheobronchitis; or the thumb sign of a swollen epiglottis on the lat-

TABLE 31–3. SYMPTOMS ASSOCIATED WITH LARYNGEAL OBSTRUCTION

Subglottis	Voice husky or normal
	Stridor biphasic
	Cough (barking)
	Feeding normal
Glottis	Voice hoarse or aphonia
	Stridor
	Inspiratory early
	Expiratory late
	No cough
	Feeding normal
Supraglottis	Voice muffled
	Stridor inspiratory
	No cough
	Feeding difficult

eral view in acute epiglottitis. There may be a radiopaque foreign body in either the airway or the esophagus, causing obstruction. High kV and coronal tomograms have been superseded by computerized axial tomography (CT).

The *chest roentgenogram* demonstrates cardiomegaly or abnormal pulmonary vasculature in congenital heart disease; it may show lobar emphysema or pneumonia from the presence of a foreign body. Inspiratory and expiratory films are obtained to demonstrate the air trapping on expiration from a foreign body.

Barium swallow may be diagnostic in vascular compression and may demonstrate an H-type tracheoesophageal fistula or gross gastroesophageal reflux.

Fluoroscopy may demonstrate a bronchial foreign body and shows abnormal movement of the supraglottic larynx in laryngomalacia.

Xeroradiography gives excellent delineation of soft tissues of the neck but involves high radiation levels.

CT scanning is used to evaluate laryngeal trauma, neck and mediastinal masses, and laryngeal tumors. In cases of trauma, examination of the cervical spine can be made at the same time. In laryngeal tumors, involvement of the cartilage framework and of lymph nodes may be demonstrated.

Magnetic resonance imaging is the investigation of choice in vascular compressions of the trachea as regional anatomy is demonstrated well. There is excellent soft tissue contrast in assessment of laryngeal tumors, and multiplanar images are possible.

Endoscopy

Advances in optical instruments have made endoscopic examination the standard for evaluation of airway obstruction. In children, a general anesthetic is often necessary, and cooperation with the anesthesia staff is obviously essential. Instruments of the appropriate size are used, and a careful, sequential inspection is made of the pharynx, larynx, trachea, bronchi, and esophagus. In infants with a congenital malformation of the larynx, more than one abnormality is found in up to 45 percent of cases, and in adults there may be more than one primary cancer of the upper aerodigestive tract.

Dynamic assessment is made for laryngomalacia, for vocal cord paralysis, and for pulsatile compression of the trachea by an abnormal vessel. If the vocal cords are immobile, the cricoarytenoid joint is tested for fixation.

Anatomic assessment includes an estimate of the caliber of the subglottis by the size of the bronchoscope that will readily pass through it as well as documentation of congenital abnormalities such as webs and cysts in children, or of tumors. Foreign bodies are removed, appropriate biopsies performed, and purulent secretions aspirated and sent for culture.

MANAGEMENT

When the airway and the diagnosis are established, a plan of management can be made.

Neonates

Laryngomalacia is a flaccidity of the supraglottic structures with collapse of the aryepiglottic folds and arytenoids into the airway on inspiration; severe obstruction is uncommon, and feeding and weight gain are normal. The clinical diagnosis should be confirmed on endoscopy as other lesions may also be present. This condition is usually self-limited by 2 years of age, with growth and maturing of the laryngeal cartilages. In severe cases, a tracheostomy may be required; surgery to remove redundant mucosa or an epiglottopexy may allow earlier decannulation (Otherson, 1991; Becker et al, 1989).

Tracheomalacia, like laryngomalacia, may be self-limited, but some cases require tracheostomy and positive-pressure ventilation to maintain the lumen. Cartilage grafts have been used to reinforce the tracheal cartilage and maintain the airway (Otherson, 1991; Bluestone and Stool, 1990).

Vocal cord paralysis is bilateral in 50 percent of cases, and 50 percent of these resolve spontaneously over the next few weeks to months. The most common cause is central nervous system disease such as hydrocephalus, meningomyelocele, and Arnold-Chiari malformation. Unilateral vocal cord paralysis is associated with birth injury, cardiac abnormalities, and other laryngeal malformations. Some are acquired as the result of injury to the vagus or recurrent laryngeal nerves during surgery for central nervous system and cardiac anomalies (Otherson, 1991; Bluestone and Stool, 1990; Blitzer et al, 1992).

Other *congenital abnormalities of the larynx and trachea* include agenesis, atresia, stenosis, webs, and cysts; anterior and posterior laryngeal clefts are less common. Benign tumors such as hemangiomas and lymphangiomas also occur.

Vascular anomalies causing airway obstruction are uncommon, although 3 percent of the population has some malformation of the great vessels in the mediastinum. The most symptomatic are the complete rings, which occur in double aortic arch and right aortic arch. Surgical treatment involves division of a complete ring, suspension of vascular slings from the sternum, or reimplantation of vessels into the aorta. Postoperatively there may be persistent tracheomalacia (Otherson, 1991).

Subglottic stenosis may be congenital, diagnosed in an infant with a subglottis that will not allow the passage of the 3.5 bronchoscope, and who has no history of trauma or intubation. The stenosis may be caused either by fibrous tissue and hyperplastic glands or by thick deformed cartilage (Otherson, 1991; Bluestone and Stool, 1990). Tracheostomy is required in 40 percent of cases, but many improve with the growth of the child, and decannulation is achieved by 3 years of age. Less severe subglottic stenosis may present in an older child with recurrent laryngotracheobronchitis. Acquired subglottic stenosis, which is usually more severe and more difficult to treat, occurs especially after long-term intubation and ventilation. The cricoid is the narrowest part of the neonatal airway, and ulceration of the mucosa may lead to destruction of the cricoid cartilage, with subsequent scarring and narrowing. Contributing factors to the development of subglottic stenosis include poor fixation of the tube, frequent reintubation, infection, and gastroesophageal reflux. The treatment for subglottic stenosis is evolving, and in addition to airway maintenance with a tracheostomy tube there are several surgical options. The purpose of the surgery is to allow decannulation and also to permit phonation. Endoscopic surgery and open surgery have been used, and for more severe stenoses, a laryngotracheal reconstruction is performed with augmentation of the lumen using an autologous cartilage graft (Otherson, 1991; Bluestone and Stool, 1990).

Subglottic hemangiomas present by 6 months of age, more commonly in females, characteristic symptoms being stridor and a harsh cry. The natural history is characterized by growth in the first 18 months, often requiring a tracheostomy, and then regression. Steroids have been used to reduce the size of the hemangioma, and if it has not resolved by 3 years of age, it is removed with laser surgery.

Recurrent respiratory papillomatosis rarely presents before 6 months of age. There is an association with the human papilloma virus types 6 and 11, which are also found in venereal condylomata. These children present with progressive hoarseness and stridor, and there is often a protracted course requiring multiple endoscopic procedures. Although usually in the larynx, they also extend into the trachea, bronchi, lung parenchyma, and esophagus. Rarely, they become malignant, especially in the irradiated larynx or if the patient starts to smoke. Many treatments have been used including the CO_2 laser, but long-term control is difficult to establish.

Older Children

In older children, upper airway obstruction is most commonly from inflammation and trauma; the etiology and management of vocal cord paralysis is similar to that in adults. Episodic laryngeal dysfunction is characterized by stridor caused by intermittent paradoxic motion of the vocal cords, with adduction on inspiration (Loginoff et al, 1990; Rogers, 1980; Christopher et al, 1983). The diagnosis is made from the typical findings on flexible fiberoptic laryngoscopy and from exclusion of a bronchospastic component because there is no improvement in the pulmonary function tests after inhaled bronchodilators. Speech therapy and psychotherapy are often helpful.

Inflammation

Epiglottitis is characterized by the rapid onset of severe illness with progressive dysphagia, dyspnea, drooling, and stridor; it is accompanied by septicemia with fever and other foci of infection. The organism is almost always *Haemophilus influenzae* in children, but other organisms such as *Streptococcus pneumoniae* and *beta hemolytic streptococcus* have also been cultured. The incidence has been reduced dramatically with the widespread use of the vaccine against *Haemophilus influenzae*. The peak age is 2 to 3 years, but it occurs in all ages. Management includes securing the airway in the operating room; in most centers a nasotracheal tube is left in place, although a tracheostomy is sometimes performed. After intubation, cultures are taken and intravenous therapy with a β-lactamase stable antibiotic is started.

Acute laryngotracheobronchitis (croup) nearly always occurs as part of an upper respiratory tract infection and presents as fever, barking cough, hoarseness, and biphasic stridor. It is most common between the ages of 6 months and 3 years, and especially in males. The usual viral isolate is *parainfluenza* types 1 and 2, but also *respiratory syncytial virus* and *adenovirus*. Treatment includes humidification and hydration; in more severe cases racemic epinephrine and dexamethasone are administered. Intubation or tracheostomy is required in only 5 percent of those children whose condition is severe enough to be admitted to the hospital and is indicated if there is fatigue, hypercarbia, and failure to respond to the medical measures.

Spasmodic croup is characterized by the sudden onset of cough and stridor in a child with no history of fever or of a preceding upper respiratory tract infection. It may be from gastroesophageal reflux or from an allergic diathesis. Antihistamines are not efficacious, but corticosteroids and racemic epinephrine are; the condition often resolves spontaneously or in response to warm humidification.

Tracheitis is a more severe form of croup, with thick purulent secretions in the trachea. The organisms cultured vary and include *Staphylococcus aureus, group A hemolytic streptococcus* and *Moraxella catarrhalis*; there is often a preceding viral infection, which predisposes to the bacterial invasion. Management of tracheitis includes an artificial airway, frequent suctioning, and intravenous antibiotics.

Trauma

Internal trauma may be the result of intubation, inhalation or thermal damage, caustic ingestion, or aspirated foreign body (Bluestone and Stool, 1990; Bailey, 1993). *External* trauma may result from blunt injuries, as in motor vehicle accidents, or from penetrating injuries. In young children the cartilages are deformable and so are unlikely to fracture; laryngotracheal disruption, however, is more common owing to the immature cartilaginous connections. There will generally be a history of trauma and there are varying degrees of respiratory distress with stridor, cough, hemoptysis, hoarseness, aphonia, dysphagia and drooling. Immediate management requires evaluation of other injuries—especially of the cervical spine, head, and chest—and measures to secure the airway in the operating room. Once this has been achieved, further investigation with endoscopy, CT scanning, and arteriography as needed may be performed (Otherson, 1991; Bluestone and Stool, 1990; Bailey, 1993; Wood et al, 1986).

Adults

In adults, *laryngeal trauma* is managed as for children. *Epiglottitis* may occur and may require intubation. The causes of *vocal cord paralysis* in adults differ from those in children (Table 31–4). However, the diagnostic and management decisions are similar. If the cause is not evident from the history, an organized work-up is necessary and includes a CT scan of the head, neck and chest, and a thyroid scan if there is any thyroid enlargement. Panendoscopy may also be indicated. In adults, unilateral cord paralysis does not cause obstruction, but in bilateral paralysis a tracheostomy is frequently required. If spontaneous recovery does not occur, surgery to lateralize one cord is possible to allow decan-

TABLE 31–4. CAUSES OF VOCAL CORD IMMOBILITY

Cerebral cortex and supranuclear	
Medulla	Motoneuron disease
	Arnold-Chiari malformation
	Brain stem stroke or tumor
	Syringomyelia
Laryngeal nerves	Inflammatory
	Tuberculosis
	Sarcoid
	Postviral
	Metabolic
	Diabetes
	Rheumatoid arthritis
	Drug toxicity
	Neoplastic
	Lung
	Thyroid
	Laryngeal
	Trauma
	Thyroid surgery
	Endotracheal intubation
	Idiopathic/unknown
Cricoarytenoid joint	
Fixation	Rheumatoid arthritis
Disarticulation	Trauma

nulation. The operations available include cordectomy, arytenoidectomy, or reinnervation procedures. Paradoxic vocal cord movement also occurs in adults, but may be in association with underlying asthma and emphysema, and so the diagnosis of pulmonary disease may then be difficult (Christopher et al, 1983; Wood et al, 1986; Ward et al, 1981). The abnormal movement is seen on laryngoscopy, and patients may benefit from speech therapy and laryngeal and neck relaxation techniques.

Laryngeal tumors are most commonly malignant in adults. Therapy depends on the histologic diagnosis and the extent of disease (staging), and may include surgery, radiotherapy, and chemotherapy (Bailey, 1993; Becker et al, 1989; Bailey and Biller, 1985).

Granulomatous diseases such as tuberculosis and Wegener's granuloma are complicated by fibrosis and laryngeal stenosis. Tracheostomy and reconstructive surgery, as for subglottic stenosis, may be required (Bailey, 1993; Bailey and Biller, 1985).

One of the roles of the otolaryngologist in the patient with airway obstruction is to aid in the diagnosis and management of conditions such as foreign bodies, anatomic abnormalities of the trachea and bronchi and vascular compressions, and paradoxic vocal cord movement, all of which may masquerade as asthma.

REFERENCES

Bailey BJ. Head and Neck Surgery—Otolaryngology. Philadelphia, JB Lippincott, 1993.

Bailey BJ, Biller HF. Surgery of the Larynx. Philadelphia, WB Saunders, 1985.

Becker W, Naumann HH, Pfaltz CR. Ear, Nose and Throat Diseases. New York, Thieme Medical Publishers, 1989.

Blitzer A, Brin MF, Sasaki CT, Fahn S, Harris KS. Neurological Disorders of the Larynx. New York, Thieme Medical Publishers, 1992.

Bluestone CD, Stool SE. Pediatric Otolaryngology. 2nd ed. Philadelphia, WB Saunders, 1990.

Christopher K, Wood R, Eckert C, Blager F, Raney R, Souhadra J. Vocal cord dysfunction presenting as asthma. N Engl J Med 308:1566–1570, 1983.

Loginoff MM, Lau KY, Weinstein DB, Chandra P. Episodic stridor in a child secondary to vocal cord dysfunction. Pediatr Pulmonol 9:46–48, 1990.

Otherson HB. The Pediatric Airway. Philadelphia, WB Saunders, 1991.

Rogers JH. Functional inspiratory stridor in children. J Laryngol Otol 94:669–670, 1980.

Ward P, Hanson D, Berci G. Observations on central neurologic etiology for laryngeal dysfunction. Ann Otol Rhinol Laryngol 90:430–431, 1981.

Wood RF, Jafek BW, Cherniack RM. Laryngeal dysfunction and pulmonary disorder. Otolaryngol Head Neck Surg 94:374–378, 1986.

Section Six
ASTHMA

Chapter 32
Etiology of Asthma: Pathology and Mediators

David J. Fraenkel, B.M., B.S., FRACP, and
Stephen T. Holgate, M.D., D.Sc., FRCP

The last decade has seen a series of major changes in our understanding of the pathology of asthma. The limitations of autopsy material, often from cases of fatal asthma, have been overcome by the widespread use of the fiberoptic bronchoscope for the biopsy and lavage of asthmatic airways. The application of this technology to groups of subjects with more moderate disease has firmly established inflammation as the basic pathology of asthma. The investigation of the dual phase response to allergen has provided important insights into the pathogenesis of the inflammatory response, with bronchoscopy providing a means for both challenging and sampling the airway.

Simultaneous developments in immunology and molecular biology have found their application in the study of the asthmatic airway. The more sophisticated analysis of inflammatory cells and their associated mediators has demonstrated that a broad range of cell types are important in asthma and that no single mediator is responsible for the bronchospasm and bronchial hyperresponsiveness that characterize the disease. The regulatory factors that control and coordinate this process are a major area of investigation with interdependent roles for cytokines, adhesion molecules, and neural mechanisms in the development of inflammation in the asthmatic airway.

INVESTIGATION OF PATHOLOGY AND MEDIATORS IN ASTHMA

Bronchial Mucosal Biopsy

The use of fiberoptic bronchoscopy in asthmatic subjects has revolutionized approaches to basic and clinical research, and has hastened the acceptance of the inflammatory model that has been developed over the last decade.

Early autopsy studies gave a histologic picture of the airways in asthma-associated deaths. This was typified by hypertrophy of smooth muscle and increased numbers of mucous glands and goblet cells. Inflammatory cell infiltrates in the submucosa were characteristically eosinophilic, and there was loss of epithelial tissue. The airway lumen was frequently occupied by mucus, cellular debris, and exuded plasma proteins (Dunill, 1960).

This early work did not provide any basis for distinguishing the morphology of the less catastrophic grades of asthma. The subsequent studies that used rigid bronchoscopy to obtain a biopsy from asthmatic airways tended to focus on the degree of epithelial disruption and the presence of "basement membrane thickening," rather than on the nature of the cellular infiltrate in the epithelium and submucosa. However, a recent study has combined the techniques of rigid bronchoscopy and an electron microscopic "montage" to carefully examine biopsies in patients with newly diagnosed asthma compared with a small control group (Laitinen et al, 1993). In the epithelium there were increased numbers of mast cells, eosinophils, lymphocytes, and macrophages. The submucosa contained increased numbers of eosinophils, lymphocytes, macrophages, and plasma cells.

Initial studies using fiberoptic bronchoscopy were of great importance in extending the range of patients studied to include those with mild and moderate asthma (Beasley et al, 1989). Quantitative measurements confirmed submucosal eosinophilic infiltration and were complemented by qualitative demonstrations of increased mast cell and eosinophil degranulation, vascular margination of leukocytes, and collagen deposition beneath the basement membrane. Features of mast cell activation demonstrated by electron microscopy included varying degrees of degranulation, rather than the normal "lattice and scroll" pattern of granule organization, and the presence of degranulation channels. Eosinophils often showed an inverted pattern of staining in which the normally darker core of the granules appeared lighter than the surrounding matrix, with a variable degree of granule heterogeneity. These findings were not uniformly reported in other studies, with some investigators reporting increased "irregular lymphocytes" in the lamina propria and submucosa, and others finding only increased numbers of mast cells in the same regions. Variations may have been due to patient selection and the use of electron microscopy for quantitative estimations of cell populations.

The application of specific monoclonal antibodies for immunohistochemistry has been a useful technique for the identification and quantification of cell types as well as subpopulations expressing activation and other surface markers. This has allowed a more definitive demonstration of increased eosinophil numbers in the epithelium and submucosa, and has identified an increase in the number of interleukin-2 receptor (IL-2R, CD25) positive cells in the submucosa (Djukanović et al, 1990b; Azzawi et al, 1990). Most of the $CD25^+$ cells were subsequently identified as T lymphocytes. An increased number of eosinophils ($EG2^+$ cells) was also demonstrated in atopic nonasthmatic subjects, although there remained a difference between these and atopic asthmatic subjects. A relationship between the cellular markers of inflammation and airway function was demonstrated by stratifying the subjects by their airway reactivity to methacholine and finding that this correlated with the numbers of $CD25^+$ and $EG2^+$ cells (Azzawi et al, 1990; Bradley et al, 1991). In addition there were positive correlations between the numbers of lymphocytes ($CD3^+$), eosinophils, and $CD25^+$ cells, providing circumstantial evidence for the interdependency of certain inflammatory cell types in asthma.

There has been one immunohistochemical study that also demonstrated increased numbers of macrophages in the mucosa, using a range of monoclonal antibodies that identified monocyte-like phenotypes among the infiltrating macrophages, suggesting a process of active recruitment of these cells from the circulation (Poston et al, 1992).

Examination of bronchial biopsies from nonatopic patients with intrinsic asthma has revealed a broad spectrum of changes. There was a marked increase in the total number of leukocytes identified, with the increases being partitioned between macrophages and $CD4^+$ lymphocytes. Both intrinsic and extrinsic asthmatics shared an increased number of eosinophils and $CD25^+$ cells. When both groups of asthmatics were combined, there was a loose correlation between eosinophil numbers and methacholine hyperresponsiveness or a clinical symptom score.

The same techniques have been used in the examination of airway histology before and after intervention with inhaled beclomethasone dipropionate. This has provided further corroboration of the previously reported increases in inflammatory cell numbers and demonstrated their reduction with a broad-spectrum anti-inflammatory agent. The number of mast cells and eosinophils in both epithelial and submucosal sites was reduced by 6 weeks of moderate-dose therapy, with a corresponding improvement in airway function. There was also a reduction in submucosal T cell numbers; however, there remained electron microscopic evidence of mast cell and eosinophil degranulation (Djukanović et al, 1992).

The immunohistochemical and quantitative techniques used in the recent biopsy studies have been so successful that these more rigorous standards are now being used to reevaluate the findings in autopsy material from asthma deaths (Fig. 32–1). This has reconfirmed the eosinophilic nature of the infiltrate and demonstrated a high degree of cellular activation, as well as a significant T lymphocyte infiltrate.

Early and Late Asthmatic Responses

Exposure to appropriate allergen in sensitized individuals produces an almost immediate episode of bronchoconstriction, often referred to as the early asthmatic response (EAR), which begins to decrease after about half an hour and is resolved within 1 to 2 hours. Approximately half of such individuals progress to develop a second phase of bronchoconstriction known as the late asthmatic response (LAR), beginning about 4 hours after the initial challenge and resolving in 8 to 12 hours. Both responses are of interest because of insights revealed by similarities and differences in their inflammatory pathogenesis. However, the late asthmatic response is accompanied by an increase in bronchial hyperresponsiveness that is thought to be a useful model of asthma *in vivo*.

Early Asthmatic Response

Traditionally the EAR is attributed to the rapid release of mediators provided by mast

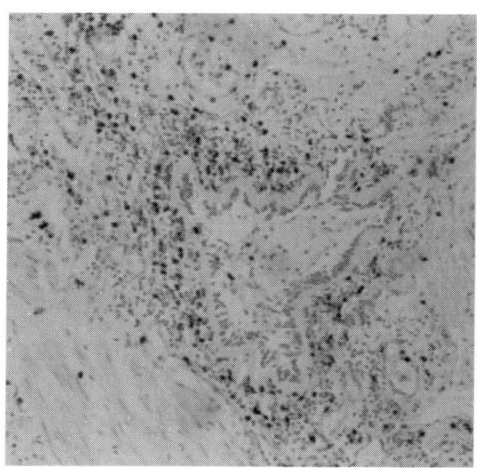

FIGURE 32–1. Eosinophilic inflammatory infiltrate in the airway wall and lumen, in an autopsy specimen from a subject with fatal asthma. Eosinophils are particularly numerous in the bronchial submucosa (EG2, immunoperoxidase, magnification ×100). (Courtesy Dr. M. Synek.)

cell activation and degranulation. Histamine and tryptase levels are elevated in the bronchoalveolar lavage (BAL) fluid of atopic asthmatics, and are increased still further within minutes of a localized endobronchial challenge (Wenzel et al, 1988). Large changes in the BAL fluid histamine content have been associated with greater methacholine sensitivity. In the peripheral blood the levels of histamine and the mast cell–derived serum high-molecular-weight neutrophil chemotactic activity (HMW-NCA) are elevated after inhalational challenge (Durham et al, 1984). Other studies using BAL soon after inhalational and local endoscopic challenge to produce an EAR have demonstrated increases in the lipid-derived mediators prostaglandin (PG)D_2, 9α11β-PGF$_2$, thromboxane, leukotriene (LT)C_4 and 15-hydroxyeicosatetraenoic acid (15-HETE), as well as kinins (Liu et al, 1991). The importance of these mediators is further emphasized by the ability of pharmacologic antagonists—such as antihistamines, leukotriene antagonists, and "mediator release inhibitors" like sodium cromoglycate and nedocromil sodium—to diminish the EAR.

However, there has been a failure to demonstrate any increase in BAL fluid cellularity in association with the EAR (Liu et al, 1991). This is perhaps not surprising if one considers the speed of the response and the presumed dominance at this stage of mediator release from cells resident in the epithelium and submucosa rather than an influx from the circulation. There have been some changes reported in BAL lymphocyte populations suggesting that subjects with only a single phase response have a decrease in BAL $CD4^+$ cells and an increase in $CD8^+$ cells, some 6 hours after challenge (Gonzalez et al, 1987). It has therefore been suggested that the $CD8^+$ cells may have had a regulatory role in preventing cytokine elaboration and inflammatory cell activation, and were therefore not as well represented in patients developing a late-phase response.

Late Asthmatic Response

The nature of the late asthmatic response has been partially characterized by the effect of pharmacologic intervention. Although albuterol and sodium cromoglycate, acting as "mast cell stabilizers," had a major effect on bronchoconstriction and mediator release during the EAR, the late response was better prevented by corticosteroids, and to a lesser extent by cromoglycate (Cockcroft and Murdock, 1987). This was early evidence for the involvement of a different range of cells and mediators in the LAR.

This has received further support from the analysis of BAL fluid during the late phase response, which usually contained increased numbers of eosinophils (Djukanović et al, 1990a). In some studies there have also been increased numbers of neutrophils and lymphocytes in response to both inhaled and endobronchial challenge, whereas no such changes were seen in subjects with an EAR only (Metzger et al, 1987; Liu et al, 1991). The presence of increased levels of eosinophil-derived major basic protein (MBP) and neurotoxin (EDN) was common to both responses, although an increase in LTC_4 was seen only in those in whom a LAR occurred. A decrease in mast cell numbers was noted and speculated to be due to continuing mast cell activation and degranulation in the bronchial tissue, as histamine levels remained elevated. Ultrastructural changes were consistent with mast cell and eosinophil activation with partial degranulation and loss of core granule material respectively. Macrophage activation was indicated by an increased number of complement rosettes, changes in cytoplasmic and membrane morphology, and occasional phagocytosed granules from eosinophils and mast cells.

In the peripheral blood the LAR has been associated with an early eosinopenia and a late eosinophilia. The magnitude of the eosinopenia correlated with the size of the LAR and the degree of hyperreactivity to histamine (Cookson et al, 1989).

The model of asthma provided by the LAR has led some investigators to develop similar physiologic and cellular pathologies in animals for more intensive study. The most successful and far reaching of these has been the adult male cynomolgus monkey exposed to inhaled *Ascaris suum* extract, as developed by Gundel, Wegner, and Letts (Wegner et al, 1990). They initially demonstrated that regular inhaled antigen produced hyperresponsiveness to methacholine with an associated increase in eosinophils in BAL fluid. Subsequent experiments demonstrated that the level of BAL eosinophil-derived peroxidase (EPO) was also increased, and was perhaps a more sensitive measure of eosinophilic pathology as its levels fell more quickly than eosinophil numbers during the recovery phase. A similar model of polymyxin-induced bronchial neutrophilia failed to demonstrate any effect on airway function or hyperresponsiveness. When the *Ascaris* sensitized monkeys were divided into single and dual responder groups, certain differences became apparent (Gundel et al, 1992). The dual responders had a higher baseline airway eosinophilia, which decreased slightly 6 hours after antigen challenge but with an associated increase in BAL fluid EPO. However, the number of BAL neutrophils actually increased at the same time as the LAR, and this increase was of greater magnitude than that observed in monkeys with the EAR only. Thus, the model provides some evidence for an interaction between the eosinophil and the neutrophil in the generation of the LAR.

Control mechanisms and cellular responses are increasing in complexity as our understanding of the EAR and LAR has been extended. It is becoming clear that there is a degree of overlap between the two responses, as was suggested by the observation that the evoked LAR was, to a degree, dose dependent. However, the characteristics of the LAR have provided a useful model for extending our understanding of the immunopathology of hyperreactive airways.

INFLAMMATORY CELLS AND MEDIATORS

Eosinophils

Eosinophils and Asthma

Although long regarded as a defense against parasitic infection and a moderator of allergic reactions, the eosinophil has gained recognition as one of the major effector cells in the airway inflammatory state we recognize as asthma (Fig. 32–2). Early indications of the importance of this cell type were provided by the association between asthma and peripheral eosinophilia, in addition to the identification of eosinophils and their products in the sputum of asthmatics in Creola bodies and Charcot-Leyden crystals. Peripheral eosinophil levels have been found to correlate with the clinical severity of asthma, as do levels of eosinophils and their products in the BAL fluid (Bousquet et al, 1990). Furthermore, the peripheral blood eosinophil level has been correlated with the degree of nonspecific bronchial responsiveness. This was supported by the description of an initial peripheral eosinopenia in response to allergen challenge, thought to be due to their rapid egress from the circulation to airway sites, followed by a later eosinophilia in subjects who developed a LAR (Cookson et al, 1989). Other studies of the effect of oral or inhaled corticosteroids have demonstrated a relationship between falling numbers of eosinophils and improvements in hyperresponsiveness. As the wider application of bronchoscopic biopsy and lavage have further emphasized the eosinophilic nature of asthmatic inflammation, there has been a broadening of investigation to include the mechanisms of eosinophil recruitment and signaling, as well as their ability to cause local toxicity.

Eosinophil Mediators

The eosinophil is well equipped to cause local inflammatory changes. Its granules contain a series of four major chemical protagonists. Major basic protein (MBP) has demonstrated bronchial cytotoxicity in animal *in vivo* and human *in vitro* models. In addition, MBP has been co-localized to sites of epithelial damage in the asthmatic bronchial mucosa. Levels of MBP in sputum and in BAL have been correlated with the severity of disease (Wardlaw et al, 1988). Increased levels of MBP have been detected in the BAL fluid of symptomatic asthmatics compared to those with asymptomatic status, and correlated with an elevated yield of eosinophils. The level of MBP was also correlated with the degree of hyperresponsiveness, and the hyperresponsive patients demonstrated increased epithelial cell counts in the lavage fluid.

Eosinophil cationic protein (ECP) is also detected in the sputum in association with asthmatic episodes and in the serum in the setting of allergen challenge. ECP has been demonstrated in the bronchial submucosa in areas of inflammation, being readily detected by the monoclonal antibodies EG1 and EG2, directed against the "stored" and "secreted" forms of ECP respectively (Djukanović et al, 1990b; Azzawi et al, 1990). Increased BAL fluid levels of ECP are found in asthmatics and correlate with serum ECP levels, and may be more readily suppressed by corticosteroid therapy than are the eosinophil numbers themselves. Eosinophil-derived neurotoxin (EDN) and eosinophil peroxidase (EPO) are also inflammatory mediators that have been utilized as indices of eosinophil activity. EDN is increased in the BAL fluid of subjects with either a single- or dual-phase response to allergen. In the primate model of asthma, BAL fluid EPO levels serve as a more sensitive measure of inflammation than eosinophil numbers (Gundel et al, 1992).

In addition to these toxic arginine-rich proteins, eosinophils are able to generate the proinflammatory metabolites of arachidonic acid,

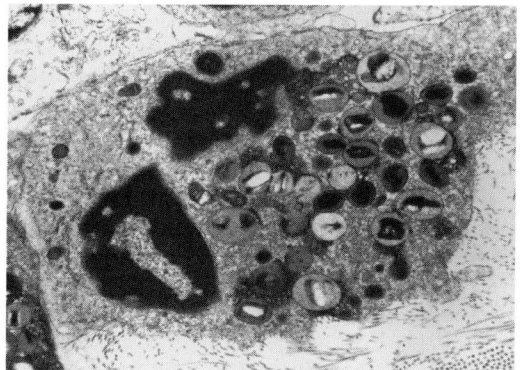

FIGURE 32–2. Transmission electron micrograph of an activated eosinophil, demonstrating granule heterogeneity with some granules having an electron lucent core compared to the surrounding matrix (Uranyl acetate-lead citrate stain, magnification ×17.5k). (Courtesy S. Wilson.)

particularly LTC$_4$ and LTD$_4$, as well as platelet activating factor (PAF). By these means and by the production of toxic superoxide anions, the eosinophil is further enabled to produce vasodilatation, microvascular leakage, and bronchial smooth muscle contraction.

Circulating eosinophils are known to vary in their metabolic state as measured by stimulated superoxide production. Eosinophils of lower than usual density demonstrate increased oxidative metabolism, morphologic evidence of degranulation, and possibly changes in the surface expression of Fc-IgG, complement receptors or the integrin common β-chain (CD18). The proportion of such low-density eosinophils was previously demonstrated to be increased in patients with asthma and during the late-phase response. By contrast, more recent studies have found that eosinophil density does not accurately reflect cell activation and surface receptor expression, and that while there was evidence for the priming of eosinophils in asthmatic subjects, there was no increase in the low-density eosinophil fraction (Hartnell et al, 1990; Bruijnzeel et al, 1993).

Eosinophil Recruitment and Activation

The accumulation, priming, and activation of eosinophils is an area of intense study and probable therapeutic yield. Production of colonies of eosinophils within the bone marrow and their subsequent maturation are stimulated by the circulating cytokines interleukin (IL)-3, IL-5 and granulocyte macrophage colony-stimulating factor (GM-CSF). This corresponds with part of the cytokine profile produced by airway inflammatory cells, particularly that of the T$_H$2-like "helper" (CD4$^+$) lymphocytes. *In vitro* experimentation suggests that these cytokines have additional importance in maintaining eosinophils in the airway site. Thus the production of GM-CSF by macrophages, epithelial cells, and fibroblasts assumes a new relevance, as does the production of GM-CSF, IL-3 (Kita et al, 1991) and IL-5 (Desreumaux et al, 1992) by the eosinophils themselves. Additional cytokine production recently attributed to eosinophils includes transforming growth factor α (TGF-α) and TGF-β, tumor necrosis factor α (TNF-α), and IL-6.

Chemoattractants for circulating eosinophils include complement component C5a, LTB$_4$, PAF, GM-CSF, IL-3, IL-5, IL-8, and regulated on activation, normal T expressed and presumably secreted (RANTES). IL-5 and RANTES are chemotactic for eosinophils rather than neutrophils. In addition, lymphocyte chemoattractant factor (LCF) and IL-2 are potent chemotactic factors that selectively act on eosinophils and not neutrophils. LCF is a glycoprotein product of CD8$^+$ cells stimulated with either histamine or antigen. CD4 is the receptor for LCF, and CD4$^+$ lymphocytes respond to the lymphokine with enhanced migration, increased expression of MHC class II (HLA-DR), and IL-2 receptors (IL-2R, CD25). However, monocytes and eosinophils also express the CD4 receptor, and it was recently demonstrated that recombinant LCF produced eosinophil migration at very low concentrations, in a fashion that was inhibited by an anti-CD4 antibody (Rand et al, 1991a). There was no evidence for increased eosinophil activation following exposure. IL-2 is well known as a T lymphocyte activating and growth factor and is chemoattractant for lymphocytes. Identification of the high-affinity heterodimeric IL-2 receptor on eosinophils accompanied the demonstration of the chemotactic ability of IL-2 for eosinophils (Rand et al, 1991b). Eosinophils exposed to GM-CSF, IL-3, or IL-5 *in vitro* demonstrate an increased chemotactic response to PAF, LTB$_4$, formyl-methionyl-leucyl-phenylalanine (FMLP) and IL-8, and this is mirrored by similar chemotactic responsiveness in eosinophils taken from asthmatic individuals (Bruijnzeel et al, 1992). RANTES is a member of the emergent family of chemokines and demonstrates clear properties of eosinophil but not neutrophil chemotaxis; it is likely to be more important than IL-8 in promoting eosinophil infiltration (Kameyoshi et al, 1992).

The initial step in eosinophil migration relies on the adherence of the cell to the endothelial cells of vessels near the inflammatory site, as mediated by the leukocyte adhesion molecules (Fig. 32–3). Eosinophils express a range of adhesion molecule ligands including the β2 integrins LFA-1 (αLβ2, CD11a/CD18) and Mac-1 (αMβ2, CD11b/CD18), the β1 integrin VLA-4 (α4β1), and the oligosaccharide sialyl Lewis X. These ligands bind in turn with the endothelial adhesion molecules intercellular adhesion molecule-1 (ICAM-1, CD54), vascular cell adhesion molecule-1 (VCAM-1) and E-selectin (previously known as endothelial leukocyte adhesion molecule-1, ELAM-1) respectively. The expression of the leucams is

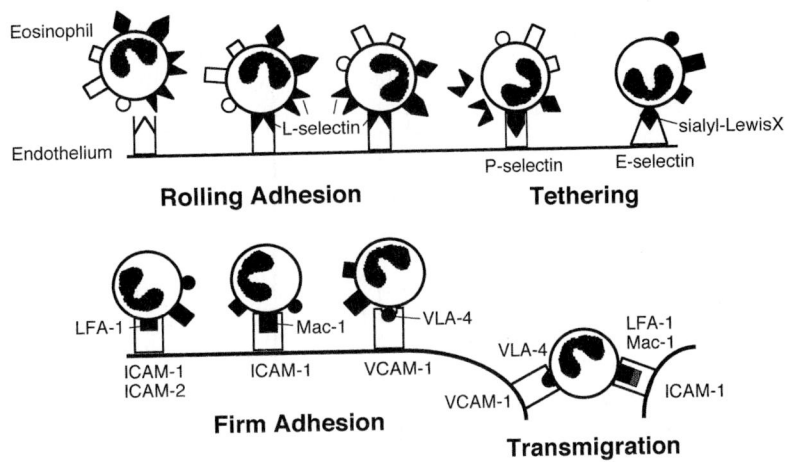

FIGURE 32-3. Diagram depicting the sequence of events in eosinophil adhesion and endothelial transmigration. Initial rolling adhesion and tethering are mediated by the selectins, with subsequent shedding of L-selectin. Increased avidity of the integrins is represented by a change from open to closed symbols. Interactions of the integrins with ICAM-1 and VCAM-1 lead to firm adhesion, diapedesis, and transendothelial migration.

under cytokine control, and induction occurs under the influence of IL-1 and TNF-α. In addition, interferon-γ (IFN-γ) induces the expression of ICAM-1 and IL-4 induces VCAM-1. The particular importance of the VLA-4–VCAM-1 interaction lies in the lack of VLA-4 expression on neutrophils, thereby conferring a degree of selectivity for eosinophil and lymphocyte recruitment, as cells on which the molecule is represented (Bochner et al, 1991). The expression of the Mac-1 ligand on the eosinophil is subject to cytokine regulation from IL-3, IL-5, GM-CSF, TNF-α and PAF (Thorne et al, 1990). The expression of VLA-4 does not appear to be so affected.

Initial "rolling adhesion" of eosinophils is the first step in their adherence to the vessel wall under conditions of flow. This is mediated in part by L-selectin on the eosinophil surface binding relatively weakly and in a repetitive fashion with its ligands on the endothelial surface. Further "tethering" is performed by endothelial P-selectin and E-selectin, which also stimulates the activation of Mac-1 and LFA-1, together with shedding of L-selectin. Interactions between ICAM-1 and LFA-1, ICAM-1 and Mac-1, and VCAM-1 and VLA-4 create firm adhesion between the eosinophil and endothelium. This is followed by diapedesis and transmigration between endothelial cells and thus across the vessel wall. Exposure of a human umbilical vein endothelial cell (HUVEC) monolayer to IL-1 and TNF-α promotes transmigration of eosinophils by mechanisms dependent on ICAM-1 and the β2 integrins (Ebisawa et al, 1991). The chemoattractant RANTES stimulates transmigration across IL-1 stimulated endothelium in a fashion that is dependent on VLA-4 (Ebisawa et al, 1993). Eosinophils from allergic donors have demonstrated an inherent transmigration capability that was reproduced by incubating eosinophils from nonallergic donors with IL-3, IL-5, and GM-CSF, leading to the conclusion that eosinophils from allergic donors had already been cytokine primed (Moser et al, 1992).

Once within the tissue matrix, a further series of interactions between Mac-1 and fibrinogen, VLA-4 and fibronectin, and CD44 and hyaluronic acid help ensure continued progress toward the eosinophils' target. The interaction between VLA-4 and fibronectin has recently been shown to prolong eosinophil survival, probably by stimulating the autocrine production of IL-3 and GM-CSF (Anwar et al, 1993).

Once "on site," a number of leukocyte-induced eosinophil surface proteins may offer the eosinophil a direct role in regulating eosinophilic inflammation. ICAM-1 and HLA-DR have been demonstrated on sputum eosinophils. Blood eosinophils will demonstrate ICAM-1 after incubation with TNF-α and the eosinophil "survival factors" GM-CSF, IL-3, or IL-5. HLA-DR is expressed following eosinophil incubation with GM-CSF, IFN-γ, or IL-4. Other eosinophil surface molecules expressed under the influence of GM-CSF and IL-3 include CD4, the IL-5 receptor (IL-5R), and IL-2R. By these means the eosinophil is able to maintain eosinophil-lymphocyte and eosinophil-eosinophil interactions to directly influence the accumulation and activity of its own and other inflammatory cell types (Hansel and Walker, 1992).

Priming of the eosinophils is represented by increased metabolic activity as a prelude to the subsequent release of mediators by the activated eosinophil. The same cytokines that are responsible for eosinophil production also have a major role here. This is best demonstrated by the increased production of LTC_4 within the primed eosinophils and by their increased oxidative metabolism in response to IL-3, IL-5, and GM-CSF. TNF-α, PAF, LTB_4, PGD_2, and histamine have a similar priming effect and will be encountered in the microenvironment of the airway submucosa. IFN-γ has a delayed priming effect that is not evident for 24 hours.

The processes of activating eosinophil mediator release are poorly understood, but they are likely to be related to binding with a selection of the antibody Fc receptors and complement receptors that have been identified on the cell surface. The low-affinity IgE receptor (FcϵR2), the carbohydrate binding protein Mac-2 (another IgE receptor), the low-affinity IgG receptor (FcγR2), IgA, and complement component receptors have variously been described, and may individually influence the release of different mediators (Tomassini et al, 1991).

Mast Cells

The contribution of the mast cell to airway inflammation dominated earlier studies of asthma. The wealth of preformed and newly synthesized mediators, together with the presence of the high-affinity IgE receptor (FcϵR1) to signal the presence of antigen, made this a cell type of obvious and primary importance. Despite subsequent confirmation of the multiplicity of cell types fulfilling fundamental roles, the new developments in cytokine signaling have maintained research interest in the significance of the mast cell.

Mast Cells and Mediators in Asthma

The cross-linkage of FcϵR1 molecules by antigen stimulates the secretion and synthesis of mediators by the mucosal mast cell. The relevance of the mast cell in asthma has been supported by the elevated numbers of mast cells found within BAL fluid from asthmatic subjects (Djukanović et al, 1990a). The proportion of mast cells and the histamine content of BAL fluid have been correlated with the degree of airflow obstruction and level of hyperresponsiveness (Wardlaw et al, 1988).

The population of mast cells within the bronchial tissue is more controversial, but in general most studies have failed to identify an increase in their numbers in the submucosa and epithelium (Djukanović et al, 1990b; Bradley et al, 1991) while some more recent studies have identified an increase in the epithelial layer (Laitinen et al, 1993; Pesci et al, 1993). However, mast cells within the asthmatic airway wall are more likely to be in an activated state (Fig. 32–4) (Beasley et al, 1989; Djukanović et al, 1990b; Pesci et al, 1993).

There is also an increase in histamine and tryptase concentrations in BAL fluid following bronchoalveolar allergen challenge (Wenzel et al, 1988). Increased levels of PGD_2 and LTC_4 have also been detected in BAL following allergen challenge (Murray et al, 1986; Wenzel et al, 1990). Plasma histamine levels have been observed to follow changes in airflow obstruction during the early- and late-phase response to allergen (Durham et al, 1984). Associations between different mast cell mediators, such as histamine, tryptase, and HMW-NCA, are taken as circumstantial evidence that these mediators are secreted by mast cells rather than by basophils.

The BAL-derived mast cells of symptomatic asthmatic subjects display increased spontaneous histamine release, but diminished IgE-stimulated release, which has been taken as evidence of ongoing mast cell degranulation (Broide et al, 1991b). This is supported by an earlier study, which demonstrated higher

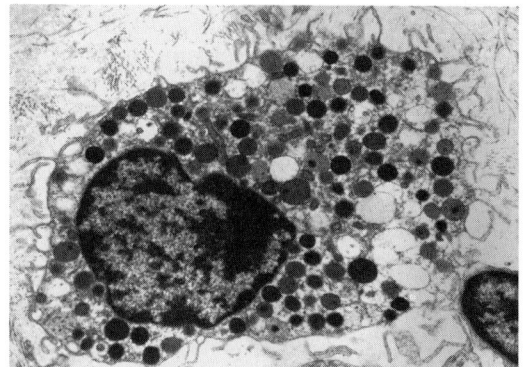

FIGURE 32–4. Transmission electron micrograph of an activated mast cell demonstrating some loss of granules and others of varying electron lucency (Uranyl acetate–lead citrate stain, magnification ×14.3k). (Courtesy S. Wilson.)

spontaneous histamine release and lavage fluid histamine levels in asthmatics with airway hyperreactivity (Wardlaw et al, 1988).

Histamine is the archetypal mast cell mediator with its well-established bronchoconstrictor effects directly on smooth muscle supplemented by its vasodilator action and increased vascular permeability. These effects are mediated by H_1 receptors, while histamine also produces increased mucus secretion by stimulation of H_2 receptors.

The only neutral protease so far identified in the bronchial epithelial mast cell is tryptase. Tryptase further enhances bronchial hyperresponsiveness by its enzymatic actions on would-be bronchoactive precursors including kinins and neuropeptides and is able to activate complement. Mast cells at other connective tissue sites, around bronchial submucosal glands and deep blood vessels, also contain chymase and carboxypeptidase A. This has led to a nomenclature in which mucosal mast cells are referred to as "MC_T" while the deeper connective tissue mast cells are designated "MC_{TC}" (Irani et al, 1986). The MC_{TC} is also in part distinguished by being activated by a number of non-IgE-related stimuli including C3a, C5a, MBP, and substance P, and such stimulation leads to a very rapid release of preformed mediators with relatively less eicosanoid generation. However, the precision of this classification is open to question. There is increasing evidence for a range of activation and degranulation of mast cells within the bronchial tissue, which increases toward the epithelium, and this may be responsible for the variety of protease contents (Pesci et al, 1993).

The activation of the mucosal mast cells leads to the production of eicosanoids from arachidonic acid. The most prolific prostaglandin is PGD_2, a mediator that has been demonstrated to increase in BAL fluid concentration after local endobronchial challenge (Wenzel et al, 1991; Liu et al, 1991). Increased levels of its bronchoconstrictor metabolite $9\alpha 11\beta PGF_2$ are also significant (Liu et al, 1991). While the disulphidopeptide leukotrienes are undoubtedly produced, it seems likely that the eosinophil is a quantitatively more important source of these agents including LTC_4.

The simultaneous suppression of both the acute airway response and some mediators by mast cell inhibitory pharmacotherapy, such as albuterol and cromolyn sodium, is further evidence for the role of mast cells in acute bronchoconstriction. The ability of nedocromil sodium, cromolyn sodium, and long-acting or high-dose β agonists to modify the LAR is taken as circumstantial evidence for a role for mast cells in the late phase. However, they are relatively less effective in the second part of the dual response, suggesting that "stabilizing" the mast cell is not by itself enough to prevent the late-phase reaction. A wide range of specific mast cell mediator inhibitors and antagonists have been demonstrated to produce modification of the response to allergen challenge. These include selective H_1 antagonists, thromboxane TP1 receptor antagonists, LTD_4 antagonists, and cyclooxygenase inhibitors. In addition, the therapeutic effect of inhaled corticosteroids is accompanied by a reduction in epithelial and submucosal mast cell numbers, together with reductions in eosinophils and T lymphocytes (Djukanović et al, 1992).

Mast Cells and Cytokines

Stem cell factor (SCF), also known as c-*kit* ligand, is a recently identified haemopoietic growth factor that supports mast cell development in rodents and, to some extent, in humans. This new cytokine has now been shown to enhance the IgE-dependent mediator release of human lung mast cells and is the first cytokine to demonstrate a regulatory effect over mast cell activation (Bischoff and Dahinden, 1992a). In addition SCF by itself has induced mediator release from cultured human mast cells. Hence, SCF is a potentially important pro-inflammatory cytokine with mast cell modulating and mediated effects.

Human dermal mast cells of the MC_{TC} phenotype have been demonstrated to contain large amounts of stored TNF-α, which is rapidly released on degranulation. One of the effects of the locally released cytokine is to increase endothelial expression of E-selectin, thus increasing the inflammatory infiltrate. As most of the identifiable TNF-α in the dermis was localized to the mast cells, it has been proposed that human mast cells may serve a "gatekeeper" function over the microvasculature (Walsh et al, 1991).

The techniques of *in situ* hybridization and immunohistochemistry have been used on asthmatic bronchial biopsies to demonstrate the presence of a range of cytokines. IL-4 has been demonstrated in mast cells in nasal biopsies from allergic rhinitic subjects and also in the bronchial biopsies of atopic asthmatics. Asthmatic and normal bronchial biopsies have also been demonstrated to contain mast cells that elaborate IL-4, IL-5, IL-6, and TNF-α, and there may be upregulation of the expression of TNF-α and IL-4 in the asthmatic mast cells (Figs. 32–5 and 32–6) (Bradding et al, 1994).

The demonstration of an active role for human mast cells in the elaboration of cytokines extends the potential importance of this cell type beyond the provision of mediators for the early or late phase of allergen response. It implicates this cell type in the initiation and regulation of the inflammatory infiltrate

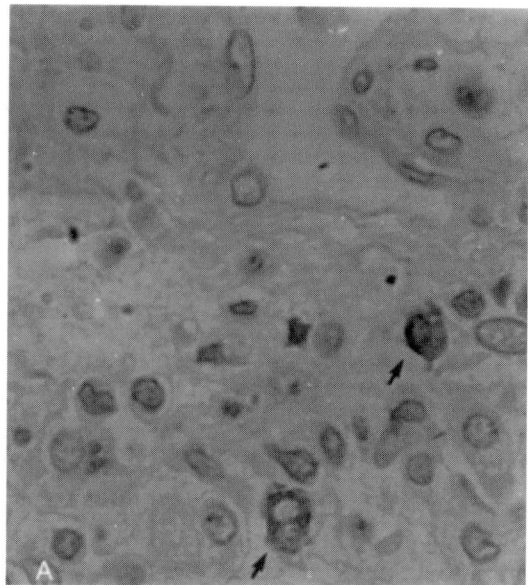

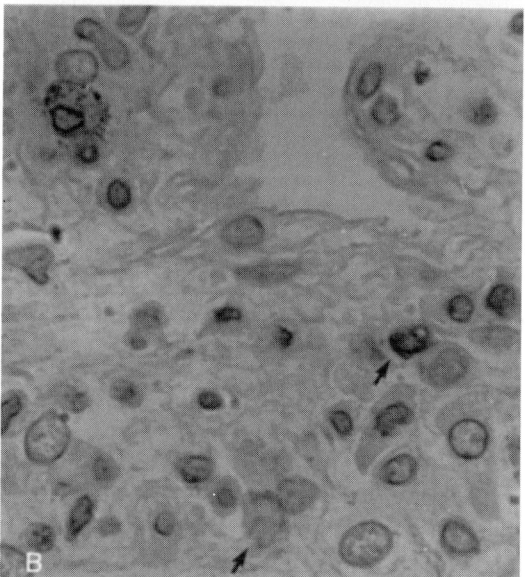

FIGURE 32–6. Immunohistochemical staining of sequential 2-μm sections demonstrating the co-localization of TNFα to mast cells in a nasal mucosal biopsy from a rhinitic subject. *A*, mAb 52B83 to TNFα. *B*, mAb AA1 to mast cell tryptase (Immunoperoxidase, magnification ×630). (Courtesy Dr. P. Bradding.)

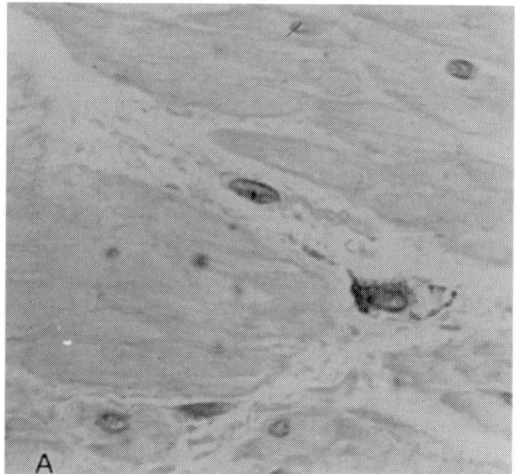

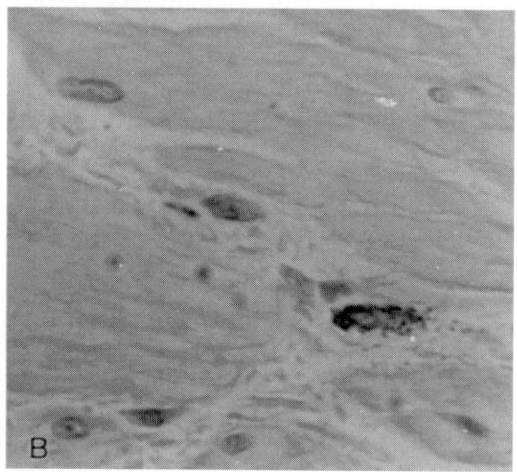

FIGURE 32–5. Immunohistochemical staining of sequential 2 μm sections demonstrating the co-localization of IL-4 to mast cells in a bronchial mucosal biopsy from an asthmatic subject. *A*, mAb 4D9 to IL-4. *B*, mAb AA1 to mast cell tryptase (Immunoperoxidase, magnification ×400). (Courtesy Dr. P. Bradding.)

following allergen exposure, with influences on accumulation and activation of T lymphocytes and eosinophils, together with the production of IgE.

Basophils

The basophil was initially regarded as a histamine-containing, circulating precursor to the tissue mast cell, particularly in view of the surface expression of high-affinity IgE receptors. Its association with allergic disease was well recognized, and both elevated numbers in the peripheral blood and increased sensitivity to stimulation *in vitro* correlated with the presence and severity of allergic rhinitis and asthma. Basophils were also identified in the nasal and bronchial secretions in allergic disease. However, the development of methodology to purify and study tissue mast cells shifted the focus of attention from their circulating relatives. While the heterogeneity of mast cells was being studied and their cytokine profile explored, new findings with regard to basophil function and response were also emerging (Massey and Lichtenstein, 1992).

Basophil Recruitment and Activation

Basophil chemotaxis is demonstrated most potently by IL-3 and GM-CSF. Other chemoattractants include C5a, LTB_4, PAF, IL-5, and IL-8 (Tanimoto et al, 1992). Basophil endothelial adherence is mediated, at least in part, by the same VLA-4-VCAM dependent mechanism as eosinophils and lymphocytes, and will therefore also be subject to cytokine control involving IL-1, TNF-α and IL-4 (Bochner et al, 1991).

There are a wide range of basophil priming and activating factors. Anti-IgE and FMLP directly stimulate basophil histamine and leukotriene release, whereas C5a will cause only histamine release. C3a and PAF require cytokine priming of the basophils (Dahinden et al, 1991). The predominant priming factors are IL-3, IL-5 and GM-CSF. At high concentrations IL-3 and GM-CSF will also cause histamine release from the basophils of some atopic subjects. SCF is also a priming factor for anti-IgE mediated release (Kuna et al, 1993).

Multiple histamine-releasing factors (HRF) have been identified within the chemokine group of cytokines (Kuna et al, 1993). Monocyte chemotactic and activating factor (MCAF, MCP-1) is the most potent of these, followed by RANTES. Connective tissue–activating peptide-III (CTAP-III) and neutrophil-activating peptide-2 (NAP-2) are less potent HRFs. While IL-8 has performed as an HRF in some studies of IL-3 primed basophils, others have found, somewhat paradoxically, that IL-8 prevents histamine release to the above chemokines when used in pre-incubation, and so IL-8 is thought to be the histamine release inhibitory factor (HRIF). In addition, there remains an uncharacterized cytokine, best categorized as an IgE-dependent HRF, that requires a particular form of IgE on the basophil surface, as is found in some atopic subjects.

Basophils are capable of IL-4 production. Murine basophils were initially identified as non-B, non-T cells in spleen suspensions and bone marrow that produced IL-4 following cross-linkage of the high-affinity IgE receptor. This effect was enhanced in the presence of IL-3 and by parasitic infection or polyclonal stimulation. Subsequent morphologic examination of the isolated cells has shown that this population consists of a high proportion of basophils. These observations have since been extended to human basophils, with the demonstration of IL-4 production by IgE receptor stimulation of basophils cultured with IL-3 (Brunner et al, 1993). This is particularly significant in view of the recently enlarged range of activities of IL-4 including VCAM-1 upregulation and T_H2 lymphocyte differentiation. By such means, basophils would be able to contribute to the cytokine signaling of an allergic infiltrate.

Basophil Mediators and Asthma

In common with mast cells, basophils will release histamine in response to the cross-linking of FcεR1. However, basophil eicosanoid production is limited to LTC_4, and not the range of prostaglandins associated with mast cells, including the BAL mast cell, which produces rather more PGD_2 than LTC_4. This different mediator profile has been used to try to separate the different potential roles of the two cell types.

As discussed earlier, the association of histamine with HMW-NCA, tryptase, and PGD_2 has been used to implicate the mast cell as the major effector cell of the acute response to allergen, with synchronous elevations being reported in both blood and BAL fluid (Durham et al, 1984; Wenzel et al, 1988, Liu et al, 1991). In studying the LAR, elevated levels of histamine and PGD_2 were also found in BAL fluid taken at 19 hours, although the levels were somewhat reduced on those found earlier, particularly the levels of PGD_2. However, there was a large increase in the number of Alcian blue–positive cells (the majority of which were basophils) in the late

BAL fluid, and these were postulated to be contributing to the histamine content (Liu et al, 1991).

A range of studies have been performed using the model of a dual-phase response to allergen in the nose and also in the skin. The acute response to upper airway allergen exposure with nasal congestion and sneezing was accompanied by mediators such as histamine, tryptase, and PGD_2 with low levels of LTC_4. In the late-phase response, there were lower levels of histamine and no PGD_2 or tryptase, but detectable levels of LTC_4, and a lavage cell population that included neutrophils, eosinophils, and basophils. A similar pattern of mediator release and cell infiltration was seen in the delayed cutaneous response to allergen, and in each of these models there was a correlation between basophil numbers and histamine levels (Massey and Lichtenstein, 1992).

This pattern of mediator response is circumstantial evidence for a role for the basophil as a major effector cell in the LAR, supported by the identification of a basophil infiltrate in the lavage fluid in small but significantly increased numbers. This must obviously be tempered by the large number of lavage and biopsy studies that have failed to identify a basophil infiltrate and the possibility that continued mast cell degranulation is responsible for the residual histamine levels.

Lymphocytes

The continuing attention directed to the role of the lymphocyte remains focused on the ability of the cell type to direct and coordinate the inflammatory response. The burgeoning diversity of influential variables and responses is reflected in the increasing number and complexity of cell surface proteins and cytokines expressed.

Lymphocytes and Asthma

In contrast to eosinophils and mast cells, there has been little information to suggest that increased absolute numbers of lymphocytes are present in asthma. However evidence is rapidly accumulating to indicate that T cell activation and subtypes display important differences. Studies in acute severe asthma have shown that $CD4^+$ cells displayed increased levels of IL-2R, HLA-DR, and VLA-1 compared with controls. These surface markers of T cell activation were not increased on $CD8^+$ cells. There was also an increase in the levels of the soluble IL-2R (sIL-2R) and IFN-γ in the asthmatic patients. $CD4^+$ cells and sIL-2R levels were said to be inversely correlated with measures of airflow obstruction (Corrigan and Kay, 1990). Increased expression of peripheral blood T cell activation markers has not been a uniform finding in studies of less severely symptomatic asthmatics (Wilson et al, 1992). However, increased activation markers on T lymphocytes have been reported with increased proportions of IL-2R positive $CD4^+$ cells in the circulation of extrinsic and intrinsic asthmatics. A correlation was found between increased IL-2R expression by T cells and the degree of eosinophilia. Also, the cytokines GM-CSF, IL-3, and IL-5 were identified in both T cell supernatants and the serum of the asthmatics and were demonstrated to be responsible for prolonging eosinophil survival *ex vivo* (Walker et al, 1991).

Similarly, examination of BAL fluid has generally failed to identify changes in absolute lymphocyte numbers, although with flow cytometry the T lymphocytes have demonstrated significantly elevated markers of activation including HLA-DR and IL-2R (Wilson et al, 1992). The activated $CD4^+$ cells in BAL from asthmatics are predominantly of a memory phenotype and correlate with symptoms and airway function. In another study on BAL fluid from allergic asthmatics, increased expression of IL-2R on $CD4^+$ cells has been shown to correlate with the number of B cells expressing the low-affinity IgE receptor, suggesting a link between T cell activation and increased expression of an atopic phenotype, with a similar observation being made on peripheral blood. The nonallergic asthmatics differed in displaying increased expression of IL-2R, HLA-DR, and VLA-1 on both $CD4^+$ and $CD8^+$ cells in both BAL and peripheral blood (Walker et al, 1992).

In the setting of local bronchoalveolar allergen challenge, BAL fluid taken some 10 minutes after challenge identified a fall in the levels of $CD3^+$, $CD4^+$, and $CD8^+$ cells, with a fall in the CD4:CD8 ratio. This may reflect the rapid acquisition of $CD4^+$ cells into the bronchial wall, or at least increased adhesion to the epithelium, in response to allergen exposure. There were no changes in the T cell surface markers of activation (Gratziou et al, 1992). However, other investigators performing BAL at 48 hours after inhalation allergen challenge found a rise in the proportion of CD4$^+$ cells in BAL, in association with a fall in peripheral blood CD4$^+$ cells (Metzger et al, 1987). The late accumulation of CD4$^+$ cells in the airway therefore coincides with the acquisition of bronchial hyperresponsiveness in the LAR. Changes in the CD4:CD8 ratio may be implicated in determining the nature of the asthmatic response. Significantly reduced proportions of CD4$^+$ cells and a greatly reduced CD4:CD8 ratio were found in BAL fluid 6 hours after allergen challenge in the patients who developed an EAR only, compared with those who had a dual response. This suggested that the early predominance of CD8$^+$ cells in the airways may protect against further subsequent bronchoconstriction by down-regulating subsequent inflammatory changes (Gonzalez et al, 1987).

The recent recognition of the role of dendritic cells as "professional" antigen-presenting cells (APCs) has further emphasized the early role of the T cell in antigen recognition and tolerance. Dendritic cells in the lung are equivalent in function to Langerhans cells in the skin and initially occupy intraepithelial sites, forming a fine network of cell processes within the epithelial layer. After contact with aeroallergens, they migrate to regional lymph nodes where they come into contact with a population of predominantly memory T cells (CD45RO$^+$). They may also be particularly important as the primary APC for the sensitization of naive T cells (CD45RA$^+$). The regional lymph nodes probably contain the majority of IgE-secreting plasma cells. These regional nodes have also been identified as the location of IgE T helper cells and the relevant T suppressor population (Holt et al, 1991).

T_H1- and T_H2-like Lymphocytes in Asthma

One of the most interesting developments in the elaboration of T cell subsets and their control over the inflammatory response emanates from the description by Mossman and colleagues of the T_H1 and T_H2 T cell groups in the mouse (Mossman and Coffman, 1989). Stimulation of the "type 1" mouse CD4$^+$ T cell clone yielded IL-2, IFN-γ, and TNF-β. By contrast "type 2" or T_H2 clones characteristically produced IL-4, IL-5, IL-6, and IL-10, thereby offering support for murine mast cell and eosinophil maturation, recruitment, and activation, together with the elaboration of IgE. Both T cell types were able to secrete GM-CSF and IL-3. The cytokine spectrum of the T_H1 cells is interpreted as being more in keeping with the generation of a delayed hypersensitivity response, with IFN-γ suppressing IgE production in favor of IgG and also suppressing B cell proliferation. Production of IFN-γ is thought to inhibit proliferation and cytokine production by T_H2 cells and induces differentiation into T_H1 cell types. Similarly, the elaboration of IL-10 by the T_H2 cells inhibits T_H1 cytokine production while IL-4 encourages T_H2 differentiation.

The extrapolation of these findings into human immunology was initially hampered by the failure to identify such phenotypes among existing panels of human T cell clones (TCC). However, examination of the cytokine phenotype of T cells from varying immunodeficiency states identified a series of similar clones. In addition, TCCs specific for the allergens of purified protein derivative (PPD) and *Toxocara canis* demonstrated T_H1 and T_H2 cytokine profiles respectively. Clones from atopic subjects sensitive to *Dermatophagoides pteronyssinus* have also demonstrated a predominantly T_H2 phenotype. Endobronchial biopsies following grass-pollen bronchoprovocation of sensitive asthmatic subjects were used to produce CD4$^+$ clones, of which 40 percent demonstrated T_H2 cytokine release, compared with 17 percent from patients with toluene diisocyanate–induced nonatopic asthma (Del Prete, 1992).

The patterns of cytokine production found in human T_H1-like and T_H2-like TCCs do not correspond precisely to those of murine derivation. While IFN-γ and TNF-β remain relatively T_H1 specific, and IL-4 and IL-5 are produced in large amounts by the T_H2 clones, both phenotypes are able to produce variable quantities of IL-2, IL-3, IL-6, IL-10, TNF-α and GM-CSF. IFN-γ and IL-4 promote the proliferation and cytokine production of T_H1 and T_H2 clones respectively. However, in contrast to murine TCCs, IL-10 inhibited these responses in both types of clones. Functionally, T_H1 but not T_H2 clones demonstrate cytolytic activity, and T_H2 clones induce IgE synthesis from autologous B cells in the presence of specific antigen. Further studies on peripheral blood mononuclear cell cultures from normal individuals have suggested that IL-4 and IFN-γ will help determine *in vitro* development of human $CD4^+$ T cells into T_H1- and T_H2-like clones (Romagnani et al, 1991).

Naturally there has been some interest in attempting to demonstrate a T_H2 involvement in atopic asthma more directly. Bronchial biopsies from asthmatic subjects have been shown to elaborate mRNA for IL-5 in six out of ten cases, as demonstrated by *in situ* hybridization, by comparison with normal controls (Hamid et al, 1991). Bronchial biopsies taken 24 hours after inhalation allergen challenge have shown increases in the number of cells containing mRNA for IL-5 and GM-CSF (Bentley et al, 1993). BAL-derived cells from mild asthmatic subjects were examined by *in situ* hybridization and shown to express increased mRNA for IL-2, IL-3, IL-4, IL-5, and GM-CSF compared with nonasthmatic controls. Immunofluorescent co-staining and immunomagnetic cell separation were used to demonstrate that the mRNA localized predominantly to the T lymphocyte population (Robinson et al, 1992). While this pattern is similar to that of the T_H2 phenotype, it is clearly not identical and further work is awaited.

Neutrophils

The neutrophil is a potent inflammatory cell, and its participation in the asthmatic inflammatory response has been the source of some study and much speculation. The granules contain a wide range of enzymes including lysosomal hydrolases, neutral serine proteases, lysozyme, myeloperoxidase, and type I collagenase. When activated, the neutrophil generates superoxide metabolites and a range of eicosanoids, including thromboxane, LTB_4, and PAF.

The neutrophil also responds to a range of mediators and cytokines that we have come to expect in the environment of the inflamed airway. Chemotactic and activating factors for neutrophils include C5a, LTB_4, PAF, FMLP, and IL-8. Other members of the chemokine family with neutrophil chemotactic properties are NAP-2 and the GRO proteins (MGSA/Groα, Groβ, TROτ) (Baggiolini, 1992).

Neutrophil recruitment involves initial attachment to the endothelium mediated by the selectin family of adhesion molecules, characterized by "rolling" of the neutrophil along the vessel wall under shear stresses. Firm adhesion of the neutrophil requires activation of the $\beta2$ integrins on the neutrophil cell surface, which is mediated by factors on the endothelium such as IL-8, PAF, and E-selectin. This "triggering" step is accompanied by the shedding of L-selectin from the neutrophil (Smith et al, 1991). Endothelial proteoglycans such as CD44 may be critical in the presentation of cytokines like IL-8 to the leukocyte as triggers for the functional activation of the integrins (Tanaka et al, 1993). Firm adhesion to the vascular endothelium is mediated by the activated $\beta2$ integrins and ICAM-1, which is upregulated in inflamed tissues. Migration through the endothelium is also dependent on the $\beta2$ integrins and ICAM-1.

Neutrophils and Asthma

Circumstantial evidence for a role for neutrophils in asthma follows the investigation of a range of serum substances referred to as "neutrophil chemotactic activity" (NCA). Serum NCAs of various molecular sizes have been identified in association with the EAR and LAR of challenged asthmatics, in association with exercise-induced asthma and in the setting of acute severe asthma. While high-molecular-weight NCA is thought to originate from mast cells, the low- and intermediate-weight forms of NCA are thought to be produced by T lymphocytes and monocytes and to be distinct from IL-8, but may still originate from the IL-8/CXC subfamily of chemokines.

Some of the evidence for a role for neutrophils in asthma is generated by animal models. In the cynomolgus monkey, a chronic bronchial neutrophilia induced by inhalation of polymyxin B was not associated with BHR. However, in the *Ascaris*-sensitized monkey model of the LAR, following a single episode of allergen exposure, there was an associated neutrophil influx in the BAL fluid that fell spontaneously to baseline after 7 days, unlike the eosinophil numbers that were higher at baseline in dual responders and failed to change significantly thereafter. These events were prevented by pretreatment with dexamethasone for a 7-day period (Gundel et al, 1992).

Direct evidence for neutrophil involvement comes from a variety of other studies. In the setting of the LAR some investigators have identified increased numbers of neutrophils in the BAL fluid from dual responders (Metzger et al, 1987). The relevant adhesion molecules, ICAM-1 and E-selectin, have been shown to be upregulated in the response to bronchial allergen challenge in association with increased numbers of neutrophils in the affected airway submucosa (Montefort et al, 1994).

Macrophages

The position of monocytes and macrophages in asthmatic inflammation is uncertain. The early finding of FcεR2 on a proportion of peripheral blood monocytes (PBM) and pulmonary alveolar macrophages (PAM) suggested an influential role in the response to allergen. However, their well-established role as antigen-presenting cells to the immune system may not necessarily have the same significance in extrinsic allergic asthma. It appears that the dendritic cells are the more important antigen-presenting cells for naive T cells, and that monocyte/macrophage function is confined to the reactivation of memory T cells. Furthermore, it seems likely that mature PAMs can actually function as immunomodulators and suppress T cell responses to antigen, whereas a shift toward the less mature monocytic phenotype of PAM may increase T cell responses (Holt, 1993).

Macrophages are able to release eicosanoids including thromboxane A_2 and LTB_4, PAF, complement fragments, and cytokines including TNF-α, IL-1, IL-6, GM-CSF, platelet derived growth factor (PDGF), and TGF-β. They produce a range of toxic substances including superoxide metabolites and proteolytic enzymes. However, their precise activity and patterns of mediator release in asthma have been difficult to establish, and there is continuing uncertainty as to whether such changes are a cause or a consequence of airway inflammation.

Peripheral blood monocytes from asthmatics demonstrate increased expression of FcεR2, complement receptor (CR)-1, CR-3, and HLA-DR, and increased rosette formation after allergen challenge. Cultured PBM from asthmatics also produce more TNF-α, IL-1β, IL-8, and GM-CSF. A novel monocyte-derived factor known as neutrophil priming activity (NPA) increases LTB_4 and superoxide production by neutrophils. The failure of corticosteroids to inhibit NPA production appears to correspond with the presence of steroid resistance in asthmatic patients (Lane et al, 1992).

Pulmonary alveolar macrophages obtained at bronchoalveolar lavage from asthmatic subjects demonstrated increases in the generation of toxic oxygen species, and BAL fluid obtained after allergen challenge had higher levels of β-glucuronidase (Murray et al, 1986). PAM from such subjects also produce higher levels of TNF-α, IL-1, IL-6 and GM-CSF. However, only one major study has identified increased numbers of macrophages in BAL at 48 hours after antigen challenge (Metzger et al, 1987).

Similarly, relatively few histologic studies have provided evidence of increased macrophage numbers in the mucosa of extrinsic asthmatics. In one such study, however, the cells demonstrated the phenotypic characteristics of blood monocytes (Poston et al, 1992).

Epithelium

Initial observations on the bronchial epithelium in asthmatic airways have been concerned with morphologic changes that reflected tissue damage from the inflammatory process. It is now becoming apparent that the epithelial cell layer has an integral role in directing and determining the pathobiology of asthma.

Epithelial Damage

Speculation that increased bronchial reactivity might be due to epithelial damage was derived in part from work in animal models and in humans after exposure to mucosal toxins such as nitrogen dioxide and ozone. In addition, it has been suggested that the epithelial changes associated with viral infections such as *influenza* might elucidate the cause of the reactivity commonly associated with viral upper respiratory infection. Proposed mechanisms included the disruption of intercellular tight junctions, thereby allowing easy allergen penetration, and the exposure of nerve endings with invoked axon reflexes.

Biopsies taken with the rigid bronchoscope demonstrated epithelial damage at all airway levels in an uncontrolled study of a small group of asthmatic patients with varying degrees of hyperresponsiveness (Laitinen et al, 1985). The range of epithelial changes included complete epithelial desquamation, a residual basal cell layer, and cleavage of the basal and more superficial columnar cells. Ciliated cells demonstrated vacuolization and the malalignment of the central ciliary filaments. In some biopsies it was possible to demonstrate neural tissue in a superficial location. In a fiberoptic biopsy study, three out of four symptomatic asthmatic subjects had a complete loss of surface epithelium, providing the basis for a correlation between epithelial loss and hyperresponsiveness to methacholine (Jeffery et al, 1989). However, a subsequent study in patients with mild asthma failed to demonstrate significant morphologic changes at a light and electron microscopic level, in comparison to normal controls (Lozewicz et al, 1990). This was an important demonstration of asthma and increased hyperresponsiveness despite minimal morphologic abnormalities, emphasizing that other factors, such as inflammatory cell infiltration and epithelial inflammatory and relaxant mediator generation, were likely to be important. The artifactual epithelial damage caused by the biopsy forceps has also been emphasized by a morphologic study in normal volunteers (Soderberg et al, 1990).

Several studies have demonstrated that asthmatics have an increased number of epithelial cells in BAL fluid, in a fashion that broadly correlates with hyperresponsiveness (Wardlaw et al, 1988; Beasley et al, 1989). However, this does not establish a causal relationship between epithelial damage and hyperresponsiveness, as inflammation in the submucosa would be expected to affect epithelial integrity, owing particularly to the released products of eosinophils such as MBP, ECP, and eosinophil peroxidase. The opening of tight junctions between ciliary cells and the widening of intercellular spaces has been shown to correlate with bronchial reactivity and increased numbers of eosinophils (Ohashi et al, 1992).

The presence of clumps of epithelial cells in the Creola bodies of asthmatic sputum was one of the early hallmarks of epithelial damage in asthmatic airways. Closer examination of the shed epithelial cells, performed using electron microscopy of cell pellets from BAL samples, has demonstrated a preponderance of columnar cells and a relative deficit of basal cells. In combination with biopsy-based observations, this has supported the concept of a cleavage plane between the basal and more superficial cells. Ultrastructural studies have demonstrated that the basal cells, but not the columnar cells, are linked to the basement membrane by hemidesmosomes (Fig. 32–7A). The columnar cells are adherent to the basal

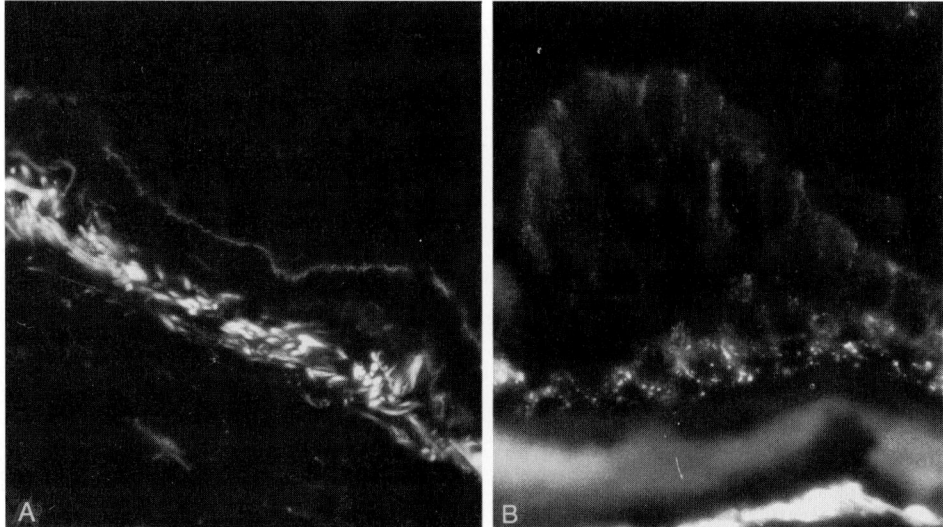

FIGURE 32–7. *A*, Frozen section of human bronchial epithelium, 5 μm in thickness. The integrin subunit α6, which is a component of hemidesmosomes, is located by indirect immunofluorescence (mAb GoH3). Immunoreactivity is localized to the junction of the basal cell layer with the basement membrane. The diffuse staining of the underlying collagen is nonspecific (magnification ×738). (Courtesy J. Baker.) *B*, Frozen section of human bronchial epithelium, 5 μm in thickness. Desmosomal proteins 1 and 2 (dp 1 and 2) are located by indirect immunofluorescence. Immunoreactivity is seen throughout the thickness of the epithelium in a characteristic punctate pattern with a concentration at the interface between basal cells and columnar cells. The diffuse staining of the basal lamina is nonspecific (magnification ×738). (Courtesy J. Baker.)

cell layer and to each other through a series of desmosomes, intermediate junctions, tight junctions, and gap junctions (Fig. 32–7B) (Montefort et al, 1992a).

Although thickening of the basement membrane was detected in early pathologic studies, it is only recently that this phenomenon has been more accurately described as "subepithelial fibrosis" (Fig. 32–8). The area immediately beneath the basement membrane is infiltrated with fibrils of collagens III and V, together with fibronectin. The lack of any epithelial cell–derived connective tissue types in the fibrotic layer, together with a lack of correlation with epithelial shedding, is circumstantially against an epithelial cell origin for this collagen layer. Rather, it has been considered more likely that this may be a fibroblast reaction to cytokine secretion from nearby inflammatory cells (Roche et al, 1989).

Epithelial Mediators and Cytokines

Human epithelial cells are able to metabolize arachidonic acid to produce a variety of eicosanoid mediators. The products of cultured tracheal and bronchial epithelial cells include 12-, 14-, and 15-HETE. The 15-HETE can increase mucus production in animal models and enhance the production of leukotrienes by isolated mast cells; it can also increase the acute response to allergen challenge in asthmatics. Bronchial epithelial cells from asthmatic subjects demonstrate increased release of 15-HETE. Epithelial cells are also able to produce the cyclooxygenase products PGE_2 and $PGF_{2\alpha}$, thereby potentially influencing bronchial smooth muscle tone in either direction, depending on their relative levels of production, which may in turn be influenced by other factors such as bradykinin, histamine, and PAF (Proud, 1993).

Endothelins are a recently discovered family of three structurally related peptides that have vasoconstrictor, growth stimulating, and bronchoconstrictor properties. They were initially considered to be endothelial products, as suggested by their nomenclature. However, endothelin-1 has been identified in a number of different tissues as well as tracheobronchial cell cultures, while binding sites exist on human airway smooth muscle. Increased levels of endothelin-1 were identified in the plasma and BAL fluid during severe asthma attacks. Immunohistochemical studies have detected

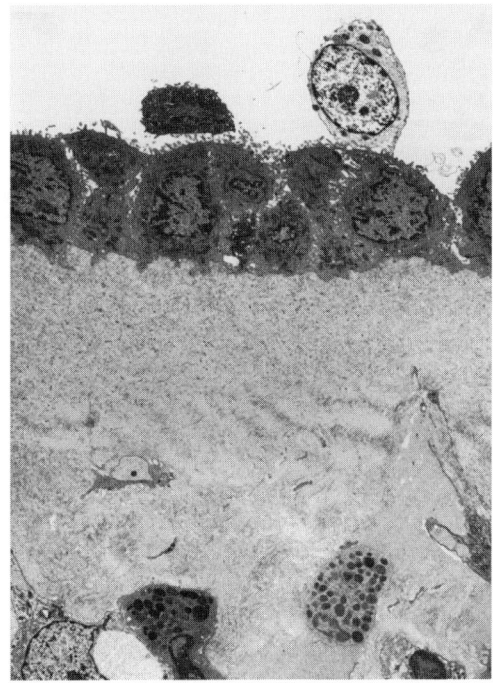

FIGURE 32–8. Transmission electron micrograph of bronchial epithelium from an asthmatic subject. The basal cell layer remains firmly adherent; however, only one overlying columnar cell remains. Subepithelial fibrosis is present with considerable thickening of the sub-basement membrane collagen layer. Two eosinophils are seen in the underlying submucosa (Uranyl acetate-lead citrate stain, magnification ×4k). (Courtesy Dr. H. Makker.)

endothelin-1 in the bronchial epithelium of 70 percent of the asthmatic subjects studied, compared with 10 percent of controls (Fig. 32–9) (Springall et al, 1991). In situ hybridization has identified mRNA for preproendothelin in bronchial epithelial cells of symptomatic asthmatics, and during subsequent culture they were able to release large amounts of endothelin. The addition of hydrocortisone to the culture medium significantly reduced the levels of endothelin release. In addition to the directly bronchoconstrictor effects of this peptide, it may further contribute to inflammatory changes by enhancing 15-lipoxygenase activity and stimulating fibroblast division.

Nitric oxide (NO) is assuming prominence as a powerful contributor to the human neural bronchodilator response. NO synthase is found in the bronchial epithelium, and an inducible form of the enzyme is found more commonly in asthmatic subjects (Springall et al, 1993). Increased activity of NO synthase

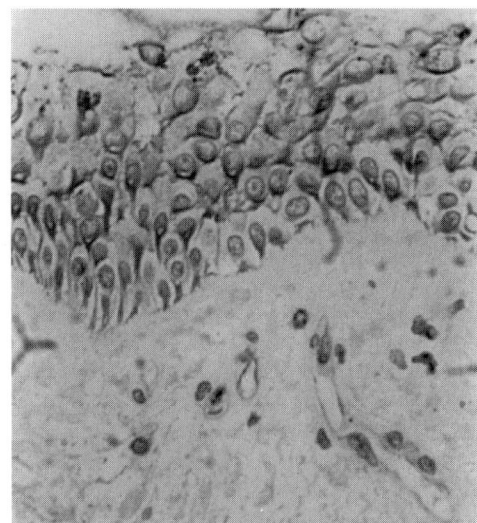

FIGURE 32–9. Immunohistochemical staining of a bronchial mucosal biopsy from an asthmatic subject demonstrating the presence of endothelin-1 in the epithelium and in the submucosal endothelium (Immunoperoxidase, magnification ×400). (Courtesy Dr. T. Redington.)

may contribute to hyperemia and cytotoxicity in the inflamed airway. Alternatively, NO may be playing a counter-regulatory role in the presence of increased levels of bronchoconstrictors such as endothelins and may be dampening cholinergic transmission (Barnes, 1993b).

Neutral endopeptidase (NEP) is found in basal epithelial cells and has an important function in degrading tachykinins in the airway. It is considered to have a major role in the regulation of neurogenic aspects of inflammation (Nadel, 1992). Perturbation of the epithelium by mechanical means, by NEP inhibitors, and by viral infections has been demonstrated to increase the effects of the tachykinins on the airway. Corticosteroids may reduce neurogenic inflammation by inducing NEP in the bronchial epithelium.

Epithelial expression of adhesion molecules is strongly implicated in the pathogenesis of asthma. Notable studies in a primate model of eosinophilic inflammation with bronchial hyperresponsiveness revealed an increased expression of ICAM-1 on the epithelium as well as on submucosal vessels (Wegner et al, 1990). Daily intravenous administration of antibody to ICAM-1 was shown to markedly diminish the BAL concentration of eosinophils and the degree of hyperresponsiveness. Initial studies in human bronchial biopsies have demonstrated expression of ICAM-1 in the epithelium of both asthmatics and normal controls, while both ICAM-1 and E-selectin were detected in the endothelium (Montefort et al, 1992b). This is an area of special interest as ICAM-1 is the epithelial receptor for the major group of human rhinoviruses, and soluble forms of blocking antibody are under investigation (Staunton et al, 1989).

The bronchial epithelium is another potentially rich source of cytokines. *In vitro* experiments on cultured human bronchial epithelial cells have shown that GM-CSF, IL-6, and IL-8 can be produced in response to a variety of stimuli including IL-1 and lipopolysaccharide (LPS). By examining bronchial biopsies from asthmatic subjects and using immunohistochemistry, PCR, and ELISA on subsequent culture supernatants, it has been possible to confirm the increased production of GM-CSF, IL-6, and IL-8 by the bronchial epithelium in patients with symptomatic asthma (Marini et al, 1992). Corticosteroids subsequently prevented the production of those cytokines from the cultured epithelial cells. Nasal epithelium has demonstrated high constitutive levels of mRNA for IL-8, together with the identification of the cytokine by immunohistochemistry. Increased IL-8 production followed stimulation with respiratory syncytial virus, IL-1, and TNF (Becker et al, 1993).

Platelet Activating Factor

Platelet activating factor (PAF) has been proposed to have a central role in the inflammatory process, although recently this has been the subject of some dissent. Initially it was identified as a leukocyte-derived factor that stimulated platelets to aggregate and to release histamine. When chemically identified it was found to be a small family of unique phosphoglycerides with wide-ranging biologic properties on an equally wide range of cells. The synthesis and precise molecular form of PAF will vary between cell types, with the derivation from membrane phospholipid by the action of phospholipase A_2 probably dominating in inflammatory cells.

The most important property relevant to asthma is the potency of PAF as a bronchoconstrictor in the human airway; however, a number of its additional effects gave rise to speculation as to a primary role for this mediator in the pathogenesis of asthma (Spencer, 1992). These include its activity as a chemotactic factor for eosinophils and, to a lesser extent, for neutrophils and basophils. PAF can stimulate endothelial adhesion of eosinophils and activate them to produce LTC_4 and further PAF. Neutrophils demonstrate endothelial adhesion following "triggering" with endothelial PAF and also activation with increased superoxide generation. Airway mucus production is enhanced and so is microvascular permeability, but mucociliary clearance is reduced. Although there are multiple mechanisms for PAF to increase bronchial hyperresponsiveness (BHR), this has generally not been observed to be the case. Initial suggestions that PAF produced BHR in normal subjects have subsequently lacked further support, with no increases in BHR following administration in asthmatic subjects (Spencer, 1992). PAF antagonists have failed to protect against allergen-induced bronchoconstriction or BHR in asthmatics.

DETERMINANTS OF THE INFLAMMATORY RESPONSE

Cytokines

The number of cytokines involved in the initiation and regulation of the asthmatic inflammatory response continues to increase. However, it is equally important to recognize that the spectrum of cells that are both susceptible to their effects and responsible for their secretion has extended well beyond T lymphocytes and macrophages to include eosinophils, mast cells, basophils, neutrophils, fibroblasts, and epithelial cells. As a result it becomes increasingly difficult to discuss cellular and cytokine functions separately, and the role of several cytokines is discussed elsewhere in the chapter. In this section we will deal with the central aspects of cytokine networking in asthma.

IL-3, IL-5, and GM-CSF

There is a continuing emphasis on the role of cytokines in eosinophil production and function. It was a series of relatively early discoveries that identified IL-3, IL-5, and GM-CSF as cytokines responsible for the bone marrow production of eosinophils. Subsequent work established that the importance of these cytokines extended beyond the production of eosinophils by the bone marrow progenitor cells. IL-3, IL-5, and GM-CSF were able to produce in the eosinophils a state of increased metabolic activity and potentiation referred to as "priming" or "early activation," recognized by morphologic changes, increased oxidative metabolism, and superoxide production. Increased cytotoxicity of eosinophils exposed to these cytokines was also recorded. Furthermore, they were found to enhance the survival of eosinophils *in vitro*, suggesting that they could have a further local function in preserving and thus increasing eosinophil numbers as an influx of inflammatory cells occurred.

The same cytokines have been demonstrated to be important in the transmigration of eosinophils across IL-1 and TNF-α–stimulated endothelial cell layers. Whereas neutrophil adherence is inevitably followed by transmigration, only eosinophils co-cultured with GM-CSF, IL-3, and IL-5 would cross the monolayers. Eosinophils from allergic asthmatic patients already demonstrated this ability, suggesting that they had already undergone *in vivo* priming. The use of blocking monoclonal antibodies has suggested that this effect is mediated through the β2 integrins and ICAM-1 (Ebisawa et al, 1991; Moser et al, 1992).

The special significance of IL-5 was quickly appreciated as it showed specificity for the eosinophil lineage and did not promote the production of neutrophils or macrophages, unlike IL-3 and GM-CSF. IL-5 was also found to be a selective chemotactic factor for eosinophils *in vitro*. In addition, it has been shown that IL-5 selectively increases eosinophil adherence to cultured endothelial cells in a β2 integrin-dependent fashion (Walsh et al, 1990).

The production of these cytokines by T lymphocytes is perhaps the best studied, but it is now established that eosinophils and mast cells are also contributors to the presence of cytokines in the inflamed airways. Eosinophils have been shown to produce eosinophil survival-enhancing activity that is due to the release of GM-CSF, IL-3, and IL-5 (Kita et al, 1991; Desreumaux et al, 1992). In response to IgE receptor stimulation *in vitro*, murine mast cells have demonstrated similar production, with the additions of IL-4 and IL-6 (Plaut et al, 1989). More recently, the presence of IL-4, IL-5, IL-6, and TNF-α has been demonstrated by immunohistochemistry in mast cells in biopsies from rhinitic and asthmatic patients, with the suggestion that

IL-4 and TNF-α secretion by mast cells may be increased in asthmatics (Bradding, 1994).

IL-3, IL-5, and GM-CSF in Asthma

Evidence for a pivotal role for IL-5 in human allergic states is mounting, largely through the demonstration of mRNA for IL-5 by the technique of *in situ* hybridization. When applied together with immunohistochemistry, in double staining techniques, it has been possible to show increases in IL-5 mRNA in areas of increased lymphocytic accumulation and activation, in association with mild extrinsic asthma and the late-phase cutaneous response to allergen, and in bronchial biopsies from asthmatics after inhalational allergen challenge (Hamid et al, 1991; Kay et al, 1991; Bentley et al, 1993). In the bronchial biopsies from atopic asthmatics, there was a good correlation between IL-5 mRNA and the numbers of activated lymphocytes and eosinophils, with a tendency toward worsening airway function in the six out of ten asthmatics positive for IL-5 mRNA. In the late-phase cutaneous reactions, mRNA was also detected for IL-2, IL-3, IL-4, and GM-CSF. The allergen-challenged asthmatics demonstrated increases in mRNA for GM-CSF as well as IL-5.

In an analysis of cells derived from BAL fluid of asthmatics, there was evidence for increased expression of mRNA for IL-2, IL-3, IL-4, IL-5, and GM-CSF (Robinson et al, 1992). The mRNA for IL-4 and IL-5 was localized predominantly to T lymphocytes. The increased expression of IL-2 in the BAL-derived T cells of asthmatics is not entirely in keeping with the increased expression of a T_H2-like gene cluster. In a separate study that compared cytokine expression in the BAL fluid from extrinsic and intrinsic asthmatics, the former group were characterized by increased levels of IL-4 and IL-5 in keeping with a pattern of T_H2 activation. However, the intrinsic asthmatics had elevated levels of IL-2 and IL-5, suggesting a pattern of T cell activation not in keeping with a T_H1 or T_H2 phenotype. In both groups there was a close correlation between IL-5 levels and eosinophilia (Walker et al, 1992).

IL-5 has been demonstrated in the BAL taken 48 hours after segmental bronchial challenge in a group of atopic subjects. The "eosinophil survival activity" of the lavage correlated with eosinophil numbers and eosinophil granule proteins in the BAL, and was neutralized by anti-IL-5 antibodies or by their combination with anti-GM-CSF antibodies in some cases (Ohnishi et al, 1993).

Endobronchial allergen challenge has also been used to demonstrate increased levels of GM-CSF in the airways of asthmatics who respond with a BAL eosinophilia. There was a large increase in lavage GM-CSF levels 24 hours after the allergen challenge. The techniques of dual staining were again used to demonstrate that allergen stimulation had increased the mRNA expression, predominantly in lymphocytes, but also in macrophages (Broide and Firestein, 1991a). The same group has demonstrated elevated levels of a broad range of cytokines in the BAL fluid of symptomatic asthmatics, when compared with asymptomatic controls. These included TNF, GM-CSF, IL-1β, IL-2, and IL-6. However, the relevance of these findings is difficult to estimate given the technical difficulties of BAL retrieval and cytokine measurement (Broide et al, 1992).

IL-3, IL-5, and GM-CSF have been identified in asthmatic T cell supernatants and sera by the use of neutralizing antibodies (Walker et al, 1991). IL-5 has been identified in the serum of 8 out of 15 patients with moderate to severe asthma exacerbations and could not be detected following their treatment with corticosteroids. Once again there was a close correlation with blood eosinophil levels (Corrigan et al, 1993).

IL-4 and IFN-γ

IL-4 has in the past been primarily associated with the isotype differentiation of B cells and can selectively increase IgE synthesis by human B cells following their contact with appropriately stimulated T cells. In addition to increasing the expression of IgE surface receptors and HLA-DR, IL-4 also increases the expression of B cell IL-4 receptors.

Localized effects of IL-4 may be of equal importance in allergic disease and would be facilitated by the production of IL-4 by mast cells and basophils. The development and cytokine expression of T_H2-like cells is promoted by IL-4. In addition, IL-4 is able to increase endothelial cell binding of lymphocytes, basophils, and eosinophils by increasing the endothelial expression of VCAM-1, which does not bind with neutrophils as they do not express the β1 integrin VLA-4 (Bochner et al, 1991).

By this mechanism, IL-4 production can contribute to the characteristically eosinophilic nature of the infiltrate in extrinsic asthma. This action of IL-4 is further enhanced by the presence of TNF-α, again through a VCAM-dependent mechanism. Finally, IL-4 stimulates fibroblast proliferation and may thereby play a role in the formation of subepithelial fibrosis in asthma.

IFN-γ is assuming increasing importance as an immune regulator in asthma and functionally behaves as an antagonist to IL-4. At the same time as IL-4 was identified as a requisite for B cell IgE synthesis it was also established that the release of IFN-γ or its addition to T cell culture suppressed this activity. This reciprocal role is also clearly seen in the ability of IFN-γ to encourage T cells to differentiate into a T_H1 phenotype and simultaneously suppress the growth of T_H2 cells (Del Prete, 1992). In the bronchial biopsy and lavage experiments performed so far, levels of IFN-γ mRNA have been similar between asthmatics and controls.

Chemokines

An interesting new group of cytokines are referred to collectively as the chemokines and are functionally distinguished by their leukocyte-selective chemotactic activity. They are structurally distinguished by their low molecular weight and the presence of a conserved group of four cysteines, and the two subfamilies are identified by the spacing of the first two cysteine residues, expressed as either CXC or CC. IL-8 is a CXC chemokine and is a chemotactic factor for neutrophils and T lymphocytes, and under some conditions for eosinophils, but not for monocytes. Other members of the CXC subfamily are MGSA/Groα, CTAP-III, and NAP-2, and they display similar chemotactic activities. IL-8 is also chemotactic for basophils and is proposed to be the histamine release inhibitory factor, while CTAP-III and NAP-2 are histamine releasing factors (HRF) (Kuna et al, 1993).

The CC subfamily contains a number of proteins that are chemotactic for monocytes but not neutrophils. One such cytokine is RANTES, which was originally identified as an inducible gene in a T cell culture line and was shown to be chemoattractant for memory T cells. The eosinophil-chemoattractant product of thrombin-stimulated platelets has been sequenced and found to be almost identical with the RANTES produced by recombinant techniques (Kameyoshi et al, 1992). RANTES stimulates the migration of eosinophils across IL-1–stimulated endothelium, by a VLA-4–dependent mechanism (Ebisawa et al, 1993). This suggests an important role for RANTES as a selective chemoattractant pathway for eosinophils and memory T cells in asthma. RANTES and another CC chemokine MCP-1 are also potent HRFs (Kuna et al, 1993).

Adhesion Molecules

The increased appreciation of cytokine actions and interactions in inflammation has been accompanied by increased investigation of adhesion molecules and their role in directing the inflammatory traffic, often also under cytokine control.

Intercellular Adhesion Molecules (ICAMs)

ICAM-1, -2, and -3 are members of the immunoglobulin gene superfamily. ICAM-1 has five immunoglobulin-like domains in contrast to the two of ICAM-2, and it would appear that the latter is not cytokine-inducible and is responsible for binding the integrin ligand LFA-1 on noninflamed endothelium. ICAM-3 has five domains, and high levels of expression are found on resting lymphocytes, but it is not present on epithelial or endothelial cells. ICAM-3 is thought to be the major LFA-1 ligand responsible for initiating interactions with other leukocytes.

The increased expression of ICAM-1 on vascular endothelium at inflammatory sites can be induced by LPS, IL-1, TNF-α, and IFN-γ. ICAM-1 interacts with cells displaying the β2 integrins LFA-1 (lymphocytes, monocytes, granulocytes) and Mac-1 (granulocytes including eosinophils) resulting in firm endothelial adhesion and subsequent transmigration. β2 integrin expression on leukocytes can be increased by a range of cytokines and mediators; however, their functional activation by direct contact interactions occurs more rapidly. LFA-1 is activated by a conformational change in interactions with the T cell receptors CD2 and CD3. Endothelial PAF, IL-8, and E-selectin will trigger functional activation of the β2 integrins with particular emphasis on Mac-1 (Tanaka et al, 1993).

A significant role for ICAM-1 in eosinophil

migration *in vivo* has been supported by the ability of ICAM-1 antibodies to prevent allergen-induced eosinophilia and hyperresponsiveness in *Ascaris*-sensitized monkeys, with an effect that is presumed to be due to inhibition of eosinophil influx to the airway (Wegner et al, 1990). Although established airway eosinophilia could not be reversed by anti-ICAM antibody alone, it did prevent the relapse of BAL fluid eosinophilia and hyperresponsiveness that followed the cessation of an otherwise effective regimen of dexamethasone.

The epithelial expression of ICAM-1 has attracted attention since it was demonstrated that this was the binding site of a major group of human rhinoviruses, which are associated with up to 70 percent of asthma exacerbations in children. *In vitro* infection of HeLa cells with rhinovirus is associated with an increase in ICAM-1 expression. Up-regulation of ICAM-1 on airway epithelium by the virus *in vivo*, perhaps mediated by IFN-γ, could enhance the asthmatic epithelial inflammatory infiltrate; at the same time, increased ICAM-1 expression in asthma could predispose to such infection. Increased levels of epithelial ICAM-1 have been noted in the sensitized primate airway following multiple allergen inhalations (Wegner et al, 1990), although such observations have yet to be confirmed in humans.

VCAM-1, VLA-4, and Selective Cell Recruitment

Mechanisms for the specificity of cell recruitment are included within the system of adhesion molecules. Of particular interest has been the interaction between the immunoglobulin superfamily member VCAM-1 and the $\beta 1$ integrin VLA-4. It has been clearly demonstrated that while VLA-4 is expressed on eosinophils and lymphocytes, this is not a property shared by neutrophils (Bochner et al, 1991), and that VLA-4 is the eosinophil receptor for VCAM-1. So the expression of VCAM-1 on the endothelial surface will favor the development of an eosinophilic and lymphocytic infiltrate. Furthermore, the degree to which VCAM-1 is expressed is influenced not only by the cytokines IL-1 and TNF-α, which also control ICAM-1 expression, but also by IL-4, which expands the potential role of mast cells and basophils in controlling infiltration by lymphocytes and eosinophils. RANTES stimulates endothelial transmigration of eosinophils by a VLA-4–dependent mechanism (Ebisawa et al, 1993).

E-selectin

Endothelial cells exposed to IL-1 or TNF-α will express E-selectin maximally at about 4 hours, this effect being controlled at the level of protein synthesis, compared with the maximal expression at 24 hours of the transcription-limited ICAM-1. E-selectin does not demonstrate the same constitutive level of expression as ICAM-1 and has usually returned to basal levels by 24 hours. The ligand for E-selectin is a specific determinant on granulocyte surface glycoproteins known as sialyl Lewis X. Together with other members of the selectin family, its major function is thought to be in granulocyte recruitment, particularly in the initial rolling adhesion or tethering required under conditions of shear stress, which allows for subsequent and firmer adhesion through ICAM-integrin interactions (Bevilacqua and Nelson, 1993). In addition to providing this initial attachment, the E-selectin–granulocyte interaction functionally activates the integrin molecules, with similar triggering being exhibited by PAF and IL-8 (Zimmerman et al, 1992).

In the primate airway model of the late phase response, acute allergen exposure in the sensitized animals caused an increase in E-selectin expression by the vascular endothelium, an effect that was found not to exist for ICAM-1. The administration of E-selectin monoclonal antibodies prior to allergen exposure significantly inhibited the late-phase response, an effect that was associated with a decrease in the total leukocyte and neutrophil numbers found in the BAL fluid taken at 6 hours after allergen exposure (Gundel et al, 1991). No such effect was seen from pretreatment with an anti-ICAM monoclonal, suggesting a specific role for the E-selectin, particularly in the recruitment of neutrophils associated with the LAR in this animal model.

Adhesion Molecules in Asthma

Initial immunohistochemical studies in bronchial mucosa from asthmatic subjects displayed staining for ICAM-1 and E-selectin in the vascular endothelium, together with some ICAM-1 staining in the epithelium. However, the levels of staining were not significantly different between normal and asthmatic subjects, and expression in the asthmatics did not appear to be affected by treatment with inhaled corticosteroids, despite an accompanying decrease in mucosal eosinophilia (Montefort et al, 1992b).

In allergic perennial rhinitis it has been possible to demonstrate increased expression of endothelial ICAM-1 and VCAM-1 compared with nonatopic control subjects. An increase in the number of LFA-1 positive cells correlated with the ICAM-1 expression, and the number of neutrophils correlated with E-selectin expression, although E-selectin itself was not significantly increased (Montefort et al, 1992). It is attractive to propose that the increase in VCAM-1 in rhinitics is mediated at least in part by local release of TNF-α and IL-4, perhaps from mucosal mast cells.

Utilizing endobronchial allergen challenge in asthmatic individuals, it was possible to detect an increase in endothelial ICAM-1 and E-selectin, although not VCAM-1, and once again with a correlating increase in LFA-1 positive cells (Montefort et al, 1994). The accompanying infiltrate included T lymphocytes, eosinophils, neutrophils, and mast cells. The lack of increased VCAM-1 levels may have been related to the time of biopsy at 6 hours after antigen challenge, and increases in VCAM-1 are seen at 24 hours after exposure, with an associated lymphocytic and eosinophilic infiltrate.

Neurogenic Inflammation

Neural mechanisms of asthmatic bronchoconstriction have always been of interest, and this now includes the contribution that they may make toward the inflammatory pattern of the airway. Suggested neural mechanisms of asthma have ranged between increased exposure and sensitivity of the afferent component of airway reflexes, to abnormalities of neural distribution, neurotransmitter content and release, and imbalances of pre- and postjunctional receptor numbers or function. It is unlikely that a fundamental neural abnormality is the primary pathogenesis of asthma. However, there is a continuing view that there is an important relationship between neural and immunologic mechanisms of inflammation. Additional concepts have utilized the expanding knowledge of nonadrenergic noncholinergic (NANC) neural pathways with peptide neurotransmitters, suggesting that abnormalities within this complex system contribute to the inflammation and pathophysiology of the airway (Daniele et al, 1992; Barnes, 1993a).

Autonomic Nerves and Receptors

The cholinergic innervation of airway smooth muscle is the only direct autonomic innervation of the airway musculature, as the sympathetic α and β receptors must rely on circulating or administered catecholamines for their stimulation. The cholinergic nerves are the dominant neural bronchoconstrictor pathway.

An abnormality of cholinergic tone has been a popular proposal, especially when it has been demonstrated that some asthma triggers such as cold air, sulfur dioxide, and esophageal reflux lead to reflex cholinergic bronchoconstriction. Furthermore, the demonstration of asthma induced by pilocarpine, a muscarinic agonist, and the relief of asthma with anticholinergics, such as ipratropium bromide, would lend further support to such a proposal. However, there is little supporting evidence for an overall increase in vagal tone in asthmatics, although this is still potentially relevant for nocturnal bronchoconstriction (Barnes, 1993a).

Alternatively, mediators such as histamine, prostaglandins, and particularly bradykinin may stimulate sensory receptors in the airway and hence induce reflex bronchoconstriction, particularly if axons are exposed by epithelial damage or are hypersensitive in the inflammatory tissue. Cholinergic overactivity may also be caused by the modulatory effects of the adrenergic and NANC systems.

Increased smooth muscle responsiveness to cholinergic stimulation has not been demonstrated to be a specific effect for cholinergic agonists, and a primary abnormality of muscarinic receptor numbers or coupling on smooth muscle is thought to be unlikely. However, the characterization of the muscarinic receptor subtypes into ganglionic pirenzepine-sensitive M_1, inhibitory prejunctional M_2, and excitatory smooth muscle M_3 receptors has opened the way for further more specific investigation. The mutually antagonistic effects of dual stimulation of the M_2 "autoreceptors," which reduce acetylcholine release from the nerve ending, and the M_3 receptor, producing smooth muscle contraction, may provide an explanation for the relative lack of efficacy of agents such as atropine and ipratropium, which are pharmacologically active at both sites. In fact, pilocarpine turns out to act as a selective agonist at M_2 autoreceptors and will inhibit the reflex cholinergic bronchoconstriction produced by sulfur dioxide. However, this is only true for normal subjects, and the lack of such an effect in asthmatics has suggested that they may have an abnormality of this muscarinic receptor subtype, providing a mechanism for enhanced cholinergic reflexes in asthma following the reduction of this negative feedback loop. The basis for this abnormality may lie in the receptors' vulnerability to damage and attenuation from oxidants, virally sourced enzymes during respiratory infection, and other cogeners of airway inflammation such as eosinophil MBP (Barnes, 1993a).

The lack of sympathetic innervation of the airway smooth muscle, the failure to demonstrate abnormal levels of circulating catecholamines, together with the dramatic symptomatic and physiologic relief offered by β agonists, have meant that investigation of possible abnormalities of the adrenergic system have concentrated on possible malfunctions at the receptor level. However, there has not been any convincing demonstration of primary abnormalities of receptor numbers or function, but rather suggestions that down-regulation of receptor numbers is a result of the inflammatory state or its pharmacologic therapy. Uncoupling of the β receptors is unlikely as a general mechanism in asthma, given the therapeutic efficacy of the agonist medications at relieving airflow obstruction.

Inhibitory NANC Neurotransmitters

The peptide neurotransmitters have provided a further direction for investigation, with their effects complicated by their status as "co-transmitters," being stored and released from nerve endings that have a more classic primary function as cholinergic or adrenergic neurones. The "inhibitory NANC" pathway achieved early recognition of its importance as the only neural bronchodilator pathway. A series of neuropeptides such as peptide histidine isoleucine (PHI), galanin, and peptide histidine valine-42 have all been co-localized to the cholinergic nerves, but the dominant neurotransmitter was initially thought to be vasoactive intestinal polypeptide (VIP), which was localized to the cholinergic nerves and ganglia around airways and vessels, with receptors predominantly in the smooth muscle of the larger airways (Barnes et al, 1991).

VIP and PHI are the most abundant lung peptides and are potent bronchodilators and vasodilators, although their bronchodilator effect when inhaled is limited by degradation. VIP may also have a regulatory role in ion and mucus transport and inhibits the release of mediators from pulmonary mast cells. Excessive and particular patterns of stimulation of cholinergic nerves induce VIP release, creating a regulatory role for VIP in areas of excessive bronchoconstriction and possibly improving the blood flow to affected areas, ensuring effective clearance of mediators. VIP also inhibits the further release of acetylcholine from the relevant nerve endings. Mast cell tryptase is highly effective at degrading VIP and may account for early reports of the absence of this neurotransmitter in asthmatic airways (Fig. 32–10). However, studies using chymotrypsin to diminish any VIP bronchodilator effect have failed to support the importance of this neuropeptide in human airways (Barnes et al, 1991; Barnes, 1993a).

It now appears that nitric oxide (NO) is the most important inhibitory NANC neurotransmitter. Inhibitors of NO synthase abolish the neural bronchodilator response in human airways *in vitro*, and characteristically increase the cholinergic neural response. NO may act as a functional antagonist to acetylcholine. Several forms of NO synthase contribute to its production, some of which are inducible and are altered in the asthmatic state (Spring-

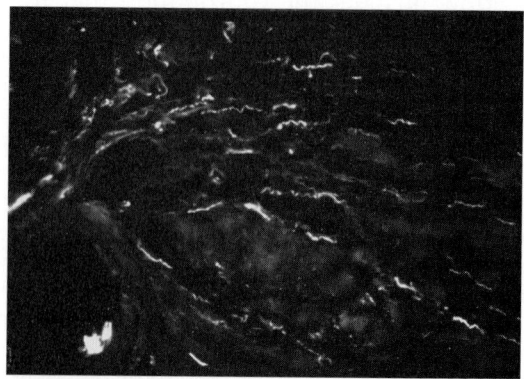

FIGURE 32–10. Frozen section of a human bronchial biopsy immunostained for VIP by indirect immunofluorescence. Staining is evident in nerve fibers in bronchial smooth muscle (magnification ×360). (Courtesy Dr. D. Springall.)

all et al, 1993), together with increased degradation of NO by oxidants in the inflamed tissue. Production of NO by epithelium, endothelium, macrophages, and neutrophils may paradoxically contribute to airway inflammation by increasing blood flow and capillary plasma leakage. These adverse effects of high concentrations of NO may be prevented by the inhibition of inducible NO synthase by corticosteroids (Barnes, 1993b).

Excitatory NANC Neurotransmitters

The candidate "excitatory NANC" neurotransmitters are co-localized to the nerve endings of unmyelinated sensory (afferent) nerves, or C-fibers, and include the tachykinins—substance P (SP), neurokinin A (NKA), and neurokinin B (NKB)—together with calcitonin gene–related peptide (CGRP) and gastrin-releasing peptide. SP is localized to sensory nerve endings in the airways of several species and is thought to be transported down these capsaicin-sensitive nerves from its site of synthesis in the nodose ganglion of the vagus. There may be an increased population of SP-containing nerves identified in the airways of asthma fatalities, suggesting a degree of neural tropism in the face of chronic inflammation. However, the significance of tachykinins in the human airway is uncertain (Barnes, 1993a).

Calcitonin gene–related peptide is co-stored and co-localized with substance P. It is a potent vasodilator with a long duration of action and may be the dominant bronchial arterial dilator, but in contrast to SP it has no effect on vascular leakage.

The effects of SP, NKA, and NKB are mediated through different receptors known as NK1, NK2, and NK3, respectively. Their mechanism of action upon smooth muscle may be indirect, but ultimately they stimulate phosphoinositide hydrolysis and increase the formation of IP_3, leading to increased intracellular release of calcium ions. SP is a potent factor in causing microvascular leakage. It stimulates goblet cell mucus secretion and also has degranulating effects on skin mast cells and on eosinophils. NKA is the more potent bronchospastic agent, while both NKA and SP cause an increase in airway blood flow. SP may facilitate cholinergic transmission through postganglionic terminals and may also inhibit the NANC bronchodilator pathway (Barnes et al, 1991).

The tachykinins are degraded near their sites of release and activity by either angiotensin converting enzyme in vascular endothelial cells or by neutral endopeptidase (NEP, enkephalinase) found in the basal epithelial cells, smooth muscle, and glandular sites. The importance of this second enzyme is demonstrated by the disruption of the airway epithelium, either mechanically or by a respiratory viral infection, which enhances the bronchoconstrictor potency of the tachykinins, presumably by limiting their degradation (Nadel, 1992). This effect can be simulated by the use of NEP inhibitors such as phosphoramidone and thiorphan, as has been demonstrated in human airways *in vivo* (Cheung et al, 1992). NEP may be a critical step at which a variety of stimuli, most notably viral infections, predispose the airways to increased neurogenic inflammation. NEP was induced by glucocorticoid treatment of human epithelial cells in tissue culture, and it has been demonstrated to be the mechanism by which steroids may reduce neurogenic inflammation in an animal model (Nadel, 1992).

The release of the excitatory NANC neuropeptides is thought to be the result of local axon reflexes. Sensory nerve endings in the inflamed airways may be both physically exposed, by epithelial shedding and tissue damage, and chemically sensitized, by the local release and activity of mediators and cytokines. Such hypersensitivity or "hyperesthesia" has been demonstrated to be induced by inhaled bradykinin, and it is suggested that symptoms of chest tightness and coughing may be the subjective corollary of such increased neural activity. Stimulation of the sensory nerve endings is accompanied by a degree of antidromic or retrograde conduction, leading to the release of the neuropeptides co-localized within the C-fibers (Barnes, 1993a).

The potential for pharmacologic manipulation of these pathways is of biologic and therapeutic interest. Tachykinin antagonists are under development. Another approach is to exploit the existing neuromodulatory pathways offered by prejunctional receptors for NPY, VIP, adenosine, and catecholamines, which may be mediated by a common potassium channel. Enkephalins inhibit NANC transmission via μ-opioid receptors at the sensory nerve endings. Drugs such as cromoglycate, nedocromil, and even furosemide may have a role in preventing the activation of sensory nerves, hence their effectiveness in reducing reflex-mediated bronchoconstriction precipitated by stimuli such as exercise and metabisulfite (Barnes, 1993a).

CONCLUSION

Our knowledge and understanding of asthma has advanced rapidly. This has been facilitated by the improved techniques of investigation available in laboratory and clinical areas, together with a merging of interests and activities shared between investigators from biologic, immunologic, and medical fields.

The roles of particular inflammatory cells and mediators are continually being expanded and clarified. This is clearly important work. However, it is ever more apparent that no single abnormality of cell, mediator, or neurotransmitter will be sufficient to describe the pathogenesis of asthma. An improved understanding of the interactions of the various elements of the inflammatory response is developing. The control and coordination administered by cytokines, adhesion molecules, and neurogenic mechanisms offer future directions for further insights into the pathology of asthma.

REFERENCES

Anwar ARF, Moqbel R, Walsh GM, et al. Adhesion to fibronectin prolongs eosinophil survival. J Exp Med 177:839–843, 1993.

Azzawi M, Bradley B, Jeffery PK, et al. Identification of activated T lymphocytes and eosinophils in bronchial biopsies in stable atopic asthma. Am Rev Respir Dis 142:1407–1413, 1990.

Baggiolini M. Neutrophil activation and the role of interleukin-8 and related cytokines. Int Arch Allergy Appl Immunol 99:196–199, 1992.

Barnes PJ. Neural mechanisms in asthma. In Holgate ST, Austen KF, Lichtenstein LM, Kay AB (eds). Asthma: Physiology, Immunopharmacology, and Treatment. Fourth International Symposium. London, Academic Press Limited, 1993a.

Barnes PJ. Nitric oxide and airways. Eur Resp J 6:163–165, 1993b.

Barnes PJ, Baraniuk JN, Belvisi MG. Neuropeptides in the respiratory tract. Am Rev Respir Dis 144:1187–1198, 1991.

Beasley R, Roche WR, Roberts JA, et al. Cellular events in the bronchi in mild asthma and after bronchial provocation. Am Rev Respir Dis 139:806–817, 1989.

Becker S, Koren HS, Henke DC. Interleukin-8 expression in normal nasal epithelium and its modulation by infection with respiratory syncytial virus and cytokines tumor necrosis factor, interleukin-1, and interleukin-6. Am J Respir Cell Mol Biol 3:20–27, 1993.

Bentley AM, Meng Q, Robinson DS, et al. Increases in activated T lymphocytes, eosinophils, and cytokine mRNA expression for interleukin-5 and granulocyte/macrophage colony-stimulating factor in bronchial biopsies after allergen inhalational challenge in atopic asthmatics. Am J Respir Cell Mol Biol 8:35–42, 1993.

Bevilacqua MP, Nelson RM. Selectins. J Clin Invest 91:379–387, 1993.

Bischoff SC, Dahinden CA. c-*kit* ligand: A unique potentiator for mediator release by human lung mast cells. J Exp Med 175:237–244, 1992.

Bochner BS, Luscinskas FW, Gimbrone MA, et al. Adhesion of human basophils, eosinophils, and neutrophils to interleukin-1–activated human vascular endothelial cells: Contributions of endothelial cell adhesion molecules. J Exp Med 173:1553–1556, 1991.

Bousquet J, Chanez P, Lacoste JY, et al. Eosinophilic inflammation in asthma. N Engl J Med 323:1033–1039, 1990.

Bradding P, Roberts JA, Britten KM, et al. Interleukins (IL)-4, -5, -6 and TNFα in normal and asthmatic airways: Evidence for the human mast cell as an important source of these cytokines. Am J Respir Cell Mol Biol 10:471–480, 1994.

Bradley BL, Azzawi M, Jacobson M, et al. Eosinophils, T lymphocytes, mast cells, neutrophils, and macrophages in bronchial biopsies from atopic subjects with asthma: Comparison with biopsy specimens from atopic subjects without asthma and normal control subjects and relationship to bronchial hyperresponsiveness. J Allergy Clin Immunol 88:661–674, 1991.

Broide DH, Firestein GS. Endobronchial allergen challenge in asthma. J Clin Invest 88:1048–1053, 1991a.

Broide DH, Gleich GJ, Cuomo AJ, et al. Evidence of ongoing mast cell and eosinophil degranulation in symptomatic asthma airway. J Allergy Clin Immunol 88:637–648, 1991b.

Broide DH, Lotz M, Cuomo AJ, et al. Cytokines in symptomatic asthma airways. J Allergy Clin Immunol 89:958–967, 1992.

Bruijnzeel PLB, Rihs S, Virchow JC, et al. Early activation or "priming" of eosinophils in asthma. Schweiz Med Wochenschr 122:298–301, 1992.

Bruijnzeel PLB, Virchow JC, Rihs S, et al. Lack of increased numbers of low-density eosinophils in the circulation of asthmatic individuals. J Allergy Clin Immunol 23:261–269, 1993.

Brunner T, Heusser CH, Dahinden CA. Human peripheral blood basophils primed by interleukin 3 (IL-3) produce IL-4 in response to immunoglobulin E receptor stimulation. J Exp Med 177:605–611, 1993.

Cheung D, Bel EH, Hartigh JD, et al. The effect of an inhaled neutral endopeptidase inhibitor, thiorphan, on airway responses to neurokinin A in normal humans in vivo. Am Rev Respir Dis 145:1275–1280, 1992.

Cockcroft DW, Murdock KY. Comparative effects of inhaled salbutamol, sodium cromoglycate, and beclomethasone dipropionate on allergen-induced early asthmatic responses, late asthmatic responses, and increased bronchial responsiveness to histamine. J Allergy Clin Immunol 79:734–740, 1987.

Cookson WCOM, Craddock CF, Benson MK, et al. Falls in peripheral eosinophil counts parallel the late asthmatic response. Am Rev Respir Dis 139:458–462, 1989.

Corrigan CJ, Haczku A, Gemou-Engesaeth V, et al. CD4 T-lymphocyte activation in asthma is accompanied by increased serum concentrations of interleukin-5. Am J Respir Cell Mol Biol 147:540–547, 1993.

Corrigan CJ, Kay AB. CD4 T-lymphocyte activation in acute severe asthma. Am Rev Respir Dis 141:970–977, 1990.

Dahinden CA, Bischoff SC, Brunner T, et al. Regulation of mediator release by human basophils: Importance of the sequence and time of addition in the combined action of different agonists. Int Arch Allergy Appl Immunol 94:161–164, 1991.

Daniele RP, Barnes PJ, Goetzl EJ, et al. Neuroimmune interactions in the lung. Am Rev Respir Dis 145:1230–1235, 1992.

Del Prete G. Human T_{H1} and T_{H2} lymphocytes: Their role in the pathophysiology of atopy. Allergy 47:450–455, 1992.

Desreumaux P, Janin A, Colombel JF, et al. Interleukin-5 messenger RNA expression by eosinophils in the intestinal mucosa of patients with coeliac disease. J Exp Med 175:293–296, 1992.

Djukanović R, Roche WR, Wilson JW, et al. State of the art: Mucosal inflammation in asthma. Am Rev Respir Dis 142:434–457, 1990a.

Djukanović R, Wilson JW, Britten KM, et al. Quantitation of mast cells and eosinophils in the bronchial mucosa of symptomatic atopic asthmatics and healthy control subjects using immunohistochemistry. Am Rev Respir Dis 142:863–871, 1990b.

Djukanović R, Wilson JW, Britten KM, et al. Effect of an inhaled corticosteroid on airway inflammation and symptoms in asthma. Am Rev Respir Dis 145:669–674, 1992.

Dunill MS. The pathology of asthma, with special reference to changes in the bronchial mucosa. J Clin Pathol 13:27–33, 1960.

Durham SR, Lee TH, Cromwell O, et al. Immunologic studies in allergen-induced late-phase asthmatic reactions. J Allergy Clin Immunol 74:49–60, 1984.

Ebisawa M, Bochner BS, Georas SN, et al. Eosinophil transendothelial migration induced by cytokines.1. Role of endothelial and eosinophil adhesion molecules in IL-1β–induced transendothelial migration. J Immunol 149:4021–4028, 1991.

Ebisawa M, Yamada T, Klunk D, et al. Regulation of eosinophil and neutrophil transendothelial migration by cytokines and chemokines. J Allergy Clin Immunol 91:313, 1993. (Abstract)

Gonzalez C, Diaz P, Galleluillos F, et al. Antigen-induced recruitment of bronchoalveolar helper (OKT4) and suppressor (OKT8) T-cells in asthma. Am Rev Respir Dis 136:600–604, 1987.

Gratziou C, Carroll M, Walls A, et al. Early changes in T lymphocytes recovered by bronchoalveolar lavage after local allergen challenge of asthmatic airways. Am Rev Respir Dis 145:1259–1264, 1992.

Gundel RH, Wegner CD, Letts LG. Antigen-induced acute and late-phase responses in primates. Am Rev Respir Dis 146:369–373, 1992.

Gundel RH, Wegner CD, Torcellini CA, et al. Endothelial leukocyte adhesion molecule-1 mediates antigen-induced acute airway inflammation and late-phase airway obstruction in monkeys. J Clin Invest 88:1407–1411, 1991.

Hamid Q, Azzawi M, Ying S, et al. Expression of mRNA for interleukin-5 in mucosal bronchial biopsies from asthma. J Clin Invest 87:1541–1546, 1991.

Hansel TT, Walker C. The migration of eosinophils into the sputum of asthmatics: the role of adhesion molecules. Clin Exp Allergy 22:345–356, 1992.

Hartnell A, Moqbel R, Walsh GM, et al. Fcγ and CD11/CD18 receptor expression on normal-density and low-density human eosinophils. Immunology 69:264–270, 1990.

Holt PG. Macrophage: Dendritic cell interaction in regulation of the IgE response in asthma. Clin Exp Allergy 23:4–6, 1993.

Holt PG, McMenamin C, Schon-Hegrad MA, et al. Immunoregulation of asthma: control of T-lymphocyte activation in the respiratory tract. Eur Resp J 4(Suppl 13):6s–15s, 1991.

Irani AA, Schechter NM, Craig S, et al. Two types of human mast cells that have distinct neutral protease compositions. Proc Natl Acad Sci USA 83:4464–4468, 1986.

Jeffery PK, Wardlaw AJ, Nelson FC, et al. Bronchial biopsies in asthma: An ultrastructural, quantitative study and correlation with hyperreactivity. Am Rev Respir Dis 140:1745–1753, 1989.

Kameyoshi Y, Dorschner A, Mallet AI, et al. Cytokine RANTES released by thrombin-stimulated platelets is a potent chemoattractant for human eosinophils. J Exp Med 176:587–592, 1992.

Kay AB, Ying S, Varney V, et al. Messenger RNA expression of the cytokine gene cluster, IL-3, IL-4, IL-5 and GM-CSF in allergen-induced late-phase cutaneous reactions in atopic subjects. J Exp Med 173:775–778, 1991.

Kita H, Tsukasa O, Okubo Y, et al. Granulocyte/macrophage colony-stimulating factor and interleukin 3 release from human peripheral blood eosinophils and neutrophils. J Exp Med 174:745–748, 1991.

Kuna P, Reddigari SR, Schall TJ, et al. Characterization of the human basophil response to cytokines, growth factors, and histamine-releasing factors of the intercrine/chemokine family. J Immunol 150:1932–1943, 1993.

Laitinen LA, Heino M, Laitenen A, et al. Damage of the airway epithelium and bronchial reactivity in patients with asthma. Am Rev Respir Dis 1985:599–606, 1985.

Laitinen LA, Laitinen A, Haahtela T. Airway mucosal inflammation even in patients with newly diagnosed asthma. Am Rev Respir Dis 147:697–704, 1993.

Lane SJ, Soh C, Hallsworth MP, et al. Monocytes and macrophages in asthma. Int Arch Allergy Immunol 99:200–203, 1992.

Liu MC, Hubbard WC, Proud D, et al. Immediate and late inflammatory responses to ragweed antigen challenge of the peripheral airways in allergic asthmatics. Am Rev Respir Dis 144:51–58, 1991.

Lozewicz S, Wells C, Gomez E, et al. Morphological integrity of the bronchial epithelium in mild asthma. Thorax 45:12–15, 1990.

Marini M, Vittori E, Hollemberg J, et al. Expression of the potent inflammatory cytokines, granulocyte-macrophage-stimulating factor and interleukin-6 and interleukin-8, in bronchial epithelial cells of patients with asthma. J Allergy Clin Immunol 89:1001–1009, 1992.

Massey WA, Lichtenstein LM. Role of basophils in human allergic disease. Int Arch Allergy Appl Immunol 92:184–188, 1992.

Metzger WJ, Zavala D, Richerson HB, et al. Local allergen challenge and bronchoalveolar lavage of allergic asthmatic lungs. Am Rev Respir Dis 135:433–440, 1987.

Montefort S, Feather IH, Wilson SJ, et al. The expression of leukocyte-endothelial adhesion molecules is increased in perennial allergic rhinitis. Am J Respir Cell Mol Biol 7:393–398, 1992.

Montefort S, Gratziou C, Goulding D, et al. Bronchial biopsy evidence for leukocyte infiltration and up-regulation of leukocyte-endothelial cell adhesion molecules 6 hours after local allergen challenge of sensitized asthmatic airways. J Clin Invest 93:1411–1421, 1994.

Montefort S, Herbert CA, Robinson C, et al. The bronchial epithelium as a target for inflammatory attack in asthma. Clin Exp Allergy 22:511–520, 1992a.

Montefort S, Roche WR, Howarth PH, et al. Intercellular adhesion molecule-1 (ICAM-1) and endothelial leucocyte adhesion molecule-1 (ELAM-1) expression in the bronchial mucosa of normal and asthmatic subjects. Eur Resp J 5:815–823, 1992b.

Moser R, Fehr J, Olgiati L, et al. Migration of primed human eosinophils across cytokine-activated endothelial cell monolayers. Blood 79:2937–2945, 1992.

Mossman TR, Coffman RL. Th1 and Th2 cells: Different patterns of lymphokine secretion lead to different functional properties. Annu Rev Immunol 7:145–173, 1989.

Murray JJ, Tonnel AB, Brash AR, et al. Release of prostaglandin D2 into human airways during acute allergen challenge. N Engl J Med 315:800–804, 1986.

Nadel JA. Regulation of neurogenic inflammation by neutral endopeptidase. Am Rev Respir Dis 145:S48–S52, 1992.

Ohashi Y, Motojima S, Takeshi F, et al. Airway hyperresponsiveness, increased intracellular spaces of bronchial epithelium, and increased infiltration of eosinophils and lymphocytes in bronchial mucosa in asthma. Am Rev Respir Dis 145:1469–1476, 1992.

Ohnishi T, Kita H, Weiler D, et al. IL-5 is the predominant eosinophil-active cytokine in the antigen-induced pulmonary late-phase reaction. Am Rev Respir Dis 147:901–907, 1993.

Pesci A, Foresi A, Bertorelli G, et al. Histochemical characteristics and degranulation of mast cells in epithelium and lamina propria of bronchial biopsies from asthmatic and normal subjects. Am Rev Respir Dis 147:684–689, 1993.

Plaut M, Pierce JH, Watson CJ, et al. Mast cells produce lymphokines in response to cross-linkage of FcϵRI or to calcium ionophores. Nature 339:65–67, 1989.

Poston RN, Chanez P, Lacoste JY, et al. Immunohistochemical characterization of the cellular infiltration in asthmatic bronchi. Am Rev Respir Dis 145:918–921, 1992.

Proud D. The epithelial cell as a target and effector cell in airway inflammation. In Holgate ST, Austen KF, Lichtenstein LM, Kay AB (eds). Asthma: Physiology, Immunopharmacology and Treatment. Fourth International Symposium, London, Academic Press Limited, 1993.

Rand TH, Cruikshank WW, Center DM, et al. CD4-mediated stimulation of human eosinophils: Lymphocyte chemoattractant factor and other CD-4 binding ligands elicit eosinophil migration. J Exp Med 173:1521–1528, 1991a.

Rand TH, Silberstein DS, Kornfeld H, et al. Human eosinophils express functional interleukin-2 receptors. J Clin Invest 88:825–832, 1991b.

Robinson DS, Hamid Q, Ying S, et al. Predominant TH2-like bronchoalveolar T-lymphocyte population in atopic asthma. N Engl J Med 326:298–304, 1992.

Roche WR, Beasley R, Williams JH, et al. Subepithelial fibrosis in the bronchi of asthmatics. Lancet 2:520–524, 1989.

Romagnani S, Del Prete G, Maggi E, et al. Human Th1 and Th2 Subsets. Int Arch Allergy Appl Immunol 99:242–245, 1991.

Smith CW, Kishimoto TK, Abbass O, et al. Chemotactic factors regulate lectin adhesion molecule 1 (LECAM-1)-dependent neutrophil adhesion to cytokine-stimulated endothelial cells in vitro. J Clin Invest 87:609–618, 1991.

Soderberg M, Hellstrom S, Sandstrom T, et al. Structural characterization of bronchial mucosal biopsies from healthy volunteers: A light and electron microscopical study. Eur Resp J 3:261–266, 1990.

Spencer DA. An update on PAF. Clin Exp Allergy 22:521–524, 1992.

Springall DR, Hamid QA, Buttery LKD, et al. Nitric oxide synthase induction in airways of asthmatic subjects. Am Rev Respir Dis 147:A515, 1993.

Springall DR, Howarth PH, Counihan H, et al. Endothelin immunoreactivity of airway epithelium in asthmatic patients. Lancet 337:697–701, 1991.

Staunton DE, Merluzzi VJ, Rothlein R, et al. A cell adhesion molecule, ICAM-1, is the major surface receptor for rhinoviruses. Cell 56:849–853, 1989.

Tanaka Y, Adams DH, Shaw S. Proteoglycans on endothelial cells present adhesion-inducing cytokines to leukocytes. Immunology Today 14:111–115, 1993.

Tanimoto Y, Takahashi K, Kimura I. Effects of cytokines on human basophil chemotaxis. Clin Exp Allergy 22:1020–1025, 1992.

Thorne KJI, Richardson BA, Mazza G, et al. A new method for measuring eosinophil activating factors, based on the increased expression of CR3 α chain (CD11b) on the surface of activated eosinophils. J Immunol Methods 133:47–54, 1990.

Tomassini M, Tsicopoulos A, Tai PC, et al. Release of granule proteins by eosinophils from allergic and nonallergic patients with eosinophilia on immunoglobulin-dependent activation. J Allergy Clin Immunol 88:365–375, 1991.

Walker C, Bode E, Boer L, et al. Allergic and nonallergic asthmatics have distinct patterns of T-cell activation and cytokine production in peripheral blood and bronchoalveolar lavage. Am Rev Respir Dis 146:109–115, 1992.

Walker C, Virchow JC, Bruijnzeel PLB, et al. T cell subsets and their soluble products regulate eosinophilia in allergic and nonallergic asthma. J Immunol 146:1829–1835, 1991.

Walsh GM, Hartnell A, Wardlaw AJ, et al. IL-5 enhances the in vitro adhesion of human eosinophils, in a leukocyte integrin (CD11/18)-dependent manner. Immunology 71:258–265, 1990.

Walsh LJ, Trinchieri G, Waldorf HA, et al. Human dermal mast cells contain and release tumour necrosis factor alpha, which induces endothelial leukocyte adhesion molecule 1. Proc Natl Acad Sci USA 88:4220–4224, 1991.

Wardlaw AJ, Dunnette S, Gleich GJ, et al. Eosinophils and mast cells in bronchoalveolar lavage in subjects with mild asthma. Relationship to bronchial hyperreactivity. Am Rev Respir Dis 137:62–69, 1988.

Wegner CD, Gundel RH, Reilly P, et al. Intercellular adhesion molecule-1 (ICAM-1) in the pathogenesis of asthma. Science 247:456–459, 1990.

Wenzel SE, Fowler AA, Schwartz LB. Activation of pulmonary mast cells by bronchoalveolar allergen challenge: In vivo release of histamine and tryptase in atopic subjects with and without asthma. Am Rev Respir Dis 137:1002–1008, 1988.

Wenzel SE, Larsin GL, Johnston K, et al. Elevated levels of leukotriene C4 in bronchoalveolar lavage fluid from atopic asthmatics after endobronchial allergen challenge. Am Rev Respir Dis 142:112–119, 1990.

Wenzel SE, Westcott JY, Larsen GI. Bronchoalveolar lavage fluid mediator levels 5 minutes after allergen challenge in atopic patients with asthma: Relationship to the development of late asthmatic responses. J Allergy Clin Immunol 87:540–584, 1991.

Wilson JW, Djukanović R, Howarth PH, et al. Lymphocyte activation in bronchoalveolar lavage and peripheral blood in atopic asthma. Am Rev Respir Dis 145:958–960, 1992.

Zimmerman GA, Prescott SM, McIntyre M. Endothelial cell interactions with granulocytes: Tethering and signalling molecules. Immunology Today 13:93–100, 1992.

Chapter 33

Asthma Epidemiology: Risk Factors and Natural History

Scott T. Weiss, M.D., M.S.

Asthma, a chronic obstructive airway disease that affects 10 million Americans, is primarily a disease of childhood; 30 percent of all asthmatics are under the age of 18, and roughly half of all these asthma cases are diagnosed by age 5. Adult asthma is also extremely common and often occurs in combination with chronic obstructive lung disease. It is estimated that 60 to 80 percent of all patients with chronic obstructive lung disease also have reversible airflow obstruction. There is evidence that the prevalence of asthma and its rate of hospitalization have increased over the past 20 years. The overall costs of asthma care in the United States currently exceed $4 billion per year. Primary preventable costs relate to hospitalizations and emergency room visits. This chapter will review common definitions of asthma, and particularly how these definitions impact on the epidemiology of the disease. We will also consider trends in asthma prevalence and incidence, and factors that may have an impact on disease occurrence. There have been changes in the role of airway responsiveness and atopy in their relationship to the asthma syndrome. Thus, the relationship of airway responsiveness to asthma and the relationship of atopy to asthma will be discussed. A variety of factors may modify the risk of getting asthma as a disease. These will also be considered. Finally, asthma mortality and asthma severity will be discussed.

DEFINITIONS

Asthma is a clinical syndrome that is characterized by: (1) airway inflammation, (2) increased airway responsiveness, and (3) variable airflow obstruction (National Asthma Education Program, 1991). Unfortunately, this syndromic definition does not allow clinicians to clearly define subgroups of patients with unique natural histories and clinical courses. In addition, this definition begs the issue of how inflammation and airway responsiveness are related. This is currently controversial and unclear based on the existing literature. Clinically, it is important to recognize that the heavy overlap of symptoms traditionally associated with both chronic obstructive lung disease and asthma seriously compromises identification of asthmatic subjects by symptoms alone. Because asthma is a syndrome, traditional clinical relationships suggest that wheezing in a nonsmoking atopic subject is likely to be asthma, whereas wheezing in a nonatopic older smoker with cough is more likely to be chronic obstructive lung disease. These findings suggest that, because of the vagueness of current definitions, significant observational bias may be present in a doctor's diagnosis of asthma as a disease. In general, epidemiologists have tended to rely on historical or questionnaire sources to identify patients with asthma. Cases have been identified either by physicians or by surveys of population groups in which the definition of who is asthmatic has been left to the patients themselves, parents of patients, or the report of the diagnosis having been made by the patient's physician. Clearly, each of these methods of identifying asthma patients has inherent weaknesses. One must assume that some bias in the reporting of cases is present in each group, and it is more likely that the biases in each method of gathering data are different. Clearly, comparisons among different countries, regions, and population groups that depend on different diagnostic criteria must be tentative, at best. The advantages and disadvantages of clinical, questionnaire, and physiologic approaches to identifying persons with asthma are summarized in Table 33–1.

ASTHMA PREVALENCE

In 1970, as part of the Health Interview Survey, a national sample of 116,000 people from 37,000 randomly selected households in the United States were asked if they had seen a physician for asthma in the preceding 2 weeks. The overall disease prevalence was 3 percent, with slightly higher rates reported for younger (<6 years) and older (>65 years) males. Some regional variation of the disease was also reported, with the southern (4.4 percent) and western (2.3 percent) parts of the country reporting slightly more asthma than the northeast (2.0 percent) (Weiss et al, 1993). Since that 1970 report, NHIS survey data suggest that, for children and adolescents (under 17 years of age), there has been a 23 percent increase in asthma prevalence, from 3.1 to 3.8 per 100 population, from 1970 to 1980. Based on data on 6- to 11-year-old children from the National Health and Nutrition Survey (NHANES Study), asthma prevalence has increased from 4.8 per 100,000 in NHANES I (1971 to 1974) to 7.6 per 100,000 population in NHANES II (1976 to 1980), a 58 percent increase (Fig. 33–1). The reasons for these increases in asthma prevalence are unclear. However, it is known that increased survival of infants with prematurity, increased cigarette smoking by women of childbearing age, and poverty are all factors that have contributed to the increase in asthma prevalence in children. It is also possible that increased physician awareness and changes in diagnostic and prescribing patterns may also have influenced physicians' attitudes toward this important public health problem.

RELATIONSHIP OF AIRWAY RESPONSIVENESS TO ASTHMA

Airway responsiveness is traditionally measured using some bronchoconstrictive stimulus and then looking at progressive decline in pulmonary function. The most common pharmacologic stimuli are histamine and methacholine. Increasing bronchoconstrictor doses of histamine or methacholine are given, and when the patient's FEV_1 decreases by 20 percent of baseline, the dose at which this drop occurs is considered the PD_{20}. In general, asthmatic subjects are more responsive than nonasthmatic subjects. Cockcroft and co-workers (1977) originally defined a PD_{20} of 8 mg or less as being the asthmatic range for increased airway responsiveness. Recently, population-based studies have begun to examine more closely the relationship of airway responsiveness to asthma. A variety of population-based surveys of children and adults, conducted in many different countries and using many different techniques for measuring airway responsiveness, defined extremely high prevalences of airway responsiveness in the general population (Table 33–2). The prevalence of airway responsiveness exceeds the prevalence of asthma two- to fivefold.

TABLE 33–1. APPROACHES FOR IDENTIFYING PERSONS WITH ASTHMA

Method	Problems
Clinical evaluation	Nonstandardization of physician criteria for diagnosis; bias toward more severe cases; bias by access to physician.
Questionnaire history of diagnosis	Same as above, plus recall bias subjects.
Questionnaire history of symptoms	Possibly influenced by frequency of other symptoms; less specific than physician's diagnosis.
Response to bronchodilator	May be influenced by level of FEV_1 correlation with bronchodilator; may lack sensitivity.
Bronchoconstrictor response	Influenced by level of FEV_1; may be nonspecific.

Modified from Samet J. Epidemiologic approaches for the identification of asthma. Chest 91:745, 1987.

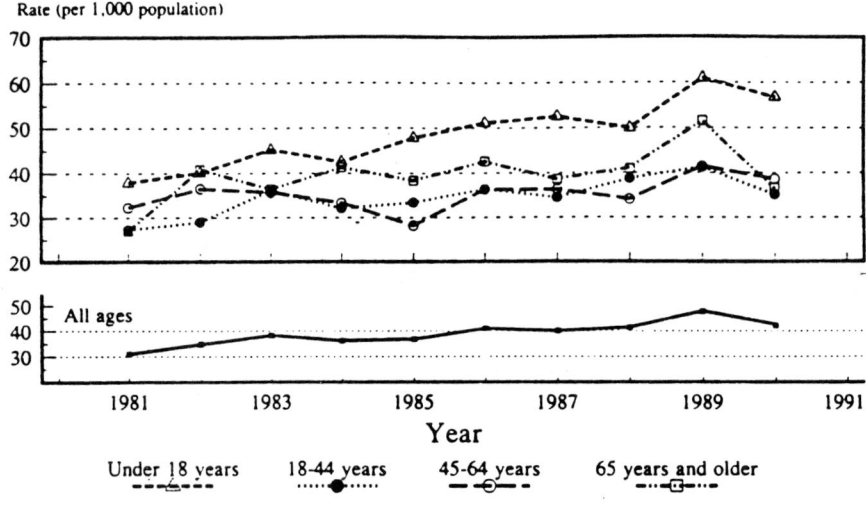

FIGURE 33–1. Trends in asthma prevalence in the United States, 1981 to 1990. (From Weiss KB, Gergen PJ, Wagener DK. Breathing better or wheezing worse? The changing epidemiology of asthma morbidity and mortality. Annu Rev Publ Health 14:494, 1993.)

These studies also demonstrated that increased airway responsiveness was log-normally distributed in populations. An example of this is given in Figure 33–2. In this population-based distribution of histamine airway responsiveness, symptomatic subjects appear at the more responsive end of the distribution, but there is considerable overlap with asymptomatic subjects. This phenomenon has been repeatedly demonstrated in population-based studies, in which a large number of asymptomatic subjects have been found in prevalence surveys (Fig. 33–3).

In addition, a variety of studies in both children and adults have demonstrated that airway responsiveness precedes and predicts

TABLE 33–2. PREVALENCE OF INCREASED AIRWAY RESPONSIVENESS (AR) IN RANDOM POPULATION SAMPLE

Country	Population	Test	% Prevalence of AR	Prevalence of Asymptomatic AR % Total Population	% of all AR Subjects
United States (Weiss et al, 1984)	Random Ages 6–24	Cold air	22	11	51
Australia (Woolcock et al, 1987)	Random Ages 8–11	Histamine	17.9	6.7	37
New Zealand (Sears et al, 1986)	Random Age 9	Methacholine	22	8	30
Australia (Salome et al, 1987)	Random Adults >21	Histamine	11	2	19
Netherlands (Rijcken et al, 1987)	Random Ages 14–64	Histamine	24.5	14	58.5
United States (Sparrow et al, 1987)	Health-screened Ages 40–80	Methacholine	29.9	—	—
England (Burney et al, 1987)	Random Ages 18–64	Methacholine	14	—	—

Adapted from Weiss ST, O'Connor GT, Sparrow D. The role of allergy and airway responsiveness in the natural history of chronic airflow obstruction. *In* Weiss ST, Sparrow D (eds). Airway Responsiveness and Atopy in the Development of Chronic Obstructive Lung Disease. New York, Raven Press, 1989, p 220.

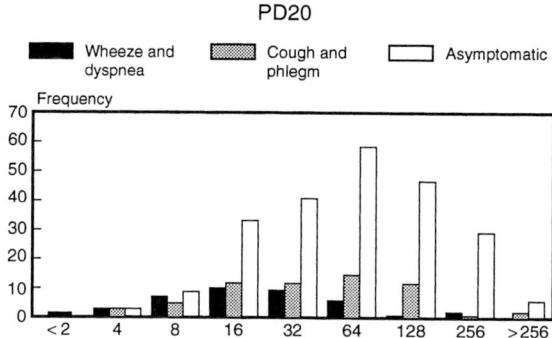

FIGURE 33–2. Distribution of PD_{20} by symptom group: Vlaardingen, The Netherlands, 1984. (Adapted from Rijcken B, Schouten JP, Weiss ST, Meinesz AF, de Vries K, van der Lende R. The distribution of nonspecific bronchial responsiveness in symptomatic and asymptomatic subjects: A population-based analysis of various indices of responsiveness. Am Rev Respir Dis 140:620, 1989.)

the development of asthma. One of the more interesting studies was a case-cohort study performed by Zhong et al (1992), in which 80 subjects with increased airway responsiveness but no asthma symptoms were matched with 80 controls, and followed up 4 years later with regard to their asthma risks. Subjects with increased airway responsiveness had a four- to fivefold greater risk of developing asthma in the follow-up interval when compared to subjects without increased airway responsiveness. These findings suggest that there are three potential models for the relationship between inflammation and airway responsiveness and their relationship to asthma. These three models are presented in Figure 33–3. The series model suggests that airway responsiveness and inflammation are separate characteristics and do not interact with regard to the development of asthma. The parallel model, which is the most commonly accepted model, suggests that all airway responsiveness is a result of inflammation and that the airway responsiveness is not an independent factor in the pathophysiologic chain predicting asthma. The third model, the combined model, suggests that there is some interrelationship between inflammation and airway responsiveness, but both are separate factors predicting the development of asthma as a disease. On the basis of current data, it is unclear which of these three models is the most appropriate for considering the relationship of airway responsiveness and inflammation to the development of asthma. It would appear, from the existing epidemiologic data, that the combined model is the most appropriate, although no studies to date have looked at both inflammation and airway responsiveness independently as predictors of disease.

Based on existing epidemiologic data, however, it would appear that a variety of indigenous host characteristics and environmental exposures can change an individual's airway responsiveness and move it in a more responsive direction.

RELATIONSHIP OF ALLERGY TO ASTHMA

Allergy refers to immediate (type 1) hypersensitivity to an antigen encountered by inhalation, ingestion, or cutaneous contact (Hopp et al, 1984). Increased production of antigen-specific immunoglobulin (IgE) by sensitized

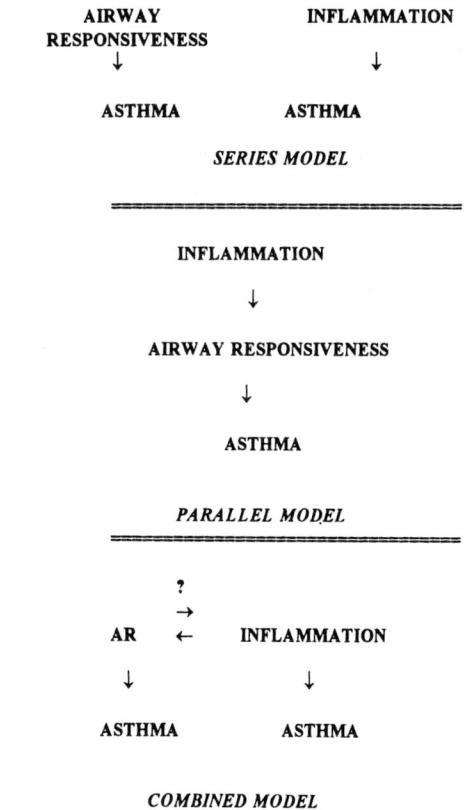

FIGURE 33–3. Three models of relationship of airway responsiveness to asthma (see text).

lymphocytes plays an essential role in the pathophysiology of this process. Atopy is a more narrowly defined condition than allergy. It is characterized by clinical manifestations, such as immediate-type hypersensitivity, immediate wheal and flare skin reactions to common environmental antigens, and familial aggregation. Atopic subjects represent a subset of all allergic subjects. Allergy or atopy can be detected in clinical studies by measuring serum total or specific IgE level, or by measuring cutaneous immediate hypersensitivity to common environmental aeroallergens. The pathophysiology of the allergic response is discussed elsewhere. Briefly, serum levels of IgE antibody are regulated by two distinct T cell populations. Helper/inducer T cells induce and enhance IgE synthesis, whereas suppressor T cells inhibit IgE synthesis. These T cell regulators are controlled by a variety of self-signaling cytokines and by the level and mode of presentation of the relevant environmental antigen. Serum total and specific IgE measurements are useful markers of allergy in clinical and epidemiologic research. Skin testing—prick, scratch, or intradermal—has been utilized as an additional clinical technique to identify the presence of hypersensitivity to environmental allergens. Currently, prick tests are the standard for clinical and epidemiologic investigations, although intradermal tests are more sensitive. Both serum IgE levels and skin test reactivity test sensitization as well as recent exposure to environmental antigens. Skin test reactivity is dependent on at least three separate factors: (1) an intact immune system, (2) the presence of a mast cell–basophil complex that can combine with IgE and release mediators when exposed to antigen, and (3) skin that can respond to histamine with the development of an inflammatory response, including erythema and induration. It is likely that the manifestation of an allergic response is dependent on the level of the relevant environmental antigen, the intrinsic activity of the immune system, and perhaps on other environmental exposures that may act as haptens or primers for the immune response. These markers of the allergic state and existing clinical and epidemiologic data do not take into account the levels of exposure to environmental antigens. In evaluating the relationship of allergy to asthma, several specific issues need to be addressed. The first issue is the underlying heritability of both allergy and airway responsiveness. The second issue is the complex interrelationship involving allergen exposure, genetics, and the development of sensitization and, ultimately, symptoms in the genetically susceptible individual. The third issue is the interrelationship between dose and duration of exposure in the development of clinical disease. Family and twin studies clearly demonstrate the familial aggregation of serum IgE levels and intradermal skin test reactivity (Mendell et al, 1978). Twin studies suggest a heritability of at least 0.6 for total serum IgE (Hopp et al, 1984). What remains at issue is the exact mode of inheritance for the allergic diathesis. Current data suggest that inheritance of the atopic state is polygenetic, segregation analysis suggesting that the mixed model of recessive inheritance of high levels of IgE is most appropriate, with approximately 36 percent of the total variation in IgE due to genetic factors, equally divided between the mendelian and the polygenetic component (Marsh et al, 1981). Cookson and Hopkins (1988) have suggested a dominant vertical transmission model for the inheritance of atopy. These investigators have also established linkage to a polymorphism on chromosome 11Q. However, four different groups were unable to confirm the initial linkage reported by the Oxford group (Amelung et al, 1992; Hizawa et al, 1992; Lympany et al, 1992; Rich et al, 1992).

The development of sensitization to environmental antigens is a function of at least four factors: genetic susceptibility, dose, timing, and duration of exposure. It has been hypothesized that foreign antigens encountered during the first 12 months of life are more likely to induce IgE-mediated hypersensitivity than antigens encountered later in life. Infant exposure to allergic foods in the diet, either directly or through breast milk, is believed to be important in the sensitization of the genetically susceptible child. It remains unclear whether avoidance of allergic foods, either by the mother or the infant, and breast-feeding influence the development of atopy (Arshad et al, 1992; Zeiger, 1985).

Relatively few studies have examined the relationship of exposure to allergen and its relationship to the development of disease. Sporik et al (1990) studied 67 children of atopic parents, 35 of whom were atopic as assessed by allergy skin testing to common aeroallergens, and 32 were initially nonatopic. Of the 17 children who developed active asthma in 11 years of follow-up, 16 were atopic, all of whom were sensitized to house dust mite. The level of house dust mite in the home at age 1 correlated directly with degree of sensitization at age 11. However, level of house dust mite in the home at birth did not correlate with the degree of sensitization at age 5. All but one of the children with asthma at age 11 have been exposed at 1 year of age to more than 10 micrograms of house dust mite per gram of dust, with a relative risk of developing asthma of 4.8. In addition, the age at which the first episode of wheezing occurred was inversely related to the level of exposure at age 1 year for all children, but especially for atopic children. What remains unclear from this study is the interrelationship between house dust mite exposure early in life and other relevant exposures and their relationship to the subsequent development of asthma.

Cockcroft and co-workers (1979) have examined the relationship of allergen exposure sensitization and underlying airway responsiveness to the development of acute asthma episodes in 25 young adult atopic asthmatic subjects. These investigators found a poor correlation between histamine PC_{20} and cutaneous sensitivity to allergen (r = 0.03, p >0.1). However, there were relatively good correlations between allergen PC_{20} and histamine PC_{20} (r = 0.52, p <0.02), and a better correlation between allergen PC_{20} and skin test reactivity to allergen (r = 0.60, p <0.01). The use of multiple linear regression of the allergen PC_{20} as a function of histamine PC_{20} and skin test reactivity to allergen gave the best correlation (r = 0.78, p <0.001). These investigators concluded that underlying airway responsiveness to allergen was a function of three factors: the dose of allergen to which the individual is exposed; the level of circulating IgE antibody to that allergen; and the underlying degree of nonspecific airway responsiveness. Burrows has shown that asthma is more closely correlated with serum IgE level than skin test reactivity (Burrows et al, 1989). Sears has extended the asthma findings by demonstrating that airway responsiveness, even in nonasthmatic children, is strongly correlated with total serum IgE level (Sears et al, 1991). It is important, however, in examining these data to realize that the relationship between serum IgE level and airway responsiveness is hardly monolithic. If one examines the Sears data in Figure 33–4,

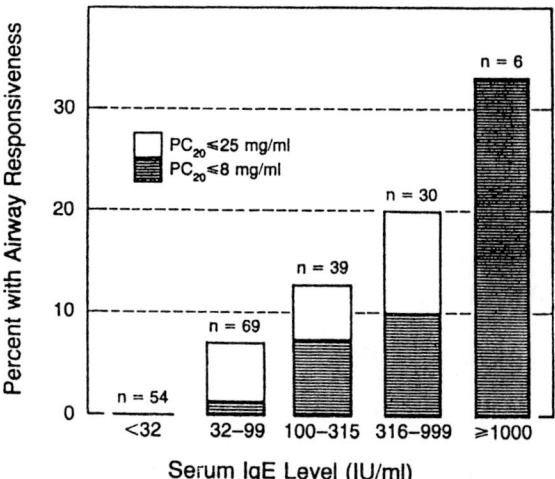

FIGURE 33–4. Proportion of children with no reported history of asthma, wheezing hay fever, or eczema who had airway responsiveness to methacholine, according to serum IgE level (P<0.001 by the chi-square test for trend). (From Sears MR, Burrows B, Flannery EM, Herbison GP, Hewitt CJ, Holdaway MD. Relation between airway responsiveness and serum IgE in children with asthma and in apparently normal children. N Engl J Med 325:1070, 1991.)

it can easily be seen, even though a dose-response relationship exists between serum IgE level and airway responsiveness, that even in the highest category of IgE, less than half of all subjects have increased airway responsiveness.

Controversy still exists as to whether atopy and airway responsiveness are separate factors determining the asthma diathesis or whether all airway responsiveness is dependent on the atopic state. Clearly, for childhood asthma, over 80 percent of childhood asthmatics are atopic. In young adults, however, although these two factors are interrelated, they appear to be independent, as there is a large group of people who have airway responsiveness without atopy, and vice-versa.

In addition, no single phenotypic marker (i.e., skin test, IgE level, or eosinophil count) completely defines the atopic state. The prevalence of increased airway responsiveness in general populations varies from 15 percent to 25 percent, depending on the age and gender distribution of the population and the definition of responsiveness. The prevalence of allergy, as measured by skin test reactivity, varies from 15 percent to 35 percent, depending on age, gender, and definition of skin test reactivity. Given these facts, the association between atopy and airway responsiveness may simply result from two separate and distinct genetic predispositions. They may be independently heritable but occur at relatively high frequency (penetrance) in the population.

OTHER FACTORS MODIFYING ASTHMA RISK

Mechanical Factors

The lower the level of prechallenge lung function, the greater the likelihood that the individual will have increased airway responsiveness (Rijcken et al, 1988). This relationship between prechallenge level of pulmonary function and degree of airway responsiveness is at least partly explained by a number of geometric, mathematical, and anatomic factors. From a mathematical point of view, an individual with a 5-liter lung will be required to drop his prechallenge level of lung function by 1 liter to achieve a PD_{20} for FEV_1. In contrast, an individual with a 500-ml lung will only need to drop his FEV_1 by 100 ml to achieve a comparable $PD_{20}FEV_1$. Thus, on a purely mathematical basis, level of lung function will be linked to the degree of airway responsiveness. In addition to this mathematical relationship, geometric factors are also important. With airflow obstruction there is a more central distribution of inhaled aerosol, emphasizing the greater importance of the central airway diameter. Airflow is inversely proportional to the fourth power of the airway radius; thus small changes in airway radius can have profound effects on airflow. Finally, most individuals with increased airway responsiveness have a heightened response to bronchodilators, suggesting that baseline bronchomotor tone may be increased, possibly because of an individual's airway responsiveness, which may in turn be responsible for decreased prechallenge pulmonary function. The final mechanical factor that can influence the relationship of airway responsiveness and baseline level of lung function is the relative relationship between lung size and airway size. Mead (1980) hypothesized that variations in airway size relative to lung size were an important source of variability in flow limitation.

It is important to recognize that the relationship of airway responsiveness and level of lung function is likely to be bidirectional. Specifically, airway responsiveness may be a factor predictive of lower level and accelerated decline in lung function. Conversely, level of lung function may influence or confound the relationship of other risk factors to airway responsiveness.

Age as Factor

Both asthma and airway responsiveness are increased in the very young and the very old. A substantial portion of this relationship may be explained by mechanical factors, as described above (Sparrow et al, 1991). Specifically, individuals at the extreme of age have lower levels of lung function, so that milder degrees of airway responsiveness and inflammation may precipitate the diagnosis of asthma. Virtually no studies have examined the relationship of age to asthma, independent of level of lung function.

Gender as Factor

Asthma in early life tends to be predominantly a male disease, whereas asthma in later life tends to be more common in females. This clinical observation tends to be confirmed by epidemiologic data. The sex ratio for male to female doctor-diagnosed asthma is approximately 2 to 1, until age 10, at which time the gender ratio is equal until about age 14 (Weiss and Speizer, 1993). Following puberty, asthma incidence is greater in females. Roughly 25 percent of all asthma subjects are diagnosed after age 40, and the majority of these subjects are female. The reasons for the gender differences in asthma incidence are unknown but are likely to relate to both hormonal and mechanical factors, as well as differing host responses to environmental exposures. Diagnostic bias on the part of physicians may also play a role.

Respiratory Illness

There is little question that, in established asthma, both viral and bacterial respiratory infections contribute to clinical exacerbations of the disease. However, data conclusively linking viral respiratory infection to the onset of asthma in previously normal individuals is not available. Theoretically, viral respiratory illness could be linked to the development of asthma by directly inducing a change in airway responsiveness by a variety of physiologic mechanisms and/or by inducing an atopic response. Airway responsiveness in normal nonasthmatic individuals increases with a viral upper respiratory tract infection (Empey et al, 1976). Atropine will inhibit this response, suggesting that damage to airway epithelium by the respiratory infection sensitizes airway receptors to be more responsive to environmental stimuli (Empey et al, 1976). Decreased beta-adrenergic sensitivity to viral respiratory infections may contribute in some individuals (Busse, 1977). Increased mucosal permeability may also play a role. A number of retrospective studies have documented the high prevalence of airway responsiveness in children following croup or bronchiolitis. Zack and co-workers followed 110 of 331 children initially hospitalized for croup (Zach et al, 1981). Nine years after the initial episode, 21 percent of these children had increased airway responsiveness. Gurwitz and co-workers (1981) reported on 96 children from a group of 229 children initially hospitalized for croup, again finding 35 percent with increased airway responsiveness 8.5 years after the hospitalization episode. Gurwitz has also reported similar results for bronchiolitis. Several important flaws may have biased these results. The hospital-based nature of these populations means that one can generalize these data only in relation to other children who may have been hospitalized at the time of the study. One cannot be sure whether factors that determine need for hospitalization would be generally applicable to the population at large. Because only one third of the original group was subsequently evaluated, there was significant potential for bias and outcome with the previously mentioned studies. Sicker children are more likely to maintain contact with the hospital, and therefore, for purposes of follow-up, these children will be most readily identified for further study. There is little question that viral respiratory illness, particularly respiratory syncytial virus, is associated with IgE production, airway inflammation, and increased airway responsiveness (Welliver and Ogra, 1987; Welliver et al, 1981).

Race

Asthma prevalence is significantly higher in blacks than in whites (Weiss et al, 1993). In addition to this increased asthma prevalence, hospitalization and mortality rates are also consistently higher in blacks than in whites. It appears that the effects of race are independent of the effects of socioeconomic status, although this finding is somewhat controversial. Recently it has been reported that African-American women have increased airway responsiveness and higher IgE levels than whites, but that the increases in airway responsiveness disappear when one controls for baseline level of lung function, which is lower in blacks than in whites (Sherman et al, 1993). To date, it remains unknown whether the racial differences in asthma prevalence, hospitalization, and mortality are due to environmental factors or whether there are inherent biologic characteristics that may contribute to these differences.

Socioeconomic Status

In the United States, it appears that low socioeconomic status (SES) is clearly associated with an increase in asthma prevalence (Weiss et al, 1993). Lower SES may also be associated with urban crowding, increases in indoor air pollution, maternal cigarette smoking, and decreased access to medical care, all of which may contribute to significant asthma morbidity.

Prematurity

Prematurity is associated with the occurrence of bronchopulmonary dysplasia, a disease characterized by increased airway responsiveness and asthma symptoms. Independent of any relationship to bronchopulmonary dysplasia, prematurity carries roughly a fourfold risk for the development of asthma (Von Mutius et al, 1993). Increasing numbers of preterm infants are surviving to maturity. Analyses independent of gestational age have looked at low birth weight and confirmed the relationship of low birth weight to asthma. It is important to note that blacks have lower birth weights and higher rates of prematurity, and this may also contribute to racial differences in asthma prevalence and severity.

Cigarette Smoking

A variety of studies have clearly linked active cigarette smoking to increased airway responsiveness (O'Connor et al, 1989). Active cigarette smoking is also related to increased serum IgE levels and eosinophilia. Burns and co-workers (1989) have postulated that increased epithelial permeability may be a mechanism by which cigarette smoking leads to an increase in serum IgE level. Epidemiologic data on the relationship of cigarette smoking to the development of asthma in adults is scant. Fletcher and co-workers (1976), in their longitudinal study of London transport workers, found 17 asthmatic adult males, all but two of whom were current or former smokers. Dodge and Burrows (1980) found that, in young adults (age 10 to 39) followed prospectively for 3 years, those who developed asthma were twice as likely to have smoked relative to those who did not develop asthma.

Passive cigarette smoke exposure exacerbates asthma symptoms in children. O'Connor and co-workers (1987) showed that asthmatic subjects exposed to maternal cigarette smoke were more likely to have increased airway responsiveness than asthmatic subjects who were not exposed to maternal cigarette smoke. Similar results have been obtained by Murray and Morrison (1986; 1989), using a clinic-based population. The bulk of the studies that have examined the relationship of parental cigarette smoking to wheezing symptoms and asthma episodes in children have found a positive association. O'Connell and Logan (1974) identified 37 asthmatic children who were "bothered" by parental cigarette smoke. Parents of 20 of these children stopped smoking, and 18 (90 percent) of the 20 children had an improvement in symptoms. A control group consisted of 15 children whose parents did not stop smoking; only four (27 percent) of these 15 children improved. In addition to possible bias in selection of cases and the reporting of symptoms by parents, subjective criteria for improvement and an unclear duration of follow-up flaw this study. British workers demonstrated an increased incidence of wheezing over a 5-year period among nonasthmatic children who had two parents who smoke when compared to children who had two nonsmoking parents. However, when controlling for other variables, parental smoking was not a significant predictor of the occurrence of wheeze or the future occurrence of asthma. In a subgroup of this cohort, 861 children of asymptomatic parents, Leeder and colleagues (1976) were unable to show a significant trend in asthma wheeze symptoms by increasing level of parental smoking over a 5-year period. In contrast, in a study of 650 children aged 5 to 10 years, Weiss and co-workers (1980) showed a significant trend in the reported prevalence of chronic wheezing with current parental cigarette smoking. Rates were 1.85 percent, 6.85 percent, and 11.8 percent for 0, 1, and 2 smoking parents, respectively. In all likelihood the age of the child is a significant factor. At least three studies have documented a strong association of maternal cigarette smoking to the development of asthma during the first year of life (Arshad et al, 1992; Martinez et al, 1992; Weitzman et al, 1990). In two of these studies, general population samples placed the estimated risk at about twofold (Martinez et al, 1992; Weitzman et al, 1990). Of interest are the data of Arshad and co-workers (1992), examining a high risk population of children of allergic parents. In this subgroup, maternal cigarette smoking carried a fourfold risk of the development of asthma in the first year of life relative to children of nonsmoking mothers. Hanrahan has also examined the relationship of maternal cigarette smoking to wheezing during the first year of life (Hanrahan et al, 1992). His is the only investigation that clearly separates prenatal from postnatal maternal cigarette smoking and its relationship to chronic wheeze symptoms in early childhood. These data suggest that the bulk of the maternal cigarette smoking effect occurs *in utero* rather than postnatally. The observation that *in utero* cigarette smoke exposure is associated with lower flows and decreased pulmonary function at 1 month of age suggests the hypothesis that maternal cigarette smoking during pregnancy may influence mechanical factors that subsequently are important throughout the life of the child.

PROGNOSIS

The first important fact to be appreciated about the prognosis of asthma is that pulmonary function tracks throughout life with a very high tracking correlation. In the short term, an individual's pulmonary function at two time points correlates on the order of 0.8 to 0.9. Thus, knowing an individual's value today gives one a high probability of knowing what this patient's value will be in subsequent years. Asthmatic subjects track in a fashion similar to that of normal subjects. Although there is some increase in variability of their pulmonary function values, the bulk of asthmatic patients are relatively mild (normal lung function and only intermittent symptoms); thus, relationships are not distorted in this disease group.

An additional factor to be appreciated is that pulmonary function increases with age until early adolescence, at which point it stabilizes until the mid-thirties, when it begins to decline. Since respiratory symptoms are loosely linked to level of pulmonary function, it is not surprising that some of the improvement in childhood asthma is simply a function of growth of the lung. Thus, childhood asthmatics may seem to "outgrow their asthma" as a result of mechanical factors (i.e., increases in lung size), yet they may still fall at the lower end of the population distribution and be at increased risk for the development of accelerated decline in FEV_1 in adult life. Roughly half of all childhood asthmatics will have their symptoms remit by early adulthood (Anderson et al, 1986; Gerritsen et al, 1989; Kelly et al, 1985; Martin et al, 1980; Ogilvy, 1962; Park et al, 1986; Rackerman and Edwards, 1952). Despite this remission of symptoms, atopy and increased airway responsiveness may still be present. In addition, current cohort studies and the long-term follow-up of asthma patients have a number of flaws. First, all or most are over 30 years old and may not clearly relate to current patterns of disease. None of the existing studies incorporates physiologic tests of airway responsiveness, and many do not examine the role of atopic status in the natural history of the disease. All are hospital or clinic based, leading to potential selection bias with choice of more severely ill patients. Most do not examine other risk factors, such as respiratory infection, active and passive cigarette smoking, socioeconomic status, or race, which may be highly relevant to disease natural history. It is currently unknown whether the presence of atopy increases disease severity or changes disease natural history. Williams and McNichol (1969) stratified their sample of children by age and examined the relationship of skin test reactivity to disease severity, and found atopy, as assessed by skin test reactivity, was associated with increased disease severity. In general, males with asthma seem to have a better prognosis than females (Anderson et al, 1986; Gerritsen et al, 1989; Kelly et al, 1985; Martin et al, 1980; Ogilvy, 1962; Park et al, 1986; Rackerman and Edwards, 1952). Weiss and co-workers (1992) analyzed the relationship of asthma to lung growth in a cohort of 5- to 9-year-old children from a population sample in East Boston over a 13-year period. The effect of asthma on lung growth was different for boys and girls. Boys with asthma had a larger growth in vital capacity than boys without asthma. They also had a normal FEV_1. Asthmatic girls, however, had reductions in FEV_1, and also reductions in FEF_{25-75}, relative to nonasthmatic girls. In addition, the girls were more likely to be hospitalized for asthma than boys, although the prevalence of asthma was twice as great in boys. Asthma that presents initially in adult life is less likely to remit. Clinical studies of the relationship of asthma to decline in FEV_1 and the development of fixed obstructive airway disease may be biased by the select nature of the patients and inadequate statistical methods. Fletcher and co-workers (1976), in their previously mentioned study, found that the rate of decline in FEV_1 adjusted for the mean value over an 8-year period was significantly more rapid (22 ml per year greater) when compared with asymptomatic nonsmokers. Schachter and co-workers (1984) studied a rural white population of 1303 subjects in Connecticut over a 6-year period. Subjects were considered to have asthma if they responded affirmatively to the question, "Have you ever had asthma?" Asthmatic adults experienced a more rapid decline in FEV_1 than did nonasthmatic adults. These data were not adjusted for age, smoking status, or initial level of FEV. Peat and colleagues (1987) examined data from the Busselton Study and found an accelerated rate of decline in asthmatic subjects relative to nonasthmatics, although there appears to be no additional effect of cigarette smoking. Buist and Vollmer (1987) studied a small group of 35 asthmatic subjects drawn from a young working population and health-screened older cohort. Subjects were considered to have asthma if a physician had ever informed them of that diagnosis. The results were presented as rate of decline of FEV_1 without adjustment of age or initial level, but stratified by cohort of origin and smoking status. No consistent accelerated decline in FEV_1 was observed. On balance, these data are consistent with the hypothesis that a doctor's diagnosis of asthma is associated with an increased risk of accelerated decline in FEV_1.

REFERENCES

Amelung PJ, Panhuxsen LIM, Postma DS, et al. Atopy and bronchial hyperresponsiveness: Exclusion of linkage to markers on chromosomes 11Q and 6P. Clin Exp Allergy 22:1074–1084, 1992.

Anderson HR, Bland JM, Patel S, et al. The natural history of asthma in childhood. J Epidemiol Commun Health 40:121–129, 1986.

Arshad SH, Matthews S, Gant C, et al. Effective allergen avoidance from development of allergic disorders in infancy. Lancet 339:1493–1497, 1992.

Buist AS, Vollmer WM. Prospective investigations in asthma. What have we learned from longitudinal studies about lung growth and senescence in asthma? Chest 91(suppl):119S–121S, 1987.

Burney PGJ, Britton JR, Chinn S, et al. Descriptive epidemiology of bronchial reactivity in an adult population: results from a community study. Thorax 42:38–44, 1987.

Burns AR, Hosford SP, Dunn LA, et al. Respiratory epithelial permeability after cigarette smoke exposure in guinea pigs. J Appl Physiol 66:2109–2116, 1989.

Burrows B, Martinez FD, Halonen M, et al. Association of asthma with serum IgE levels and skin test reactivity to allergens. N Engl J Med 320:271–277, 1989.

Busse WW. Decreased granulocyte response to isoproteranol in asthma during upper respiratory infections. Am Rev Respir Dis 115:783–788, 1977.

Cockcroft DW, Killian DN, Mellon JJA, et al. Bronchial reactivity to inhaled histamine: A method in clinical survey. Clin Allergy 7:235–243, 1977.

Cockcroft DW, Ruffin RE, Frith PA, et al. Determinants of allergen-induced asthma: Dose of allergen, circulating IgE antibody concentration, and bronchial responsiveness to inhaled histamine. Am Rev Respir Dis 120:1053–1058, 1979.

Cookson WOCM, Hopkin JN. Dominant inheritance of atopic immunoglobulin-E responsiveness. Lancet 1:86–88, 1988.

Dodge RR, Burrows B. The prevalence and incidence of asthma and asthma-like symptoms in a general population sample. Am Rev Respir Dis 122:567–575, 1980.

Empey DW, et al. Mechanisms of bronchial hyperreactivity in normal subjects after upper respiratory tract infection. Am Rev Respir Dis 113:131–136, 1976.

Fletcher CM, Pedo R, Tinker C, et al. The Natural History of Chronic Bronchitis and Emphysema. An Eight-Year Study of Early Chronic Obstructive Lung Disease in Working Men in London. New York, Oxford University Press, 1976.

Gerritsen J, Koeter GH, DeMonchy JGR, et al. Allergy in subjects with asthma from childhood to adulthood. J Allergy Clin Immunol 85:116–125, 1989.

Gurwitz D, Mindorff C, Levinson H. Increased incidence of bronchial reactivity in children with a history of bronchiolitis. J Pediatr 98:551–558, 1981.

Hanrahan JP, Tager IB, Segal MR, et al. The effect of maternal smoking during pregnancy on early infant lung function. Am Rev Respir Dis 145:1129–1135, 1992.

Hizawa N, Yamaguchi E, Ore M, et al. Lack of linkage between atopy and locus 11Q13. Clin Exp Allergy 22:1065–1069, 1992.

Hopp RJ, Bewtra AK, Watt GD, et al. Genetic analysis of allergic disease in twins. J Allergy Clin Immunol 73:265–270, 1984.

Kelly WJW, Hudson I, Phelan PD, et al. Childhood asthma in adult life. The further study at 28 years of age. Br Med J 294:1059–1062, 1985.

Leeder SR, et al. Influence of family factors on asthma and wheezing during the first five years of life. Br J Prev Soc Med 30:213–218, 1976.

Lympany P, Welsh K, MacCochrane GM, et al. Genetic analysis using DNA polymorphism of the linkage between chromosome 11q13 and atopy and bronchial hyperresponsiveness to methacholine. J Allergy Clin Immunol 89:619–628, 1992.

Marsh DG, Meyers DA, Bias WB. Epidemiology and genetics of atopic allergy. N Engl J Med 305:1551–1559, 1981.

Martin HA, McClennan LA, Landau LI, et al. Natural history of childhood asthma to adult life. Br Med J 2:1395–1400, 1980.

Martinez FD, Cline M, Burrows B. Increased incidence of asthma in children of smoking mothers. Pediatrics 89:21–26, 1992.

Mead J. Dysanapsis in normal lungs assessed by the relationship between maximal flow, static recoil, and vital capacity. Am Rev Respir Dis 121:339–342, 1980.

Mendell NR, Blumenthal MM, Amos TB, et al. Ragweed sensitivity: Segregation analysis and linkage to HLA-B. Cytogenet Cell Genet 22:330–334, 1978.

Murray AB, Morrison BJ. Passive smoking by asthmatics: Its greater effect on boys than on girls and on older than on younger children. Pediatrics 84:451–459, 1989.

Murray AB, Morrison BJ. The effect of cigarette smoking from the mother on bronchial hyperresponsiveness and severity of symptoms in children with asthma. J Allergy Clin Immunol 77:575–581, 1986.

National Asthma Education Program. Expert Panel Report. Guidelines for the diagnosis and management of asthma. US Department of Health and Human Services, Pub. No. 91–3042, 1991.

O'Connell EJ, Logan GB. Parental smoking and childhood asthma. Ann Allergy 32:142–146, 1974.

O'Connor GT, Sparrow D, Weiss ST. The role of allergy in nonspecific airway hyperresponsiveness and the pathogenesis of chronic obstructive pulmonary disease. Am Rev Respir Dis 140:225–252, 1989.

O'Connor GT, Weiss ST, Tager IB, et al. Effect of passive smoking on pulmonary function and nonspecific bronchial responsiveness in a population-based sample of children and young adults. Am Rev Respir Dis 135:800–804, 1987.

Ogilvy AG. Asthma: The study and prognosis of 1,000 patients. Thorax 17:183–189, 1962.

Park ES, Goldin GJ, Carswell F, et al. Preschool wheezing and prognosis at age 10. Arch Dis Child 61:642–646, 1986.

Peat JK, Woolcock AJ, Collen K. Rate of decline of lung function in subjects with asthma. Eur J Respir Dis 70:171–176, 1987.

Rackerman FM, Edwards MC. Asthma in children: A follow-up study of 688 patients after an interval of 20 years. N Engl J Med 246:815–823, 1952.

Rich SS, Roitman-Johnson B, Greenberg B, et al. Genetic analysis of atopy in three large kindreds: No evidence of linkage to D11S97. Clin Exp Allergy 22:1070–1076, 1992.

Rijcken B, Schouten JP, Weiss ST, et al. The relationship between airways responsiveness to histamine and pulmonary function level in a random population sample. Am Rev Respir Dis 137:826–832, 1988.

Rijcken B, Schouten JP, Weiss ST, et al. The relationship

of nonspecific bronchial responsiveness to respiratory symptoms in a random population sample. Am Rev Respir Dis 136:62–68, 1987.

Salome CM, Peat JK, Britton WJ, et al. Bronchial hyperresponsiveness in two populations of Australian schoolchildren. I. Relation to respiratory symptoms and diagnosed asthma. Clin Allergy 17:271–281, 1987.

Schachter EN, Doyle CA, Beck GJ. A prospective study of asthma in a rural community. Chest 85:623–628, 1984.

Sears MR, Burrows B, Flannery EM, et al. Relation between airway responsiveness and serum IgE in children with asthma and apparently normal children. N Engl J Med 325:1067–1071, 1991.

Sears MR, Jones DT, Holdaway MD, et al. Prevalence of bronchial reactivity to inhaled methacholine in New Zealand children. Thorax 41:283–289, 1986.

Sherman CB, Tollerud DJ, Heffner LJ, et al. Airways responsiveness in young black and white women. Am Rev Respir Dis 148:98–102, 1993.

Sparrow D, O'Connor G, Colton T, et al. The relationship of nonspecific bronchial responsiveness to the occurrence of respiratory symptoms and decreased levels of pulmonary function. The Normative Aging Study. Am Rev Respir Dis 135:1255–1260, 1987.

Sparrow D, O'Connor GT, Segal M, et al. The influence of age and level of pulmonary function on nonspecific bronchial responsiveness. Am Rev Respir Dis 143:978–982, 1991.

Sporik R, Holgate ST, Platts-Mills TAE, et al. Exposure to house dust mite allergen (der P I) and development of asthma in childhood. N Engl J Med 323:502–507, 1990.

Von Mutius E, Nicolai T, Martinez FD. Prematurity as a risk factor for asthma in preadolescent children. J Pediatr 123:223–229, 1993.

Weiss KB, Gergen PJ, Wagener DK. Breathing better or wheezing worse? The changing epidemiology of asthma morbidity and mortality. Annu Rev Publ Health 14:491–513, 1993.

Weiss ST, et al. The effect of asthma on lung growth in children: A longitudinal study of male-female differences. Am Rev Respir Dis 145:58–63, 1992.

Weiss ST, Speizer FE. Asthma epidemiology natural history. In Weiss E, Stein M (eds). Bronchial Asthma: Mechanisms and Therapeutics. 3rd ed. Boston, Little Brown, 1993, pp 15–25.

Weiss ST, Tager IB, Speizer FE, et al. Persistent wheeze: Its relation to respiratory illness, cigarette smoking, and level of pulmonary function in a population sample of children. Am Rev Respir Dis 122:697–707, 1980.

Weiss ST, Tager IB, Weiss JW, et al. Airways responsiveness in a population sample of adults and children. Am Rev Respir Dis 129:898–902, 1984.

Weitzman M, Gortmaker S, Walker DK, et al. Maternal smoking and childhood asthma. Pediatrics 85:505–511, 1990.

Welliver RC, Ogra PL. Respiratory syncytial virus-specific IgE antibody responses at the mucosal surface: Predicted value for recurrent wheezing and suppression by ribovirin. Adv Exp Biol Med 216B:1701–1708, 1987.

Welliver RC, Wong DT, Sun M, et al. The development of respiratory syncytial virus-specific IgE and the release of histamine in nasopharyngeal secretions after infection. N Engl J Med 305:841–846, 1981.

Williams H, McNichol KN. Prevalence, natural history and relationship of wheezy bronchitis and asthma in children: An epidemiologic study. Br Med J 4:321–326, 1969.

Woolcock AJ, Peat JK, Salome CM, et al. Prevalence of bronchial hyperresponsiveness and asthma in a rural adult population. Thorax 42:361–368, 1987.

Zach M, Erban A, Olinsky A. Croup, recurrent croup, allergy, and airways hyperreactivity. Arch Dis Child 56:336–339, 1981.

Zeiger RS. Atopy in infancy and early childhood: Natural history and role of skin testing. J Allergy Clin Immunol 75:633–645, 1985.

Zhong NS, Chen RC, Yang MO, et al. Is asymptomatic bronchial hyperresponsiveness an indication of potential asthma? A two-year follow-up of young students with bronchial hyperresponsiveness. Chest 102:1104–1109, 1992.

ACKNOWLEDGMENT: Supported by research grants HL50811, HL36474, HL36002, HL34645, HL49460, and SCOR HL19170, all from the National Heart, Lung, and Blood Institute.

Chapter 34

Asthma (Bronchial Asthma): Principles of Diagnosis and Treatment

David S. Pearlman, M.D., and Robert F. Lemanske, Jr., M.D.

Asthma is a chronic, variably obstructive disorder of the tracheobronchial tree characterized by paroxysmal episodes of respiratory distress generally interspersed with periods of apparent complete well-being. Typically, there are wide variations in the degree of obstruction over relatively short periods of time; the obstruction may subside spontaneously or only as a result of therapy. The obstruction may be mild to severe, transient, or chronic and incompletely reversible. The hallmark of the disease is *wheezing*, a squeaky sound made by air rushing through the larger but narrowed airways. Cough also is a characteristic part of the disorder and may constitute the major symptom with which an asthmatic patient presents. A patient with asthma may even present with subtle symptoms of bronchopulmonary obstruction *without wheezing* (McFadden, 1975a and 1975b; Corrao et al, 1979). The more subtle symptoms and signs of asthma often are unappreciated, and asthma is a commonly underdiagnosed disorder. Because of this underdiagnosis and the prevalence of erroneous concepts of the etiology, course, and prognosis, asthma also tends to be a greatly undertreated disorder in childhood and adulthood (Speight et al, 1983; Pearlman, 1989), resulting in excessive mortality and needless morbidity (NAEP, 1991).

There is a steep price to society for this escalating dysfunction. Physician and medication costs for asthma are high, and they are heavily weighted by inpatient and emergency room encounters, which should be largely preventable through patient education regarding pathogenesis and disease control. Quality of life is negatively affected by loss of school and work days as well as missed leisure opportunities.

These issues of escalating numbers affected, adversely affected life style, and rising mortality paved the way for a major national effort at reversing these trends supported by the National Heart, Lung, and Blood Institute. The creation of a National Asthma Education Program resulted in guidelines for disease control which have been widely read by physicians caring for patients with asthma. A National Asthma Education Prevention Program continues to produce educational materials and innovative programs for physicians, families, and patients.

PATHOLOGY

In asthma, airflow obstruction is produced by a combination of pathogenic abnormalities (Table 34–1). The precise contribution of each of these abnormalities varies among asthmatic patients and no doubt contributes to the diversity in clinical manifestations such as triggering factors, chronicity and severity of the disease, and the therapeutic response to various medications.

TABLE 34–1. FACTORS CONTRIBUTING TO AIRWAY OBSTRUCTION IN ASTHMA

Airway smooth muscle spasm
Edema of airway mucosa
Increased mucus secretion
Inflammation: resident cell (epithelium, macrophage, mast cells) participation
Inflammatory cell infiltration/activation

Factors Contributing to the Airway Obstruction in Asthma

AIRWAY SMOOTH MUSCLE SPASM. The ability to produce symptomatic improvement with the use of bronchodilators and the remarkable airway hyperresponsiveness to a wide variety of stimuli seen in asthmatic patients have indicated that bronchial smooth muscle spasm contributes significantly to airway obstruction. These features suggest that either the quantity or the function of bronchial smooth muscle in asthma is abnormal. Autopsy specimens obtained from asthmatic patients who died of their disease have demonstrated hypertrophy of the smooth muscle lining the airways. *In vitro* examinations by some, but not all, investigators have demonstrated a greater maximal response to contractile agonists and an impaired relaxation to beta-agonists and theophylline (Bai, 1990; Bai et al, 1992). The airway contains a number of resident cells (mast cells, alveolar macrophages, airway epithelium, and endothelium) as well as migrating inflammatory cells (eosinophils, lymphocytes, neutrophils, basophils, platelets), which are capable of generating a wide variety of mediators that can induce bronchospasm. These include histamine; platelet activating factor; and a number of derivatives of the arachidonic acid cascade such as prostaglandin D_2 and leukotrienes C_4, D_4, and E_4 (slow-reacting substances of anaphylaxis). Thus, it is likely that infiltration of inflammatory cells into the airway walls contributes to bronchial smooth muscle tone through the local effects of these various mediators.

EDEMA OF THE AIRWAY MUCOSA. Edema of the airway mucosa is due to increased capillary permeability with leakage of serum proteins into interstitial areas. A number of cell-derived mediators are capable of inducing edema formation including histamine, prostaglandin E, leukotriene C_4 (LTC_4), leukotriene D_4 (LTD_4), platelet activating factor (PAF), and bradykinin. Although the precise contribution of edema to the episodic airway obstruction seen in asthma is unknown, it has been demonstrated that one of the striking immediate features of local airway allergen challenge is extensive mucosal edema (Metzger et al, 1987). Further, increased bronchovascular permeability occurs after local allergen exposure in sensitive asthmatic patients (Frick et al, 1987). Finally, using mathematical modeling, it has been shown that both edema and cellular inflammation result in an increased airway wall thickness that contributes to the mechanics of airway narrowing in asthma (Wiggs et al, 1992; James et al, 1989).

ALTERATIONS IN RESPIRATORY SECRETIONS WITH MUCUS PLUGGING OF SMALLER AIRWAYS. One of the characteristic pathologic features seen in status asthmaticus is the formation of tenacious mucus plugs within the airways. Increased mucus secretion contributes to both hyperinflation and focal atelectasis and may be the result of both hyperplasia and metaplasia of goblet cells lining the airway. The pathogenesis of mucus hypersecretion is complex, with multiple mediators and cells capable of influencing this particular aspect of the airway obstruction in asthma. Factors important in this regard have recently been extensively reviewed by Lundgren and Shelhamer (1990).

INFLAMMATION. Airway inflammation has long been recognized as a major feature of the histopathologic findings in many patients dying in status asthmaticus (McFadden and Gilbert, 1992). Significant findings include denudation of the airway epithelium, mucus plugging of segmental bronchi and bronchioles, so-called thickening of the epithelial basement membrane, edema of the submucosa, infiltration by polymorphonuclear leukocytes (predominantly eosinophils), and smooth muscle hypertrophy. These findings differ from those seen in other forms of chronic lung disease, such as cystic fibrosis in both children and adults or chronic bronchitis in adults, in which significant airway neutrophilia is more characteristic (Thompson et al, 1989; Salvato, 1968). Eosinophil degranulation (Lacoste et al, 1993) and plasma cell infiltration of the lamina propria and thickening of the basement membrane (Salvato, 1968) are more characteristic of asthma.

Of equally important clinical relevance, however, has been the more recent observations that significant tissue inflammation can be noted in bronchial biopsy specimens even in patients whose symptoms can be readily controlled clinically with intermittent bronchodilator therapy. Cutz et al (1978) were among the first groups to observe these changes in their evaluation of lung biopsies from two children with bronchial asthma in remission compared with two children dying in status asthmaticus. Bronchial changes, such as goblet cell hyperplasia, mucus plugging, and increased collagen deposition beneath the epithelial basement membrane were comparable in the two groups. Interestingly, the only differences were the presence of a larger number of submucosal eosinophils and more extensive denudation of the epithelium in fatal asthma.

Since these early observations, the use of various procedures (bronchial alveolar lavage, bronchial biopsy, and analysis of induced sputum) and techniques (immunohistochemistry, in situ hybridization, and polymerase chain reactions) to analyze airway inflammation has been aggressively applied to the asthmatic population. Indeed, in the past 5 years, there has been a virtual explosion of publications in which authors have evaluated the presence and participation of a number of resident (e.g., mast cells, epithelial cells, alveolar macrophages) and inflammatory (eosinophils, lymphocytes, neutrophils, basophils) cells, mediators, cytokines, and adhesion molecules (McFadden and Gilbert, 1992). Although not observed uniformly, the following changes have been reported in patients with mild to moderate asthma: denudation of the airway epithelium, collagen deposition beneath the basement membrane, mast cell degranulation, and lymphocyte and eosinophil infiltration and activation. Many of the cells present in the airway appear to be in an activated state (e.g., lymphocytes, eosinophils, epithelial cells), supporting a direct role for them in asthma pathogenesis through the release of various preformed or generated mediators.

The presence of various cytokines such as tumor necrosis factor (TNF), interleukin-1_β (IL-1β), interleukin-5 (IL-5), interleukin-6 (IL-6), granulocyte-macrophage colony-stimulating factor (GM-CSF) (Broide et al, 1992), and endothelin (Vittori et al, 1992) in bronchoalveolar lavage fluid, or the demonstration of intracellular mRNA coding for them, has provided further evidence for an ongoing inflammatory response in the asthmatic airway. Since these cytokines are elaborated by, and can have multiple effects on, a number of resident and inflammatory cells, the autocrine, paracrine, and endocrine cytokine networks are obviously complex and, in many cases, redundant. The ability of cytokines to induce the expression of various adhesion molecules—such as intercellular adhesion molecule (ICAM), vascular cell adhesion molecule (VCAM), and endothelial leukocyte adhesion molecule (ELAM)—no doubt provides a mechanism for inflammatory cell adhesion and migration from the circulation into the lamina propria, the epithelium, and, in many cases, the airway lumen itself (Leff et al, 1991).

Although the recognition of inflammation even in mild-to-moderate asthma has influenced our traditional therapeutic approach to asthma management, much remains to be learned. It is unclear when this inflammatory process starts and how the characteristics of it may change over time, in response to either various triggering mechanisms or therapeutic intervention. Since many lung diseases are characterized by airway inflammation, the patterns of cell migration, cell location, cell activation patterns, cytokine elaboration, and adhesion molecule expression that are specific and/or pathognomonic of asthma need to be established. Finally, determining the relationships of these immunohistopathologic alterations to airway physiologic changes such as airway hyperresponsiveness needs further exploration and definition.

EPIDEMIOLOGY

Asthma commonly begins in childhood and has been considered mistakenly to be a disorder confined largely to early life. In many cases, childhood asthma persists through adulthood; in almost half of all adults with asthma, the disease began in childhood. In the vast majority of cases, childhood asthma begins before the age of 8 years, in most of these, before the age of 6 years, and in about half, before the age of 3 years. Until puberty, males are affected twice as frequently as are females. In the teens and in early adulthood, there is a reversal of this trend, so that by mid- to late-adult life, females are affected more frequently than males.

Asthma is a deceptively common disorder; the exact figures on incidence and prevalence vary from study to study, related at least in part to different criteria for diagnosis and different methodologies used in the studies (see Chapter 33). In addition, the incidence and prevalence are increasing. Approximately 7 percent of the pediatric population in the United States, with over 10 percent cumulative prevalence in adulthood, are considered to have asthma (see Chapter 5), but this undoubtedly is an underestimate (Speight et al, 1983; Pearlman, 1989). The mortality rate among asthmatics is less than 0.1 percent per year, a relatively low yet significant rate, and has increased in many Western countries (Asthma Deaths, 1986). However, the morbidity in asthma is extraordinarily high. It is a source of chronic fatigue and may interfere with sleep, with school and work performance, and with normal exercise and physical development. Asthma may affect a child's psychologic growth and development. At all ages it may affect interactions with family and peers, disturb family life, and cause economic hardship—because of medical costs as well as time lost from work by the patient or by the parent who cares for the child with asthma. In 1990, asthma accounted for 1 percent of costs of health care in the United States (Weiss et al, 1992).

NATURAL COURSE

It is a common belief that childhood asthma generally is "outgrown" by adulthood. Indeed, in various studies, 30 to 50 percent of asthmatic children have been reported to be symptom-free at puberty. Remissions occur somewhat earlier in girls than in boys, as do pubertal changes. Patients who are not symptom-free at puberty are not likely to outgrow their symptoms as young adults (Blair, 1977). In addition, many children who have "outgrown" asthma in puberty develop recurrent asthmatic symptoms in later adult life, as is clearly shown in a series of studies by Flensborg (1945) and Ryssing (1959).

Asthmatic children and adults examined during "symptom-free" periods frequently have clinically significant evidence of obstruction by objective testing. In addition, pharmacologic hyperresponsiveness of the airways in asthmatic individuals generally persists for many years, even in the absence of overt asthmatic attacks (Townley et al, 1975), and evidence of pulmonary obstruction can be found in patients many years after the apparent cessation of asthmatic symptoms. Although many asthmatic children improve significantly by puberty, a small subpopulation may actually develop more severe asthma. It is clear also that in only a relatively small proportion does asthma completely disappear. More often ". . . it is the pediatrician rather than the disease that is outgrown" (Levison et al, 1974). The natural history of asthma in adults is unclear, but it appears to take the same form as does asthma in children, becoming chronically or frequently symptomatic in some and episodic and occasional in others. In some cases, it may be lost altogether; remissions are said to occur at a rate of 1 percent per year (Nelson, 1991).

PHYSIOLOGY

An extraordinary tracheobronchial hyperresponsiveness to acetylcholine, histamine, and other neurotransmitters and mediators of inflammation is characteristic of symptomatic asthma and occurs regardless of whether allergic mechanisms can be demonstrated. Bronchial hyperresponsiveness is considered to be a basic element in asthma and is the basis for diagnostic tests for asthma (methacholine and histamine bronchial challenges) (see Chapter 13). Responsiveness to these agents correlates imperfectly with responsiveness to other more natural stimuli, such as exercise and hyperventilation in cold air.

The fact that chemical mediators to which the tracheobronchial tree is hyperresponsive can be liberated by various mechanisms, immune and nonimmune, may explain the observation that in most asthmatic individuals numerous factors such as inhalant irritants, allergens, exercise, infections, and possibly psychologic factors can act as a trigger of bronchoconstriction. Moreover, the degree of reactivity can vary from time to time, creating an inconsistency in the susceptibility or tolerance of the airways to various potential asthmogenic stimuli (Cockroft, 1983).

Bronchial hyperresponsiveness is thought to be related to inflammation characteristic of asthma, which is found to some extent even in mild, asymptomatic asthma. However, the relationships among bronchial hyperresponsiveness as measured by histamine or methacholine challenge, airway inflammation, and clinical asthma severity is highly variable. Not only is the heightened *sensitivity* to a bronchoconstrictor stimulus an important common feature of asthma, but the degree of airway *reactivity* manifested as the extent of airway obstruction inducible by a stimulus also is characteristically heightened in asthma, the degree related in large part to the severity of asthma. Whereas in normal individuals, methacholine or histamine challenges result in bronchial obstruction, which plateaus at about a 30 percent fall in FEV_1, that plateau is heightened with more severe asthma and may be relatively unlimited in severe disease.

An important mechanism by which sensitivity, as well as reactivity, to bronchoconstrictive stimuli is greatly exaggerated is through the physical changes in the bronchial airways induced by airway wall thickening by various components of the inflammatory process (James et al, 1989). Changes responsible for this include vascular engorgement, vascular leakage with edema, serosal edema interfering with the natural parenchymal counterbalancing forces that help to keep the airways open, epithelial hyperplasia, and an increase in the volume of airway smooth muscle. Deposition of connective tissue below the basement membrane probably plays a role as well. Additionally, viscid intraluminal secretions contribute to the alterations in the dynamics of airflow obstruction. This thickening of the airway wall serves to greatly exaggerate the effects of bronchoconstriction so that a relatively small degree of bronchial smooth muscle contraction can induce a marked degree of bronchial obstruction. Any stimulus that causes airway wall thickening predisposes to an exaggeration of bronchoconstrictive stimuli regardless of the cause of thickening (James et al, 1989). This may include various and variable components of thickening that may be differentially responsive to different forms of treatment. A common pathway by which bronchial hyperresponsiveness may be produced by potentially diverse etiologic agents is through activation of the inflammatory cascade. Once set in motion by any single agent, various other stimuli may act to propagate the inflammation, airway wall thickening, and bronchial hyperresponsiveness (Fig. 34–1).

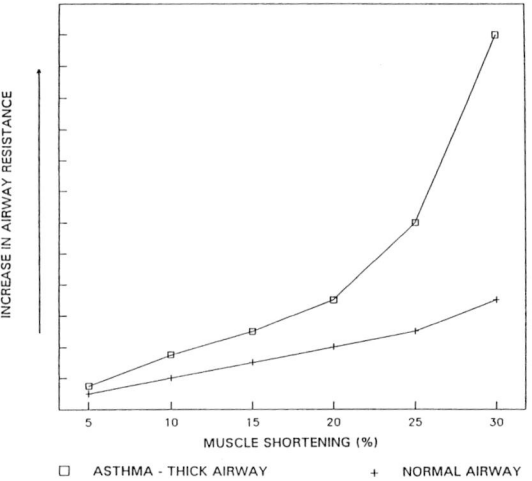

FIGURE 34–1. Airway narrowing in asthma. Calculated changes in relative resistance of cartilaginous airways in normals and asthmatics. (Adapted from James AL, et al. Am Rev Respir Dis 139:242, 1989.)

It is likely that bronchial hyperresponsiveness has various etiologies (Wanner et al, 1990). The basis for one form of pharmacologic hypersensitivity in asthma may be genetic. There is a familial association between clinical asthma and bronchial hyperresponsiveness and, separately, a familial association of heightened IgE antibody responsiveness. The coexistence of asthma, bronchial hyperresponsiveness, and IgE antibody production is striking (Cockroft et al, 1984), but each is a separable phenomenon and seems to be genetically independent. Within a given family constellation, some members may have asthma and also manufacture large amounts of IgE; others may manufacture IgE antibody extraordinarily well but have no evidence of bronchial hyperresponsiveness (Townley et al, 1976; Sibbald et al, 1980). The mode of inheritance of asthma is still not clear. Although in twin studies concordance for asthma generally has been greater for identical twins than for nonidentical twins or other non-twin siblings, concordance nevertheless is lower than 50 percent (Bias, 1973).

ETIOLOGY

Environmental factors play a critical role in the expression of asthma. Some environmental exposures have been identified as risk factors for the development of asthma. Principal among these are prolonged exposure to critical levels of allergens such as house dust mite, cat and dog dander, cockroach, possibly mold, and occupational allergen (Sporik et al, 1992). In childhood as well as in adulthood, the onset of asthma frequently is associated with a viral respiratory tract infection (Cypcar et al, 1992). Certain viruses (respiratory syncytial virus [RSV], adenovirus, parainfluenza virus, possibly corona virus, influenza virus) and *Mycoplasma* are particularly associated with wheezing episodes, and some, such as RSV, are commonly responsible for the first wheezing episode early in life. Whether or not these infections are etiologic in the development of asthma is unclear (Cypcar et al, 1992). Wheezing with RSV or other viral infections, even when recurrent early in life, does not necessarily lead to chronic asthma (Wilson, 1994). Maternal smoking appears to be another risk factor for the occurrence of childhood asthma (McConnochie and Roghmann, 1986).

The presumption that all asthma was "allergic" or had an immune basis led to the concept of "extrinsic" asthma owing to exogenous allergens and "intrinsic" asthma owing to "normal" bacterial antigens from the respiratory tract (Rackemann, 1940). However, no evidence can be found that allergic mechanisms are operative in many individuals with asthma. Moreover, the presence of IgE antibody to a specific allergen may not appear to be relevant to the disease (Aas, 1970). On the other hand, in the presence of even small amounts of IgE antibody, acute asthma can be provoked by inhalation of allergen with clinical reactivity a factor of the combined variables of the amount of antibody present, the amount of allergen exposure, and the degree of bronchial irritability (Cockroft et al, 1979) (Fig. 34–2). Furthermore, allergic sensitization, particularly that which results in the production of "late" asthmatic responses, which have been associated with activation of an inflammatory reaction, may be the critical initiating process of asthma in many patients. These late responses have been associated with the induction of bronchial hyperresponsiveness, which may persist for weeks following exposure (Lemanske and Kaliner, 1993). In allergic individuals, withdrawal of allergen exposure is by far the most potent means by which clinical disease can be attenuated.

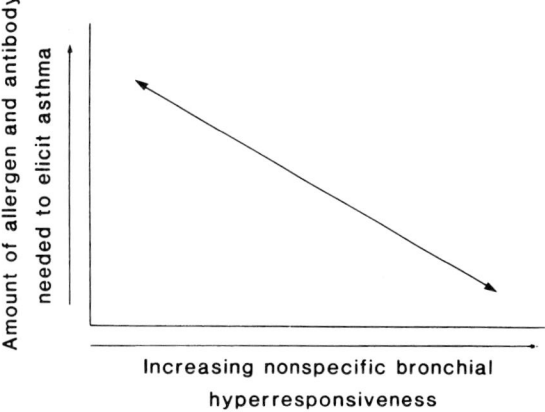

FIGURE 34–2. Relationship between bronchial hyperreactivity and amount of allergen exposure required to induce bronchial obstruction. As the degree of nonspecific bronchial responsiveness increases, the amount of antigen-antibody reacting required to induce obstruction diminishes. Thus, casual encounter with allergen in a highly sensitive individual with marked nonspecific bronchial hyperresponsiveness may induce asthma, but intense antigen exposure may be required to do so in the asthmatic with relatively little IgE antibody or relatively little nonspecific bronchial hyperresponsiveness. (Modified from Cockroft DW, et al. Determination of allergen-induced asthma: Dose of allergen, circulating IgE antibody concentration, and bronchial responsiveness to inhaled histamine. Am Rev Respir Dis 120:1053, 1979.)

PRECIPITATING AND AGGRAVATING FACTORS IN ASTHMA

ALLERGENS. In many individuals with asthma, allergens to which IgE antibody can be demonstrated play a major identifiable or strongly suspected role in the disease. In others, allergens may play an ancillary or negligible role. Allergic reactions may induce bronchoconstriction and obstruction directly, may increase tracheobronchial sensitivity in general, and may be obvious or subtle precipitating factors and may propagate the disease by prolonged exposure through clinically inapparent reaction (Pearlman, 1989). In addition, the role played by an allergen may appear to be inconsistent. Although "immediate" responses to allergens via IgE antibody-induced mediator release are striking, it may be that "late" reactions (which occur 4 to 12 hours after antigen contact, usually after an immediate reaction has subsided) are more important in the disease. Allergens that can induce asthma include foods (mainly in early life), animal proteins, mold spores, pollens, acarids (dust mites), insects (mainly by inhalation but also by sting), infectious agents (especially fungi but perhaps viruses, as discussed subsequently), chemicals, and occasionally drugs (Lemanske and Kaliner, 1993).

IRRITANTS. Numerous upper and lower respiratory irritants have been implicated as precipitants of asthma. These include paint odors, hair sprays, perfumes, chemicals, air pollutants, cigarette smoke (also cigar and pipe smoke), cold air, cold water, cough, and positive ions. Some allergens may act as irritants. As indicated previously, some irritants such as ozone and industrial chemicals also may initiate bronchial hyperresponsiveness. Active and passive exposure to cigarette smoke, in addition to acting as a precipitant and aggravator of asthma, also can be associated with an accelerated irreversible loss of pulmonary function (Barter and Campbell, 1976).

WEATHER CHANGES. Atmospheric changes commonly are associated with an increase in asthmatic activity. The mechanisms of this effect have not been defined (Robuschi et al, 1987).

INFECTIONS. By far, the most common infectious agents responsible for precipitating or aggravating asthma, especially in young children, are viral respiratory pathogens (Cypcar et al, 1992). In some instances, however, fungal infections (e.g., bronchopulmonary aspergillosis), bacterial infections (e.g., pertussis), and parasitic infestations (e.g., toxocariasis and ascariasis) can be important triggers. The importance of viral infections as precipitants and possible initiators of asthma in children and adults is clear. Various mechanisms have been implicated to explain the role of viruses in asthma and other allergic diseases, including IgE-mediated mechanisms (Cypcar et al, 1992; Cypcar and Busse, 1993).

EXERCISE. Strenuous exercise ordinarily associated with breathlessness, such as running, uphill bicycle riding, and cross-country skiing (downhill skiing generally is not associated with this problem), may induce bronchial obstruction (exercise-induced bronchospasm [EIB]) in the vast majority (at least 70 to 80 percent) of individuals with asthma. In some instances, exercise is a major asthmatic precipitant, whereas in others it is a minor or an insignificant one altogether (McFadden and Gilbert, 1992) (see Chapter 36). Although some patients present only with EIB, exercise rarely is an isolated stimulus in asthma, and obstruction from other precipitating factors may not have been recognized.

EMOTIONAL FACTORS. The influence of the psyche on asthma is unquestioned, and in some instances suggestion has been shown to alter airway resistance significantly. Emotional upsets clearly aggravate asthma in some individuals. However, there is no evidence indicating that psychologic factors are the basis for asthma. The studies of Kinsman and associates (1977) strongly indicate that coping styles of patients, their families, and their physicians can intensify or lead to more rapid amelioration of asthma. Conversely, denial of asthma by patients, parents, or physicians may delay therapy to the point that reversibility of obstruction is more difficult. Psychologic factors have been implicated in deaths from asthma in children (Strunk et al, 1985). The influence of psychosocial factors on compliance and the effect of hostility or fear on the ability or propensity to comply are yet other important facets of treatment failure or success.

Just as psychologic factors may influence the course of asthma in a given patient, it is important to recognize that asthma itself can strongly influence the emotional state of the patient, of the family, and of other individuals associated with the patient. Indeed, asthma probably is more frequently "somatopsychic" than it is "psychosomatic" (see Chapter 18).

GASTROESOPHAGEAL REFLUX. Reflux of the gastric contents into the tracheobronchial tree can aggravate asthma in some children and adults and is one of the causes of nocturnal asthma. There also is suggestive information that gastroesophageal reflux (GER) may increase airway reactivity.

ALLERGIC RHINITIS, SINUSITIS, AND UPPER RESPIRATORY TRACT INFLAMMATION. Acute or chronic sinusitis can be associated with aggravation of asthma and can be a cause of recalcitrant asthma (Slavin, 1986). Evidence from experimental animal studies also suggests that sinusitis may be capable of increasing bronchial responsiveness. It is probable that allergic rhinitis also aggravates asthma; improvement of rhinitis by topical nasal steroids has been reported to lead to improvement of asthma (Reed et al, 1988). Irritation of the upper respiratory tract by any of a variety of mechanisms appears to be capable of triggering asthmatic symptoms.

NONALLERGIC HYPERSENSITIVITY TO DRUGS AND CHEMICALS. Though allergic sensitivity to aspirin has been reported on occasion with manifestations that include asthma, aspirin and nonsteroidal anti-inflammatory drugs (NSAIDs), such as indomethacin and ibuprofen, are more likely to exacerbate asthma on a nonallergic basis. Aspirin ingestion may diminish pulmonary functions in up to one third of children and adolescents with steroid-dependent asthma (Rachelefsky et al, 1975). In many instances, this effect may be subtle. Consequently, as a general rule, it is wise to restrict aspirin and aspirin-containing products for all individuals who have asthma. Patients who react to aspirin are likely to react to other NSAIDs that should be avoided, but most are able to tolerate acetaminophen. Metabisulfite can be an important precipitant or aggravator of asthma, both by allergic and nonallergic mechanisms (Bush et al, 1986) (see Chapter 38). This interaction is much more likely to occur in the steroid-dependent asthmatic patient.

ENDOCRINE FACTORS. Aggravation of asthma occurs in some patients in relation to the menstrual cycle, beginning shortly before menstruation. Whether this reflects changes in water and salt balance, irritability of bronchial and smooth muscle, or other factors is unknown. The use of birth control pills occasionally also aggravates asthma. Hyperthyroidism has been reported to worsen or precipitate asthma severely in an occasional patient. Treatment of hyperthyroidism usually ameliorates the asthma.

SLEEP OR NOCTURNAL ASTHMA. Sleep or nocturnal asthma is a risk factor for asthma severity and even death in some asthmatics. Although nocturnal asthma may result from late-phase reactions to earlier allergen exposure, GER, or sinusitis in some patients, these conditions are not present in most patients with severe nocturnal asthma. Nocturnal asthma does not consistently appear to be related to recumbency or to sleep per se. One possible explanation is an exaggeration of a normal circadian variation in bronchomotor tone (Barnes, 1986). Abnormalities in central nervous system control of respiratory drive, in particular with defective hypoxic drive, also may be present in some patients and can pose serious risks to those with asthma (Martin, 1993). Nocturnal asthma per se should not be considered a unique disease. The patient who manifests increased symptoms at night is likely to have some symptoms in the daytime also, reflecting inflammatory changes in the pulmonary tree around the clock. Consequently, anti-inflammatory therapy in conjunction with bronchodilator is more appropriate than is only symptomatic bronchodilator therapy at night.

INTERACTION OF VARIOUS PRECIPITATING FACTORS. Not infrequently, concurrent exposure to various precipitating or aggravating factors may induce additive effects in asthma. For example, some individuals experience exercise-induced asthma only when exercising in cold air or during a pollen allergy season. Others recognize increased symptoms from specific allergen exposure after respiratory infections. As indicated previously, this may be due to increased bronchial responsiveness caused by inflammation (allergic or infectious).

ASTHMATIC PATTERNS

In some asthmatics, most of the factors listed previously appear to play important roles in asthma, whereas in other asthmatics, only some appear to be important. For example, one patient's asthma may be precipitated by each of the factors listed, whereas for another patient, allergic triggers are of predominant influence in the disease, and other factors are of minor influence. A third patient may have nonallergic asthma precipitated mainly by viral respiratory infection. The estimated importance of each of the precipitating factors in the asthmatic population is noted in the table. Table 34–2 relates the importance of various asthmatic precipitants to age. For example, viral infections are of great importance in precipitating asthma early in the child's life, become relatively less important as the child grows older, and assume a major role again in the adult.

Since the development of allergy is dependent on duration and intensity of exposure to allergens, allergy to foods in infancy generally precedes allergy to inhaled substances. Thereafter, inhaled allergens become progressively more important, as prolonged exposure to such perennial factors as epidermals from domestic animals, house dust mite and cockroach antigens, and airborne mold spores results in allergic sensitization. As the child grows older, repeated pollen exposure results in "pollen" and seasonal mold-induced asthma. In later childhood and in adulthood, exercise becomes an important factor as the patient participates in more strenuous activities, including competitive sports. In later

TABLE 34–2. PRECIPITANTS OF ASTHMATIC SYMPTOMS IN VARIOUS AGE GROUPS

	INFANCY	EARLY CHILDHOOD	LATER CHILDHOOD	ADOLESCENCE AND ADULTHOOD
Viral infections	+ + + +*	+ + +	+ (+)	+ + +
Exercise	+	+ +	+ + +	+ + +
Irritants	+	+ +	+ + +	+ + +
Foods	+ +	+	(+)	(+)
Indoor inhalants	+ (+)	+ + +	+ + +	+ + +
Pollens		+ +	+ + +	+ + (+)
Emotions†		(+)	+	+

*Relative importance denoted, in order, by + + + +, + + +, + +, + + (+), +, + (+), and (+).
†See text.

adulthood, allergens tend to assume much less or no importance, possibly because of age-related waning of immune responsiveness.

THE PRESENTATION OF ASTHMA

A patient with asthma may present with any or all of a variety of symptoms, which can include wheezing, cough, shortness of breath, and complaints of "chest congestion," "tight chest," exercise intolerance, and recurrent "bronchitis" or recurrent "pneumonia." Often asthma appears subtly as coughing without overt wheezing, especially in conjunction with colds or during pollen seasons. On the one hand, the adage attributed to Chevalier Jackson that ". . . not all that wheezes is asthma" has been well publicized, and indeed causes for wheezing other than asthma are numerous (Table 34–3). On the other hand, it has become apparent also that ". . . not all asthma wheezes" (at least not overtly), a presentation in fact that is not uncommon, especially in childhood. In many instances, cursory physical examination fails to reveal evidence of obvious pulmonary obstruction (although careful examination might do so), and obstructive disease of the lower respiratory tract may be overlooked unless pulmonary function is tested. Thus, the physician should consider the diagnosis of asthma not only when the patient has recur-

TABLE 34–3. DIFFERENTIAL DIAGNOSIS OF ASTHMA

CONDITION	RELATIVE FREQUENCY OF OCCURRENCE			
	Infancy	Childhood	Adolescence	Adulthood
Laryngomalacia-tracheomalacia-bronchomalacia	+ +	±	−	−
Cystic fibrosis	+ + +*	+*	±	±†
Chronic viral infection	+ + +	+ +		
Foreign body	+ +	+ + +	±	±
Croup	+ +	+	−	−
Epiglottitis	+ + +	+	−	−
Pertussis	+ + +	+	−	−
Congenital anomalies	+ + +	+	−	−
Hyperventilation syndrome	−	+	+ +	+ +
Bronchiectasis	+	+	+	+
Laryngeal (physical or psychologic) dysfunction	−	−	−	+
Tumors (extra- or intraluminal)	−	−	−	+
COPD (includes emphysema, chronic bronchitis)	−	−	−	+ + *
Cardiac abnormalities	−	−	−	+
Pulmonary embolism	−	−	−	±
Collagen-vascular	−	−	±	±
Aspiration syndromes	+	±	±	+

*Often coexists with an element of "asthma."
†Many patients with cystic fibrosis are now living into adulthood.
The minus sign denotes never or extremely rare.

rent wheezing but when there are repeated complaints referable to the lower respiratory tract even in the absence of wheezing.

"Wheezing" may be a late sign in asthma. It is caused by air rushing past a narrowed portion of the airway in sufficient force to generate air vibrations perceived as sound, and *it occurs only in the larger airways where airflow is turbulent. The small airways are "silent,"* since the air flow there is laminar rather than turbulent. Consequently, marked small airway obstruction can be present but may not be recognized on physical examination. In most instances, airway narrowing in asthma is sufficiently generalized that large and small airway obstruction coexist, so that wheezing is audible either overtly or by auscultation. Before wheezing is perceptible to the patient or the patient's parent, however, there are generally more subtle symptoms of obstruction, such as cough or a feeling of chest discomfort. *Moreover, in many patients, there may not be signs or symptoms until airflow limitation, easily measured by spirometry, is moderately severe (forced expiratory volume in 1 second or FEV_1 below 50 percent of normal). It cannot be overemphasized that auscultation is a useful but highly imperfect device for determining whether or not there is any airflow limitation and, if so, the degree that exists.*

This phenomenon may be more readily appreciated using as an analogy the concept of an iceberg (Fig. 34–3). By this analogy, the ocean floor represents completely normal pulmonary function, and the ocean surface the point at which pulmonary obstruction is obvious clinically. Wheezing, in other words, is the tip of the iceberg. Just as most of the iceberg is not evident, pulmonary obstruction begins well before wheezing is heard and lasts after wheezing is gone (McFadden et al, 1973; Levison et al, 1974). In some instances, the slope of the tip of the iceberg is slight, and obstruction progresses slowly (days); in others, it is steep, and pulmonary obstruction advances rapidly to overt symptoms in minutes to hours. Auscultation may detect wheezing or prolonged expiration before wheezing is overt, and sensitive pulmonary function measurements may detect obstruction before wheezing can be heard by auscultation. Some patients never wheeze despite significant pulmonary obstruction; the obstruction may not be recognized unless pulmonary function tests are performed. "Patterns" can vary substantially from time to time, influenced by treatment and/or natural exposure to allergens or irritants.

Any classification of asthma severity is problematic since asthma is such a heterogeneous disease and functionally dynamic, varying not only between individuals but often in the same individual over time. Nevertheless, a functional classification formulated by the National Asthma Education Program and International Consensus Report on Diagnosis and Management of Asthma will be adopted here because of the importance of accepting

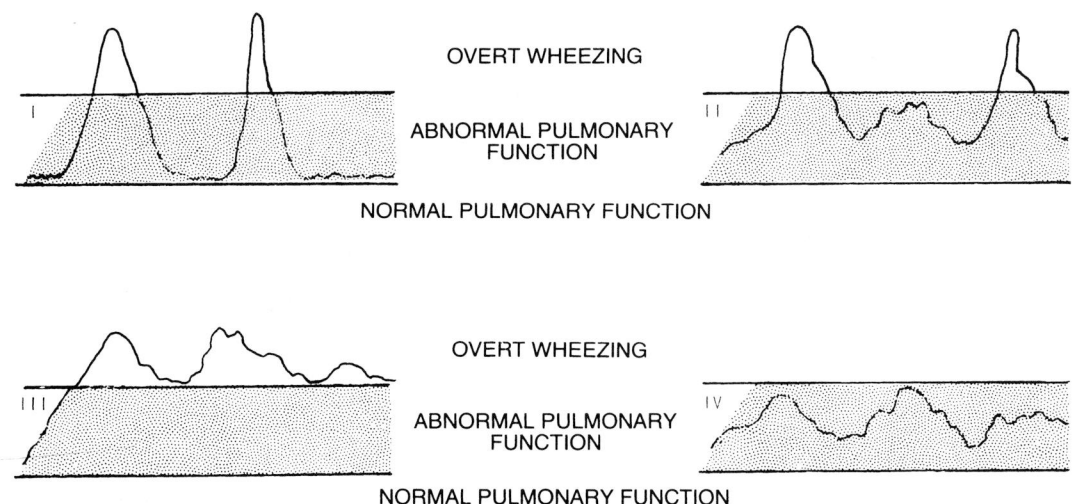

FIGURE 34–3. Iceberg concept of asthma. The "ocean floor" represents pulmonary normality; the surface of the ocean, the point at which asthmatic symptoms (e.g., wheezing) are obvious.

common classifications for a discussion of therapeutic approaches to asthma (Table 34–4).

Recognition of various asthmatic patterns has important therapeutic implications. First, early treatment of asthma is more successful than is late treatment, and even subtle signs of pulmonary obstruction should be signals to institute therapy. In the patient who wheezes with upper respiratory tract infection, the characteristic cough that precedes overt wheezing should be a signal to initiate therapy. In addition, pharmacologic therapy should be continued, even when overt symptoms of asthma have cleared, until pulmonary obstruction has reversed or pulmonary functions have become stable at an acceptable functional level.

In asthmatics who have chronic pulmonary obstruction, pharmacologic treatment must be continuous. *Asthma is a chronic disorder that may surface periodically but in which chronic obstruction may be more severe than frequently is appreciated.*

PROGNOSIS

In children and adolescents, asthma frequently is a completely "reversible" obstructive airway disease, and indeed no abnormalities in pulmonary function can be detected in many asthmatic patients when they become symptom-free. However, there is a significant subpopulation of asthmatic children and adults who, even in the absence of symptoms for prolonged periods of time, have persistent abnormalities in pulmonary function, with chronic hyperinflation, decreased pulmonary flow rates, or both, with or without mild hypoxemia. The potential reversibility of abnormal pulmonary function—even in severely asthmatic children—toward normal by intensive therapy was demonstrated by Tooley and colleagues (1965). However, it is clear that in many children and adults with severe asthma, normal pulmonary function cannot be maintained without continuous intensive therapy, including oral corticosteroids. Reversibility of pulmonary function

TABLE 34–4. ASTHMA SEVERITY

ASTHMA SEVERITY	TREATMENT

Mild asthma
  Brief episodes up to twice a week
  Asymptomatic between episodes
  Brief if any exercise-related symptoms
  Little (less than twice a month) or no nocturnal symptoms
  FEV_1 or peak flow at least 80% of "normal"*
	Inhaled $beta_2$-agonist p.r.n. (i.e., every 4–6 hours). (For very young children, an oral $beta_2$ agent can be used.)
	Inhaled $beta_2$-agonist, cromolyn sodium or both before exercise if needed

Moderate asthma
  Episodes greater than twice a week
  Episodes last for hours to days
  Emergency care, if necessary, infrequent
  FEV_1 or peak flow 60–80% of normal (without medication)
	Inhaled $beta_2$-agonist p.r.n. If needed daily,† other than for exercise, probable need for daily maintenance "anti-inflammatory" (inhaled corticosteroid, cromolyn sodium or nedocromil). A trial of cromolyn sodium is encouraged first in children.†
	Theophylline, oral or long-acting inhaled $beta_2$ can be added to the above agents, but are not considered "anti-inflammatory"

Severe asthma
  Symptoms more or less continuous in the absence of medication
  Frequent asthma exacerbations
  Frequent nocturnal symptoms
  Activity generally limited
  Periodic emergency treatment; occasional hospitalization
  Any life-threatening episodes
  FEV_1 or peak flow less than 60% without medication
	Inhaled $beta_2$-agonist p.r.n.
	Inhaled corticosteroid; possibly at higher dosage
	Cromolyn sodium or nedocromil sodium, theophylline and/or long-acting oral or inhaled† $beta_2$ agents may be used as steroid-sparing or for added control of nocturnal or other symptoms
	Consideration of oral corticosteroids at lowest dose possible if other therapy not adequate

*Defined as the best function achievable for the child or, until that is established, "predicted" (average) for a normal population.
†Authors' modification.
Adapted from NAEP Guidelines for the Diagnosis and Management of Asthma, 1991, and the International Consensus Report on Diagnosis and Management of Asthma, 1992.

abnormalities with therapy is transient in that withdrawal of constant therapy usually leads to the return of pulmonary function to initial abnormal baselines (Cade and Pain, 1973).

As noted previously, even severe asthma generally does not progress to emphysema. However, asthma appears to progress to chronic nonreversible obstructive disease in some individuals with the disorder. Chronic mucus plugging, tracheobronchial ciliary dysfunction, smooth muscle hyperplasia, and persistent hyperinflation among other factors may lead to pulmonary abnormalities in adult life. Findings of residual pulmonary function abnormalities following respiratory viral infections early in life (Cypcar and Busse, 1993) and the fact that viral respiratory tract infections occur more commonly in asthmatic children than in their nonasthmatic siblings are other contributing factors. Similarly, one may see similar irreversible pulmonary changes in asthmatic adults. In addition, passive or active smoking has been shown to be related to more rapid decline in the small airways function in comparison with nonasthmatics (Barter and Campbell, 1976). Thus, it is not clear to what extent asthma per se leads to irreversible pulmonary changes and what accounts for the great variability, even among patients with seemingly similar severity of clinical disease. This variability undoubtedly is a reflection, in part, of the fact that asthma is a heterogeneous disease with sufficient clinical and pathologic similarities to warrant its inclusion in a common syndrome. Evidence suggests, however, that asthma significantly predisposes patients to irreversible damage from various noxious environmental agents (Pearlman, 1989).

Since the natural course of continued bronchial obstruction is not known, a therapeutic dilemma arises about the extent to which asthma should be treated. Should the patient be treated until pulmonary function is totally normal or until he or she can function reasonably and normally even though pulmonary function is abnormal? There is suggestive evidence that prolonged treatment of asthma with anti-inflammatory agents in the form of inhaled corticosteroids (Dompeling et al, 1993) can slow the rate of decline in baseline lung function, and that a delay in initiating inhaled corticosteroid therapy may diminish the ultimate improvement in lung function that can be achieved (Agertoft and Pedersen, 1994). Whether intensive therapy early in the course of asthma or persistent therapy to achieve constant pulmonary normality can prevent any irreversible changes or can optimize lung growth needs to be confirmed. Evidence from removal of adults with occupational asthma from the workplace early in the course of the development of their disease (Chan-Yeung et al, 1982) and asthmatic patients sensitive to dust mites from dust mite–laden environments (see Chapter 15) *strongly suggests that the most favorable prognosis for ameliorating or eliminating asthma results from the identification of causative allergen(s) and early elimination of exposure to the allergen.*

Information on the relationships among age of onset, severity of asthma, and ultimate prognosis is conflicting. It appears, however, that a patient with asthma that begins before 2 years of age and is allergic may have a worse prognosis (Wilson, 1994) in terms of severity and longevity than one with asthma that begins later in childhood. Those with *severe* asthma earlier in life also appear to have less favorable prognoses than those with mild asthma. Asthma in childhood tends to be more severe, and the patient is less likely to become symptom-free if allergic mechanisms are involved in the disease. Conversely, there is some suggestion that infants and young children with symptoms precipitated only by viral respiratory tract infections ("wheezy bronchitis" or "asthmatic bronchitis") more likely will become symptom-free in later childhood. Indeed, it is not clear that episodic wheezing induced only by viral infection early in life necessarily is "asthma" (Wilson, 1994). Nonallergic asthma in adulthood, however, has a significantly worse prognosis than does allergic asthma.

Asthma tends to be more severe in general and occurs earlier if there is a family history of atopic disease in close relatives or if there is a personal history of other atopic disorders (atopic dermatitis or allergic rhinitis).

Although morbidity from asthma is high, mortality from asthma fortunately occurs at a low rate. Nevertheless, deaths from asthma do occur, attributable to a variety of causes and occurring mainly in patients with severe asthma. Foremost among these causes are the failure by patient, physician, or both to appreciate the severity of asthma and to treat it appropriately. Deaths have been attributed to overuse of inhaled $beta_2$ bronchodilators.

However, by far the greatest contributor to death from the disease is undertreatment. The underdiagnosis of the severity of asthma by physicians and health care workers in general undoubtedly contributes to the fact that an emergency room constitutes a risk factor for death in asthmatics! The lability of asthma, regardless of severity, also is a risk factor, as are respiratory infections, nocturnal asthma, history of respiratory failure, and marked diurnal variation in airflow limitation with low pulmonary function in the morning ("morning dippers"). *It is important to recognize that some patients cannot perceive severe airflow obstruction, especially when it occurs gradually.* Such patients must be taught to recognize warning signs of airflow obstruction. A simple device for measuring airflow, such as a portable peak flow meter, will help the patient to recognize the development of severe asthma. Psychologic factors have also been implicated in sudden deaths, particularly in asthmatic adolescents (Strunk et al, 1985; Asthma Deaths, 1986; Benatar, 1986).

REFERENCES

Aas K. Bronchial provocation tests in asthma. Arch Dis Child 45:221, 1970.

Agertoft L, Pedersen S: Effects of long-term treatment with an inhaled corticosteroid on growth and pulmonary function in asthmatic children. Respir Med 88:373–381, 1994.

Asthma Deaths. N.E.R. Allergy Proc 7:421–470, 1986.

Bai TR. Abnormalities in airways smooth muscle in fatal asthma. Am Rev Respir Dis 141:552–557, 1990.

Bai TR, Mak JCW, Barnes PJ. A comparison of beta-adrenergic receptors and *in vitro* relaxant responses to isoproterenol in asthmatic airway smooth muscle. Am J Respir Cell Molec Biol 6:647–651, 1992.

Barnes PJ. Nocturnal asthma: Underlying mechanisms and implications for therapy. Immunol Allergy Pract 3:9–15, 1986.

Barter CE, Campbell AH. Relationship of constitutional factors and cigarette smoking to decrease in 1-second forced expiratory volume. Am Rev Respir Dis 113:305–314, 1976.

Benatar SR. Fatal asthma. N Engl J Med 314:423–488, 1986.

Bias WB. The genetic basis of asthma. *In* Austen KF, Lichtenstein LM (eds). Asthma. New York, Academic Press Inc., 1973.

Blair H. Natural history of childhood asthma. Arch Dis Child 52:613–619, 1977.

Broide DH, Lotz M, Cuomo AJ, Coburn DA, Federman EC, Wasserman SI. Cytokines in symptomatic asthma airways. J Allerg Clin Immunol 89:958–967, 1992.

Bush RK, Taylor SL, Busse W. A critical evaluation of clinical trials in reactions to sulfites. J Allergy Clin Immunol 78:191–201, 1986.

Cade JF, Pain MCF. Pulmonary function during clinical remission of asthma. How reversible is asthma? Aust N Z J Med 3:545–551, 1973.

Chan-Yeung M, Lam S, Koener S. Clinical features and natural history of occupational asthma due to Western Red Cedar (Thuja plicata). Am J Med 72:411–415, 1982.

Cockroft DW. Mechanism of perennial allergic asthma. Lancet 2:253–255, 1983.

Cockroft DW, Murdock KY, Berscheid BA. Relationship between atopy and bronchial responsiveness to histamine in a random population. Ann Allergy 53:26–29, 1984.

Cockroft DW, Ruffin RE, Frith PA, Cartier A, Juniper EF, Dolovich J, Hargreave FE. Determinants of allergen-induced asthma: Dose of allergen circulating IgE antibody concentration and bronchial responsiveness to inhaled histamine. Am Rev Respir Dis 120:1053–1058, 1979.

Corrao WM, Braman SS, Irwin RS. Chronic cough as the sole presenting manifestation of bronchial asthma. N Engl J Med 300:633–637, 1979.

Cutz E, Levison H, Cooper DM. Ultrastructure of airways in children with asthma. Histopathology 2:407–421, 1978.

Cypcar D, Busse WW. Role of viral infections in asthma. Immunol Allergy Clin North Am 13:745–767, 1993.

Cypcar D, Stark J, Lemanske RF Jr. The impact of respiratory infections on asthma. Pediatr Clin North Am 39:1259–1276, 1992.

Dompeling E, van Schayck CP, van Grunsven PM, van Herwaarden CL, Akkermans R, Molema J, Folgering H, van Weel C. Slowing the deterioration of asthma and chronic obstructive pulmonary disease observed during bronchodilator therapy by adding inhaled corticosteroids. A 4-year prospective study. Ann Intern Med 118:770–778, 1993.

Flensborg EW. The prognosis for bronchial asthma arisen in infancy after the nonspecific treatment hitherto applied. Acta Paediatr 33:4–23, 1945.

Frick RB, Metzger WJ, Richerson HB, Zavala DC, Moseley P, Schoderbek WE, Hunninghake GW. Increased bronchovascular permeability after allergen exposure in sensitive asthmatics. J Appl Physiol 63:1147–1155, 1987.

James AL, Pare PD, Hogg JC. The mechanics of airway narrowing in asthma. Am Rev Respir Dis 139:242–246, 1989.

Kinsman RA, Dahlein NW, Spector S, Studenmayer H. Observations on subjective symptomatology, coping behavior, and medical decision in asthma. Psychosomat Med 39:102–119, 1977.

Lacoste J-Y, Bousquet J, Chanez P, Van Vyve T, Simony-Lafontaine J, Lequeu N, Vic P, Enander I, Godard P, Michel F-B. Eosinophilic and neutrophilic inflammation in asthma, chronic bronchitis, and chronic obstructive pulmonary disease. J Allergy Clin Immunol 92:537–548, 1993.

Leff AR, Hamann KJ, Wegner CD. Inflammation and cell-cell interactions in airway hyperresponsiveness. Am J Physiol 260:L189–L206, 1991.

Lemanske RF Jr, Kaliner M. Late-phase allergic reactions. *In* Middleton E Jr, Reed CE, Ellis EF, Adkinson NF Jr, Yunginger JW, Busse WW (eds). Allergy: Principles and Practice. 4th ed. St. Louis, Mosby–Year Book, 1993, pp 320–361.

Levison H, Collins-Williams C, Bryan AC, Reilly BJ, Orange RP. Asthma: Current concepts. Pediatr Clin North Am 21:957–965, 1974.

Lundgren JD, Shelhamer JH. Pathogenesis of airway mucus hypersecretion. J Allergy Clin Immunol 85:399–417, 1990.

Martin RJ. Insights into the management of nocturnal asthma. Immunol Allergy Clin North Am 13:803–818, 1993.

McConnochie KM, Roghmann KJ. Breast feeding and maternal smoking as predictors of wheezing in children age 6 to 10 years. Pediatr Pulmonol 2:260–268, 1986.

McFadden ER Jr. Exertional dyspnea and cough as preludes to acute attacks of bronchial asthma. N Engl J Med 292:555–559, 1975a.

McFadden ER Jr. The chronicity of acute attacks of asthma—mechanical and therapeutic implications. J Allergy Clin Immunol 56:18–26, 1975b.

McFadden ER Jr, Gilbert IA. Asthma. N Engl J Med 327:1928–1937, 1992.

McFadden ER Jr, Kisser R, DeGroot WJ. Acute bronchial asthma: Relations between clinical and physiological manifestations. N Engl J Med 288:221–228, 1973.

Metzger WJ, Zavala D, Richerson HB, Moseley P, Iwamota P, Monick M, Sjoerdsma K, Hunninghake GW. Local allergen challenge and bronchoalveolar lavage of allergic asthmatic lungs. Description of the model and local airway inflammation. Am Rev Respir Dis 135:433–440, 1987.

NAEP Guidelines for the diagnosis and management of asthma. US Dept of Health and Human Services. Public. No. 91–3042, 1991.

Nelson H. The natural history of asthma. Ann Allergy 66:196–204, 1991.

Pearlman DS. Bronchial Asthma. A perspective from childhood through adulthood—update. Pediatr Asthma Allergy Immunol 3:191–205, 1989.

Rachelefsky GS, Coulson A, Siegel SC, Stiehm ER. Aspirin intolerance in chronic childhood asthma: Detected by oral challenge. Pediatrics 56:443–448, 1975.

Rackemann FM. Intrinsic asthma. J Allergy 11:147, 1940.

Reed CE, Marcoux JP, Welsh PW. Effects of topical nasal treatment on asthma symptoms. J Allergy Clin Immunol 81:1042–1047, 1988.

Robuschi M, Vaghi A, Simone P. Prevention of fog-induced bronchospasm by nedocromil sodium. Clin Allergy 17:69–75, 1987.

Ryssing E. Continued follow-up investigation concerning the fate of 298 asthmatic children. Acta Pediatr 48:255–260, 1959.

Salvato G. Some histologic changes in chronic bronchitis and asthma. Thorax 23:168–172, 1968.

Sibbald B, Horn MEC, Brain EA, Gregg L. Genetic factors in childhood asthma. Thorax 35:671–674, 1980.

Slavin RG. Recalcitrant asthma: Have you looked for sinusitis? J Resp Dis 7:61–68, 1986.

Speight ANP, Lee DA, Hey EN. Underdiagnosis and undertreatment of asthma in childhood. Br Med J 286:1253–1256, 1983.

Sporik R, Chapman MD, Platts-Mills TAE. House dust mite exposure as a cause of asthma. Clin Exper Allergy 22:897–906, 1992.

Strunk RD, Mrazek DA, Fuhrmann GS, LaBreoque JF. Physiologic and psychological characteristics associated with deaths due to asthma in childhood. JAMA 254:1193–1198, 1985.

Thompson AB, Daughton D, Robbins RA, Ghafouri MA, Oehlerking M, Rennard SI. Intraluminal airway inflammation in chronic bronchitis. Am Rev Respir Dis 140:1527–1537, 1989.

Tooley WH, DeMuth C, Nadel JA. The reversibility of obstructive changes in severe childhood asthma. J Pediatr 66:517–524, 1965.

Townley RG, Guirgis H, Bewtra A, Watt G, Burke K, Carney K. IgE levels and methacholine inhalation responses in monozygous and dizygous twins. J Allergy Clin Immunol 57:227, 1976. (Abstract)

Townley RG, Ryo UY, Kolokin BM, Kang B. Bronchial sensitivity to methacholine in current and former asthmatic and allergic rhinitis patients and control subjects. J Allergy Clin Immunol 56:429–432, 1975.

Vittori E, Marini M, Fasoli A, de Franchis R, Mattoli S. Increased expression of endothelin in bronchial epithelial cells of asthmatic patients and effect of corticosteroids. Am Rev Respir Dis 146:1320–1325, 1992.

Wanner A, Abraham WM, Douglas JS, Drazen JM, Richerson HB, Sri Ram J. Modes of airway hyperresponsiveness. NHLBI Workshop Summary. Am Rev Respir Dis 141:253–257, 1990.

Weiss KB, Gergen PJ, Hodgson TA. An economic evaluation of asthma in the United States. N Engl J Med 326:862–866, 1992.

Weitzman M, Gortmaker S, Walker DR, Sobol A. Maternal smoking and childhood asthma. Pediatrics 85:505–511, 1990.

Wiggs BR, Bosken C, Pare PF, James A, Hogg JC. A model of airway narrowing in asthma and in chronic obstructive pulmonary disease. Am Rev Respir Dis 145:1251–1258, 1992.

Wilson NM. The significance of early wheezing. Clin Exper Allergy 24:522–529, 1994.

Chapter 35

Evaluation and Treatment of the Patient with Asthma

Pediatric Asthma

C. Warren Bierman, M.D., and Gail G. Shapiro, M.D.

Adult Asthma

Deborah Ortega Carr, M.D., Robert K. Bush, M.D., and William W. Busse, M.D.

EVALUATION

There are three important elements in the evaluation of the patient with asthma: the history, the physical examination and measurement of pulmonary function.

History

The history should uncover the evolution of symptoms over days, months, or years, specific days of the week, and time of day, with a view toward associations such as seasonality, visits to homes with pets, times of respiratory infections, and physical activity. The history should answer the following questions: Is the problem episodic or continual? If episodic, how often are the episodes, and are they truly isolated or rather acute bursts connected by more subtle symptoms of disease? Since all but the mildest asthma involves chronic pulmonary inflammation, it is likely that the situation is also chronic, if one delves under the surface exacerbations. Are there specific cause and effect associations or trigger factors? These should be clarified so that their avoidance can be incorporated in a management plan. The severity of the symptoms will largely influence therapy. Have there been emergency room visits, hospitalizations, need for intubation and assisted ventilation? Have these problems occurred in the face of appropriate medication, or has the patient been undertreated?

Symptoms vary with age. The infant and young child may have histories of recurrent bronchitis or pneumonia, persistent coughing with colds, recurrent "croup," or just a chronic "chest rattle." Older children and adolescents and adults often develop "tight" chests with colds, recurrent "chest congestion," "bronchitis," or persistent coughing or wheezing. Respiratory symptoms may be precipitated or exacerbated also by exposure to animals, moldy or dusty areas, tobacco smoke, or cold air, or by exercise.

The past medical history and review of systems often clarifies the picture presented by the history of the present illness. If the patient had food allergy and eczema in infancy, allergy will probably remain an important factor. One needs to inquire about such allergic manifestations as gastrointestinal problems, including vomiting or diarrhea; skin conditions, such as atopic dermatitis or hives; and the presence or absence of factors such as recurrent colds, perennial nasal obstruction, hay fever, ear infections, sinus infections, bronchitis, pneumonia, and exercise tolerance. One needs to ask specifically about factors that may aggravate symptoms such as exposure to house dust, animals, grass cuttings, and irritants such as aerosol sprays and cigarette smoke, or reactions to outdoor pollutants. Drug reactions are particularly important, especially idiosyncratic or allergic reactions to antibiotics, aspirin, and other nonsteroidal antiinflammatory drugs, bronchodilators, or antihistamines. One should also inquire about unusual reactions to insect stings and about hospitalizations. Details about whether the patient had previously had an allergy-related work-up, with studies for specific IgE identification and immunotherapy (hyposensitization), lung functions, and response to medication should be recorded.

The environmental history is a unique and important element in the patient with suspected asthma or other respiratory allergies, since many of the symptoms may be exacerbated by factors found in the surroundings, whether home, school, work, or play. The environmental history is of importance primarily because it provides information on potential allergens to which the patient is exposed, and it is the cornerstone of therapy in terms of avoidance of specific factors that may be identified by allergy testing. The patient's environment includes the home, neighborhood, and work or school. Materials used in hobbies or at work may prove to be of significance in inducing symptoms (see Chapters 8 and 37). In patients of all ages, it is important to ask about cigarette smoking or exposure to second-hand tobacco smoke.

Physical Examination

The physical examination may be dramatic or unrevealing. It begins with an overall visual impression and should include at least an assessment of the head, neck, chest and skin, but other systems as well, if indicated by the history. If the patient is experiencing an acute episode of airway obstruction, it is common to note anxiety, dyspnea, and increased respiratory rate in both children and adults. There may be audible wheezing and probably cough. None of this may be apparent between acute episodes. In children, if chronic obstruction has been longstanding, one may see a bowing of the ribs and an increased anterior-posterior diameter of the chest, since growth and bony remodeling will accommodate chronic pulmonary hyperinflation. On auscultation, one may notice increased expiratory phase of respiration. There may be wheezing on expiration or on both inspiration and expiration; coarse wheezes may take on the quality of rhonchi. Rales usually indicate parenchymal disease (e.g., pneumonia); however, they may also be present if there is localized atelectasis, not uncommon with asthma. Sudden deterioration and absence of breath sounds suggest the rare complication of pneumothorax. More common is crepitus and extrapulmonary dissection of air with apparent edema extending upward from the chest into the neck and face due to dissecting pneumomediastinum, usually a spontaneously resolving event, but one that suggests severe obstruction.

The head and neck examination is often abnormal in patients with asthma. Children may show evidence of middle ear disease (which may be a complication of allergic rhinitis): middle ear fluid, otitis, or ventilating tubes. In both children and adults, the eyes may show conjunctival edema and injection compatible with allergic disease. There may be periorbital edema and discoloration due to the venous and lymphatic stasis that may accompany allergic rhinitis (so-called "allergic shiners"). The nose may show the pallor, edema, and clear secretions of allergic rhinitis or erythema and purulent secretion from infectious rhinitis or sinusitis. The presence of nasal polyps in children suggests cystic fibrosis, whereas in the adolescent and adult it suggests nonallergic eosinophilic disease (possibly with aspirin sensitivity), which may involve the upper and lower airway. Since sinusitis and viral upper respiratory infections both exacerbate asthma, it is important to diagnose and treat those problems that are likely to be bacterial. Skin manifestations of atopy, such as the lichenification and flexor crease rash of atopic dermatitis (eczema), frequently precede the onset of chronic asthma.

Laboratory Evaluation (See Table 35–1)

LUNG FUNCTION TESTS. Lung function tests are objective, noninvasive, and cost-effective

TABLE 35–1. LABORATORY TESTS IN ASTHMA

Tests	Possible Abnormalities in Asthma	Comments
Complete blood count	Leukocytosis (occasionally)	Induced by infection, epinephrine administration, "stress" (?)
	Eosinophilia (frequently)	Varies with medication, time of day, adrenal function; not necessarily related to "allergy" (often higher in "intrinsic" than "extrinsic" asthma)
Sputum examination	Eosinophils	In both "intrinsic" and "extrinsic" asthma
White or "clear" and small yellow plugs	Charcot-Leyden crystals	Derived from eosinophils
	Creola bodies	Clusters of epithelial cells
	Curschmann's spirals	Threads of glycoprotein
Nasal smear	Eosinophils	Suggests probably concomitant nasal allergy
	Lymphocytes, PMNs, macrophages	Sometimes replace eosinophils in upper respiratory infection
	PMNs with ingested bacteria	Bacterial rhinitis or sinusitis
Serum tests	IgG, IgA, IgM	Often normal; may be abnormal; various patterns seen
	IgE	Sometimes elevated in "allergic" asthma; markedly elevated in active bronchopulmonary aspergillosis; often normal
	Aspergillus-precipitating antibody	Suggestive, not diagnostic of bronchopulmonary aspergillosis
Sweat test	Normal in asthma	Cystic fibrosis and asthma can coexist
	Perform to rule out cystic fibrosis	
Chest film	Hyperinflation, infiltrates, pneumomediastinum, pneumothorax	Indicated once in all patients with asthma; should be considered on hospitalization for asthma
Lung function tests	↓ FEV_1, ↓ $FEF_{25-75\%}$, ↓ PEFR; FEV_1/FVC ↓	Useful for following course of disease, response to treatment
Response to bronchodilators	>15% improvement FEV_1, PEFR	Safest diagnostic test for asthma
Exercise tests	Decreased lung function after 6 minutes of exercise	Useful to diagnose asthma; often abnormal when resting lung function is normal
	PEFR and FEV_1 >15% ↓	
	$FEF_{25-75\%}$ >25% ↓	
Methacholine inhalation test (mecholyl test); histamine inhalation test	20% fall in lung function with dose tolerated by "normal" subjects	Should be performed by specialist only
Antigen inhalation test	20% fall in lung function immediately after challenge; may cause delayed response 6–8 hours later	Potentially dangerous; should be performed by specialist only
Allergy skin tests	Identifies allergic factors that *might* be causative factors	Test likely factors only; select by history
Serologic tests for IgE antibody (e.g., RAST)	Same significance as skin tests	More expensive than skin tests

in the diagnosis and follow-up of the patient with asthma. A simple mechanical spirometer, from which an FEV_1 and forced vital capacity (FVC) can be calculated, or a Wright Peak Flow Meter (pediatric meters are available for younger children) is useful in office practice. Children as young as 4 years old can be taught to perform pulmonary function maneuvers with birthday party favors that make whistle sounds to reinforce forced expiration. Results can be compared with normal standards (Chapter 12).

Spirometry involves certain pitfalls, but adequate results generally can be obtained from children over 5 years of age. The best of three forced expiratory tracings should be used as the best estimate of a patient's pulmonary function. Coaching and teaching are required for the patient to achieve good technique. If the curves that are generated do not fit the clinical picture, one must look at the quality of data entry and technique before assuming that there is lung disease. Spirometry may be expressed with flow-volume curves rather than time-volume curves. Flow-volume loops include a tracing for inspiratory flow. This is helpful for distinguishing extrathoracic from intrathoracic obstruction. Normal configurations for flow-volume loops and time-volume spirometry are described in Chapter 12. When patients are uncooperative or unable to learn proper spirometric technique, body plethysmography, which is generally available in hospital pulmonary function laboratories, can be used.

RESPONSE TO BRONCHODILATORS. The safest diagnostic test for asthma is to look for an improvement in lung function before and after administration of bronchodilators, preferably β_2-agonists (inhalation of two actuations of albuterol or equivalent) by pressurized metered-dose inhaler or 0.1 to 0.15 mg/kg aerosol solution of albuterol (5 mg maximum), or epinephrine injections (epinephrine hydrochloride 1:1000, 0.01 ml/kg up to a maximum dose of 0.3 ml subcutaneously). A greater than 15 percent improvement is virtually diagnostic of asthma. If there is a lack of improvement in FEV_1, it does not necessarily rule out asthma. With severe airway inflammation, a 1- to 2-week course of oral corticosteroids may be necessary to demonstrate a reversible component to airflow obstruction.

EXERCISE TOLERANCE TESTS. In older children and adolescents, a free-running exercise tolerance test is simple to perform and requires little equipment (see Chapter 36). One may also use a treadmill in a pulmonary function laboratory. A fall greater than 15 percent in FEV_1 or peak flow, or alternatively a 30 percent fall in forced expiratory flow between 25 to 75 of vital capacity (FEF_{25-75}) is diagnostic of exercise-induced asthma.

CHEMICAL CHALLENGE TESTS. Chemical challenges are valuable for the adult patient with presumptive asthma and/or chronic cough when baseline pulmonary function is normal and therapeutic trials with anti-asthma medications are inconclusive. Patients with asthma have airways that are overly sensitive to bronchoconstrictors (see Chapter 13). Methacholine and histamine challenges can be performed with standardized protocols that have high specificity and sensitivity for airway hyperresponsiveness and asthma (Williams and Shapiro, 1995). Methacholine is commercially available as an FDA-approved product, Provocholine. Patients inhale increasing concentrations of methacholine according to a standardized protocol and perform spirometry after inhaling each concentration of the drug. The challenge is complete when FEV_1 has dropped 20 percent or more from baseline or when one completes inhalation of a dosage of 25 mg/ml. A decline in FEV_1 of 20 percent indicates bronchial hyperresponsiveness. When this information is melded with a supporting clinical history, the diagnosis of asthma becomes likely (Holgate et al, 1987). On the other hand, a negative challenge usually excludes asthma (see Chapter 13).

Distilled water inhalation, eucapneic hyperventilation of cold air, and hypertonic water inhalation are alternative challenge procedures. These are less well standardized than methacholine and exercise challenge. Inhalation challenge of specific antigens would seem to offer valuable diagnostic information regarding asthma triggers; however, in practice, antigen challenge has severe limitations. Antigen inhalation may produce bronchospasm in the laboratory whereas only rhinitis occurs after natural inhalation. Also, late phase reactions are common and may occur after the patient leaves the laboratory. *All bronchial challenge tests are potentially dangerous. They should be performed only by specialists who have had special training in their use and experience in this technique.*

NASAL AND SPUTUM CYTOLOGY. These may be helpful in patient evaluation. The patient blows his or her nose or coughs into plastic wrap; the secretions are then applied to a glass slide, heat-fixed, and stained with Hansel's stain, an eosin-methylene blue combination that stains eosinophils distinctively. Alternatively, a tiny nasal brush or rhino-probe device can be used to obtain a specimen from the wall of the nasal vault. The presence of greater than 5 to 10 percent eosinophils is suggestive of allergic inflammatory disease but not necessarily asthma. Hyperplastic nonallergic rhinosinusitis with eosinophilia also can be seen in patients in whom sinus disease and asthma coexist. The presence of large numbers of neutrophils and bacteria suggests infection. If the problem has been longstanding, the possibility of subacute or chronic sinusitis, which serves to aggravate bronchial hyperresponsiveness, should be considered (Rachelefsky et al, 1984). When dealing with sputum, fresh sputum is placed in a thin layer on a slide with a platinum loop, is stained, and then examined in the same fashion. In sputum, one may also see "Curschmann's spirals," which are threads of glycoprotein; "creola bodies," which are clusters of epithelial cells; or "Charcot-Leyden crystals," which are derived from eosinophils.

TOTAL SERUM IgE. Total serum IgE determination may be helpful at times although it is nonspecific and there are overlaps in the serum levels of normal and allergic individuals. Approximately 80 percent of children with allergen-induced asthma and 50 percent of adults will have a total serum IgE greater than two standard deviations from the nonallergic population mean. The presence of an elevated IgE suggests allergic bronchopulmonary aspergillosis (ABPA) or an environmental allergy that may be an important trigger factor for asthma (see Chapter 40). More helpful, however, is evaluation of antigen-specific IgE (see Chapter 11).

CHEST X-RAY EXAMINATION. All patients with asthma should have chest roentgenograms at some time to rule out parenchymal disease, congenital anomaly, and foreign body. A chest film should be considered for every patient admitted to a hospital with asthma, depending on the presentation and severity of asthma and any suspicion of complications, such as pneumonia and pneumothorax. Roentgenographic findings in asthma may range from normal to hyperinflation with peribronchial interstitial infiltrate and atelectasis. In a 3-year study of children hospitalized for asthma, the following abnormalities were seen: 76 percent had hyperinflation with increased bronchial markings; 20 percent had infiltrates, atelectasis, pneumonia, or a combination of the three; and 5.4 percent had pneumomediastinum, often with infiltrates (Eggleston et al, 1974). Pneumothorax occurs rarely and did not occur in this study. Paranasal sinus films also should be considered in patients with persistent nocturnal coughing, postnasal mucus, and headaches (see Chapter 30).

ALLERGY TESTING. Allergy testing (skin testing or serologic testing, such as radioallergosorbent testing or RAST) is indicated in patients in whom specific allergic factors are believed to be important. Testing is done with extracts of selective allergen based on history and known or potential allergen exposure (see Chapter 11). Asthma in children and adults is frequently exacerbated by exposure to environmental allergens through mechanisms that are described in Chapter 15. In a given patient, the same antigen-specific IgE that can trigger inflammatory events in the airway can be detected in the skin. Antigen applied to the skin reacts with specific mast cell–bound antibody, which induces mediator release. Histamine will create local vasodilation with wheal and flare within 15 minutes, and a variety of chemotactic factors may create a delayed inflammatory response hours later. Although true positive skin tests indicate that a patient has antigen-specific IgE, it does not prove that exposure will create clinically significant disease. The predictive value of a positive skin test is enhanced if the reactivity is intense and occurs in conjunction with a positive provocative history.

Allergens may play a significant role in asthma pathogenesis in many adult patients. Up to 85 percent of asthma patients have positive skin test reactions to common aeroallergens (Kaliner and Lemanske, 1992). The control of outdoor allergens usually relies on medication and immunotherapy, whereas control of indoor allergens involves elimination of the offending antigen, particularly in the case of house dust mite, fungi, and animal dander (see Chapter 15) (Platts-Mills and Chapman, 1987).

As an alternative to allergen-specific skin tests, serum IgE against a specific antigen can be measured with serologic tests such as the radioallergosorbent (RAST) test, as noted in Chapter 11. In this procedure, antigens are coupled to an inert carrier such as latex or cellulose and mixed with the patient's serum, after which binding of antigen and patient's antibody is measured. In general, RAST testing is less sensitive and more expensive than skin testing (AAAI Position Statement, 1983). Its use may be needed in specific situations such as when severe skin disease or dermatographism precludes skin testing, or when the subject is taking an agent such as an antihistamine, which will suppress skin tests.

THERAPEUTIC CONSIDERATION

PHILOSOPHY OF MANAGEMENT. A comprehensive approach to treatment of asthma requires an understanding of the disease, the manner in which patients present, and how the disease may affect physical and psychological growth and development in children and interfere with work and normal interpersonal relationships in adolescents and adults. *The ultimate goals are to prevent disability and to minimize physical and psychological morbidity.* These include facilitating social adjustment of the patient with the family, school, work, and community, including normal participation in recreational activities and sports. This adjustment is achieved in steps and should begin with early diagnosis and appropriate management of acute episodes. Irritant and allergic factors should be identified and eliminated from the patient's environment. *Education of the patient's parents, the patient, or both to the long-term course of asthma, to the management of exacerbations, and to the importance of ongoing therapy to minimize acute exacerbations is an essential part of asthma treatment.* Unnecessary and illogical restriction of the patient's and family's life styles should be avoided. Associated conditions that exacerbate asthma and predispose the patient to school or work absenteeism or interfere with school or work performance must be recognized and treated. The ultimate goal should be "functional" normality, in which maximal benefit is achieved from total therapy with the fewest detrimental effects.

Achieving these goals requires time, knowledge, and experience. The demands on the physician will vary depending on the severity of the disease, the age of the patient, and the resources of the patient or family. The family physician, internist, or pediatrician *who is willing to devote the time* can care adequately for the patient with mild or moderate asthma. Allergens and irritants that may be driving this disease should be investigated thoroughly in patients with all forms of asthma. However, the patient with moderate and severe asthma will benefit from referral to an allergist who has the knowledge and experience to modify therapy for special situations, to educate the patient about asthma, to follow the patient's progress, and to act as a co-manager with the primary care physician. Such a referral should help to minimize acute attacks and the need for hospitalization or, when hospitalization is necessary, to reduce the length of hospital stay. A team approach that includes regular communication between the primary care physician and the specialist is essential for consistent and comprehensive long-term care.

Compliance by patient, family, or both is the keystone of any therapy. Compliance is influenced by many factors: the physician's attitude; the family's and the patient's understanding of the disease; and peer pressure. It is in relation to *compliance* that psychological factors are of overwhelming importance. The attitude of the patient toward the disease is paramount in his or her willingness to follow the physician's recommendations. The patient's attitude toward asthma and willingness to comply with recommendations reflect the parents' or peers' attitudes toward the disease. The physician's guidance can prevent overprotection or neglect by helping the family of a younger child to cope with such aspects of asthma as the inconvenience of a round-the-clock medication schedule and environmental control. In older children and adults, the physician should place the responsibility for taking medication on the patient. When medication is needed in school or at work, the patient should be permitted to take it privately without embarrassment. The physician should aid the patient in making decisions on such activities as sports, camping trips, traveling, and other activities requiring the patient to be away from the home environment while ensuring appropriate control of asthma.

Finally, when a patient fails to comply, the physician should try to find out the reasons and should work out a reasonable solution acceptable to the patient and/or the family. *Noncompliance in the face of severe disease, particularly in an adolescent or geriatric patient, places him or her at great risk with regard to both morbidity from the disease and death.*

Environmental Control

Exposure to allergen and irritants at vulnerable times may significantly increase bronchial reactivity and adversely influence asthma control. The antigens most commonly implicated in chronic asthma are house dust mite and/or cockroaches, pet-derived antigenic proteins (with cat being the most common), and airborne molds and pollens. Murray reported on the beneficial influence of bedroom dust control measures in 1983 (Murray and Ferguson, 1983), and subsequent studies add to the information implicating dust mite antigen as a major factor in asthma. Certain environmental efforts are most successful for limiting mite antigen, whereas others that have been traditionally valued are not particularly helpful.

Dust mites are microscopic creatures that feed on human skin scales, require humidity greater than 50 percent, and tend to seek darker environments. They are found in carpets, mattresses, and stuffed furniture in homes where the ambient climate is moderate and not too dry. They are not removed by traditional dusting and vacuuming. Encasing mattresses in airtight covers, washing pillows and bedding weekly in hot water (over 130°), and removing carpeting, particularly if laid on concrete slab floors, will reduce house dust mite levels in the home; other measures include reducing the humidity to less than 50 percent and using acaricides (to kill the mites). When carpets cannot be removed, acaricides such as benzyl benzoate and products that denature mite antigen such as 3 percent tannic acid spray to the carpet and stuffed furniture are helpful, as is reducing humidity to less than 50 percent (see Chapter 15). Most physicians concentrate efforts on education that relates to keeping the bedroom and family area as free as possible of house dust mite antigens.

It is unfortunate that pet removal is necessary to effect major improvement in asthma symptoms for some highly atopic patients, but that carrying out this removal is so difficult. Families are often unable to deal with the loss of a pet, putting asthma lower on the priority list than other psychosocial issues. If a pet to which a patient is sensitive cannot be removed from the home, certain temporizing measures are worthwhile: keeping the pet out of the bedroom, using tannic acid spray on carpets and furniture to denature pet antigen, and considering an electrostatic or HEPA filter. Studies have shown that a weekly washing of cats reduces the amount of allergen deposited on carpet and furnishings (Kruszynska et al, 1987), but this is controversial. Many pet antigens are tenacious molecules that travel easily and are difficult to eliminate from the home. The part-time indoor pet may produce the same antigen load as the full-time indoor pet, and it may take months after the pet is removed from the environment for residual allergen to decrease to nonproblematic levels. Also, the chronic inflammatory changes that occur with asthma often prevent patients and families from being able to appreciate improvement in asthma control with a brief period of pet avoidance.

Cockroach antigen is a problem primarily in the eastern and southern United States. Antigen concentration appears to be related in part to lower socioeconomic populations. Cockroach antigen may be more important than dust mite among this population. Attempts at environmental control include removing uncovered food sources and exterminating these insects.

Irritant exposure should also be limited to achieve best asthma control. Tobacco smoke exposure has been linked to asthma exacerbations, decreased lung growth, and age of onset of asthma (Wright et al, 1991). Therefore, smoking in the home should be forbidden. Wood stove heat has been linked to increased emergency room visits for asthma and should be avoided in favor of cleaner heating fuels. Atmospheric levels of ozone and SO_2 may be related to asthma exacerbations, although correlations are modest (Chilmonczyk et al, 1993).

The amount of counseling that one offers concerning the environment depends largely on historical issues, level of allergy skin test relativity, and the ability of a family to make changes in their surroundings. The physician should offer firm counseling regarding environmental control if it is pertinent to a specific situation and then show flexibility when there are impasses. This approach is preferable to assuming that a family will not deal with avoidance and failing to provide appropriate information.

HOME PEAK-FLOW MONITORING. Another area of management is home peak-flow monitoring, which is important in reviewing the overall asthma control. Instruction in the peak-flow recording draws in the patient, or parent, as an active manager of his/her disease. Home peak-flow monitoring is particularly suited to a subset of patients with asthma: (1) patients with fairly severe disease who may not appreciate early deterioration because they do not sense obstruction and hypoxemia, (2) children whose parents are unclear about symptoms and would respond better to objective cues than to vague symptoms, (3) patients who are not communicative regarding symptoms, and (4) patients who need objective cues to spur compliance with medication regimens. To increase the ease of monitoring, a color-coded system has evolved. A patient's chart contains colored forms where the "green" zone means 80 to 100 percent of best personal peak-flow rate, "yellow" is 50 to 79 percent, and "red" is below 50 percent. The patient is instructed to exercise caution and use supplemental medication when in the yellow zone and to notify the physician for further instructions when in the red zone. Some peak-flow meters are color-coded, which aids the subject's assessment (see Chapter 12).

These nonpharmacologic management techniques should be part of an ongoing educational process that involves physician, patient, family, and other health educators such as nurses and respiratory therapists. Education should begin with an explanation of asthma as an inflammatory disease, including an explanation of asthma trigger factors in and outside of the home, and should emphasize environmental control. It should stress the importance of monitoring pulmonary function. Pharmacologic intervention should be posed as an important element in the equation of optimal control, but not as the sole desirable intervention.

Pharmacologic Management

The goal of pharmacologic therapy is to improve pulmonary function and decrease lability in order to allow patients to have a "normal" life style. Drugs available in the United States are noted in Table 35–2. Rarely should patients need to be satisfied with missing school or work time due to asthma or with limiting physical activity or sleeping poorly due to nocturnal exacerbations of their disease. This optimal life style requires compliance with medication as well as avoidance of environmental trigger factors.

The National Heart, Lung, and Blood Institute has supplied guidelines for the management of asthma which serve as an excellent foundation for treatment today (Expert Panel

TABLE 35–2. CURRENT DRUGS FOR MANAGEMENT OF ASTHMA IN THE UNITED STATES

Name	Notes
Beta-agonist bronchodilating drugs	
Metaproterenol sulfate (liquid, tablets, MDI)	2–3 hours duration
Albuterol sulfate (tablets, MDI, Nebules solution, Rotacaps for inhalation)	4–6 hours duration
Pirbuterol acetate (MDI)	4–6 hours duration
Terbutaline sulfate (tablets, MDI, SC solution)	4–6 hours duration
Bitolterol mesylate (MDI, inhalation solution)	4–6 hours duration
Salmeterol (MDI)	12 hours duration
Nonsteroidal anti-inflammatory agents	
Cromolyn sodium (ampules and MDI)	Begin q.i.d.—reduce gradually to b.i.d. if possible
Nedocromil (MDI)	Begin q.i.d.—reduce gradually to b.i.d. if possible
Oral corticosteroids	
Prednisone (tablets/liquid)	Give as single morning dosage
Prednisolone (tablets/liquid)	Give as single morning dosage
Methyl prednisolone (tablets)	Give as single morning dosage
Aerosolized steroids	
Beclomethasone dipropionate	Administer every 8–12 hours
Triamcinolone acetonide	Administer every 8–12 hours
Flunisolide	Administer every 8–12 hours
Theophylline	
Various S.R. products available	Administer every 8–24 hours
	Serum levels 5–15 µg/ml therapeutic
Other agents	
Anticholinergic (ipratropium bromide) (MDI + nebulizer solution)	May increase albuterol bronchodilation
Methotrexate sodium (antimetabolite) (IM, oral preps)	Experimental only, no pediatric trials performed
Troleandomycin (TAO) (macrolide antibiotic)	Prolongs half-life of methylprednisolone, no pediatric trials performed

MDI, metered dose inhaler

Guidelines, 1991). These guidelines stress the concept of inflammation in asthma and suggest that patients who require bronchodilator therapy more than twice a week for non–exercise-related asthma should have chronic anti-inflammatory therapy. A schematic view (Table 35–3) of a step approach to asthma care describes the ascent from use of a simple bronchodilator to use of cromolyn-like or steroidal anti-inflammatory medication, depending on disease severity.

APPROACHES TO CARE

TREATMENT OF ACUTE ASTHMA. An acute exacerbation of asthma poses an urgent medical problem, as noted in Table 35–4. The best strategy for management is early recognition. Evaluation and treatment prevent worsening and abort further exacerbation and respiratory compromise. Early recognition by the patient and prompt communication between the patient and the health care provider are essential components of the process. This allows the physician to modify the individual patient's medication regimen and to control his or her asthma more effectively.

The intensity of the acute attack and its outcome are influenced by a number of factors: (1) the patient's age (with the elderly having the greatest risk), (2) the duration of the episode, (3) a history of previous life-threatening asthma exacerbations requiring hospitalization, intubation, and intensive care, or a history of complications secondary to hypoxia, (4) recent and frequent emergency room visits, and (5) either systemic corticosteroid usage or recent withdrawal from corticosteroids.

Each patient should have available and be familiar with a "plan of action" to follow for acute asthma exacerbations. Peak-flow measurements by the patient are important in this

TABLE 35–3. MANAGEMENT OF CHRONIC ASTHMA

	CLASSIFICATIONS	ASSESSMENT OF LUNG FUNCTION	THERAPY

Mild	Asymptomatic	PEFR ≥80% of baseline	Children <5 years
			  Nebulized cromolyn
			Children >5 years to adulthood
			  Cromolyn or nedocromil

	Symptomatic	20% reduction in baseline	Children <5 years
			  Nebulized or oral β_2-agonist
			Children >5 years to adulthood
			  Inhaled β_2-agonist—2 puffs every 3–4 hours if needed

Moderate	Asymptomatic	60–80% of baseline	Children <5 years
			  Nebulized or inhaled β_2-agonist t.i.d. or q.i.d. as needed and nebulized cromolyn
			Children >5 years to adulthood
			  Anti-inflammatory agents or theophylline

	Symptomatic	Variation more than 30%	Oral corticosteroid burst plus nebulized or oral β_2-agonists

Severe	Asymptomatic	<60% baseline	Children <5 years
			  Nebulized cromolyn and β_2-agonist up to q.i.d.
			Children >5 years to adulthood
			  Inhaled β_2-agonist q.i.d.
			  Inhaled corticosteroids 2–6 puffs b.i.d. to q.i.d.

	Symptomatic	50% variation	Children
			  Prednisone 30–40 mg/day × 2 days, then taper to every other day dosage that stabilizes lung function
			Adults
			  60 mg/day up to 1 week, then taper

From Expert Panel on the Management of Asthma. Guidelines for the diagnosis and management of asthma. National Asthma Education Program. National Institutes of Health. J Allergy Clin Immunol 88:425, 1991.

TABLE 35-4. MANAGEMENT OF ACUTE ASTHMA

Step	Treatment	Assessment
1 (After initial assessment) 0–40 minutes	Inhaled (nebulized) β_2-agonist $\times$ 2, then β_2-agonist every 20 minutes $\times$ 1 hour; systemic corticosteroids if no immediate response or if patient is currently on or recently has been on oral taper; oxygen 2–6 L/min; consider subcutaneous epinephrine 0.3 cc (1:1000)	Peak flow, FEV_1, FVC, physical exam, O_2 sat if warranted
2 (FEV_1 >50–70% predicted), 40–120 minutes	If not already initiated, administer systemic corticosteroids. Continue treatment with inhaled or injected (SC epinephrine, 0.3 cc 1:1000) q3h if patient is improving	Peak flow, FEV_1, FVC, physical exam
2 (FEV_1 <50% predicted) 40–120 minutes	Inhaled β_2-agonist hourly or continuous; begin IV corticosteroids (methylprednisolone 60–120 mg IV); oxygen 6 L/min or as required	Peak flow, FEV_1, continuous O_2 sat or ABG, physical exam (with severe symptoms, look for hypoxia, hypercarbia)
3 (FEV_1 >70%) 120–180 minutes	Consider disposition: *for discharge home* Patient to continue frequent inhaled β_2-agonist every 3–4 hours as needed, and a short course of oral corticosteroids 40 mg PO $\times$ 3–7 days, then either taper by 5 mg/day or give 10–20 mg PO OD $\times$ 3–7 days; also include patient education on treatment plan and schedule medical follow-up	Home peak-flow monitoring
3 (FEV_1 <70%) 120–180 minutes	For poor or incomplete response; *hospital admission* Consider intravenous aminophylline, respiratory support with O_2, continue inhaled β_2-agonist hourly (every 1–3 hours) or continuously	FEV_1, FVC, continuous O_2 sat or ABG
	Disposition and appropriate follow-up must be determined on an individual basis. A patient with a pertinent medical history such as prolonged symptoms prior to visit, previous severe exacerbations, or pertinent psychosocial history may require closer observation. In addition, any suggestion of deterioration throughout the course of treatment with increasing P_{CO_2} merits intensive care monitoring.	

From Expert Panel on the Management of Asthma. Guidelines for the diagnosis and management of asthma. National Asthma Education Program. National Institutes of Health. J Allergy Clin Immunol 88:425, 1991.

early assessment process and provide a more precise quantitation of airflow obstruction. The basic goal of treatment is to achieve a rapid reversal of airflow obstruction. The first line of therapy in this setting is repetitive inhalation of β_2-agonists. Poor or minimal response to β_2-agonists is an indication for an emergent evaluation by medical personnel. Parents or patients should be instructed to administer a beta-agonist, for example albuterol, either by nebulizer at 0.1 mg/kg/dose (5 mg maximum) or 2 actuations of a metered-dose inhaler. If the patient's asthma is stable, these regimens can be repeated every 20 minutes up to three times as needed. If the initial response to treatment is good, based on PEFR ≥70 percent of the patient's personal best, the beta-agonist should be continued every 3 to 4 hours along with routine medications. If the patient responds only partially, he or she or the parent should contact the health care provider without further delay, who could initiate oral prednisone therapy at 1 to 2 mg/kg/dose and arrange for the patient to be seen in an emergency care setting. A β_2-agonist may be given by inhalation every 2 hours over the next 6 hours.

When caring for a patient with acute asthma in the emergency room or clinic, the interaction should begin with a quickly obtained pertinent history and physical examination. It is important to ascertain the presence of relevant environmental exposures and infectious triggers such as otitis and sinusitis.

Physical examination often reveals wheezing, accessory muscle use, and tachycardia. These findings are helpful to confirm the diagnosis of acute asthma; unfortunately, they do not reliably indicate the severity of the asthma episode. In the child under 3 years of age, one may hear only coughing or signs of croup. Objective measurements include pulmonary functions, such as spirometry or peak expiratory flow rate. In severe asthma with lung function less than 50 percent of predicted normal, one should attempt pulse oximetry or arterial blood gas measurements. Early administration of oral or systemic corticosteroids in adults and children should allow for more rapid improvement of pulmonary function. Close monitoring of the patient during treatment, with repeated measures of lung function, is essential for optimal management of the exacerbation and directions for changes in therapy. While paying attention to chest movement and sounds, one must remember that pulmonary function may tell more than auscultation. If the child is too young for pulmonary function, and dyspnea is severe, one should consider obtaining pulse oximetry. Supplemental oxygen should be administered so as to keep oxygen saturation above 95 percent. Nebulized albuterol should be administered at 0.15 mg/kg/dose every 20 minutes (maximum 5 mg/dose) for up to an hour. Prednisone at a loading dose of 1 to 2 mg/kg should be administered orally. If the patient responds well, beta-agonist therapy should continue every 4 hours until symptoms and peak-flow measurements show that the patient has reached his or her normal baseline, but can be administered every 1 to 2 hours if lung function continues to be poor until the response to prednisone is evident. The patient should continue prednisone therapy for at least 4 to 10 days to ensure adequate anti-inflammatory benefit. Some physicians will give the same total prednisone dose daily for 4 days; others will recommend a tapering dose over 4 to 10 days. Prednisone can be used as a single morning dose or can be divided during the day. However, the initial loading should be administered as a single dose. Patients with peak-flow rates between 40 and 70 percent of baseline and O_2 saturation between 91 and 95 percent should be observed for several hours to assess response. The more severe the obstruction, the longer the patient needs to be watched. If the patient continues to demonstrate severe symptoms or if poor peak-flow rate continues (<40 percent of predicted) or O_2 saturation (<91 percent) in room air is diminished, hospitalization should be considered. Clinical findings indicating the need for hospitalization include the use of accessory muscles, the presence of pulsus paradoxus, and increasing dyspnea or cyanosis.

As an alternative to nebulizer therapy, epinephrine 1:1000 can be injected subcutaneously (0.01 ml/kg up to 0.3 ml) and repeated every 15 to 20 minutes for as many as three treatments along with supplemental oxygen. This therapy is adequate but involves the pain of injections and cardiovascular side effects of epinephrine that are often unpleasant.

ACUTE SEVERE ASTHMA IN CHILDREN REQUIRING HOSPITALIZATION. If hospitalized because of poor response to treatment, the child should be managed in a facility where vital signs and overall condition can be monitored closely. The PEFR, O_2 saturation, and degree of dyspnea should be assessed frequently. Generally, if the peak flow is above 30 percent of predicted and the O_2 saturation is above 90 percent, the child with moderate dyspnea can be managed in an intermediate unit.

Children with more severe airway obstruction should be admitted to an intensive care unit and should have arterialized or arterial blood gases assessed. Supplemental oxygen should be continued and nebulized albuterol should be administered every 15 to 60 minutes as necessary with the administration of intravenous fluids. However, it is important not to overload the patient with fluids because of the danger of causing pulmonary edema. Further doses of systemic corticosteroids should be administered as oral prednisone or intravenous methylprednisolone or equivalent at 1 to 2 mg/kg/dose every 6 hours. For the patient who is slow to respond, one may consider the use of intravenous aminophylline, although its beneficial effects are now controversial in children. A loading dose of 6 mg/kg over 20 minutes followed by a continuous infusion of 0.9 mg/kg per hour may be administered. The loading dose should be eliminated or reduced substantially if the patient has been maintained on therapeutic levels of theophylline pending a stat theophylline serum level. Theophylline serum concentration should be obtained 1½ hours after the loading dose, several hours later, and then as indicated by the patient's course, and should be maintained at peak concentrations of less than 15 µg/ml.

If the patient fails to improve and there are signs of respiratory failure, such as PEFR less than 25 percent of predicted, P_{CO_2} greater than 45 mm Hg, and a falling pH value, continuous nebulization of a β_2-agonist should be considered. It should be noted that patients with severe asthma usually have carbon dioxide tensions less than 35 mm mercury. Mechanical ventilation should be considered in the child with persistent hypercarbia (Simons et al, 1977). Antibiotics should be used only when there are signs of a bacterial infection. Sedatives should be avoided, and food and fluid by mouth should be given only when the patient wants them.

As the child improves, preparation for hospital discharge should include a medication plan with emphasis on chronic medication and a short course of prednisone. The use of peak-flow monitoring at home should be continued, and a follow-up clinic visit should be planned for shortly after discharge.

TREATMENT OF THE HOSPITALIZED ADULT ASTHMATIC PATIENT. The decision to hospitalize should not be delayed unnecessarily. If a patient's asthma is severe and does not improve substantially after a few hours of treatment in the emergency room, more intensive monitoring should be strongly considered. This is particularly true in individuals with a poor response to β_2-agonists, hypoxia, hypercarbia ($CO_2 > 45$ mg Hg), previous history of respiratory failure, advanced age, or multiple medical problems.

Hospital management of asthma should continue to address the same goals as those initiated with emergency management, that is, relieve airflow obstruction with intensive bronchodilator therapy and reduce inflammation with corticosteroids. Initial assessment of lung function with spirometry or peak-flow monitoring is essential. Arterial blood gases may be required to monitor the consequence of airflow obstruction on pulmonary gas exchange. Special caution must be exercised when the patient with clinically moderately severe obstruction and arterial blood gas values indicating hypoxemia has "normal" $PaCO_2$ and pH values. In such circumstances, the arterial $PaCO_2$ and pH values are not "normal." Rather, these values suggest that the patient's condition has deteriorated or that he or she is in a transition phase to eventual hypercarbia and respiratory failure. If respiratory failure occurs with a progressive increase of $PaCO_2$ greater than 45, the patient may require endotracheal intubation and mechanical ventilation. Early aggressive and well-monitored therapy can usually prevent respiratory failure.

Nebulized β_2-agonist therapy should be continued in the hospitalized patient. Initially β-agonists are administered hourly and then reduced to every 3 to 4 hours as airflow obstruction becomes less severe. Subcutaneous administration of β_2-agonists may supplement inhaled therapy in adolescents and adults; however, intravenous administration should be avoided because of the risk of myocardial injury.

Therapy with corticosteroids should be initiated, if not already started in the emergency room. An initial dose of methylprednisolone, 1 mg/kg/every 6 hours (60 mg IV every 6 to 8 hours) or hydrocortisone 2 mg/kg bolus every 4 hours is recommended (Horst et al, 1990). Intravenous dosing is continued until the patient shows improvement in pulmonary function; this usually requires 24 to 48 hours. At that point oral prednisone or its equivalent may be substituted (10 to 15 mg four times daily); some experts may prefer a single morning dosing regimen. Oral corticosteroids are usually given at high doses for 7 days and then tapered as necessary, and inhaled corticosteroids are added.

Methylxanthines could be considered in most hospitalized adolescent and adult patients with asthma, especially in those who have received benefit from theophylline therapy in the past. Although they are often part of the routine care of patients hospitalized with severe asthma, the precise benefit that they afford is not clear, as noted in the previous section on pediatrics (Siegel et al, 1985). For patients not receiving theophylline, an intravenous loading dose of 5 to 6 mg/kg is followed by an infusion appropriate for the age and condition of the patient (Webb-Johnson and Andrews, 1977). Patients should have plasma theophylline levels monitored, with subsequent adjustment of dosages to achieve peak levels of 10 to 15 μg/ml.

Patients who have received theophylline prior to hospital admission should have plasma theophylline levels determined; if there are no signs of clinical toxicity, and if the theophylline serum concentration is low, patients may be given a loading dose of 2.5 mg/kg over 30 minutes followed by constant intravenous infusion. A plasma theophylline level should be obtained approximately 60 minutes after the loading dose to ascertain whether additional theophylline is required (one strives for a peak level of 10 to 15 µg/ml). Intravenous theophylline is continued until (or 24 hours after) intravenous corticosteroids are discontinued. At that time, the patient may be placed on an oral sustained-release theophylline preparation. An estimated dosage may be calculated from the total theophylline requirement in a 24-hour period that produced a therapeutic plasma theophylline concentration. The role of theophylline in the hospitalized patient continues to undergo reevaluation.

Supplemental oxygen is an integral part of therapy. Although it is commonly recommended that hydration is essential, there is little evidence to support this recommendation; in fact, overhydration may predispose some patients to pulmonary edema. Unless an infectious complication such as sinusitis, pneumonia, or bronchitis is found, antibiotics are not needed. Sinusitis should be strongly considered in a patient with an asthma exacerbation, especially one following a cold.

Morbidity in asthma is increased in the elderly and in those with previous episodes of respiratory failure. Morbidity also is greater when sedatives are administered or when corticosteroid therapy is withheld. Status asthmaticus is a medical emergency that should have a favorable outcome with proper treatment. To accomplish this goal, the physician and patient must recognize and heed the warnings of severe disease, intervene with bronchodilators and corticosteroids appropriately but aggressively, and monitor pulmonary functions and levels of arterial oxygenation and carbon dioxide tension carefully.

Weaning from acute treatment, discharge, and follow-up are much the same for children and adults.

COMPLICATIONS OF SEVERE ASTHMA

Complications of asthma may be pulmonary or extrapulmonary. Pulmonary complications include (1) acute respiratory failure, (2) atelectasis, (3) pneumomediastinum and pneumothorax, and (4) superimposed infections (pneumonia, empyema). Extrapulmonary complications include (1) vasopressin excess, (2) flaccid paralysis of an arm or leg, (3) sudden alteration in theophylline metabolism with toxicity, (4) cardiac arrhythmia, (5) hypoxic brain damage and hypoxic seizures, and (6) death. Pulmonary and extrapulmonary factors may combine to cause acute respiratory failure, resulting in brain damage or death.

Pulmonary Complications

RESPIRATORY FAILURE. Respiratory failure occurs in a small but significant number of patients admitted to the hospital with status asthmaticus (Simons et al, 1977). It often is the result of failure by the physician, patient, or family to recognize the severity of the patient's asthma. Clinical signs of overt respiratory failure include decreased or absent pulmonary breath sounds, severe intercostal retractions, pulsus paradoxus, use of accessory muscles of respiration, cyanosis with treatment with a final oxygen concentration (FIO_2) of 40 percent, reduced response to pain, poor skeletal muscle tone, and profuse diaphoresis. The use of accessory muscles of respiration, as previously noted, is one of the early signs of respiratory failure.

These signs indicate an extreme emergency and mandate immediate treatment for acute respiratory failure.

Arterial blood gas tension and pH must be monitored frequently in a distressed patient. Impending respiratory failure cannot be diagnosed from clinical signs alone. For example, a rise of $PaCO_2$ from 39 to 44 mm Hg in 1 hour in an exhausted patient who is receiving maximal therapy should be considered progressive respiratory failure and treated as discussed previously (Simons et al, 1977).

ATELECTASIS. Up to one third of all hospitalized asthmatic children have had pulmonary complications, such as pneumonia and atelectasis, and 20 percent have had pulmonary infiltrates involving multiple lobes (Eggleston et al, 1974). Perihilar interstitial infiltrates will vary in severity from increased bronchovascular markings to shaggy, diffuse peribronchial viral pneumonia. Atelectasis of all or part of a lobe, the next most common complication, will occur in 10 percent of admissions. The right middle lobe is most frequently involved because of anatomic factors, for example, the right main stem bronchus tends to twist with hyperinflation, resulting in its partial occlusion. Why right middle lobe atelectasis develops more frequently in girls than in boys is not clear (Dees and Spock, 1966).

The treatment of atelectasis should be conservative. In most cases it will resolve when the asthma is controlled. Respiratory therapy consisting of postural drainage and clapping as tolerated clinically is helpful. Intermittent positive pressure breathing (IPPB) therapy should be avoided, since it is likely to induce pneumomediastinum or pneumothorax (Bierman, 1967). If atelectasis persists, the presence of a foreign body, an anatomic defect, or an obstructing peribronchial lymph node should be considered. Fiberoptic bronchoscopy may be useful if a foreign body is suspected.

Pneumomediastinum and Pneumothorax. In status asthmaticus, 5 percent of patients may develop extrapulmonary air (Eggleston et al, 1974). Shearing forces from coughing and bronchospasm, superimposed on hyperinflation, also related to atelectasis or pneumonia and possible structural weakness, cause air to rupture alveolar bases and to dissect along blood vessel sheaths (Bierman, 1967) (Fig. 35–1). These effects result in pulmonary interstitial emphysema. It manifests as a worsening clinical course associated with reduced venous return, cardiac output, and blood pressure. Air dissects along the great vessel sheaths to the mediastinum and pericardium and along the aorta to the intestinal wall or along the fascial planes into the neck (Fig. 35–2). While this air remains under high pressure, asthma symptoms worsen and precardiac dullness disappears. Air may escape into the relatively low-pressure subcutaneous tissue of the neck and axilla, resulting in crepitant subcutaneous emphysema.

Rarely, pneumothorax complicates childhood asthma. It may be self-limited if small, or tension pneumothorax can occur that may severely compromise breathing. Bilateral pneumothorax can be the cause of sudden death in asthma (Jorgensen et al, 1963). Tension pneumothorax that results from the rupture of a pleural bleb needs decompression with a chest tube and underwater suction (Fig. 35–3). A pneumothorax secondary to air rupturing through parietal pleura into the pleural space from a pneumomediastinum is less serious and may be treated conserva-

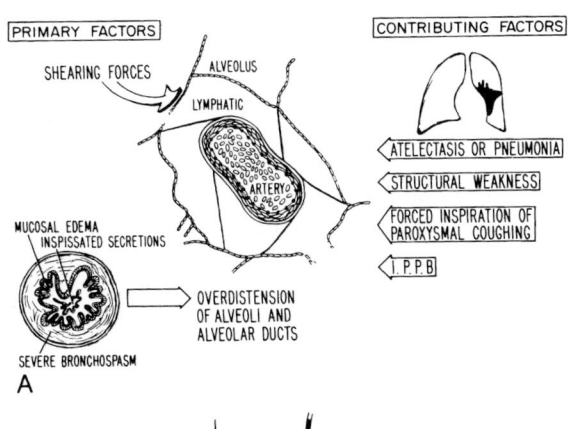
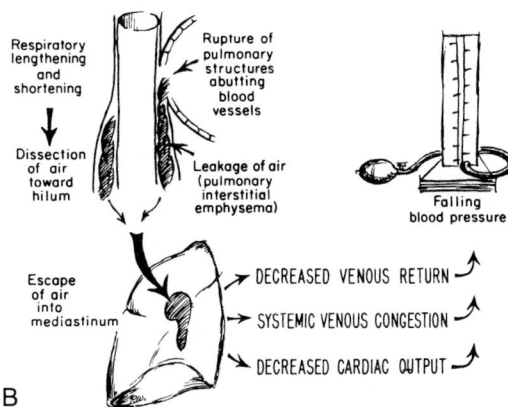
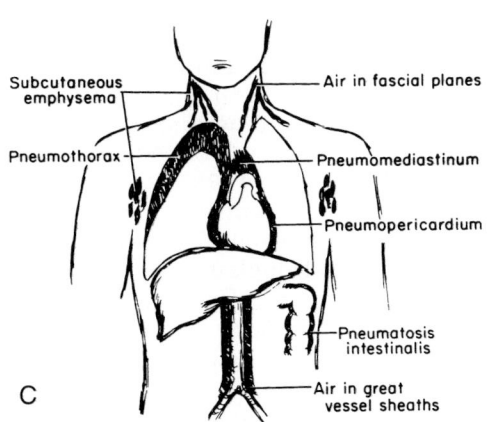

FIGURE 35–1. Mechanism of pneumomediastinum in acute asthma.

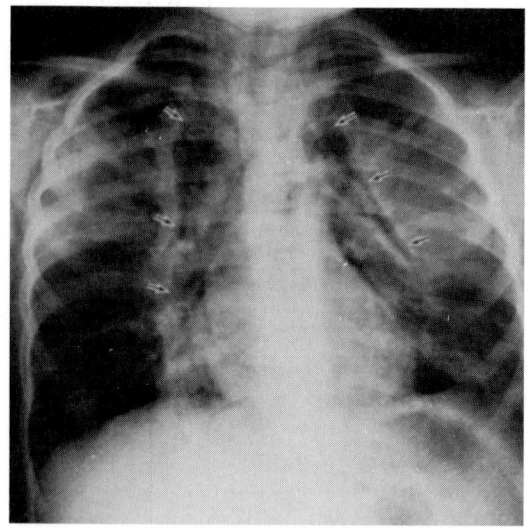

FIGURE 35–2. Massive pneumomediastinum complicating asthma.

tively. Often it will clear with treatment of the asthma.

Extrapulmonary Complications

VASOPRESSIN EXCESS (INAPPROPRIATE ADH SECRETION). The release of ADH is regulated through mechanisms such as (1) pain, fear, and drugs acting on higher central nervous system centers; (2) drops in arterial pressure; (3) increases in plasma concentration (0.280 mOsm/L) of nondiffusible solute perfusing the hypothalamus, and (4) decreases in stimulation of stretch receptors in the left atrium.

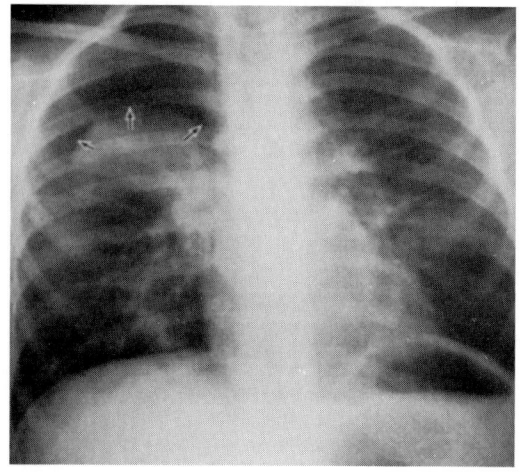

FIGURE 35–3. Pneumothorax secondary to paroxysmal coughing in asthma.

When filling of the left atrium is reduced, the vagus nerve stimulates the hypothalamus to secrete vasopressin. In severe asthma, vasopressin levels are elevated regardless of the serum sodium concentrations, apparently because of the effect of severe asthma on the pulmonary circulation. Vasopressin levels fall as the patient's condition improves (Benfield et al, 1982; Segar and Cheyne, 1981).

Criteria for the diagnosis of vasopressin excess are as follows:
1. Hyponatremia that is associated with plasma hypo-osmolarity.
2. Continuing renal excretion of sodium in the presence of hyponatremia.
3. Absence of any evidence of dehydration.
4. Urinary osmolality value that is greater than plasma osmolality value.
5. Normal kidney and adrenal function.

The treatment of excessive vasopressin involves three general principles. First, severe asthma must be corrected with appropriate therapy. Second, water intake and body weight, plasma electrolyte concentration and osmolarity, and urine volume and osmolality must be monitored closely; fluid intake should be restricted to the minimal amount compatible with control of asthma. Third, complications such as water intoxication with seizures should be treated with hypertonic saline and furosemide. Hypertonic saline and furosemide are rarely needed if the underlying asthma is treated successfully.

NEUROMYOPATHY. In 1974, Hopkins reported ten children with flaccid paralysis after acute asthma severe enough to require hospitalization (Commentary, 1980). The paralysis developed during the recovery phase from asthma, and all had been immunized for poliomyelitis. In all patients, paralysis was permanent and involved one arm or one leg. To date, over 20 children with this syndrome from Australia, England, Sweden, and the United States have been reported in the medical literature, including one case of areflexic tetraplegia in a 10-year-old girl (Kaplan et al, 1986; Shapiro et al, 1979). Severe myopathy appears to be an element in certain of these pediatric cases as well as in several cases involving adults (Douglass et al, 1992).

Transient phrenic nerve paralysis also has been reported in status asthmaticus, possibly as a complication of assisted ventilation (Rohatigi et al, 1980).

CARDIORESPIRATORY ARREST WITH BRAIN

DAMAGE. Permanent hypoxic brain damage due to cardiorespiratory arrest can be a complication of severe asthma and is particularly unfortunate because it is preventable with appropriate therapy. In the majority of these patients, it has been the result of the parent's or the physician's failure to recognize the severity of asthma and to institute appropriate therapy (Bierman et al, 1975). More recently there has also been a description of sudden asphyxic asthma in which there has been sudden progression to severe hypercarbia with severe mixed acidoses and coma. Usually these patients have had massive allergen exposure, emotional stress, or respiratory infection (Wasserfallen et al, 1990).

DEATH. Table 35–5 lists the causes of death associated with asthma in children. Virtually all are potentially preventable and can be avoided with appropriate education and treatment (Strunk and Mrazek, 1986).

MANAGEMENT OF CHRONIC ASTHMA

It is important to recognize that chronic asthma may not be obvious in its presentation. Although there may be recurrent episodes of wheezing and shortness of breath, the presentation may be more subtle. Chronic cough may be the sole manifestation of asthma. When cough persists after each upper respiratory infection and when exercise tolerance diminishes markedly with each infection, asthma is a consideration. Patients may complain of exercise intolerance and become noticeably more winded than teammates during sports or may choose a sedentary life style. The patient with a history of "recurrent bronchitis" or "pneumonia" may also have asthma. Both diagnoses are used as euphemisms to diminish anxiety, but this practice actually prevents families and patients from dealing with the very manageable reality of asthma. Drugs useful in the treatment of asthma are noted in Table 35–2.

For patients with intermittent episodes of mild bronchospasm who appear to be free of wheezing for days or weeks between problem times, intermittent therapy may be appropriate. One may choose an inhaled beta agonist for children over 5 years of age or an oral one for children under 5 years of age. An alternative for the young child or older adult is a motor-driven nebulizer, which can be used to provide β_2-agonists in saline or cromolyn sodium solution as an aerosol that can be delivered by face mask.

Metered-dose inhalers are effective for children above 4 years of age and throughout adulthood. As the world moves away from Freon-containing propellants, more variations on "classic" metered-dose inhalers (MDIs) are appearing, including breath-activated aerosol devices, dry powder devices, and dry powder capsules for puncture and inhalation.

Spacer devices used with metered-dose inhalers should be considered for (1) lowering the age that MDIs are usable to about 4 years, (2) increasing their use in the geriatric population, (3) decreasing the amount of Freon inhaled, and (4) increasing drug effect by improving lung deposition of drug. Certain spacers that are also holding chambers (i.e., Inspirease or Aerochamber) eliminate the need to synchronize the actuation and inhalation processes. When a spacer is used, the increased transit time of the aerosol results in lower velocity of particles and smaller diameter due to evaporation of propellant. This allows for more efficient deposition of the drug in the pulmonary tree. Some physicians report success with an inhaled corticosteroid

TABLE 35–5. CAUSES OF DEATH FROM ASTHMA

Failure of physician or patient to appreciate severity
  Lack of objective measurements
  Lack of intensified therapy

Inappropriate therapy given
  Too late due to delay by patient or physician
  Too little (e.g., low steroid dose or recent discontinuation)
  Too much (e.g., beta-agonists, theophylline, sedative abuse)

Progressive unresponsive asthma

Prolonged attack

Pulmonary complications
  Infection (often undiagnosed)
  Pneumothorax
  Barotrauma
  Aspirations of gastric contents
  Malfunction of ventilator

Cardiac complications
  Arrhythmias
  Hypotension
  Myocardial toxicity
  Sudden cardiac arrest

Underlying cardiopulmonary disease

Hemodynamic
  Hypovolemia, shock
  Pulmonary edema

and an aerochamber with face mask in small children. After each actuation, the mask is kept loosely over the child's face, and several inspirations and expirations are allowed before the next actuation. Usually, these children continue to use nebulizer therapy with cromolyn and a beta-agonist several times daily.

With an increasing incidence of symptoms, the patient requires a regular regimen. Obvious clues to this are frequent visits for emergent care and episodes that affect sleep and school or work attendance. The use of home peak-flow monitoring may well indicate that PEFR is chronically less than 80 percent of the patient's best baseline, that drops of 20 to 30 percent are taking place with some regularity, and/or that there is considerable variability between morning and evening peak flow. At the milder end of this spectrum, patients may do well with bronchodilator alone. However, as asthma becomes more severe, patients should be placed on chronic anti-inflammatory therapy (Spitzer et al, 1992). Many younger patients (under 5 years of age) do well with cromolyn by nebulizer, whereas patients over 5 years of age can use cromolyn by metered-dose inhaler and nedocromil if over 12 years of age. Therapy usually begins with an ampule of cromolyn or two actuations of cromolyn or nedocromil on a regular three or four times per day basis, depending on the patient's particular need and age (nedocromil is not approved by the FDA for use in patients under 12 years of age). Cromolyn can be tapered successfully to twice daily in many cases (Furukawa et al, 1984).

Cromolyn-like nonsteroidal anti-inflammatory agents appear to prevent release of mediators from mast cells which induce acute bronchoconstriction and chronic inflammatory airway changes. In addition, these drugs may modulate the activity of neuropeptides and other inflammatory molecules that upregulate airway hyperresponsiveness. Cromolyn is useful as a maintenance, prophylactic agent for mild-to-moderate chronic asthma. In addition, cromolyn can be used intermittently to decrease exercise-induced asthma and to prevent antigen-induced episodes. Much of the data concerning cromolyn's anti-inflammatory potential are based on studies using the no-longer-available 20-mg capsule delivered by Spinhaler device. Whether the currently available formulation by metered-dose inhaler (1 mg/actuation) provides equivalent action in the recommended dosage of two actuations is unclear. Cromolyn is administered by inhalation from the metered-dose inhaler or nebulizer. The nebulizer ampule contains 20 mg/2 ml and probably provides more therapeutic efficacy per dose than the recommended two actuations of the MDI, but no comparative studies have been published.

Nedocromil is a pyranoquinoline that has specific anti-inflammatory effects on the airway. It has been shown to be effective in clinical trials of children and adults with chronic asthma (Schwartz et al, 1993). It appears to have prophylactic properties when used prior to antigen challenge as well as a variety of other challenges including sulfur dioxide, cold air, and exercise (Schwartz et al, 1993). It appears to be similar to cromolyn in anti-asthma potency. Whether its onset of action is faster, whether it is more potent, and whether it has steroid-sparing properties have not yet been determined. Approximately 13 percent of patients strenuously object to its taste and refuse to use it, whereas another subset found it unpleasant but tolerable. Nedocromil for asthma is currently available in the United States in metered-dose inhaler form.

If a one-month trial of a cromolyn-like nonsteroidal anti-inflammatory drug is not beneficial, aerosolized corticosteroid therapy should be initiated. When the patient is stabilized with this, cromolyn or nedocromil can usually be discontinued, since there are no data to support their steroid-sparing potential. Beta-agonist bronchodilators should be continued. If they continue to be needed several times a day and if nocturnal asthma continues to be a concern, the long-acting beta-agonist salmeterol can be added in hopes of stabilizing the patient's condition without needing a high dose of inhaled corticosteroid. If patients need a beta-agonist mainly in the day or mainly at night, salmeterol can be used just once a day, either in the morning or evening. There may be an advantage to avoiding 24-hour beta-agonist therapy, which could possibly increase bronchial hyperresponsiveness or tachyphylaxis (Cheung et al, 1992; Ullman et al, 1990). A long-term study is currently under way to test this observation.

Patients with severe asthma are those who have such problems as frequent symptoms affecting sleep and activity as well as emergent visits and occasional hospitalizations. When untreated, their peak-flow rates are markedly depressed and labile. These will require regular use of a beta-agonist and an aerosolized steroid, if the child is old enough to use a metered-dose inhaler (MDI). Short-acting beta-agonist by nebulizer or MDI can be used as often as every 4 hours. In patients who can use an MDI, salmeterol, a long-acting β-agonist drug, administered at night may prevent nocturnal asthma and may simplify the beta-agonist regimen (Twentyman et al, 1990). Albuterol can then be used as needed during the day (Holgate et al, 1992). Children unable to use an MDI may respond to an inhaled steroid delivered from an MDI into an aerochamber with face mask. Others may require oral steroid therapy. If so, a short-acting drug such as prednisone or methylprednisolone used in the morning on alternate days will minimize steroid-induced adverse effects.

Theophylline is another bronchodilator that had great popularity in the United States until the late 1980s. It has lost its popularity for treating asthma because it is relatively difficult to use, its safety and efficacy being related to serum levels, which must be monitored regularly for optimal risk-benefit ratio. Theophylline may be used as an adjunctive bronchodilator (Hendeles and Weinberger, 1983).

Essential points to know concerning theophylline are that: (1) in general, children over 1 year and under 9 years of age require a higher theophylline per-kilogram dose than do older children, nonsmoking adolescents, or adults, (2) the ideal therapeutic range for maximizing effectiveness and decreasing adverse effects has been modified to 5 to 15 μg/ml in order to lessen the risk of adverse effects, and (3) diseases and drugs that affect the P450 cytochrome system in the liver can decrease theophylline clearance, as can febrile infections such as influenza, and thus markedly elevate the serum theophylline levels.

ORAL CORTICOSTEROIDS. Corticosteroids are potent anti-inflammatory drugs that are available for asthma therapy in oral and inhalable formulations. Steroids are used in a variety of situations: (1) short-term, systemic oral therapy, usually in high doses is essential for treating acute asthma exacerbations; (2) short-term high-dose intravenous therapy is useful in status asthmaticus, though high-dose oral therapy can be sometimes used; (3) inhaled topical corticosteroids are used as chronic maintenance therapy for moderate-to-severe chronic asthma; and (4) low-dose oral daily or alternate-morning therapy is used in severe asthma when inhaled steroids have not been adequate or when children are too young to use the aerosolized formulations. For oral use, short half-life steroids such as prednisone and methylprednisolone are preferable, since they are less likely than the longer-acting drugs to affect pituitary-adrenal axis function.

Inhaled corticosteroids, in the usually recommended doses, are unlikely to cause significant systemic adverse effects, but mild complications such as throat irritation, hoarseness, or pharyngeal candidiasis (often asymptomatic) occur occasionally. As these agents have become more popular for the treatment of asthma and as primary care doctors have been encouraged to become comfortable with prescribing them, there has been more discussion of potential risks such as growth retardation, hypothalamic-pituitary-adrenal axis dysfunction, and possibly posterior subcapsular cataracts (Toogood, 1990). With dosages that are usual for moderate disease (e.g., 400 to 800 μg/day beclomethasone equivalent), clinically significant adverse effects are uncommon (Barnes and Pedersen, 1993). Although higher-dose therapy does increase the possibility of clinically significant evidence of systemic absorption, it is less than one would expect from oral steroid dosage for equivalent disease control.

Aerosolized agents currently available in the United States include beclomethasone diproprionate, triamcinolone acetonide, and flunisolide. Their relative potency is difficult to assess. Some pharmacologists attempt to equate them on the basis of weight per actuation: beclomethasone 50 μg, triamcinolone 100 μg, flunisolide 250 μg. Since there are no direct comparative trials, these relationships are difficult to verify. More potent inhaled steroids for asthma, including fluticasone and budesonide, are under investigation in the United States. Budesonide is being evaluated in a dry powder formulation to be delivered by a breath-actuated device as well as in a suspension for nebulizer delivery (Toogood et al, 1982). The current absence in the United States of a nebulizer aerosol preparation poses a problem in caring for the very young child with severe chronic asthma. Some physicians have used an aerochamber spacer with a face mask for children who need inhaled steroid and have had varying degrees of success with this delivery system.

Adding to difficulties in winning compliant

behavior in the use of corticosteroids, the U.S. Food and Drug Administration (FDA) has added labeling to topical steroid preparations regarding possible increased risk of disseminated varicella in children who use any systemic or topical preparation for asthma or rhinitis. The association between topical steroid use and such increased risk is speculative, while the association between infrequent oral steroid "bursts" for acute asthma and disseminated varicella is statistically real but clinically remote (AAAI Position Statement, 1993). Accordingly, many physicians now institute treatment with oral acyclovir when patients who are receiving or have recently received oral prednisone are exposed to varicella. Such therapy may also be used when patients being treated with inhaled steroid develop varicella lesions. Since patients who use oral or inhaled steroids may be more vulnerable to stress, if they are scheduled for surgery or have experienced severe physical trauma, they are candidates for oral or parenteral corticosteroid replacement until the high-risk situation has passed.

ALLERGEN IMMUNOTHERAPY. Immunotherapy may be used as adjunctive therapy in patients who have an IgE-mediated component to asthma (see Chapter 17). Allergen immunotherapy has been shown to reduce the symptoms of asthma in double-blind studies with a variety of allergens including house dust mite (Aas, 1971), cat dander (Ohman et al, 1984), grass pollen (Reid et al, 1986), and Alternaria (Horst et al, 1990). Recent studies have also shown that allergen immunotherapy reduces the late pulmonary reaction to allergen in the lungs (Van Bever and Stevens, 1989). Maintenance immunotherapy appears to be safe in the pregnant patient with asthma (Turner et al, 1980); however, initiation of immunotherapy should be reserved until after the birth of the child. Since immunotherapy modifies the allergic reaction to antigen, it is possible that its use might be most effective if administered early in the course of asthma; such an approach needs to be evaluated (see Chapter 17). Since immunotherapy does carry risk of anaphylaxis, this approach to therapy should be considered in highly specific situations and should be carried out by specifically trained physicians.

PREGNANCY. Retrospective analyses suggest that approximately one third of women will have more severe asthma during pregnancy, another third will have improvement, and the other third remains unchanged. Peak severity of asthma usually occurs at 29 to 36 weeks of gestation. Asthma becomes less severe during the last 4 weeks of pregnancy and usually returns to pre-pregnancy levels 4 weeks postpartum (Schatz et al, 1988a). Poorly controlled asthma has an adverse effect on the fetus, resulting in increased perinatal mortality, increased prematurity, and low birth weight. Therefore, optimal perinatal asthma control is essential.

During pregnancy, inhaled medications are preferred. Terbutaline (Brethaire) is the preferred β_2-agonist because there is no evidence from animal studies that teratogenicity occurs. For most drugs used to treat asthma and rhinitis—with the exception of brompheniramine, hydroxyzine, and epinephrine—there is little evidence to suggest increased risk to the fetus (Schatz et al, 1988b; Greenberger and Patterson, 1985). All of the new nonsedating antihistamines should be omitted in pregnancy, astemizole 6 weeks before becoming pregnant. Because beclomethasone is the only inhaled steroid that has been used in well-controlled studies during pregnancy, it is generally prescribed when such treatment is indicated. Oral β-agonists should be stopped near term since they inhibit uterine contraction. Theophylline dosage should be reduced and serum concentration monitored in the third trimester because of decreased metabolic rate.

Acute exacerbations of asthma should be treated aggressively in order to avoid fetal hypoxia. The use of epinephrine acutely has been a subject of controversy. Schatz and associates, quoting studies indicating an epinephrine-induced decrease in utero-placental blood flow and its association with congenital malformations, prefer to use parenteral terbutaline in acute asthma (Schatz et al, 1992). Others have not confirmed the findings of epinephrine's teratogenicity (Greenberger and Patterson, 1985). In general, acute asthma treatment should include the nebulized β-agonist, such as terbutaline or albuterol, and oxygen; systemic corticosteroids should be instituted when necessary (see Chapter 53).

SURGERY. Primary care physicians and asthma specialists are often asked to participate in the preoperative evaluation of their asthmatic patients (see Chapter 54). This involves assessing the risk of anesthesia and the surgical procedure itself as well as taking measures to minimize any risk. Preoperative assessment includes careful evaluation of the patient's current respiratory status. Integral to this evaluation is measurement of pulmonary function and its comparison with the patient's recent best values. This comparison allows the physician to determine the degree of improvement that may be required to optimize the patient's lung function. Should the patient have increased asthma or worsening of airway obstruction on spirometry, attempts should be made to improve lung function prior to surgery. This may require a short burst of corticosteroids. The possible adverse effects of systemic corticosteroids on wound healing and suppressive effects on the adrenal-pituitary axis are not a contraindication to their preoperative use.

Immediately prior to surgery, inhaled β_2-agonists are recommended; this approach will minimize the risk of bronchoconstriction during endotracheal intubation. Inhaled bronchodilators may be maintained intraoperatively. In mechanically ventilated patients, parameters such as peak inspiratory airway pressures may signal changes in airway resistance requiring modifications in ventilatory management as well as administration of inhaled bronchodilators. For patients who regularly take theophylline, intraoperative aminophylline may be used to maintain its therapeutic effects. A usual maintenance dose is 0.5 mg/kg/hour by continuous infusion; rates are modified depending on the individual metabolism of the patient. For patients with a therapeutic blood level (5 to 15 µg/ml) on their oral regimen, aminophylline infusion may be calculated as 1.25 × total daily theophylline dose over 24 hours.

Patients with moderately severe or severe asthma may be on chronic corticosteroid administration at the time of surgery. These patients should be considered to have a decreased adrenal-pituitary response to stress. To prevent the complications of adrenal insufficiency with surgery, patients should be supplemented intraoperatively and perioperatively with corticosteroids.

The routine dose of corticosteroids for replacement during stress is 300 mg of hydrocortisone per day (Expert Panel Guidelines, 1991), given as 100 mg intravenously preoperatively, 100 mg intraoperatively, and 100 mg by intravenous bolus postoperatively. Systemic corticosteroids may then be tapered over the next few days, depending on the patient's postoperative course. Patients should be treated with stress-dose corticosteroids if they have been treated with corticosteroids for more than 2 weeks within the last 6 months. They are also at risk if they have taken inhaled corticosteroids at greater-than-recommended doses.

COPD AND ASTHMA

Some patients with chronic obstructive lung disease have a component of reversible airway obstruction. These individuals generally fall into two groups of patients. First, there are individuals who have smoked and have either emphysema or, more commonly, chronic bronchitis. Tests of their lung function usually indicate a significant degree of permanent airflow obstruction that does not respond to either bronchodilators or anti-inflammatory therapy. The second group are individuals who have never smoked but have had longstanding asthma and apparently have developed a component of fixed airflow obstruction. In both groups of adult patients, lung function values are significantly compromised even with optimal therapy. Furthermore, both groups of patients may also have a component of reversible airflow obstruction that usually occurs with respiratory tract infection and is associated with an increase in symptoms of cough, shortness of breath, and wheeze. At this time, their already compromised lung function becomes worse. Although the absolute changes in lung function may not appear to be great (i.e., a decrease of 300 to 400 ml), this reduction is significant in the face of already reduced lung function.

Treatment of these individuals requires that the physician maximize bronchodilator therapy. In addition, oral corticosteroids are often helpful. Usual dosing regimens include prednisone, 15 mg three times daily for one week, then a lower dose (i.e., 10 mg daily for one week) before stopping. In addition, these individuals usually have purulent sputum; broad-spectrum antibiotic therapy is beneficial. With this therapeutic approach, the intensity of the exacerbation can be diminished and a return to baseline, albeit compromised, lung function will follow. The physician needs to keep in mind that, although the absolute changes in lung function in these individuals are small, the relative compromises in airflow limitation are considerable.

Other conditions in which wheezing may occur are bronchopulmonary dysplasia (see Chapter 42), cystic fibrosis (see Chapter 41), and allergic bronchopulmonary aspergillosis (ABPA) (see Chapter 40). In these conditions also, the patients will benefit from bronchodilators and anti-inflammatory medication.

PSYCHOSOCIAL ISSUES

Psychosocial issues inevitably influence chronic asthma management. For best results in caring for children, physicians must be listeners and educators. The therapeutic regimen should be simplified when possible to encourage compliance. Families should be counseled periodically on giving the child responsibility for his disease and its treatment without putting unrealistic expectations on those who are too young to assume it. Educational materials available through groups such as the Asthma and Allergy Foundation of America, Allergy and Asthma Network/ Mothers of Asthmatics, and the American Lung Association can be helpful resources to adult and pediatric patients, as can support groups also identifiable through these national organizations.

GOALS

The goal of asthma therapy should be a normal life style for the patient, as free of restrictions as possible. Usually, this can be achieved with appropriate therapy. Patients often benefit from home peak-flow monitoring, objective data being helpful to the patient (and parents) and physician. Most disability from asthma is avoidable with appropriate monitoring and therapy.

References

Aas K. Controlled trial of hyposensitization to house dust. Acta Paediatr Scand 60:264–268, 1971.

American Academy of Allergy and Immunology. Position Statement: Skin testing and RAST for diagnosis of specific allergens responsible for IgE-mediated disease. J Allergy Clin Immunol 72:515–517, 1983.

American Academy of Allergy and Immunology. Position Statement: Inhaled steroids and severe viral infections. J Allergy Clin Immunol 92:223, 1993.

Barnes PJ, Pedersen S. Efficacy and safety of inhaled corticosteroids in asthma. Am Rev Respir Dis 148:S1–26, 1993.

Benfield QF, Odoherty K, Davies BH. Status asthmaticus and the syndrome of inappropriate secretion of antidiuretic hormone. Thorax 37:147–148, 1982.

Bierman CW. Pneumomediastinum and pneumothorax complicating asthma in children. Am J Dis Child 114:42, 1967.

Bierman CW, Pierson WE, Shapiro GG, Simons FER. Brain damage from asthma in children. J Allergy Clin Immunol 55:126, 1975.

Cheung D, Timmers MC, Zwinderman AH, Bel EH, Dijkman JH, Sterk PJ. Long-term effects of a long-acting B_2 adrenoceptor agonist, salmeterol, on airway hyperresponsiveness in patients with mild asthma. N Engl J Med 327:1198–1203, 1992.

Chilmonczyk B, Salmun LM, Megathlin KN, Neveux LM, Palomaki GE, Knight GJ, Pulkkinen AJ, Haddow JE. Association between exposure to environmental tobacco smoke and exacerbations of asthma in children. N Engl J Med 328:1665–1669, 1993.

Commentary: Post-asthmatic pseudopolio in children. Lancet 1:860, 1980.

Dees SC, Spock A. Right middle lobe syndrome in children. JAMA 197:8, 1966.

Douglass JA, Tuxen DV, Horne M, Scheinkestel CD, Weinmann M, Czarny D, Bowes G. Myopathy in severe asthma. Am Rev Respir Dis 146:517–519, 1992.

Eggleston PA, Ward BH, Pierson WE, Bierman CW. Radiographic abnormalities in acute asthma in children. Pediatrics 54:442–449, 1974.

Expert Panel on the Management of Asthma. Guidelines for the diagnosis and management of asthma. National Asthma Education Program, National Institutes of Health. J Allergy Clin Immunol 88:425, 1991.

Furukawa CT, Shapiro GG, Kraemer MJ, Pierson WE, Bierman CW. A double-blind study comparing the effectiveness of cromolyn sodium and sustained-release theophylline in childhood asthma. Pediatrics 74:453–459, 1984.

Greenberger PA, Patterson R. The management of asthma during pregnancy and lactation. Clin Rev Allergy 5:317–324, 1985.

Hendeles L, Weinerger M. Theophylline: A state of the art review. Pharmacotherapy 3:2–44, 1983.

Holgate ST, Baldwin CJ, Tattersfield AE. β-adrenergic agonist resistance in normal human airways. Lancet 2:375–377, 1992.

Holgate ST, Beasley R, Twentyman OP. The pathogenesis and significance of bronchial hyperresponsiveness in airways disease. Clin Sci 73:561–572, 1987.

Hopkins IJ. A new syndrome: Poliomyelitis-like illness associated with acute asthma in childhood. Aust Pediatr J 10:273, 1974.

Horst M, Hejjaoui A, Horst V, Michel FB, Bousquet J. Double-blind, placebo controlled rush immunotherapy with a standardized Alternaria extract. J Allergy Clin Immunol 85:460–472, 1990.

Jorgensen JR, Fallure CJ, Bukantz SC. Pneumothorax and mediastinal and subcutaneous emphysema in children with bronchial asthma. Pediatrics 3:824, 1963.

Kaliner MA, Lemanske RL. Rhinitis and asthma. JAMA 268:2807–2829, 1992.

Kaplan PW, Rocha W, Sanders DB, D'Souza B, Spock A. Acute steroid-induced tetraplegia following status asthmaticus. Pediatrics 78(1):121–123, 1986.

Konig P. Inhaled corticosteroids: Their present and future role in the management of asthma. J Allergy Clin Immunol 82:297–306, 1988.

Kruszynska YT, Greenstone M, Home PD, et al. Effect

of high-dose inhaled beclomethasone dipropionate on carbohydrate and lipid metabolism in normal subjects. Thorax 42:881–884, 1987.

Murray AB, Ferguson AC. Dust-free bedrooms in the treatment of asthmatic children with house dust or house dust mite allergy: A controlled trial. Pediatrics 71:418–422, 1983.

Ohman JL Jr., Findlay SR, Leiterman KM. Immunotherapy in cat-induced asthma: A double-blind trial with evaluation of in vivo and in vitro responses. J Allergy Clin Immunol 74:230–239, 1984.

Platts-Mills TAE, Chapman MD. Dust mites: Immunology, allergic disease, and environmental control. J Allergy Clin Immunol 80:755–779, 1987.

Rachelefsky GS, Katz RM, Siegel SC. Chronic sinus disease with associated reactive airway disease in children. Pediatrics 73:526–529, 1984.

Reid MJ, Moss RB, Hsu YP. Seasonal asthma in northern California: Allergy causes and efficacy of immunotherapy. J Allergy Clin Immunol 78:590–600, 1986.

Rohatigi N, Fields A, Sly RM. Status asthmaticus complicated by phrenic nerve paralysis. Ann Allergy 45:177–178, 1980.

Schatz M, Harden KM, Forsythe A, Chilingar L, Hoffman C, Sperling W, Zeiger RS. The course of asthma during pregnancy, post-partum, and with successive pregnancies: A prospective analysis. J Allergy Clin Immunol 81:509, 1988a.

Schatz M, Zeiger RS, Harden KM, Hoffman CP, Forsythe AB, Chilingar KM, Porreco RP, Benenson AS, Sperling WL, Saunders BS, Kagnoff MC. The safety of inhaled β-agonist bronchodilators during pregnancy. J Allergy Clin Immunol 82:686, 1988b.

Schatz M, Hoffman CP, Zeiger RS, Falkoff R, Macy E, Mellon M. The course and management of asthma and allergic diseases during pregnancy. In Middleton E, Reed CE, Ellis EF, Adkinson NF Jr, Yunginger JW, Busse WW (eds). Allergy: Principles and Practice. 4th ed. St. Louis, Mosby–Year Book 1301–1342, 1992.

Schwartz HJ, Kemp JP, Bianco S, Bone M, Bruderman I, Rebuck AS, Bergmann K. Highlights of the nedocromil sodium clinical study presentation. J Allergy Clin Immunol 92:204–209, 1993.

Segar WE, Cheyne RW. Disorders of electrolyte metabolism. Pediatr Ann 10:288, 1981.

Shapiro GG, Chapman JI, Pierson WE, Bierman SW. Poliomyelitis-like illness after acute asthma. J Pediatr 94:767–768, 1979.

Siegel D, Sheppard D, Gelb A, Weinberg PF. Aminophylline increases the toxicity but not the efficacy of an inhaled beta adrenergic agonist in the treatment of acute exacerbations of asthma. Am Rev Respir Dis 132:283–286, 1985.

Simons FER, Pierson WE, Bierman CW. Respiratory failure in childhood status asthmaticus. Am J Dis Child 131:1097, 1977.

Spitzer WO, Suissa S, Ernest P, Horowitz RI, Habbick B, Cockcroft D, Boivin JF, McNutt M, Buist AS, Rebuck AS. The use of beta-agonists and the risk of death and near death from asthma. N Engl J Med 326(8):501–506, 1992.

Strunk RC, Mrazek DA. Deaths from asthma in childhood. Can they be predicted? N Engl Reg Allergy Proc 7:454–461, 1986.

Toogood JH, Baskerville JC, Jennings B, Lefcoe NM, Johanssen SA. Influence of frequent dosing schedule on the response of chronic asthmatics to the aerosol steroid, budesonide. J Allergy Clin Immunol 288–298, 1982.

Toogood JH. Complications of topical steroid therapy for asthma. Am Rev Respir Dis 141:S89–96, 1990.

Turner ES, Greenberger PA, Patterson R. Management of the pregnant asthmatic patient. Ann Intern Med 93:905–918, 1980.

Twentyman OP, Finnerty JP, Harris A, Palmer J, Holgate ST. Protection against allergen induced asthma by salmeterol. Lancet 336:1338–1342, 1990.

Ullman A, Hedner J, Svedmyr N. Inhaled salmeterol and salbutamol in asthmatic patients. An evaluation of asthma symptoms and the possible development of tachyphylaxis. Am Rev Respir Dis 142:571–575, 1990.

Van Bever HP, Stevens WJ. Suppression of the late asthmatic reaction by hyposensitization in asthmatic children to house dust mites (Dermatophagoides pteronyssinus). Clin Exp Allergy 19:399–404, 1989.

Wasserfallen J, Schaller M, Feihl F, Perret CH. Sudden asphyxic asthma: A distinct entity? Am Rev Respir Dis 142:108–111, 1990.

Webb-Johnson CD, Andrews JL. Bronchodilator therapy. N Engl J Med 297:476–482, 1977.

Williams PV, Shapiro GG. Inhalation Bronchoprovocation in Children. In Spector SL (ed). Provocation Testing in Clinical Practice. New York, Marcel Dekker, 1995.

Wright AL, Holberg C, Martinez FD, Taussig LM. Relationship of parental smoking to wheezing and nonwheezing lower respiratory tract illness in infancy. J Pediatr 118:207–214, 1991.

Chapter 36

Exercise-Induced Asthma

Peyton A. Eggleston, M.D.

For centuries, physicians caring for asthmatic patients have recognized that exercise can precipitate an attack of wheezing. Sir John Floyer, in 1698, commented that "All violent exercise makes the asthmatic to breathe short." In 1864, H. H. Salter noted that the attacks were related to cold air and the "rapid passage of fresh and cold air over the bronchial mucosal membranes." We now know a great deal about the mechanisms involved in exercise-induced asthma (EIA), and the phenomenon is so well characterized that it is believed—mistakenly—to be a unique asthmatic syndrome.

ASTHMATIC RESPONSE TO EXERCISE

Most of what is known about the details of the exercise-induced asthma attack is the result of exercise challenges conducted under controlled conditions in the laboratory. EIA following such a challenge is accompanied by the coughing, wheezing, dyspnea, and chest tightness that typify any asthma attack. Symptoms generally worsen for 5 to 10 minutes after a brief (5 to 8 minutes) period of exercise and resolve spontaneously within 30 to 60 minutes. During exercise and usually immediately after brief exercise, existing obstruction actually may be relieved. However, this improvement is transient and of questionable clinical significance, since the dominant event reported by patients is obstruction. With more prolonged exercise, patients report that asthma begins during exercise and then resolves with continued exercise ("running through" the attack).

Obstruction involves both large and small airways and affects pulmonary function tests in the same way as attacks following other stimuli (Anderson, 1992). All measures of airflow are diminished to a similar extent, so that relatively simple measures such as PEFR and FEV_1 are generally used to assess the response.

Arterial Po_2 is depressed during severe attacks, probably as a consequence of spotty areas of obstruction, which lead to ventilation-perfusion abnormalities. Arterial pH is also depressed at the height of the attack; however, this metabolic (lactic) acidosis occurs in anyone who exercises strenuously and is not caused by EIA. One important difference between acute asthma induced by allergen exposure and that induced by exercise is that the late-phase obstruction is both less severe and less common following exercise than after allergen exposure (Bierman and Spiro, 1984). Even more important, airway hyperresponsiveness does not increase after an exercise-induced late-phase attack. The practical corollary of this is that allergic individuals never report that chronic asthma is induced by repeated exercise, although this commonly occurs following chronic allergen exposure.

The severity of obstruction with exercise depends on several factors. The most important factor is the severity of the airway disease at the time of exercise, whether this is determined by a history of asthma symptoms, medication requirements, resting airflow obstruction, or responsiveness to histamine or methacholine. At the same time, it should be emphasized that asthmatics with apparently mild disease may have quite significant EIA. Resting airflow obstruction at the time of exercise has a more direct effect in that the maximal severity of obstruction after exercise is greater in a person with more severe resting obstruction.

The severity of the attack also depends on the exercise conditions. The severity of an attack increases with more strenuous exercise, but its relationship to the duration of exercise is more complex. The severity increases with longer exercise, but with exercise longer than 6 minutes, severity begins to diminish as subjects begin to "run through" their attacks (Godfrey et al, 1973). Exercise in cold dry air induces more severe attacks than similar exercise in warmer air, but exercise in hot humid conditions does not diminish the attack. Exercising while breathing air contaminated with gaseous pollutants, especially SO_2, increases airway obstruction (Sheppard et al, 1981). Moreover, the response is greater during a pollen season in persons allergic to that pollen, presumably because ongoing inflammation in the lower airway increases bronchial responsiveness to all stimuli (Eggleston, 1975).

REFRACTORY PERIOD

In about 50 percent of asthma patients, EIA is followed by a refractory period of 30 to 90 minutes, during which further exercise is followed by a shorter, less severe asthmatic response (Fig. 36–1). The degree of refractoriness is related to the intensity of initial EIA; when the initial exercise is strenuous and induces more severe EIA, a second exercise period induces milder EIA even if the exercise is equally strenuous. The mechanism of the refractory period is not known, but recent experiments provide some clues. It is possible to develop a refractory period without provoking EIA. For example, exercise while breathing warm moist air will induce a refractory period without inducing EIA (Hahn et al, 1985), as will repeated brief exercise which does not induce EIA (Schnall and Landau, 1980). Airway hyperresponsiveness does not change during the refractory period. Following bronchoprovocation with aerosols of hyperosmolar saline or adenosine, a refractory period is induced both to further inhalation

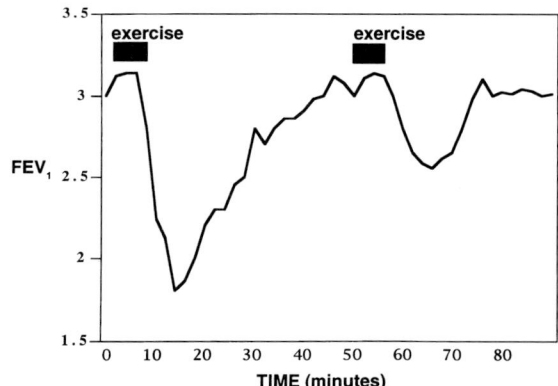

FIGURE 36–1. Change in FEV_1 associated with exercise in a single patient. Following the first 6-minute exercise period, FEV_1 fell by 43 percent, then gradually recovered to baseline by 50 minutes. A second, identical exercise at this time resulted in a fall of 18 percent with a quicker recovery to baseline, a typical refractory period.

with these agents and to exercise. Finally, indomethacin interferes with the refractory period following EIA (O'Byrne and Jones, 1988), suggesting that prostaglandin production is a necessary step.

PATHOPHYSIOLOGY

Our current understanding of the pathophysiology of EIA can be approached in four components: initiating stimulus, translational events, obstructive response, and modulating factors. The pathophysiology is reviewed in detail in several recent publications (McFadden and Gilbert, 1994; Anderson et al, 1989; Anderson, 1992).

The Initiating Stimulus

The initiating stimulus is the stress imposed on the airway to heat and humidify large volumes of air during exercise, and EIA can be mimicked by having asthmatic patients hyperventilate without exercising (Deal et al, 1986). Bronchospasm following both exercise and hyperventilation can be minimized by breathing warm moist air during exercise. Alveolar air is 37°C and fully saturated with moisture (44 mg/L). Even in summer, ambient air is cooler and rarely contains more than 25 mg/L of water; in the winter, at subfreezing temperatures, air contains as little as 2 mg/L of water. During quiet inspiration, ambient air is rapidly brought to alveolar conditions in the upper airway (nose, trachea, and bronchi). Although some of this water is recovered during expiration, net losses occur in the environment. Because of this net loss, the tracheal surface at rest is 2 to 3°C cooler than core body temperature, and the airway fluid is slightly hyperosmolar (340 to 380 mOsm/L) (Mann et al, 1979). In adapting to exercise, respiration increases quickly and may double during quiet walking or increase 30-fold with more strenuous exercise, and tracheobronchial temperatures approach those in the ambient air (McFadden et al, 1982). Airway osmolarity is likely to be high as well, and it has been calculated that airway losses during each minute of vigorous exercise are equivalent to the entire volume of the airway periciliary fluid, so that osmolarity is certainly higher than 340 to 380 mOsm/L (Anderson et al, 1989), whether heat, water loss, or both could be initiating stimuli.

Translational Events

The mechanism by which either may cause obstruction is not clear. One hypothesis states that airway water loss increases the epithelial osmolarity, thus activating pulmonary mast cells (Anderson et al, 1989). Inhaled hyperosmolar aerosols have been shown to induce obstruction that shares many characteristics with EIA (Belcher et al, 1987). Finally, hyperosmolarity activates inflammation and mast cells release histamine when placed in hyperosmolar buffers (Eggleston et al, 1987). Although there is no proof that this occurs in the lungs, dry air insufflated through the nose for 5 to 10 minutes results in secretion of histamine, prostaglandins, TAME esterase, and other mast cell mediators (Togias et al, 1985). Quantities of these mediators are similar to those found after nasal allergen challenge, as are the accompanied functional changes of increased vascular permeability. Interestingly, the osmolarity of nasal mucus increases slightly in proportion to the changes in mast cell products.

An alternative hypothesis is that airway mucosal vessels constrict when cooled during exercise (McFadden et al, 1986), and rebound vasodilation of bronchial vessels may be accompanied by interstitial edema after exercise, which narrows the airway lumen (McFadden et al, 1994). Although experiments show that obstruction can be prevented by delaying rewarming, it is difficult to reconcile this with evidence that drugs, such as beta-adrenergic agonists or cromolyn, which have minimal vascular effects, are effective in preventing or decreasing EIA.

Obstructive Response

Since these pathophysiologic changes occur in persons without asthma, EIA must be related to bronchial hyperresponsiveness. EIA is most severe in the most severe asthmatics. The severity of EIA is related to airway sensitivity to inhaled histamine or methacholine (Eggleston et al, 1979). Hyperventilation-induced asthma also correlates with response to these stimuli. The increased severity of EIA that occurs during a pollen season or following a cold may be explained by increased airway responsiveness, which accompanies these conditions.

Modulating Factors

Other exercise-related changes could also increase airway obstruction. Core body temperatures increase by 1°C or more during exercise and might increase water loss or interfere with airway cooling. Lactic acid, adenosine, and other metabolites from exercising skeletal muscle may modify the asthmatic response to exercise. Moderate exercise is associated with a mild lactic acidosis, and arterial pH may fall as low as 7.0 during maximal exercise (after a marathon for instance) and remain there for 15 to 30 minutes. Sympathetic neural tone is increased during exercise, and plasma catecholamine concentrations increase five- to tenfold, returning to baseline in 10 minutes (Larsson, 1983). Since bronchial smooth muscle preparations become less responsive to beta-adrenergic stimulation when cooled or when placed in acidic conditions, airway responsiveness to beta-adrenergic stimulation may decrease. This may be the mechanism by which alpha-adrenergic antagonists inhibit EIA (Walden et al, 1984).

Certain pollutants also increase obstruction during exercise. Sulfur dioxide at levels of 0.5 ppm can increase obstruction twofold (Sheppard et al, 1981).

EPIDEMIOLOGY AND DIAGNOSIS

Because exercise is a stimulus for asthma that is encountered in daily living, and because the asthmatic response is so comparable to those seen with allergen exposure and other daily triggers of asthmatic episodes, exercise challenges have been suggested as a preferred method for the epidemiologic surveys for asthma and for clinical diagnosis. Using as a threshold response a 10 percent fall in PEFR or 15 percent fall in FEV_1, 70 to 75 percent of persons with asthma have EIA. In a study published in 1976, 78 percent of children studied had a positive history of EIA, but 54 percent had a negative history and yet all had EIA (Kawabori et al, 1976). However, EIA is also seen in children with chronic cough, in relatives of asthmatics, and in patients with cystic fibrosis, allergic rhinitis, or a past history of asthma or bronchiolitis.

DRUG EFFECTS

Many drugs have been shown to affect EIA when given immediately before exercise. In Table 36–1 are listed those drugs whose effects have been documented with placebo-controlled challenges. Comparison to a placebo control is important because placebo treatment itself may reduce EIA by 20 to 30 percent.

Orally administered adrenergic agonists are effective bronchodilators, but the reported studies on the effects of oral treatment with metaproterenol, terbutaline, and albuterol on EIA are conflicting, with some showing clear inhibition of airflow obstruction with exercise and others showing only bronchodilation at similar doses (Anderson et al, 1989). Inhibition, when seen, generally lasts for 2 hours. Inhaled doses of the same agents will inhibit EIA in over 90 percent of persons, will have a more rapid onset of action (minutes), and will have a comparable duration of action at one twentieth of the dose (Konig et al, 1981). The lower effective dose is obviously associated with less severe toxicity, which may be an especially important advantage when cardiovascular risks must be minimized. Salmeterol and formoterol, new adrenergic agonists with an extraordinarily long duration of action, have been shown to prevent EIA for 12 hours and promise to become the drugs of choice for treating EIA, especially with children and adolescents in school who will not have to use a bronchodilator before participating in physical education or sports (Simons et al, 1992).

Methylxanthines partially inhibit EIA and also act as weak bronchodilators. Although some effect of theophylline may be seen with serum levels less than 10 μ/ml, protection is significantly greater at higher levels (Eggleston et al, 1981). Protection is additive with combined theophylline and beta-adrenergic agonist therapy.

Cromolyn has no bronchodilatory properties, but pretreatment with a 20-mg dose can decrease EIA for up to an hour. The metered dose inhaler, which delivers 1-mg doses of the drug, is somewhat less effective. The effect is not increased with chronic therapy, and the drug is not effective if given during or immediately after exercise. Cromolyn is not uniformly effective, and most studies show that EIA is not significantly inhibited in 25 to 30 percent of asthmatics. However, its effects are additive with beta-adrenergic agonists, so that it may be added to beta-adrenergic drugs, especially in the small number of patients whose EIA is not controlled by a single drug. Nedocromil sodium is also effective and, in comparative studies, is as effective as cromolyn in the 20-mg doses delivered by the older Spinhaler device (Konig et al, 1987).

Cholinergic antagonists (atropine, ipratropium bromide) are potent bronchodilators but generally are less effective inhibitors of EIA compounds discussed above; however, they are effective in a subgroup (20 to 25

TABLE 36–1. DRUG TREATMENT PROVED TO BE EFFECTIVE IN CONTROLLED TRIALS

Beta-adrenergic agonists
   Albuterol, 0.2 mg by inhalation
   Terbutaline, 1.25 mg by inhalation
   Bitolterol, 0.5 mg by inhalation
   Salmeterol, 0.8 mg by inhalation
Theophylline
   Orally with serum level above 10 μg/ml
Alpha-adrenergic agonists
   Phentolamine, 100 mg orally three times a day
Cromolyn
   MDI 1 mg/inhalation
   Spinhaler 20 mg/inhalation
Nedocromil
   2 mg/inhalation
Corticosteroids
   Prednisone, 20–35 mg orally for 4 days
   Budesonide, 200–400 μg inhaled twice a day for 4 days
Antihistamines
   Terfenadine, 60 mg twice a day orally

percent) of asthmatics. These subjects exhibit predominantly large airway obstruction after exercise.

Although antihistamines and corticosteroids are generally said to have little effect on EIA, only recently have blinded controlled studies of either class of drug been published. Moderate doses of terfenadine, clemastine, and chlorpheniramine partially inhibit EIA (Patel, 1984). However, these drugs are associated with sedation and/or cardiac conductive defects at effective doses, and so they cannot be recommended for clinical care. In a controlled study (Konig et al, 1974), prednisone, 12.5 to 40 mg daily for 1 week, caused a modest decrease in the percentage change in FEV_1 after exercise but a striking improvement in baseline FEV_1 and the severity of obstruction. Chronic treatment with inhaled steroids improves resting obstruction and partially inhibits EIA; the effects of treatment with beta-adrenergic agonists is also increased. Interestingly, treatment with intranasal corticosteroids is also modestly effective, presumably by allowing patients to decrease mouth breathing during exercise (Henrickson et al, 1984).

Recent studies demonstrating inhibition by inhaled furosemide, which inhibits chloride and water flux across epithelium (Bianco et al, 1988), and by LTD_4 antagonists (Manning et al, 1990) contribute to our understanding of the pathophysiology of EIA and may someday provide important therapeutic options.

Alpha-adrenergic antagonists cause moderate bronchodilation and partially inhibit EIA (Sly et al, 1967; Walden et al, 1984). Calcium channel blockers weakly inhibit EIA by inhalation. Nonsteroidal anti-inflammatory agents have no effect on EIA, but indomethacin blocks the exercise-induced refractory period (O'Byrne and Jones, 1988). This could have practical implications for athletes who may be receiving this drug for pain relief and use a warm-up routine that is designed to induce a refractory state prior to an athletic event.

CLINICAL MANAGEMENT

Diagnosis

Exercise-induced asthma is simple to diagnose. Coughing or wheezing that is related to exercise by a person with asthma or allergic rhinitis should be considered to be EIA, especially if symptoms can be prevented with an inhaled beta-adrenergic agonist before exercise. In doubtful cases, an exercise challenge may be helpful with 6 to 8 minutes of free running, treadmill exercise, or cycloergometer exercise. Airway function is determined before and for 20 minutes after exercise, employing spirometry and/or peak flow measurements (see Table 36–3). The effectiveness of inhaled beta-adrenergic treatment is so predictable that this is a useful therapeutic trial to confirm a suspected diagnosis.

The real clinical issue is recognizing that exercise is an essential part of normal daily activity and that a major goal of asthma therapy is to allow the patient to achieve normal daily activity. Therefore, EIA is an indication that additional treatment is required. The additional treatment may be as simple as adding an inhalation of beta-adrenergic agonist before exercise. If this is not completely effective or if many additional treatments are required each day, chronic anti-inflammatory therapy should be added or increased.

Table 36–2 lists the differential diagnosis of EIA. The most commonly confused condition is exercise-related hyperpnea in patients unaccustomed to exercise. Here the most important historical point is that dyspnea and noisy breathing occur during exercise and improve quickly after resting—the opposite of EIA timing. Dyspnea related to other lung disease (for example, tuberculosis, sarcoidosis, or idiopathic pulmonary fibrosis) follows a similar pattern.

Hyperventilation syndrome may be confused with EIA. This diagnosis should be considered in persons who have hyperventilation attacks with associated paresthesia, cramps, or faintness.

Exercise-induced anaphylaxis presents with skin lesions (urticaria, maculopapular rash, flushing), hypotension, and airway symptoms, which might include cough or sneeze (Kaplan et al, 1981) (see Chapter 26). Cholinergic urticaria is a form of physical urticaria

TABLE 36–2. DIFFERENTIAL DIAGNOSIS OF EXERCISE-INDUCED ASTHMA

Normal hyperpnea related to exercise
Dyspnea with other lung or heart disease
Hyperventilation syndrome
Exercise-induced anaphylaxis
Exercise-induced laryngospasm

in which typically small urticarial lesions occur on the trunk and face and may occasionally be associated with chest symptoms and hypotension. Attacks occur during exercise, but they also occur with any condition that warms the skin and causes vasodilation.

Finally, exercise-induced laryngospasm is a condition of unknown mechanism in which airway obstruction occurs abruptly during exercise. Typically, the patient loses his/her voice and experiences inspiratory stridor as well as expiratory obstruction. This syndrome has a different time course from EIA, since it begins abruptly during exercise and stops quickly afterward. It responds poorly to inhaled adrenergic treatment.

In the unusual case in which EIA is not well controlled or the diagnosis of EIA is doubted, an exercise challenge may be indicated. The methods for a clinical challenge are outlined in Table 36–3. The safety of the patient should be a major concern, and patients who have severe unstable asthma or who are potential cardiovascular risks, such as those unaccustomed to exercise or those older than 35 years, should not be exercised in an office setting. Figure 36–2 shows the relation of maximal heart rate to age. The results of the challenge may be interpreted as follows: a fall of FEV_1 of 15 percent or greater should be considered diagnostic of EIA; 20 to 40 percent is a moderately severe response, and greater than 40 percent represents severe EIA.

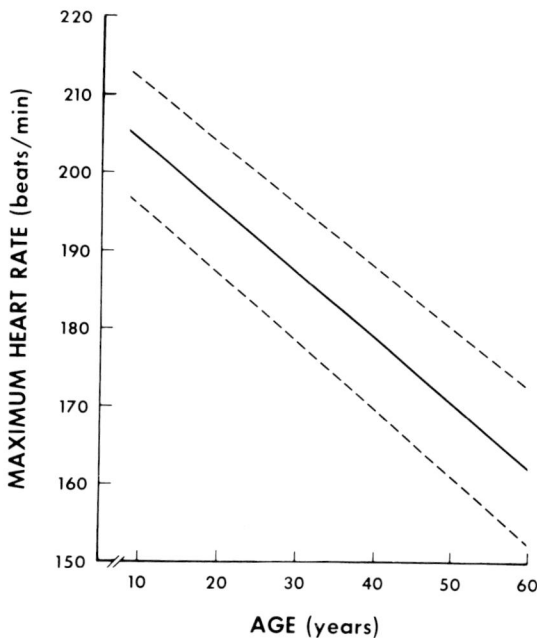

FIGURE 36–2. The relation of maximal heart rate to age. Solid line is drawn at the mean, while the dotted lines represent one standard deviation. (Adapted from Lange Anderson K, Shephard RJ, Denolin H, et al. Fundamentals of Exercise Testing. Geneva, World Health Organization, 1971.)

The medication of choice for EIA is currently a beta-adrenergic agonist taken by inhalation 5 to 30 minutes before exercise, depending on the agent. Whenever inhaled

---

TABLE 36–3. CLINICAL EXERCISE CHALLENGE PROCEDURE

Equipment:
1. Spirometer
2. Exercise space (stairway, sidewalk, treadmill)
3. Stopwatch
4. Standard resuscitation equipment
5. Cardiac monitor

Procedure:
1. This procedure is appropriate for 7- to 35-year-old patients who are otherwise healthy. Some older patients may participate safely if they are accustomed to vigorous exercise.
2. MD or RN should supervise test.
3. Measure resting pulse, blood pressure.
4. FEV_1, PEFR should be within 80% of predicted or personal best.
5. Exercise:
    6–8 min duration
    60–80% predicted aerobic capacity. This may be estimated by measuring pulse rate every minute during the procedure. Percent of maximal pulse and percent maximal aerobic capacity correlate closely. Age adjusted maximal heart rate as shown in Figure 36–2.
    Usual exercise rate:
    Up and down 1 or 2 floors per minute in stairway
    500 yards per minute in free-range running
6. Repeat FEV_1, PEFR at 1, 5, 15 minutes.
7. Abnormal result is 10% fall FEV_1, 20% fall PEFR.

drugs are used, observe how the patient uses them. To avoid complicating the treatment of an asthmatic patient already taking one bronchodilator, however, it is better to adjust the dose or timing of that medication rather than adding another drug. Cromolyn or nedocromil is usually prescribed as first drug only when there is a concern about the cardiovascular side effects of bronchodilators during exercise. If there is a problem with coordination, the use of a spacer or such preparations as Ventolin Rotocaps or Maxaire Autohaler should be used. On the other hand, when treatment with a beta-adrenergic agonist is only partially effective, the addition of cromolyn or nedocromil as a second drug just before exercise may produce additive inhibition.

The presence of EIA indicates that a patient's asthma is poorly controlled. It is important to remember that exercise is part of the normal life style, especially in the child, and one of the major goals of asthma therapy is to restore the patient to normal function. The physician should encourage children and adolescents to participate to their ability in gym class and play activities and/or competitive athletics, but should make it possible by prescribing appropriate premedication. Premedication, even if required on a regular basis, is preferable to avoidance of exercise at the risk of exclusion from a peer group or to establishing sedentary habits that may increase health risks later in life. It may be helpful to give examples of successful athletes with asthma to provide the child with a role model.

For recreation, patients should be advised to pursue activities that are less likely to induce asthma, such as swimming. A porous mask (3M Cold Weather Mask) increases the humidity of inspired air and reduces EIA (Schachter et al, 1981); a muffler probably has the same effect, but is more cumbersome. Consciously breathing through the nose reduces EIA, and many patients can train themselves to use this technique in mild and modest exercise. Patients should be aware that they may experience more severe EIA during a pollen season, following a cold or recent asthma attack, or when air pollution is present. Scuba diving may induce asthma through pathways similar to EIA. Although the balance of data suggests that asthmatics are not at increased risk when scuba diving, this should remain an individual decision for each patient (Schanker and Spector, 1992).

The Asthmatic Athlete

In athletes with asthma, special educational problems are encountered. Coaches, as well as team physicians, must be made aware of the diagnosis; the athlete will usually turn to them for advice before asking his or her own physician. Athletes and their coaches should be aware of the potential danger of abusing adrenergic aerosols in a subject who is likely to be both acidotic from maximal exercise and hypoxic from asthma. Similarly, the coach should be aware that performance will be suboptimal on certain days, when the air is cold, during pollen seasons, or when the athlete is recovering from a cold; the athlete should certainly not be penalized or derided as a malingerer.

On the other hand, the competitive drive of athletes must be acknowledged. Whether driven by team spirit or by their own personal desire, most athletes have a strong desire to excel and view EIA as an obstacle to be ignored or overcome. If these drives can be enlisted by providing the athlete with an understanding that performance can be enhanced with proper treatment, treatment will be more successful.

Drugs are officially restricted at the Olympic level of competition. Inhaled beta-adrenergic agonists (albuterol, bitolterol, and terbutaline), cromolyn, and theophylline are allowed. Inhaled corticosteroids are allowed, but written notification must be given to the International Olympic Committee Medical Commission or the U. S. Olympic Committee Drug Control Program (U. S. Olympic Committee, 1989–1992). At the National Collegiate Athletic Association and scholastic levels, any drugs recommended by physicians are allowed.

Several general measures can be recommended. Early in an athletic child's career, it may be possible to select sports in which EIA will create less disadvantage, such as swimming or those that emphasize skill, hand-eye coordination, or strength (e.g., baseball, golf, field events) rather than endurance (e.g., track, soccer, football, basketball, hockey). Later it may be possible to select a position that requires less endurance (e.g., goalie). Aerobic conditioning appears to have little effect on EIA per se, but a given exercise in a well-conditioned person will induce less hyperventilation and will therefore be less likely to cause EIA. In addition to being aware of

TABLE 36–4. WARM-UP ROUTINE FOR ASTHMATIC ATHLETES

1. Begin within 1 hour of event.
2. Begin by inhaling albuterol, 200 µg, or cromolyn, 4 mg (salmeterol or nedocromil if not an Olympic event).
3. Warm-up with 10–15 minutes of stretching.
4. Slow jog for 5–10 minutes. If wheezing begins, inhale albuterol.
5. Run ten 30-second sprints in sequence. If wheezing develops, inhale albuterol.
6. Use drugs sparingly during event.

the benefit of nasal breathing and conditioning, athletes should be aware of the refractory period of EIA. Repeated short sprints (seven successive 30-second sprints performed every 2 minutes) are an effective way of inducing this refractory period without first inducing asthma (Schnall and Landau, 1980). A warm-up routine is outlined in Table 36–4, which utilizes both premedication and repeated exercise to generate a refractory period before a competitive event. A portable peak flow meter is substantially less expensive than a pair of athletic shoes and can provide invaluable feedback to the athlete in designing a warm-up program or adjusting medication.

REFERENCES

Anderson SD. Exercise-induced asthma. *In* Middleton E Jr, Reed CE, Ellis EF, et al (eds). Allergy: Principles and Practice. 4th ed. St. Louis, CV Mosby, 1992, p 1005.

Anderson SD, Daviskas E, Smith CM. Exercise-induced asthma: a difference in opinion regarding the stimulus. Allergy Proc 10:215, 1989.

Anderson SD, Seale JP, Rozea R, et al. Inhaled and oral salbutamol in exercise-induced asthma. Am Rev Respir Dis 114:493, 1976.

Belcher NG, Rees PJ, Clark TJH, et al. A comparison of the refractory periods induced by hypertonic airway challenge and exercise in bronchial asthma. Am Rev Respir Dis 135:822, 1987.

Bianco S, Vagh A, Robuschi M, et al. Prevention of exercise-induced bronchoconstriction by inhaled furosemide. Lancet 2:252, 1988.

Bierman CW, Spiro SG. Characteristics of the late response in exercise-induced asthma. J Allergy Clin Immunol 74:701, 1984.

Deal EC Jr, McFadden ER Jr, Ingram RH Jr, et al. Hyperpnea and heat flux: Initial reaction sequence in exercise-induced asthma. J Appl Physiol 46:476, 1986.

Eggleston PA, Beasly PP, Kindley RT. The effects of oral doses of theophylline and fenoterol on exercise-induced asthma. Chest 79:399, 1981.

Eggleston PA, Kagey-Sobotka A, Lichtenstein LM. A comparison of the osmotic activation of basophils and human lung mast cells. Am Rev Respir Dis 135:1043, 1987.

Eggleston PA, Rosenthal RR, Anderson SA, et al. Guidelines for the methodology of exercise challenge testing of asthmatics. Study Group on Exercise Challenge, American Academy of Allergy. J Allergy Clin Immunol 46:42–45, 1979.

Eggleston PA. A comparison of the asthmatic response to methacholine and exercise. J Allergy Clin Immunol 63:104, 1979.

Eggleston PA. Exercise-induced asthma in children with intrinsic and extrinsic asthma. Pediatrics 56:856, 1975.

Godfrey S, Silverman M, Anderson SD. Problems of interpreting exercise-induced asthma. 59:199, 1973.

Hahn AG, Nogrady SG, Burton GR, et al. Absence of refractoriness in asthmatic patients after exercise with warm humid inspirate. Thorax 40:418, 1985.

Henrickson JM, Wenzel A. Effects of an intranasally administered corticosteroid (budesonide) on nasal obstruction, mouth breathing and asthma. Am Rev Respir Dis 130:1014, 1984.

Kaplan AP, Natbony SF, Tawil AP, et al. Exercise-induced anaphylaxis as a manifestation of cholinergic urticaria. J Allergy Clin Immunol 68:319, 1981.

Kawabori I, Pierson WE, Conquest LL, et al. Incidence of exercise-induced asthma in children. J Allergy Clin Immunol 58:447, 1976.

Konig P, Eggleston PA, Serby CW. Comparison of oral and inhaled metaproterenol for prevention of exercise-induced asthma. Clin Allergy 11:597, 1981.

Konig P, Hordvig NL, Kreuttz C. The preventive effect and duration of action of nedocromil sodium and cromolyn sodium on exercise-induced asthma (EIA) in adults. J Allergy Clin Immunol 7:64, 1987.

Konig P, Jaffe P, Godfrey S. Effect of corticosteroids on exercise-induced asthma. J Allergy Clin Immunol 45:14, 1974.

Lange Anderson K, Shephard RJ, Denolin H, et al. Fundamentals of Exercise Testing. Geneva, World Health Organization, 1971.

Larsson K, Hjemdahl P, Martinsson A. Sympathoadrenal reactivity in exercise-induced asthma. Chest 82:560, 1983.

Mann SFP, Adams GK III, Proctor DF. Effects of temperature, relative humidity and mode of breathing on canine airway secretions. J Appl Physiol 46:205, 1979.

Manning PJ, Watson PM, Mangolskee DJ, et al. Inhibition of exercise-induced bronchoconstriction by MK-571, a potent leukotriene D_4 receptor antagonist. N Engl J Med 323:1736, 1990.

McFadden ER Jr, Lenner KA, Strohl KP. Post exertional airway rewarming and thermally induced asthma: New insights into pathophysiology and possible pathogenesis. J Clin Invest 78:18, 1986.

McFadden ER Jr, Denison DM, Aller JF, et al. Direct recording of the temperature in the tracheobronchial tree in normal man. J Clin Invest 69:700, 1982.

McFadden ER Jr, Gilbert IA. Current concepts: Exercise-induced asthma. N Engl J Med 330:1362–1367, 1994.

O'Byrne POM, Jones GL. The effect of indomethacin in exercise-induced bronchoconstriction and refractoriness after exercise. Am Rev Respir Dis 134:69, 1988.

Patel JR. Terfenadine in exercise-induced asthma. Br Med J 288:1496, 1984.

Schachter EN, Lach E, Lee M. The protective effect of a cold weather mask on exercise-induced asthma. Ann Allergy 46:12, 1981.

Schanker HMJ, Spector SL. Exercise-induced asthma and scuba diving. Insights in Allergy 7:1, 1992.

Schnall RP, Landau LI. Protective effects of repeated short

sprints in exercise-induced asthma. Thorax 35:828, 1980.

Sheppard D, Saisho A, Nadel J, Boushey HA. Exercise increases sulfur-dioxide-induced bronchoconstriction in asthmatic subjects. Am Rev Respir Dis 123:286, 1981.

Simons FER, Soni NR, Wade TAW, et al. Bronchodilator and bronchoprotective effect of salmeterol in young patients with asthma. J Allergy Clin Immunol 90:840, 1992.

Sly RM, Heimlich EM, Busser RJ, et al. Exercise-induced bronchospasm: Effect of adrenergic and cholinergic blockade. J Allergy 40:93, 1967.

Togias AG, Naclerio RA, Proud DA, et al. Nasal challenge with cold dry air results in release of inflammatory mediators. Possible mast cell involvement. J Clin Invest 76:1375, 1985.

U. S. Olympic Committee. Drug Free 1989–1992. Pages 34–35.

Walden SM, Bleecker ER, Chahal K, et al. Effect of alpha-adrenergic blockade on exercise-induced asthma and conditioned cold air. Am Rev Respir Dis 130:357, 1984.

Chapter 37

Occupational Asthma

Jonathan A. Bernstein, M.D., David I. Bernstein, M.D., and I. Leonard Bernstein, M.D.

Asthma in the workplace was recognized as early as 460 B.C.E., when Hippocrates first described respiratory symptoms in metal workers, tailors, horsemen, farm hands, and fishermen (Bernstein DI, 1992). In modern history, the most germane contributions were made by Bernardino Ramazzini, who published a collection of descriptive articles on work-related respiratory diseases in 1713. The interest in occupational asthma (OA) has grown exponentially over the past three decades to the point where there are now well over 200 recognized causative agents (Bernstein JA, 1992). As industrial technology becomes more sophisticated, the number of etiologic agents is projected to rise, highlighting the need for early recognition and diagnosis of workers with OA. Some countries have therefore established government-supported programs to compile information about the prevalence, causes, and natural course of OA (Bernstein IL, 1982; Meredith et al, 1991). This has enhanced the opportunity to evaluate and monitor large populations of workers in a variety of industries (Bernstein DI, et al, 1993). Currently, it is estimated that OA may account for 2 to 15 percent of all new cases of asthma (Bernstein IL, 1992). These estimates fluctuate between countries owing to differences in reporting systems that document new cases of OA. In the United Kingdom, physicians have instituted a program referred to as "Surveillance of Work-Related and Occupational Respiratory Disease" (SWORD) (Meredith et al, 1991). This surveillance program involves the voluntary reporting of occupational respiratory illnesses from a variety of industries by pulmonologists and occupational physicians (Meredith et al, 1991). During its first year of operation, SWORD reported that 26.4 percent of all work-related respiratory diseases were due to OA, with the most frequent cause (22 percent) being diisocyanates. This study, however, used only case definitions of OA and did not require objective tests to confirm reported cases (Meredith et al, 1991). Attempts are currently being made to compile more information about work-related respiratory diseases in the United States. Beginning in the early 1980s, the National Institute for Occupational Safety and Health (NIOSH) has initiated the Sentinel Health Notification System for Occupational Risks (SEHNSOR) (Becklake, 1992). This system, which is currently operational in ten states, was devised to identify and characterize new case reports of OA. Its efficacy as a national public health surveillance tool is still being assessed (Becklake, 1992). In Finland there is a national registry for identification of all new cases of occupational respiratory diseases and their specific causes (Becklake, 1992). This registry has compiled enough data so that the estimated yearly incidence of OA and hypersensitivity pneumonitis can be reported. Registries in Finland and the United States may provide the opportunity to identify risk factors for developing OA in specific industries, thereby allowing precautionary measures to be taken to reduce or prevent the occurrence of OA (Becklake, 1992).

Other national programs such as the United States National Occupational Exposure Survey (NOES) data base have been created to facilitate the reporting of workplace exposures by workers to their physicians (Seta and Young, 1993). In France, a Telematic Information Service (MINITEL) on OA has been created to aid primary practitioners in the diagnosis of OA (Perrin et al, 1993). The ultimate intent of NOES and MINITEL is to improve the diagnosis and reporting of OA cases by primary care physicians, which may directly contribute to more accurate prevalence statistics in the future (Perrin et al, 1993; Seta and Young, 1993).

DEFINITION

Recently, the following definition of OA was agreed upon and published by a group of experts after careful consideration of all previous attempts:

A disease characterized by variable airflow limitation and/or airway hyperresponsiveness due to causes and conditions attributable to a particular occupational environment and not to stimuli encountered outside the workplace. (Bernstein IL, et al, 1993).

The definition was expanded to include two categories of OA distinguished by the presence or absence of a latency period of exposure prior to the onset of symptoms. In the presence of a defined latency period, the causes of occupational asthma can be accounted for by an underlying IgE-mediated mechanism, but in other instances an immunologic mechanism has not been identified. The second category of OA without a latency period includes irritant-induced asthma or the Reactive Airways Dysfunction Syndrome (RADS) (Bernstein IL, et al, 1993).

Irritant-induced asthma or RADS occurs after a single exposure to high concentrations of toxic chemicals, such as anhydrous ammonia or chlorine gas, which results in acute-onset bronchial hyperresponsiveness (BHR) and asthmatic symptoms (Boulet, 1988; Brooks and Bernstein, 1993). The RADS syndrome is histopathologically similar to asthma. However, the underlying mechanism(s) for this syndrome has not been proved. RADS is characterized by absence of a latency period and is treated the same as asthma. Nonspecific bronchial hyperresponsiveness (NSBH) and asthma symptoms may persist in affected individuals for months to years after exposure (Boulet, 1988; Brooks and Bernstein, 1993). Asthma-like disorders that are not included in the latter definition of OA are reserved to describe work-related obstructive syndromes in which BHR and eosinophilia are not associated features. An example of such a disorder is byssinosis, which occurs in textile workers exposed to a variety of dusts from cotton, flax, hemp, or jute (Bernstein IL, et al, 1993).

PATHOPHYSIOLOGY

For decades the pathophysiology of OA has been defined primarily by specific bronchoprovocation studies performed on workers with OA induced by high-molecular-weight (HMW) or low-molecular-weight (LMW) agents. More recently our understanding has been greatly enhanced from studies that have utilized bronchoalveolar lavage (BAL) and transbronchial biopsy techniques in evaluation of workers with diisocyanate asthma (Chan-Yeung et al, 1988; DeMonchy et al, 1985). Specific inhalation challenge tests typically correspond well with the worker's occupational history and histopathologic changes demonstrated by BAL and transbronchial biopsy (Chan-Yeung et al, 1988; DeMonchy et al, 1985). Workers sensitized to HMW substances primarily exhibit immediate or dual airway responses, whereas LMW chemical agents induce more diverse patterns of bronchospastic reactions. For example, workers with diisocyanate or red cedar OA manifest not only isolated early asthmatic reactions (EAR) 10 to 20 percent of the time, but also isolated late asthmatic reactions (LAR) in 30 to 50 percent of cases; the remainder exhibit dual asthmatic reactions (DAR) (Fabbri and Ciaccia, 1993). The LAR, which occurs 4 to 12 hours after exposure to toluene diisocyanate (TDI), is associated with an influx of inflammatory cells into the airways (Fabbri and Ciaccia, 1993); following resolution of the LAR, there is a measurable increase in NSBH. Recent studies have demonstrated that the increase in NSBH actually precedes the LAR as early as 2 hours after TDI or antigen challenge (Durham et al, 1987; Steinberg et al, 1987). Figure 37–1 shows a characteristic dual asthmatic response after a TDI inhalation challenge in a worker with OA (Bernstein DI, 1992). Methacholine responsiveness increased 24 hours after challenge from the measured prechallenge baseline (Bernstein DI, 1992).

The pathologic findings in the airways of patients with occupational asthma are similar to those of nonoccupational asthma and therefore serve as a useful model for studying airway inflammation in asthma. These in-

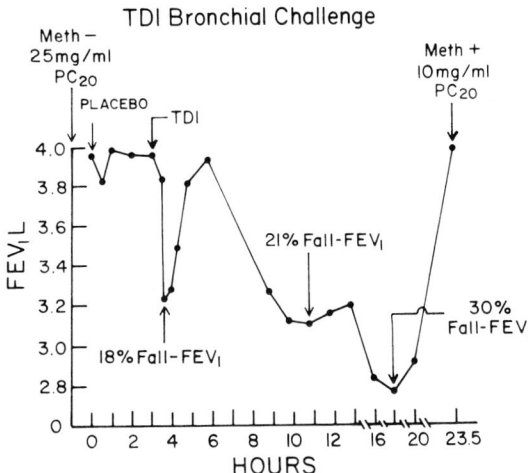

FIGURE 37–1. A dual-phase response in a polyurethane foam worker after bronchial provocation with toluene diisocyanate (TDI). Early-phase bronchospasm is followed by spontaneous recovery, which in turn is followed by late-phase bronchospasm. The concentration of methacholine required to reduce the forced expiratory volume in 1 second (FEV_1) by 20 percent (PC_{20}) fell from a baseline normal of 25 mg/ml to 10 mg/ml the day after TDI challenge. (From Bernstein DI, Bernstein IL: New developments in the diagnosis and management of occupational asthma. Resident and Staff Physicians, July 1988. Copyright © 1988 by Romaine Pierson Publishers, Inc; with permission.)

clude bronchial mucosal edema, smooth muscle hypertrophy, and basement membrane thickening, part of which is due to subepithelial deposition of collagen under the lamina reticularis (Beasley et al, 1989; Fabbri and Ciaccia, 1993; Roche et al, 1989). The BAL fluids from patients with asymptomatic nonoccupational asthma and subjects with inactive occupational asthma have similar distributions of inflammatory cells (90 to 95 percent alveolar macrophages, 5 to 10 percent lymphocytes, and <1 percent leukocytes and epithelial cells) (Fabbri and Ciaccia, 1993). However, the number of inflammatory cells (i.e., eosinophils and neutrophils) is dramatically increased in the BAL of individuals with persistent bronchial hyperreactivity or active OA (Fabbri and Ciaccia, 1993). Saetta et al examined serial bronchial biopsies in workers with TDI-OA and found increased numbers of inflammatory cells (i.e., eosinophils, mast cells, and lymphocytes) compared with normal nonasthmatic subjects (Bentley et al, 1992; Saetta et al, 1992a). The reticular basal membranes were also thickened due to deposition of collagen (types I, III, and V) (Saetta et al, 1992a; 1992b). Electron microscopy revealed widened spaces between basal epithelial cells, which the authors speculated may be associated with loss of intracellular adhesion, thereby potentiating inflammatory cell migration into the airways (Wagner et al, 1990). Bronchial biopsies of patients with OA have demonstrated increased numbers of eosinophils and activated T cells (Saetta et al, 1992a; 1992b). The numbers of eosinophils correlated with expression of mRNA for IL-5, the cytokine responsible for growth, differentiation, and activation of eosinophils (Saetta et al, 1992a). BAL has also been used to demonstrate the presence of a variety of bioactive mediators released by inflammatory cells into the airways. Histamine and leukotriene E_4 (LTE_4) have been detected in BAL immediately after plicatic acid inhalation challenges but disappear during the LAR (Chan-Yeung et al, 1989). LTB_4 and LTE_4 have been found in BAL and urine respectively after TDI challenges (Zocca et al, 1990). Other mediators such as platelet activating factor and prostaglandins have not yet been measured in BAL obtained from subjects with OA (Chan-Yeung et al, 1989).

MECHANISMS OF OCCUPATIONAL ASTHMA

OA has been described in many different work environments including the pharmaceutical, textile, automobile manufacturing, food processing, hair care, printing, farming, smelting, soldering, metal plating, tanning, and brewing industries (Bernstein JA, 1992). The numerous causes of OA have typically been classified by their molecular weights and biologic sources. Separating the etiologic agents associated with OA into HMW and LMW categories has allowed a clearer distinction of the underlying mechanisms of these disorders (Table 37–1) (Bernstein JA, 1992).

The HMW substances from numerous sources including animal and plant by-products induce OA primarily through IgE-mediated mechanisms (Bernstein DI, 1992). High-molecular-weight agents that induce OA are proteins, polysaccharides, or glycoproteins that possess multivalent allergenic determinants capable of inducing allergic sensitization and production of specific IgE antibodies (Tables 37–1 and 37–2) (Bernstein DI, 1992; Bernstein JA, 1992). The pathogenic role of specific IgG_4 or short-term sensitizing anti-

TABLE 37-1. CLASSIFICATION OF OCCUPATIONAL ASTHMA MECHANISMS

Nonimmunologic mechanisms
   Reflex bronchoconstriction
   Irritant bronchoconstriction (i.e., reactive airways dysfunction syndrome)
   Pharmacologically induced bronchoconstriction
Immunologic mechanisms
   Immediate hypersensitivity response (IgE-mediated)
      High-molecular-weight allergens
      Low-molecular-weight allergens
      Mixed (immunologic and nonimmunologic) allergens
   IgG antibody and/or immune (antigen-antibody) complex response
   Complement pathway activation
   Cell-mediated response

From Bernstein JA. Occupational asthma. "My job is making me sick." Postgrad Med 92:109, 1992.

body in OA has not been proved (Nielsen et al, 1988). Once sensitized, the specific IgE antibodies are bound to high-affinity IgE receptors on mast cells and basophils (Bernstein JA, 1992). Upon re-exposure to the workplace allergen, cross-linking of cell-bound specific IgE by antigen leads to activation and release of an array of preformed and newly synthesized bioactive mediators as well as cytokines, which result in the physiologic events associated with OA. Workers with IgE-mediated asthma characteristically exhibit either an EAR (onset of symptoms within one hour) or dual response (immediate asthmatic responses followed by recovery within 2 hours, with LAR occurring after 4 to 12 hours) (Pepys, 1975). Isolated LARs can occur but are uncommonly seen in IgE-mediated forms of asthma (Pepys, 1975).

Low-molecular-weight agents can induce IgE-mediated responses by acting as haptens, which form linkages with autologous protein carriers (i.e., albumin) to form complete antigens (Bernstein DI, et al, 1993). This haptenation reaction may result in formation of new antigenic determinants (NAD), which themselves act as allergenic epitopes (Bernstein DI, et al, 1993; Bernstein DI, et al, 1984). Such mechanisms have been clearly demonstrated in the induction of IgE-mediated responses by acid anhydride chemicals (i.e., phthalic and trimellitic anhydrides) (Bernstein DI, et al, 1984; Maccia et al, 1976).

Low-molecular-weight substances can induce OA by both immunologic and nonimmunologic mechanisms (Bernstein JA, 1992). The mechanisms associated with OA caused by LMW agents are more diverse than those caused by HMW agents (Table 37-1) (Bernstein JA, 1992). Immunologic mechanisms responsible for OA caused by LMW agents have been categorized according to the Gell-Coombs classification. Type I IgE-mediated immune response has been demonstrated to occur with OA caused by acid anhydrides, polyisocyanates, and other reactive chemical agents (Table 37-3) (Bernstein IL, 1992; Gallagher et al, 1981; Patterson et al, 1982). A type II or cytotoxic mechanism involving complement-fixing IgM or IgG antibodies directed against specific tissue antigens has been used to explain the occurrence of hemolytic anemia and pulmonary hemorrhage in workers exposed to high concentrations of trimellitic anhydride (TMA) fumes (Zeiss et al, 1982). The "late respiratory systemic syndrome" (LRSS) also reported in TMA workers—characterized by cough, wheezing, shortness of breath, and systemic symptoms such as chills, myalgias, and arthralgias—resembles a type III immune complex reaction (Bernstein IL, 1992). Finally, although classic type IV delayed hypersensitivity responses had not been previously recognized as a factor in the immunopathogenesis of OA, there is now an abundance of evidence suggesting that T cells may play a major role in elicitation of non-OA and OA, especially in those affected with diisocyanate asthma (Bernstein IL, 1992; Solway et al, 1991). It is possible that epitopes formed by hapten protein antigens could be processed by antigen-presenting cells (APC) and presented in association with major histocompatibility (MHC) molecules to receptors on T cells. Ultimately this process could result in T cell activation and release of lymphokines, which could perpetuate the inflammatory cascade associated with asthma (Solway et al, 1991). Early evidence for cellular involvement in TDI-induced OA was demonstrated by Gallagher et al, who found *in vitro* leukocyte inhibitory factor in peripheral blood leukocytes from the majority of affected workers stimulated with TDI-HSA (Gallagher et al, 1981). Subsequently, investigators have demonstrated increased CD8+ cells in the peripheral circulation of workers with OA after TDI challenge. Increased CD8+ cells and eosinophils have also been found in BAL fluids of workers with confirmed TDI asthma (Fabbri and Ciaccia, 1993; Finotto et al, 1991). In workers suspected of having nickel- and cobalt-induced

TABLE 37–2. CAUSES OF OCCUPATIONAL ASTHMA: ALLERGIC MECHANISM; HIGH-MOLECULAR-WEIGHT COMPOUNDS

Agents	Occupations	No. of Subjects	Prevalence	Skin Test	Specific IgE	Precipitin	Broncho-provocation Test
Animal products, insects, others	Laboratory workers						
	Veterinarians	1,487	3.1%				
Laboratory animals: rats, mice, rabbits, guinea pigs	Animal handlers	399	7.5%	+			+ (12/12)
		179	11.7%	+		−	
		130	30.4%	+			
		146	10.3%	+			
		5		+	+	−	+ (5/5)
		11					
Birds: Pigeon, budgerigar, chicken	Pigeon breeders	10		+			+ (9/10)
	Poultry workers	14		+	+		+ (L/1)
	Bird fanciers						
Insects							
Grain mite	Grain workers	1		+		+	+
Locust	Research laboratory	119	26%	+	+		
River fly	Power plant along rivers	1,284	3.1%	+			
Screw worm fly	Flight crews	182	70%	+			
Cockroach	Laboratory workers	10		+			+ (4/10)
Cricket	Field contact	1		+	−	−	+
Bee moth	Fish bait breeders	18	5.5%	+		−	+
Moth and butterfly	Entomologists	2		+			
Plants							
Grain dust	Grain handlers	17		+		+	+ (8/15)
		22		−	−	−	+ (6/22)
		11		+		+	+ (5/11)
Wheat/rye flour	Bakers, millers	1		+	+	−	+
		2		+		+	+ (2/2)
		4		+	+		+ (L/2)
		7		+	+		+ (4/7)
		31		+	+		+ (22/31)
Buckwheat	Bakers	3		+			+
Coffee beans	Food processors	6		+		+	+ (2/3)
Castor bean	Oil industry	5			+		
Tea	Tea worker	1		+			+
Tobacco leaf	Tobacco manufacturing	1		+			+
Hops (*Humulus lupulus*)	Brewery chemist	1		+			
Biologic enzymes							
B. subtilis	Detergent industry	3		+	+		+ (3/3)
		98	50%	+			
		38	66%	+	+	+	+ (9/10)
Trypsin	Plastic, pharmaceutical	14	29%	+	+	−	+ (3/4)
Pancreatin	Pharmaceutical	5					
Papain	Laboratory	1		+	+	+	
	Packaging	33	46%	+	+	−	+ (8.9)
Pepsin	Pharmaceutical	1		+	+		+
Flaviastase	Pharmaceutical	3		+	+	+	+ (2/2)
Bromelin	Pharmaceutical	2		+			
Fungal amylase	Manufacturing, bakers	5		+			
Vegetable gums							
Gum acacia	Printers	2		+			+ (1/1)
		63					
Gum tragacanth	Gum manufacturing	1	51%	+			
Others							
Crab	Crab processing	303	16%	+	+		+ (33/57)
Prawns	Prawn processing	50	36%	+	+	+	+ (2/2)
Hoya	Oyster farm	1,413	29%	+	+		
Larva of silkworm	Sericulture	5,519	0.2%	+	+		+ (9/9)

Adapted from Chan-Yeung M, et al. Occupational asthma—state of the art. Am Rev Respir Dis 133:686, 1986.

TABLE 37–3. CAUSES OF OCCUPATIONAL ASTHMA: ALLERGIC OR POSSIBLY ALLERGIC MECHANISM; LOW-MOLECULAR-WEIGHT

Agents	Occupations	No. of Subjects	Prevalence	Skin Test	Specific IgE	Precipitin	Broncho-provocation Test
Diisocyanates							
Toluene diisocyanate	Polyurethane industries, plastics, varnish	4					+ (4/4)
		21	38%	−		−	
		112	12.5%	+	−	−	+ (5/11)
		23	17.4%		+		
		15		+	−		
		26			+		+ (26/26)
		17			−		+ (14/17)
		195					
Diphenylmethane diisocyanate			28%		+		+ (12/17)
	Foundries	57	5%	−			
		1		−	+		
		11			+		+ (6/11)
Hexamethylene diisocyanate	Automobile spray painting	1		−		+	+
Anhydrides							
Phthalic anhydride	Epoxy resins, plastics	4					+ (3/3)
		1		+	+		+
Trimellitic anhydride	Epoxy resins, plastics	14	29%	+	+		+ (1/1)
		14	36%		+		
Tetrachlorophthalic anhydride	Epoxy resins, plastics	5		−	−		+ (3/3)
Wood dust							
Western red cedar (*Thuja plicata*)	Carpenter, construction, cabinet maker, sawmill worker	6					
		1320	3.4%	+			+ (18.22)
		22		+		−	+ (185/185)
		185			+		
California redwood (*Sequoia sempervirens*)		2		−		−	+ (2/2)
Cedar of Lebanon (*Cedra libani*)		6		−		−	
Cocabolla (*Dalbergia resusa*)		2		−			
Iroko (*Chlorophora excelsa*)		1		+	+		+
Oak (*Quercus robur*)		1		−	+		+
Mahogany (*Shorreal* sp)		1		−	+		+
Abiruana (*Pouteria*)		2		+	−		+ (2/2)
African maple (*Triplochiton scleroxylon*)		2		+	+		+ (2/2)
						−	
Tanganyika aningre		3		+	−		+ (3/3)
Central American walnut (*Juglans olanchana*)		1		−	−	−	+
Kejaat pterocarpus angolensis		1		+		−	
African zebrawood (*Microberlinia*)		1		+	+		+
Metals							
Platinum	Platinum refinery	91	57%	+			
		16		+			+ (10/16)
Nickel	Metal plating	1		+	−	−	+
		1		+	−		+
		1		+	+	+	+
Chromium	Tanning	1	−	+		+	
		1	+				
		1	+				
Cobalt	Hard metal industry	4		+		+	+ (2/4)
Vanadium	Hard metal industry	12	33%				
Tungsten carbide	Hard metal industry	1					

TABLE 37-3. CAUSES OF OCCUPATIONAL ASTHMA: ALLERGIC OR POSSIBLY ALLERGIC MECHANISM; LOW-MOLECULAR-WEIGHT Continued

Agents	Occupations	No. of Subjects	Prevalence	Skin Test	Specific IgE	Precipitin	Broncho-provocation Test
Fluxes							
Aminoethyl ethanolamine	Aluminum soldering	3					+ (3/3)
		2		−			+ (2/2)
Colophony	Electronic	51					+ (34/51)
Drugs							
Penicillins	Pharmaceutical	4		−			+ (3/4)
Cephalosporins	Pharmaceutical	2		+			+ (2/2)
Phenylglycine acid chloride	Pharmaceutical	24	29%	+	+		+ (2/2)
Piperazine hydrochloride	Chemist	2		+			+ (2/2)
Psyllium	Laxative manufacturer	3		+			+ (2/3)
Methyl dopa	Pharmaceutical	1		−			+
Spiramycin	Pharmaceutical	1		+			+
Salbutamol intermediate	Pharmaceutical	1					+
Amprolium HCl	Poultry feed mixer	1					+
Tetracycline	Pharmaceutical	1					+
Sulfone chloramides	Manufacturers, brewery	12		+			
Other chemicals							
Dimethyl ethanolamine	Spray painting	1		−			+
Persulfate salts and henna	Hairdressing	2	+				+ (2/2)
				−			+
Ethylene diamine	Photography	1	18.5%	−			
Azodicarbonamide	Plastics and rubber	151					+
Dioazonium salt	Photocopying and dye	1					+
Hexachlorophene (sterilizing agent)	Hospital staff	1	29%				
Formalin	Hospital staff	28		−			+ (2/4)
Urea formaldehyde	Insulation, resin	2					+ (2/2)
Freon	Refrigeration	1					+
Paraphenylene diamine	Fur dyers	80	37.5%	+			+
Furfuryl alcohol (furan-based resin)	Foundry mold makers	1					+

Adapted from Chan-Yeung M, et al. Occupational asthma—state of the art. Am Rev Respir Dis 133:686, 1986.

OA, proliferation of peripheral lymphocytes coincubated with nickel and cobalt metallic salts have been demonstrated (Herzog et al, 1991; Kusaka et al, 1989). Animal models have been informative in the investigation of the role of T lymphocytes in the pathogenesis of OA induced by LMW chemicals. A murine model of OA has been developed to study the differential production of cytokines by helper T cell subsets (T_{H1} and T_{H2}) after sensitization and re-exposure to different reactive chemicals (Dearman and Kimber, 1991; 1992). It has been shown that under normal conditions T_{H1} lymphocytes primarily secrete IL-2, gamma interferon (γ-IFN), and tumor necrosis factor-β (TNF-β) whereas T_{H2} lymphocytes secrete IL-4, IL-5, IL-6, and IL-10 (Mosmann and Coffman, 1989; Mosmann et al, 1991). A predominance of T_{H2} cells occurs in association with IgE immune responses, whereas a predominance of T_{H1} cells is associated with cell-mediated immune responses (Mosmann and Coffman, 1989; Mosmann et al, 1991). Dearman and Kimber have demonstrated that there was preferential activation of T cells with a T_{H2} cytokine profile in mice immunized with phthalic anhydride (PA), trimellitic anhydride (TMA), and diphenyl-methane diisocyanate (MDI) as opposed to T_{H1} profiles induced after immunization with dinitrochlorobenzene (DNCB), suggesting that chemical structure may be important in determining induction of IgE responses (Dearman and Kimber, 1991; 1992).

Nonimmunologic toxic or irritant effects can injure bronchial epithelial cells. LMW agents such as acid anhydrides, diisocyanates, colophony fumes, and plicatic acid (the organic acid responsible for red cedar OA) are examples of agents with potent irritant effects (Bernstein IL, 1982; Chan-Yeung et al, 1973). Damaged bronchial epithelial cells could permit easier access of irritants or allergens into the subepithelial tissues and lamina propria. Such chemicals could also exert direct effects on inflammatory cells and the bronchial microvasculature (Sheppard, 1989). Nonspecific bronchial hyperresponsiveness may result from stimulation of sensory vagal afferent nerves and release of pro-inflammatory cytokines, neurokinins, and/or bioactive mediators from bronchial epithelial cells (Sheppard, 1989). Sheppard et al have investigated the role of neuropeptides in OA. Guinea pig afferent nerve endings exposed to toluene diisocyanate (TDI) have been demonstrated to release the tachykinins—substance P and neurokinin A—resulting in increased airway responsiveness (Fabbri and Ciaccia, 1993; Sheppard et al, 1988). Bronchial hyperresponsiveness was abolished by depleting these nerve endings of tachykinins by pretreatment with capsaicin and potentiated by TDI's ability to inhibit neutral endopeptidase, an ectoenzyme important for tachykinin degradation (Sheppard et al, 1988). In addition, substance P itself may activate mast cells in the respiratory tract to release mediators capable of inducing neurogenic inflammation (Barnes et al, 1991a; 1991b). Phthalic anhydride (PA) also has been shown to exhibit a neurogenic effect by stimulating local release of substance P and calcitonin gene-related peptide (CGRP) from afferent nerve endings, independent of the central nervous system (Thompson et al, 1987).

It has been postulated that certain reactive chemicals may induce activation of the alternate or classic complement pathways (Chan-Yeung, 1982). Activation of either complement pathway could result in the formation of the anaphylatoxins, C3a and C5a, which can induce histamine release from mast cells and basophils. Human peripheral blood leukocytes from some workers with western red cedar OA have been shown to release histamine when incubated with low concentrations of plicatic acid. This effect could not be demonstrated in subjects without asthma or with non-OA (Chan-Yeung, 1982). Whether this reactivity is due specifically to plicatic acid or the formation of complement pathway fragments is unclear (Chan-Yeung, 1982).

"Pharmacologic" mechanisms may be responsible for airway obstructive changes occurring during the workshift in certain workers. Organophosphate insecticides are cholinesterase inhibitors that result in accumulation of acetylcholine in neuronal synaptic clefts, which can trigger bronchospasm especially in workers with preexisting NSBH (Bernstein IL, 1992). A nonspecific pharmacologic mechanism could explain bronchoconstrictive responses observed after inhalation of cotton dust by-products (Buch and Bonhuys, 1980). Both normal subjects and cotton workers exhibited dose-related airway obstruction after inhalation of cotton bract extracts, an effect possibly related to endotoxin (Merchant and Bernstein, 1992). Cross-shift decrements in lung function have been documented in pharmaceutical workers continuously exposed to opiate by-products. Opiates are known to cause direct release of histamine from mast cells (Biagini et al, 1990). Pharmacologic mechanisms have also been postulated but not proved to be involved in meat wrapper's and wood dust asthma (Chan-Yeung, 1982; Vandervort and Brooks, 1977).

EPIDEMIOLOGY AND RISK FACTORS

Epidemiologic studies have yielded invaluable information about prevalence, exposure-response relationships, and risk factors associated with OA. Most of the epidemiologic studies of OA conducted in the United States and abroad have been "cross-sectional" (Bernstein IL, 1982). These surveys have provided most of the information pertaining to prevalence within specific industries. These prevalence statistics are thought to underestimate the true incidence of OA cases in the United States because symptomatic workers often leave their jobs prior to medical identification (Becklake, 1992). Due to high cost and logistic considerations, relatively few well-designed prospective longitudinal studies have been performed (Bernstein DI et al, 1993; Gannon and Burge, 1991; Meredith et al, 1991).

Properly designed epidemiologic studies should attempt to evaluate associations between the worker's environmental exposure and clinical symptoms (Smith et al, 1989). Results of these studies may occasionally be obfuscated because symptoms suggestive of

OA may not always be provided by the worker. In addition, low levels of antigen, which can be sensitizing in susceptible individuals, may not be clinically recognized (Becklake, 1992; Smith et al, 1989). In most studies occupational questionnaires have been used to identify symptomatic individuals, but these often lack adequate specificity for OA (Malo et al, 1991). The questionnaire should elicit detailed information related to previous work history, current job description, previous or current exposures, asthma and rhinitis symptoms, and smoking history as well as the personal and familial atopic histories (Smith et al, 1989). The questionnaire should also seek to define whether a temporal relationship exists between symptoms and exposure. However, it has been demonstrated that questionnaires alone are not reliable for diagnosing OA (Becklake, 1992). Those workers who satisfy a case definition based on questionnaire responses must be evaluated further using physiologic lung function tests at work and immunologic methods (if appropriate) to objectively confirm suspected diagnoses of OA. In this manner, reliable conclusions can eventually be made with respect to disease prevalence and risk factors. Such information can be used to make recommendations regarding which workers should be reassigned to different jobs and whether certain process modifications can be undertaken to prevent new cases of OA (Bernstein DI et al, 1993).

One of the advantages of well-designed epidemiologic investigations is identification of risk factors for OA. Numerous studies have demonstrated that the degree of exposure to causative agents increases the risk for development of OA (Becklake, 1992). This relationship between exposure and OA has been demonstrated for laboratory animal handlers, locust research workers, snow crab and prawn processors, bakers, papain workers, electronic and steel coating workers, and TDI production workers (Bernstein DI et al, 1987; Bernstein IL, 1982; Bernstein IL et al, 1993).

Atopy, defined by cutaneous reactivity to environmental aeroallergens, has been implicated as an important risk factor for development of OA in workers exposed to certain HMW (>1000kD) compounds such as detergent enzymes and laboratory animal proteins. A similar relationship has not been demonstrated consistently for LMW (<1000kD) compounds (Mitchell and Gandevia, 1971; Slovak and Hill, 1981). OA is more common among atopic individuals who are laboratory animal handlers, locust research workers, oyster farm workers, prawn processors, electronic workers exposed to colophony fumes, and psyllium processors (Becklake, 1992; Burge et al, 1979).

In certain studies, cigarette smoking has been identified as a risk factor among workers who develop OA (Burge et al, 1979; Chan-Yeung et al, 1982; Venables et al, 1985). Smoking is associated with an increased prevalence of OA in platinum workers and snow crab processors (Becklake, 1992). Venables reported that cigarette smoking and atopy were co-associated as risk factors for IgE-mediated sensitization to tetrachlorophthalic anhydride (TCPA) (Venables et al, 1985). In a subsequent study, Liss and co-workers found just the opposite association; that is, nonsmokers were more likely to become sensitized to TCPA (Liss et al, 1993). Chan-Yeung et al found that OA due to red cedar wood dust is more common among nonsmokers, suggesting that this group is more susceptible to red cedar asthma (Chan-Yeung et al, 1982). Finally, NSBH has not yet been demonstrated as a risk factor for OA, although more prospective studies are needed to address this question. Currently, it is believed that NSBH occurs as the result of exposure to allergens or irritants and does not appear to enhance susceptibility for development of OA (Lam et al, 1979).

CLINICAL APPROACH TO THE DIAGNOSIS OF OCCUPATIONAL ASTHMA

The diagnosis of OA first requires a careful occupational history. This should be focused on identifying a relationship between respiratory symptoms and work. On initial presentation, symptoms may consist of dyspnea, chest tightness, wheezing, and cough. Upper airway symptoms—such as rhinorrhea, nasal congestion, and ocular pruritus—which precede or begin concurrently with lower respiratory symptoms are highly suggestive of an IgE-mediated mechanism. Symptoms may begin minutes, hours, or days after one comes to work and typically improve when one is away from work only to recur upon re-exposure (Bernstein DI, 1992; Bernstein DI, et al, 1993). There are several instances in which a history may fail to identify the relationship between asthma symptoms and work. For example, workers who manifest primarily a LAR may not have symptoms until they are at home. If OA is very severe and chronic, demonstrable improvement of symptoms may not occur with cessation of work exposure after weeks, months, or even years.

A diagnosis of OA can mistakenly be made in an individual with preexisting asthma who was introduced into a workplace where factors such as irritants or exercise simply aggravated those symptoms (Bernstein DI, 1992). However, it should be emphasized that preexisting asthma does not always preclude a diagnosis of OA (Bernstein DI, 1992). OA must be distinguished from other diseases such as chronic obstructive lung disease, occupational pneumoconioses, and bronchiolitis obliterans. Other pulmonary syndromes, which are characterized by systemic symptoms of fever, malaise, myalgias, headaches, cough, and chest tightness, include grain fever, metal fume fever, mill fever, or byssinosis. These disorders are induced by either vegetable or textile dusts, bacterial endotoxin, mold spores, or fumes and can be difficult to distinguish from OA. A chest film is essential in all patients being evaluated for OA. Diffusing capacity of the lung for carbon monoxide (DLCO), which is typically normal in asthmatics, may be helpful for distinguishing some of these disorders from OA (Bernstein DI, 1992; Bernstein DI, et al, 1993).

A detailed environmental employment history must be obtained to identify all of the worker's direct and indirect exposures. The work process description should be in sufficient detail to ascertain whether exposure is occurring from fumes, dusts, or aerosols. Any accidental spills or toxic exposures to fumes, smoke, or chemicals that would predispose the worker to develop OA should be determined (Bernstein DI, 1992; Bernstein DI, et al, 1993). Material safety data sheets (MSDS), which by federal law must be accessible to employees in their work areas, are often useful for determining the most likely agent(s) responsible for inducing OA. Industrial hygienists, who routinely perform air sampling measurements in the workplace in compliance with NIOSH standards, may be helpful in providing information about the worker's level of exposure (Bernstein DI, 1992; Bernstein DI, et al, 1993).

Confirmation of OA should utilize an algorithmic approach, as outlined in Figure 37–2 (Bernstein DI, 1992). Administration of a validated occupational questionnaire to the worker(s) should ideally be followed by objective assessment of NSBH in the workplace. A negative methacholine or histamine inhalation test can be helpful in excluding OA in workers actively exposed at work due to the high negative predictive value of these tests. However, if a test of NSBH is positive, it is necessary to demonstrate improvement of symptoms and lung function after removal from the workplace combined with deterioration after reintroduction into the workplace. Serial peak expiratory flow rates (PEFR) are the most frequently used objective methods to measure lung function both at work and away from work. Peak expiratory flow rates should be recorded for 2 weeks at work and 2 to 3 weeks away from work. The patient must be instructed to measure and record the peak expiratory flow rate every 2 to 3 hours while at work and at home, documenting work exposure and asthma medication usage. While at work, 24-hour peak expiratory flow rate variability greater than 15 to 20 percent, together with a reversal of variability while away from work, is considered an abnormal response compatible with OA. One of the shortcomings of PEFR measurements is that patients can falsify their readings (Bernstein DI, 1992). Therefore, workers must be supervised and checked for compliance. Furthermore, while PEFR variability can assist in confirming OA, it cannot identify the specific causative agent. Cross-shift changes in FEV_1, although frequently used, have been shown to lack sensitivity for the diagnosis of OA (Bernstein DI, 1992). Serial PD_{20} measurements (provocative dose of methacholine or histamine required to cause a 20 percent decrease in FEV_1) in and away from the workplace are useful in demonstrating changes in NSBH. Although these tests do not enhance the diagnostic sensitivity and specificity of information obtained from previous serial PEFR studies, they are useful adjuncts in the overall diagnosis of OA (Bernstein DI, 1992; Cote et al, 1990).

The specific inhalation challenge test is considered to be the gold standard for diagnosing OA (Cartier and Malo, 1993). If a suspect substance in the workplace can be identified, a specific inhalation challenge may often be performed at work to confirm this relationship. Before a controlled challenge is per-

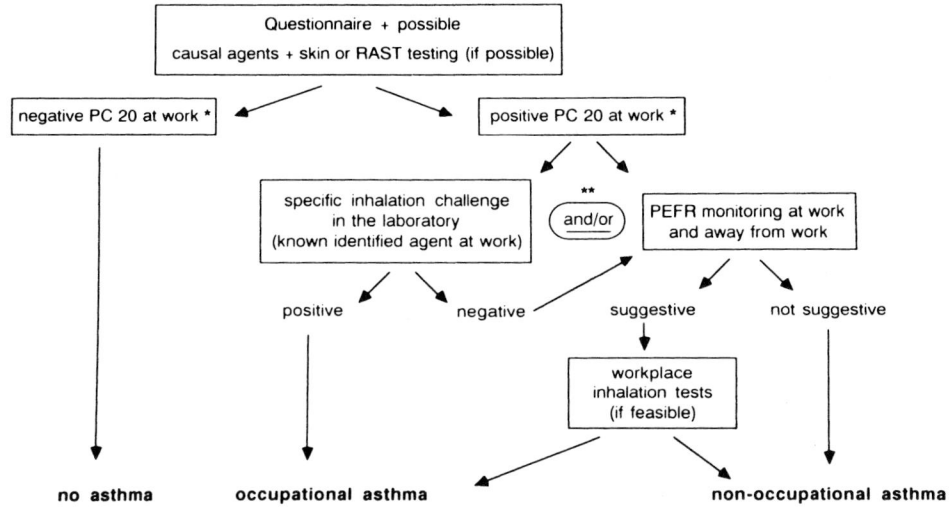

FIGURE 37–2. An algorithmic approach for the confirmation of occupational asthma. (From Bernstein DI. Clinical assessment and management of occupational asthma. *In* Bernstein IL, Chan-Yeung M, Malo JL (eds). Asthma in the Workplace. New York, Marcel Dekker, 1992, p 103.)

formed in the laboratory, prior determination of methacholine or histamine PD_{20} is useful in estimating the initial dose of a challenge agent (Cartier and Malo, 1993). These challenges should not be performed on workers with severe cardiac or pulmonary disease or with an FEV_1 <70 percent. Specific inhalation challenge tests have been reserved to document index cases of new causative substances causing OA or for medicolegal purposes such as proving a worker's eligibility for workmen's compensation or disability benefits (Cartier and Malo, 1993). They can also be done when there is uncertainty about the diagnosis. If positive, specific challenge tests provide a definitive diagnosis of OA. However, a negative challenge study does not always exclude the diagnosis as sensitivity to a suspect agent can decrease in workers removed from the workplace for a period of time (Cartier and Malo, 1993). It is therefore important to perform specific challenge tests before or soon after the worker is removed from the workplace (Cartier and Malo, 1993). Standardized approaches for performing specific allergen inhalation challenges to LMW chemicals as well as HMW allergens have been published (Cartier and Malo, 1993). It is impossible to reproduce exactly work exposure conditions in the laboratory while controlling for technical factors such as temperature and atmospheric pressure. The concentration of the challenge agent must also be controlled in order to ensure a safe exposure (Cartier and Malo, 1993). Moreover, the exposure during challenge may underestimate the actual exposure in the workplace, resulting in a false-negative study. Because of the risks and technical problems inherent in challenge testing, these procedures should only be performed by experienced individuals and only at specialized centers (Cartier and Malo, 1993).

Immunologic studies may be helpful in establishing a diagnosis of OA. It is important to determine a worker's atopic status by skin testing with common aeroallergens as this could represent a risk factor for OA (Bernstein DI, 1992; Bernstein DI, et al, 1993). Extracts of nonchemical agents can be used as skin prick test reagents to detect allergic sensitization. Examples of such substances are listed in Table 37–2 and include cereal proteins in flour, coffee beans, castor beans, *Bacillus subtilis*-derived enzymes, and egg white proteins (Bernstein DI, 1992; Bernstein DI, et al, 1993). *In vitro* assays to measure specific IgE to these proteins can also be performed but are less sensitive than *in vivo* skin testing (Bernstein DI, et al, 1993). It should be emphasized that the presence of either cutaneous reactivity or elevated serum-specific IgE indicates sensitization but does not confirm a diagnosis of OA in an individual worker (Bernstein DI, et al, 1993). In various epidemiologic studies, cutaneous reactivity to HMW agents is significantly associated with atopy, variability in PEFRs at work, and a confirmed diagnosis of OA.

Serum-specific IgE assays using RAST or ELISA methods are useful as screening tests in the identification of OA in workers exposed to acid anhydrides (Bernstein DI, 1992; Sarlo et al, 1990). Elevated serum-specific IgE antibodies are detectable in only a minority of workers (10 to 30 percent) diagnosed with diisocyanate OA confirmed by inhalational challenge (Cartier et al, 1989). IgG antibodies, when present, may represent markers of exposure to either chemical or HMW antigens but usually do not distinguish between those workers with OA and those without OA. *In vitro* techniques, such as leukocyte histamine release and leukocyte inhibitory factor are sometimes useful for research purposes (Bernstein DI, 1992; Bernstein DI, et al, 1993). Table 37–3 summarizes the LMW agents for which either positive skin tests or serum-specific IgE and/or specific IgG responses have been documented in association with OA (Chan-Yeung, 1993).

SPECIFIC CAUSES OF OCCUPATIONAL ASTHMA

HIGH-MOLECULAR-WEIGHT AGENTS. These agents account for most of the known causes of OA in a number of industries (see Table 37–2) (Bernstein DI, et al, 1993). Emanations from saliva, urine, skin, and dander are animal sources of workplace allergen (Bernstein DI, et al, 1993). Atopic individuals who work in professions that routinely come into frequent contact with these by-products (e.g., laboratory technicians, veterinarians, farmers, and other animal handlers) are often at greater risk (Bernstein DI, et al, 1993). It has been estimated that asthma and/or rhinitis symptoms affect approximately 10 to 15 percent of animal handlers, 50 percent of whom develop OA (Bernstein DI, et al, 1993). Other occupations at risk for developing OA due to animal allergens include poultry workers, shellfish (e.g., snow crab, oyster, prawn) processors, and silkworm farmers (Bernstein DI, et al, 1993). Cutaneous reactivity to these animal allergens correlates well clinically with OA (Bernstein DI, 1992).

OA associated with exposure to insects or their by-products (i.e., dust) has been diagnosed in grain workers, insect breeders, entomologists, and fish bait handlers (e.g., mealworm larvae) (Bernstein DI, et al, 1983; Matthews, 1989). Storage mites (e.g., *Lepidoglyphus destructor, Acarus siro,* and *Tyrophagus putrescentiae*), which contaminate grain and flour, have been identified as possible sources of occupational allergens that could induce OA in handlers and farmers (Bernstein DI, et al, 1993). Grain dust asthma may occur as the result of sensitization to grain dust or one of these storage mites (Chan-Yeung et al, 1993). Inhalational challenge studies to crude grain dust or grain dust mite extracts have been used to confirm a diagnosis (Chan-Yeung et al, 1993).

Plant products were also recognized to cause OA as early as 1713 when Ramazzini described asthma in bakers exposed to flour (Bernstein DI, 1992). Flour allergy, manifested by upper and lower respiratory symptoms, has been estimated to occur in 10 to 30 percent of bakers (Thiel and Ulmer, 1980). Nasal symptoms precede OA in approximately 10 percent of these workers (Musk et al, 1989). Flour dust contains a diversity of allergens including cereal proteins, mold spores, grain mites, and microbial enzymes—all or some of which could act as sensitizing agents. Sensitization to both soluble and insoluble wheat fractions has been demonstrated in workers with baker's asthma, with albumin considered the most important allergen. In affected bakers, sensitization has also been demonstrated to barley, rye, oat, and triticale cereal proteins (Bernstein DI, et al, 1993). Buckwheat and soy flour proteins are less frequent causes of OA (Bernstein DI, et al, 1993). Baker's asthma has also been shown to be induced by sensitization to α-amylase and hemicellulase enzymes, which are used as dough conditioners (Baur et al, 1986).

Recently, allergenic proteins in latex gloves derived from the rubber plant, *Hevea brasiliensis,* have been recognized as a frequent cause of OA among approximately 6 percent of exposed health professionals (Tarlo et al, 1990).

OA has also been described in food processing industries. Workers with inhalational exposure to egg white proteins (i.e., conalbumin, ovalbumin, and ovomucoid), coffee beans, spices, and soy proteins are at risk (Bernstein DI, et al, 1987; Edwards et al, 1983; Smith et al, 1987). A study evaluating workers in two egg-breaking and processing plants found that the prevalence of OA due to sensitization to egg proteins was 7 percent. The prevalence was higher (10 to 12 percent) in egg-breaking areas where there was exposure to aerosolized egg whites (Bernstein DI, et al, 1987; Smith et al, 1987). A variety of other food agents such as tea dust, garlic dust, pectin, mushroom powder, green coffee, and beans have been reported to cause OA (Bernstein DI, et al, 1993). Specific IgE antibodies have been identified in workers with OA induced by all of the above agents except tea dust (Bernstein DI, et al, 1993).

Animal or plant-derived enzymes are important causes of OA. OA caused by microbial detergent enzymes was first described in 1969 and subsequently found to occur in as many as 30 percent of exposed workers (Pepys et al, 1969). These enzymes are derived primarily from *Bacillus subtilis* and *Aspergillus* species. Sensitization occurs with higher frequency among atopic workers (Franz et al, 1971; Quirce et al, 1992). Other enzymes used in food and pharmaceutical industries, such as egg lysozyme, have recently been shown to induce OA by inhalational exposure (Bernstein JA, et al, 1993).

Vegetable gums are high-polymer carbohydrate products commonly used as thickening agents in foods such as salad dressings, ice cream, soup, emulsifying agents in lotions and creams, as substrates in pills, and as sizing material for paper and textiles (Bush, 1990). The prototype for OA-induced vegetable gums is "printer's asthma" caused by gum acacia (Fowler, 1952). Gum acacia was used extensively in the printing industry before it was replaced by other materials in the late 1950s (Bush, 1990; Fowler, 1952). Other vegetable gums include guar gum used in the textile industry (Lagier et al, 1990). Malo et al found that 5 percent of workers in a carpet factory exhibited positive skin prick tests to guar gum and that 2 percent of these individuals had confirmed OA (Malo et al, 1990).

LOW-MOLECULAR-WEIGHT AGENTS. A variety of LMW substances have been shown to induce OA (Table 37–3) (Bernstein JA, 1992). In one survey, diisocyanates were identified as responsible for more cases of OA than other classes of LMW chemicals (Bernstein IL, 1982). It is estimated that 5 to 10 percent of workers exposed to diisocyanates develop OA. These compounds, which have reactive $N=C=O$ side groups, are used in the production of polyurethane foams, plastimers, adhesives, varnishes, coatings, and paint hardeners in numerous industries (Bernstein IL, 1982). The three major commonly used diisocyanate compounds are hexamethylene diisocyanate (HDI), 4-4-diphenylmethylene diisocyanate (MDI), and toluene diisocyanate (TDI) (Kennedy and Brown, 1992). Although the chemical properties of diisocyanates vary, workers sensitized to one compound may exhibit significant bronchial cross-reactivity to other diisocyanate chemicals (Baur, 1983; Kennedy and Brown, 1992). The natural history of diisocyanate-induced OA is variable in that some workers may have a complete remission following cessation of exposure whereas others have symptoms and NSBH persist for years after removal from workplace exposure (Moller et al, 1986a). Risk factors for development of diisocyanate-induced OA have not been identified. In humans there are many reports of OA developing after excessive exposure to chemicals during accidental spills (Mapp et al, 1988). Workers with diisocyanate OA demonstrate variability in serum-specific antibody responses to diisocyanate antigens (Baur, 1983; Kennedy and Brown, 1992; Moller et al, 1986b). Specific IgG antibodies to diisocyanate conjugates are observed in as many as 70 percent of HDI- and MDI-exposed workers with OA, whereas TDI workers frequently fail to elicit any specific antibody responses (Grammer et al, 1988; Liss et al, 1990; Lushniak et al, 1990). Serum-specific antibody assays with diisocyanate-HSA conjugates are of limited value in the diagnosis of diisocyanate OA as increased antibody levels can be detected in workers with either positive or negative inhalational diisocyanate challenges (Butcher et al, 1993). Skin testing with diisocyanate conjugates is less sensitive than assays for serum-specific IgE (Butcher et al, 1993; Gallagher et al, 1981). Diisocyanates have also been demonstrated to cause RADS and hypersensitivity pneumonitis syndromes (Gallagher et al, 1981; Luo et al, 1990).

Acid anhydrides are a group of reactive organic compounds that are constituents of alkyl and epoxy resins (Venables, 1989). These chemicals are found in paints, varnishes, and plastics. TMA has been useful as a plasticizer in the production of wire and cable coatings and has wide applications in the manufacturing of other products such as paints, textiles, and paper goods (Venables, 1989). Acid anhydrides cause a variety of clinical reactions in which several immunologic mechanisms have been implicated (Venables, 1989). Many of the acid anhydride compounds have been associated with a type I IgE-mediated mechanism for inducing OA. These include phthalic (PA), trimellitic (TMA), hexahydrophthalic (HHPA), himic (HA), and tetrachlorophthalic (TCPA) anhydrides. In some workers anhydrides have been associated with causing a syndrome characterized by anemia with pulmonary hemmorhage, presumably on the basis of a type II cytotoxic immune response. The late respiratory systemic syndrome (LRSS), which resembles some of the clinical symptoms of hypersensitivity pneumonitis, has been postulated to be a type III immune complex response (Leach et al, 1987; Zeiss et al, 1987). This syndrome begins 4 to 12 hours after TMA exposure and is associated with a nonproductive cough and systemic symptoms including fever, chills, arthralgias, and myalgias (Zeiss et al, 1987). Because workers exposed to acid anhydrides frequently produce IgE antibodies to either haptenic determinants (acid anhydrides) or new antigenic determinants formed by conjugation of the chemical to a protein carrier, *in vitro* assays such as the radioallergosorbent test (RAST) and enzyme-linked immunosorbent assay (ELISA), in conjunction with skin testing to acid anhydride conjugates, have served as sensitive markers of exposure and development of OA (Zeiss et al, 1990).

Wood dusts are responsible for a variety of occupation-related lung disorders including hypersensitivity pneumonitis, organic dust syndrome, asthma, chronic bronchitis, and a mucous membrane irritation syndrome (Chan-Yeung et al, 1973; Enarson and Chan-Yeung, 1990). Disorders related to western red cedar wood dust (*Thuja plicata*) have been the most extensively studied (Chan-Yeung et al, 1973). Longitudinal studies of workers exposed to western red cedar dust have found that approximately 5 percent develop OA (Chan-Yeung et al, 1987). Western red cedar wood dust contains a variety of chemicals including tannin, dyes, pitch, resins, and gums (Chan-Yeung et al, 1973). These chemicals are extracted by steam distillation from the cedar wood to form volatile and nonvolatile components (Chan-Yeung et al, 1973). The volatile components contain a variety of agents such as tropolones and natural fungicides, which protect the wood from decay. Nonvolatile residues consist primarily of plicatic acid, which is the organic component responsible for red cedar OA (Chan-Yeung et al, 1973). In these workers, preexisting atopy and nonspecific bronchial hyperresponsiveness have not been found to be risk factors for developing OA. As alluded to earlier, nonsmokers or ex-smokers have demonstrated a greater propensity for developing red cedar OA compared to active smokers (Chan-Yeung et al, 1987). Specific inhalation tests to plicatic acid typically reveal dual asthmatic responses or an isolated LAR (Chan-Yeung et al, 1987). Since immediate skin testing and serum IgE antibodies are not diagnostically useful, specific bronchial challenge with plicatic acid is often necessary to confirm a diagnosis of OA (Paggiaro and Chan-Yeung, 1987). Several other wood dusts that have been recognized as causes of OA include African maplewood and zebrawood, mahogany, and *Quillaja* bark (Chan-Yeung, 1993).

Microbial contaminants of wood dusts have been identified as causes of hypersensitivity pneumonitis disorders including maple bark disease, sequoiosis, suberosis, and wood pulp worker's disease. These diseases are caused by immunologic responses to a variety of fungi including *Cryptostroma corticale* (maple bark disease), *Alternaria* species (wood pulp worker's disease), *Aspergillus* species, and *Thermoactinomyces vulgaris* (sawmill workers disease), which contaminate the wood dust or bark of the tree (Chan-Yeung, 1993). Wood dusts have also been implicated in causing other nonrespiratory symptoms including allergic conjunctivitis, rhinitis, dermatitis, and adenocarcinoma of the nasal pharynx (Chan-Yeung, 1993).

Metallic salts cause a variety of pulmonary reactions in addition to OA including chemical pneumonitis, bronchitis, pulmonary emphysema, and adult respiratory distress syndrome (ARDS) (Nemery, 1990). Metallic salts cause respiratory diseases through immunologic and nonimmunologic mechanisms (Bernstein IL, et al, 1993). The metallic salts that have been most extensively studied include platinum, nickel, chromium, and cobalt salts (Bernstein IL, et al, 1993). Platinum salts are highly allergenic and have a high prevalence of skin sensitization compared to other metallic salts (Brooks et al, 1990). Although platinum salt cutaneous reactivity is present more frequently in those workers with rhinitis and asthma, it is not itself a predictor of OA (Biagini et al, 1985). Cigarette smoking has been implicated as a significant risk factor for cutaneous sensitization to platinum (Biagini et al, 1985). The immunopathogenesis of platinum salt–induced OA has been demonstrated to be primarily IgE mediated. Platinum-HSA–specific reaginic IgG_4 antibody has also been reported (Biagini et al, 1985). Although nickel is widely used in mining, milling, smelting, and refinishing processes and can be extremely toxic to the central nervous system, nickel-induced OA is very rare (Bernstein IL, et al, 1993). Nickel-specific IgE antibodies have been found in a few individual case reports (Bernstein IL, et al, 1993; Malo et al, 1982). Chromium is used in electroplating processes, in leather tanning, and in the production of cement (Burrows, 1984). Exposure to hexavalent chromium salts has been associated with OA (Moller et al, 1986a). Both IgE specific antibody and cell-mediated immune responses are thought to be involved in the pathogenesis of asthma (Burrows, 1984; Moller et al, 1986a). Cobalt salts are responsible for inducing OA in approximately 5 percent of exposed workers and should be distinguished from hard metal diseases, which can result in interstitial pneumonia and pulmonary fibrosis (Gheysens et al, 1985; Shirakawa et al, 1989). Workers who are exposed to cobalt and subsequently develop OA have been documented to produce specific IgE antibodies (Shirakawa et al, 1988). Exposure to a variety of other metals—including vanadium pentoxide, zinc oxide, cadmium, and aluminum (potroom asthma)—has been associated with respiratory diseases (Bernstein IL, et al, 1993). Individuals with metal fume fever and potroom asthma both may present with shortness of breath, wheezing, and chest tightness with coughing, which occurs hours after exposure (Bernstein IL, et al, 1993). Symptoms of metal fume fever usually subside 1 to 2 days after removal from the workplace, whereas potroom asthma may persist long after removal from exposure (Bernstein IL, et al, 1993).

Exposure to colophony fumes may cause OA in electronic soldering workers (Burge, 1982a; 1982b). Colophony is derived from pine tree resin and contains abietic, pumaric, and dihydroabietic acids, which are believed to be the causative compounds responsible for OA (Burge, 1982a; 1982b). Atopic workers with preexisting asthma are at an increased risk for developing OA due to colophony fumes (Burge, 1982a; 1982b). Because immune mechanisms have not been demonstrated, confirmation of OA may depend on specific inhalational challenges or serial PEFR studies performed at work. Persistence of BHR and asthma symptoms is common among affected workers once they have been removed from the workplace (Burge, 1982a; 1982b).

Finally, a number of other LMW chemicals have been identified or suspected as causes of OA. These include: primary, secondary, tertiary, and quaternary amines (Belin et al, 1983; Bernstein JA et al, 1994); formaldehyde; sulfone chloramide (chloramine T); azo dyes; persulfates; diazonium salts; and a variety of pharmaceutical agents (i.e., β-lactam, macrolide and tetracycline antibiotics, hydralazine, isoniazid, penicillamine, and methyldopa) (Malo and Bernstein, 1993; Cooper et al, 1986a; 1986b). In addition, pyrolysis fumes of polyvinyl chloride (PVC) have been associated with meat wrapper's asthma (Brooks et al, 1977; Pauli et al, 1980; Vandervort et al, 1977). Other chemicals that have been incriminated with OA, but for which immune mechanisms have not been defined, include methyl methacrylates, Freon, hexachlorophene, furan, styrene, machining fluid, and noxious fumes from concentrated acids (Malo and Bernstein, 1993).

TREATMENT

Once the diagnosis of OA has been confirmed, treatment should be directed toward removing the worker from further potentially harmful exposure (Reports of the Working Groups, 1990). Studies evaluating the clinical course of workers after removal from exposure have found that the persistence of asthma after leaving work is directly related to the duration of symptoms prior to diagnosis (Bernstein DI, 1992). Individuals who are diagnosed earlier in the course of their disease, have relatively normal lung function, and have a lesser degree of airway hyperresponsiveness at initial diagnosis are more likely to have a remission after removal from the workplace (Reports of the Working Groups, 1990). Individuals with red cedar asthma who remained in the workplace with continuous exposure to the offending agent were stable on medication only 50 percent of the time, whereas the remainder experienced deterioration of their lung function with a significant increase in symptoms and medication requirements (Bernstein DI, 1993). The pharmacologic treatment of acute or chronic OA is similar to the treatment of non-OA which may include β_2 selective agonists, theophylline, cromolyn sodium, and inhaled and systemic corticosteroids in various combinations, depending on the severity of the worker's symptoms (Bernstein DI, 1992). Pharmacotherapy should not be considered a suitable alternative to elimination of exposure. An initial successful response to medications, which could prolong exposure to harmful agents, may have a deleterious long-term result. Immunotherapy has been successful in treating laboratory animal workers with the offending allergen(s) and in shellfish handlers with sea squirt asthma (Armentia et al, 1992; Bernstein DI, 1992).

PREVENTION

The prevention of OA depends on the future cooperation between management and labor to organize comprehensive immunosurveillance programs for detecting and monitoring workers at increased risk for exposure to known inducers of OA (Venables, 1992). When appropriate, employees should be screened for risk factors that place them at greater risk for certain jobs (e.g., atopy in enzyme workers). Every attempt should be made to minimize a worker's exposure to potentially causative agent(s) by implementing good industrial hygiene (Venables, 1992). Information about the level of exposure necessary to initiate or perpetuate sensitization is not available for most allergens (Reed et al, 1992). For reactive chemicals such as diisocyanates, the levels eliciting sensitization range between 1 and 30 ng/m^3 (Reed et al, 1992). Most protein allergens are also believed to fall in this same range. Exposure can be minimized by careful handling procedures of toxic chemicals to avoid accidents such as large chemical spills. Workers should be continually educated about the importance of adhering to these procedures (Venables, 1992). Exposure may also be minimized by upgrading of the ventilation and filtration systems in the work area. In the appropriate setting, special air-fed body suits can substantially reduce a worker's exposure to potentially sensitizing agents (Bernstein JA et al, 1993). Use of respirators in the work environment generally does not reduce exposure or prevent clinical deterioration (Bernstein DI, et al, 1993). Some studies have suggested that certain types of respirators, such as well-fitting airstream helmets, may offer adequate protection for the worker from the offending agent. However, barrier protective devices are not considered better than absolute avoidance measures (Bernstein DI, et al, 1993). Encapsulation of enzymes has been one example where it has been possible to modify a product in order to reduce the worker's risk for sensitization. Encapsulation of enzymes in conjunction with improved efficient dust removal has significantly reduced the incidence of enzyme-induced OA (Liss et al, 1984). Longitudinal studies have already demonstrated that implementation of comprehensive immunosurveillance programs in the workplace can significantly reduce the incidence of OA (Bernstein DI, et al, 1993).

CONCLUSIONS

The incidence of OA may be increasing as modern industry introduces new processes into the work environment and the utilization of potentially asthmagenic compounds. Medical surveillance programs should be instituted to identify workers at risk for developing OA early in the course of the disease. Timely removal from the workplace within months after the onset of symptoms may prevent disability associated with chronic asthma. The diagnosis of OA requires a standardized, stepwise approach, which includes a thorough history and physical examination, objective measurements of lung function in the workplace, and immunologic testing when appropriate. Prospective studies of large populations of exposed workers will enhance our understanding of the natural course and pathogenesis of OA. Environmental monitoring studies of work environments are necessary to establish safe ambient levels of exposure, which could minimize or prevent development of OA due to reactive chemicals or HMW allergens.

REFERENCES

Armentia A, Arranz M, Martin JM, et al. Evaluation of immune complexes after immunotherapy with wheat flour in baker's asthma. Ann Allergy 69(5):441, 1992.

Barnes PJ, Baraniuk JN, Belvisi MG. Neuropeptides in the respiratory tract. Part II. Am Rev Respir Dis 144:1187, 1991a.

Barnes PJ, Baraniuk JN, Belvisi MG. Neuropeptides in the respiratory tract. Part II. Am Rev Respir Dis 144:1391, 1991b.

Baur X. Immunologic cross-reactivity between different albumin-bound isocyanates. J Allergy Clin Immunol 71:197, 1983.

Baur X, Fruhmann G, Haug B, et al. Role of aspergillus amylase in baker's asthma. Lancet 1:43, 1986.

Beasley R, Roce WR, Roberts JA, et al. Cellular events in the bronchi in mild asthma and after bronchial provocation. Am Rev Respir Dis 139:806, 1989.

Becklake MR. Epidemiology: Prevalence and determinants. In Bernstein IL, Chan-Yeung M, Malo JL (eds). Asthma in the Workplace. New York, Marcel Dekker, 1992, p 29.

Belin L, Wass U, Audnusson G, et al. Amines: Possible causative agents in the development of bronchial hyperreactivity in workers manufacturing polyurethanes from isocyanates. Br J Ind Med 40:251, 1983.

Bentley AM, Maestrelli P, Saetta M, et al. Activated lymphocytes-T and eosinophils in the bronchial mucosa in isocyanate-induced asthma. J Allergy Clin Immunol 89:821, 1992.

Bernstein DI. Occupational asthma. Clin Allergy 76:917, 1992.

Bernstein DI. Clinical assessment and management of occupational asthma. In Bernstein IL, Chan-Yeung M, Malo JL (eds). Asthma in the Workplace. New York, Marcel Dekker, 1993, p 103.

Bernstein DI, Bernstein IL: Occupational asthma. In Middleton E, Reed CE, Ellis EF (eds). Allergy: Principles and Practice. 4th ed. St. Louis, Mosby–Year Book, 1993, p 1369.

Bernstein DI, Gallagher JS, Bernstein IL. Meal worm asthma: Clinical and immunologic studies. A new occupational disease. J Allergy Clin Immunol 72:475, 1983.

Bernstein DI, Gallagher JS, D'Souza L, et al. Heterogeneity of specific-IgE responses in workers sensitized to acid anhydride compounds. J Allergy Clin Immunol 74:794, 1984.

Bernstein DI, Korbee L, Stauder T, et al. The low prevalence of occupational asthma and antibody-dependent sensitization to diphenylmethane diisocyanate (MDI) in a plant engineered for minimal exposure to diisocyanates. J Allergy Clin Immunol 92:387, 1993.

Bernstein DI, Smith AB, Moller DR, et al. Clinical and immunologic studies among egg-processing workers with occupational asthma. J Allergy Clin Immunol 80:791, 1987.

Bernstein DI, Malo JL. High-molecular-weight agents. In Bernstein IL, Chan-Yeung M, Malo JL (eds). Asthma in the Workplace. New York, Marcel Dekker, 1993, p 373.

Bernstein IL. Isocyanate-induced pulmonary diseases: A current perspective. J Allergy Clin Immunol 70:24, 1982.

Bernstein IL. Pulmonary hypersensitivity disorders. In Newcombe DS, Rose NR, Blood JC (eds). Pulmonary Hypersensitivity Disorders. New York, Raven Press, 1992, p 191.

Bernstein IL, Brooks SM. Metals. In Bernstein IL, Chan-Yeung M, Malo JL (eds). Asthma in the Workplace. New York, Marcel Dekker, 1993, p 459.

Bernstein IL, Chan-Yeung M, Bernstein DI. Definition and classification of asthma. In Bernstein IL, Chan-Yeung M, Malo JL (eds). Asthma in the Workplace. New York, Marcel Dekker, 1993, p 1.

Bernstein JA. Occupational asthma. "My job is making me sick." Postgrad Med 92:109, 1992.

Bernstein JA, Kraut A, Bernstein DI, et al. Occupational asthma induced by inhaled egg lysozyme. Chest 103:532, 1993.

Bernstein JA, Stauder T, Bernstein DI, et al. A combined respiratory and cutaneous hypersensitivity syndrome induced by work exposure to quaternary amines. J Allergy Clin Immunol 94:257, 1994.

Biagini RE, Bernstein IL, Gallagher JS, et al. The diversity of reaginic immune responses to platinum and palladium metallic salts. J Allergy Clin Immunol 76:794, 1985.

Biagini RE, Klincewicz SL, Henningsen GM, et al. Antibodies to morphine in workers exposed to opiates at a narcotic manufacturing facility and evidence for similar antibodies to heroin abusers. Life Sci 47:897, 1990.

Boulet LP. Increases in airway hyperresponsiveness following acute exposure to respiratory irritants. Reactive airways dysfunction syndrome or occupational asthma. Chest 94:47, 1988.

Brooks SM, Baker DB, Gann PH, et al. Cold air challenge and platinum skin reactivity in platinum refinery workers. Chest 97:1401, 1990.

Brooks SM, Bernstein IL. Reactive airways dysfunction syndrome or irritant-induced asthma. In Bernstein IL, Chan-Yeung M, Malo JL (eds). Asthma in the Workplace. New York, Marcel Dekker, 1993, p 533.

Brooks SM, Vandervort R. Polyvinyl chloride film thermal decomposition products as an occupational illness. 2. Clinical studies. J Occ Med 19:192, 1977.

Buch MG, Bonhuys A. Airway constriction response to cotton bract. Lung 150:25, 1980.

Burge PS. Occupational asthma due to soft soldering fluxes containing colophony (rosin, pine, resin). Eur J Respir Dis 63:65, 1982a.

Burge PS. Occupational asthma in electronics workers caused by colophony fumes: Follow-up of affected workers. Thorax 37:348, 1982b.

Burge PS, Perks WH, O'Brien IM, et al. Occupational asthma in an electronics factory: A case control study to evaluate etiological factors. Thorax 34:300, 1979.

Burrows D. The dichromate problem. Int J Dermatology 23:215, 1984.

Bush RK. Occupational asthma from vegetable gums. J Allergy Clin Immunol 86:443, 1990.

Butcher BT, Mapp CE, Fabbri LM. Polyisocyanates and their prepolymers. In Bernstein IL, Chan-Yeung M, Malo JL (eds). Asthma in the Workplace. New York, Marcel Dekker, 1993, p 415.

Cartier A, Grammer L, Malo JL, et al. Specific serum antibodies against isocyanates. J Allergy Clin Immunol 84:507, 1989.

Cartier A, Malo JL. Occupational challenge tests. In Bernstein IL, Chan-Yeung M, Malo JL (eds). Asthma in the Workplace. New York, Marcel Dekker, 1993, p 215.

Chan-Yeung M. Immunologic and nonimmunologic mechanisms in asthma due to western red cedar (Thuja plicata). J Allergy Clin Immunol 70:32, 1982.

Chan-Yeung M. Western red cedar and other wood dusts. *In* Bernstein IL, Chan-Yeung M, Malo JL (eds). Asthma in the Workplace. New York, Marcel Dekker, 1993, p 503.

Chan-Yeung M, Barton G, MacLean L, et al. Occupational asthma and rhinitis due to western red cedar (*Thuja plicata*). Am Rev Respir Dis 108:1094, 1973.

Chan-Yeung M, Chan H, Tse KS, et al. Histamine and leukotriene release in bronchoalveolar lavage fluid during plicatic acid induced bronchoconstriction. J Allergy Clin Immunol 84:762, 1989.

Chan-Yeung M, Kennedy S, Enarson D. Grain dust–induced lung diseases. *In* Bernstein IL, Chan-Yeung M, Malo JL (eds). Asthma in the Workplace. New York, Marcel Dekker, 1993, p 577.

Chan-Yeung M, Lam S, Koerner S. Clinical features and natural history of occupational asthma due to western red cedar, *Thuja plicata*. Am Rev Respir Dis 72:411, 1982.

Chan-Yeung M, Leriche J, MacLean L, et al. Comparison of cellular and protein changes in bronchial lavage fluid of symptomatic and asymptomatic patients with red cedar asthma on follow-up examination. Clin Allergy 18:359, 1988.

Chan-Yeung M, MacLean L, Paggiaro PL. Follow-up study of 232 patients with occupational asthma caused by western red cedar (*Thuja plicata*). J Allergy Clin Immunol 79:792, 1987.

Cooper JAD Jr, White DA, Matthay RA. Drug-induced pulmonary disease. Part 1: Cytotoxic drugs. Am Rev Respir Dis 133:321, 1986a.

Cooper JAD Jr, White DA, Matthay RA. Drug-induced pulmonary disease. Part 2: Noncytotoxic drugs. Am Rev Respir Dis 133:488, 1986b.

Cote J, Kennedy S, Chan-Yeung M. Sensitivity and specificity of PC_{20} and peak expiratory flow rate in cedar asthma. J Allergy Clin Immunol 14:592, 1990.

Dearman RJ, Kimber I. Differential stimulation of immune function by respiratory and contact chemical allergens. Immunology 72:563, 1991.

Dearman RJ, Kimber I. Divergent immune responses to respiratory and contact chemical allergens: Antibody elicited by phthalic anhydride and oxazolone. Clin Exp Allergy 22:241, 1992.

DeMonchy GR, Kauffman HF, Venge P, et al. Bronchoalveolar eosinophils following allergen-induced late-phase asthmatic reactions. Am Rev Respir Dis 131:373, 1985.

Durham SR, Graneck BJ, Hawkins R, et al. The temporal relationship between increases in airway responsiveness to histamine and late asthmatic responses induced by occupational agents. J Allergy Clin Immunol 79:398, 1987.

Edwards JH, McComchie K, Trotman DM, et al. Allergy to inhaled egg material. Clin Allergy 13:427, 1983.

Enarson DA, Chan-Yeung M. Characterization of health effects of wood dust exposures. Am J Ind Med 17:33, 1990.

Fabbri LM, Ciaccia A. Pathophysiology of occupational asthma. *In* Bernstein IL, Chan-Yeung M, Malo JL (eds). Asthma in the Workplace. New York, Marcel Dekker, 1993, p 61.

Finotto S, Fabbri LM, Rado V, et al. Increase in numbers of CD8+ lymphocytes and eosinophils in peripheral blood of subjects with late asthmatic reactions induced by toluene diisocyanate. Br J Ind Med 48:116, 1991.

Fowler PBS. Printer's asthma. Lancet 2:755, 1952.

Franz T, McMurrain KD, Brooks S, et al. Clinical, immunologic and physiologic observations in factory workers exposed to *B. subtilis* enzyme dust. J Allergy 47:170, 1971.

Gallagher JS, Tse CST, Brooks SM, et al. Diverse profiles of immunoreactivity in toluene diisocyanate (TDI) asthma. J Occ Med 23:610, 1981.

Gannon PFG, Burge PS. A preliminary report of a surveillance scheme of occupational asthma in the West Midlands. Br J Ind Med 48:579, 1991.

Gheysens B, Auwerx J, Van den Eeckkhout A, et al. Cobalt-induced bronchial asthma in diamond polishers. Chest 88:740, 1985.

Grammer LC, Eggum P, Silverstein M, et al. Prospective immunologic and clinical study of a population exposed to hexamethylene diisocyanate. J Allergy Clin Immunol 82:627, 1988.

Herzog CH, Villiger B, Braun P. Nickel-specific T cell clones in asthma—preferential use of V-beta 14 in T cell receptor beta chain. Eur Respir J 4:4255, 1991.

Kennedy AL, Brown WE. Isocyanates and lung disease: Experimental approaches to molecular mechanisms. Occ Med 7:301, 1992.

Kusaka Y, Nakona Y, Shirakawa T, et al. Lymphocyte transformation with cobalt in hard metal asthma. Ind Health 27:155, 1989.

Lagier F, Cartier A, Somer J, et al. Occupational asthma caused by guar gum. J Allergy Clin Immunol 85:785, 1990.

Lam S, Chan-Yeung M. Ethylenediamine-induced asthma. Am Rev Respir Dis 121:151, 1980.

Lam S, Wong R, Chan-Yeung M. Nonspecific bronchial reactivity in occupational asthma. J Allergy Clin Immunol 63:28, 1979.

Leach CL, Hatoum NS, Ratjczak HV, et al. The pathologic and immunologic response to inhaled trimellitic anhydride in rats. Toxicol Appl Pharmacol 87:67, 1987.

Liss GM, Bernstein DI, Genesove L, et al. Assessment of risk factors for IgE mediated sensitization to tetrachlorophthalic anhydride. J Allergy Clin Immunol 92:237–247, 1993.

Liss GM, Bernstein DI, Moller DR, et al. Pulmonary and immunologic evaluation of foundry workers exposed to methylene diphenyldiisocyanate (MDI). J Allergy Clin Immunol 85:1076, 1990.

Liss GM, Kominsky JR, Gallagher JS, et al. Failure of enzyme encapsulation to prevent sensitization of workers in the dry bleach industry. J Allergy Clin Immunol 73:348, 1984.

Luo JD, Nelsen KG, Fischbein A. Persistent reactive airway dysfunction syndrome after exposure to toluene diisocyanate. Br J Ind Med 47:239, 1990.

Lushniak BD, Reh CM, Gallagher JS, et al. Indirect assessment of exposure to MDI by evaluation of specific immune responses to MDI-HSA in foam workers. J Allergy Clin Immunol 85:251, 1990.

Maccia CA, Bernstein IL, Emmett EA, et al. In vitro demonstration of specific IgE in phthalic anhydride hypersensitivity. Am Rev Respir Dis 113:701, 1976.

Malo JL, Bernstein IL. Other chemical substances causing occupational asthma. *In* Bernstein IL, Chan-Yeung M, Malo JL (eds). Asthma in the Workplace. New York, Marcel Dekker, 1993, p 481.

Malo JL, Cartier A, L'Archeveque J, et al. Prevalence of occupational asthma and immunological sensitization to guar gum among employees at a carpet manufacturing plant. J Allergy Clin Immunol 86:562, 1990.

Malo JL, Cartier A, Doepner M, et al. Occupational asthma caused by nickel sulfate. J Allergy Clin Immunol 69:55, 1982.

Malo JL, Ghezzo H, L'Archeveque J, et al. Is the clinical history a satisfactory means for diagnosing occupational asthma? Am Rev Respir Dis 143:528, 1991.

Mapp CE, Boschetto P, Dal Vecchio, et al. Occupational asthma due to isocyanate. Eur Resp J 1:273, 1988.

Matthews KP. Inhalant insect-derived allergens. Immunol Allergy Clin North Am 2:2, 1989.

Merchant JA, Bernstein IL. Cotton and other textile dusts. In Bernstein IL, Chan-Yeung M, Malo JL (eds). Asthma in the Workplace. New York, Marcel Dekker, 1992, p 551.

Meredith SK, Taylor VM, McDonald JC. Occupational respiratory disease in the United Kingdom 1989: A report to the British Thoracic Society and the Society of Occupational Medicine by the SWORD project group. Br J Ind Med 48:292, 1991.

Mitchell CA, Gandevia B. Respiratory symptoms and skin sensitivity in workers exposed to proteolytic enzyme in detergent industry. Am Rev Respir Dis 104:1, 1971.

Moller DR, Brooks SM, Bernstein DI, et al. Delayed anaphylactoid reaction in a worker exposed to chromium. J Allergy Clin Immunol 77:451, 1986a.

Moller DR, McKay RT, Bernstein IL, et al. Persistent airways disease caused by toluene diisocyanate. Am Rev Respir Dis 134:175, 1986b.

Mosmann TR, Coffman RL. Heterogeneity of cytokine secretion patterns and functions of helper T cells. Adv Immunol 46:111, 1989.

Mosmann TR, Schumacher JH, Street NF, et al. Diversity of cytokine synthesis and function of mouse CD4+ T cells. Immunol Rev 123:209, 1991.

Musk AW, Venables KM, Crook B, et al. Respiratory symptoms, lung function and sensitization to flour in a British bakery. Br J Ind Med 46:636, 1989.

Nemery B. Metal toxicity and the respiratory tract. Eur Respir J 3:202, 1990.

Nielsen J, Welinger H, Schutz A, et al. Specific serum antibodies against phthalic anhydride in occupationally exposed subjects. J Allergy Clin Immunol 82:126, 1988.

Paggiaro PL, Chan-Yeung M. Pattern of specific airway response in asthma due to western red cedar (*Thuja plicata*): Relationship with length of exposure and lung function measurements. Clin Allergy 17:333, 1987.

Patterson R, Zeiss CR, Pruzansky JJ. Immunology and immunopathology of trimellitic anhydride pulmonary reactions. J Allergy Clin Immunol 70:19, 1982.

Pauli G, Bessot JC, Kopferschitt MC, et al. Meat wrapper's asthma: Identification of the causal agent. Clin Allergy 10:263, 1980.

Pepys J. Inhalation challenge tests in asthma. N Engl J Med 293:758, 1975.

Pepys J, Longbottom JL, Hargreave FE, et al. Allergic reactions of the lungs to enzymes of *Bacillus subtilis*. Lancet 1:1811, 1969.

Perrin B, Dhivert H, Godard P, et al. The telematic information service (MINITEL) on occupational asthma in France. In Bernstein IL, Chan-Yeung M, Malo JL (eds). Asthma in the Workplace. New York, Marcel Dekker, 1993, p 635.

Quirce S, Cuevas M, Diez-Gomez M, et al. Respiratory allergy to Aspergillus-derived enzymes in baker's asthma. J Allergy Clin Immunol 90:970, 1992.

Reports of the Working Groups. Workshop on Environmental and Occupational Asthma. Chest 96:240S, 1990.

Reed CE, Swanson MC, Li JTC. Environmental monitoring of protein aeroallergens. In Bernstein IL, Chan-Yeung M, Malo JL (eds). Asthma in the Workplace. New York, Marcel Dekker, 1992, p 249.

Roche WR, Beasley R, Williams JH, et al. Subepithelial fibrosis in the bronchi of asthmatics. Lancet 1:520, 1989.

Saetta M, Di Stefano A, Maestrelli P, et al. Airway mucosal inflammation in occupational asthma induced by toluene diisocyanate. Am Rev Respir Dis 145:160, 1992a.

Saetta M, Maestrelli P, De Stefano A, et al. Effect of cessation of exposure to toluene diisocyanate (TDI) on bronchial mucosa of subjects with TDI-induced asthma. Am Rev Respir Dis 145:169, 1992b.

Sarlo K, Clark ED, Ryan CA, et al. ELISA for human IgE antibody to subtilisin. A (Alcalase): Correlation with RAST and skin test results with occupationally exposed individuals. J Allergy Clin Immunol 83:393, 1990.

Seta JA, Young RO. The United States National Occupational Exposure Survey (NOES) Data Base. In Bernstein IL, Chan-Yeung M, Malo JL (eds). Asthma in the Workplace. New York, Marcel Dekker, 1993, p 627.

Sheppard D. Airway hyperresponsiveness mechanisms in experimental models. Chest 96:2265, 1989.

Sheppard D, Thompson JE, Scypinski L, et al. Toluene diisocyanate increases airway responsiveness to substance P and decreases airway neutral endopeptidase. J Clin Invest 81:1111, 1988.

Shirakawa T, Kusaka Y, Fukimura N, et al. Occupational asthma from cobalt sensitivity in workers exposed to hard metal dust. Chest 95:29, 1989.

Shirakawa T, Kusaka Y, Fujimura N, et al. The existence of specific antibodies to cobalt in hard metal asthma. Clin Allergy 18:451, 1988.

Slovak AMJ, Hill RN. Laboratory animal allergy: A clinical survey of an exposed population. Br J Ind Med 38:38, 1981.

Smith AB, Bernstein DI, Tar-Ching AW, et al. Occupational asthma from inhaled egg protein. Am J Ind Med 12:205, 1987.

Smith AB, Castellan RM, Lewis D, et al. Guidelines for the epidemiologic assessment of occupational asthma. J Allergy Clin Immunol 94:794, 1989.

Solway P, Fish S, Passmore H, et al. Regulation of the immune response to peptide antigens: Differential induction of immediate-type hypersensitivity and T cell proliferation due to changes in either peptide structure or major histocompatibility complex haplotype. J Exp Med 174:847, 1991.

Steinberg DR, Bernstein DI, Bernstein IL, et al. Bronchial reactivity increases early in both immediate and dual phase responders to allergen. J Allergy Clin Immunol 79:249, 1987.

Tarlo SM, Wong L, Roos J, et al. Occupational asthma caused by latex in a surgical glove manufacturing plant. J Allergy Clin Immunol 85:626, 1990.

Thiel H, Ulmer WT. Baker's asthma: Development and possibility for treatment. Chest 78:400, 1980.

Thompson JE, Scypinsky LA, Gorton T, et al. Tachykinins mediate the acute increase in airway responsiveness caused by toluene diisocyanate in guinea pigs. Am Rev Respir Dis 136:43, 1987.

Vandervort R, Brooks SM. Polyvinyl chloride film thermal decomposition products as an occupational illness. 1. Environmental and experimental toxicology. J Occ Med 10:263, 1977.

Venables K. Low-molecular-weight chemicals, hypersensitivity and direct toxicity: The acid anhydrides. Br J Ind Med 46:222, 1989.

Venables KM. Preventing occupational asthma. Br J Ind Med 49:817, 1992.

Venables KM, Topping MD, Howe W, et al. Interaction of smoking and atopy in producing specific IgE antibody against a hapten protein conjugate. Br Med J 290:201, 1985.

Wagner CD, Gundel RH, Reilly P, et al. Intercellular adhesion molecule-1 (ICAM-1) in the pathogenesis of asthma. Science 247:456, 1990.

Zeiss CR, Mitchell JH, Van Peenen PFD, et al. A twelve-year clinical and immunologic evaluation of workers involved in the manufacture of trimellitic anhydride (TMA). Allergy Proc 11:71, 1990.

Zeiss CR, Patterson R, Pruzansky JJ, et al. Trimellitic anhydride-induced airway syndromes: Clinical and immunologic studies. J Allergy Clin Immunol 60:96, 1987.

Zeiss CR, Wolkonsky P, Pruzansky JJ, et al. Clinical and immunologic evaluation of trimellitic anhydride workers in multiple industrial settings. J Allergy Clin Immunol 70:15, 1982.

Zocca E, Fabbri LM, Boschetto P, et al. Leukotriene B4 and late asthmatic reactions induced by toluene diisocyanate. J Appl Physiol 68:1576, 1990.

Chapter 38

Drug-Induced Asthma

Ronald A. Simon, M.D., and James L. Baldwin, M.D.

Asthma can be provoked and aggravated by a number of pharmacologic agents. It has been estimated that up to 10 percent of acute asthmatic episodes may, in fact, be drug-induced. Certainly any IgE-mediated drug reaction can result in asthma in the susceptible individual; however, there are several agents that have been implicated in drug-induced asthma via non–IgE-mediated mechanisms. In many cases the mechanisms involved are poorly understood. This chapter will review the most common agents implicated in drug-induced asthma and discuss, where possible, the mechanisms involved, prevention, and treatment strategies.

ASPIRIN (ASA) AND OTHER NONSTEROIDAL ANTI-INFLAMMATORY DRUGS (NSAIDs)

ASA and other NSAIDs are capable of evoking several adverse effects including gastrointestinal irritation, nephropathy, hepatitis, erythema multiforme, Stevens-Johnson syndrome, salicylism, and a variety of hematologic abnormalities. However, these drugs can also be responsible for four types of idiosyncratic adverse effects: urticaria and angioedema, anaphylaxis, selective NSAID-induced hypersensitivity pneumonitis, and rhinosinusitis and asthma. Only the ASA/NSAID-sensitive rhinosinusitis and asthma will be discussed below.

Presentation and Clinical Features

ASA-sensitive rhinosinusitis and asthma typically present during adulthood, often following an upper respiratory tract illness that resembles a typical viral infection, but persists and evolves into a chronic eosinophilic rhinosinusitis, often with nasal polyps and pansinusitis. Nasal cytology reveals eosinophils in over 90 percent of cases and metachromatic cells in over 50 percent. Cutaneous tests for common allergens are positive in up to 50 percent, though in less than 25 percent do these appear to clinically account for the respiratory disease. Occasionally, only the upper respiratory tract is involved, but more commonly lower respiratory tract inflammation and asthma are also present. This "intrinsic" asthma is often progressive and severe, requiring chronic corticosteroid therapy in order to maintain adequate respiratory function. Although a triad of rhinitis with nasal polyps, asthma, and ASA sensitivity was first described, a quartet of symptoms is more common: rhinitis with or without nasal polyps, sinusitis, asthma, and ASA sensitivity. The ASA/NSAID sensitivity is first suspected by the patient, usually with the appearance of facial or generalized flushing, nasal and ocular congestion and watering, and an acute severe bronchospastic episode 20 minutes to 3 hours following a usual dose of one of these agents. β-adrenergic agonists, subcutaneous epinephrine, oxygen, aminophylline, corticosteroids, and even intubation with mechanical ventilation may be required as dictated by the severity of such an episode.

Prevalence

The reported prevalence of ASA/NSAID-sensitive asthma varies, depending on the study design and population in question. Historical studies in general underestimate ASA/NSAID sensitivity as many asthmatics with the disease may not have associated asthma exacerbations with ASA/NSAIDs. Furthermore, more widespread awareness of this condition and its potential severity has prompted many physicians to recommend avoidance of ASA/NSAIDs uniformly to their asthmatic patients. Since this will not prevent the sensitivity from developing, but only an acute episode from occurring, as the population of asthmatics avoiding ASA/NSAIDs increases, so do the numbers of unrecognized ASA/NSAID-sensitive asthmatics. The prevalence is estimated to be approximately 10 percent in adult asthmatic populations and considerably less in childhood asthmatic populations. In asthmatics without previous history of ASA sensitivity but with rhinosinusitis and nasal polyps, the prevalence of ASA sensitivity increases to 30 percent as confirmed by oral challenge. In fact, the presence of normal sinus roentgenograms (Waters view) essentially rules out ASA sensitivity. Should this same population also give a history of ASA-induced bronchospasm, the prevalence rises to 66 percent or more, although certainly not 100 percent.

Diagnosis

The diagnosis of ASA-induced asthma is based on history, physical examination, and ASA challenge results. Currently, no *in vitro* diagnostic method exists. Challenge may be either by the oral or by the inhalational route. Although inhalation challenge with lysine-ASA has been used for diagnosis of ASA-induced asthma in other countries, this agent is not approved in this country. Consequently, ingestion challenge is the standard technique used in the United States. The details of oral challenge are outlined in Chapter 14. It should be stressed that the standard protocols involving challenge with increasing doses of ASA are capable of provoking severe bronchospasm. Consequently, these procedures should only be attempted by experienced physicians in an area close to an intensive care unit, with emergency personnel capable of intubation and initiation of mechanical ventilation readily available.

Cross-Sensitivities

Several cross-sensitivities in ASA-sensitive asthmatics have been proposed. There is significant cross-sensitivity among cyclooxygenase inhibitors (Table 38–1) in ASA-sensitive asthmatics. Virtually all NSAIDs that inhibit cyclooxygenase cross-react with ASA, and the degree of cross-reactivity correlates with the concentration of drug necessary to inhibit cyclooxygenase *in vitro*. Even ophthalmic indomethacin in one patient induced bronchospasm requiring intubation and mechanical ventilation (Sheehan et al, 1989). Other ophthalmic NSAIDs available include diclofenac, flurbiprofen, ketorolac, and suprofen, though no ASA/NSAID-induced asthma has yet been reported with these ophthalmic preparations.

Acetaminophen and salsalate are weaker cyclooxygenase inhibitors that at higher doses (1000 mg and 2 g respectively) have been reported to provoke bronchospasm in some ASA-sensitive asthmatics. However, challenges with less than 650 mg of acetaminophen and less than 1500 mg of salsalate have

TABLE 38–1. NONSTEROIDAL ANTI-INFLAMMATORY DRUGS

CARBOXYLIC ACIDS
Acetic acids
   Diclofenac (Voltaren, Voltaren*)
   Indomethacin (Indocin)
   Profenal (Suprofen*)
   Sulindac (Clinoril)
   Tolmetin (Tolectin)
Propionic acids
   Ibuprofen (Motrin, Rufen, Advil)
   Fenoprofen (Nalfon)
   Flurbiprofen (Ansaid, Ocufen*)
   Ketoprofen (Orudis)
   Naproxen (Naprosyn)
   Naproxen sodium (Anaprox)
   Oxaprozin (Daypro)
ENOLIC ACIDS
Oxicams
   Piroxicam (Feldene)
Fenamates
   Meclofenamate (Meclomen)
   Mefenamic acid (Ponstel)
Pyranocarboxylates
   Etodolac (Lodine)
Salicylates
   Acetylsalicylic acid
   Choline magnesium trisalicylate (Trilisate)
   Diflunisal (Dolobid)
   Salsalate (Disalcid)
Pyrazoles
   Ketorolac (Toradol, Accular*)
   Oxyphenylbutazone (Tandearil)
   Phenylbutazone (Butazolidin)
NAPHTHALKANONES
   Nabumetone (Relafen)

*Signifies ophthalmic preparations.

failed to provoke asthma in ASA/NSAID-sensitive asthmatics. It should be noted that other weaker cyclooxygenase inhibitors, including choline magnesium trisalicylate and diflusinal, have been inadequately studied but would be expected to cross-react with ASA and other NSAIDs at higher doses.

Other non-cyclooxygenase-inhibiting agents that have been suspected of cross-reacting with ASA in ASA-sensitive asthmatics include tartrazine, sulfites, monosodium glutamate, and corticosteroids. We have no data at Scripps regarding the suspicion that cross-reactivity between ASA/NSAIDs and any of these non-cyclooxygenase-inhibitors exists. Aside from a single uncontrolled case report (Mendleson et al, 1974), all cases of "corticosteroid-induced asthma" occurred with intravenous sodium succinate–containing preparations (Fulcher and Katelaris, 1991). In a double-blind placebo-controlled study done at Scripps (Feigenbaum et al, 1994), only one of 53 asthmatic subjects suspected of having aspirin-sensitive asthma consistently experienced a significant fall in FEV_1 with two different intravenous sodium succinate–containing corticosteroid preparations, both prior to and following ASA desensitization. The phenomenon of "corticosteroid-induced asthma" appears actually to be a sensitivity to sodium succinate, unrelated to ASA/NSAID sensitivity.

Mechanisms

The mechanism by which ASA/NSAID-induced asthma occurs is incompletely understood. Because of the high cross-sensitivity with all the cyclooxygenase-inhibiting agents, the focus of study has been on products of the arachidonic acid pathway (Fig. 38–1). ASA, by preferentially blocking cyclooxygenase, inhibits the production of prostaglandins and thromboxanes, but not the leukotrienes, which are under the control of the 5-lipoxygenase arm. These leukotrienes include LTB_4, which is a potent chemotactic factor, and LTC_4, LTD_4, and LTE_4, which are potent bronchoconstrictors and secretagogues. Consequently, it was theorized that with ASA inhibiting cyclooxygenase, preferential shunting down the 5-lipoxygenase arm with resultant production of leukotrienes might account for ASA-induced asthma. Evidence supporting this theory includes increased calcium ionophore A23187-induced release of LTB_4 and LTC_4 from peripheral blood mononuclear cells of ASA-sensitive asthmatics compared with controls (Juergens et al, 1991). Following ASA challenge, further increase in LTB_4 significantly greater than controls occurs, and after desensitization, A23187-stimulated release of these mediators is blunted further, supporting the shunting theory (Juergens et al, 1992). Also, baseline urinary LTE_4 levels in ASA-sensitive asthmatics are greater than levels in non-ASA-sensitive asthmatics, and urinary LTE_4 increases further after ASA-induced bronchospasm (Christie et al, 1990). In addition, this increase also has been shown to be blunted following challenge of desensitized patients. No increases were noted in the following groups: (1) asthmatics with negative challenges, (2) ASA-sensitive asthmatics challenged with placebo, or (3) following methacholine-induced bronchospasm. In addition, pretreatment with either the LTD_4 antagonist SKF 104353 (Christie et al, 1991) or the 5-lipoxygenase inhibitor zileuton (Israel et al, 1993) effectively protects against ASA-induced bronchospasm in the majority of ASA-sensitive asthmatics studied.

Other data suggest that ASA-sensitive asthmatics may have increased sensitivity to LTE_4 compared with non-ASA-sensitive asthmatics or ASA-sensitive asthmatics challenged with histamine (Arm et al, 1989). In the same report, following desensitization, a significant decrease in LTE_4 hyperresponsiveness is noted, whereas no decline in histamine responsiveness is noted. Furthermore, after discontinuing ASA ingestion the LTE_4-induced hyperresponsiveness returns. This decreased sensitivity to LTE_4 following ASA desensitization in ASA-sensitive asthmatics may represent inhibition or down-regulation of LTE_4 receptors (Arm et al, 1989).

Evidence for mast cell activation during ASA-induced reactions includes elevated serum tryptase levels in a few patients with naso-ocular and bronchospastic response to ASA challenge (Bosso et al, 1991) accompanied by flushing and either nausea or diarrhea. Increase in neutrophil chemotaxis following ASA-induced bronchospasm (Hollingsworth et al, 1984) and increase in basophil histamine release to platelet activating factor in ASA-sensitive asthmatics (Okuda et al, 1990) have also been described.

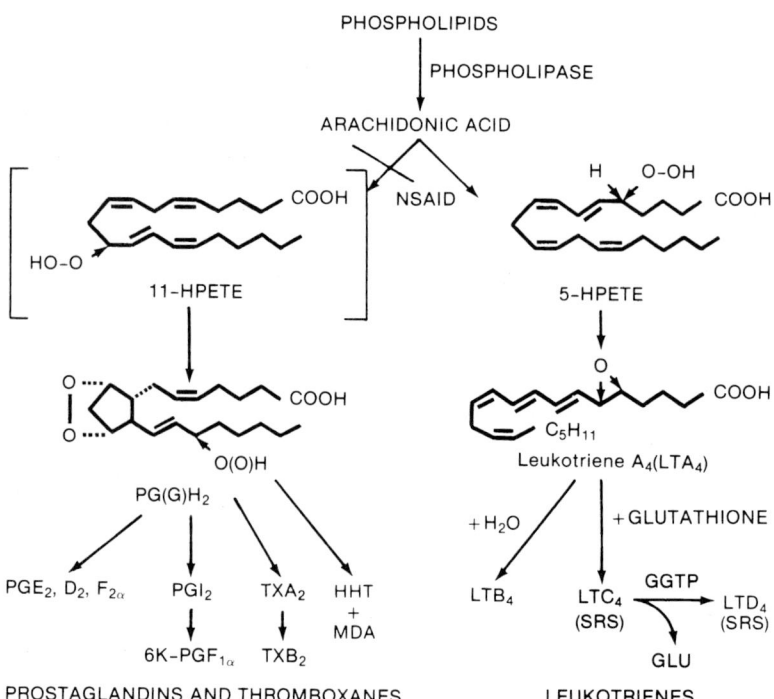

FIGURE 38–1. Metabolic cascade of arachidonic acid. The cyclooxygenase pathway leads to prostaglandins and thromboxanes (left column); aspirin (ASA) and other nonsteroidal anti-inflammatory drugs (NSAIDs) inhibit the cyclooxygenase pathway. The lipoxygenase pathway leads to leukotrienes; ASA and NSAIDs may enhance formation of these metabolites. (From Manning ME, et al. Reactions to aspirin and other nonsteroidal anti-inflammatory drugs. Immunol Allergy Clin North Am 12:611, 1992.)

Therapy

Although avoidance of ASA/NSAIDs can prevent life-threatening bronchospasm resulting from exposure to these agents in the susceptible host, this will not result in an amelioration of the disease. For subjects whose rhinosinusitis/asthma cannot be managed with conventional therapy utilizing reasonable doses of systemic corticosteroids, long-term therapy for ASA-sensitive rhinosinusitis and asthma consists of ASA desensitization and continued ASA therapy. ASA desensitization is basically a continuation of the challenge protocol. After one dose is tolerated, gradually increasing challenge doses are given until 650 mg ASA produce no signs, symptoms, or significant drop in FEV_1. ASA desensitization is universally attainable. However, it can be accomplished more quickly in those patients who react at a higher threshold ASA dose. Once ASA desensitization has been accomplished, cross-desensitization to all NSAIDs exists and can be maintained indefinitely, provided the patient continues to ingest at least 325 mg ASA per day. The desensitized state begins to wane 2 days after discontinuation of ASA, and a full reactivity state occurs in most by 7 days after ASA discontinuation (Pleskow et al, 1982).

Several studies have shown the efficacy of desensitization and treatment in ASA-sensitive rhinosinusitic/asthmatic patients. The largest study of the efficacy and long-term benefits of ASA desensitization and treatment in this population was reported by Sweet et al (1990). This retrospective study compared 35 desensitized and treated patients, 42 ASA-sensitive patients who avoided ASA/NSAIDs, and 30 initially desensitized and treated patients who discontinued ASA therapy after a mean of 2 years. Results showed that the continuously treated patients had highly statistically significant differences in many clinical parameters measured including a decrease in hospitalizations per year, emergency room visits, outpatient visits, antibiotic-requiring upper respiratory tract/sinus infections, nasal/sinus surgeries, corticosteroid bursts per year, and overall corticosteroid dependence compared to the control groups. The patients who discontinued ASA (usually due to gastrointestinal irritation) noted statistically significant improvement in respiratory disease while they maintained ASA therapy. The role of the rhinosinusitis in determining corticosteroid dose and asthma status cannot be overemphasized. This usually requires surgical intervention to establish adequate aeration and drainage. Most often this should be accomplished prior to desensitization.

BETA-ADRENERGIC ANTAGONISTS

Beta blocking drugs are used in the management of a wide variety of disorders, including angina pectoris, hypertension, migraine headaches, glaucoma, tremors, and hyperthyroidism. Beta blocker–induced bronchospasm, however, often precludes the utilization of this class of drugs in those with hyperreactive airways. Beta blockers neither precipitate bronchospasm nor increase bronchial reactivity to methacholine in normal populations. Even in four cases of propranolol overdose, bronchospasm was not observed. In patients with airway hyperreactivity, however, beta blockers may induce life-threatening asthma. This occurs most often in patients with a previous history of hyperreactive airways but occurs, though rarely, in those without such a previous history. In at least one of these cases, however, a subsequent positive methacholine challenge was documented. It should be noted that asthma may result from ophthalmic beta blocking agents as well (Dunn et al, 1986). In these situations, symptoms may result within minutes of administration (Prince and Carlener, 1983) and peak by 2 hours (Schoene et al, 1981).

There are several mechanisms by which beta blockers might induce bronchospasm. It has been documented that beta agonists modulate acetylcholine release and beta blockade may enhance cholinergic tone. Beta blockers may also enhance mast cell mediator release, as β-adrenergic receptors are present on the surface of mast cells. Although elevation in serum histamine levels following propranolol-induced bronchospasm has not been documented, pretreatment with disodium cromoglycate does inhibit propranolol-induced bronchospasm. Since there is little direct sympathetic innervation to bronchial smooth muscle, β-adrenergic receptors are stimulated primarily by circulating catecholamines. Although these catecholamines are thought to be protective bronchorelaxants, which help maintain stable airways in asthmatics, plasma catecholamine levels in normal subjects have not been shown to differ from those measured in stable asthmatics. Furthermore, no correlation between the severity of airway obstruction and plasma catecholamine levels has been documented. For these reasons, the mechanisms underlying beta blocker–induced asthma are still incompletely understood.

Although the so-called cardioselective beta blockers (e.g., atenolol, metoprolol) and those beta blockers with intrinsic sympathomimetic activity (e.g., pindolol) have resulted in less bronchospasm in susceptible hosts, bronchospasm can be produced at higher doses. Furthermore, 10 percent of the population metabolizes metoprolol less efficiently, effectively increasing the dose in this population (Lennard et al, 1982). Although asthmatics clearly are at risk for beta blocker–induced bronchospasm, there is evidence to suggest that all chronic obstructive pulmonary disease patients may not be at increased risk and may be identified by utilizing carbachol bronchial challenge (Popio et al, 1983).

The treatment of choice for beta blocker–induced bronchospasm is inhaled anticholinergics (e.g., atropine, ipratopium) (Ind et al, 1984; 1989), though 30 percent may not respond to this therapy. Inhaled β-agonists are generally not as effective. Finally, it should be noted that anaphylaxis in the presence of beta blockade is more frequent and more severe, and often responds poorly to treatment. In addition to withdrawing the offending agent and administering epinephrine and intravenous fluids, administration of intravenous glucagon may be beneficial in these difficult cases.

INTRAOPERATIVE AGENTS

The most commonly implicated agents in intraoperative systemic reactions with accompanying bronchospasm are the thiobarbiturate intravenous induction agents (e.g., thiopental, thioamylal), intravenous muscle relaxants (e.g., succinylcholine), and latex.

Incidence and Clinical Features

The incidence of systemic reactions to thiobarbiturates is estimated to be 1 in 15,000 to 30,000 administrations, and to muscle relaxants, approximately 1 in 5000. Bronchospasm occurs in over 50 percent of these cases. Although there is a slight female predominance in intraoperative systemic reactions, and atopy and previous drug exposures have been implicated by some as predisposing risk factors, at least 30 percent of reactions occur in patients not previously exposed. Other than a prior systemic reaction during anesthesia or to latex, no predisposing risk factor has been identified for either muscle relaxants or thiobarbiturates.

The incidence of latex allergy is increased in health care workers (5 to 10 percent), those with previous industrial exposure (11 to 12 percent), and those with spina bifida (18 to 28 percent). However, less than 25 percent of latex reactions actually fit into one of these risk factor groups. Although latex gloves are the most common source of intraoperative latex exposure, other sources including stoppers from multi-dose vials, injection sites in intravenous tubing, rectal and bladder catheters, adhesives, and disposable syringes should not be overlooked (Slater, 1989; Slater et al, 1990).

Mechanisms

The specific mechanisms involved in intraoperative systemic reactions with accompanying bronchospasm are still under investigation. Evidence supporting an IgE-mediated mechanism exists for the thiobarbiturates, muscle relaxants, and latex. However, it should also be noted that thiobarbiturates and muscle relaxants are capable of producing direct non-IgE-mediated histamine release as well.

Diagnosis and Prevention

Skin testing protocols for the thiobarbiturates and muscle relaxants have been established (Moscicki et al, 1990). Generally these consist of prick testing followed by intradermal testing using 0.02 cc of appropriate dilutions. *In vitro* testing has not been consistently helpful. While skin testing for latex is sensitive, standardized extracts are not currently available in this country. When intravenous anesthesia is deemed necessary in the presence of a prior history of intraoperative systemic reaction, skin testing should be done with the thiobarbiturate(s) and muscle relaxant(s) used previously, as well as alternatives. Should skin testing be negative, a search for another cause of the intraoperative reaction should be initiated (e.g., antibiotics, protamine, blood products, opiates, dextran, radiocontrast). If this search fails to identify the culpable agent(s), we recommend the use of alternative thiobarbiturates and muscle relaxants, other than those used during the previous reaction, and pretreatment with diphenhydramine, 50 mg, 1 hour prior to anesthesia, as well as prednisone, 50 mg every 6 hours for three doses, with the last dose 1 hour prior to anesthesia (Moscicki et al, 1990). In the presence of a prior history and positive skin tests, alternative methods of anesthesia are recommended, as pretreatment alone without avoiding the culpable agent(s) may not be efficacious (Moscicki et al, 1990).

Other Intraoperative Agents

Cough and bronchospasm have been described in association with propofol and enflurane administration (Martin and Miller, 1990). Significant elevation of peak airway pressures and resultant ventilation difficulty have also been documented. The mechanism is somewhat obscure, and no testing protocol exists. Consequently, in the setting of a previous reaction to these agents, avoidance is recommended.

DIPYRIDAMOLE

Intravenous dipyridamole–induced bronchospasm has been reported in six patients in a series of 3911 undergoing dipyridamole thallium myocardial perfusion imaging. All bronchospastic episodes occurred acutely. Nearly all were in patients with a history of asthma or wheezing, and all were successfully treated with administration of intravenous aminophylline (Ranhosky and Kempthorne-Rowson, 1990). Similar cases of bronchospasm attributed to oral dipyridamole have not been reported.

Although the mechanism for dipyridamole-induced bronchospasm is not certain, the best hypothesis appears to be that dipyridamole blocks endogenous adenosine uptake, transiently raising levels available for interaction with adenosine receptors. Exogenously inhaled adenosine has been shown to induce bronchospasm in certain susceptible subjects and can be prevented by administration of either antihistamine or cromolyn. This suggests that adenosine's effect is executed through mediator release.

In addition to instituting standard therapy for acute bronchospasm, treatment of dipyridamole-induced bronchospasm includes administration of aminophylline, an adenosine receptor antagonist.

ANGIOTENSIN CONVERTING ENZYME (ACE) INHIBITORS

Although ACE inhibitors do not cause asthma, they can result in a persistent nonproductive cough that may be mistaken for so-called cough-equivalent asthma. ACE inhibitor–induced cough occurs in up to 30 percent of patients, with a 3:1 predilection for women. Asthmatics do not appear to be at increased risk, and ACE inhibitor–induced cough does not represent hyperreactive airways as measured by methacholine challenge, nor does it result in pulmonary dysfunction. The onset of the cough usually occurs within weeks of initiating the drug, although delayed onset of up to 6 months has been described and does not appear to be dose-dependent (Israili and Hall, 1992).

Several mechanisms for ACE inhibitor–induced cough have been proposed. It has been shown that doses of aerosolized capsaicin (an irritant with a protussive effect) required to elicit cough are lower in the presence of ACE inhibitor (Morice et al, 1989), suggesting an increased sensitivity of the cough reflex. It has been proposed that accumulation of bradykinin and substance P (both normally degraded by angiotensin converting enzyme) while on ACE inhibitor induces the cough reflex via C fibers (Semple and Herd, 1986). However, neither consistently elevated bradykinin nor substance P serum levels have been shown following ACE inhibitor therapy. Other possible involved mediators include histamine, prostaglandins, leukotrienes, and thromboxanes.

ACE inhibitor–induced cough responds poorly to the usual antitussive approaches and often necessitates discontinuation of therapy. The cough usually resolves within 1 to 4 days following ACE inhibitor removal, although it may persist for as long as 4 weeks (O'Hollarien and Porter, 1990). It should be noted that rechallenge with any ACE inhibitor is likely to result in recurrent cough; therefore, substitution of an alternative antihypertensive class is the preferred approach.

RADIOCONTRAST MEDIA (RCM)

Systemic reactions to RCM with accompanying bronchospasm have been well documented. Patients with a strong history of allergic disease or asthma appear to be at increased risk.

Intravascular procedures, particularly intravenous rather than nonvascular or intra-arterial procedures, present the greatest risk. The older, higher osmolar RCM are much more likely to induce a RCM reaction than the newer, lower osmolar agents. In fact, the risk of subsequent reaction following a previous reaction with a higher osmolar agent can be reduced from approximately 30 percent to less than 1 percent by both substituting a lower osmolar agent and pretreating with prednisone (50 mg every 6 hours for three doses, with the last dose 1 hour prior to the procedure) and diphenhydramine (50 mg 1 hour prior to procedure), with or without ephedrine (25 mg 1 hour prior to procedure) (Greenberger and Patterson, 1991). Either substitution of a lower osmolar agent or pretreatment alone reduces risk to approximately 5.5 percent.

The pathogenesis of RCM reactions is still not clear. Several mechanisms have been proposed, including complement activation, nonspecific mast cell/basophil mediator release, and activation of factor 12 with resultant kinin formation. Evidence for an IgE-specific mechanism is lacking (Lieberman, 1992).

PENTAMIDINE

Pneumocystis carinii pneumonia (PCP) prophylaxis in patients with AIDS can be accomplished by either oral trimethoprim-sulfamethoxazole (TMP-SMX) or aerosolized pentamidine. Intolerance of TMP-SMX in this population is frequent, due to the high prevalence of cutaneous reactions and to hematologic toxicity, especially with concurrent AZT therapy. Consequently, aerosolized pentamidine is often relied upon for PCP prophylaxis. Cough and bronchospasm resulting from aerosolized pentamidine are not uncommon (Montgomery et al, 1987), and one case of bronchospasm resulting from intravenous pentamidine has even been reported (Gearheart and Bhutani, 1991). Although a history of smoking or of previous asthma has been implicated by some as a risk factor, cough and bronchospasm have been described in patients without either history.

Several proposed mechanisms have been implicated in pentamidine-induced cough and bronchospasm including nonspecific irritation, histamine release, and cholinesterase inhibition. None of these mechanisms has been conclusively shown to be solely operative, however.

In most cases, pretreatment with either a β-agonist or anticholinergic agent effectively diminishes symptoms but may not be fully protective (Montgomery et al, 1987).

DRUG ADDITIVES

Numerous drug additives have been suspected of producing and aggravating asthma (Simon and Stevenson, 1993). These include benzoates and parabens, which are used as preservatives in local anesthetics and corticosteroid preparations, sulfites found in epinephrine, Bronkosol and total parenteral nutrition solutions, benzalkonium chloride used as a preservative in beclomethasone, flunisolide and saline nasal preparations, albuterol nebulization solutions, and azo dyes used widely as coloring agents.

Benzoates and Parabens

Rare reports of systemic or bronchospastic reactions to parabens can be found in the literature. There is one report of recurrent anaphylaxis in a normal individual secondary to parabens contained in local anesthetic preparations (Aldrete and Johnson, 1969). However, bronchospasm is not listed as a component of these reactions. In another report, bronchospasm and pruritus were induced by an intravenous hydrocortisone preparation containing parabens, which was administered to an asthmatic child. Although sodium benzoates in foods have reportedly produced bronchospasm in known asthmatics, only one positive double-blind placebo-controlled challenge to date has been documented, and there was no improvement in this subject's asthma when parabens were removed from the diet. Furthermore, no case of drug-induced asthma attributed to this agent has been described.

Sulfites

Although the ingestion of sulfites in foods has been associated with severe—even life-threatening—asthma, fortunately this is not often the case with sulfites in drugs. The quantity of sulfite contained in epinephrine preparations, even when administered in the absence of epinephrine, is insufficient to provoke asthma, even in the most sulfite-sensitive asthmatic. However, the dose contained in Bronkosol is sufficient, when administered alone, to produce asthma in some sulfite-sensitive individuals and may counteract the beneficial effect of the isoetharine in another portion of patients. One case of paradoxical bronchospasm from the sulfite in Bronkosol has been reported (Koepke et al, 1984); however, neither the solutions commonly used in hand-held nebulizers nor the metered-dose inhalers contain any sulfites. To date, there are no reports of asthma exacerbations associated with total parenteral nutrition solutions.

Benzalkonium Chloride

Although distinctly uncommon, cases of paradoxical bronchoconstriction with nebulized bronchodilators have been attributed to benzalkonium chloride contained in some of these preparations (Ponder and Wray, 1993). Enhanced response to inhaled histamine with this agent has also been described. Proposed mechanisms include direct mast cell release, IgE-dependent mast cell release, and irritant effect mediated through neural C fibers.

Tartrazine

Tartrazine is the first and most commonly reported dye implicated in inducing asthma. This agent is often cited in association with aspirin-sensitive asthma. The majority of these reports, however, were poorly controlled. Despite numerous previous reports, in our studies of over 250 aspirin-sensitive asthmatics, not a single case of tartrazine-induced asthma has been documented by double-blinded challenge at Scripps Clinic.

MISCELLANEOUS AGENTS

There are several agents that can aggravate asthma by interfering with the efficacy of medications used to treat asthma or by provoking exacerbating conditions. Thyroid excess, be it natural or iatrogenic, phenytoin, and barbiturates induce rapid metabolization and elimination of corticosteroids and theophylline, and can therefore exacerbate asthma. Other agents that decrease theophylline plasma levels include rifampin, tobacco, and charbroiled foods. Several agents can aggravate asthma by lowering the lower esophageal sphincter amplitude and predisposing to gastroesophageal reflux, which in turn aggravates the asthmatic condition. Agents in this class include tobacco, fats, chocolates, xanthines, calcium channel antagonists, anticholinergics, PGE_2, alcohol, peppermints, carminatives, and tomatoes.

REFERENCES

Aldrete JA, Johnson DA. Allergy to local anesthetics. JAMA 207:356, 1969.

Arm JP, O'Hickey SP, Spur BW, et al. Airway responsiveness to histamine and leukotriene E_4 in subjects with aspirin-induced asthma. Am Rev Respir Dis 140:148, 1989.

Bosso JV, Schwartz LB, Stevenson DD. Tryptase and histamine release during aspirin-induced respiratory reactions. J Allergy Clin Immunol 88:830, 1991.

Christie P, Arm JP, Tagari P, et al. Leukotriene E_4 release after aspirin challenge in aspirin-sensitive subjects. J Allergy Clin Immunol 85:264, 1990.

Christie PE, Smith C, Lee TH. The potent selective sulfidopeptide leukotriene antagonist SKF 104353 inhibits aspirin-induced asthma. Am Rev Respir Dis 144:957, 1991.

Dunn TL, Gerber MJ, Shen AS, et al. The effect of topical ophthalmic instillation of timolol and betaxolol on lung function in asthmatic subjects. Am Rev Respir Dis 133:264, 1986.

Feigenbaum BA, Stevenson DD, Simon RA. Lack of cross-sensitivity to IV hydrocortisone in aspirin-sensitive subjects with asthma. J Allergy Clin Immunol 93:242, 1994. (Abstract)

Fulcher DA, Katelaris CH. Anaphylactoid reaction to intravenous hydrocortisone sodium succinate: A case report and literature review. Med J Australia 154:210, 1991.

Gearhart MO, Bhutani MS. Intravenous pentamidine-induced bronchospasm. Chest 102:1891, 1991.

Greenberger P, Patterson R. Beneficial effects of lower osmolality contrast media in pretreated high-risk patients. J Allergy Clin Immunol 87:867, 1991.

Hollingsworth HM, Downing ET, Braman SS, et al. Identification and characterization of neutrophil chemotactic activity in aspirin-induced asthma. Am Rev Respir Dis 130:373, 1984.

Ind PW, Barnes PJ, Durham SR, et al. Propranolol-induced bronchoconstriction in asthma: Beta-receptor blockage and mediator release. Am Rev Respir Dis 129(suppl):A10, 1984.

Ind PW, Dixon CMS, Fuller RW, et al. Anticholinergic blockage of beta-blocker-induced bronchoconstriction. Am Rev Respir Dis 139:1390, 1989.

Israel E, Fischer AR, Rosenberg MA, et al. The pivotal role of 5-lipoxygenase products in the reaction of aspirin-sensitive asthmatics to aspirin. Am Rev Respir Dis 148:1447, 1993.

Israili ZA, Hall DW. Cough and angioneurotic edema associated with angiotensin-converting enzyme inhibitor therapy. Ann Intern Med 117:234, 1992.

Juergens UR, Christiansen SC, Stevenson DD, et al. Arachidonic acid metabolism in monocytes of aspirin (ASA)-sensitive asthmatic patients before and after oral aspirin challenge. J Allergy Clin Immunol 90:636, 1992.

Koepke JW, Christopher KL, Chai H, et al. Dose-dependent bronchospasm from sulfites in isoetharine. JAMA 251:2982, 1984.

Lennard MS, Silas JH, Freestone S, et al. Oxidation phenotype: A major determinant of metoprolol metabolism and response. N Engl J Med 307:1558, 1982.

Lieberman P. Anaphylactoid reactions to radiocontrast material. Immunol Allergy Clin North Am 12:49, 1992.

Martin CS, Miller CD. Recurrent bronchospasm during anesthesia. Anesthesia 45:373, 1990.

Mendleson L, Meltzer EO, Hamburger P. Anaphylaxis-like reactions to corticosteroid therapy. J Allergy Clin Immunol 54:125, 1974.

Montgomery AB, Debs RJ, Luce JM, et al. Aerosolized pentamidine as sole therapy for *Pneumocystis carinii* pneumonia in patients with acquired immunodeficiency syndrome. Lancet 2:480, 1987.

Morice AH, Brown MJ, Higenbottam T. Cough associated with angiotensin converting enzyme inhibition. J Cardiovasc Pharmacol 13(suppl 3):S59, 1989.

Moscicki RA, Sockin SM, Corsello BF, et al. Anaphylaxis during induction of general anesthesia: Subsequent evaluation and management. J Allergy Clin Immunol 86:325, 1990.

O'Hollarien MT, Porter GA. Angiotensin converting enzyme inhibitors and the allergist. Ann Allergy 98:1133, 1990.

Okuda Y, Hattori H, Takashima T, et al. Basophil histamine release by platelet activating factor in aspirin-sensitive subjects with asthma. J Allergy Clin Immunol 86:548, 1990.

Pleskow WW, Stevenson DD, Mathison DA, et al. Aspirin desensitization in aspirin-sensitive asthmatic patients: Clinical manifestations and characterization of the refractory period. J Allergy Clin Immunol 69:11, 1982.

Ponder RD, Wray BB. A case report: Sensitivity to benzalkonium chloride. J Asthma 30:22, 1993.

Popio KA, Jackson DH Jr, Utell MJ, et al. Inhalation challenge with carbachol and isoproterenol to predict bronchospastic response in COPD. Chest 83:175, 1983.

Prince DS, Carliner NH. Respiratory arrest following first dose of timolol ophthalmic solution. Chest 84:640, 1983.

Ranhosky A, Kempthorne-Rawson J. The safety of intravenous dipyridamole thallium myocardial perfusion imaging. Circulation 81:1205, 1990.

Schoene RB, Martin TR, Charan NB, et al. Timolol-induced bronchospasm in asthmatic bronchitis. JAMA 245:1460, 1981.

Semple PF, Herd GW. Cough and wheeze caused by inhibitors of angiotensin converting enzyme. N Engl J Med 314:61, 1986.

Sheehan GJ, Kutzner MR, Chin WD. Asthma attack due to ophthalmic indomethacin. Ann Intern Med 111:337, 1989.

Simon RA, Stevenson DD. Adverse reactions to food and drug additives. *In* Middleton E, Reed CE, Ellis EF, et al (eds). Allergy: Principles and Practice. 4th ed. Mosby–Year Book, St. Louis, 1993, p 1687.

Slater JE. Rubber anaphylaxis. NEJM 320:1126, 1989.

Slater JE, Mostello LA, Shaer C, et al. Type I hypersensitivity to rubber. Ann Allergy 65:411, 1990.

Sweet JM, Stevenson DD, Simon RA, et al. Long-term effects of aspirin desensitization-treatment for aspirin-sensitive rhinosinusitis-asthma. J Allergy Clin Immunol 85:59, 1990.

Section Seven
IMMUNE AND NONIMMUNE CHRONIC PULMONARY DISEASE

Chapter 39
Hypersensitivity Pneumonitis

Michael C. Zacharisen, M.D., and Jordan N. Fink, M.D.

Hypersensitivity pneumonitis, or extrinsic allergic alveolitis, is an immunologic non-IgE-mediated, diffuse inflammatory interstitial and alveolar pulmonary disease that follows repeated exposures to diverse organic dusts or low-molecular-weight chemicals usually present in the work, home, or hobby environment. The antigens reach the alveoli by inhalation (organic dusts) or through the blood stream (drugs), and the clinical, immunologic, and pathophysiologic features are similar in susceptible individuals despite the multiple antigens incriminated.

Although pulmonary disease resembling hypersensitivity pneumonitis was first alluded to in 1713 by Ramazzini, the classic example, farmer's lung, was not described until 1932 by Campbell, when farmers exposed to moldy hay developed symptoms of pneumonitis. The reaction, initially believed to be of infectious etiology, was later found to be due to hypersensitivity to *Thermoactinomyces vulgaris*, a microorganism that proliferates in hay and compost as it becomes overheated and decomposes.

The major features include peripheral airway involvement with associated constitutional symptoms on acute exposure without hilar adenopathy or systemic organ involvement. The interstitial lung infiltrates are characterized by activated macrophages and CD8 T lymphocytes and a granulomatous reaction. Elevated levels of immunoglobulins of all isotypes except IgE, and specific IgG-precipitating antibodies are found in both serum and alveolar lavage. Lymphokines are produced by T cells of symptomatic patients.

ETIOLOGY

A number of organic antigens derived from bacteria, fungi, protozoa, and plant and animal proteins of the appropriate size to reach the terminal airways (about 5 microns and smaller) have been shown to cause hypersensitivity pneumonitis. As almost any organic dust may result in hypersensitivity pneumonitis, only a partial list is presented in Table 39–1. Volatile chemicals including diisocyanates and anhydrides used in plastic production and paint refinishing have caused both hypersensitivity pneumonitis and occupational asthma. Drugs including amiodarone, gold, and procarbazine have also been associated with interstitial lung diseases resembling hypersensitivity pneumonitis.

The common form of hypersensitivity pneumonitis is related to inhalation exposure, particularly to thermophilic actinomycetes (Fink, 1984). These bacteria are ubiquitous, having been found in decomposing vegetable matter, sugar cane, mushroom compost, soil, manure, grain, and hay. It is this organism, which thrives at 50°C in compost and moldy hay, that is responsible for farmer's lung.

TABLE 39–1. SELECTED CAUSATIVE AGENTS OF HYPERSENSITIVITY PNEUMONITIS

ANTIGEN	SOURCE	DISEASE
Bacteria		
Thermophilic actinomycetes		
Micropolyspora faeni	Moldy hay, grain or compost	Farmer's lung
Thermoactinomyces vulgaris	Moldy sugar cane	Bagassosis
T. sacharii	Humidifier or air conditioner	Ventilation pneumonitis
T. candidus	Mushroom compost	Mushroom worker's lung
T. viridis		
Fungi		
Aspergillus species	Moldy malt dust	Malt worker's lung
Alternaria species	Moldy wood dust	Woodworker's lung
Penicillium caseii	Cheese mold	Cheese worker's lung
Cryptostroma corticale	Wet maple bark	Maple bark stripper's disease
Penicillium frequentans	Moldy cork dust	Suberosis
Pullularia species	Moldy redwood dust	Sequoiosis
Trichosporum cutaneum	Japanese house mold	Summer type
Animal Proteins		
Avian serum proteins	Avian dust	Bird breeder's disease
Bovine and porcine protein	Pituitary snuff	Pituitary snuff user's lung
Rat urinary protein	Rat urine	Laboratory worker's lung
Oyster/mollusk shell protein	Shell dust	Oyster shell lung
Insect Proteins		
Sitophilus granarius	Infested wheat flour	Wheat weevil disease
Silkworm larvae	Cocoon fluff	Sericulturist's lung disease
Amoebae		
Naegleria gruberi	Contaminated ventilation system	Ventilation pneumonitis
Acanthamoeba castellani		
Medication		
Amiodarone, gold, and procarbazine	Drugs	Drug-induced
Chemicals		
Toluene diisocyanate (TDI)	Paint catalyst	Paint refinisher's disease
Diphenylmethane diisocyanate	Paint catalyst	Bathtub refinisher's lung
Phthalic anhydride	Epoxy resin	Epoxy resin worker's lung
Trimellitic anhydride	Plastics industry	Plastic worker's lung

These organisms may also contaminate stagnant water in residential or commercial air conditioning, humidification, and forced air heating systems, resulting in ventilation pneumonitis. A second common form of hypersensitivity pneumonitis and the most common pediatric hypersensitivity pneumonitis is bird breeder's disease. It has been associated particularly with exposure to pigeons, but also to chickens, parrots, doves, and parakeets. Susceptible individuals develop disease following inhalation of avian proteins in serum, bird dander and feathers or excrement from birds kept as pets for racing or showing. Disease has been described in wives and children of pigeon breeders exposed to antigen (Pitcher, 1990).

Hypersensitivity pneumonitis occurs relatively infrequently, and diagnostic accuracy is limited. Its exact incidence is not known but is thought to vary between 5 and 15 percent in an exposed population. There does not appear to be an increase in the IgE mast cell–mediated diseases in such individuals, and levels of IgE in pulmonary lavage and peripheral blood are usually normal, unless the individual is also atopic (Fink, 1992).

PATHOGENESIS

Although the exact pathogenetic mechanism is unclear, hypersensitivity pneumonitis is believed to be secondary to the combination of an immune-complex and cell-mediated immune response. Abnormalities in immunoregulation pertaining specifically to the function of suppressor T lymphocytes may play a role as well (Salvaggio, 1990).

The presence of high titers of specific serum-precipitating antibodies (usually IgG, but also IgM and IgA in lower titers) observed by gel diffusion or immunoelectrophoresis is clinically significant and confirms the diagnosis as they can be detected in nearly all ill individuals. However, approximately 50 percent of exposed but asymptomatic individuals also have specific serum antibodies, making such tests less helpful in diagnosis. Although the IgG antibodies are capable of fixing complement, complement studies are generally normal, and rarely has vasculitis or hemorrhagic pneumonitis typical of antigen-antibody interaction occurred. Elevated complement fragments have been identified in lavage fluid in patients with the acute form and correlate with chemotactic activity of neutrophils and disease activity. Since specific antibodies can be elevated in exposed asymptomatic patients and serum complement levels remain normal, the exact role of the immune complex response is unclear.

Much evidence points to an important role of cell-mediated hypersensitivity in the disease. In the lungs of affected individuals, activated T lymphocytes are often greater than 70 percent of the total cells and over 40 percent of these are of the CD8 T cell subset. These cells have decreased suppressor activity, which may influence T or B cell proliferation, cytokine secretion, and antibody formation, resulting in ongoing inflammation.

Other activated pulmonary cells that may be important include mast cells, which are found in increased numbers, and alveolar macrophages. The alveolar macrophages may be important in initiating the inflammatory phase of hypersensitivity pneumonitis by releasing a wide array of active products such as eicosanoids, particularly lipoxygenase products, and reactive oxygen species, including superoxide anions and hydroxyl radicals. Specific immune complexes or antigen alone may induce early activation of such alveolar macrophages, with subsequent release of the pro-inflammatory cytokines TNF-alpha, macrophage migration inhibition factor, IL-1, and IL-6, resulting in an early neutrophilic influx followed by lymphocyte predominance. Interferon-gamma may play a bidirectional role, with the potential for both pro- and anti-inflammatory properties. This may set the stage for T cell–dependent mechanisms, which provide the primary immunoregulatory response for both propagation and suppression of the inflammatory response of hypersensitivity pneumonitis.

CLINICAL FEATURES

Although hypersensitivity pneumonitis is a syndrome with a broad spectrum of signs and symptoms, the clinical features are typically separated into the more common acute form and the chronic form in less than 5 percent of cases. The type or nature of the inhaled organic dust is probably less important than is the intensity and frequency of inhalation or the immune response of the patient. Also, a concomitant pulmonary insult such as a lower respiratory infection may be important in inducing sensitization. Sensitization of a susceptible individual occurs after inhalation or, in some cases, ingestion of appropriate antigens. After a variable latent period, the symptoms occur either acutely after subsequent intermittent exposures or insidiously if exposure to small amounts of antigen persists over long periods (Fink, 1992).

In the acute form of the disease, explosive symptoms of fever up to 104°F, chills, headache, malaise, myalgia, minimally productive cough, and dyspnea usually occur approximately 4 to 6 hours after inhalation of the antigen, may persist for up to 18 hours, and are followed by spontaneous recovery. However, these attacks repeatedly recur following exposure to the offending antigen or particular environment. On physical examination, the patient appears acutely ill and dyspneic. Bibasilar end-inspiratory crepitant rales are prominent and can persist for weeks. Wheezing is not a prominent sign. One study demonstrated that up to half of patients with pigeon breeder's disease have digital clubbing at the time of diagnosis.

The most common pulmonary function abnormalities are a restrictive pattern with a decrease in the forced vital capacity (FVC), forced expiratory volume in 1 second (FEV_1), diffusing lung capacity for carbon monoxide (DL_{CO}), and oxygen saturation. These abnormalities often parallel the acute episode and are accentuated with exercise. Expiratory flow rates and the FEV_1/FVC ratio show little change. If sufficient pulmonary damage has occurred secondary to repeated acute episodes, decreases in volume and flow may be found during the asymptomatic period. A dual response similar to the early- and late-phase reactions of asthma may be seen in patients purposely exposed to the offending antigen. However, the late phase of asthma manifests as an obstructive change, whereas the late phase of hypersensitivity pneumonitis presents as a primarily restrictive ventilatory defect. The chest radiograph during an acute attack reveals diffuse, bilateral, soft, patchy parenchymal densities that tend to coalesce. Between attacks the radiograph may be normal or, more commonly, show reticulations and fine sharp nodulations with coarsening of the bronchovascular markings, with sparing of the apices.

Routine laboratory tests are usually normal between attacks and after corticosteroid treatment, but during acute episodes, a moderate leukocytosis with a marked left shift and, rarely, eosinophilia up to 10 percent may be present. Except for IgE, all immunoglobulin isotypes are frequently elevated. Serum-specific precipitating antibodies are detectable (Fig. 39–1). Rheumatoid factor may be moderately high in some patients, reflecting a nonspecific inflammatory response.

Bronchoalveolar lavage specimens reveal elevations of total protein related to elevated immunoglobulins with specific IgG and IgA antibody, albumin, and adhesive glycoproteins, including vitronectin and fibronectin. A fivefold increased recovery of cellular constituents includes neutrophils, followed by T lymphocytes expressing CD8 and natural killer cell markers CD56 and CD57, but not CD16, with reversal of the normal CD4 to CD8 ratio, large foamy macrophages, mast cells, and eosinophils. Lung biopsies demonstrate lymphocytic infiltration of the alveolar walls, while plasma cells and macrophages occlude the alveolar spaces. With disease progression, the alveolar space becomes obliterated and interstitial fibroblast infiltration is observed. Histologically, the presence of histiocytes with foamy cytoplasm surrounded by many mononuclear cells, which may be activated macrophages, may be a unique feature of hypersensitivity pneumonitis.

In the chronic form of hypersensitivity pneumonitis, antigen exposure is less intense but may be continuous and result in an intense inflammatory reaction in the lung, with irreversible pulmonary damage occurring

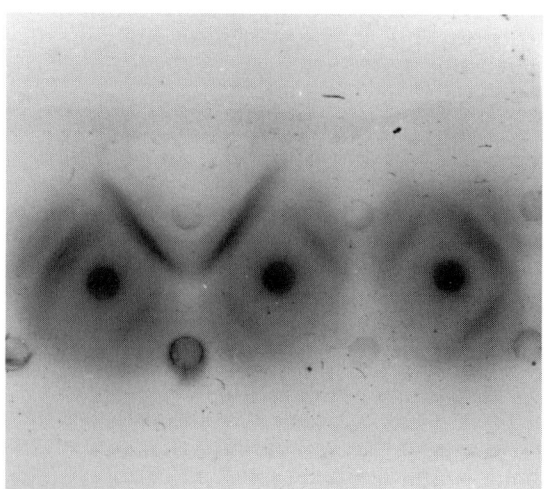

FIGURE 39–1. Precipitin arcs between patient sera (peripheral wells) and pigeon proteins (central wells) as seen in double-gel immunodiffusion.

without the presence of acute episodes. This form is more likely to occur in ventilation pneumonitis, farmer's lung, or bird breeder's disease where the birds are kept in the home. The symptoms include progressive dyspnea with cyanosis on exertion, chronic cough, weakness, malaise, and anorexia with occasional weight loss and often without fever. Physical examination may reveal fine bibasilar rales and clubbing of the fingers. Pulmonary function tests reveal a predominately restrictive ventilatory impairment with a decreased diffusing capacity. Chest radiographs are typically abnormal with a reticulonodular infiltrate (Fig. 39–2). With advanced disease, diffuse infiltrative fibrosis with honeycombing is common. Routine laboratory evaluation is generally unrewarding, as with the acute form. Lavage fluid compared to the acute stage reveals slightly lower percentage of lymphocytes, less protein and immunoglobulin, increased basophils, and fewer neutrophils. Lung biopsy may show interstitial fibrosis, small noncaseating granulomas, alveolitis with wall thickening secondary mainly to lymphocytes, but also monocyte, macrophage, and plasma cell infiltration and intra-alveolar foamy macrophages (Fig. 39–3). Eosinophils and other polymorphonuclear leukocytes are less common (Kawanami et al, 1983).

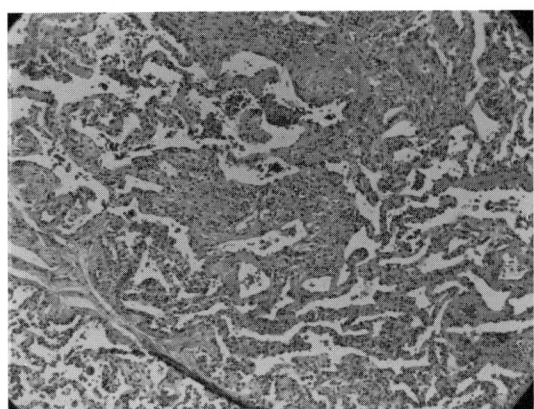

FIGURE 39–3. Lung biopsy revealing lymphocytic infiltrate, thickened alveolar walls, and early granuloma formation.

DIAGNOSIS

The diagnosis of hypersensitivity pneumonitis is suggested by the clinical history of intermittent pulmonary and systemic symptoms temporally associated with an environmental exposure. A detailed history regarding occupation, medication, hobbies, forced air equipment, and ventilation systems is invaluable. An improvement of symptoms after avoidance of the suspected environment is an important clue to implicating the allergen or environment (Salvaggio, 1990).

In asymptomatic individuals, routine laboratory tests are frequently nonspecific. Supporting evidence is the presence of serum-precipitating antibodies against the suspected antigen; however, this indicates exposure and not necessarily disease. The clinical picture must therefore be correlated with the presence of antibodies. Percutaneous skin testing is not helpful and intradermal skin testing is limited as standardized extracts are not available and crude extracts tend to irritate. Skin testing with avian serum in pigeon breeder's disease can reveal an immediate wheal and flare reaction followed by erythema and edema at 4 to 8 hours in most ill patients and in some exposed asymptomatic subjects. Amiodarone has been reported to induce a skin reaction at 6 hours in a patient with low-dose amiodarone-induced pneumonitis. Pulmonary function testing and chest radiog-

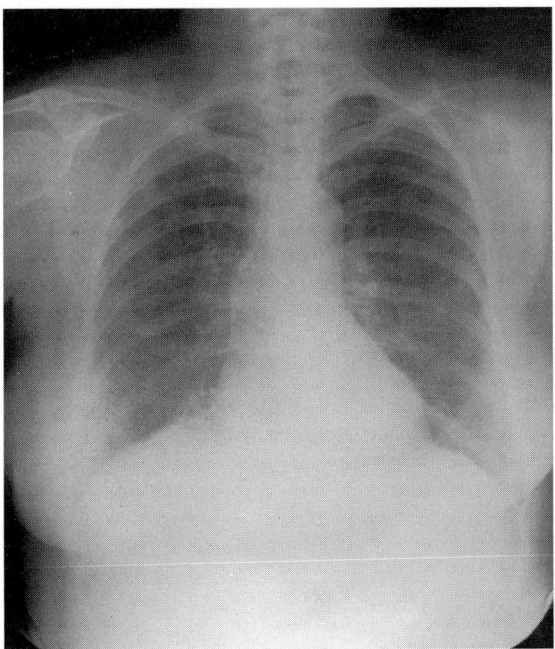

FIGURE 39–2. Chest radiograph showing bibasilar reticular and nodular infiltrates.

raphy may be helpful immediately after an acute exposure or in the chronic phase of the disease, but may be normal if obtained during an asymptomatic period.

If further evidence is needed to support the diagnosis, bronchial inhalation challenge may be performed in a laboratory using suspected antigen material. Repeated pulmonary function studies, white blood cell counts, and temperature measurement follow a characteristic course, which normalizes within 24 hours. Although now rarely required for diagnosis, lung biopsy in patients with chronic or subacute disease may reveal histopathologic features, which may be nonspecific or may aid in diagnosis by eliminating other possibilities.

The differential diagnosis of hypersensitivity pneumonitis includes many interstitial pulmonary disorders, which can be progressive and have constitutional symptoms. The acute form may be mistaken for community-acquired infectious pneumonias, usually mycoplasma or influenza, but also disseminated tuberculosis, as well as building-related infections such as legionnaires' disease, psittacosis, and Q fever. Microbial pneumonias cause single attacks of severe illness and lack recurrent similar attacks after recent exposures to an offending antigen or particular environment. The lack of serum precipitins also suggests an alternative diagnosis. Drug-induced reactions that involve the lung parenchyma have been described in association with antibiotics, cytotoxic agents, anticonvulsants, and antirheumatic drugs. The antibiotics most commonly implicated are nitrofurantoin and sulfonamides. Generally these reactions involve other organ systems and show peripheral eosinophilia and elevated levels of serum IgE. A condition that may be difficult to distinguish clinically from hypersensitivity pneumonitis is the organic dust toxic syndrome. This acute febrile noninfectious illness occurs 2 to 12 hours after exposure to high levels of organic dust contaminated with bacteria and fungi, and occurs in a variety of situations. Although most episodes are associated with agricultural exposure such as mill fever, silo unloader's disease, pulmonary mycotoxicosis, and grain fever, contaminated ventilation systems have been described as causative, as in humidifier fever. The pathogenesis of this group of disorders is unclear, but they may be due to inhalation of airborne bacterial endotoxin. In contrast to hypersensitivity pneumonitis, many individuals who are similarly exposed will develop symptoms. Other characteristics include absence of a sensitizing exposure or symptoms on repeated low-dose exposure, less frequent radiographic and pulmonary function abnormalities, lack of relevant precipitins, and a shorter course without permanent pulmonary impairment. Acute toxic gas exposure to either sulfur dioxide or nitrogen dioxide can occur in a variety of occupational and industrial settings. The resulting bronchiolitis is characterized by an increased number of neutrophils rather than lymphocytes in the alveolar lavage fluid. One example, silo filler's disease, is acute pulmonary edema caused by the inhalation of nitrogen oxides generated by fresh silage (Parker et al, 1992).

Chronic hypersensitivity pneumonitis should be differentiated from other causes of progressive dyspnea with interstitial infiltrates and pulmonary fibrosis. Chronic aspergillosis, sarcoidosis, chronic granulomatous infections, chronic bronchitis, drug reactions, collagen vascular diseases, building-related illnesses, and inorganic respiratory dust syndromes including berylliosis, silicosis, and asbestosis need to be considered.

Distinguishing features of allergic bronchopulmonary aspergillosis include a history of atopy, asthma, immediate skin test reactivity to *Aspergillus*, eosinophilia, abnormal sputum with mycelia, obstructive ventilatory defect on pulmonary function testing, and central bronchiectasis. The diagnosis of pneumoconioses or "inorganic dust" respiratory disorders is usually established by a careful environmental history. Nonpulmonary manifestations distinguish the collagen vascular diseases. Sarcoidosis may present with pulmonary symptoms but is differentiated from hypersensitivity pneumonitis by the presence of bilateral hilar adenopathy, lack of exposure to inciting agents, presence of several affected organ systems, and CD4 helper T lymphocytes predominating in the lavage fluid. "Sick-building syndrome," which manifests as irritative ocular and respiratory symptoms in exposed individuals, is probably due to increased concentrations of fungal spores, carbon monoxide, and formaldehyde after energy-conserving practices are instituted. With adequate ventilatory exchanges the problem is usually resolved. Idiopathic pulmonary fibrosis has clinical features similar to those of chronic hypersensitivity pneumonitis but is a diagnosis of exclusion (Fink, 1993).

THERAPY

As with other allergic, occupational, and environmental respiratory diseases, removal or avoidance of the offending antigen is the most effective therapy. Many patients, especially those with acute illness, will spontaneously improve after avoidance measures are implemented. After identification of the antigen, avoidance techniques may include air-filtering systems, personal protective masks, or changes in the cooling and forced air system. A change of habit, hobby, or occupation may be necessary for some individuals. Elevated levels of bird antigen may be detectable for months in the home environment, even after removal of the birds and environmental clean-up.

When avoidance cannot be carried out immediately, oral corticosteroids can dramatically improve acute disease. Single morning dosing should be used with a gradual daily tapering regimen as pulmonary functions stabilize. When long-term therapy is needed, alternate-day dosing should be used, and careful environmental investigations should be repeated to totally eliminate antigen exposure. Cromolyn sodium and inhaled corticosteroids have been tried but are believed to be of little benefit. Allergen immunotherapy, as performed in atopic disease, should be avoided as the potential exists for toxic immune complex formation, resulting in vasculitis or serum sickness.

PROGNOSIS

The prognosis is related to the reversibility of the disease, which depends on the degree of permanent respiratory impairment, the patient's ability to avoid re-exposure, and the patient's age. Over four episodes of recurrent acute symptoms or low-grade exposure may result in progressive pulmonary disease with irreversible pulmonary fibrosis and, rarely, early demise. Digital clubbing, which is associated with fibrosing interstitial lung disorders, has been proposed as a prognostic clinical tool. In one study of adults with pigeon breeder's disease, clubbing appeared to be related to a worse prognosis without relation to age, exposure time, or duration of disease. Chest radiographs and pulmonary function should be monitored carefully. A reduced diffusing capacity appears to be the most sensitive index of impaired lung function, but any abnormalities persisting for at least 6 months are suggestive of the chronic stage of hypersensitivity pneumonitis.

REFERENCES

Fink JN. Hypersensitivity pneumonitis. J Allergy Clin Immunol 74:1–9, 1984.

Fink JN. Hypersensitivity pneumonitis. Clin Chest Med 13:303–309, 1992.

Fink JN. Hypersensitivity pneumonitis. In Middleton RJ, Reed CE, Ellis EF, et al (eds). Allergy: Principles and Practice. St. Louis, Mosby–Year Book 1993, pp 1415–1431.

Kawanami O, Basset F, Barrios R, et al. Hypersensitivity pneumonitis in man. Light and electron microscope studies of 18 lung biopsies. Am J Pathol 110:275–289, 1983.

Parker JE, Petsonk EL, Weber SL. Hypersensitivity pneumonitis and organic dust toxic syndrome. Immunol Allergy Clin North Am 12:279–290, 1992.

Pitcher WD. Southern Internal Medicine Conference: Hypersensitivity Pneumonitis. Am J Med Sci 300:251–266, 1990.

Salvaggio JE. Recent advances in pathogenesis of allergic alveolitis. Clin Exp Allergy 20:137–144, 1990.

Chapter 40
Allergic Bronchopulmonary Aspergillosis

Cynthia Steichen Kabalin, M.D., and Paul A. Greenberger, M.D.

DEFINITION

Allergic bronchopulmonary aspergillosis (ABPA) is an immune-mediated pulmonary disease that complicates asthma. ABPA is the most common of the allergic bronchopulmonary fungoses and is usually attributable to *Aspergillus fumigatus* (Af). This disease was described first in 1952 in three adults in England, and then identified in cystic fibrosis patients in 1965. The initial patient to be diagnosed with ABPA in the United States was reported in 1968. In 1970, ABPA was identified in a 9-year-old child by Slavin et al. ABPA is more common than initially believed and has been identified in 1 to 2 percent of patients with chronic asthma and up to 11 percent of patients with cystic fibrosis (Imbeau et al, 1977; Slavin, 1985; Turner et al, 1989; Wang et al, 1979). ABPA may begin in infancy or childhood but may remain latent or unrecognized for years. Pulmonary infiltrates tend to occur with the progression of disease but are transient (Richeson and Stander, 1990). Thus, the child with ABPA may be difficult to diagnose if one waits for an episode of "pulmonary eosinophilia." If unrecognized and untreated, repeated pulmonary infiltrates have resulted in end-stage bronchiectasis with fibrotic and cavitary lung disease by the third or fourth decade of life. When diagnosed and treated early, significant fibrosis and bronchiectasis may be avoided.

CLINICAL FEATURES

The patient suspected of having ABPA, by definition, has a history of bronchial asthma, and most have other atopic conditions. At presentation, the patient is usually under 40 years of age. In classic cases, a patient will present with a productive cough with solid, golden-brown sputum plugs. On physical examination, wheezing is common if asthma is active. Crackles are common over areas of pulmonary infiltration. However, according to Saferstein et al (1973), as many as one third of patients may have no clinical findings despite consolidation on chest roentgenograms. Basic laboratory studies reveal peripheral blood eosinophilia, usually greater than 1000/mm^3, as well as an elevated total serum IgE with rare extremes to 80,000 ng/ml in a patient with coexistent atopic dermatitis. Microscopic evaluation of the sputum may reveal fungal mycelia and large numbers of eosinophils in patients who have not received oral corticosteroids.

A few patients have been reported by Glancy et al (1981) with roentgenographic infiltrates and peripheral blood eosinophilia consistent with ABPA. Surprisingly, the patients were not previously recognized as having asthma, although limited clinical information was provided. For example, one patient had symptoms of recurrent bronchitis, which perhaps could have been cough-equivalent asthma.

DIAGNOSTIC CRITERIA

The diagnostic criteria for ABPA are listed in Table 40–1. When all eight of the major criteria are present, the diagnosis is made easily and is known as ABPA-CB (central bronchiectasis). When central bronchiectasis is not present or not identified, the term ABPA-S (seropositive) is used (Greenberger and Miller, 1993). Because any asthmatic patient may have ABPA, the diagnosis should be considered in all patients with chronic asthma. The classic patient will meet the major criteria, but some patients may require periodic evaluation over several years until sufficient criteria for diagnosis are present.

Skin Testing

All patients with ABPA will demonstrate an immediate cutaneous response to skin testing with Af, which is manifested by a wheal and erythema reaction. A negative skin test will rule out the diagnosis of ABPA if performed appropriately with reactive extracts of Af. However, an immediate cutaneous reaction is not by itself diagnostic. Twenty-five percent of asthmatic patients have positive skin tests to Af. As reported by Laufer et al (1984), 53 of 100 patients with cystic fibrosis had positive immediate reactions to skin testing with Af. Of these, only ten were diagnosed with confirmed or probable ABPA.

Precipitins

An IgG-precipitating antibody to Af is present in the serum of most patients with ABPA at the time of diagnosis in the absence of oral corticosteroids. According to Hoehne et al (1973), precipitating antibody by itself is not diagnostic of ABPA as it has been found in 9 percent of hospitalized patients, 3 percent of healthy office workers, 12 percent of allergic asthmatic patients, 27 percent of patients with farmer's lung, and almost all patients with aspergilloma (Hoehne et al, 1973). Also, in patients with cystic fibrosis, various studies reveal precipitins to Af in 31 to 51 percent of patients. This finding implies that the host was exposed to Af by inhalation and that sensitization occurred.

IgE Antibodies

Patients with ABPA have high concentrations of total serum IgE, which are much higher than those found in uncomplicated cases of extrinsic asthma. Also, serum IgE and IgG antibodies against Af (IgE and IgG-a-Af) are elevated in the patient with ABPA as compared with patients with asthma, immediate cutaneous reactivity to Af, but without ABPA.

According to Laufer et al (1984), patients with cystic fibrosis and ABPA commonly have elevated total serum IgE levels to 5524 ± 3682 ng/ml. Also, serum IgE and IgG antibod-

TABLE 40–1. DIAGNOSTIC CRITERIA FOR ABPA

Major Criteria	ABPA-S	ABPA-CB	CF	ABPA+CF
1. Asthma	Essential	Essential	Possible	Probable
2. Immediate cutaneous reactivity to Af	Essential	Essential	Possible	Essential
3. Precipitating antibodies to Af	Essential	Essential	Probable	Essential
4. Elevated total serum IgE	Essential	Essential	Possible	Essential
5. Elevated serum IgE-a-Af and IgG-a-Af	Essential	Essential	Possible	Essential
6. Chest roentgenographic infiltrate	Probable	Probable	Probable	Probable
7. Peripheral blood eosinophilia	Probable	Probable	Possible	Probable
8. Central bronchiectasis	Not present	Essential	Probable	Essential
Other Findings				
9. Positive sputum culture for Af	Doubtful	Probable	Possible	Probable
10. History of golden-brown sputum plugs	Doubtful	Probable	Infrequent	Probable
11. Sputum eosinophilia	Possible	Possible	Possible	Probable
12. Atopic status	Essential	Essential	Possible	Essential
13. Fall in total IgE post-prednisone	Essential	Essential	N/A	Essential

ABPA-S (seropositive ABPA; have no bronchiectasis by CT examination) = criteria 1–7.
ABPA-CB (ABPA with central bronchiectasis; have bronchiectasis by CT examination or chest roentgenogram) = criteria 1–8.
CF = cystic fibrosis.
ABPA+CF = (ABPA plus cystic fibrosis) = criteria 1–6 plus clinical history.

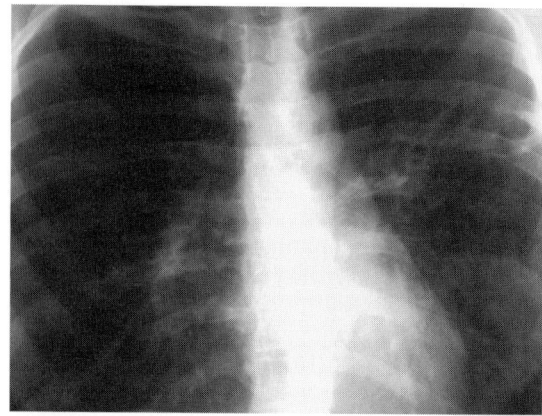

FIGURE 40–1. Exacerbation of ABPA in a 27-year-old patient whose only symptom was a nonproductive cough. There is a cavitary infiltrate extending to the periphery in the left upper lobe. The total serum IgE was 5904 ng/ml and precipitins to *A. fumigatus* were present. The serum IgE-a-Af was 3.62 and IgG-a-Af was 9.06 times sera from asthmatic patients with immediate skin reactivity to *A. fumigatus*.

ies against Af were higher in patients with either ABPA or suspected ABPA than in patients with cystic fibrosis alone or in patients with extrinsic asthma. The serum IgE-a-Af and IgG-a-Af were higher than in patients with asthma in 80 percent and 60 percent, respectively, of the patients with cystic fibrosis suspected of having ABPA. This is in contrast to a 20 percent prevalence of sharply increased serum IgE-a-Af and a 10 percent prevalence of increased serum IgG-a-Af in cystic fibrosis patients with asthma alone. In patients with cystic fibrosis without asthma or ABPA, serum IgE-a-Af and IgG-a-Af are not elevated.

Roentgenographic Findings (Figs. 40–1 to 40–3)

Central bronchiectasis is the most important radiographic finding in ABPA and is pathognomonic for ABPA in the absence of cystic fibrosis. The radiographic findings may be permanent or transient. The acute changes may range from lobar or whole lung consolidation to patchy atelectasis. There may be homogeneous shadows caused by bronchi filled with secretions, "tram lines" indicating dilated bronchi, and "toothpaste" shadows representing secretions in dilated bronchi. The chronic, permanent findings include ring shadows due to dilated bronchi and circular shadows due to proximal, saccular bronchiectasis. Ring shadows are 1 to 2 cm in diameter

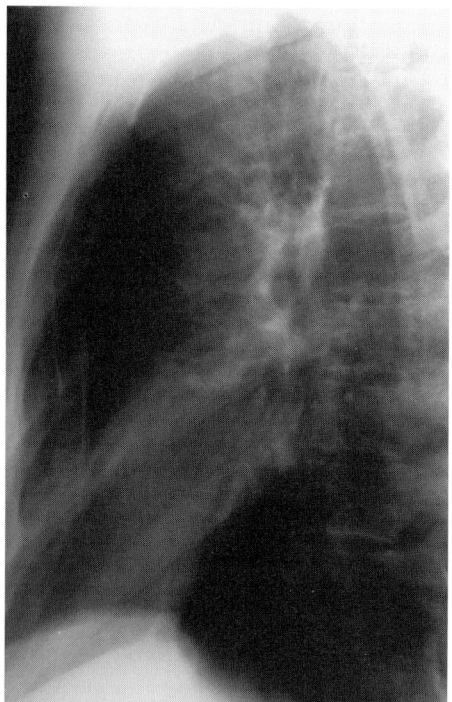

FIGURE 40–2. Lateral view of patient in Figure 40–1.

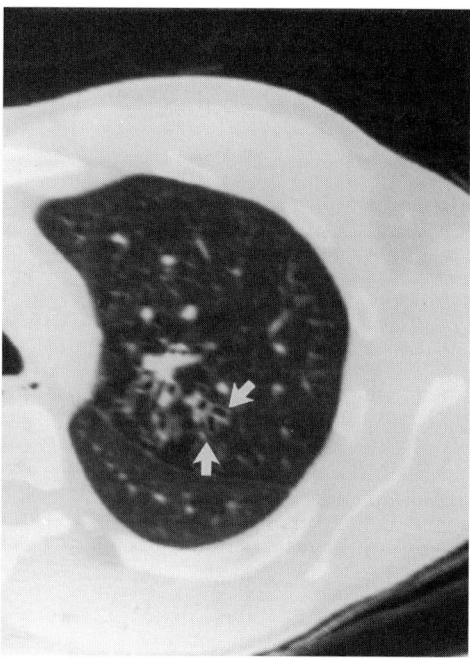

FIGURE 40–3. Computerized tomographic examination demonstrating proximal bronchiectasis in the left lung in a 29-year-old male with allergic bronchopulmonary aspergillosis. The arrows show widened ectatic bronchi.

and, on PA roentgenograms or hilar (coronal) tomograms, represent dilated bronchi *en face*. Dilated bronchi have been detected on high-resolution (1.5-mm thickness cuts) computerized tomography (CT), which provides an axial view of the lung. The CT may reveal additional areas of consolidation from mucoid impaction, which are not present on conventional PA and lateral chest roentgenograms. Late findings may include fibrosis, cavitations, and contracted upper lobes. All findings are most common in the upper lobes. As in pulmonary tuberculosis (non-AIDS cases), posterior segments of upper lobes are involved in ABPA.

CYSTIC FIBROSIS AND ABPA

ABPA in cystic fibrosis may be a difficult diagnosis because both diseases have similar clinical findings. Often, each is associated with hyperinflation, peribronchial thickening, nodular densities of bronchial mucoid impaction, atelectasis, infiltrates, upper lobe disease prominence, and central bronchiectasis. However, when the infiltrates do not respond to antibiotic therapy, are transient, or respond to steroid treatment, the diagnosis of ABPA may be more highly suspected.

It appears that Af frequently colonizes the respiratory tract of patients with cystic fibrosis (Nelson et al, 1979; Voss et al, 1982). An increased incidence of cutaneous reactivity to *Aspergillus,* elevated total serum IgE, presence of precipitins to Af, positive sputum cultures, and the presence of bronchiectasis are commonly found in cystic fibrosis patients. Thus, according to Laufer et al (1984), the presence of an elevated total serum IgE, an elevated serum IgG-a-Af and IgE-a-Af, along with a compatible clinical history seem to be the best screening method for ABPA in patients with cystic fibrosis.

PATHOPHYSIOLOGY

Aspergillus fumigatus is a 2- to 3.5-micron-sized spore that is found in soil, air, sewage, decaying vegetation (including compost piles that undergo organic heating), swimming pool water, basements, and bedding. This fungus is able to grow in a wide temperature range of 12°C to 53°C. Af spores are inhaled and colonize bronchial secretions of the constricted large bronchi of the asthmatic patient or other suitable host. They grow as hyphae and expose the patient to antigen and probably proteolytic enzymes synthesized by Af. Antigen-antibody interaction results in the immunologically mediated reactions of Gell and Coombs' types I, III, and IV. Possibly a similar immune response occurs in the lung with involvement of lymphocytes, their cell products, eosinophils, and activated macrophages. Cell-mediated immunity probably contributes, as evidenced by the presence of mononuclear cell infiltrates, granulomas, and sensitized lymphocytes. Localized complement activation also may occur. The end result of the immune response is localized bronchial wall destruction, replacement by collagen, eosinophilic pneumonia, granulomatous bronchiolitis, and central bronchiectasis, usually of the upper lobes of the lung. The viscid secretions that develop in ABPA are not easily cleared, and continued colonization and immune lung destruction lead to further areas of infiltration. Bronchiectasis occurs in areas of prior infiltrates.

Findings from lung biopsy or autopsy specimen reveal areas of mucoid impaction and fungal hyphae as well as the aforementioned histologic findings. Some patients have had several histologic diagnoses present in different areas of lung, such as eosinophilic pneumonia and mucoid impaction syndrome. At end stage, there is evidence of pulmonary fibrosis and bronchiolitis obliterans, which emphasizes that ABPA is not confined to the first few orders of bronchi.

STAGING

A staging system developed by Greenberger and Patterson (1986) classifies ABPA into five stages. Stage I (acute) ABPA is characterized by the presence of the classic findings (Table 40–2). Stage II (remission) ABPA is defined as prolonged or permanent remission after treatment of stage I with corticosteroids. There are no subsequent roentgenographic lesions, and the total serum IgE concentration declines and is stable for at least 6 months in the absence of prednisone. Inhaled corticosteroids may be used for control of asthma. Stage III (exacerbation) ABPA resembles the acute stage, with roentgenographic infiltrates, sharply elevated total serum IgE, and eosinophilia. A greater than twofold rise in total

TABLE 40-2. FEATURES OF FIVE STAGES OF ALLERGIC BRONCHOPULMONARY ASPERGILLOSIS

Stage	Total Serum IgE	Precipitins	Peripheral Blood Eosinophilia	Chest X-Ray Abnormalities	Serum IgE-Af	Serum IgG-Af
I (Acute)	+++	+	+	+	+	+
II (Remission)	+	±	−	−	±	±
III (Exacerbation)	+++	+	+	+	+	+
IV (Corticosteroid-dependent asthma)	++	±	±	±	±	±
V (Fibrotic)	+	±	−	+	±	±

From Greenberger PA, Patterson R. Diagnosis and management of allergic bronchopulmonary aspergillosis. Ann Allergy 56:444–448, 1986.

serum IgE and the presence of pulmonary infiltrates characterize an exacerbation. Stage IV (corticosteroid-dependent asthma) ABPA is diagnosed when the prednisone taper results in a significant exacerbation or recurrence of pulmonary infiltrates or worsening of asthma. The total serum IgE may be normal or elevated; precipitins are present, and serum IgE-a-Af and IgG-a-Af usually are elevated. Finally, stage V (fibrotic) ABPA is characterized by permanent pulmonary fibrosis on roentgenogram and irreversible restrictive and obstructive pulmonary function. The findings in this stage may include an elevated total serum IgE as well as the presence of serum precipitins and IgE-a-Af and IgG-a-Af. Some stage V patients show little or no improvement when placed on corticosteroids and often require high-dose alternate-day steroids to prevent exacerbations. Death may occur secondary to cor pulmonale. New infiltrates are frequently bacterial in origin rather than from ABPA.

TREATMENT

Once the diagnosis of ABPA is made, prednisone therapy should be initiated at a dose of 0.5 mg/kg/day, given as a single morning dose for 2 weeks. If there is improvement in the chest roentgenogram and clinical status, the same dose should be changed to an alternate-day schedule. Serial total IgE levels should be monitored monthly. If, at the end of 3 months, there is at least a 35 percent reduction in the total serum IgE and the chest roentgenogram remains improved, a rapid steroid taper may be attempted. Pulmonary function tests may be obtained yearly or after a change in the clinical status. The total serum IgE concentration should be monitored every 4 to 6 weeks for one year, then every 2 months. If there is a twofold increase in the total serum IgE without other cause, a roentgenographic exacerbation should be excluded by obtaining a chest radiograph. If typical infiltrates are present, prednisone, 0.5 mg/kg/day, should be reinstated. Repeat the radiograph in 1 month. Therapy with prednisone results in the stabilization of asthmatic symptoms, resolution of the infiltrates on chest roentgenogram, decreased sputum production, and decreased total serum IgE levels. Corticosteroid therapy does not prevent development of stage IV ABPA but appears to prevent emergence of end-stage pulmonary fibrosis—stage V.

Prednisone or similar short-acting corticosteroids administered in this manner (primarily alternate-day) does not cause superinfection by bacterial or fungal organisms growing saprophytically in bronchial mucus. In patients with cystic fibrosis (age 1–12 years), prednisone (2 mg/kg alternate-day) has been considered helpful in preventing a decline in vital capacity, peak expiratory flow rates, and FEV_1 over a 4-year period. This study by Auerbach et al (1985) did not mention whether or not ABPA was present. In addition, the incidence of hospitalization for cystic fibrosis–related respiratory problems was 35 in 24 placebo-treated patients and only 9 in 21 prednisone-treated patients. Inhaled corticosteroids can be used for control of asthma but do not prevent new roentgenographic infiltrates from APBA.

REFERENCES

Auerbach HA, Williams M, Kirkpatrick JA, Colten HR. Alternate-day prednisone reduces morbidity and improves pulmonary function in cystic fibrosis. Lancet 2:686–688, 1985.

Glancy JJ, Elder JL, McAleer R. Allergic bronchopulmonary fungal disease without clinical asthma. Thorax 36:345–349, 1981.

Greenberger PA, Miller TP, Roberts RN. Allergic bronchopulmonary aspergillosis in patients with and without evidence of bronchiectasis. Ann Allergy 70:333–338, 1993.

Greenberger PA, Patterson R. Diagnosis and management of allergic bronchopulmonary aspergillosis. Ann Allergy 56:444–448, 1986.

Hoehne J, Reed C, Dickie H. Allergic bronchopulmonary aspergillosis is not rare. Chest 63:177–181, 1973.

Imbeau SA, Cohen M, Reed CE. Allergic bronchopulmonary aspergillosis in infants. Am J Dis Child 131:1127–1130, 1977.

Laufer P, Fink JN, Bruns WT, et al. Allergic bronchopulmonary aspergillosis in cystic fibrosis. J Allergy Clin Immunol 73:44–48, 1984.

Nelson LA, Callerane ML, Schwartz RH. Aspergillosis and atopy in cystic fibrosis. Am Rev Respir Dis 120:863–873, 1979.

Richeson RB, Stander PE. Allergic bronchopulmonary aspergillosis. Postgrad Med 88:217–223, 1990.

Saferstein BH, D'Souza MF, Simon G, et al. Five-year follow-up of allergic bronchopulmonary aspergillosis. Am Rev Respir Dis 108:450–459, 1973.

Slavin RG. Allergic bronchopulmonary aspergillosis. Clin Rev Allergy 3:167–182, 1985.

Slavin RG, Laird TS, Cherry JD. Allergic bronchopulmonary aspergillosis in a child. J Pediatr 76:416–421, 1970.

Turner ES, Greenberger PA, Sider L. Complexities of establishing an early diagnosis of allergic bronchopulmonary aspergillosis in children. Allergy Proc 10:63–69, 1989.

Voss MJ, Bush RK, Mischler E, et al. Association of allergic bronchopulmonary aspergillosis and cystic fibrosis. J Allergy Clin Immunol 60:539–546, 1982.

Wang JLF, Patterson R, Mintzer R, et al. Allergic bronchopulmonary aspergillosis in pediatric practice. J Pediatr 94:376–381, 1979.

ACKNOWLEDGMENT: Supported by USPHS Grants NIAID AI 11403, and the Ernest S. Bazley Grant to Northwestern Memorial Hospital and Northwestern University

Chapter 41

Chronic Pulmonary Disease in Children: Including Cystic Fibrosis and Primary Ciliary Dyskinesia

Robert H. Schwartz, M.D.

Primary care physicians and specialists frequently see patients with bronchial asthma, the most common chronic pulmonary condition of childhood and adolescence. However, other nonallergic chronic pulmonary diseases share many signs and symptoms with asthma, and physicians must consider these conditions in the differential diagnosis of pediatric chronic pulmonary disease (Table 41–1) when abnormal signs and symptoms recur or last 3 or more months. This chapter discusses two chronic conditions characterized by impaired mucociliary clearance in the bronchial tree. The first, cystic fibrosis (CF), results from thick viscous endobronchial mucus due to a defect in chloride, sodium, and water transport. The second condition, primary ciliary dyskinesia (PCD), results from a failure of respiratory tract cilia to beat effectively because of ultrastructural abnormalities. CF and PCD are multisystem diseases; the basic defects are expressed in the lungs and in other organs. This situation is similar to asthma, which frequently is considered to be part of a generalized atopic diathesis. CF and PCD also are inherited, another similarity to asthma. In contrast, bronchopulmonary dysplasia (BPD), also an important chronic pulmonary disease of childhood, is an acquired condition. It is discussed in the next chapter.

In the last decade, medicine has witnessed an explosive growth in knowledge about the pathogenesis and pathophysiology of disease in general. Genetic insights, made possible by recombinant DNA molecular technology, are now being transcribed into new modalities for the diagnosis and treatment of chronic diseases affecting the lungs. Examples include (1) genotyping for the common and less common mutations of the cystic fibrosis transmembrane conductance regulator (CFTR) gene on chromosome seven, (2) enzyme inhibitor replacement with intravenous alpha-1-proteinase inhibitor (Prolastin) for the treatment of panacinar emphysema due to congenital deficiency of alpha-1-antitrypsin, (3) enzyme replacement with intravenous modified β-glucocerebrosidase (Ceredase) for the treatment of type 1 Gaucher disease, and (4) enzyme therapy with aerosolized recombinant human deoxyribonuclease I (rhDNase-Pulmozyme) for the treatment of the viscous mucus endobronchial inflammatory condition in cystic fibrosis. It is hoped that, in the next decade, further insights will translate into therapeutic cures, either through the use of other new innovative recombinant DNA-derived drugs or by the replacement of disease-producing genetic mutations with normal genes. Even now, it is possible to test

TABLE 41–1. CHRONIC PULMONARY DISEASES IN CHILDREN AND ADOLESCENTS

Allergic	Infectious	Idiopathic
Bronchial asthma*	Chronic tuberculosis	Pulmonary hemosiderosis
Allergic bronchopulmonary aspergillosis (ABPA)*	Atypical mycobacterial infection	Pulmonary fibrosis
Hypersensitivity pneumonitis	Histoplasmosis	Fibrosing alveolitis (usual interstitial pneumonia, UIP)
Hypersensitivity reactions to drugs and chemicals	Other mycoses	Desquamative interstitial pneumonia (DIP)
	Cytomegalic inclusion disease	
Hereditary	*Chlamydia*, including psittacosis and ornithosis	Lymphoid interstitial pneumonia (LIP)
Cystic fibrosis (CF)*	*Pneumocystic carinii* infection	Giant cell interstitial pneumonia (GIP)
Primary ciliary dyskinesia (PCD) and Kartagener syndrome*	Visceral larva migrans	Bronchiolitis obliterans with interstitial pneumonia (BIP)
Alpha-1-antitrypsin deficiency	Postinfectious	Pulmonary alveolar microlithiasis
Ectodermal dysplasia	Bronchiectasis*	
Familial dysautonomia	Bronchiolitis obliterans	
Immune deficiency disorders	Unilateral hyperlucent lung syndrome	
Williams-Campbell syndrome	Interstitial fibrosis	
Fucosidosis	Associated with underlying systemic disease	
Congenital	Collagen diseases	
Anomalies of the lung (cysts and sequestration)	Malignancy	
Congenital lobar emphysema	Reticuloendothelioses	
Complicating management of preexisting conditions	Liporeticuloses	
Bronchopulmonary dysplasia (BPD)	Gaucher disease	
Acquired immune deficiency disease syndrome (AIDS)	Niemann-Pick disease	
Radiation pneumonitis	Histiocytosis-X	
Musculoskeletal disorders	Letterer-Siwe disease	
Central nervous system disorders	Hand-Schüller-Christian disease	
	Eosinophilic granuloma	
	Sarcoidosis	
	Wegener granulomatosis	

*Discussed in this chapter.

pharmacologic and gene therapy protocols in genetic mouse models of cystic fibrosis and in genetic pig and dog models of primary ciliary dyskinesia (Roperto et al, 1993; Edwards et al, 1992).

CYSTIC FIBROSIS

Cystic Fibrosis (CF) is the most common life-shortening autosomal recessive genetic disease of white children. Its incidence varies among different populations, ranging from one in 1700 live births in Northern Ireland to one in 7700 in Sweden, and implying a carrier frequency of about one in 20 to one in 44. It is rare in Orientals and in African Blacks (less than one in 100,000). CF is lethal because of chronic bronchopulmonary infection and progressive lung destruction. However, in recent years, its prognosis has improved. From 1990 to 1992 the proportion of adult (18 years or older) CF patients in the United States was 33 percent, a fourfold increase since 1969 (8 percent). The median survival age in 1992 was 29.4 years, a twofold increase since 1969 (14 years).

Because CF is a chronic multisystem disease, there are many secondary complicating features (Table 41–2). Allergy and CF can coexist. The child with phenotypically mild CF who remains undiagnosed while being treated for atopic asthma is one example. Wheezing occurs in both conditions. Also, CF's gastrointestinal manifestations can mimic non-respiratory allergic conditions such as food allergy. Most frequently, allergy occurs as a complication of CF. Examples include the CF child who develops allergic bronchopulmonary aspergillosis (ABPA) and the CF child who develops β-lactam antibiotic allergy. Also, certain complications of CF resemble other immune diseases (Table 41–3).

Diagnosis of Cystic Fibrosis

The diagnosis of CF is suspected on clinical grounds. It is confirmed by sweat testing, which can be supplemented with DNA analysis (genotyping). The diagnostic hallmarks of

TABLE 41–2. CLINICAL FEATURES AND COMPLICATIONS OF CYSTIC FIBROSIS

Integument and external areas
  Pallor
  Failure to thrive
  Purpura
  Telangiectasia
  Erythema nodosum
  Digital clubbing
  Protuberant abdomen
  Emphysematous chest
  Short stature
  Delayed puberty
  Cyanosis
  Angular stomatitis
  Salt crystals on face
  Paronychia
  Edema
Head
  Sinusitis
  Nasal polyposis
  Optic neuritis
  Nyctalopia
  Enlarged submaxillary glands
Thorax and pulmonary system
  Bronchiolitis
  Bronchitis
  Bronchiectasis
  Pneumonia
  Staphylococcus organisms in sputum
  Pseudomonas organisms in sputum
  Allergic bronchopulmonary aspergillosis
  Pulmonary cysts and abscesses
  Atelectasis
  Pneumomediastinum
  Pneumothorax
  Massive hemoptysis
  Botryomycosis
  Pulmonary insufficiency
  Pulmonary failure
Thorax and cardiac system
  Pulmonary hypertension
  Right ventricular hypertrophy
  Cor pulmonale
  Right ventricular failure
  Myocardial fibrosis
Abdomen and gastrointestinal tract
  Pancreatic enzyme deficiency
  Steatorrhea
  Azotorrhea
  Pancreatitis
  Meconium ileus
  Intestinal atresia
  Fecal impaction
  Intussusception
  Duodenitis and ulceration
  Mucocele of appendix
  Biliary cirrhosis of liver
  Hepatomegaly
  Splenomegaly
  Portal hypertension
  Esophageal varices
  Ascites
  Gallbladder stones
  Pneumatosis intestinalis
  Pneumatosis coli
  Pseudomembranous colitis
  Rectal prolapse
  Inguinal hernia
  Diabetes mellitus
Genitourinary system
  Absence of vas deferens
  Male sterility
  Thick cervical mucus
  Cervical polyps
  Female decreased fertility

TABLE 41–3. ALLERGIC COMPLICATIONS OF CYSTIC FIBROSIS AND COMPLICATIONS THAT RESEMBLE OTHER IMMUNE DISEASES

Asthma-airway hyperreactivity due to inflammation
Allergic bronchopulmonary aspergillosis (ABPA)
Drug hypersensitivity
Gastrointestinal allergy to cow's milk
Protein-losing gastroenteropathy
Systemic amyloidosis with renal involvement
Vascular purpura and cutaneous vasculitis
Arthritis of pulmonary osteoarthropathy
Transient episodic polyarticular or monarticular arthritis

CF are (1) pancreatic enzyme deficiency with intestinal maldigestion and malabsorption, (2) chronic progressive obstructive pulmonary disease, (3) chronic pulmonary infection (with *Staphylococcus* and/or *Pseudomonas*), and (4) electrolyte loss through sweat. Any pulmonary condition should also be suspected of being CF if there is (1) a history of intestinal obstruction or meconium ileus at birth, (2) a family history of CF, (3) male infertility due to azoospermia, and/or (4) nonallergic nasal polyposis. Sweat tests should also be considered in children with unexplained chronic cough, with recurrent or chronic pneumonia, with *Staphylococcus* or *Pseudomonas* (especially mucoid form) cultured from sputum, with nasal polyps, and with unexplained recurrent respiratory symptoms and digital clubbing. These and other indications for sweat testing are listed in Table 41–4. False-positive sweat tests may occur in adrenal insufficiency, diabetes insipidus, glycogen storage disease, and the hypohidrotic form of ectodermal dysplasia.

Confirmation of the diagnosis of CF requires two positive sweat test results, done on different days, by quantitative pilocarpine iontophoresis, according to methods approved by the Cystic Fibrosis Foundation

TABLE 41–4. INDICATIONS FOR SWEAT TESTING

Pulmonary
  Chronic cough
  Recurrent or chronic pneumonia
  Staphylococcal pneumonia
  Recurrent bronchiolitis
  Atelectasis
  Hemoptysis
  Mucoid Pseudomonas infection
Gastrointestinal
  Meconium ileus
  Steatorrhea
  Malabsorption
  Childhood cirrhosis (portal hypertension or bleeding esophageal varices)
  Hypoprothrombinemia beyond newborn period
Other
  Family history of cystic fibrosis
  Failure to thrive
  Salty sweat, salty taste when kissed, salt frosting of skin
  Nasal polyps
  Heat prostration, hyponatremia, and hypochloremia, especially in infants
  Pansinusitis
  Aspermatism

Center Committee and Guidelines Subcommittee. A positive test result is defined by sweat chloride measurements in excess of 60 mM/l in an adequate sample of sweat (a minimum of 75 mg collected on 2 × 2 gauze or filter paper or 15 μl collected in Macroduct coils during a 30-minute period). Repeated borderline measurements (40 to 60 mM/l) require clinical correlation for diagnosis, preferably confirmed by DNA genotyping for the common and uncommon mutations. Most (98 percent) CF sweat chlorides fall between 60 mM/l and 160 mM/l (FitzSimmons, 1993). Less than 2 percent are below 60 mM/l. These are associated with a novel mutation in the cystic fibrosis gene (Highsmith et al, 1994).

Genetics of Cystic Fibrosis

Our understanding of the etiology, pathophysiology, and genetics of CF has changed considerably since the original familial description by Guido Fanconi in 1936, since the original pathologic description by Dorothy Anderson in 1938, and since the recognition of the sweat chloride reabsorption defect by Paul A. diSant'Agnese in 1953. In 1989, the CF gene was found on the long arm of chromosome 7 (Kerem et al, 1989; Rommens et al, 1989; Riordan et al, 1989). The CF gene consists of about 250 kb of DNA containing 27 exons. The mRNA transcript contains about 6500 base pairs encoding a protein of 1480 amino acids. This protein is called the cystic fibrosis transmembrane regulator (CFTR). It forms the major electrochemical apparatus, a channel for Cl^- ion transport regulated by cyclic AMP. RNA transcripts of the CFTR gene are found in lung, pancreas, sweat glands, liver, nasal polyps, salivary glands, and colon. The CFTR protein is expressed on the apical surface of pancreatic and sweat gland epithelial cells and in submucosal glands lining the airways. The proposed functions of CFTR and the relationship of abnormal CFTRs to CF pathophysiology are described below (Collins, 1992).

More than 300 mutations of the CF gene have been described (Tsui, 1992b). The most common mutation (ΔF_{508}) consists of a three-basepair *inframe deletion* in exon 10 at codon 508 resulting in a deletion (Δ) of phenylalanine (F). Other types of mutations include *missense* (substitution of a single amino acid), *nonsense* (premature termination leading to a nonfunctional CFTR), *frameshift* (deletions or additions of basepairs), and *splicing* (involving splice junctions) mutations (Table 41–5).

The ΔF_{508} mutation is present on about 67 percent of CF chromosomes worldwide (82 percent of CF patients in the United States; 1992 CF Foundation Patient Registry Annual Data Report). ΔF_{508} homozygotes and most ΔF_{508} compound heterozygotes (ΔF_{508} plus another mutation) usually have pancreatic insufficiency of early onset with markedly elevated sweat chloride concentrations. In one important study (n = 798 CF patients; The Cystic Fibrosis Genotype-Phenotype Consortium, 1993), compound heterozygotes having the genotype R117H/ΔF_{508} (n = 23) had lower sweat chloride concentrations (80 ± 18 vs 108 ± 14 mM/l, P<0.001) than age-matched more common ΔF_{508} homozygotes (n = 399). Also, they more often had pancreatic sufficiency (87 percent versus 4 percent, P<0.001). Meconium ileus was not seen in this group (n=23). This study of genotype-phenotype relationships has genetic counseling, therapeutic, and prognostic implications (Tsui, 1992). Patients with R117H/ΔF_{508} can expect long-term pancreatic sufficiency. Those with other genotypes can expect early onset of pancreatic insufficiency. However, this first report found no statistically significant differences in the incidence of common features of CF such as *Pseudomonas* colonization, nasal polyps, pancreatitis, diabetes mellitus, distal intestinal obstruction syndrome, rectal prolapse, cirrhosis, and gallbladder disease. Obviously, additional genetic and environmental factors influence the phenotypic expression of CF. Nutritional factors are probably of importance since other nongenetic studies (Gaskin et al, 1982) suggest that CF patients with pancreatic sufficiency have milder lung disease. Also, in one study (Campbell et al, 1992), poor pulmonary clinical status of ΔF_{508} homozygotes (n = 44) was associated with heavy exposure to tobacco smoke. The studies of genotypes and phenotypes continue.

There are differences in the frequency of various mutations among different national, ethnic, and racial groups. These variations need to be considered to allow precise carrier detection and prenatal diagnosis. The frequency of ΔF_{508} is found to be 65 to 80 percent in North American, British, Swiss (Liechti-Gallati et al, 1991), and Dutch patients but only 51 to 58 percent in Spanish and Italian populations and 37 percent of

TABLE 41–5. SELECTED COMMON AND UNCOMMON CYSTIC FIBROSIS MUTATIONS

MUTATION	MUTATION TYPE	LOCATION	FREQUENCY USA*	FREQUENCY WORLD†
ΔF_{508}	Inframe deletion	Exon 10	82.1	67.2
G542X	Nonsense	Exon 11	3.5	3.2
G551D	Missense	Exon 11	3.4	2.4
N1303K	Missense	Exon 21	1.8	1.8
W1282X‡	Nonsense	Exon 20	1.6	2.1
R553X	Nonsense	Exon 11	1.3	1.3
621+1G—>T	Splice site	Intron 4	1.0	1.3
R117H‡‡	Missense	Exon 4	0.7	0.8
3848(9)+10kbC—>T§	Splice site	Intron 19	0.6	1.4
1717-1G—>A	Splice site	Intron 10	0.4	1.1
M1101K§§	Missense	Exon 17b	Rare	Rare

*Cystic Fibrosis Foundation. Patient Registry 1992 Annual Report, Bethesda, Maryland, October 1993.
†CF Genetics Analysis Consortium (Tsui, 1992a).
‡Most common (60%) mutation in the CF Ashkenazi Jewish population of Israel.
‡‡Associated with pancreatic sufficiency.
§Associated with normal sweat chloride concentration.
§§Most common (69%) mutation among CF Hutterites of North America.

black American patients. Among the French-Canadians in Saquenay-Lac St. Jean, Quebec province, the frequency is 56 percent (Rosen et al, 1990). The frequency of the ΔF_{508} mutation is only 22 percent in the Ashkenazi Jewish population in Jerusalem whereas the W1282X nonsense mutation is the most common (60 percent of CF chromosomes). The ΔF_{508} mutation accounts for only 31 percent of mutations in CF families representing the three endogamous subdivisions (Dariusleut, Lehrerleut, and Schmiedeleut) of the Hutterite population of North America (Fujiwara et al, 1989). A rare missense mutation (M1101K) has been found on the other 69 percent of CF chromosomes (Zielenski et al, 1993). These two mutations account for all of the CF mutations among Hutterites, making it possible to offer the Hutterites accurate carrier testing and genetic counseling of adults and early diagnosis and treatment of CF infants (Miller and Schwartz, 1992).

Further caution is needed if carrier screening and genetic counseling of populations other than at-risk families is to be undertaken because the less common mutations may account for phenotypic variations such as milder disease in CF patients with pancreatic sufficiency, less severe CF in black persons, and other very mild forms of the disease. These associations are only beginning to be identified and understood. For example, in a group of 23 non-CF patients with congenital absence of the vas deferens, 11 were heterozygous for the ΔF_{508} mutation (Gervais et al, 1993). Among patients with congenital absence of the vas deferens without unilateral renal agenesis, the frequency of the R117H mutation of exon 4 was found to be high (4 of 18). These unrelated patients in their thirties had normal chest films and FEV_1. Their sweat chloride values were elevated (62 to 90 mM/l). A novel mutation (3849+10kbC—>T) in the cystic fibrosis gene in patients with pulmonary disease but normal sweat chloride concentrations also has recently been described (Highsmith et al, 1994). They do not have obstructive azoospermia.

Structure and Function of the Cystic Fibrosis Transmembrane Regulator (CFTR); Relationship to the Pathogenesis of CF

CF is caused by mutations in the cystic fibrosis transmembrane conductance regulator (CFTR) gene; its product has been shown to be a cAMP-regulated chloride channel. The CFTR structure consists of 12 membrane-spanning regions (transmembrane domains TM1 to TM12), two ATP-binding domains (nucleotide binding folds NBF1 and NBF2), and a regulatory domain (R domain). Perturbation of CFTRs normal structure results in abnormal transport of chloride ions across sweat duct epithelial cells and across mucosal surface epithelial cells. In the sweat gland there is abnormal reabsorption of chloride and sodium, accounting for the elevation of these ions in sweat and providing the genetic pathophysiologic basis for the diagnostic sweat test. At the respiratory, pancreatic, and hepatic organ levels, there is a block in chloride channel transport to the luminal surface of epithelial cells, resulting in a decrease in sodium and water transport to the mucus sol layer. A dehydrated thickened viscous mucus impairs mucociliary clearance and contributes to obstruction of bronchioles, bronchi, pancreatic ducts, and bile canaliculi. In the respiratory tract, mucus viscosity is increased even more by large amounts of DNA from the neutrophilic response to infection and to a lesser extent by exopolysaccharides from infecting mucoid strains of *Pseudomonas aeruginosa*.

There are at least four mechanisms by which mutations disrupt CFTR function. Their elucidation and enumeration will have implications for understanding the many phenotypic variations in CF and for developing therapeutic strategies to correct different degrees of CFTR dysfunction. Class I mutations (defective production) produce no CFTR protein; class II (defective protein processing) results in defective trafficking of CFTR protein from the endoplasmic reticulum to the Golgi, where normally it would be glycosylated and then move to the plasma membrane (Yang et al, 1994); class III mutations have defective regulation at the nucleotide binding folds; class IV mutants have defective conduction through the CFTR chloride channel. Defective trafficking (class II mutation) accounts for 60 to 80 percent of CF alleles (ΔF_{508}). Therapeutic strategies (Table 41–6) currently include gene therapy to restore normal CFTR structure and function (Olsen et al, 1992) and pharmacologic therapy to correct abnormal CFTR function (Knowles et al, 1991).

Clinical Presentation of Cystic Fibrosis

External Manifestations of Internal Disease

The potential external manifestations of internal disease in CF are numerous. The child who tastes salty when kissed or who has white powdery salt crystals across the bridge of the nose, forehead, and hairline manifests the CF eccrine sweat abnormality. He or she may appear fair skinned and pale because of decreased subcutaneous fat, decreased carotenoid pigmentation of the skin, and subcutaneous blood vessels close to the surface of the skin. Besides chronic cough and sputum production, clubbing of the fingers and cyanosis become apparent and progress with increasing pulmonary disease. Short stature, protuberant abdomen, thin extremities, barrel chest, pectus carinatum, pulmonary osteoarthropathy, and kyphosis are other secondary external manifestations of internal chronic pulmonary infection and intestinal maldigestion. Palmar erythema and spider angiomas may accompany severe multinodular biliary cirrhosis. Purpura, ecchymoses, and bleeding may develop in young children with vitamin K deficiency caused by malabsorption. A deficiency of vitamin K–dependent coagulation factor II (prothrombin) activity also may result from liver disease. Vascular purpura (described as cutaneous necrotizing

TABLE 41–6. NEW STRATEGIES FOR THE TREATMENT OF CYSTIC FIBROSIS

Reconstitution of normal CFTR expression	Gene therapy
	Transfer of normal CFTR cDNA
	Recombinant adenovirus
	Adeno-associated virus (AAV)
	Retroviruses
	Cationic liposomes
	DNA-protein complexes
	Receptor-mediated endocytosis gene transfer
	Relocate (activate) CFTR in class II mutations (trafficking defect)
Repair of decreased chloride secretion and increased sodium reabsorption defects	Pharmacologic therapy
	Alter impaired chloride secretion
	Aerosolized UTP (uridine triphosphate)—secretagogue that activates non-CFTR chloride channels
	Alter excessive sodium reabsorption
	Aerosolized amiloride—sodium channel inhibitor
	Alter chloride and sodium transport defects
	Amiloride and UTP

venulitis and erythema nodosum) may occur, presumably as a result of immune complex phenomena. Transient episodic polyarticular or monarticular arthritis, usually involving large joints, also has been described in association with a nodular rash. Goiters have been described in those CF patients receiving chronic expectorant therapy with iodides. Large goiters have been observed in those CF patients in whom the rare complication of secondary systemic amyloidosis develops. Pitting edema is observed when right heart failure occurs or in young untreated CF children with hypoproteinemia, edema, and anemia resulting from nutritional protein deficiency. Angular stomatitis may be seen secondary to vitamin B (riboflavin) deficiency. Other features and complications of CF are listed in Table 41–2. However, it is important to note that the infant, child, and adult with CF may appear entirely normal and may exhibit none of these external manifestations of internal disease.

Pulmonary Manifestations

The first respiratory symptom of CF is usually cough. However, wheezing can occur early and mimic either bronchiolitis or asthma. The first sign of pulmonary involvement is chest hyperexpansion or increased radiolucency of the lung fields on chest roentgenogram. These are due to the earliest lesion of CF, which occurs as bronchiolar obstruction with mucus, predisposing the lung to infection, neutrophilic inflammation, and hyperplasia of goblet cells, progressing with time to the larger airways and destruction of airway walls. Mucociliary clearance becomes impaired. Progressive involvement begins with bronchiolitis and is followed by bronchitis, bronchiectasis, peribronchial pneumonia, peribronchial fibrosis, and large cystic bronchial dilation that eventually involves all subsegmental bronchi. Alveolar destruction ensues, with infection of atelectatic areas or with episodes of patchy pneumonia and hemorrhagic pneumonia. There is progressive loss of pulmonary function, with possible complications from massive hemoptysis, recurrent pneumothorax, hypoxemia, pulmonary hypertension, and cor pulmonale, all of which are poor prognostic signs. The presence of mucoid strains of *Pseudomonas aeruginosa* or *Pseudomonas cepacia* seem to separate the more severe cases from the milder ones. Although these pathogens occur in elderly adult non-CF patients with bronchiectasis and in immunocompromised patients, their presence in the lower respiratory tracts of children or in sputum is almost unique to CF.

Gastrointestinal Manifestations

The earliest postnatal presentation of CF is meconium ileus, which occurs in 16 to 18 percent of patients. Today this is managed medically but may require surgical correction if prenatal obstructive events have led to intestinal obstruction, perforation, sterile peritonitis, and secondary intestinal atresia. Scrotal calcification or peritoneal calcification, seen on abdominal roentgenogram, are clues to the early diagnosis of these complications. Pancreatic exocrine function may be completely ablated, partially active, or normal. About 30 to 40 percent of patients initially present with failure to thrive/malnutrition and steatorrhea/abnormal stools. Eventually most patients will have pancreatic insufficiency. However, compared with their counterparts with severe maldigestion (steatorrhea and azotorrhea), patients with near-normal pancreatic function (normal fat absorption without oral pancreatic enzyme replacement) have milder symptoms, lower mean chloride concentration values in sweat, and less lung involvement with better pulmonary function. This seems to emphasize the primary relationship between pancreatic sufficiency and genotypes and the secondary connection between good nutrition and resistance to infection. Alternative explanations include phenotypic differences in mucus viscosity secondary to genotypic variation and a spectrum of electrolyte and mucus transport abnormalities or additional genetic factors not yet defined.

Early obstruction and destruction of the exocrine pancreas and its progressive functional deterioration is usually observed clinically. It can be followed by measurement of serum immunoreactive trypsinogen (high levels early and very low levels later). Seventy-two hour stool fat measurements can be used to estimate pancreatic function and to adjust oral pancreatic enzyme replacement. Secretin and pancreozymin tests currently are used less frequently than in the past. The goal of pancreatic enzyme replacement is weight gain or maintenance, and nonfatty stools—one to two per day—without abdominal pain or other evidence suggestive of distal intestinal obstruction syndrome (meconium ileus equivalent in older patients).

The pancreatic destructive process eventually affects the endocrine function of islet tissue. Glucose intolerance caused by insulinopenia ensues (30 to 75 percent of reported cases). Overt clinical diabetes (hyperglycemia, glycosuria, polyuria, polydipsia, and weight loss) occurs in approximately 5 percent of cases, mostly during the teenage years. Ketonuria and ketoacidosis, as occur in juvenile diabetes mellitus, are not seen in CF.

Allergic Complications of Cystic Fibrosis and Other Relationships

Asthma and Allergy Skin Tests

Immediate wheal and flare skin test reactions can be demonstrated in 25 to 50 percent of patients with CF. However, the development of these immune phenomena does not imply a pathogenic significance. When "atopy" was defined as positive immediate skin test reactions to five or more allergens, we found 46 percent of CF patients to be atopic (Nelson et al, 1979). Significantly more ($p<0.025$) severely affected (63 percent) CF patients (T-K score <80) were atopic when compared to a healthier group (T-K score >80) of CF (30 percent) patients. Although the incidence of atopy was much higher in a non-CF asthmatic control group (87 percent) than in CF patients (46 percent), the incidence of mold sensitivity alone and predominant mold sensitivity (three or more molds than pollens) was much higher than in the non-CF asthmatic control group. These findings have been confirmed by Wilmott (1991), who also found that skin test positivity correlated with *Pseudomonas* colonization of the respiratory tract, which in turn was associated with more severe disease. Thus, damage of the respiratory epithelium due to infection probably contributes to allergen sensitization. Neither study supports a previously reported notion that CF patients with asthma or hayfever have milder disease (Rachelefsky et al, 1974).

Although asthma and CF can coexist, the frequently observed airway hyperreactivity in CF is probably based on nonimmune mechanisms and not on the presence of allergy or atopy (Mitchell et al, 1978). Airway hyperreactivity can be demonstrated by histamine (Mellis and Levison, 1978; Holzer et al, 1981; Van Asperen et al, 1981) and methacholine (Mitchell et al, 1978) inhalation challenges and by exercise testing (Day and Mearns, 1973). Increased bronchomotor tone has been demonstrated by its reversibility with isoproterenol, theophylline (Pan et al, 1989), and ipratropium bromide (Sanchez et al, 1992). If either airway hyperreactivity or rhinitis occurs in CF on a specific immune basis, this relationship has yet to be proved by inhalation challenge or provocative nasal challenge with specific allergens. It should be noted that bronchodilator responsiveness (to theophylline and β_2-agonists) in CF tends to undulate with pulmonary exacerbations of the disease (Hordvik et al, 1985) and that expiratory flow rates may improve in some patients but can get worse in others (Landau and Phelan, 1973; Shapiro et al, 1976; Zach et al, 1985; Eber et al, 1988). Perhaps this adverse response is due to enhanced airway compressibility and decreased peripheral expiratory airflow. Several investigators have warned that adrenergic and methylxanthine drugs be used with caution in patients with CF. Bronchodilators may reduce the efficacy of cough by increasing large airway collapse. Thus, the clinical long-term effectiveness of bronchodilators has not been demonstrated. Pulmonary function testing with bronchodilators should be done to identify patients with a clearly negative response (Tepper and Eigen, 1990). When bronchodilators seem helpful to relieve symptoms, they can be used.

Thus, pharmacotherapy should be individualized and used in those patients who demonstrate significant improvements in airway obstruction with oral or inhaled bronchodilators. Sodium cromoglycate has not been shown to be of any benefit in CF patients with bronchial hyperreactivity (Sivan et al, 1990). Immunotherapy is not warranted unless there are symptoms present that are associated with clear-cut allergen exposure, as with seasonal allergic asthma or allergic rhinitis. Immunotherapy with allergenic extracts of *Aspergillus fumigatus* is probably contraindicated because it stimulates IgG antibodies thought to be essential to the ABPA process. Because lung destruction is partly due to inflammatory processes, alternate-day prednisone (2 mg/kg) has been used to treat CF patients with mild-to-moderate pulmonary disease. In a 4-year study (Auerbach et al, 1985), the prednisone-treated group had better growth (height and weight), FVC, FEV_1, and erythrocyte sedimentation rate, and fewer hospitalizations than the placebo-treated group. There were no observed steroid-induced side effects. However, in a later study of close to 3 years (Rosenstein and Eigen, 1991), patients in a high-dose group (2 mg/kg every other day) had a higher frequency of cataracts, growth retardation, and glucose abnormalities (intermittent hyperglycemia and glycosuria) than low-dose (1 mg/kg every other day) and placebo groups. Therefore, although glucocorticosteroid therapy can be beneficial in individual cases, these CF patients should be carefully monitored.

Nasal Polyps and Chronic Sinusitis

Pansinusitis occurs in almost 100 percent of CF cases. Ethmoidal and maxillary nasal polyposis complicates chronic sinusitis in 10 to 15 percent of all patients, approaching 50 percent in the adult CF population. CF nasal polyps differ morphologically from allergic polyps. In contrast to allergic polyps, CF polyps have a thin subepithelial hyaline layer and lower eosinophil infiltrates in the polyp stroma (Miller et al, 1994). These differences may be useful when deciding which patients with nasal polyps should have sweat tests. Since nasal polyps from other causes are rare in childhood and CF can present in extremely mild forms, sweat testing should be performed on children with unexplained nasal polyps. In CF, there is no association between nasal polyps and aspirin idiosyncrasy (Noritake et al, 1981). Management of chronic sinusitis and nasal polyposis is usually medical. When severe nasal obstruction and anosmia occur, polypectomy is indicated. The sinus condition can be complicated by mucoceles or mucopyoceles, which can erode the sinus wall into the orbit or central nervous system. Then surgery is indicated. More aggressive medical and surgical therapy for chronic sinusitis, including endoscopic surgery with serial antimicrobial lavage, is currently being evaluated at several centers.

Allergic Bronchopulmonary Aspergillosis (ABPA)

An association between CF and ABPA has been known since 1965 (Mearns et al, 1965). Thirty percent of CF patient groups in the United States (Schwartz et al, 1970) and in London, England (Mearns et al, 1965) have been reported to have serum precipitins to *Aspergillus* antigens. This high prevalence, verified in other studies, indicates a ubiquitous exposure to *Aspergillus* and suggests that ABPA might be anticipated as a frequent complication of CF. As can occur in asthma, *Aspergillus* mold spores are easily trapped by mucus in the proximal bronchi, thus providing a milieu for germination, hyphal growth, and stimulation of local and systemic immune responses. In Rochester, New York, we reported that 57 percent of 46 CF patients were colonized with *Aspergillus fumigatus*; 37 percent had serum precipitins to antigenic extracts of this fungus; 39 percent had positive immediate skin test reactions; and 22 percent had elevated total serum IgE concentrations (Nelson et al, 1979). Seven of 46 (15 percent) patients developed ABPA (Schwartz and Hollick, 1981), according to the accepted diagnostic criteria (Rosenberg et al, 1977). Other studies have reported a similar high incidence (Laufer et al, 1984). However, the incidence was only 1.6 percent (272 in 17,068) of patients seen at CF care centers in 1992. The true incidence of ABPA in CF is difficult to determine because of variations in mold exposure in different locales (urban versus rural) and sporadic case-finding among clinics. Nevertheless, ABPA should be anticipated as a complication of CF and, in the milder cases, treated with oral glucocorticosteroids. In the more severe cases, concomitant bacterial antibiotic therapy is usually necessary. Response to therapy is evidenced by a fall in total serum IgE concentrations. Exacerbations are heralded by a rise in serum total IgE, although this is not always the case (Nelson et al, 1979; Schwartz and Hollick, 1981). The best screening test for ABPA in CF is the prick skin test with *Aspergillus fumigatus* antigens. A negative test has excellent negative predictive value. If positive, the skin test should be supplemented with other tests to satisfy the diagnostic criteria for making a diagnosis of ABPA. Because ABPA is a potential complication of either CF or asthma, it is wise to obtain skin prick tests with *Aspergillus fumigatus* antigens and total serum IgE levels on all children with these conditions.

Complications Resembling Other Immune Diseases

In early infancy, CF has been mistaken for gastrointestinal allergy to cow's milk, especially protein-losing enteropathy. However, in CF, a syndrome of hypoproteinemia, hypoalbuminemia, edema, anemia, and failure to thrive is due to protein maldigestion and malabsorption and not to protein loss through the gut. The erroneous use of soybean formulas compound the problem. Prompt resolution occurs with the introduction of pancreatic enzymes or the use of cow's milk hydrolysate formulas, preferably with medium-chain triglycerides rather than whole fat. Amyloidosis (Ristow et al, 1977) and conditions for which immune complexes have been implicated are listed in Table 41–3.

Altered Immune Processes

Chronic pulmonary *Pseudomonas* infections cause most of the morbidity and mortality in CF. Significant local colonization occurs in the CF host who rarely develops sepsis or metastatic foci of infection such as brain abscess, and who can develop hypergammaglobulinemia and a vigorous antibody response to bacterial, viral, and fungal antigens, even in the more severe cases. Aberrations in the immune system, not yet proved to be related to the primary genetic defect, have been proposed to account for the inability of CF patients to clear *Pseudomonas* (Berger et al, 1989; Tosi et al, 1990; Berger et al, 1994). Within the milieu of the *Pseudomonas*-infected and inflamed lung, proteases are released into tissues and secretions. There is evidence to suggest that protease-antiprotease imbalance plays a role in the pathogenesis of chronic lung disease in CF (Birrer et al, 1994). Excessive amounts of neutrophil elastase, unopposed by alpha-1-antitrypsin and secretory leukoprotease inhibitor, cleave anti-*Pseudomonas* IgG, rendering it opsonically ineffective. Elastase also cleaves antigen-bound IgG, interfering with the activation of phagocytic cells by immune complexes, and it removes CR1, an important complement receptor of polymorphonuclear neutrophils (but not alveolar macrophages), impairing their ability to kill opsonized *Pseudomonas aeruginosa*. In addition, proteases also remove iC3b, an important opsonin, from bacteria. It has also been shown that CF sera and lung IgG antibodies actually "block" phagocytosis, especially by alveolar macrophages, which express a high-affinity IgG receptor, Fc γRI, not contained on blood or alveolar neutrophiles (both have Fc γRII and Fc γRIII). The Fc γRI alveolar macrophage IgG receptor is saturated by low concentrations of IgG antibodies. IgG1 and IgG3 antibodies may be blocked from the high-affinity Fc γRI receptor by enzymatically altered or degraded IgG Fc or by an excess of other IgG subclass antibodies, resulting in decreased phagocytosis. Thus, there is a rationale for the use of glucocorticosteroids to modulate the neutrophil inflammatory response and to decrease the local production of elastase. There is also a rationale for intravenous and aerosolized alpha-1-antitrypsin (anti-protease, anti-elastase) therapy. Intravenous gamma globulin or *Pseudomonas* immunoglobulin to replace damaged autogenous antibodies is also a potential strategy. Clinical trials, using all these modalities, are currently under way.

Another observation that may be relevant to the development of effective immunotherapy for CF is that there is a subset of CF patients who remain clear of colonization with *Pseudomonas aeruginosa*. In contrast to those who are colonized, the noncolonized patients develop specific opsonic antibodies to the mucoid exopolysaccharide coat of *Pseudomonas aeruginosa* (Pier et al, 1987). A mucoid exopolysaccharide (MEP) vaccine has been prepared, and phase I studies are under way in CF patients to test the safety and pharmacology of intravenously administered hyperimmune IgG prepared from normal human donors. Therapeutic potentials include active immunization with the vaccine early in young CF patients to prevent *Pseudomonas* colonization and passive immunotherapy with hyperimmune gammaglobulin for the treatment of older CF patients already colonized and infected with *Pseudomonas*.

Pulmonary Complications of Cystic Fibrosis and of Other Conditions

Clubbing of the Fingers and Toes

The association of clubbing of the fingers and toes with lung disease has been recognized since the time of Hippocrates. Finger clubbing is common in cystic fibrosis (CF) but unusual in asthma. Clubbing in asthmatics should always prompt a search for other conditions more commonly associated with it (Table 41–7). Clubbing can be ameliorated when the conditions are successfully treated. Dramatic improvement has been noted after lung transplantation in CF.

TABLE 41-7. CONDITIONS ASSOCIATED WITH CLUBBING

Pulmonary
   Cystic Fibrosis (CF)
   Bronchiectasis of other etiologies
   Pulmonary abscess
   Empyema
   Chronic interstitial pneumonitis
   Alpha-1-antitrypsin deficiency with lung disease
   Primary and metastatic pulmonary neoplasms
   Cavitary tuberculosis

Cardiac
   Congenital cyanotic heart disease
   Subacute bacterial endocarditis

Hepatic
   Hepatic cirrhosis
      Postinfectious
      Associated with alpha-1-antitrypsin deficiency
      Associated with cystic fibrosis
   Intrahepatic biliary atresia
   Thalassemia

Gastrointestinal
   Chronic ulcerative colitis
   Regional enteritis
   Multiple intestinal polyposis
   Chronic dysentery (amebic or bacillary)

Other
   Thyrotoxicosis

Accurate clinical assessment of finger clubbing is helpful both in detecting serious lung disease and in following its course. Clubbing occurs in the following order:

1. *Development of a floating nail.* This sign can be demonstrated by pressing the mantle (nail root) with the examining finger and finding it soft and mushy.

2. *A diminution in the angle the nail makes with the extrapolated axis of the digit.* This change is often accompanied by an increased longitudinal curvature of the nail.

3. *An increase in the DPD/IPD* (see following discussion). This change is accompanied by broadening of the terminal phalanx as viewed from the palmar surface, leading to a "drumstick" finger.

A metric micrometer or caliper is used to measure the finger depth at the nail base. This is called the distal phalangeal depth (DPD). The depth of the finger is also measured at the interphalangeal fold. This measurement is the interphalangeal depth (IPD). A ratio of the DPD/IPD greater than 1.0 is considered indicative of clubbing. The left index finger should be used, as the normal ratio may be different for other fingers.

Progressive fingertip deformity is accompanied by increased blood flow to the digits, overgrowth of vascular elements, hyperplasia of fibrous tissue, and edema. The pathophysiologic mechanisms that induce these changes are not well understood. A variety of factors implicated include hypoxemia, vasoactive substances (prostaglandin E, serotonin, and bradykinin), and autonomic reflexes. Clubbing also has been observed in association with vascular abnormalities leading to differences in blood flow to the extremities (arteriovenous fistulas of the subclavian artery and aortic aneurysms).

Clubbing usually is painless. However, it may be accompanied by hypertrophic pulmonary osteoarthropathy (HPO), which is manifested by stiffness, swelling, and arthralgia of the fingers, wrists, ankles, and knees. Formation of new periosteal bone most frequently occurs along distal portions of the tibia, fibula, radius, and ulna. Less commonly, the humerus, femur, metacarpal, and metatarsal bones may be involved. Pain and tenderness are exacerbated by cold and relieved by warmth and rest. Nonsteroidal anti-inflammatory drugs are also helpful.

Hemoptysis

Hemoptysis is defined as the spitting or coughing of blood, ranging from streaks of blood admixed with sputum to massive exsanguination originating from a lesion anywhere in the respiratory tract. Although hemoptysis is uncommon in children, when it occurs it is a frightening experience for the patient and parent and should be considered with alarm by the physician because it usually implies either significant trauma or serious pulmonary disease. Bleeding of esophageal or gastric origin (hematemesis) may be mistaken for hemoptysis. In some infants, blood from the bronchopulmonary tree is swallowed without coughing and then vomited; therefore, when one encounters unexplained hematemesis in an infant with abnormal chest findings, a pulmonary source of bleeding should be considered. History and careful physical examination of the nose, mouth, and throat will usually provide clues to bleeding from the gums or other oral lesions. Blood originating from the trachea and distal bronchopulmonary areas may occur under a variety of circumstances (Table 41–8).

Bronchiectasis is one of the most frequent causes of hemoptysis. In CF patients, acute

TABLE 41–8. CONDITIONS ASSOCIATED WITH HEMOPTYSIS

Infections
  Bronchitis/bronchiectasis
  Tuberculosis (adult)
  Lung abscess
  Intracavitary fungus balls (aspergillomas)
  Certain pneumonias *(Pseudomonas, Staphylococcus, Klebsiella)*
  Fungal diseases (the mycoses)
  Parasitic infections (e.g., paragonimiasis)
Neoplasms
  Tracheal tumors
  Bronchial adenomas
  Bronchogenic cancer
  Endobronchial metastases
Vascular disorders
  Arteriovenous malformations
  Pulmonary embolism and infarction
  Mitral stenosis
  Cardiac failure with pulmonary edema
	Vasculitic disorders
	  Churg-Strauss syndrome
	  Systemic lupus erythematosus
	  Wegener granulomatosis
	Coagulation and bleeding disorders
	  Primary (inherited)
	  Secondary (acquired)
	Trauma
	  Lung contusion
	  Rib fracture
	  Foreign bodies
	Other
	  Cystic fibrosis
	  Neonatal pulmonary hemorrhage
	  Pulmonary sequestration
	  Idiopathic and primary pulmonary hemosiderosis
	  Goodpasture syndrome
	  Myocarditis
	  Cow's milk sensitivity

arterial bleeding originates from erosion of destroyed lung parenchyma, which erodes into enlarged tortuous blood vessels and bronchopulmonary arterial anastomoses adjacent to bronchiectatic airways. In CF, *Pseudomonas aeruginosa* may also cause hemorrhagic pneumonitis. Blood streaking of mucus is frequent in CF, in which widespread bronchiectasis is the rule. Fifty percent of adult patients with CF have such minor bleeding. Massive hemoptysis (>240 cc in 24 hours) is life threatening (Schidlow et al, 1993). Major hemoptysis (>100 cc/day over 3 to 7 days) may threaten life due to asphyxiation; produce airway obstruction, hypotension, anemia, and chemical pneumonitis; and trigger a pulmonary exacerbation. About 1 percent of CF patients and 5 percent of adult patients have major bleeding each year.

Blood streaking of sputum requires no specific treatment other than antibiotics for pulmonary infectious exacerbations. Contributing factors such as bleeding diatheses and use of nonsteroidal anti-inflammatory drugs (NSAID) should be ruled out. The management of major and massive hemoptysis is more complex, but the essentials have been published and are easily available (Schidlow et al, 1993). Patients may be able to identify the area of the lung that is bleeding by describing a feeling of warmth or a gurgling sensation in their chests. The best diagnostic tests to localize the site of bleeding are bronchoscopy and arteriography during or immediately after an acute episode. Conservative medical management (antibiotics, rest, oxygen, blood replacement, correction of bleeding diathesis) usually is adequate to treat minor episodes. Coagulation defects should be corrected with vitamin K, fresh frozen plasma, or specific factors. Relentless bleeding may cease with intravenous pitressin or premarin. Endobronchial tamponade may be necessary. Bronchial artery embolization with gelatin sponge (Gelfoam) has been successful in patients with life-threatening hemoptysis and in patients with lesser bleeds that interfere with their life styles. Transverse myelitis and paralysis may complicate this procedure if the spinal arteries are inadvertently embolized. Pulmonary infarction and embolization of the mesenteric arteries also may occur. This procedure should be done by an experienced angiographer who is usually available at one of the CF care centers.

Bronchiectasis

Cylindric, tubular, and pseudobronchiectasis (absence of normal bronchial tapering) frequently follows acute lower respiratory infections and is reversible. Saccular bronchiectasis (irregular bronchial dilatations and narrowings) is irreversible. Large dilatations are referred to as cystic bronchiectasis. Proximal or central bronchiectasis is a late complication of allergic bronchopulmonary aspergillosis (ABPA). Bronchiectasis is usually acquired, occurring commonly in disorders such as CF, immune deficiency disorders, Kartagener syndrome, alpha-1-antitrypsin deficiency, and, rarely, severe chronic asthma. Postinfectious bronchiectasis is seen less frequently than in former years. The decreased incidence is due to the decline in rubeola and pertussis infections, the effective use of antibiotics in lingering lower respiratory infections, the control of influenza by current vaccines, the decrease in primary tuberculosis in infancy and childhood, and the better management of atelectasis and chronic bronchial inflammation. Acquired bronchiectasis may be a sequela of viral infection, such as influenza and adenovirus, particularly types 3, 7, and 21. For instance, acute adenoviral infections induce a necrotizing bronchiolitis, which may proceed to bronchiolar obliteration (bronchiolitis obliterans). The consequences of this include atelectasis and inflammation in areas of stagnant secretions, both thought to be the main causes of bronchiectasis. Chronic airway obstruction due to mucus plugging, foreign body aspiration, and compression or erosion of bronchi by tuberculous lymph nodes also can lead to bronchiectasis.

The cardinal clinical feature of bronchiectasis is chronic cough productive of mucopurulent sputum, which on culture usually yields *Haemophilus influenzae* or *Streptococcus pneumoniae*. Gram-negative organisms, such as *Escherichia coli, Proteus,* and *Klebsiella*, also may be cultured after multiple courses of antibiotics. *Staphylococcus* and *Pseudomonas aeruginosa* are the predominant organisms in CF. Bronchiectasis should be anticipated when acute lower respiratory illnesses are slow to resolve, when there is a history of recurrent pulmonary infections, or when there is persistent atelectasis. Lesions may be localized or diffuse. Localized lesions most commonly involve the left lower lobe except with foreign body aspiration, which commonly involves the right lower lobe. For unknown reasons, the right upper lobe commonly is the first and most severely involved in CF. Physical examination usually reveals rales and crackles in the affected areas. Digital clubbing usually occurs with diffuse disease but may occur with localized lesions and has been noted to disappear when these are resected. The spectrum of bronchiectasis may range from almost asymptomatic localized disease to full-blown chronic diffuse disease. Malnutrition, clubbing, hypoxemia, pulmonary hypertension, and cor pulmonale are late complications. Pneumonia and atelectasis are frequent complications. Bronchopleural fistula and metastatic brain abscess are less common complications since the advent of antibiotics.

Chest roentgenograms may appear normal or may exhibit increased linear markings ("tramline" tracks and ring shadows) due to peribronchial thickening and inflammation. If disease is allowed to progress, small cystic and nodular lesions show a honeycomb-like pattern. Large cysts and bullae occur with most advanced disease and predispose to pneumothorax. The cysts may be filled with air or with air/fluid and predispose to aspergillomas (mycetomas). Today, computerized tomography of the chest is used to diagnose and evaluate the extent of bronchiectasis to assist both in medical and surgical management.

Medical management is preferred for patients with minimal disease who are asymptomatic, patients with early disease that may be reversible, and patients with advanced diffuse disease who are unable to tolerate surgery because of greatly impaired pulmonary function or are awaiting lung transplantation. Medical management should include chest physiotherapy, bronchodilators, and appropriate antibiotics. Respiratory bacterial and viral vaccination should be kept current. Proper nutrition is important. Surgical treatment is reserved for those patients whose disease is localized to one segment or lobe with (1) a persistent or recurrent obstruction, (2) an infection uncontrolled by antibiotic therapy, (3) an uncontrolled recurrent hemoptysis from a localized source, or (4) a foreign body that cannot be removed by bronchoscopy. In CF, prognosis may be improved by resection when one segment or lobe has far-advanced bronchiectasis and the remaining lung involvement is mild. This situation is unusual, however. Resection should be an elective procedure, if possible. Double-lung transplantation is the corrective procedure for diffuse severe disease.

Pneumothorax

Pneumothorax is another frequent complication of chronic obstructive lung disease with bronchiectasis. In 1992, pneumothorax requiring chest tube treatment occurred in 0.6 percent of 17,068 patients seen at CF care centers in the United States. It occurs more commonly in advanced disease caused by rupture of subpleural blebs through the visceral pleura and resulting in air in the pleural space. Approximately 16 to 20 percent of adults (over 18 years) with CF will experience a pneumothorax at some time in their lives (Schidlow et al, 1993).

Although spontaneous pneumothorax may be "silent" and discovered only on chest roentgenogram, patients are usually symptomatic, experiencing sudden onset of chest pain and dyspnea. This event may be associated with a paroxysm of cough, too vigorous physical activity, or overzealous physical therapy. However, more frequently the triggering event cannot be identified or anticipated. Tachypnea, tachycardia, pallor, and cyanosis are common signs. Decreased excursion, hyperresonance, decreased vocal fremitus, and decreased breath sounds of the affected hemithorax are found on physical examination. Deviation of the trachea from the midline and shift of the mediastinum are signs of tension pneumothorax. Subcutaneous emphysema and circulatory compromise are signs of advanced tension pneumothorax. Localization and evaluation of the size of the pneumothorax is made by chest roentgenograms including inspiratory, expiratory, and lateral decubitus views.

Symptomatic patients and those with a pneumothorax of 20 percent or more should be first given oxygen and soon thereafter have a chest tube inserted. The recommendations for chest tube management have recently been summarized (Schidlow et al, 1993).

Sclerosing agents—including quinacrine, tetracycline, and talcum powder—have been used in the treatment of pneumothorax in patients with CF. Open thoracotomy or thoracoscopy and mechanical or CO_2 laser abrasion, with or without stapling of blebs or instillation of chemical agents, are other options for patients with pneumothorax unresponsive to chest tube drainage and those with recurrent pneumothorax. Previous trauma to the pleural space by chest tubes, pleurodesis, or thoracotomy increases the complexity of future lung transplantation because of increased perioperative blood loss through vascularized scar tissue. However, this is not now a contraindication to lung transplantation.

Principles of Management for Cystic Fibrosis

Proper management of patients with CF requires a broad understanding of the pathology of CF; a knowledge of its secondary physical and psychological manifestations, and its social, and financial implications; and a multidisciplinary approach. The most capable physician should no longer be the sole provider of the multiple services needed.

The task of keeping up with the CF literature is a job in itself. One can expect one article per month to appear in pediatric journals. Because approximately one third of CF patients are now adults, recent advances in knowledge and therefore in management also are published in internal medicine journals and other subspecialty journals. The Cystic Fibrosis Foundation (6931 Arlington Road, Bethesda, Maryland 20814) serves as a clearing house for medical information. The medical director and staff members are equipped to answer or redirect all inquiries and to direct the health care professional or patient to his or her nearest CF care, teaching, and research center where comprehensive services are provided (Table 41–9).

The CF specialist is trained to make or confirm the diagnosis and to coordinate ongoing care of the chronically ill patient in the context of his or her family and community. The health care professional should be prepared and open minded; communication with the specialist and coordination of the patient's nutritional, pulmonary, and psychological care are vital. The open, inquisitive minds of primary physician and the CF specialist and their attitudes toward the patient and family

TABLE 41–9. SERVICES PROVIDED BY CYSTIC FIBROSIS CENTERS

Sweat testing and confirmation of diagnosis
Evaluation and outline of therapeutic and prophylactic programs
Education of the patient and the entire family
Instruction in pulmonary physiotherapy and inhalation therapy
Instruction in nutrition, diet, and enzyme replacement
Genetic counseling and prenatal diagnosis
Vocational counseling
Financial counseling
Teenage, adult, and parent discussion and support groups
Other consultative services (allergy, otolaryngology, psychiatry, surgery)
Hospitalization and treatment for complications
Hospitalization for lung transplantation
Voluntary research by patients and relatives

Adapted and modified from Cystic Fibrosis Foundation guidelines for patient services, evaluation, and monitoring in cystic fibrosis centers. Am J Dis Child 144:1311–1312, 1990.

from the time of diagnosis often determine their future adjustments and attitudes to the vicissitudes of CF. An informed case manager—whether the primary physician, CF specialist, nurse practitioner, family counselor, or other health professional—is a necessity. These persons have the difficult task of providing information, advice, and access to old and newer modes of management. The ability of these patient-advocates to function effectively in the face of many uncertainties of CF has been bolstered in recent years by the exciting breakthroughs in genetics and molecular biology that have provided a new optimism and momentum for progress.

Traditionally and historically, the management of CF has included pancreatic enzyme replacement; vitamin A and K supplementation; attention to nutrition; chest percussion to improve clearance of infected secretions; and oral, intravenous, and aerosolized antibiotics to treat *Staphylococcus* and *Pseudomonas* endobronchial infection. Today, therapy for CF has come of age (Table 41–10). It is less controversial than in the past; it is buttressed by basic scientific fact and controlled clinical trials. Aerosolized recombinant human DNase (rhDNase; Pulmozyme) has been shown to reduce pulmonary exacerbations, reduce hospitalizations, and improve pulmonary function in patients with cystic fibrosis (Hubbard et al, 1992; Ramsey et al, 1993). It is now part of the CF therapeutic armamentarium. Tomorrow, other new innovative therapies will provide further hope for a cure. These strategies have been summarized in Table 41–6.

Lung Transplantation for Cystic Fibrosis

Lung transplantation is now an acceptable option for the management of end-stage pulmonary disease including cystic fibrosis, chronic obstructive pulmonary disease, alpha-1-antitrypsin deficiency, pulmonary fibrosis, primary pulmonary hypertension, Eisenmenger's syndrome, sarcoidosis, bronchiectasis, and bronchiolitis obliterans. CF patients with a forced expiratory volume in one second (FEV_1) less than 30 percent of the predictive value, a partial pressure of arterial oxygen below 55 mm Hg, or a partial pressure of arterial carbon dioxide above 50 mm Hg had two-year mortality rates above 50 percent (Kerem et al, 1992). These patients should consider the transplant option. Successful transplantation results in a marked improvement in functional capacity and quality of life. The first successful heart-lung transplant for patients with CF occurred in England in 1985 (Jones et al, 1988). Heart-

TABLE 41–10. APPROACHES TO CYSTIC FIBROSIS THERAPY

Abnormality	Solution	Approach
Abnormal CF gene ↓	Provide normal gene	Gene therapy
Abnormal CFTR protein ↓ ↓	Provide normal protein Activate mutant form	Protein therapy ?
Abnormal salt transport ↓	Block sodium ion uptake Increase chloride ion efflux	Amiloride ATP/UTP
Viscid pancreatic duct mucus Abnormal respiratory mucus ↓	Replace enzymes Decrease viscosity	Oral pancreatic enzymes DNAase (Pulmozyme)
Impaired clearance ↓ ↓	Augment ciliary action	Chest percussion
Pseudomonas infection ↓ ↓	Reduce bacterial count Prevent colonization	Antibiotics Hyperimmune globulin Pseudomonas vaccines
Inflammatory response ↓	Decrease host reaction	Glucocorticosteroids Other mediator inhibitors Alpha-1-antitrypsin
Bronchiectasis	Replace irreversibly damaged lung	Lung transplantation

Adapted from Collins FS. Cystic fibrosis: Molecular biology and therapeutic implications. Science 256:774–779, 1992.

lung, double-lung, and sequential lung transplants have been done at a number of CF centers in North America and Europe. One-year survival results have ranged from 58 to 88 percent. The sequential bilateral lung transplant has emerged as the procedure of choice. Five-year survival rates will probably approach 50 to 60 percent. CF patients now constitute half of all bilateral lung transplant grafts. Inclusion and exclusion guideline criteria have been established at different transplant centers. The entire process, ranging from the first consideration of transplantation by the patient and care givers, coming to terms with the concept, through the evaluation process at one of the transplant centers, waiting in turn for a compatible transplant organ, and into the procedure itself with its immediate and long-term postoperative course and multiple potential complications, is a tour de force made possible only by modern medicine in a supportive modern society based on the strengths of the human condition. Currently, the limiting problem is bronchiolitis obliterans, which develops in approximately 50 percent of transplant cases. Problems, somewhat unique to CF patients, including infected lungs, previous thoracic surgery, nutrition, donor shortage, lung size matching, anastomotic complications, and immunosuppression of infected hosts, have not been insurmountable (Egan and Detterbeck, 1992). For a more thorough synopsis of the issues and factors surrounding lung transplantation, the reader is directed to published consensus reviews (American Thoracic Society Statement, 1993) and discussions of limited resources in the face of high-tech capabilities (Fiel, 1991).

PRIMARY CILIARY DYSKINESIA (PCD) AND KARTAGENER SYNDROME

Primary ciliary dyskinesia (PCD), with or without dextrocardia and situs inversus, is an inherited disorder characterized by recurrent respiratory tract infections related to abnormal ciliary ultrastructure and function. It also has been called the immotile cilia syndrome (ICS) and the dysmotile cilia syndrome. Its prevalence in the Caucasian population is approximately one in 12,500 (Kroon et al, 1991). The same ultrastructure abnormalities are found in Kartagener syndrome, which consists of a triad of dextrocardia with situs inversus totalis, chronic sinusitis or agenesis of the frontal sinuses, and bronchiectasis. The prevalence of Kartagener syndrome has been estimated at one per 50,000 population, whereas the prevalence of situs inversus is one per 8000 (Adams and Churchill, 1937). Bronchiectasis, which occurs in less than 0.5 percent of the general population, is found in up to 25 percent of patients with situs inversus (Olsen, 1943). Kartagener syndrome has been reported among family members; in these cases, the mode of inheritance is thought to be autosomal recessive. Penetrance is variable, as siblings may have bronchiectasis without situs inversus (see subsequent discussion), reflecting the similarities being the result of an inherited disorder, primary ciliary dyskinesia (PCD). An important component of this syndrome is male infertility. Women with Kartagener syndrome have borne children, however.

It should be noted that not all people with dextrocardia and situs inversus have Kartagener syndrome, PCD, or male infertility. Also, dextrocardia with or without situs inversus may be associated with other anomalies, such as single ventricle, arterial transposition, pulmonary stenosis, ventricular and atrial septal defects, and asplenia. However, associations of other congenital heart defects and esophageal anomalies with PCD have been reported (Engesaeth et al, 1993).

Pathogenesis

Ciliated epithelia are present in the respiratory tract, paranasal sinuses, eustachian tubes, oviducts, and vas efferentia. Inborn errors of cilia structure and ciliary function explain upper respiratory tract pathology in PCD. Mucociliary transport is maintained by the rhythmic beating of cilia. Cilia and sperm tails each contain nine microtubular doublet filaments, which are arranged symmetrically and radially around a central doublet and are connected to each other by nexin links and to the central sheath by radial spokes. Energy for the shortening of the outer microtubular filaments is provided by the hydrolysis of ATP by ATPase contained in dynein arms, which are attached to one of each doublet. The bending motion and the direction of ciliary beating occurs because of the orientation of the outer microtubules to the central tubules. Absence of dynein arms, radial spokes, or shortening of central tubules has been detected by electron microscopy in patients with inherited (primary) functional immotile cilia, dysmotile cilia, and Kartagener syndrome. Similar structural and functional abnormalities also may be found in bronchitis and other non-inherited bronchial inflammatory conditions. However, in these cases, the percent of abnormal cilia is much less than in PCD; the abnormalities are transient, reverting to normal when inflammation subsides.

Immotile cilia also may be one important factor accounting for situs inversus (Afzelius, 1976). Unidirectional embryonic ciliary beating determines organ spiral orientation. There is an even chance of rotation to either side in the absence of ciliary movement. Thus, situs inversus occurs by chance. Dysmotile cilia and sperm may be found in patients without situs inversus, and 50 percent of those with this defect will have normal organ orientation.

Respiratory Manifestations

Impaired removal of secretions results in sinusitis, otitis media, and recurrent bronchitis. Children with PCD may present with neonatal respiratory distress. Symptoms of cough, rhinitis, wheezing, and other respiratory difficulties may begin in the first year of life or later. *Haemophilus influenzae* and *Streptococcus pneumoniae* cause recurrent pneumonia in contrast to *Staphylococcus* and *Pseudomonas* organisms, which are common pathogens of CF. Chronic pulmonary changes resemble postinfectious interstitial pneumonitis and cylindric, follicular, and saccular bronchiectasis. Persistent cough, sputum production, and recurrent fevers ensue when bronchiectasis becomes severe. Patients with situs inversus may develop left middle lobe pneumonia, atelectasis, and bronchiectasis.

Diagnosis

Situs inversus should be diagnosed in the newborn period. As many as 25 percent of these infants will develop bronchiectasis. The diagnosis of PCD syndrome should be suspected in the child with recurrent or chronic otitis media, sinusitis, bronchitis, and pneumonia. When chronic and recurrent bacterial infections occur in multiple organ sites, an immunodeficiency should be considered first. Immunoglobulin deficiency, antibody deficiency, complement deficiency, and phagocytic defects should be ruled out. The occurrence of chronic otitis media and the absence of *Pseudomonas* pathogens are unusual in CF. Atopic respiratory disease should be considered. After immune deficiency, CF, and atopy are ruled out by history, physical examination, and appropriate diagnostic tests, the PCD syndrome can be considered. Family history should be verified to include bronchiectasis, Kartagener syndrome, cardiac anomalies, and esophageal problems.

Functional and ultrastructural examinations of respiratory ciliated epithelium specimens are necessary to make the diagnosis of PCD. The validity of these tests is highly dependent on a number of factors including: (1) the absence of active infection when nasal or bronchial brush or punch biopsies are obtained, (2) adequate size of the biopsy sample with a large number of cilia for analysis, (3) the technical and interpretive skills of the electron microscopist or the light microscopist who examines ciliary beating, and (4) the frequency with which the testing is done. Standardized testing procedures have not been developed and testing is not readily available to the practicing physician, although most university medical centers can offer these services. Samples for ciliary study can be obtained from either nasal or bronchial epithelium. When most of the cilia are abnormal and dynein arm (DA) defects are predominant, a nasal sample should be enough to conclude an inherited disorder (Verra et al, 1993). When a small percentage of cilia are abnormal with various axonemal ultrastructural abnormalities (AUA = absence of outer dynein arms, absence of inner dynein arms, abnormal central complex, abnormal peripheral linkages, abnormal peripheral microtubules) or predominant central complex (CC = central microtubules and central sheath) defects associated with clinical suspicion of inherited disease, a bronchial sample should be studied. The presence of the same ultrastructural abnormalities at both levels confirms the presence of a congenital defect.

Management

Anticipatory and preventive measures should be started at the time of diagnosis. These should include immunizations against respiratory pathogens—rubeola, pertussis, influenza, *Haemophilus influenzae* type B and pneumococci—according to age and dosage recommendation; early detection of bacterial infection by culture and treatment with antibiotics; and postural drainage and chest percussion to prevent pooling of secretions. Functional endoscopic sinus surgery (FESS) may be necessary, but good studies of outcome have not been done in these disorders (Parsons et al, 1993). Reproductive and genetic issues must be addressed. With proper treatment, these disorders are compatible with normal life expectancies (Rott, 1979).

THE YOUNG SYNDROME

In addition to CF and PCD, mucociliary clearance is also impaired in patients with Young syndrome, which is characterized by obstructive azoospermia and chronic sinopulmonary infections (Young, 1970; Hendry et al, 1978; Handleman et al, 1984). A thorough study of ciliary beat frequency and ultrastructure has not revealed any functional abnormality or microtubular defects in these patients (n = 20) when compared to normal controls (de Iongh et al, 1992). It is still not possible to exclude the chance that this syndrome is a genetic variant of CF. The pediatric respiratory aspects of Young syndrome have not been characterized because a prepubertal genetic or functional marker has not yet been identified.

REFERENCES

Adams R, Churchill ED. Situs inversus, sinusitis, bronchiectasis: Report of five cases including frequency statistics. J Thorac Surg 7:206, 1937.

Afzelius BA. A human syndrome caused by immotile cilia. Science 193:317, 1976.

American Thoracic Society Board of Directors' Statement. Lung transplantation. Report of the ATS workshop on lung transplantation. Am Rev Respir Dis 147:772–776, 1993.

Auerbach HS, Kirkpatrick JA, Williams M, Colten HR: Alternate-day prednisone reduces morbidity and improves pulmonary function in cystic fibrosis. Lancet 2:686–688, 1985.

Berger M, Sorensen RU, Tosi MF, Dearborn DG, Doring G. Complement receptor expression on neutrophiles at an inflammatory site, the pseudomonas-infected lung in cystic fibrosis. J Clin Invest 84:1302–1313, 1989.

Berger M, Norvell TM, Tosi MF, Emancipator SN, Konstan MW, Schreiber JR. Tissue-specific Fcγ and complement receptor expression by alveolar macrophages determines relative importance of IgG and complement in promoting phagocytosis of *Pseudomonas aeruginosa*. Pediatr Res 35:68–77, 1994.

Birrer P, McElvaney NG, Rudenberg A, Wirz Zommer C, Liechti-Gallati S, Kraemer R, Hubbard R, Crystal RC. Protease-antiprotease imbalance in the lungs of children with cystic fibrosis. Am J Respir Crit Care Med 150:207–213, 1994.

Campbell PW, Parker RA, Roberts BT, Krishnamani MRS, Phillips JA. Association of poor clinical status and heavy exposure to tobacco smoke in patients with cystic fibrosis who are homozygous for the F508 deletion. J Pediatr 120:261–264, 1992.

Collins FS. Cystic fibrosis: Molecular biology and therapeutic implications. Science 256:774–779, 1992.

Cystic Fibrosis Foundation. Patient Registry 1992 Annual Data Report, Bethesda, Maryland, October 1993.

Cystic Fibrosis Genotype-Phenotype Consortium. Correlation between genotype and phenotype in patients with cystic fibrosis. N Engl J Med 329:1308–1313, 1993.

Day G, Mearns MB: Bronchial lability in cystic fibrosis. Arch Dis Child 48:355–359, 1973.

de Iongh R, Ing A, Rutland J. Mucociliary function, ciliary ultrastructure, and ciliary orientation in Young's syndrome. Thorax 47:184–187, 1992.

Eber E, Oberwaldner B, Zach MS. Airway obstruction and airway wall instability in cystic fibrosis: The isolated and combined effect of theophylline and sympathomimetics. Pediatr Pulmonol 4:205–212, 1988.

Edwards DF, Patton CS, Kennedy JR. Primary ciliary diskinesia in the dog. Probl Vet Med 4:291–319, 1992.

Egan TM, Detterbeck FC. Technique and results of double lung transplantation. Chest Surg Clin North Am 3:89–111, 1992.

Engesaeth VG, Warner JO, Bush A. New associations of primary ciliary dyskinesia syndrome. Pediatr Pulmonol 16:9–12, 1993.

Fiel SB. Heart-lung transplantation for patients with cystic fibrosis. Arch Intern Med 151:870–872, 1991.

FitzSimmons SC. The changing epidemiology of cystic fibrosis. J Pediatr 122:1–9, 1993.

Fujiwara TM, Morgan K, Schwartz RH, Doherty RA, Miller SR, Klinger K, Stanislovitis P, Stuart N, Watkins PC. Genealogical analysis of cystic fibrosis families and chromosome 7q RFLP haplotypes in the Hutterite Brethren. Am J Hum Genet 44:327–337, 1989.

Gaskin K, Gurwitz D, Durie P, Corey M, Levison H, Forstner G. Improved respiratory prognosis in patients with cystic fibrosis with normal fat absorption. J Pediatr 100:857–862, 1982.

Gervais R, Dumer V, Rigot J-M, Lafitte J-J, Roussel. High frequency of the R117H cystic fibrosis mutation in patients with congenital absence of the vas deferens. N Engl J Med 328:446–447, 1993.

Handleman DJ, Conway AJ, Boylan LM, Turtle JR. Young's syndrome: Obstructive azoospermia and chronic sinopulmonary infections. N Engl J Med 310:3, 1984.

Hendry WF, Knight RK, Whitfield HN, Stansfield AG, Pryse-Davies J, Ryder TA, Pavia D, Bateman JRM, Clarke SW. Obstructive azoospermia: Respiratory function tests, electron microscopy, and results of surgery. Br J Urol 50:598, 1978.

Highsmith EW, Burch LH, Zhou Z, Olsen JC, Boat TE, Spock A, Gorvoy JD, Quittel L, Friedman KJ, Silverman LM, Boucher RC, Knowles MR: A novel mutation in the cystic fibrosis gene in patients with pulmonary disease but normal sweat chloride concentrations. N Engl J Med 331:974–980, 1994.

Holzer FJ, Olinsky A, Phelan PD. Variability of airways

hyper-reactivity and allergy in cystic fibrosis. Arch Dis Child 56:455–459, 1981.

Hordvik NL, Konig P, Morris D, Kreutz C, Barbero GJ. A longitudinal study of bronchodilator responsiveness in cystic fibrosis. Am Rev Respir Dis 131:889–893, 1985.

Hubbard RC, McElvaney NG, Birrer P, Shak S, Robinson WW, Jolley C, Wu M, Chernick MS, Crystal RG. A preliminary study of aerosolized recombinant deoxyribonuclease I in the treatment of cystic fibrosis. N Engl J Med 326:812–815, 1992.

Jones K, Higgenbattam T, Wallwork J. Successful heart-lung transplantation for CF. Chest 93:644–645, 1988.

Kerem B, Rommens JM, Buchanan JA, et al. Identification of the cystic fibrosis gene: Genetic analysis. Science 245:1073–1080, 1989.

Kerem E, Reisman J, Corey M, Canny GJ, Levison H. Prediction of mortality in patients with cystic fibrosis. N Engl J Med 326:1187–1191, 1992.

Knowles MR, Clarke LL, Boucher RC. Activation by extracellular nucleotides of chloride secretion in the airway epithelia of patients with cystic fibrosis. N Engl J Med 325:533–638, 1991.

Kroon AA, Heij JM, Kuijper WA, Veerman AJ, van der Baan S. Function and morphology of respiratory cilia in situs inversus. Clin Otolaryngol 16:294–297, 1991.

Landau LI, Phelan PD. The variable effect of a bronchodilating agent on pulmonary function in cystic fibrosis. J Pediatr 82:863–868, 1973.

Laufer P, Fink JN, Bruns T, Unger GF, Kalbfleisch JH, Greenberger PA, Patterson R. Allergic bronchopulmonary aspergillosis in cystic fibrosis. J Allergy Clin Immunol 73:44–48, 1984.

Liechti-Gallati S, Malik N, Alkan M, Maechler M, Morris M, Thonney F, Sennhauser F, Moser H. Association between haplotypes and specific mutations in Swiss cystic fibrosis families. Pediatr Res 30:304–308, 1991.

Mearns M, Young W, Batten J: Transient pulmonary infiltrations in cystic fibrosis due to allergic aspergillosis. Thorax 20:385–392, 1965.

Mellis CM, Levison H. Bronchial reactivity in cystic fibrosis. Pediatrics 61:446–450, 1978.

Miller CH, Hatem F, Metlay LA, Schwartz RH, Hengerer AS. Can histologic criteria of nasal polyps be used to screen for cystic fibrosis? Pediatr Asthma Allerg Immunol 8:51–56, 1994.

Miller SR, Schwartz RH. Attitudes toward genetic testing of Amish, Mennonite, and Hutterite families with cystic fibrosis. Am J Public Health 82:236–242, 1992.

Mitchell I, Corey M, Woenne R, Krastins IRB, Levison H. Bronchial hyperreactivity in cystic fibrosis and asthma. J Pediatr 93:744–748, 1978.

Nelson LA, Callerame ML, Schwartz RH. Aspergillosis and atopy in cystic fibrosis. Am Rev Respir Dis 130:863–873, 1979.

Noritake D, Hen J, Dolan TF. Effects of aspirin on pulmonary function in patients with cystic fibrosis. Cystic Fibrosis Club Abstracts, 22nd Annual Meeting. San Francisco, CA 22:144, 1981.

Olsen AM. Bronchiectasis and dextrocardia: Observations on etiology of bronchiectasis. Am Rev Tuberc 47:435, 1943.

Olsen JC, Johnson LG, Stutts MJ, Sarkadi B, Yankaskas JR, Swanstrom R, Boucher RC. Correction of the apical membrane chloride permeability defect in polarized cystic fibrosis airway epithelia following retroviral-mediated gene transfer. Hum Gene Ther 3:253–266, 1992.

Pan S-H, Canafax DM, Le CT, Cipolle RJ, Uden DL, Warwick WJ. Bronchodilation in patients with cystic fibrosis: results of a blinded placebo-controlled crossover clinical trial. Pediatr Pulmonol 6:172–179, 1989.

Parsons DS, Greene BA. A treatment for primary ciliary dyskinesia: Efficacy of functional endoscopic sinus surgery. Laryngoscope 103:1269–1272, 1993.

Pier GB, Saunders JM, Ames P, Edwards MS, Auerbach H, Goldfarb J, Speert, Hurwitch S. Opsonophagocytic killing antibody to *Pseudomonas aeruginosa* mucoid exopolysaccharide in older noncolonized patients with cystic fibrosis. N Engl J Med 317:793–798, 1987.

Rachelefsky GS, Osher A, Dooley RE, Ank B, Stiehm ER. Coexistent respiratory allergy and cystic fibrosis. Am J Dis Child 128:355–359, 1974.

Ramsey B, et al. Efficacy and safety of short term administration of aerosolized recombinant human deoxyribonuclease in patients with cystic fibrosis. Am Rev Respir Dis 148:145–151, 1993.

Riordan JR, Rommens JM, Kerem B, et al. Identification of the cystic fibrosis gene: Cloning and characterization of complementary DNA. Science 245:1066–1073, 1989.

Ristow SC, Condemi JJ, Stuard ID, Schwartz RH, Bryson MF. Systemic amyloidosis in cystic fibrosis. Am J Dis Child 131:886–888, 1977.

Rommens JM, Iannnuzzi MC, Kerem B, et al. Identification of the cystic fibrosis gene: Chromosome walking and jumping. Science 245:1059–1065, 1989.

Roperto F, Galati P, Rossacco P. Immotile cilia syndrome in pigs, a model for human disease. Am J Pathol 143:643–647, 1993.

Rosenberg M, Patterson, Minter R, et al. Clinical and immunologic criteria for the diagnosis of allergic bronchopulmonary aspergillosis. Ann Intern Med 86:405–414, 1977.

Rosenstein BJ, Eigen H. Risks of alternate-day prednisone in patients with cystic fibrosis. Pediatrics 87:245–246, 1991.

Rott HD. Kartagener's syndrome and the syndrome of immotile cilia. Hum Genet 46:541, 1979.

Rozen R, Schwartz RH, Hilman BC, Stanislovitis P, Horn GT, Klinger K, Daigneault J, De Braekeleer M, Kerem B, Tsui L-C, Fujiwara TM, Morgan K. Cystic fibrosis mutations in North American populations of French ancestry: Analysis of Quebec French-Canadian and Louisiana Acadian Families. Am J Hum Genet 47:606–610, 1990.

Sanchez I, Holbrow, Chernick V. Acute bronchodilator response to a combination of beta-adrenergic and anticholinergic agents in patients with cystic fibrosis. J Pediatr 120:486–488, 1992.

Schidlow DV, Taussig LM, Knowles MR. Cystic fibrosis foundation consensus conference report on pulmonary complications of cystic fibrosis. Pediatr Pulmonol 15:187–198, 1993.

Schwartz RH, Johnstone DE, Holsclaw DS, Dooley RR. Serum Precipitins to *Aspergillus fumigatus* in cystic fibrosis. Am J Dis Child 120:432–433, 1970.

Schwartz RH, Hollick GE. Allergic bronchopulmonary aspergillosis with low serum IgE. J Allergy Clin Immunol 68:290–294, 1981.

Shapiro GG, Bamman J, Kanarek P, Bierman CW. The paradoxical effect of adrenergic and methylxanthine drugs in cystic fibrosis. Pediatrics 58:740–743, 1976.

Sivan Y, Arce P, Eigen H, Nickerson BG, Newth CJL. A double-blind, randomized study of sodium cromoglycate versus placebo in patients with cystic fibrosis and bronchial hyperreactivity. J Allergy Clin Immunol 85:649–654, 1990.

Tepper RS, Eigen H. Airway reactivity in cystic fibrosis. Clin Rev Allergy Cystic Fibrosis 9:24–33, 1990.

Tosi MF, Zakem H, Berger M. Neutrophil elastase cleaves C3bi on opsonized pseudomonas as well as CR1 on neutrophils to create a functionally important receptor mismatch. J Clin Invest 86:300–308, 1990.

Tsui L-C. Mutations and sequence variations detected in the cystic fibrosis transmembrane conductance regulator (CFTR) gene: A report from the cystic fibrosis genetic analysis consortium. Human Mutation 1:197–203, 1992a.

Tsui L-C. The spectrum of cystic fibrosis mutations. Trends in Genetics 8:392–398, 1992b.

Van Asperen P, Mellis CM, South RT. Bronchial reactivity in cystic fibrosis with normal pulmonary function. Am J Dis Child 135:815–819, 1981.

Vera F, Fleury-Feith J, Boucherat M, Pinchon M-C, Bignon J, Escudier E. Do nasal ciliary changes reflect bronchial changes? An ultrastructural study. Am Rev Respir Dis 147:908–913, 1993.

Wilmott RW. The relationship between atopy and cystic fibrosis. Clin Rev Allergy 9:29–46, 1991.

Yang Y, Engelhardt JF, Wilson JM. Ultrastructural localization of variant forms of cystic fibrosis transmembrane conductance regulator in human bronchial epithelia of xenografts. Am J Respir Cell Mol Biol 11:7–15, 1994.

Young D. Surgical treatment of male infertility. J Reprod Fertil 23:541, 1970.

Zach MS, Oberwaldner B, Forche G, Polgar G. Bronchodilators increase airway instability in cystic fibrosis. Am Rev Resp Dis 131:537–543, 1985.

Zielenski J, Fujiwara TM, Markiewicz D, Paradis AJ, Anacleto I, Richards B, Schwartz RH, Klinger KW, Tsui L-C, Morgan K. Identification of the M1101K mutation in the cystic fibrosis transmembrane conductance regulator (CFTR) gene and complete detection of cystic fibrosis mutations in the Hutterite population. Am J Hum Genet 52:609–615, 1993.

Chapter 42
Bronchopulmonary Dysplasia

Denise M. Coleman, M.D., and Shirley Murphy, M.D.

Bronchopulmonary dysplasia (BPD) is a chronic lung disease that develops in infants following acute lung injury in the neonatal period. The most common cause of acute lung injury in the neonate is hyaline membrane disease, which is a disease of premature infants characterized by surfactant deficiency, a marked decrease in lung compliance, airway inflammation, and an abnormal permeability of the alveolar-capillary membrane (O'Brodovich and Mellins, 1985; Watterberg et al, 1993). Respiratory failure may develop in these premature infants, necessitating mechanical ventilation with supplemental oxygen. Iatrogenic injury from barotrauma and oxygen toxicity compound the initial lung injury, causing further lung damage. BPD may also follow acute lung injury secondary to meconium aspiration, pneumonia, persistent fetal circulation, and apnea requiring mechanical ventilation (Edwards, 1988).

For the purposes of this discussion, BPD will be defined as a chronic lung disease that develops in the neonatal period and is characterized by a requirement for supplemental oxygen at one month of age with an abnormal chest radiograph (hyperinflation and streaky densities interspersed with cystic changes). BPD was first described in 1967 by Northway and co-workers in a group of premature infants who developed a "chronic pulmonary syndrome" following mechanical ventilation for hyaline membrane disease (Northway et al, 1967). Since that time, BPD has been recognized as an important cause of morbidity in the newborn intensive care unit. Twenty-five years after its initial description, there continues to be much disagreement regarding not only specific diagnostic criteria but also a specific definition for BPD. This may partially explain the marked differences in incidence reported in the literature, with the incidence ranging from 2.4 to 68 percent (O'Brodovich and Mellins, 1985). There is an inverse relationship between birth weight and the incidence of BPD developing in premature infants who required mechanical ventilation. The incidence of BPD in infants weighing less than 700 gm approaches 100 percent, decreasing to 25 percent in those infants with birth weights of 1000 to 1500 gm (Alpert et al, 1993).

While advances in neonatology have improved the mortality rate for hyaline membrane disease, the overall incidence of BPD has not changed in the past two decades (Northway, 1990). This may be explained in part by the improved survival of very-low-birth-weight infants today, in whom the incidence of BPD is high, as opposed to 25 years ago when this population of infants would not have survived.

PATHOGENESIS

The factors that are most often implicated in the development of BPD are closely interrelated. An initial lung injury from hyaline membrane disease, for example, is followed by oxygen toxicity, which triggers pulmonary injury not only by the host's inflammatory responses but also by barotrauma from positive pressure ventilation. Hyaline membrane disease is complicated by pulmonary edema, which is often worsened by left-to-right shunting through a patent ductus arteriosus (O'Brodovich and Mellins, 1985). Oxygen toxicity also leads to pulmonary edema, surfactant dysfunction, free-radical production, and an infiltration of polymorphonuclear leukocytes into the lung (Massaro, 1986). Barotrauma causes epithelial damage, leading to a necrotizing bronchiolitis and possibly to pulmonary air leaks that could prolong the need for mechanical ventilation.

Premature infants with hyaline membrane disease have been shown to develop an influx of alveolar macrophages and neutrophils into the airways in the first 2 to 4 days of life (Ogden et al, 1983). In those infants who eventually develop BPD, the neutrophil count remains elevated for several weeks with declining alveolar macrophages, whereas those who do not have BPD have neutrophil counts that return to normal by 4 days of life and normal macrophage counts. This influx of neutrophils into the airways may contribute to the lung injury that occurs in the development of BPD by the production of free radicals and the release of elastase. Ogden and co-workers (1983) found an elevation of elastase to alpha-1-protease inhibitor ratio in bronchoalveolar lavage of infants who developed BPD when compared to bronchoalveolar lavage of infants with uncomplicated hyaline membrane disease. Elastase has also been found in the tracheal aspirates of infants with documented infection and hyperoxic exposure (Bruce et al, 1992). Other studies have shown a decrease in protease inhibition in infants who were mechanically ventilated with an FiO_2 greater than 0.60 for more than 5 days (Bruce et al, 1982). This imbalance between elastase production and its inhibition may lead to destruction of elastic fibers in the lung. They have postulated that, since elastic fibers in the lung form the framework for alveolar septation, their destruction explains in part the pathology seen in BPD (Bruce et al, 1992).

Viscardi and co-investigators (1992) found an imbalance between coagulation and fibrinolysis in premature infants with hyaline membrane disease. By evaluating lung lavage samples in premature infants, they showed depressed fibrinolytic activity in the first 7 to 10 days of life in the face of preserved procoagulant activity, which was associated with the severity of lung disease at 24 hours of life as determined by radiographs and elevated airway resistance.

Abnormal ratios of collagen types have been reported by Shoemaker and co-investigators (1984) as having a role in the pathogenesis of BPD. An increased ratio of type I collagen to type III in infants with chronic lung disease has been found with hyaline membrane disease and pulmonary fibrosis from a variety of causes. Since type I collagen is less compliant than type III it appears to play a role in lung pathophysiology seen in infants with BPD on postmortem examination.

PATHOLOGY

BPD pulmonary pathology has largely been determined by postmortem examinations of infants and children who have died and thus represents the extreme form of this disease. Extrapolation of these data to apply to the less severely affected children with milder forms of BPD should be cautiously interpreted, since there are no reports to date of autopsies done on children with mild BPD who have died from other causes.

Northway, in 1967, in the first description of BPD, reported four stages of a disease process that progressed along a continuum beginning with hyaline membrane disease and ending with chronic lung disease (Northway et al, 1967). Because of advances in neonatal intensive care in the past 2 decades, the classic four stages originally described are no longer seen. Stage four (the chronic phase, that period beyond one month) was reported to be associated with alveolar distention, peribronchiolar smooth muscle hypertrophy, increased number of inflammatory cells, squamous metaplasia of the airways, focal thickening of alveolar basement membranes, tortuous lymphatics, and vascular medial hypertrophy.

Studies of the pathology of BPD as well as morphometric analyses through the ensuing years have reported similar findings. Bonikos and co-investigators, in 1976, found large and small airway ciliary damage, necrotizing bronchiolitis, squamous metaplasia of bronchial and bronchiolar epithelium, bronchiolar fibrosis, alveolar septal fibrosis, areas of atelectasis, and areas of overdistended alveoli. Vascular changes consisted of small to medium-sized arteries and arterioles with hyperplastic endothelial cells, medial hypertrophy, and intimal thickening. In 1991, Margraf and co-workers compared the lungs of infants and children who had died secondary to BPD with the lungs of term infants and children who had died from nonpulmonary complications. All of the children in the BPD group had heights and weights less than the fifth percentile for age as well as a decrease in the total number of alveoli when compared to children near their same age who did not have a pulmonary disease. The findings in the BPD group revealed dilated alveoli, abnormal distribution and structure of elastic fibers, decreased lung volumes, an increase in submucous glands, hypertrophy of the smooth muscle of the large and small airways, squamous metaplasia, and submucosal fibrosis.

Overall, the pathologic findings appear to be reproducible over time in infants with varying degrees of clinical severity of BPD. However, within an individual patient's lungs there can be marked variability of pathologic findings, with severely affected areas interspersed with relatively normal areas (Abman and Bancalari, 1987). The reasons are not well understood.

CLINICAL FINDINGS

The diagnosis of BPD is not usually made until the age of one month. The infant with BPD has clinical evidence of abnormal pulmonary physiology manifested as shallow, rapid respirations, persistent retractions, and a hyperinflated chest; requires supplemental oxygen; and has an abnormal chest roentgenogram. These infants often have poor growth, with weight and height measurements less than the fifth percentile for age, even after correcting for their prematurity. They may require extremely high calorie diets of greater than 150 Kcal per kilogram per day in order to grow well. Infants with BPD have abnormal gas exchange, as evidenced by hypoxia on room air and a metabolic compensated respiratory acidosis on blood gas evaluations. Radiographically there is hyperinflation with dense fibrotic-appearing streaks interspersed with cystic-appearing areas. Pulmonary function testing reveals increased airway resistance, decreased dynamic compliance, increased functional residual capacity, and bronchial hyperreactivity (O'Brodovich and Mellins, 1985; Abman and Bancalari, 1987; Northway, 1992; Northway et al, 1990). Infants with BPD often develop right ventricular hypertrophy secondary to increased pulmonary artery pressure and increased pulmonary vascular resistance that is variably responsive to supplemental oxygen therapy (Abman and Bancalari, 1987; Berman et al, 1982). This pulmonary hypertension can progress to cor pulmonale unless treated. Left ventricular hypertrophy has also been described.

MEDICAL MANAGEMENT

Prevention of BPD

SURFACTANT THERAPY. The use of exogenous surfactant in premature newborns is currently the standard of care at most centers. While widespread use of surfactant therapy has decreased the mortality from hyaline membrane disease, there has been no overall change in the incidence of BPD (Farrell and Zimmerman, 1992; Long et al, 1991; Rozycki and Kirkpatrick, 1993). The recommended dose varies, depending on which preparation is used.

CONVENTIONAL VENTILATION. Because of the high mean airway pressures and high FiO_2 that are often required to prevent hypoxia and adequately ventilate the noncompliant lungs in hyaline membrane disease, conventional mechanical ventilation is implicated in the treatment of BPD. Ideally, the infant should be ventilated with the lowest FiO_2 and peak inspiratory pressure tolerated. Guidelines for initial ventilator settings, as recommended by Viscardi and Fox (1991), can be found in Table 42–1.

High-frequency positive pressure ventilation may decrease the risk of barotrauma, but it has not been shown to decrease the incidence of BPD. Neither high-frequency jet ventilation nor high-frequency oscillatory ventilation decreased the incidence of BPD when compared to mechanical ventilation (HIFI Study Group, 1989). Clark and co-investigators (1990) studied lower-birth-weight infants using lower frequencies and a shorter inspiratory phase and found no difference in the mortality when compared to conventional ventilation, but they showed a decreased incidence of BPD from 65 percent in conventional ventilation to 30 percent in high-frequency ventilation. To date, there

TABLE 42–1. GUIDELINES FOR VENTILATOR MANAGEMENT IN RDS

INITIAL SETTINGS

1. FiO_2 as needed to keep O_2 saturation >92%
2. Flow rate 6–10 L/min
3. IMV 30–60 breaths/min
4. PIP as necessary to generate adequate breath sounds and chest excursions (typically 20–25 cm H_2O)
5. PEEP 4–5 cm H_2O
6. Inspiratory time 0.2–0.5 sec

ASSESSMENT

1. Observation of color, chest expansion, auscultation of breath sounds
2. Transcutaneous PaO_2 or pulse oximetry monitoring
3. ABG 15–20 minutes after pressure or rate change and after 5–10% change in FiO_2

RECOMMENDATION FOR VENTILATOR CHANGES

PaO_2 (torr)	$PaCO_2$ (torr)	FiO_2	PEEP	PIP	IMV
<50	<40	↑	↑		
<50	>50	↑		↑ (1)	↑ (2)
>80	<40	↓ (1)		↓ (1)	↓ (2)
>80	>50	↓	↓		

Note: Several changes may accomplish the same thing. Changes marked as (1) are usually the most effective. Rule of weaning: decrease the most harmful parameter first. In general, PIP preferentially if PIP >30; FiO_2 >0.60.

From Viscardi RM, Fox RE. Respiratory distress syndrome and related disorders. In Donn SM, Faix RG (eds): Neonatal Emergencies. Mount Kisco, Futura Publishing Company, Inc, 1991, pp 253–267.

---

have been no published studies evaluating the incidence of BPD with the use of high-frequency flow interruption.

STEROIDS. The use of steroids in the treatment of hyaline membrane disease has been theorized to be effective in the improvement of pulmonary function in infants because they may decrease inflammation and decrease the production of type I collagen (a noncompliant form of collagen found in increased ratios in the lungs of infants with BPD (Thompson et al, 1993). Cummings and co-workers (1989) performed a randomized, double-blind, controlled trial of dexamethasone therapy in premature infants with hyaline membrane disease with birth weights of 1250 gm or less. At 2 weeks of age, infants who were ventilator and oxygen dependent were assigned to a placebo group, or to an 18-day trial or a 42-day trial of dexamethasone. The longer course of steroids led to continued improvement in pulmonary function and better neurodevelopmental outcome than the other two study groups. The group that received long-term steroids had a decreased duration of mechanical ventilation and supplemental oxygen and decreased hospitalization. The treatment group had no more complications than the placebo group. Yoder et al (1991) evaluated ventilator-dependent infants with BPD. After 3 days of intravenous steroid therapy, there was an improvement in pulmonary mechanics and a decrease in pulmonary inflammation in the treatment group when compared to the placebo group. Kari and co-workers (1993) evaluated the use of a one-week course of high-dose intravenous steroids at 10 days of life in very-low-birth-weight premature infants and its effects on pulmonary status, the severity of BPD, and the incidence of side effects. There was no difference in outcome at 28 days and at one year when compared to placebo; nor was there a difference in complications such as sepsis.

Accepted treatment of BPD is dexamethasone, 0.25 mg/kg/12 hours, given orally or intravenously for 3 days, decreased to 0.3 mg/kg/24 hours for 3 days, and then tapered 10 to 20 percent every 3 days (Davis et al, 1990).

CROMOLYN SODIUM. It has been postulated that cromolyn sodium, because of its anti-inflammatory activity, might be useful in preventing the inflammation-mediated damage that occurs in the lungs in hyaline membrane disease. Watterberg and Murphy showed no difference in the incidence of BPD in two study groups of infants with birth weights less than 1000 gm and birth weights between 1000 and 2000 gm who received 20 mg of nebulized cromolyn sodium or placebo four times a day from birth to one month of age (Watterberg et al, 1993).

Acute and Chronic Management

DIURETICS. Diuretics improve pulmonary status in BPD in both acute and chronic management. In 1983, Kao and co-workers showed acute improvement in pulmonary mechanics in infants with chronic BPD one hour after furosemide administration. In 1987, Kao and co-investigators evaluated the effects of combined theophylline and diuretic therapy of spironolactone and chlorothiazide on pulmonary mechanics in infants with BPD, and found an additive effect leading to improved pulmonary function. Albersheim and co-investigators (1989) evaluated the effects of long-term hydrochlorothiazide and spironolactone therapy on pulmonary function of infants with BPD who were mechanically ventilated, and found that treatment reduced mechanical ventilation from 57 to 26 percent of infants who were discharged alive.

Commonly used doses of diuretics are listed in Table 42–2. Side effects associated with the use of these diuretics include electrolyte abnormalities such as hypokalemia, metabolic alkalosis, hypercalciuria, osteopenia, and ototoxicity (Davis et al, 1990).

BRONCHODILATORS. Bronchodilators have been used in BPD to treat the bronchospasm that often occurs in association with airway smooth muscle hypertrophy with a significant clinical response.

Wilkie and Bryan (1987) found that administration of salbutamol as well as ipratropium bromide resulted in improvement in respiratory resistance and respiratory compliance. Brundage et al (1990) evaluated the bronchodilator response to ipratropium bromide in mechanically ventilated infants with BPD as well as response to combined therapy with salbutamol. Combined therapy resulted in decreased respiratory resistance. Beta$_2$-agonist agents, by oral administration, improve gas exchange and airway conductance without adverse cardiovascular effect (Farrell and Zimmerman, 1992).

Albuterol, 2.5 mg every 2 to 4 hours, and ipratropium bromide, 0.025 to 0.05 mg/kg administered by inhalation every 6 to 8 hours, are effective, as is aminophylline administered intravenously or theophylline orally. Theophylline should be given as a loading dose of 5 mg/kg and a maintenance dose of 2 mg/kg every 8 to 12 hours for a therapeutic serum concentration of 5 to 15 mg/l (Davis et al, 1990). Serum concentrations greater than 20 µg/ml have been associated with severe side effects, such as arrhythmias, seizures, and death (Katz and McWilliams, 1988; Katz and Samet 1988).

ANTI-INFLAMMATORY MEDICATIONS. While cromolyn sodium does not decrease the incidence of BPD, it does have an anti-inflammatory action that is useful in chronic management. In any child with BPD who requires daily bronchodilator therapy, cromolyn sodium should be considered at a dose of 20 mg via nebulizer every 6 to 12 hours.

Steroids may be necessary in the treatment of patients with BPD with reactive airway disease. (See the discussion in the previous section on the use of steroids.) A child who fails to improve with the addition of cromolyn sodium to chronic medication may improve with the addition of inhaled steroids. The development of infant spacers makes this therapy practical. We recommend the use of beclomethasone, two to four puffs two to four times daily.

Chronic systemic steroids should be avoided, but short bursts of oral steroids may be needed for 3 to 5 days to treat respiratory exacerbations in BPD. (Prednisone doses: 1 mg/kg every 12 hours for one day, then 1 mg/kg every day for 2 days, then discontinue.) Steroid therapy should be individualized, with longer courses used in those patients who rebound after discontinuation of systemic steroids.

COMPLICATIONS

The list of complications associated with BPD is extensive, and a complete discussion is beyond the scope of this chapter (Table 42–3) (Alpert et al, 1993). The more com-

TABLE 42–2. COMMONLY USED DIURETICS IN BPD

Furosemide	0.5–2.0 mg/kg dose IV or PO given bid (qd in infants <31 weeks postconceptional age)
Chlorothiazide	5–20 mg/kg/dose IV or PO given bid
Spironolactone	1.5 mg/kg/dose PO given bid

From Davis JM, Sinkin RA, Aranda JV: Drug therapy for bronchopulmonary dysplasia. Pediatr Pulmonol 8:117–125, 1990.

TABLE 42-3. LONG-TERM COMPLICATIONS ASSOCIATED WITH BPD

Respiratory
    Chronic respiratory distress
    Respiratory acidosis
    Bronchospasm
    Recurrent pneumonia
    Ventilator dependency
    Tracheostomy
    Subglottic stenosis
    Tracheomegaly
    Tracheomalacia
    Bronchomalacia
    Airway granulation tissue and pseudopolyps
    Acquired lobar emphysema
    Laryngospasm
    Apnea
    Atelectasis
    Chronic hypoxemia
    Sleep hypoxemia
    Sudden death
Gastrointestinal
    Gastroesophageal reflux
    Aspiration
    Behavioral feeding disorders
    Oral movement disorder
Metabolic
    Metabolic alkalosis
    Hypokalemia
    Hypochloremia
    Elevated metabolic rate
    Failure to thrive
    Rickets of prematurity
Cardiovascular
    Pulmonary hypertension
    Right ventricular hypertrophy
    Systemic hypertension
    Left ventricular hypertrophy
    Heart failure
    Patent foramen ovale
    Occult congenital heart disease
    Systemic-to-pulmonary arterial shunts
Renal
    Nephrocalcinosis
Neurologic
    Developmental delay
    Static encephalopathy
    Progressive encephalopathy
    Movement disorders
    Seizures
    Visual impairment
    Hearing impairment
    Oromotor feeding disorders

From Alpert BE, Allen JL, Schidlow DV: Bronchopulmonary dysplasia. In Hilman BC (ed). Pediatric Respiratory Disease: Diagnosis and Treatment. Philadelphia, WB Saunders, 1993, pp 440–457.

monly seen complications include gastroesophageal reflux, pulmonary hypertension, and tracheobronchomalacia.

Gastroesophageal reflux should be suspected in those infants who are not responding to routine management of respiratory symptoms or who have a history of chronic emesis. For reflux, medical management with metoclopromide, 0.1 mg/kg/dose, given orally four times a day before meals and at bedtime, is indicated. Cisapride, a substituted piperidinyl benzamide, or bethanechol may also be tried. If medical treatment fails, a Nissen fundoplication may be needed.

Pulmonary hypertension leading to cor pulmonale can best be avoided by the use of chronic supplemental oxygen therapy. Many children are discharged home from the nursery on oxygen by nasal cannula because they exhibit hypoxemia and pulmonary hypertension on room air. Serial echocardiograms evaluating pulmonary artery acceleration times size and function of the right ventricle, tricuspid regurgitation, and presence of right ventricular hypertrophy as an indicator of pulmonary hypertension are recommended every 3 to 6 months. When serial echocardiograms have been normal and the child's transcutaneous oxygen saturation is normal on room air, weaning from oxygen therapy can begin by limiting to nocturnal use only. If no pulmonary hypertension is found on a follow-up echocardiogram and the child is growing well, oxygen may be discontinued.

An infant with a history of prolonged intubation and mechanical ventilation who persists with chronic wheezing despite bronchodilators or worsens with the use of these agents should alert the health care provider to the possibility of tracheobronchomalacia. Infants with tracheobronchomalacia may have a history of frequent bradycardic and hypoxic episodes with or without a history of stridor. Bethanechol, 2.9 mg/m^2 given orally every 8 hours, is a recommended pharmacologic treatment for tracheomalacia by Panitch and co-workers (1990). Positive pressure ventilation via a tracheostomy may be indicated should tracheobronchomalacia persist, interfere with growth, or be life-threatening.

LONG-TERM PROGNOSIS

The long-term pulmonary outcome of BPD is still evolving. The disease itself was first described 25 years ago, and today infants with much lower birth weights are surviving and developing BPD. Northway and co-workers (1990) studied infants born between 1969 and 1973. They had asymptomatic airway obstruction and bronchial hyperresponsiveness and hyperinflation.

Blayney and co-investigators (1991) studied infants born between 1977 and 1980 with mean gestational ages of 29 weeks and birth weights of 1228 grams who had been ventilated for 29 days and had 202 days of supplemental oxygen on average. They were growing well and had expected increases in total lung capacity (TLC) and forced expiratory volume at one second (FEV_1) between age 7 and age 10 years. These children did have elevated residual volumes (RV), some reduction of FEV_1, forced expiratory flow rate between 25 and 75 percent of vital capacity (FEF_{25-75}), and bronchial hyperreactivity when compared to standards for age. This study did not include the more severely ill patients who are currently surviving in the 1990s with birth weights less than 1000 gm and require months of mechanical ventilation.

Once discharged from the newborn intensive care unit, the patients with BPD continue to have significant pulmonary morbidity. In the first year after discharge from the hospital, the incidence of readmission to the hospital for respiratory distress is as high as 50 percent (Rozycki and Kirkpatrick, 1993). Katz and co-investigators (1988) found that 49 percent of patients with BPD had been hospitalized at least once, and that 17 percent had been hospitalized three or more times. These infants have little respiratory reserve and can become severely ill with minor illnesses such as viral upper respiratory tract infections. Infants with BPD are at risk for serious complications from respiratory syncytial virus infections (Groothius et al, 1988) and also are at risk of sudden unexpected death (Abman et al, 1989).

Cerebral palsy, hearing deficits, and retinopathy of prematurity are also occasionally seen in these patients. Thompson et al (1993) found that 61 percent of all births less than 1250 grams survived to discharge. Twenty-two percent had major handicaps at 2 years of age, and 37 percent of the survivors required hospitalization in their first year.

In summary, infants with BPD can have multiple sequelae following a prolonged hospitalization for prematurity. These infants may be difficult to manage medically. A multidisciplinary approach involving physicians, pediatric nurses, nutritionists, respiratory therapists, and social workers may be extremely helpful in the overall management of these infants and their many special needs.

REFERENCES

Abman SH, Bancalari E. The Aspen conference on bronchopulmonary dysplasia. Pediatr Pulmonol 3:185–196, 1987.

Abman SH, Burchell MF, Schaffer MS, Rosenberg AA. Late sudden unexpected deaths in hospitalized infants with bronchopulmonary dysplasia. Am J Dis Child 143:815–819, 1989.

Albersheim SG, Solimano AJ, Sharma AK, et al. Randomized, double-blind, controlled trial of long-term diuretic therapy for bronchopulmonary dysplasia. J Pediatr 115:615–620, 1989.

Alpert BE, Allen JL, Schidlow DV. Bronchopulmonary dysplasia. In Hilman BC (ed). Pediatric Respiratory Disease: Diagnosis and Treatment. Philadelphia, WB Saunders, 1993, pp 440–457.

Berman W Jr, Yabek SM, Dillon T, et al. Evaluation of infants with bronchopulmonary dysplasia using cardiac catheterization. Pediatrics 70:708–712, 1982.

Blayney M, Kerem E, Whyte H, O'Brodovich H. Bronchopulmonary dysplasia: Improvement in lung function between 7 and 10 years of age. J Pediatr 118:201–206, 1991.

Bonikos DS, Bensch KG, Northway WH, Edwards DK. Bronchopulmonary dysplasia: The pulmonary pathologic sequel of necrotizing bronchiolitis and pulmonary fibrosis. Hum Pathol 7:643–666, 1976.

Bruce MC, Boat TF, Martin RJ, et al. Proteinase inhibitors and inhibitor activation in neonatal airways secretions. Chest 81S:44S–45S, 1982.

Bruce MC, Schuyler M, Martin RJ, et al. Risk factors for the degradation of lung elastic fibers in the ventilated neonate. Am Rev Respir Dis 146:204–212, 1992.

Brundage KL, Mohsini KG, Froese AB, Fisher JT. Bronchodilator response to ipratropium bromide in infants with bronchopulmonary dysplasia. Am Rev Respir Dis 142:1137–1142, 1990.

Clark RH, Gertsmann DR, Null DM Jr, et al. High-frequency oscillatory ventilation reduces the incidence of severe chronic lung disease in respiratory distress syndrome. Am Rev Respir Dis 141:A686, 1990.

Cummings JJ, D'Eugenio DB, Gross SJ. A controlled trial of dexamethasone in preterm infants at high risk for bronchopulmonary dysplasia. N Engl J Med 320:1505–1510, 1989.

Davis JM, Sinkin RA, Aranda JV. Drug therapy for bronchopulmonary dysplasia. Pediatr Pulmonol 8:117–125, 1990.

Edwards DK III. The radiology of bronchopulmonary dysplasia and its complications. In Merritt TA, Northway WH, et al (eds). Bronchopulmonary Dysplasia. Boston, Blackwell Scientific, 1988, pp 185–234.

Farrell PM, Zimmerman JJ. Bronchopulmonary dysplasia. Curr Opinion Pediatr 4:410–416, 1992.

Groothius JR, Gutierrez KM, Lauer BA. Respiratory syncytial virus infection in children with bronchopulmonary dysplasia. Pediatrics 82:199–203, 1988.

HIFI Study Group. High-frequency oscillatory ventilation compared with conventional mechanical ventilation in the treatment of respiratory failure in preterm infants. N Engl J Med 320:88–93, 1989.

Kao LC, Durand DJ, Phillips BL, Nickerson BG. Oral theophylline and diuretics improve pulmonary mechanics in infants with bronchopulmonary dysplasia. J Pediatr 111:439–444, 1987.

Kao LC, Warburton D, Sargent CW, et al. Furosemide acutely decreases airways resistance in chronic bronchopulmonary dysplasia. J Pediatr 103:624–629, 1983.

Kari MA, Heinonen K, Ikonen RS, et al. Dexamethasone treatment in preterm infants at risk for bronchopulmonary dysplasia. Arch Dis Child 68:566–569, 1993.

Katz RW, McWilliams BC. Bronchopulmonary dysplasia in the pediatric intensive care unit. Crit Care Clin 4:755–787, 1988.

Katz RW, Samet J. Longitudinal study of respiratory morbidity of infants with bronchopulmonary dysplasia. Am Rev Respir Dis 137 (Suppl):A235, 1988. (Abstract)

Long W, Thompson T, Sundell H, et al. Effects of two rescue doses of a synthetic surfactant on mortality rate and survival without bronchopulmonary dysplasia in infants in 700-1350 gram infants with respiratory distress syndrome. J Pediatr 118:595–605, 1991.

Margraf LR, Tomashefski JF, Bruce MC, Dahms BB. Morphometric analysis of the lung in bronchopulmonary dysplasia. Am Rev Respir Dis 143:391–400, 1991.

Massaro D. Oxygen: Toxicity and tolerance. Hosp Pract 21(7):95–101, 1986.

Northway WH. Bronchopulmonary dysplasia: Then and now. Arch Dis Child 65:1076–1081, 1990.

Northway WH. Bronchopulmonary dysplasia: Twenty-five years later. Pediatrics 89:969–973, 1992.

Northway WH, Moss RB, Carlisle KB, et al. Late pulmonary sequelae of bronchopulmonary dysplasia. N Engl J Med 323:1793–1799, 1990.

Northway WH, Rosan RC, Porter DY. Pulmonary disease following respirator therapy of hyaline-membrane disease: Bronchopulmonary dysplasia. N Engl J Med 276:357–368, 1967.

O'Brodovich, Mellins RB. Bronchopulmonary dysplasia: Unresolved neonatal lung injury. Am Rev Respir Dis 132:694–709, 1985.

Ogden BE, Murphy S, Saunders GC, Johnson JD. Lung lavage of newborns with respiratory distress syndrome. Prolonged neutrophil influx is associated with bronchopulmonary dysplasia. Chest 5:31S–33S, 1983.

Panitch HB, Esteban NK, Motley RA, et al. Effect of altering smooth muscle tone on maximal expiratory flows in patients with tracheobronchomalacia. Pediatr Pulmonol 9:170–176, 1990.

Rozycki HJ, Kirkpatrick BV. New developments in bronchopulmonary dysplasia. Pediatr Ann 22(9):532–538, 1993.

Shoemaker CT, Reiser KM, Goetzman BW, Last JA. Elevated ratios of type I/III collagen in the lungs of chronically ventilated neonates with respiratory distress. Pediatr Res 18:1176–1180, 1984.

Thompson CM, Buccimazza SS, Webster J, et al. Infants of less than 1250 grams birth weight at Groote Schuur Hospital: Outcome at 1 and 2 years of age. Pediatrics 91:961–968, 1993.

Viscardi RM, Broderick K, Sun CJ, et al. Disordered pathways of fibrin turnover in lung lavage of premature infants with respiratory distress syndrome. Am Rev Respir Dis 146:492–499, 1992.

Viscardi RM, Fox RE. Respiratory distress syndrome and related disorders. In Donn SM, Faix RG (eds). Neonatal Emergencies. Mount Kisco, Futura Publishing Company, 1991, pp 253–267.

Watterberg KL, Murphy S, et al. Failure of cromolyn sodium to reduce the incidence of bronchopulmonary dysplasia: A pilot study. Pediatrics 91:803–806, 1993.

Wilkie RA, Bryan MH. Effect of bronchodilators on airway resistance in ventilator-dependent neonates with chronic lung disease. J Pediatr 111:278–282, 1987.

Yoder MC Jr, Chua R, Tepper R. Effect of dexamethasone on pulmonary inflammation and pulmonary function of ventilator-dependent infants with bronchopulmonary dysplasia. Am Rev Respir Dis 143:1044–1048, 1991.

Chapter 43

Chronic Obstructive Pulmonary Diseases in Adults

Eric C. Kleerup, M.D., and Donald P. Tashkin, M.D.

An imprecise clinical syndrome characterized by obstruction to expiratory airflow, chronic obstructive pulmonary disease (COPD) is an ill-defined mixture of three elements—chronic bronchitis, emphysema and small airways disease (Snider, 1989). These three disease entities can be characterized pathologically but their clinical and physiologic manifestations overlap and interact such that it is difficult to assign a single element to any patient. Combined together in varying proportions they comprise a broad spectrum of disease known as COPD. In the United States, 15 to 30 million individuals are affected by COPD, which contributes to one-fifth of all deaths. Specifically excluded from COPD are a number of well-defined disease entities such as asthma, cystic fibrosis, bronchiectasis and chronic pulmonary infections such as tuberculosis.

DEFINITIONS AND PATHOLOGY

Chronic bronchitis has been defined as the condition of subjects with chronic or recurrent excess mucus secretion into the bronchial tree (American Thoracic Society, 1987). Clinically, production of any sputum, whether expectorated or swallowed, and in most instances accompanied by chronic cough, occurring on most days for at least 3 months of the year for at least 2 consecutive years, defines chronic bronchitis. Specifically excluded from this definition are bronchiectasis and chronic bronchopulmonary infections. Pathologically, chronic bronchitis can be equated with *mucus hypersecretion*—hypertrophy and hyperplasia of the subepithelial tracheobronchial mucus glands (Thurlbeck, 1990). Accompanying this is dilation of gland ducts, inflammation and variable amounts of goblet cell metaplasia, and smooth muscle hyperplasia. Ciliary abnormalities, including replacement of ciliated epithelium with squamous metaplasia, may also be present.

Emphysema is defined pathologically as a condition of the lung characterized by abnormal permanent enlargement of the air spaces distal to the terminal bronchiole, accompanied by destruction of their walls, and without obvious fibrosis (American Thoracic Society, 1987). Destruction results not simply in overinflation, but also in nonuniformity in the pattern of air space enlargement so that the orderly appearance of the acinus and its components is disturbed and may be lost. In early emphysema, three types may be distinguished by the portion of the acinus that is involved. Late in the disease the overlap among subtypes is extensive, and distinction between them debatable. Dominant involvement of the respiratory bronchiole, or *centriacinar emphysema*, is commonly seen in cigarette smokers but is also associated with coal dust exposure from mining. Typically, smoking-related centriacinar emphysema occurs at the center of lobules *(centrilobular emphysema)* in the upper lobes. Involvement of the alveoli near the septa, or *distal acinar emphysema*, may result in spontaneous pneumothorax.

Involvement of all components of the acinus equally, or *panacinar emphysema*, is seen incidentally to some extent in older patients but occurs extensively in patients with alpha-1-antitrypsin deficiency. It may also occur at the lung bases of patients with centrilobular emphysema.

Small airway disease, also defined pathologically, is *bronchiolitis*—chronic inflammation, with subsequent fibrotic repair reaction, of the membranous and respiratory bronchioles (Wright, 1992). Membranous (terminal) bronchioles contain a complete fibromuscular wall without alveoli or cartilage; respiratory bronchioles are partially alveolated and terminate in the alveolar sacs. Inflammation results in thickening of the airway walls from inflammatory edema and cellular infiltrates. Bronchiolar fibrosis, smooth muscle hyperplasia and goblet cell hyperplasia may be present. Airway distortion may result from fibrous scarring.

ETIOLOGY AND PATHOGENESIS

By far the most common and most strongly associated risk factor for COPD is *tobacco smoking* (Fig. 43–1) (Sherrill et al, 1990). Among chronic cigarette smokers, more than 50 million in the United States, 15 to 18 percent are impaired by COPD. A small number of additional patients develop COPD as a result of occupational exposures or genetic enzyme deficiencies.

As a result of normal host defenses, the lung is constantly subjected to connective tissue proteases (elastases and collagenases). The resulting proteolysis is balanced by constant reconstruction and limited by antiproteases. According to the *protease/antiprotease hypothesis*, outside forces, particularly cigarette smoke, shift the balance toward destruction and promote irreparable damage (Gadek and Pacht, 1990). The most important protease in the lung is neutrophil elastase, which degrades both elastin and collagen. Alpha-1-antitrypsin (AAT, alpha-1-protease inhibitor) is the principal inhibitor of neutrophil elastase. Smoking has several effects on the protease-antiprotease balance. Cigarette smoke may result in increased release of neutrophil chemoattractants. Increased numbers of neutrophils and macrophages may release more proteases and overwhelm the normal antiprotease defenses.

Neutrophils also release reactive oxygen species as part of the respiratory burst to kill invading bacteria. Oxidative damage is limited and localized by antioxidants. *Oxidants and free radicals* may directly damage matrix proteins and inactivate elastin and collagen cross-linking enzymes. Likewise, oxidants may also activate connective tissue protease precursors and inactivate antiproteases. Specifically, the affinity of alpha-1-antitrypsin (AAT) is dramatically lowered by oxidation of a thioether bond at the active site methionine. By this mechanism, either directly from oxidants in smoke or indirectly from oxidants derived from increased inflammatory cell activity, the AAT of smokers is oxidatively altered to have a significantly lower affinity for neutrophil elastase. By inhibiting antiproteases, increased oxidant activity causes increased protease activity, resulting in damage to lung connective tissue or emphysema.

Clearly, not all persons who smoke develop COPD. Heritable differences in antioxidants, free radical scavenging, antiproteases, connective tissue proteins, and repair proteins may explain some of the variation and slight familial predisposition for COPD. The most dramatic example is severe AAT deficiency, which results in severe and early-onset emphysema in many homozygous patients.

Alpha-1-antitrypsin is a 52-kD protein with 394 amino acids and three carbohydrate side chains. At least 75 codominant alleles exist and are classified in the Pi (protease inhibitor) system by electrophoretic mobility. The most common allele, Pi M, is found in 90 percent of the population in the United States. The most common abnormal allele is Pi Z, a point mutation resulting in reduction of secretion from hepatocytes to 15 percent of normal. Probably originating in a single Northern European person about 4000 years ago, the current frequency of homozygotes (Pi ZZ) is 1 in 1670 to 3500 individuals in Europe and North America. It is rare in Black or Asian populations. The Pi S allele, more common in Spain and Portugal, represents a point mutation resulting in decreased serum half-life; plasma concentrations are approximately 60 percent of normal. Frame-shift mutations (Pi null) also exist but are very rare. A critical serum level of 11 μM (equivalent to 80 mg/dl) appears necessary to prevent the development of emphysema. Previous assays, reported in mg/dl, overestimated the true levels by 35 to 40 percent. Pi ZZ (2.5 to 7 μM) and Pi null,

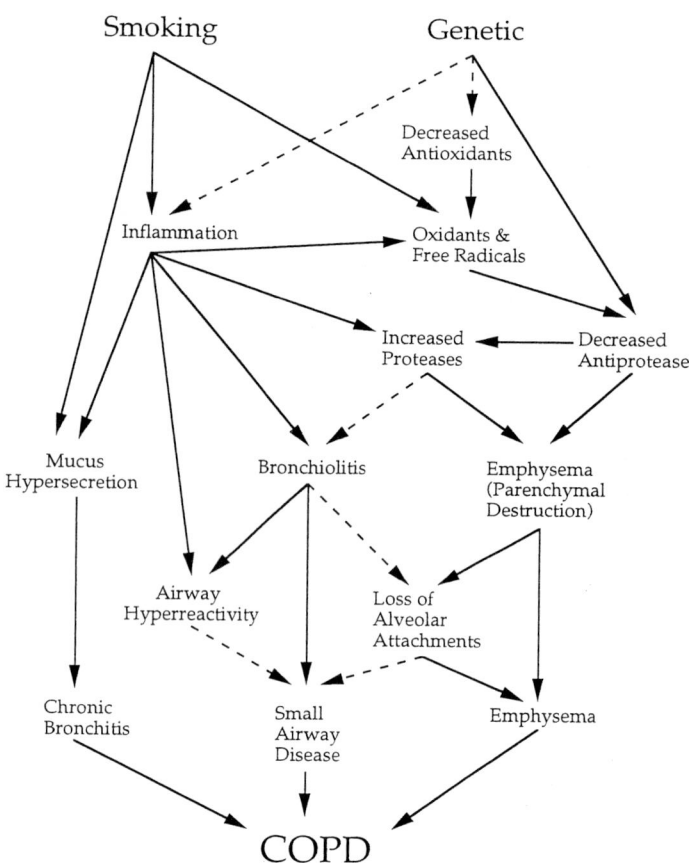

FIGURE 43–1. Model of COPD pathogenesis. Dashed lines represent possible associations.

null (0 μM) are at high risk, and Pi SZ (8 to 19 μM) are at mildly increased risk for developing emphysema. There is no increased risk associated with Pi SS (13 to 33 μM) or heterozygous Pi M combinations. Approximately 60 percent of nonsmoking Pi ZZ individuals develop emphysema. Neonatal hepatitis and cirrhosis develop in 10 to 20 percent of Pi ZZ individuals from accumulation of unsecreted protein. There is no known selection advantage to the heterozygous state. Smoking greatly increases the risk of emphysema, presumably through oxidative inactivation of the limited quantities of alpha-1-antitrypsin.

Occupational exposures from coal or gold mining or inhalation of vaporized cadmium salts may result in emphysema that is additive to that found from cigarette smoking. Small airway disease may be produced by mineral dust (coal, talc, mica, silica), aluminum oxide, iron oxide, or chrysotile and amphibole asbestos.

Airway hyperresponsiveness (AHR) is frequently found in COPD. In the Lung Health Study (a COPD prevention trial), for example, approximately 75 percent of female smokers and 50 percent of male smokers with early COPD and no history of asthma had AHR in the asthmatic range (PC_{20} ≤10 mg/ml methacholine) (Tashkin et al, 1992). In COPD, AHR is probably an *effect* of inflammation, airway narrowing, and increased epithelial permeability due to smoking and not a *cause* of COPD. It remains a matter of debate, however, whether in COPD airway narrowing develops as a consequence of primary or preexisting hyperreactivity to environmental stimulants, including tobacco smoke, in a manner similar to that of allergic asthma, as proposed by the Dutch hypothesis.

Childhood respiratory illnesses or poor lung function at birth may result in impaired development of the lung, but it is unclear how this relates to the development of COPD other than as a decline beginning from a lower maximal lung function. Adult infections do not appear to cause COPD but are more frequent in those with COPD.

Cor pulmonale, hypertrophy of the right ventricle resulting from diseases of the lung, may accompany severe COPD (Wiedemann and Matthay, 1990). Alveolar hypoxia in synergy with acidosis results in pulmonary vasoconstriction. Eventual remodeling of the muscular arteries and arterioles and vascular destruction (from emphysema) result in increased pulmonary vascular resistance (PVR). Increased PVR results in increased pulmonary artery pressures, which prevent increases in right ventricular ejection fraction due to increased afterload. After initial right ventricular hypertrophy, right-sided heart failure eventually ensues.

CLINICAL CHARACTERISTICS

Signs and symptoms typically begin in middle age and later after a long latent period of asymptomatic progressive pathologic and physiologic changes. A nonproductive smoker's cough is common early. This may soon progress to a chronic cough with sputum—chronic bronchitis. Subsequently, breathlessness develops, first only with moderate-to-strenuous exertion, then with less and less exertion, and finally at rest. Typically, nonsmokers with AAT deficiency develop dyspnea at 40 to 50 years of age, whereas smokers become breathless 10 years earlier (Turino, 1991). Physical findings with chronic bronchitis include inspiratory and expiratory wheezes and gurgles. With significant obstruction, expiratory wheezes predominate, and expiratory time is prolonged. As many as 40 percent of AAT-deficient patients present with obstruction or cough. Accessory muscles may be used at rest for inspiration, and abdominal muscles may be used for exhalation. Hyperinflation from severe obstruction and or emphysema may be manifested by a barrel-shaped chest, low diaphragms that do not descend perceptibly with percussion, hyperresonance, and diminished breath sounds. With cor pulmonale, cyanosis and peripheral edema may be present. Pulmonary hypertension may be manifested by a loud P2 heart sound. Weight loss may be evident in advanced disease.

Radiologic findings on plain films are generally not specific or sensitive. Low flat diaphragms and enlarged retrosternal air spaces indicate hyperinflation. Bullae, air spaces greater than 1 cm, and attenuated vascular shadows are associated with emphysema, but may be subtle. Chronic bronchitis may be associated with diffuse linear or reticular-nodular densities, which represent peribronchial cuffing and thickened bronchial walls, but these radiographic findings are difficult to distinguish from other causes. If the right descending pulmonary artery is greater than 16 mm, pulmonary hypertension is usually present. Although the chest roentgenogram is insensitive and correlates poorly with the severity of COPD, it may identify complications (e.g., pneumothorax), contributing morbidities (e.g., pneumonia, congestive heart failure), or other diseases related to smoking (e.g., lung cancer). High-resolution computed tomography (HRCT) correlates well with pathologic emphysema scores but is less sensitive in mild cases.

An *electrocardiogram* with right axis deviation and an R/S ratio >1 in V1 or <1 in V6 indicates right ventricular hypertrophy. Enlargement of the right atrium from pulmonary hypertension results in increased p-wave amplitude in leads II, III, aVF—P-pulmonale. Hyperinflation of the lungs results in a low-voltage QRS. Echocardiography provides an assessment of right ventricular function and hypertrophy and an estimate of pulmonary artery pressure if tricuspid regurgitation is present.

Physiologic findings of airway obstruction are the hallmark of COPD. In contrast to asthma, in COPD, obstruction inexorably increases with time and seldom varies greatly or returns to normal. In normal lungs, only approximately 25 percent of the total airway resistance is encountered in the small airways. In lungs affected by smoking, on the other hand, up to 80 percent of the total resistance may be due to small airway disease. This markedly reduces the total cross-sectional airway size (diameter), which correlates inversely with flow resistance. Inflammation and fibrosis in the small airways result in physiologic and clinical obstruction independent of emphysema. In severe emphysema, loss of elastic recoil and rupture of alveolar attachments with resultant distortion of the bronchioles may play an additional role. Bronchospasm plays a variable role in COPD. Most patients exhibit some response to bronchodilators, even if a single administration does not result in a significant increase in forced expiratory volume in one second (FEV_1) or forced vital capacity (FVC), thus providing a rationale for symptomatic bronchodilator therapy. In mucus hypersecretion, the enlarged glands with or without inflammatory edema result in thickening of the airway walls, and the excess mucus may cause intermittent narrowing of the airway; because this narrowing is relatively modest and occurs in the larger airways, however, it does not produce significant flow limitation. Although the correlation between mucus hypersecretion and obstruction is poor, mucus hypersecretion may contribute significantly to obstruction during acute exacerbations.

In nonsmokers FEV_1 peaks at an age of 19.5 years in men (18.2 in women) and then declines gradually until approximately age 42.8 in men (37.3 in women), following which the rate of decline increases (Fig. 43–2). *Decline in FEV_1* averages 24 ml/year for ages 30 to 39, 27 ml/year for ages 40 to 49, 53 ml/year for ages 50 to 59, and 31 ml/year for age 60 and over. Yearly decline in FEV_1 in women is somewhat less than in men. Smoking is associated with both an earlier onset and an accelerated rate of decline. Declines slightly larger than normal do not predict accelerated decline in smokers. Ex-smokers rapidly return to levels of decline similar to those of nonsmokers.

Nonsmoking alpha-1-antitrypsin–deficient patients have average declines of 80 ml/year, but smokers may exceed 200 ml/year. Low mid-flow rates, i.e., low forced expiratory flow from 25 to 75 percent of total lung capacity ($FEF_{25-75\ percent}$), may represent obstruction in small airways and therefore may decline early in the course of COPD. Unfortunately, the range of normal values for $FEF_{25-75\ percent}$ is wide and encompasses values as low as 65 percent of predicted, making it difficult to differentiate normal variation in mid-flow rates from early small airway disease.

Spirometry measurements in established COPD are characterized by reduced FEV_1/FVC ratio, FEV_1, and $FEF_{25-75\ percent}$. An FEV_1/FVC ratio of <70 percent predicts further decline of ≥50 ml/year in FEV_1 if asthma is excluded. Dyspnea on mild exertion typically develops below an FEV_1 of 1.5 liters (<50 percent predicted). Hypoxemia may develop in patients with an FEV_1 <1.5 liters and hypercapnia with an FEV_1 <0.75 to 1.0 liter. A low FEV_1 shows only a weak correlation with degree of emphysema graded by HRCT, suggesting that intrinsic airway disease may be a more important determinant of airflow obstruction than emphysema in most patients with COPD (Gelb et al, 1993). In contrast to COPD, diseases with restrictive ventilatory defects are characterized by a reduced TLC and FVC and a normal or increased FEV_1/FVC ratio.

Lung volumes are useful in demonstrating hyperinflation and air trapping. Total lung capacity (TLC) >120 percent predicted is consistent with hyperinflation from emphysema or severe obstruction from any cause. TLC correlates well with the pathologic emphysema score. An increase in the functional residual capacity (FRC) is consistent with hyperinflation and air trapping secondary to obstruction. Early in COPD, residual volume (RV) often increases due to air trapping behind prematurely closed airways. Areas of lung that exchange gas slowly (due to severe obstruction) or not at all (due to the presence of bullae) may result in an underestimation of lung volumes when measured by helium dilution or nitrogen washout; whole body plethysmography does not have this limitation.

Diffusing capacity (DL_{CO}, transfer factor) is affected by the surface area for gas transfer, the rate of diffusion across the alveolar membrane, and the alveolar capillary blood volume. Emphysema reduces both the surface area for gas exchange and the alveolar capillary blood volume. DL_{CO} correlates well with

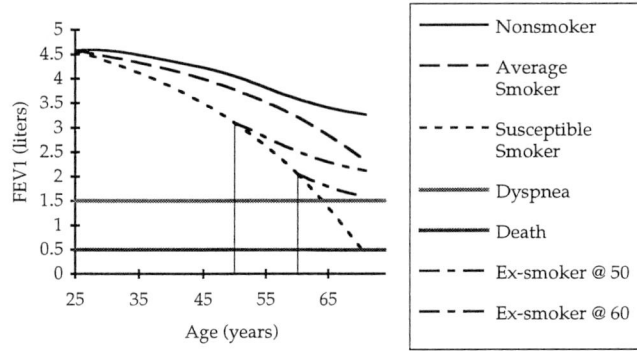

FIGURE 43–2. Decline in FEV_1 with age. In the smoker with accelerated decline in FEV_1, smoking cessation leads to a reduction in the rate of FEV_1 decline to or toward that of a nonsmoker.

emphysema if the FEV_1 is ≥1 liter but may be spuriously low if the FEV_1 is <1 liter. If the FEV_1 is normal, DL_{CO} correlates well with emphysema only if early obstruction is present, as detected by reduced flow rates at mid to low lung volumes (e.g., decreased $FEF_{25-75\ percent}$. A reduction in DL_{CO} is not specific for emphysema, however, since other diseases of the lung and pulmonary vessels reduce the diffusing capacity by altering the alveolar membrane or pulmonary capillary blood volume.

Maximal exercise performance is generally limited by mechanical ventilatory abnormality (obstruction resulting in low ventilatory reserve) or impairment in gas diffusion (resulting in desaturation), although further diminution in exercise tolerance can result from general weakness and physical deconditioning secondary to malnutrition and/or inactivity. Exercise performance can be improved by bronchodilator therapy (if impairment in mechanical ventilatory function is limiting), supplemental oxygen therapy (if exercise is limited by desaturation), and graded exercise training.

DIFFERENTIAL DIAGNOSIS

Many pulmonary diseases are characterized by obstruction, dyspnea, and cough. To distinguish COPD from other obstructive disorders requires collateral evidence and often observation over time (Burrows, 1990). In general, COPD has a gradual onset and a slow progressive course, but a careful history may be required to elicit this. In the absence of a history of smoking or AAT deficiency, COPD is unlikely. Except for smokers with AAT deficiency, symptoms due to COPD rarely begin before age 40. Cystic fibrosis and ciliary dyskinesias are usually symptomatic in childhood. Bronchiectasis, from these disorders or any infectious cause, typically results in frequent production of copious purulent sputum and may be confirmed, if necessary, with HRCT. Histiocytosis X and endobronchial sarcoidosis may be associated with obstructive ventilatory defects due to granulomatous involvement of the bronchioles, but usually can be differentiated from COPD by the appearance of the plain chest roentgenogram. Small airway disease may also be caused by constrictive bronchiolitis due to rheumatoid arthritis, chronic hypersensitivity pneumonitis, occupational mineral dust exposure, inflammatory bowel disease, drug reactions, resolved adult respiratory distress syndrome (ARDS), or idiopathic causes, and following lung, heart-lung, or bone marrow transplants (Wright et al, 1992). Most have associated clinical findings or exposure histories that are suggestive. Lymphangiomyomatosis (LAM), found only in women, is a rare disease in which smooth muscle hypertrophy results in bronchiolar obstruction and impairment of diffusion. Interstitial pulmonary fibrosis (IPF) and bronchiolitis obliterans with organizing pneumonia (BOOP) may present with dyspnea or cough but are characterized by a predominantly restrictive ventilatory defect and characteristic radiologic abnormalities. Left-sided congestive heart failure (CHF) may produce dyspnea, wheezing, and cough (particularly when patients are supine). Physical findings usually identify the presence of CHF, and treatment should be carried out prior to spirometric evaluation for possible coexistent COPD. Localized upper airway obstructions may be apparent on physical examination, with stridor or inspiratory wheezes, and can be detected by the characteristic expiratory and/or inspiratory flow-limiting plateaus on the flow-volume loop.

Asthma is generally characterized by episodic airway obstruction with interval recovery to normal or near-normal lung function. In some cases, improvement to near-normal may require maximal therapy with inhaled or oral corticosteroids and bronchodilators, for an extended period. A personal or family history of atopic manifestations may be helpful, such as allergic rhinitis, nasal polyps, specific allergen triggers, high serum IgE, and eosinophilia of the blood or sputum. Both asthmatics and, in general, COPD patients show positive responses to bronchodilators and methacholine or histamine challenge, but the responses are generally more dramatic in asthma. Importantly, asthma does not reduce the diffusing capacity. A small proportion of patients will not be classifiable on presentation. These should be treated as asthmatics and reevaluated as therapy progresses. Generally, asthma or "asthmatic bronchitis" has a better prognosis than COPD.

TREATMENT

Treatment of COPD involves a multifaceted program directed at preventing development or advancement of the disease, providing symptomatic relief, improving quality of life, preventing complications, and reducing mortality (Fig. 43–3) (Chapman, 1991; Ferguson and Cherniack, 1993). *Preventive therapy* involves the modification of risk factors. Smoking cessation is the most effective intervention to prevent progression of COPD. Smoking cessation reduces the rate of decline in FEV_1 to near the rate of nonsmokers. Smoking cessation also reduces the risk of developing respiratory tract cancer, as well as other nonpulmonary malignancies, in addition to having social, economic, and cardiovascular benefits. Continued smoking is a combination of learned behaviors, environmental influences, and chemical dependence on nicotine. The most successful smoking intervention programs combine nicotine replacement patches with behavior modification (Brunton et al, 1991).

Alpha-1-antitrypsin (AAT) deficiency should be suspected in all nonsmokers with otherwise unexplained dyspnea, smokers in their 30s and 40s with dyspnea and abnormal lung function, appropriate family members of affected individuals and of infants with liver disease in the neonatal period (American Thoracic Society, 1989). Screening should be carried out with serum AAT levels and low levels confirmed by phenotyping. It is possible to elevate AAT to adequate levels in the serum and alveolar lining fluid by infusion of human AAT (from heat-treated pooled human plasma); a recombinant form should be available in the near future. Supplementation is not curative since it does not alter the AAT gene or restore previously lost lung function. An ongoing NIH cohort study is evaluating the natural history of AAT deficiency and its alteration by AAT supplementation. Candidates for supplementation should have an AAT level <11 μM with Pi ZZ, Pi null, null, or, rarely, Pi SZ phenotype, evidence of decreased lung function and successful smoking cessation and abstinence. Supplementation is generally by weekly intravenous infusion, although longer intervals and aerosol administration are being evaluated.

Prevention of possible infections with *vacci-*

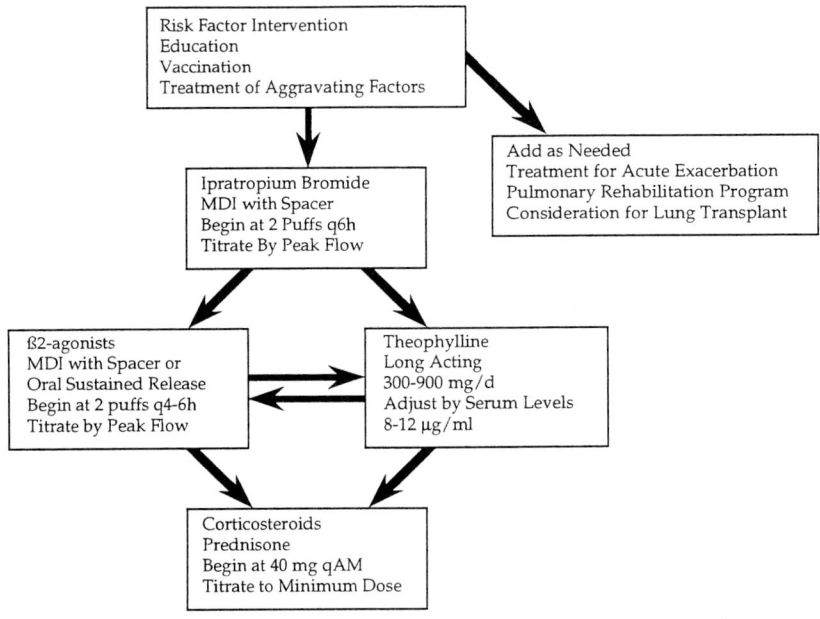

FIGURE 43–3. Model of COPD treatment.

nation may reduce the number or severity of acute exacerbations. Yearly influenza vaccination provides a 60 to 80 percent protection rate and remains a rational recommendation but has not been proved in large-scale clinical trials. Likewise, 23 serotype pneumococcal vaccine should be administered every 5 to 6 years. Chronic use of antibiotics outside of acute exacerbations is not useful.

Pharmacologic Therapy

First-line therapy for relief of dyspnea, bronchoconstriction, and exercise intolerance consists of inhaled *anticholinergics*. Ipratropium bromide and atropine methonitrate (not FDA approved) are poorly absorbed quaternary ammonium derivatives of atropine that reduce the elevated intrinsic cholinergic tone in COPD. Although slightly slower in onset than β-agonists, ipratropium has an effect equal to that of β-agonists by 15 minutes, a larger average effect by one hour, and a longer duration of action (Braun et al, 1991). Failure to improve after bronchodilator challenge on spirometry testing does not preclude the benefit of long-term bronchodilators, and some "nonresponders" to β-agonists may respond to ipratropium. Poor systemic absorption results in minimal or no systemic anticholinergic effects, such as blurred vision, significant tachycardia, or urinary retention that may be seen with nebulized atropine. Currently in the United States, ipratropium is available only in a multidose inhaler (MDI) form. Optimization of therapy can be attained with monitoring by peak-flow meter. The initial dose of two puffs every 6 hours can be increased by one to two puffs every week up to eight puffs every 6 hours. Objective evaluation of the peak-flow or spirometry measurements should show a sustained 10 to 15 percent improvement to justify continuation of the drug or a higher dose. In the future, nebulized ipratropium, a combination MDI with β-agonist and ipratropium, and longer-acting anticholinergic compounds will become available in the United States. These are currently available in many places outside the United States.

Selective *$β_2$-agonists* such as albuterol, terbutaline, and pirbuterol are a second-line option that may be additive in those patients who do not adequately respond to anticholinergics. Because of their rapid onset of action, inhaled β-agonists are also useful for PRN use for acute dyspnea between doses of anticholinergics or prior to exercise. In addition, β-agonists may augment mucociliary clearance and act as mild pulmonary vasodilators. As with ipratropium, a single trial may not identify all patients who will eventually respond to β-agonists, and dose titration over 2 to 4 weeks with monitoring of daily peak flows is appropriate. Sustained-release oral forms may be useful in controlling nocturnal symptoms but are associated with side effects more commonly than inhaled forms. Maximal oral or inhaled doses are usually limited by side effects including palpitations, nervousness, anxiety, restlessness, and tremor. More severe side effects include hypokalemia and cardiac arrhythmias, which may be more frequent with concomitant administration of theophylline. β-adrenergic tolerance (tachyphylaxis) with diminution of peak effect and reduced duration of action may occur, but the clinical significance of tachyphylaxis is unclear. Rebound bronchoconstriction can be demonstrated with very short-acting β-agonists, but its presence and clinical significance with longer-acting β-agonists is not yet clarified. In the future, salmeterol and formoterol, very long-acting β-agonists, currently available outside the United States, may be more convenient for chronic management of COPD.

Metered-dose inhalers (MDI) and hand-held nebulizers deliver active drug to the lower respiratory tract equally effectively, assuming proper technique of MDI use and dose adjustment for the loss of drug in the nebulizer. MDIs are associated with increased convenience and decreased paraphernalia, but may be difficult for some extremely dyspneic patients and patients with poor hand-lung coordination to use. Bronchodilators delivered by intermittent positive pressure breathing (IPPB) have no advantage over hand-held nebulizers and may be associated with increased complications and poor compliance (Intermittent Positive Pressure Breathing Trial Group, 1983). In all patients, careful training and retraining in the proper use of MDIs is critical. Spacer devices are recommended to maximize dose delivered to the lung and minimize oropharyngeal deposition, particularly in patients who are unable to demonstrate consistently adequate technique of MDI use. Compliance may be low for any regimen requiring frequent dosing or in asymptomatic patients.

Theophylline, another second-line drug for

COPD, has slightly less bronchodilator effect but may be additive to inhaled β-agonists (Ziment, 1990). Even without change in FEV_1, theophylline may reduce dyspnea, possibly by increasing respiratory muscle strength, collateral ventilation, mucociliary clearance, and/or central respiratory drive (Vaz Fragoso and Miller, 1993). Available long-acting oral preparations may also prevent nocturnal declines in FEV_1. Toxic and therapeutic ranges overlap considerably, with side effects common at normally "therapeutic" levels (10 to 20 μg/ml). Headache, dizziness, nervousness, insomnia, nausea, and vomiting may be present even with serum concentrations in the low therapeutic range. Hypokalemia, cardiac arrhythmias (including multifocal atrial tachycardia), agitation, and seizures may occur at higher levels, but are not reliably preceded by minor symptoms. Monitoring of blood levels is critical. Since additional bronchodilator effects are uncommon with doses above 15 μg/ml, dosage should be adjusted to maintain blood levels in the relatively low therapeutic range of 8 to 15 μg/ml. The narrow therapeutic range is further complicated by increased hepatic metabolism with concomitant use of cigarettes, phenytoin, or phenobarbital and decreased clearance in the elderly and those with hepatic dysfunction, congestive heart failure, pulmonary edema, obesity, infections, fever, and concomitant use of cimetidine, allopurinol, oral contraceptives, or macrolide antibiotics.

Corticosteroids are the third line of therapeutic agents. Theoretically, inflammation is one of the major initiating events of COPD, and corticosteroids are effective in suppressing inflammation. Unfortunately, most treatment of COPD begins at a time when irreversible fibrosis and lung destruction have already taken place. A subset of COPD patients respond significantly to corticosteroids (Hudson and Monti, 1990). Those patients with a large bronchodilator response are more likely to respond to corticosteroids, but failure to improve with bronchodilators does not preclude benefit from corticosteroids. An individualized trial is indicated if patients with disabling dyspnea have not responded adequately to, or do not tolerate, treatment with anticholinergics, β-agonists, theophylline, or combinations of these agents. During a period of clinical stability in patients receiving maximal bronchodilator therapy, a 2- to 3-week course of prednisone, 40 mg PO each morning, should be objectively evaluated. A ≥20 percent increase in FEV_1 or a significant increase in daily peak-flows or in functional tests such as a 6-minute walk is considered objective evidence of improvement. If successful, the prednisone dose may be decreased to 20 mg/day and then tapered by 2.5 to 5 mg every 3 to 7 days as tolerated by measurement of continuing response. The minimum possible maintenance dose should be used. If oral corticosteroids are successful, an attempt may be made to substitute inhaled corticosteroids or to change to an alternate-day regimen to minimize side effects. Short- and long-term side effects of oral steroids may be severe, and the risk is unwarranted unless there is significant objective response. Preventive measures to reduce the risk of steroid-induced osteoporosis should be considered. In contrast to asthma, limited data are currently available to support the use of inhaled corticosteroids in COPD. Two large-scale clinical trials are now in progress in Europe to assess the efficacy of inhaled corticosteroids in established, symptomatic COPD. In addition, a large clinical trial is planned in the United States to evaluate the effectiveness of inhaled corticosteroids in preventing progression of COPD in patients with relatively early disease.

Low-flow oxygen is indicated for the correction of severe hypoxemia. Two large studies in the United States and Great Britain have proved decreased mortality for hypoxemic patients receiving continuous oxygen therapy (>18 hours/day) (Medical Research Council Working Party, 1981; Nocturnal Oxygen Therapy Trial Group, 1980). Patients who exhibit oxygen desaturation at rest, with exercise, or with sleep should be considered for supplemental oxygen therapy. Nocturnal desaturation is more common during REM sleep and should be distinguished from sleep apnea and other sleep-disordered breathing. An arterial Po_2 of ≤55 mm Hg (SaO_2 ≤88 percent) or a Po_2 of 56 to 59 mm Hg (SaO_2 ≤89 percent) in the presence of evidence of pulmonary hypertension, cor pulmonale, or polycythemia is acceptable for reimbursement from Medicare, but the optimal cut-point remains to be established, especially during sleep and exercise. Supplementation should maintain arterial Po_2 >60 mm Hg (SaO_2 >90 percent). Those with exercise or sleep desaturation should show a reduction in symptoms as well as improvement in arterial Po_2 or saturation with supplemental oxygen therapy. Oxygen may be supplied by stationary concentrators (least expensive for sedentary patients) or by liquid or compressed gas systems. Portable capabilities for ambulatory patients should also be provided by liquid or small compressed gas tanks. Reservoir conservors or demand oxygen delivery systems may prolong the time available on portable systems compared to the usual nasal cannula. Higher oxygen requirements may be met by transtracheal oxygen catheters. Patients should be reevaluated 1 to 3 months after initiation and then every 6 to 12 months to ascertain that they are continuing to meet the criteria. As many as one third will no longer need supplemental oxygen after 1 to 3 months. For air travel, planes are typically pressurized to 2500 m (8000 ft.), and patients with arterial Po_2 <60 mm Hg will generally need continuous oxygen supplementation in flight. Patients with Po_2 >72 mm Hg at sea level will generally not require supplementation during air travel.

The underlying cause of *cor pulmonale* in COPD is usually hypoxic vasoconstriction (Wiedemann and Matthay, 1990). Oxygen is the best pulmonary vasodilator. The mortality associated with cor pulmonale can be reduced by 30 to 50 percent (to a level similar to that of obstructed patients without cor pulmonale) if hypoxemia is corrected. Reduction in pulmonary arterial pressure (PAP) after therapy with oxygen may predict survival. Other vasodilators have no proven effect on survival. With hydralazine, nifedipine, and nitroglycerin, objective measurements of PAP (decrease ≥20 percent) and cardiac output (increased or unchanged) are necessary to assess the effects in each individual. If these agents are used, catheterization should be repeated in 4 to 6 months as these effects may not be sustained. Diuretics improve cardiac output in patients with volume overload, but reduction of preload may result in systemic hypotension. Volume reduction may also reduce peribronchial edema, resulting in improved airflow. Digitalis improves right ventricular contractility but also increases pulmonary vasoconstriction. It is therefore not beneficial unless left ventricular failure is present. Exercise training results in no significant improvement in pulmonary hemodynamics due to limitation of training intensity by mechanical ventilatory abnormality. Nocturnal ventilatory support may improve cor pulmonale beyond correction of hypoxia, but more study is required.

Pulmonary Rehabilitation

Education is a vital part of the treatment of COPD and a cornerstone of *pulmonary rehabilitation*. Specific segments of pulmonary rehabilitation programs in inpatient or outpatient settings may be beneficial for different patients (Hodgkin, 1990b). In COPD, exercise is usually limited by mechanical ventilatory abnormality, and exercise tolerance can be improved by optimizing lung function with bronchodilator therapy. However, exercise may also be limited, at least in part, by physical deconditioning; exercise training and reconditioning may provide some task-specific improvements and an improved sense of well-being. Walking is probably most useful and should be carried out in a progressive program for 20 to 30 minutes three to five times/week. Pursed-lip breathing provides positive end-expiratory pressure to prevent airway collapse and reduces respiratory frequency, thus decreasing the work of breathing; it may be beneficial in coping with dyspnea along with diaphragmatic training. Patients may also be benefited by training in pacing of activities and adaptive methods of energy conservation. Malnutrition, below 90 percent of ideal body weight, is present in 25 percent of COPD patients. Caloric requirements are 15 to 17 percent underestimated by standard equations, and intake may be limited by dyspnea, bloating, fatigue, early satiety, and anorexia. Improved nutrition or caloric supplementation may increase respiratory muscle strength. Vocational rehabilitation, psychosocial support, and family or caretaker training are also important aspects of pulmonary rehabilitation.

Lung Transplantation

Lung transplantation offers a remarkable "cure" for patients with severe COPD (American Thoracic Society, 1993). Single-lung transplant, rather than double-lung or heart-lung transplant, is now generally recommended. Following single-lung transplant, FEV_1 averages 57 percent of predicted, compared to 18 percent prior to transplantation (Trulock, 1992). In addition, right ventricular function often shows remarkable recovery. Although acceptance criteria vary by center, lung transplantation should be considered for patients with severe obstruction and/or pulmonary hypertension in whom medical therapy is ineffective, activities of daily living are substantially limited, and life expectancy is limited. Candidates should be ambulatory with good rehabilitation potential and a satisfactory psychosocial and emotional support system. They should not have significant coronary artery disease (for lung transplant alone), obesity, or malnutrition. Although results vary from center to center, short-term technical successes are common, 1-year survival may be as high as 67 percent, and 2-year survival as high as 62 percent. Delays from evaluation to transplant are often long due to shortages of donors.

Other Treatment Options

Thinning of secretions may benefit selected patients (Ziment, 1990). Hydration is appropriate if the patient is dehydrated, but overhydration is not beneficial. There is little evidence of improved clearance of secretions and no consistent benefit with guaifenesin, SSKI (saturated solution of potassium iodide), iodinated glycerol, or nebulized saline. Acetylcysteine may improve clearance but does not increase FEV_1 and may induce bronchospasm. If bullae occupy greater than one third of the lung and adjacent relatively normal lung is compressed, surgical *bullectomy* may improve airflow and gas exchange, although results of bullectomy are disappointing when emphysema is extensive. It is unclear whether respiratory muscle rest by *intermittent ventilation* (nasal or tracheal positive pressure) is helpful in reducing symptoms or hypercarbia. Small doses of *narcotics* may decrease the perception of dyspnea without respiratory depression. *Carotid body resection* provides relief of dyspnea but removes hypoxic drive, an action that may be potentially life-threatening. In advanced COPD, hypercapnia may be protective against fatigue of respiratory muscles by reducing the alveolar ventilation—and hence the work of breathing—to eliminate the CO_2 of metabolism; therefore, the benefit of *respiratory stimulants* is questionable. Almitrine, available in Europe, increases hypoxic ventilatory drive and improves V/Q matching by increasing hypoxic vasoconstriction, but it also increases pulmonary vascular resistance, thus possibly worsening pulmonary hypertension.

Treatment of Acute Exacerbations

Acute respiratory infections, inhaled irritants, respiratory muscle weakness, respiratory depression, concomitant illnesses (such as congestive heart failure), or patient noncompliance may cause *acute exacerbations* or worsening of COPD (Rosen and Bone, 1990). The most common infections are viral. Bacterial pathogens, particularly *Haemophilus influenzae, Streptococcus pneumoniae*, and *Moraxella (Branhamella) catarrhalis*, may be primary or secondary (Murphy and Sethi, 1992). *Gram-staining of sputum* may be useful to identify purulence indicative of bacterial infection and direct antibiotic therapy by bacterial morphology. Sputum culture is not helpful because of the frequent presence of potentially pathogenic commensal organisms and contamination with oral flora. Chest roentgenograms are useful if pneumonia is suspected. Respiratory muscle weakness may be due to fatigue or electrolyte imbalance (Mg, PO_4, K). Respiratory depression may be due to metabolic alkalosis or the inadvertent or unrecognized overuse of narcotics or sedative-hypnotics.

Intensification of the regimen used for the maintenance therapy of COPD is the basis for acute treatment. More frequent and higher doses or the addition of *ipratropium, β-agonists*, and/or *theophylline* may be beneficial. Theophylline may be given in the oral immediate-release form or as aminophylline beginning with a bolus of 6 mg/kg (if no prior theophylline) at <25 mg/minute followed by a continuous infusion at 0.5 (0.2 to 0.8) mg/kg/hour. It is important to closely monitor theophylline blood levels to maintain a serum level between 10 and 15 μg/ml. Controlled studies of the use of oral and intravenous *corticosteroids* are conflicting, and the optimal dose is unknown. In patients with severe exacerbations, intravenous corticosteroids result in significant improvement in airflow after 12 hours, and response continues through 3 days of treatment. Methylprednisolone, 0.5 mg/kg every 6 hours, or prednisone, 40 to 60 mg by mouth each morning, is an acceptable regimen. The initial dose should be continued for 3 days or until significant clinical improvement occurs. Thereafter, the corticosteroid dose should be tapered over 2 weeks to prevent rebound of symptoms.

There is no conclusive evidence that *antibiotics* are beneficial in treating exacerbation of COPD in general; ideally, their use should be limited to treating exacerbations with purulent sputum and an increase in dyspnea and cough. Diminished severity and a shorter duration of acute exacerbations may be achieved with early initiation of antibiotic therapy when changes in sputum purulence, cough, and dyspnea are first noted. A 7- to 10-day course of trimethoprim-sulfamethoxazole, tetracycline, ampicillin, amoxicillin, or erythromycin is usually adequate; however, up to 30 percent of *H. influenzae* in the United States may be β-lactamase-positive. Amantadine may be useful in unimmunized individuals with acute influenza if begun within 48 hours of onset of symptoms.

Low-flow oxygen may be necessary to maintain Po_2 between 65 and 80 mm Hg, as indicated by serial arterial blood gases or pulse oximetry. Acute hypercarbia and ventilatory failure may occur if supplemental oxygen therapy is uncontrolled, leading to suppression of the hypoxic ventilatory drive. If severe acute exacerbations are refractory to the above measures, intubation and *mechanical ventilatory support* for respiratory failure may be necessary. Selected patients may benefit from nasal mechanical ventilation. Patients with identifiable acute causes of exacerbation should be considered for mechanical ventilation. Patients with a slowly progressive decline should be counseled regarding the possibility of prolonged ventilator dependence, and consideration should be given to advanced directives regarding intubation.

COPD may be exacerbated by many other diseases. Reflux of acidic stomach contents may cause reflex bronchoconstriction even without aspiration. Sleep-disordered breathing or sleep apnea may contribute to nocturnal hypoxemia and pulmonary hypertension. Inactivity and cor pulmonale may predispose patients to deep vein thrombosis and pulmonary emboli (PE). In acute exacerbations, PE should be considered if dyspnea is unresponsive to bronchodilators. Even relatively modest left-sided congestive heart failure combined with COPD may result in severe dyspnea and hypoxemia unresponsive to bronchodilator therapy. Pneumothorax may occur in two or three per 1000 patients. Chronically ill patients may become infected with atypical mycobacteria (e.g., *Mycobacterium kansasii, M. avium-intracellulare, M. fortuitum*), and this infection may result in slowly progressive lung destruction.

PROGNOSIS

COPD is associated with a highly variable mortality (Hodgkin, 1990a). Survival correlates well with percent predicted FEV_1, post-bronchodilator FEV_1, and age. Mild obstruction is not indicative of a progressive downhill course. Severe obstruction, as indicated by an FEV_1 <1.2 liters portends a marked acceleration in death rate; an FEV_1 <0.75 liters is associated with a 20 percent 6-year survival. Higher rates of decline in FEV_1 indicate a poorer prognosis as does poor nutritional status. Cessation of smoking results in a rapid return of the yearly rate of decline in FEV_1 to an annual decline close to that of nonsmokers, thus retarding further progression of the disease. Diffusion impairment (DL_{CO} <10 ml mm Hg) is associated with a 7-year survival of 10 percent. Alpha-1-antitrypsin–deficient patients may be severely affected (Turino, 1991). For Pi ZZ smokers, death in the sixth decade of life is typical; Pi ZZ nonsmokers usually have significant emphysema after age 60, but many remain asymptomatic. In patients with cor pulmonale, supplemental oxygen reduces mortality to that of similarly obstructed patients. In general, correction of hypoxemia with continuous low-flow oxygen results in a decrease in mortality by one half (45 percent to 25 percent at 5 years). Hypercapnia (arterial Pco_2 >52 mm Hg) is an indicator of poor prognosis—<10 percent survival at 6 years. Prognosis is not related to mucus hypersecretion.

REFERENCES

American Thoracic Society. Standards for the Diagnosis and Care of Patients with Chronic Obstructive Pulmonary Disease (COPD) and Asthma. Am Rev Respir Dis 136(1):225, 1987.

American Thoracic Society. Guidelines for the Approach to the Patient with Severe Hereditary Alpha-1-Antitrypsin Deficiency. Am Rev Respir Dis 140(5):1494, 1989.

American Thoracic Society. Lung transplantation. Am Rev Respir Dis 147(3):772, 1993.

Braun SR, Levy SF, Grossman J. Comparison of ipratropium bromide and albuterol in chronic obstructive pulmonary disease: A three-center study. Am J Med 91(suppl 4A):28S, 1991.

Brunton SA, Henningfield JE, Solberg LI. Smoking cessation: What works best?, Patient Care 25(11):89, 1991.

Burrows B. Differential diagnosis of chronic obstructive pulmonary disease. Chest 97(2):16S, 1990.

Chapman KR. Therapeutic algorithm for chronic obstructive pulmonary disease. Am J Med 91(suppl 4A):17S, 1991.

Ferguson GT, Cherniack RM. Management of chronic obstructive pulmonary disease. N Engl J Med 328(14):1017, 1993.

Gadek JE, Pacht ER. The protease-antiprotease balance

within the human lung: Implications for the pathogenesis of emphysema. Lung 168(suppl):552, 1990.

Gelb AF, Schein M, Kuei J, et al. Limited contribution of emphysema in advanced chronic obstructive pulmonary disease. Am Rev Respir Dis 147:1157, 1993.

Hodgkin JE. Prognosis in chronic obstructive pulmonary disease. Clin Chest Med 11(3):555, 1990a.

Hodgkin JE. Pulmonary rehabilitation. Clin Chest Med 11(3):447, 1990b.

Hudson LD, Monti CM. Rationale and use of corticosteroids in chronic obstructive pulmonary disease. Med Clin North Am 74(3):661, 1990.

Intermittent Positive Pressure Breathing Trial Group. Intermittent positive pressure breathing therapy of chronic obstructive pulmonary disease: A clinical trial. Ann Intern Med 99:612, 1983.

Medical Research Council Working Party. Long-term domiciliary oxygen therapy in chronic hypoxic cor pulmonale complicating chronic bronchitis and emphysema. Lancet 1:681, 1981.

Murphy TF, Sethi S. State of the art: Bacterial infection in chronic obstructive pulmonary disease. Am Rev Respir Dis 146:1067, 1992.

Nocturnal Oxygen Therapy Trial Group. Continuous or nocturnal oxygen therapy in hypoxemic chronic obstructive pulmonary disease: A clinical trial. Ann Intern Med 93:391, 1980.

Rosen RL, Bone RC. Treatment of acute exacerbations in chronic obstructive pulmonary disease. Med Clin North Am 74(3):691, 1990.

Sherrill DL, Lebowitz MD, Burrows B. Epidemiology of chronic obstructive pulmonary disease. Clin Chest Med 11(3):375, 1990.

Snider GL. Chronic obstructive pulmonary disease: A definition and implications of structural determinants of airflow obstruction for epidemiology. Am Rev Respir Dis 140:S3, 1989.

Tashkin DP, Altose MD, Bleecker ER, et al. The Lung Health Study: Airways hyperresponsiveness to inhaled methacholine in smokers with mild to moderate airflow limitation. Am Rev Respir Dis 145:301, 1992.

Thurlbeck WM. Pathology of chronic airflow obstruction. Chest 97(2):6S, 1990.

Trulock EP. Lung transplantation. Ann Rev Med 43:1, 1992.

Turino GM. Natural history and clinical management of emphysema in patients with and without alpha-1-antitrypsin inhibitor deficiency. Ann N Y Acad Sci 624:18, 1991.

Vaz Fragoso CA, Miller MA. Review of the clinical efficacy of theophylline in the treatment of chronic obstructive pulmonary disease. Am Rev Respir Dis 147:S40, 1993.

Wiedemann HP, Matthay RA. Cor pulmonale in chronic obstructive pulmonary disease. Clin Chest Med 11(3):523, 1990.

Wright JL, Cagle P, Churg A, et al. State of the art: Diseases of the small airways. Am Rev Respir Dis 146:240, 1992.

Wright JL. Small airways disease: Its role in chronic airflow obstruction. Semin Respir Med 13(2):72, 1992.

Ziment I. Pharmacologic therapy of obstructive airway disease. Clin Chest Med 11(3):461, 1990.

Section Eight
MANAGEMENT OF SKIN DISEASE

Chapter 44
Atopic Dermatitis

Allen D. Adinoff, M.D., and Richard A.F. Clark, M.D.

Atopic dermatitis is a chronic relapsing, pruritic dermatitis that usually occurs in individuals with a personal or family history of atopy. In most patients, atopic dermatitis begins during infancy. Once coordinated rubbing and scratching begin at 2 to 3 months, a more typical picture of eczema becomes manifest. It has been estimated that 65 percent of patients develop atopic dermatitis the first year of life and 90 percent before the age of 5. Onset after 30 years of age is so unusual that the diagnosis should be questioned. Most patients tend to improve with age (Vickers, 1980).

The disorder affects 0.5 to 1 percent of the general population. The prevalence in children is 5 to 10 percent. In infants and young children, the dermatitis often occurs on the scalp, face, and extensor surfaces. In older children and adults, the dermatitis tends to localize to the flexural areas, especially the antecubital and popliteal fossae and the neck. In addition, the dermatitis may affect the hands and feet, sometimes in the absence of dermatitis elsewhere. Recently, food ingestion and aeroallergen contact have been shown to initiate flares of atopic dermatitis. Therapy includes allergen avoidance, intensive skin hydration, topical glucocorticoids and tar preparations, systemic antibiotics, and systemic antihistamines. Newer immunomodulating agents offer promise for future treatment. Recent advances in the understanding of the pathobiology of this disorder strongly suggest an important role for allergens in the pathogenesis of atopic dermatitis.

CLINICAL FEATURES

Atopic dermatitis is identified by a constellation of symptoms, some of which are dis-

TABLE 44–1. DIAGNOSTIC FEATURES OF ATOPIC DERMATITIS

Major features (must have three or more)
  Pruritus
  Typical morphology and distribution
  Chronic or chronically relapsing course
  Personal or family history of atopy
Minor features (must also have three or more)
  Xerosis
  Ichthyosis/palmar hyperlinearity/keratosis pilaris
  Immediate skin test reactivity
  Elevated serum IgE
  Early age of onset
  Tendency toward cutaneous infections
  Nonspecific hand or foot dermatitis
  Nipple eczema
  Cheilitis
  Recurrent conjunctivitis
  Dennie-Morgan infraorbital fold
  Keratoconus
  Anterior subcapsular cataract
  Orbital darkening
  Facial pallor/erythema
  Pityriasis alba
  Itch when sweating
  Intolerance to wool and lipid solvents
  Perifollicular accentuation
  Food hypersensitivity
  Course influenced by environmental factors
  White dermographism/delayed blanch

Adapted from Hanifin JM, Rajka G. Diagnostic features of atopic dermatitis. Acta Derm Venereol 92(suppl):44–47, 1980.

cussed below in more detail. The criteria for the diagnosis, suggested by Hanifin and Rajka (1980), have been recognized internationally (Table 44–1). A modification of these criteria for young infants has been subsequently proposed (Table 44–2) (Seymour et al, 1987). The main features include an extremely pruritic rash, its typical morphology and distribution, and its tendency toward a chronic or relapsing course, all in the context of an atopic individual. Some features such as xerosis, immediate skin test reactivity, and orbital darkening are common but nonspecific, whereas others such as anterior subcapsular cataracts, upper lip cheilitis, and keratoconus are uncommon but relatively specific for the diagnosis of atopic dermatitis.

Morphology, Distribution, and Symptoms

The *morphology* of atopic dermatitis varies according to three relatively distinctive stages of the skin reaction: acute, subacute, and chronic. Acute eczema is characterized by extensive erosions with serous exudate or intensely pruritic, erythematous papules and vesicles on a background of erythema (Fig. 44–1). Subacute eczema is characterized by erythematous, excoriated, scaling papules or plaques grouped or scattered over erythematous skin. Often the scaling is so fine and diffuse that the skin acquires a silvery sheen (Fig. 44–2). Chronic eczema is characterized by thickened skin and increased skin markings secondary to rubbing and scratching, called lichenification (Fig. 44–3). Sometimes, chronic eczema is associated with excoriated

TABLE 44–2. MODIFIED CRITERIA FOR DIAGNOSIS OF ATOPIC DERMATITIS IN INFANTS

Three major features
  Family history of atopic disease
  Typical facial or extensor eczematous or lichenified dermatitis
  Evidence of pruritus
Three minor features
  Xerosis, ichthyosis, hyperlinear palms
  Perifollicular accentuation
  Postauricular fissures
  Chronic scalp scaling

Adapted from Seymour JL, et al. Clinical effects of diaper types on the skin of normal infants with atopic dermatitis. J Am Acad Dermatol 17:988–997, 1987.

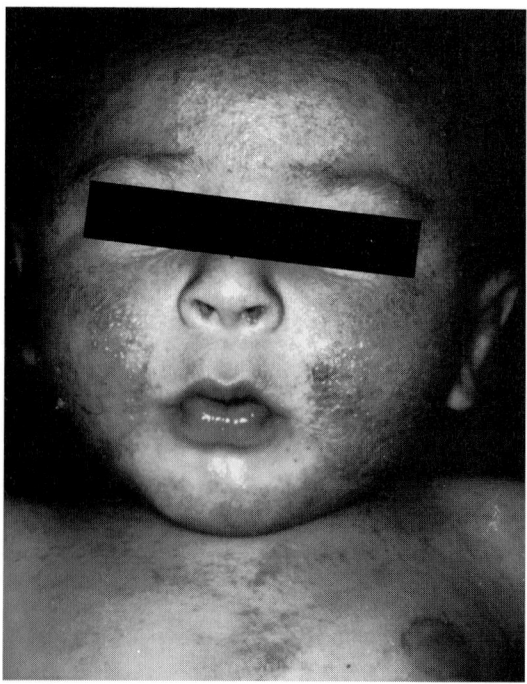

FIGURE 44–1. Acute atopic dermatitis, presenting as a weeping eruption in a typical distribution in an infant.

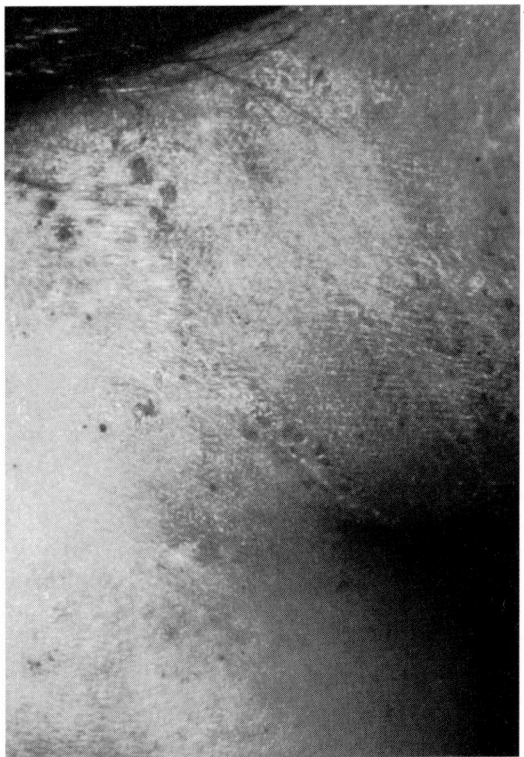

FIGURE 44–2. Subacute atopic dermatitis, presenting with papules, excoriations, and a silvery sheen on the neck.

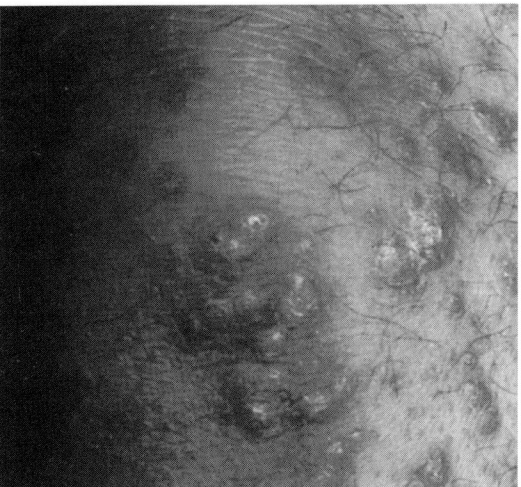

FIGURE 44–4. Prurigo nodularis, with excoriated fibrotic nodules.

papules, fibrotic papules, and nodules—called prurigo nodularis (Fig. 44–4), or post-inflammatory hyper- and hypopigmentation (Fig. 44–5). The pigmentary disorder is often observed in patients with a darker skin type. These individuals should be reassured that the dyschromia will gradually resolve over 6 to 12 months, once the dermatitis is brought under control. Since atopic dermatitis is a chronic relapsing condition, acute, subacute, and chronic dermatitis may occur together in a given patient.

The *distribution* of eczema tends to vary with the age of the patient. In infants and young children the scalp, face, and extensor surface of extremities are often involved. In older children and adults the neck, antecubital and popliteal fossae, wrists, and ankles tend to be involved. Not all flexural areas are affected, however. For example, it is distinctly unusual for axilla or groin to become involved with atopic dermatitis. In fact, if axillary, intragluteal, or groin dermatitis occurs in a patient thought to have atopic dermatitis,

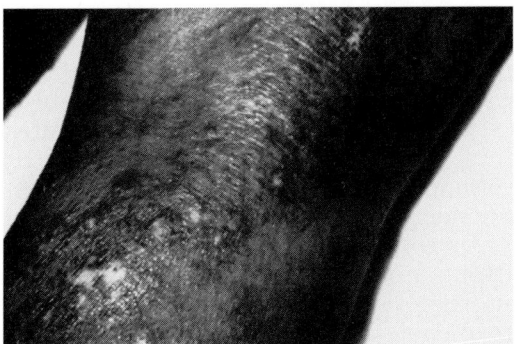

FIGURE 44–3. Chronic atopic dermatitis, with lichenification and large papules from chronic frequent scratching and rubbing.

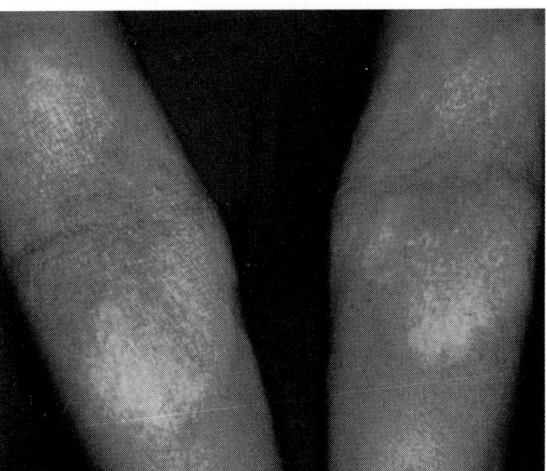

FIGURE 44–5. Post-inflammatory pigment changes and lichenification.

another cause for the dermatitis should be sought. Hand and foot dermatitis become a significant problem in some patients.

In all stages and distributions of atopic dermatitis, *pruritus* and increased cutaneous reactivity are the major hallmarks of the disease and cause the greatest morbidity. It is often said that no primary lesion exists in atopic dermatitis, but rather lesions result from scratching. Excoriation may intensify the dermatitis; it is unlikely, however, that erythematous reactions on the central back are caused by scratching alone. In addition, some infants develop an erythematous eruption before 3 months of age, a time when itch-scratch coordination has not developed. Finally, we have had the opportunity to clear the dermatitis in a number of patients and then rechallenge them with inciting allergens. Often a morbilliform eruption or, less frequently, urticaria occurs in association with intense pruritus. If the allergen is withdrawn, these eruptions are transient. However, if the allergen exposure persists, these eruptions become eczematous over 24 to 48 hours. Thus, we believe that atopic dermatitis evolves initially from an intensely pruritic erythematous, papular, or urticaria-like eruption. The eczema is propagated by excoriation, particularly if exposure to the offending allergen or irritant continues.

Associated Clinical Features and Complications

Atopic Diathesis

According to several studies, 75 to 80 percent of patients with atopic dermatitis have a personal or family history of allergic disease. Approximately 80 percent of patients develop positive reactions to one or more foods or inhalant allergens upon immediate hypersensitivity skin testing (Hoffman et al, 1975). The genetic predisposition for atopic dermatitis, given an allergic disease in one or more parents, is not readily available; rather, the risk for atopy in general (allergic asthma, hay fever, and atopic dermatitis) has been reported. Nevertheless, a personal or family history of atopic disease in a patient with severe dermatitis sways one toward the diagnosis of atopic dermatitis.

Xerosis and Ichthyosis

Dry, lackluster skin is a hallmark of atopic dermatitis and is often, but not always, associated with ichthyosis vulgaris. Xerosis is usually worse during periods of low humidity, such as winter in Northern latitudes. Xerosis in the absence of active dermatitis may aggravate pruritus. Compared to normal skin, the skin of atopic dermatitis has a reduced water-binding capacity and a higher transepidermal water loss. Although the underlying biochemical abnormality for xerosis in atopic dermatitis is unknown, clinically noninflamed, nonichthyotic skin in atopic dermatitis contains a mild inflammatory infiltrate and epidermal edema (spongiosis) (Mihm et al, 1976). Whether these pathologic findings cause the dry skin or are a result of the dry skin is unknown. Ichthyosis vulgaris, an autosomal dominant disorder of epidermal maturation, characterized by polygonal fish-like scales, is found in up to 37 percent of patients with atopic dermatitis. Other manifestations of ichthyosis vulgaris, such as hyperlinear palms and soles, have been described in one third to one half of patients with atopic dermatitis.

Cutaneous Infections

Patients with atopic dermatitis have a tendency to develop viral, bacterial, and fungal skin infections. It is not clear whether these cutaneous infections arise secondary to a disruption of normal barrier function or secondary to reduced local immunity. Cutaneous anergy is a striking immunologic dysfunction that occurs during active atopic dermatitis. However, the anergy is transient and resolves with resolution of the dermatitis (Dahl et al, 1978).

VIRAL INFECTIONS. Patients with atopic dermatitis have a propensity to infection with herpes simplex, vaccinia, molluscum contagiosum, and papilloma virus (Leyden and Baker, 1979). The most common viral infection is herpes simplex, which tends to spread locally or become generalized. When herpes is generalized, it is known as Kaposi's varicelliform eruption or eczema herpeticum. Herpes simplex infection of the lip may spread to one side of the face and be confused with herpes zoster, which appears to affect atopic patients no more seriously than normals. A misdiagnosis can result in otherwise easily preventable corneal damage. Generalized infections with herpes simplex can masquerade as an eczematous flare.

BACTERIAL INFECTIONS. Studies in adults

have shown that more than 90 percent of patients with chronic atopic dermatitis are colonized with coagulase-positive *Staphylococcus aureus*, with particularly high concentration of the organism in areas of active dermatitis (Leyden et al, 1974). The infections tend to be superficial. Septicemia generally is not a problem, and deep cutaneous infections are rare in contrast to patients with the hyper-IgE syndrome. Honey-color crusting, extensive serous weeping, folliculitis, pyoderma, and furunculosis indicate bacterial infection, usually secondary to *S. aureus*. Besides predisposing factors such as disrupted cutaneous barrier and possibly local suppression of host defenses, patients with atopic dermatitis are heavily colonized with *S. aureus*. The *S. aureus* colonization may be extremely difficult to eradicate. Interestingly, the lipophilic bacteria, which colonize normal skin, are scarce or absent from normal and uninvolved skin of patients with atopic dermatitis. Perhaps absence of normal lipophilic bacteria sets the stage for *S. aureus* colonization.

It has been suggested that *S. aureus*, through either immunologic or nonimmunologic mechanisms, may initiate the eczematous process. The recent observations that staphylococcal enterotoxins (superantigens) are potent stimulators of macrophages and T cells provides a possible mechanism by which *S. aureus* could exacerbate atopic dermatitis. Nearly 50 percent of patients with atopic dermatitis have circulating IgE directed to staphylococcal toxins. These toxins have been identified on their skin (Leung et al, 1992). Basophils from patients release histamine on exposure to the relevant toxin but not following exposure to those enterotoxins in which there is no IgE response. These findings suggest the possibility that local production of endotoxin by *S. aureus* at the skin surface could induce IgE-mediated histamine release and thereby trigger exacerbations of atopic dermatitis.

FUNGAL INFECTION. Superficial fungal infections may also appear more frequently in atopic individuals. *Trichophyton rubrum* skin infection was found to occur three times more frequently in patients with atopic dermatitis than in nonatopic controls (Jones et al, 1973a; 1973b). Not infrequently, recurrence of a dermatophyte infection may coincide with flaring of the dermatitis at sites other than that of the infection, suggesting a possible pathogenic role for this organism. Particular interest has been focused on *Pityrosporum ovale* as a pathogen in atopic dermatitis. A recent study found IgE antibodies against *P. ovale* in two thirds of patients with atopic dermatitis (Kieffer et al, 1990).

Emotional and Family Dysfunction

Anger, frustration, and anxiety are commonly experienced by patients with atopic dermatitis and often exacerbate the disorder. Atopic patients are likely to respond to stress, frustration, embarrassment, or any emotionally upsetting event with itching and scratching. Excitability and arousal of the central nervous system from an emotional upset can intensify the vasomotor and sweat responses in the skin and lead to the itch-scratch cycle. The added dimension of family hostility, rejection, and guilt can damage the family structure.

Differential Diagnosis

A number of cutaneous disorders may appear in a similar presentation with atopic dermatitis. A skin biopsy may be needed in some clinical situations to exclude these conditions. Table 44–3 reviews the differential diagnosis of atopic dermatitis.

PATHOPHYSIOLOGY

Histopathology

The histologic features of atopic dermatitis vary with the stage of the lesion but are not diagnostic for the disease. A skin biopsy, therefore, can suggest but cannot establish the diagnosis. Nevertheless, a biopsy may be helpful in excluding other conditions, which clinically may appear to resemble atopic dermatitis. A skin biopsy is essential if the dermatitis is recalcitrant to vigorous topical therapy or if the dermatitis appears hemorrhagic or excessively infiltrated. In these clinical situations, neoplastic disease such as Letterer-Siwe disease or cutaneous T cell lymphoma must be considered. Acute lesions of atopic dermatitis are characterized by intracellular edema within keratinocytes, intraepidermal vesicles, and intercellular edema (spongiosis) of the epidermis (Mihm et al, 1976). Within the dermis, a perivascular inflammatory cell infiltrate of lymphocytes, and occasional monocyte-macrophages and neutrophils, can be found.

TABLE 44–3. DIFFERENTIAL DIAGNOSIS OF ATOPIC DERMATITIS

Psoriasiform dermatoses
  Psoriasis
  Lichenified contact dermatitis
  Seborrheic dermatitis
Ichthyosis
  Ichthyosis vulgaris
  X-linked ichthyosis
  Erythrokeratodermia variabilis
  Netherton's syndrome
Infection
  Staphylococcus aureus folliculitis
  Herpes simplex
  Scabies
  Dermatophytosis
Neoplastic diseases
  Letterer-Siwe
  Histiocytosis X, Sézary syndrome
  Mycosis fungoides
Metabolic diseases
  Phenylketonuria
  Acrodermatitis enteropathica
  Tyrosinemia
  Ahistidinemia
  Hartnup disease
  Hurler's syndrome
Immune deficiency diseases
  Wiskott-Aldrich syndrome
  Selective IgA deficiency
  Ataxia telangiectasia
  Agammaglobulinemia
  Hyper-IgE (Job's) syndrome

Mast cells are frequently hypogranulated. In chronic lesions, the epidermis is acanthotic with elongation of the rete ridges and dyskeratosis. There are increased numbers of Langerhans' cells and mast cells, with fibrosis occasionally seen at all levels of the dermis.

Intact eosinophils are rarely seen in skin lesion biopsies prepared with standard counterstains. However, immunofluorescence has shown patterns of localization of the eosinophil granule major basic protein (MBP) within the dermis of patients with atopic dermatitis (Leiferman et al, 1985). In addition to the staining found within intact eosinophils, extracellular fluorescence was also seen, particularly a fibrillar pattern within the upper dermis. These results suggested that eosinophils migrate into the skin and commonly release granule products in the dermis of patients with atopic dermatitis. The histology of atopic dermatitis has been reported in two food-challenged patients after oral food challenge (Sampson, 1988). Both patients developed a pruritic morbilliform rash within 1 hour after the challenge. Skin biopsies obtained from involved sites 4 and 14 hours later revealed infiltration of eosinophils and deposition of MBP. The eosinophilic infiltrate was of a greater degree than previously seen in chronic lesions, and the deposition of MBP less. This suggests that eosinophils are quickly mobilized into lesions of atopic dermatitis following allergen exposure, with later degranulation and deposition of MBP.

Further immunohistochemical studies have shown Langerhans' cells in the epidermis and dermis, bearing high-affinity Fcϵ receptors and allergen-specific IgE on their surface in patients with atopic dermatitis (Bruynzeel-Koomen et al, 1986; Bieber et al, 1992). Although IgE-bearing Langerhans' cells and macrophages have been found in other inflammatory skin diseases such as psoriasis, these other skin conditions, unlike atopic dermatitis, are not associated with the production of allergen-specific IgE. A significant proportion of mast cells in involved skin are lymphocyte-dependent M_T type (instead of M_{TC} type) (Irani et al, 1989). The majority of infiltrating CD4+ T cells are T_{H2} cells. These T cells may be antigen-specific for antigens such as house dust mites (Sager et al, 1992). Activated T_{H2} cells secrete a variety of cytokines that promote IgE production (e.g., IL-4), increase IgE receptors on Langerhans' cells, and decrease T_{H1} activity.

An interesting series of reports have studied the histologic evolution of eczematous reactions induced by the modified patch test with aeroallergens. All have abraded the skin to remove the epidermal barrier and/or utilized high concentrations of allergens compared with those used for standard prick testing. Comparison of these studies or consolidation of the findings is difficult. Each performed patch testing in a different manner, and biopsies were obtained at different times. Nevertheless, a dermal infiltrate of mononuclear cells, neutrophils, basophils, and eosinophils has generally been found 24 to 48 hours after patch test application. Eosinophils have been noted as early as 2 to 6 hours, and many were activated (Bruynzeel-Koomen et al, 1986). Electron microscopy showed epidermal eosinophils at 24 to 48 hours in close contact with Langerhans' cells, suggesting a cell-cell interaction (Bruynzeel-Koomen and Bruynzeel, 1988). Mast cell degranulation was present at 2 to 6 hours (Bruynzeel-Koomen et al, 1986). A marked increase in mast cell numbers was observed at 6 to 10 days, a time when all other inflammatory cells were decreasing. These studies have introduced an exciting investigative tool, which is likely to aid in our understanding of the pathogenesis of atopic dermatitis.

Role of IgE, Aeroallergens, and Foods

There has been considerable controversy over whether atopic dermatitis is an allergic disorder or simply an inflammatory skin disease seen in patients with respiratory allergy. A large body of evidence exists which strongly supports the role of IgE-mediated mechanisms in the pathogenesis of atopic dermatitis (Adinoff and Clark, 1989). Recent information would indicate that atopic dermatitis is indeed an allergic disorder with important parallels with asthma and allergic rhinitis. This view has been strengthened by the recognition that the inflammatory component of asthma is probably more important than bronchospasm.

The initial studies of Coca and Cooke associating atopic dermatitis with allergic rhinitis and asthma have been extended, demonstrating that approximately two thirds of children with atopic dermatitis have positive family histories for atopic diseases (NIAID Task Force Report, 1979). Fifty to 80 percent of children with atopic dermatitis will ultimately develop allergic rhinitis and/or asthma. The long-term prognosis of childhood asthma is worsened in the presence of atopic dermatitis (Vickers, 1980). Serum IgE concentrations are elevated in approximately 80 percent of children with atopic dermatitis and tend to correlate roughly with the severity and extent of skin symptoms. The concentration of IgE may also be a useful marker of disease improvement following dietary elimination of offending foods (Sampson, 1985).

Foods

The concept that food hypersensitivity plays a pathogenic role in atopic dermatitis dates from several studies in the 1920s, when it was reported that patients with atopic dermatitis who avoided specific foods to which they were sensitive improved. A large number of reports implicating the role of foods in atopic dermatitis followed (Adinoff and Clark, 1989). These studies often were not well controlled. In addition, many of them were published during a time when the role of allergy in atopic dermatitis was minimized.

Studies over the past 15 years have clearly demonstrated a pathogenic role for food allergy in some patients with atopic dermatitis. Overall, it appears that one third of children with atopic dermatitis will have food hypersensitivity contributing to their symptoms (Burks et al, 1988). In their development of the double-blind placebo-controlled food challenge (DBPCFC), Bock and May were the first to report the association of foods and atopic dermatitis in a controlled fashion (Bock et al, 1978). Although their studies did not focus on the role of foods in atopic dermatitis, five of nine children with a history of eczematous reactions to foods developed eczema within 2 hours of administration of the challenge. Atkins and co-workers reported the results of 12 positive controlled food challenges in ten adults (Atkins et al, 1985). One patient developed "eczema" after ingestion of peanuts.

Sampson has systematically studied the role of food hypersensitivity in large numbers of children with moderately severe atopic dermatitis (Sampson, 1983). Foods chosen for challenge were based on the results of positive immediate hypersensitivity skin prick tests and/or a convincing history suggesting clinical reactivity. Approximately 55 percent of children challenged have experienced at least one positive clinical response. All reactions have occurred within 3 hours of challenge. Approximately 75 percent of reactions involved the skin and were characterized by erythema, papules, and pruritus. Often the patients scratched their skin intensely. Skin symptoms occurred most commonly in areas where the patients' eczema lesions had flared previously. Although skin symptoms induced by food challenges usually resolved within 2 to 3 hours, some patients developed pruritus and, less frequently, a macular, pruritic rash in reaction sites 6 to 8 hours after the initial response (Sampson, 1985). Patients experiencing several such reactions during a week of DBPCFCs developed eczematous skin lesions. This suggests that repeated ingestion of foods and the scratching that results from such exposure contributes to the development of atopic dermatitis skin lesions. Although many studies have suggested that children with atopic dermatitis are sensitive to a large number of food antigens, most children (78 percent) have had documented reactions to only one or two foods. Nineteen percent have reacted to three foods, and only a few children have been sensitive to four or more different foods. Six food antigens (egg, peanut, milk, wheat, fish, and soy) have accounted for approximately 90 percent of the positive reactions.

These studies clearly demonstrate that some young patients with moderate-to-severe atopic dermatitis develop immediate pruritic cutaneous reactions after the ingestion of foods. Furthermore, the intense itching and scratching can produce eczematous skin lesions, particularly when the offending food is repeatedly ingested. Thus the evidence seems quite clear that allergy to foods can precipitate eczema in many patients with atopic dermatitis.

Aeroallergens

Many patients with atopic dermatitis report worsening of their dermatitis with aeroallergen contact or experience seasonal flares. In our recent report of ten patients with atopic dermatitis, two patients experienced significant seasonal exacerbations of their eczema that correlated with positive immediate hypersensitivity skin tests and delayed patch tests to relevant aeroallergens (Adinoff et al, 1988). We also found that five of ten patients with atopic dermatitis gave impressive histories of worsening of their dermatitis with house dust exposure or when in geographic environments known to contain high loads of house dust mites. A dose-response relationship was recently demonstrated between exposure to house dust mites and risk of developing atopic dermatitis (Harving et al, 1990).

In addition to these clinical observations, experimental evidence for the role of aeroallergens in atopic dermatitis has been reported. In an interesting series of experiments by Tuft and colleagues, direct inhalation of aeroallergens was performed in an attempt to establish their role as a direct cause of eczematous changes (Tuft et al, 1950). Nasal inhalation challenges were performed in two patients with atopic dermatitis but without allergic rhinitis or asthma. Immediately after inhaling ragweed pollen, the subjects developed itching and sweating in the antecubital and popliteal fossae followed by a "mild dermatitis," which persisted for several days. One patient with atopic dermatitis developed itching, sweating, and dermatitis after repeated bronchial inhalations of house dust extract.

The clinical observations and results of inhalation challenges that suggest a role for aeroallergens in the pathogenesis of atopic dermatitis in some patients cannot be ignored. Nevertheless, the reports remain largely anecdotal and uncontrolled. It is our belief, however, that future controlled studies will validate these concepts, and the importance of aeroallergens in atopic dermatitis will be confirmed.

Skin Prick Tests and RAST

Immediate hypersensitivity skin tests and radioallergosorbent tests (RAST) to various environmental and/or food allergens are positive in approximately 80 percent of patients with atopic dermatitis, whether or not they have allergic rhinitis or asthma (Hoffman et al, 1975). It has been suggested, however, that the results of skin tests appear to correlate poorly with clinical sensitivity. Nevertheless, in a group of 123 patients with atopic dermatitis who had positive wheal and flare reactions to ragweed, 59 (49 percent) had seasonal flares of dermatitis during the fall (Tuft and Heck, 1952). The sensitivity and specificity of immediate hypersensitivity skin tests in the diagnosis of potential offending food allergens in patients with atopic dermatitis has been assessed. In studies of patients with atopic dermatitis and food sensitivity, it has been demonstrated that a negative skin prick test virtually excludes immediate food hypersensitivity (Sampson, 1983). The positive predictive accuracy of skin prick testing with food antigens was found to be poor and quite variable (25 to 75 percent). Of 63 controlled food challenges carried out in patients who had both a positive wheal and flare skin test and a history suggestive of possible food intolerance, 20 (32 percent) were positive. Therefore, although a positive skin prick test indicates the presence of allergen-specific IgE, it should be considered a suggestive indicator of immediate food sensitivity requiring confirmation with a more definitive study, such as an oral challenge.

Patch Tests

The delayed cutaneous response to substances applied to the skin is a well-accepted method of diagnosis for contact allergy, but its use as a diagnostic or investigative tool in atopic dermatitis had not been widespread prior to the 1980s. In 1982, Mitchell and colleagues described the results of patch testing in 17 patients with atopic dermatitis (Mitchell et al, 1982). After abrasion of uninvolved areas of the skin and application of concentrated solutions of allergens, 38 of 38 patch tests placed were positive 48 hours later and progressed until 72 hours. Reactions showed confluent papular erythema with stronger responses producing edema and exudation, and were seen with house dust mite, grass pollen, animal danders, and extracts of the patients' floor dust. However, application of purified house dust mite antigen (Der P1) produced positive reactions in four of six dust mite allergic patients without a history of dermatitis and one of nine nonallergic controls. Nevertheless, the intensity of the reactions was considerably less than observed in patients with atopic dermatitis.

Since then, several studies utilizing allergen patch testing in patients with atopic dermatitis have been reported (Adinoff and Clark, 1989). Most studies were designed to examine the histologic changes associated with cutaneous application of allergen in patients with atopic dermatitis. Since elicitation of a reaction was desired, allergen extracts were often concentrated many times greater than those used for standard prick testing, or the skin was abraded to remove the stratum corneum. However, Norris and colleagues applied standard concentrations of dust mite extract in 50 percent glycerine on unabraded skin of the antecubital or popliteal fossae daily for 5 consecutive days (Norris et al, 1988). Seven of 13 patients who had extract placed on mildly eczematous lesions developed significant delayed reactions, whereas only three of ten patients who had extract placed on uninvolved skin developed reactions. Interestingly, 9 of 12 dust mite prick test–positive subjects without atopic dermatitis developed local erythema and scattered pruritic, urticarial papules within 10 minutes of application, and these lasted as long as 6 hours. These reactions occurred only in the antecubital fossa and not when allergen was placed on the back.

We reported 10 subjects with moderate-to-severe atopic dermatitis and positive patch test reactions to common aeroallergens (Adinoff et al, 1988). A careful history was taken for contact with animals, pollens, dust, and irritants, and for variations in dermatitis with changes in climatic conditions and seasons. In most cases, disease activity varied with changes in environment. Removal from the home or the humid local environment resulted in marked improvement of skin symptoms in many patients. Additionally, many patients were able to associate contact with specific allergens and exacerbations of atopic dermatitis, or noted seasonal variability in disease severity. Aeroallergens that produced positive reactions on prick testing were selected for patch testing. These were performed without skin abrasion on clinically uninvolved areas of the back. Extracts of 1:20 w/v in 50 percent glycerine were occluded for 48 hours, and removed and interpreted 24 hours later. Positive reactions produced erythema and papules or vesicles. Twenty-nine percent of 91 applied patch tests were positive. Positive patch tests correlated strongly with aeroallergens identified in patients' environment or suspected by patients to be the cause of their eczema. An example of the reactions seen is illustrated by the case of a 6-year-old boy from humid Haifa, Israel, who had uncontrolled atopic dermatitis that worsened in spring and with dust contact. His eczema resolved in Denver, whether in or out of the hospital, and worsened when he returned to Israel. Reactions to three grass pollen extracts and dust mite *(D. farinae)* were observed. House dust mites are not found in significant numbers in Denver, whereas they are much more prevalent in humid geographic areas. Patch tests were placed on 32 control subjects with chronic rhinitis (19 with positive skin prick tests, 13 with negative skin tests). Only one of the 160 patch tests applied was positive.

More recently we have studied the prevalence of patch tests reactions in 40 consecutively evaluated patients with moderately severe atopic dermatitis (Clark and Adinoff, 1990). Twenty common aeroallergens (pollens, fungi, mites, cockroaches, and animal danders) were tested on each patient. Sixty-seven percent of patients had at least one positive patch test, and 51 percent had at least four positive reactions. Twenty-three percent of all patch tests placed were positive. The patch reactions seen were clinically similar to the morphology of the lesion of eczema. Skin prick tests performed with similar allergens, when positive, were not always predictive of a positive patch test.

These studies indicate that patients with atopic dermatitis can develop eczematous lesions upon cutaneous application of aeroallergens and suggest that contact sensitivity can be demonstrated to a wide variety of aeroallergens, which correlate with a history of precipitating environmental factors. Additionally, the ability to elicit reactions using a much less concentrated extract on unabraded normal-appearing skin underlines the fact that some patients can be exquisitely sensitive to topically placed aeroallergens. It demonstrates the ability of aeroallergens to penetrate normal-appearing skin and cause eczematous reactions as might likely occur with natural exposure. Thus, part of the defect in atopic dermatitis may lie in an inherent abnormality in the epidermal permeability barrier. Support for this possibility comes from a study showing that patients with atopic dermatitis had increased transepidermal water loss through both dry and clinically normal skin (Werner and Lingberg, 1985). Patch testing may be a useful provocative challenge to the skin in certain patients.

Immunologic Features

It is often stated that patients with atopic dermatitis demonstrate defects in their cellular immune system. An underlying T cell defect is suggested by their propensity to develop cutaneous viral and fungal infections. Patients with atopic dermatitis have been reported to have a reduced incidence of contact sensitization as well as decreased sensitization to *Rhus oleoresin* and DNCB (Jones et al, 1973b; Rees et al, 1990). Patients with primary T cell immunodeficiency disorders, such as Wiskott-Aldrich syndrome, frequently have elevated serum IgE levels and eczematous skin lesions indistinguishable from atopic dermatitis. Laboratory evidence of immunoregulatory abnormalities include decreased CD8+ suppressor/cytotoxic T cell number and function, increased expression of CD23 on mononuclear cells, increased production of interleukin-4 (IL-4), and decreased production of interferon-gamma. However, most of these abnormalities in immune function have been noted in patients who were symptomatic with active disease. For example, it was found that significantly fewer patients with atopic dermatitis had *Rhus oleoresin* sensitivity than normal control subjects (Jones et al, 1973b). Careful examination of the patient data revealed that 90 percent of the patients had active dermatitis at the time of patch testing. In subsequent studies, it has been demonstrated that nearly all immunologic abnormalities (*in vivo* and *in vitro*) returned to normal when the dermatitis was controlled or resolved (Dahl et al, 1978; Uehara, 1977). This suggests that many of the immunologic abnormalities associated with atopic dermatitis may be epiphenomena but nevertheless could be pathogenetically important to the disease.

However, there is considerable evidence that abnormalities of T cell regulation and cytokine production contribute to the elevated serum IgE levels and eczematous rash associated with atopic dermatitis (Leung et al, 1992). Recently recognized is an "imbalance" in the production of IL-4 and interferon-gamma (IFN-γ) in patients with atopic dermatitis. IL-4 is the first of at least two signals that activate B cells to synthesize IgE. T cells from patients with atopic dermatitis secrete increased amounts of IL-4 and express increased levels of IL-4 receptors. In contrast, IFN-γ suppresses IL-4-induced IgE synthesis. Peripheral blood mononuclear cells from patients with atopic dermatitis have been found to have a decreased capacity to produce IFN-γ (Jujo et al, 1992). Thus, the combined effects of elevated IL-4 synthesis and defective production of IFN-γ may contribute to the enhanced synthesis of IgE. In addition, these effects may contribute to the deficiency of cytotoxic/suppressor T cell function and the reduced antiviral activity and impaired delayed-type hypersensitivity reactions. Taken together, these abnormalities could then contribute to the clinical picture seen in atopic dermatitis.

As mentioned, Langerhans' cells in the epidermis and dermis, bearing high-affinity Fcϵ receptors and allergen-specific IgE on their surface, have been identified in patients with atopic dermatitis (Bruynzeel-Koomen et al, 1986; Bieber et al, 1992). In addition, the antigen-presenting role of these IgE-bearing Langerhans' cells has also been studied. It has been demonstrated that IgE-positive Langerhans' cells, but not IgE-negative Langerhans' cells, were capable of presenting house dust mite allergen to T cells (Mudde et al, 1990). Further evidence for the role of Langerhans' cells in the activation of T cells in atopic dermatitis is supported by the finding that Langerhans' cells are responsible for increased autologous T lymphocyte reactivity to lesional epidermal cells in patients with atopic dermatitis. These results suggest that cell-bound IgE on Langerhans' cells bind to relevant allergens prior to their processing and antigen presentation to T cells.

Mechanisms of Chronic Inflammation

A hypothesis for the mechanisms by which allergens may initiate and perpetuate the chronic inflammatory process seen in atopic dermatitis can be developed (Fig. 44–6). Allergens to which patients have developed specific IgE bind to either dermal mast cells or antigen-presenting Langerhans' cells. Allergen binding to these lymphocyte-dependent mast cells results in the release of inflammatory mediators, causing an immediate cutaneous response of pruritus, erythema, papular rash, and occasional urticaria. This response is clinically observed in the few hours following oral food challenges. It is unlikely, however, that this mechanism alone accounts for the chronic skin inflammation seen in atopic dermatitis. It is more likely that allergen bound to specific IgE-bearing Langerhans' cells then present antigen to T cells, which induces a delayed hypersensitivity response more characteristic of the chronic lesions of eczema. Since the majority of these T cells are T_{H2} cells, a variety of cytokines that promote ongoing inflammation are secreted. For example, IL-4 activates B cells to synthesize IgE. The deficiency of interferon-gamma fails to terminate the immune response. Cytokines and chemoattractants from T cells and mast cells recruit eosinophils, which secrete MBP and other injurious substances.

Thus, if allergen exposure is ongoing, a vicious cycle of T_{H2} stimulation, allergen-specific IgE production, eosinophil recruitment, and cutaneous inflammation is perpetuated. Just as airway inflammation contributes to the nonspecific bronchial reactivity seen in asthma, cutaneous inflammation undoubtedly plays an important role in the pathogenesis of nonspecific cutaneous hyperreactivity seen in atopic dermatitis. Once a state of increased cutaneous reactivity is established, patients find their skin more sensitive to nonallergic stimuli, such as irritants and perspiration. A breakdown in the skin barrier and the

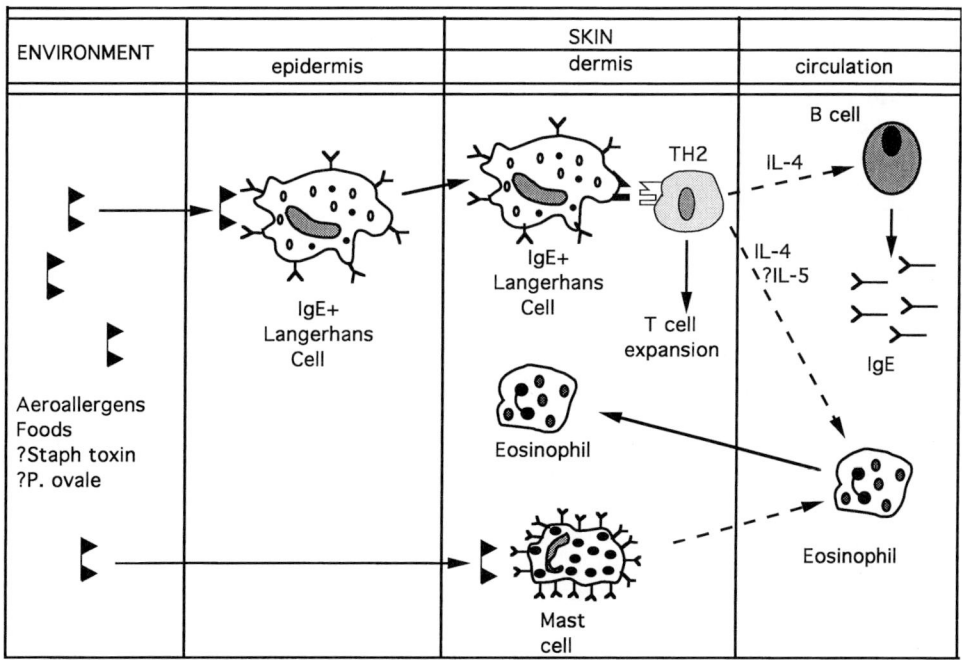

FIGURE 44–6. Immunologic events in atopic dermatitis. (Adapted from Bruynzeel-Koomen CAF, Bruynzeel PLB. A role for IgE in patch test reactions to inhalant allergens in patients with atopic dermatitis. Allergy, 43(suppl):15–21, 1988.)

cutaneous anergy that develops increase the susceptibility to infection. A state of "status eczematous" evolves, which then becomes refractory to standard therapies. These observations would suggest that treatment needs to be focused on allergen avoidance and the reduction of ongoing cutaneous inflammation.

MANAGEMENT

Atopic dermatitis is a chronic relapsing disease that can be frustrating to both patients and physicians. However, the disorder can be controlled by therapy. The therapy must be individualized and is dependent on whether the patient is experiencing an acute flare of dermatitis or dealing with chronic atopic dermatitis. It is preferable to treat acute flares at home; however, hospitalization may be necessary. Frequently, a few days of vigorous inpatient skin care can result in a dramatic clearing of the dermatitis.

Identification and Elimination of Exacerbating Factors

Allergens

The role of allergens (foods and aeroallergens) in the initiation and perpetuation of atopic dermatitis has been discussed. Once identified, the elimination and avoidance of triggering allergens becomes an essential and critical part of the management of this chronic condition.

Foods. Dietary avoidance of major food allergens in infants at high risk for atopy and elimination of foods demonstrated to exacerbate eczema in patients with known atopic dermatitis can be of great benefit to patients.

Infant Prophylaxis. Several studies suggest that strict dietary elimination of major food allergens can reduce the prevalence of atopic dermatitis in infants at high risk for atopy. A number of studies have shown that eliminating major allergens from the maternal diet during the third trimester of pregnancy does not prevent the development of atopy in their children (Falth-Magnusson and Kjellman, 1992). However, removing major food allergens from the maternal diet during lactation appears to have a beneficial effect. In a follow-up of infants whose mothers were placed on a restrictive diet (prophylactic group) and infants whose mothers consumed a normal diet, children in the prophylactic groups had significantly less atopic dermatitis at 18 months and 4 years of age than children whose mothers received a regular diet during lactation (Sigurs et al, 1992). The potential benefit of placing both the lactating mother and her infant on food allergen elimination diets has also been studied (Zeiger et al, 1989). One hundred and three high-risk infant-mother pairs were compared with 185 high-risk controls. Infants of mothers placed on strict allergen avoidance diets were found to have significantly less atopic dermatitis at 1 year of age than infants of mothers on no dietary restriction. The late addition of solid foods to the diet (after 6 months) has been shown to delay the development of atopic dermatitis (Kajosaari and Saarinen, 1983). It therefore appears that the identification and dietary counseling of pregnant mothers at high risk for bearing an atopic child can result in reducing the likelihood that atopic dermatitis will develop in that infant.

Dietary Avoidance. Once atopic dermatitis has developed, it would appear that the identification and elimination of offending foods can improve the course of illness in patients with atopic dermatitis. The clinical course of atopic dermatitis was monitored for 3 years in 27 children with the disease (Sampson, 1985). Thirteen children with documented food hypersensitivity were maintained with appropriate elimination diets (on diet). The other group was comprised of 14 children in whom no offending food was identified or eliminated (no diet). A scoring system was devised based on the patients' skin symptoms, medication requirements, physician visits, and days absent from school. The clinical symptom scores of the "on diet" group were significantly better than those of the "no diet" group. Similarly, the "on diet" group experienced a significant decrease in total IgE during the course of the study (median pre-study: 11,000 IU/ml; post-study: 4700 IU/ml), whereas the "no diet" group experienced an increase in total IgE (median pre-study: 3950 IU/ml; post-study: 7900 IU/ml).

These data strongly suggest that the elimination of foods provoking clinically documented hypersensitivity responses will favorably affect the course of atopic dermatitis. Nevertheless, dietary recommendations must be made with an understanding of their potentially disruptive effects on the patient and family as well as the nutrition of the patient. Broad-based elimination diets cannot be recommended. Dietary recommendations based on DBPCFC are ideal but often not practical in an office setting. However, dietary elimination trials based on positive prick skin tests or a highly suggestive history should be pursued. Any apparent improvement in the eczema should be confirmed by reintroduction of the food into the diet. If it has been reasonably established that food(s) do exacerbate the patient's eczema, that substance should be eliminated from the diet for at least 4 to 6 months. Reintroduction into the diet should be periodically attempted. Patients who require elimination of multiple foods or foods critical for adequate nutrition should receive dietary counseling. Educational information for patients with food hypersensitivities is available through a variety of sources. The Food Allergy Network (4744 Holly Avenue, Fairfax VA 22030) provides information regarding food allergies, nutrition, coping strategies, "how to read a label" cards, and the like. Its medical advisory board includes leading national experts in food allergy.

AEROALLERGENS. Avoidance of aeroallergens suspected to be triggers of atopic dermatitis has also been reported to be of benefit. Platts-Mills and co-workers found that 20 of 23 mite-allergic patients with atopic dermatitis, when admitted to the hospital and without changing their medical treatment, showed dramatic improvement within 10 days (Platts-Mills et al, 1983). Seven patients have shown long-term improvement after cleaning their bedrooms. We reported 10 patients with severe atopic dermatitis who demonstrated immediate prick and delayed cutaneous patch tests to aeroallergens (Adinoff et al, 1988). That aeroallergen contact might be an important etiologic factor in these patients was suggested by their histories of worsening skin symptoms with allergen contact and marked improvement when they were removed from their usual environment. The improvement often occurred with minimal changes in skin care and persisted for as long as 4 years when patients continued to avoid environments known to precipitate their disease state. Exacerbations invariably occurred within 1 to 2 days after return to the original environments. It would appear, therefore, that avoidance of aeroallergens suggested as important by the history or delayed patch test responses might improve the course of atopic dermatitis. Further controlled studies are needed, however, before the exact role of aeroallergens in atopic dermatitis can be established.

Irritants

The fact that atopic dermatitis is a condition of dry, sensitive, easily irritated skin should be stressed with patients and parents. To prevent irritation, the use of soaps, solvents, and other drying compounds should be minimized. If soaps are to be used they should have minimal defatting activity and a neutral pH; examples include Dove, Cetaphil cleanser, Eucerin cleanser, and Neutrogena. Non-soap cleansing agents are also available such as Aveeno and Emulave. The use of soap should be confined mainly to the intertriginous areas to avoid unnecessary defatting of other skin surfaces. Residual laundry detergent in clothes may also be irritating. While changing detergents may help (e.g., Cheer Free), more often adding a second rinse cycle to ensure removal of soap from clothing is more beneficial. Many atopic dermatitis patients have hand dermatitis. Irritant contact with solvents, soaps, and detergents is probably a major factor. Patients with this problem should avoid jobs that require exposure to these irritants. A non-aqueous cleansing method may be helpful for atopic patients with irritant hand dermatitis who need to wash frequently and are not able to apply emollients after every washing.

Perspiration—whether thermal, emotional, or gustatory—may cause itching. Atopic patients should modify their activities and surroundings to minimize sweating. They should work and sleep in comfortable surroundings at a fairly constant temperature (68 to 75°F) and humidity (45 to 55 percent). Occlusive clothing may be poorly tolerated, and open-weave, loose-fitting garments may be preferred. Patients intolerant of woolen or stiff fabrics may find relief with cotton or cotton blend clothing. Sunscreen should also be used on a regular basis to avoid sunburn. Swimming is an activity that is recommended and well tolerated; however, swimming pools are often treated with chloride or bromine. It is important that patients shower immediately after leaving the pool and then apply moisturizers or occlusives (see below) to the total body.

Controlling the Itch

Pruritus is the most common and least tolerated symptom of atopic dermatitis, often leading to patient frustration and exhaustion. Excoriations during episodes of severe scratching can be minimized by cutting nails and using cotton gloves at night. In our experience, baths and wet wraps (see Hydration below) are often the most effective therapy for nocturnal pruritus. Systemic antihistamines may offer some symptomatic relief. Whether this is due to an antipruritic or sedative effect remains unclear. Both sedating and nonsedating antihistamines generally have performed poorly in clinical trials (Berth-Jones and Graham-Brown, 1989). Nevertheless, one trial did demonstrate a significant clinical effect of both hydroxyzine and loratadine in patients with atopic dermatitis (Monroe, 1992). The relatively poor response to antihistamines probably relates to a number of studies investigating the antipruritic effect of these drugs, showing that histamine plays a minor role in the itchy skin of atopic dermatitis.

Other mediators (e.g., neuropeptides, cytokines) probably contribute to the pruritus. If antihistamines are to be used, hydroxyzine, loratadine, or cetirizine is a reasonable choice; all three have unique properties that may favor their use in atopic dermatitis. Not only are these drugs effective H_1 antagonists, but they also block IgE-mediated late-phase mast cell release of platelet activating factor (Michel et al, 1988) and the recruitment of neutrophils, eosinophils, and basophils into allergen-challenged skin blisters (Charlesworth et al, 1989). Increased awareness of the potent antihistamine H_1 and H_2 binding affinity of the tricyclic antidepressants has led to use of these compounds as well. Doxepin or amitriptyline may be given as a single 75-mg dose with the evening meal or in 25-mg doses three times daily. The topical use of antihistamines and local anesthetics should be avoided since they may induce hypersensitivity reactions. Sensitization could prevent future systemic use of these agents and related compounds such as sulfonamides, thiazides, and oral hypoglycemic agents. If night-time scratching is severe and continues in spite of antihistamine administration, the short-term administration of a sedative (e.g., chloral hydrate) to allow adequate rest is appropriate.

Hydration

Hydration is the key to good therapy in any stage of the disease. The primary means for correcting dryness is to add water to the skin and then apply a hydrophobic occlusive substance to retain the absorbed water. This can be accomplished by either soaking the affected area or bathing for 15 to 20 minutes in tepid water two or three times a day. Hot water should always be avoided as it often stimulates itching. Addition of substances such as oatmeal (Aveeno or sodium bicarbonate) to the bath water is soothing to a certain population of patients but does nothing to increase water absorption. Bath oils are not recommended as they give the patient a false sense of lubrication and make the bathtub very slippery. Patients leaving the bath should remove excess water by patting with a soft towel and immediately apply the appropriate topical medication. If the skin is not occluded within 3 to 5 minutes, evaporation will rapidly dry the skin and no beneficial effect will be obtained. The hydration from bathing will also increase the penetration of topical medication up to tenfold if applied immediately.

The patient may be placed in wet wraps after baths to further accentuate hydration and medicinal penetration, and to promote cooling of the skin (Nicol, 1987). Bedtime wraps are most practical. The wraps are recommended for use on severely affected or persistent areas of dermatitis. If only arms and legs need to be wrapped, wet Kerlix gauze can be applied followed by elastic bandages. For total body occlusion, double cotton pajamas can be used. One pair of pajamas is wetted, wrung out so as to be damp but not soaking wet, and placed on the patient. The second pair of pajamas is worn dry over the wet pair. To effect even greater occlusion, a plastic sauna suit is used instead of the dry pajamas. For wrapping the hands and feet, wet socks followed by dry socks can be used in the same manner as pajamas. The face can be wrapped with two layers of wet Kerlix followed by two layers of dry Kerlix, to be held in place with Spandex netting. Holes are cut out for eyes, nose, and mouth. The patient may require additional blankets or increased room heat to prevent chilling. Baths and compresses are also effective in removing crusts and reducing exudation. Burow's 1:40 solution (one packet of Domeboro powder per quart) provides astringent and antibacterial effects for localized weeping lesions. This solution should only be used for 2 to 3 days as it is extremely drying and may predispose the skin to increased itching and cracking.

Moisturizers, available as lotions or creams, help to add some moisture to the skin. Lotions contain more water than creams and thus evaporate more quickly. Eucerin, Aquaphor, Lubriderm, Vaseline Dermatology Formula, Moisturel, and Curel are some that contain water and oil. These preparations should be applied three to four times per day, including immediately after bathing. Occlusives such as petroleum jelly or vegetable shortening are effective in dry environments because they allow less evaporation. Occlusives, however, are effective only when used with hydration, since they do not contain water and only prevent water from evaporating from the skin.

Corticosteroids/Tars

Topical Corticosteroids

Topical corticosteroids are frequently needed in the therapy of acute exacerbations of atopic dermatitis. Corticosteroids possess anti-inflammatory, antipruritic, and vasoconstrictive activity when used topically. Fluorinated and/or esterified corticosteroids are more potent on a milligram-to-milligram basis than are nonfluorinated and nonesterified compounds. Table 44–4 lists many of the more common topical corticosteroids currently available by their rank order of potency. Generally it is advisable to become familiar with one or two preparations in each group. The cost of these topical agents can be considerable. Generic equivalents should be prescribed whenever possible.

Choice of agents varies according to location and extent of lesions. As a general rule, the lowest-potency corticosteroid that is effective should be used. Creams, while spreading more easily, may produce increased drying in some patients. Ointments are more occlusive; thus they provide better delivery of the medication and prevent water loss from the skin. Nevertheless, in some cases this occlusion may result in increased pruritus or folliculitis. For instance, in humid environments, creams may be better tolerated than ointments. Sprays and lotions are best used on scalp or other hairy areas. Topical steroids should be applied immediately after baths or soaks to take advantage of increased penetra-

TABLE 44–4. RELATIVE POTENCY OF TOPICAL STEROID PRODUCTS

Class	Brand Name	Generic Name
Lowest potency		
0.1%	Decadron Phosphate	Dexamethasone
1.0%*	Cort-Dome/Cortaid	Hydrocortisone
Low potency		
0.01%	Valisone	Betamethasone valerate
0.05%	DesOwen	Desonide
0.025%	Kenalog/Aristocort A	Triamcinolone acetonide
Medium potency		
0.1%	Valisone	Betamethasone valerate
0.05%	Topicort LP	Desoximetasone
0.2%	Westcort	Hydrocortisone valerate
0.025%	Halog	Halcinonide
0.1%	Kenalog/Aristocort A	Triamcinolone acetonide
High potency		
0.1%	Cyclocort	Amcinonide
0.05%	Diprosone	Betamethasone dipropionate
0.25%	Topicort	Desoximetasone
0.2%	Synalar HP	Fluocinolone
0.05%	Lidex	Fluocinonide
Ultra-high potency		
0.05%	Diprolene	Betamethasone dipropionate
0.05%	Temovate	Clobetasol propionate
0.05%	Ultravate	Halobetasol

*Now available over-the-counter.
Note: Generic creams and lotions may contain allergens (e.g., preservatives) not found in trade name preparations.

tion through hydrated skin. Topical steroids should be applied no more than twice daily, as more frequent application does not improve efficacy and can dramatically increase cost.

It is important not to use medium- to high-potency topical corticosteroids on the thin-skinned areas of the face, neck, axilla, and groin, unless done with great caution or for short periods of time. Adverse effects of topical corticosteroids include cataracts if used in the periorbital areas, skin atrophy, depigmentation, acne, and, rarely, systemic effects. When the patient is receiving three baths/day, it is recommended that after the morning and bedtime bath, a medium-potency preparation, such as triamcinolone acetonide 0.1 percent, be applied to all affected areas except the face, groin, and axilla. To affected areas on face, groin, and axilla a low-potency product such as hydrocortisone 1 percent or desonide 0.05 percent may be used. After the noon bath and to any unaffected areas after each bath, the patient should apply a water-in-oil or fatty hydrophobic base (Aquaphor, Eucerin, Eutra, white petroleum).

Systemic Corticosteroids

Systemic corticosteroids generally are not warranted in the treatment of this non-life-threatening illness. Oral steroids often have been viewed as a "quick cure," although the dramatic improvement may be followed by an equally dramatic flare once they are stopped. Additionally, the side effects of chronic systemic steroids are both unpleasant and dangerous. Nevertheless, a recent report has suggested the use of low-dose alternate-day prednisone in patients with severe atopic dermatitis refractory to potent topical corticosteroids (Sonenthal et al, 1993).

Tar

Tars and extracts of crude coal tar have been used for their anti-inflammatory properties for years and are recommended to reduce the use of topical corticosteroids in the chronic maintenance of atopic dermatitis. LCD (liquor carbonis detergens), 2.5 percent or 5.0 percent, in Aquaphor has been found to have acceptable cosmetic properties and to be minimally irritating. It may be used only at bedtime to increase compliance. Tar gel products (Estar Gel and Psorigel) are formulations of crude coal tar that are commercially available and cosmetically acceptable; however, they contain alcohol and often cause burning and irritation on eczematous skin. Tar shampoos are often helpful in patients with scalp involvement when used routinely. Side effects associated with tars include folliculitis, photosensitization, and contact dermatitis.

Antimicrobials

Acute flares of eczema, often associated with multiple excoriations and crusting, or chronic poorly controlled dermatitis should be assumed to be infected and should be treated with systemic antibiotics. Failure to recognize and treat secondary infection is likely to frustrate attempts to bring the eczema under control. *Staphylococcus aureus* causes the majority of these infections and is often penicillin-resistant. Culture and sensitivity tests are important during an acute flare to help in the selection of the appropriate antibiotic. It is also important to use the upper limits of recommended dosage to ensure that adequate levels reach the skin. Either erythromycin or cephalexin is a reasonable first choice of therapy. Erythromycin-resistant organisms occasionally account for a poor therapeutic response and necessitate the use of dicloxacillin or clindamycin. In addition, a course of dicloxacillin in combination with rifampin might be tried. Extended treatment ranging from 14 to 28 days is indicated for acute flares. Chronic maintenance therapy may be indicated in patients who repeatedly develop infections. Antibacterial cleansers cannot be recommended. The antibacterial cleansers may worsen the condition by irritating the sensitive skin of these patients. Topical antibiotics are generally not efficacious and may sensitize the patient. However, recent studies have found mupirocin (Bactroban) to be a potentially useful, though expensive, topical antibiotic (Luber et al, 1988).

Herpes simplex should be considered if crusted lesions fail to respond to antibiotics. Patients at risk for widespread dissemination or for systemic or ocular involvement should be treated with intravenous acyclovir. Less extensive involvement may be treated with topical acyclovir. Topical dermatophyte infections usually respond readily to either locally applied imidazole creams or oral griseofulvin daily for one month. *Pityrosporum ovale* may be treated with clotrimazole (Jensen-Jarolim et al, 1992).

Education/Emotional Support

Patients with atopic dermatitis share features common to all chronic diseases: the sense of frustration and anger experienced by them and their families. Unlike most diseases, however, eczema is constantly visible and obvious. Parents of infants with atopic dermatitis are often frustrated by the chronically "sick" appearance of their child. Children and adults are embarrassed by their appearance, which may lead to a poor self image and social isolation. Further frustration develops as it becomes apparent that the process is a chronic one and that quick "cures" cannot be provided. Anger may be directed toward health care providers, who do provide solutions to the problem and prescribe time-consuming treatment plans. All health care providers need to reassure the patient and family that emotional stress is common in situations involving chronic disease. Education and emotional support therefore become critical elements of any successful treatment plan. It has been demonstrated, for example, that improvement in dysfunctional parent-child relationships permits acceptance of educational recommendations and allows for normal development to be resumed and the eczema to improve (Koblenzer and Koblenzer, 1988).

Patients and families should be offered strategies for coping with the disease; these include an increased knowledge base and an understanding of therapies. Knowledge that the disease can be controlled and that the majority of patients improve with age is often reassuring. Patients need to understand the essentials of taking care of their disease. They must be taught the importance of regular skin care and the practical aspects of how it is done. The considerable time involved is usually not available to physicians. Nurses or other health care personnel are often best suited for this task. Follow-up visits to nurses for reviews of the treatment plan and ongoing education can be extremely helpful. Practical tips for skin care are available through a variety of sources (Clark et al, 1990). The Eczema Association for Science and Education (1221 SW Yamhill, #303 Portland, OR 97205) offers health providers, their patients, and patients' families a wealth of information regarding atopic dermatitis and its care. Its medical advisory board includes leading national experts in the field of atopic dermatitis. In addition to educational materials, this association provides a forum for emotional support for patients with atopic dermatitis. Locally formed support groups may also be extremely helpful. Recent research has suggested a variety of new therapeutic approaches, and patients need to be kept up to date to prevent a sense of hopelessness.

Immunomodulators

Since patients with atopic dermatitis manifest abnormalities in immune regulation, therapy directed toward modulation of their immune dysfunction has been suggested. These novel forms of therapy represent exciting alternatives for patients who are resistant to available treatment. However, most measures would not be considered standard treatment but may lead to more effective forms of therapy.

Allergen Immunotherapy

Many of the early investigators studying the role of aeroallergens in atopic dermatitis used immunotherapy for the treatment of their patients. While some claimed marked improvement as a result of therapy, others found that injections had no beneficial value. All investigators found that immunotherapy frequently led to acute flares of skin lesions. None of these early studies were performed in a controlled manner. More recently, several reports of the successful use of immunotherapy in the treatment of atopic dermatitis have appeared in the literature (Kaufman and Roth, 1974; Fuenmayor and Champion, 1979). Ring reported the results of a double-blind placebo-controlled study of the effects of immunotherapy in a pair of monozygotic twins with atopic dermatitis (Ring, 1982). These sisters with severe atopic dermatitis had noted pronounced seasonal exacerbations during the spring and early summer months and demonstrated positive prick skin tests and RAST to grass allergen. Following 2 years of preseasonal injections to grass pollen extract, the twin receiving active allergen had a lower clinical symptom score and serum IgE concentration than her placebo-treated sister. Additionally, the first twin did not experience her usual summer flare during the grass pollen season.

It would seem that there is not sufficient evidence to allow conclusions regarding the usefulness of immunotherapy in atopic dermatitis. Nevertheless, all recent studies have tended to demonstrate a beneficial effect. A clinical trial in selected allergic patients would seem reasonable. The observation that immunotherapy injections often exacerbate eczema would seem to provide further evidence regarding the role of aeroallergens in the pathogenesis of atopic dermatitis. Further controlled studies should select patients on the basis of a history of allergen-induced exacerbations or seasonal flares of atopic dermatitis.

Interferon-gamma

Interferon-gamma is a cytokine that suppresses IL-4-induced IgE synthesis and inhibits T_{H2} cell function. As mentioned above, peripheral blood mononuclear cells from patients with atopic dermatitis have been found to have a decreased capacity to produce IFN-γ (Jujo et al, 1992). In a 12-week double-blind, placebo-controlled trial of interferon-gamma patients receiving daily injections, significant improvement in physician and patient severity scores was noted when compared with placebo results (Boguniewicz et al, 1990). In addition, total circulating eosinophil counts and *in vitro* IgE synthesis by peripheral blood lymphocytes were decreased in the treated group.

Thymopentin

Thymopentin is a synthetic pentapeptide that promotes differentiation of thymocytes and enhances T lymphocyte function. In a 6-week double-blind, placebo-controlled trial of thymopentin, patients receiving daily injections showed significant relief of pruritus and erythema when compared with placebo results (Leung et al, 1990). Significant differences were not seen until the 6-week examination, suggesting a delayed onset of action.

Cyclosporine

Cyclosporine, a drug that down-regulates cytokine production, has been studied as a treatment for atopic dermatitis. In an 8-week double-blind, placebo-controlled trial of cyclosporine in adults with refractory atopic dermatitis, significant benefit was noted when compared with placebo results (Sowden et al, 1991). Because of the hepatotoxic and immunosuppressive effects of this drug, its continued use, except in the most refractory cases of adults with atopic dermatitis, seems unlikely. Early enthusiasm for the use of topical cyclosporine was not borne out in controlled trials.

Phototherapy

Ultraviolet light therapy may be a useful adjunctive modality in the treatment of chronic recalcitrant disease. Patients with a history of improvement with sunlight exposure and who are not fair complexioned should be encouraged to avail themselves of moderate amounts of natural sunlight as an initial trial. However, they should be warned against sunburn and to avoid hot or humid conditions, which may actually induce more pruritus. Ultraviolet light therapy (UVA) and psoralen photochemotherapy (PUVA) have been shown to induce remission in many patients with severe disease (Atherton et al, 1988), probably owing to its suppressive effect on Langerhan's cells and, possibly, on cutaneous mast cells. Although UVB alone provides a good response rate, the addition of UVA to UVB may improve the therapeutic response. The expense, slow response rate, almost inevitable relapse following treatment, and increased risk of skin cancer limit its usefulness.

REFERENCES

Adinoff AD, Tellez P, Clark RAF. Atopic dermatitis and aeroallegen contact sensitivity. J Allergy Clin Immunol 81:736, 1988.

Adinoff AD, Clark RAF. The allergic nature of atopic dermatitis. Immunol Allergy Prac 11:17–28, 1989.

Atkins FM, Steinberg SS, Metcalfe DD. Evaluation of immediate adverse reactions to foods in adult patients II: A detailed analysis of reaction patterns during oral food challenge. J Allergy Clin Immunol 75:356, 1985.

Atherton DJ, Cabablott F, Glover MT, et al. The role of psoralen chemotherapy (PUVA) in the treatment of severe atopic eczema in adolescence. Br J Dermatol 118:791–795, 1988.

Bieber T, de la Salle H, Wollenberg A, et al. Human epidermal Langerhans' cells express the high affinity receptor for immunoglobulin E. J Exp Med 175:1285, 1992.

Berth-Jones J, Graham-Brown RA. Failure of terfenadine in relieving the pruritus of atopic dermatitis. Br J Dermatol 121:635–637, 1989.

Bock SA, Lee WY, Remigio LK, May CD. Studies of

hypersensitivity reactions to foods in infants and children. J Allergy Clin Immunol 62:327, 1978.
Boguniewicz M, Jaffe HS, Izu A, et al. Recombinant gamma interferon therapy in treatment of patients with atopic dermatitis and elevated IgE levels. Am J Med 88:365–370, 1990.
Bruynzeel-Koomen C, vanWichen DF, Toonstra J, et al. The presence of IgE molecules of epidermal Langerhans' cells in patients with atopic dermatitis. Arch Derm Res 278:199, 1986.
Bruynzeel-Koomen C, Bruynzeel PLB. A role for IgE in patch test reactions to inhalant allergens in patients with atopic dermatitis. Allergy 43(suppl 5):15, 1988.
Burks AW, Mallory SB, Williams LW, et al. Atopic dermatitis: Clinical relevance of food hypersensitivity reactions. J Pediatr 113:447–451, 1988.
Charlesworth EN, Kagey-Sabotka A, Norman PS, et al. Effect of cetirizine on mast cell–mediator release and cellular traffic during the cutaneous late-phase reaction. J Allergy Clin Immunol 83:905–912, 1989.
Clark RAF, Adinoff AD. The relationship between positive aeroallergen patch test reactions and aeroallergen exacerbations of atopic dermatitis. J Allergy Clin Immunol 85:292, 1990. (Abstract)
Clark RAF, Nichol N, Adinoff AD. Current concepts in the management of the patient with atopic dermatitis. Mod Med 58:78, 1990.
Dahl MV, Cates KL, Quie PG. Neutrophil chemotaxis in patients with atopic dermatitis without infection. Arch Dermatol 114:544–546, 1978.
Falth-Magnusson K, Kjellman NIM. Allergy prevention by maternal elimination diet during late pregnancy—a 5-year follow-up of a randomized study. J Allergy Clin Immunol 89:709–713, 1992.
Fuenmayor MC, Champion RH. Specific hyposensitization in atopic dermatitis. Br J Dermatol 101:697, 1979.
Hanifin JM, Rajka G. Diagnostic features of atopic dermatitis. Acta Derm Venereol 92(suppl):44–47, 1980.
Harving H, Korsgaard J, Dahl R, et al. House dust mites and atopic dermatitis: A case-control study on the significance of house dust mites as etiologic allergens in atopic dermatitis. Ann Allergy 65:25, 1990.
Hoffman DR, Yamamoto FY, Geller B, et al. Specific IgE antibodies in atopic eczema. J Allergy Clin Immunol 55:256, 1975.
Irani AM, Sampson HA, Schwartz LB. Mast cells in atopic dermatitis. Allergy 44(suppl 9):31–34, 1989.
Jensen-Jarolim E, Poulsen LK, With H, et al. Atopic dermatitis of the face, scalp and neck: Type I reaction to the yeast *Pityrosporum ovale*? J Allergy Clin Immunol 89:44–51, 1992.
Jones HE, Bergbardt JH, Rinaldi MG. A clinical, mycological and immunological survey for dermatophytosis. Arch Dermatol 108:61–65, 1973a.
Jones HE, Lewis C, McMarlin SL. Allergic contact sensitivity in atopic dermatitis. Arch Dermatol 107:217, 1973b.
Jujo K, Renz H, Abe J, et al. Decreased INF-γ and increased IL-4 in atopic dermatitis. J Allergy Clin Immunol 90:323, 1992.
Kajosaari M, Saarinen UM. Prophylaxis of atopic disease by six months' total solid food elimination. Acta Paediatr Scand 72:411–414, 1983.
Kaufman HS, Roth HL. Hyposensitization with alum-precipitated extracts in atopic dermatitis: A placebo-controlled study. Ann Allergy 32:321, 1974.
Kieffer M, Bergbrant IM, Faegernann M, et al. Immune reactions to *Pityrosporum ovale* in adult patients with atopic and seborrheic dermatitis. J Am Acad Dermatol 22:739, 1990.
Koblenzer CS, Koblenzer PJ. Chronic intractable atopic eczema: Its occurrence as a physical sign of impaired parent-child relationships and psychologic development arrest: Improvement through parent insight and education. Arch Dermatol 124:1673, 1988.
Leiferman KM, Ackerman SJ, Sampson HA, et al. Dermal deposition of eosinophil-granule major basic protein in atopic dermatitis: Comparison with onchocerciasis. N Engl J Med 313:282, 1985.
Leung DYM, Hirsh RL, Schneider L, et al. Thymopentin therapy reduces the clinical severity of atopic dermatitis. J Allergy Clin Immunol 85:927–933, 1990.
Leung DYM, Harbeck R, Bina P, et al. Patients with atopic dermatitis contain IgE directed against toxins secreted by *Staphylococcus aureus* grown from their skin. J Allergy Clin Immunol 89:724, 1992.
Leyden JE, Marples RR, Kligman AD. *Staphylococcus aureus* in the lesions of atopic dermatitis. Br J Dermatol 90:52, 1974.
Leyden JE, Baker DA. Localized herpes simplex infection in atopic dermatitis. Arch Dermatol 115:311, 1979.
Luber H, Amornsiripanitch S, Lucky AW. Mupirocin and the eradication of *Staphylococcus aureus* in atopic dermatitis. Arch Dermatol 124:853–854, 1988.
Michel L, De Vos D, Rihowx JP, et al. Inhibitory effect of oral cetirizine on in vivo antigen-induced histamine and PAF-acether release and eosinophil recruitment in human skin. J Allergy Clin Immunol 82:101–109, 1988.
Mihm MC, Soter NA, Dvorak HF, et al. The structure of normal skin and the morphology of atopic eczema. J Invest Dermatol 67:305, 1976.
Mitchell EB, Crow J, Chapman MD, et al. Basophils in allergen-induced patch test sites in atopic dermatitis. Lancet 1:127, 1982.
Monroe EW. Relative efficacy and safety of loratadine, hydroxyzine, and placebo in chronic idiopathic urticaria and atopic dermatitis. Clin Ther 14:17–21, 1992.
Mudde GC, Van Reijsen FC, Boland GJ, et al. Allergen presentation by epidermal Langerhans' cells from patients with atopic dermatitis is mediated by IgE. Immunology 69:1077, 1990.
NIAID Task Force Report. Dermatologic Allergy: Asthma and the Other Allergic Diseases. NIH Publication No. 79–387, May 1979, p 375.
Nicol NH. Atopic dermatitis: The (wet) wrap-up. Am J Nursing 87:1560–1563, 1987.
Norris PG, Schofield O, Camp RDR. A study of the role of house dust mite in atopic dermatitis. Br J Dermatol 118:435, 1988.
Platts-Mills TAE, Mitchell EB, Rowntree S, et al. The role of dust mite allergens in atopic dermatitis. Clin Exp Dermatol 8:233, 1983.
Rees J, Friedmann PS, Matthews JNS. Contact sensitivity in dinitrochlorobenzene is impaired in atopic subjects. Arch Dermatol 126:1173, 1990.
Ring J. Successful hyposensitization treatment in atopic eczema: Results of a trial in monozygotic twins. Br J Dermatol 107:597, 1982.
Sager N, Feldman A, Schilling G, et al. House dust mite-specific T cells in the skin of subjects with atopic dermatitis: Frequency and lymphokine profile in the allergen patch test. J Allergy Clin Immunol 89:801–810, 1992.
Sampson HA. Role of immediate food hypersensitivity in the pathogenesis of atopic dermatitis. J Allergy Clin Immunol 71:473, 1983.

Sampson HA, McCaskill CC. Food hypersensitivity and atopic dermatitis: Evaluation of 113 patients. J Pediatr 107:669, 1985.

Sampson HA. The role of food allergy and mediator release in atopic dermatitis. J Allergy Clin Immunol 81:635, 1988.

Seymour JL, Kewick BH, Hanifin JM, et al. Clinical effects of diaper types on the skin of normal infants and infants with atopic dermatitis. J Am Acad Dermatol 17:988–997, 1987.

Sigurs N, Hattevig G, Kjellman B. Maternal avoidance of eggs, cow's milk, and fish during lactation: Effect on allergic manifestations, skin prick tests, and specific IgE antibodies in children at age 4 years. Pediatrics 89:735–739, 1992.

Sonenthal KR, Grammer LC, Patterson R. Do some patients with atopic dermatitis require long-term oral steroid therapy? J Allergy Clin Immunol 91:971–973, 1993.

Sowden JM, Berth-Jones J, Ross JS, et al. Double-blind, controlled, crossover study of cyclosporin in adults with severe refractory atopic dermatitis. Lancet 338:137–140, 1991.

Tuft L, Tuft HS, Heck VM. Atopic dermatitis II. Role of the sweating mechanism. J Invest Dermatol 15:333, 1950.

Tuft L, Heck VM. Studies in atopic dermatitis IV. Importance of seasonal inhalant allergens, especially ragweed. J Allergy 23:528, 1952.

Uehara M. Atopic dermatitis and tuberculin reactivity. Arch Dermatol 113:1226–1228, 1977.

Vickers CFH. The natural history of atopic eczema. Acta Derm Venereol (Stockh) 92(suppl):113, 1980.

Werner Y, Lingberg M. Transepidermal water loss in dry and clinically normal skin in patients with atopic dermatitis. Acta Derm Venereol (Stockh) 65:102, 1985.

Zeiger RS, Heller S, Mellon MH, et al. Effect of combined maternal and infant food allergen avoidance on development of atopy in early infancy: A randomized study. J Allergy Clin Immunol 84:72–89, 1989.

ACKNOWLEDGMENT: We would like to thank Barbara R. Reed, M.D., Denver Skin Clinic, Denver, Colorado, for her thoughtful and critical review of this chapter.

Chapter 45

Contact Dermatitis

John L. Aeling, M.D.

IMMUNOLOGY

Contact dermatitis occurs when a substance contacts the skin and elicits an inflammatory reaction. This reaction can be secondary to cutaneous exposure to an irritant or an allergen. Irritant reactions are common and include diaper dermatitis, hand dermatitis, and dermatitis from exposure to strong acids and alkalis. There is a marked variability from person to person in response to irritants. Atopic patients tend to be especially sensitive to irritants such as wool, soaps, detergents and other common chemicals. It is difficult to distinguish irritant dermatitis from allergic contact dermatitis solely on the basis of history and clinical appearance. Irritant dermatitis usually occurs within minutes or hours of exposure, is sharply localized to the area of exposure, and is often painful.

Allergic contact dermatitis occurs 24 to 48 hours after exposure, may spread beyond the areas of contact, progresses for several days, and itches more than it hurts. Both types of contact dermatitis may show erythema, scaling, papules, and blisters. This chapter will concentrate primarily on allergic contact dermatitis.

IMMUNOPATHOGENESIS

In 1895, Jadassohn first described contact allergy to mercury. Since that time much has been learned about the pathogenesis of allergic contact sensitivity. The skin is a unique and complex immune organ that can react in a multitude of ways to an immune stimulus.

Most contact allergens are low-molecular-weight substances of less than 500 daltons, which can easily penetrate the stratum corneum and combine with an epidermal protein to form a complete antigen of greater than 5000 daltons. This protein probably represents a constituent of cell membrane, and the conjugation with an antigen probably occurs as an antigen-processing function by Langerhans' cells.

T lymphocytes cannot interact directly with potential antigens, which must first be processed and presented on the surface of a unique cell to an appropriate lymphocyte. This antigen-processing cell (Langerhans' cell) is a dendritic epidermal cell that can move within the epidermis, from the epidermis to the dermis, and eventually to regional lymph nodes. Langerhans' cells express alloantigens (Ia antigens), receptors for the FC fragment of IgG immunoglobulin and complement (C3) on their cell surface. Only a small subpopulation of T lymphocytes having receptors for a specific antigen are available to interact with antigen-presenting cells. When this interaction occurs, interleukin-1 (lymphocyte-activating factor) is released by the Langerhans' cells and also by keratinocytes. This cytokine triggers T lymphocytes to release interleukin-2 (lymphocyte-proliferating factor). These specific activated lymphocytes migrate to regional lymph nodes, where they stimulate the production of a specific clone of lymphocytes, which are able to recognize and interact with a specific antigen. The latter cells enter the circulation and are capable of migrating through skin and will interact with the specific antigen when it is contacted on the cutaneous surface. When recognition and interaction occur, a host of cytokines are released including chemotactic factors, macrophage-activating and migration-inhibitory factors, transfer factors, and cytotoxic factors. Gamma

634—MANAGEMENT OF SKIN DISEASE

interferon is important in this complex reaction. Langerhans' cells are an early and important participant in the induction of allergic contact dermatitis, as demonstrated by the fact that ultraviolet light interferes with Langerhans' cell function and inhibits the induction of allergic contact dermatitis (Okamoto and Horio, 1981).

CLINICAL PRESENTATIONS AND EVALUATION

The history is extremely important when evaluating a clinical presentation suggesting an allergic contact dermatitis. All potential contact antigens have a variable potential to elicit contact allergy. For instance, exposure to dinitrochlorobenzene will sensitize almost 100 percent of patients, whereas contact allergy to water is almost 0 percent. Therefore, when a history is taken, specific questions focusing on the most common antigens associated with allergic contact dermatitis should be asked. For example, it is not sufficient to ask a woman if she breaks out when her skin is in contact with metal. Specific questions that seek to implicate or exclude contact metal sensitivity should be addressed, including the following:

1. "Did your ears become infected after ear piercing or do you break out from the metal button on your jeans during the summer months?" (Induction of metal contact sensitivity most commonly occurs after ear piercing, and perspiration will leach potential antigens from wearing apparel.)

2. "Have you ever broken out from contact with cement or from a leather hat band, wallet, or shoes?" (These are common sources of chromate sensitivity (Fig. 45–1).)

3. "Have you had poison ivy or lived in an area where poison ivy is common?"

4. "Have you ever broken out in reaction to hair dye?" (This is the most common source of contact allergy to paraphenylenediamine (Fig. 45–2).)

5. "Have you ever broken out in reaction to the elastic in your undergarments, rubber gloves, or adhesives?" (These are common sources of rubber chemicals that can be directed at natural rubber antigens or additives in synthetic rubber. Mercaptobenzathiazole and thiurams are the most common antigens in synthetic rubbers.)

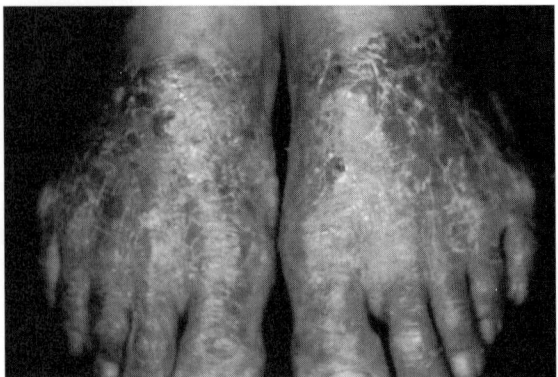

FIGURE 45–1. Bilaterally symmetric dorsal foot dermatitis is an allergic dermatitis from a shoe allergen until proven otherwise.

These questions cover five of the most common contact antigens as noted in Table 45–1 (Rudner et al, 1973).

Almost all patients who have chronic or recurrent dermatitis will self-treat with over-the-counter products or with their family's and friends' topical prescription medications. Subsequently, it is common for patients to

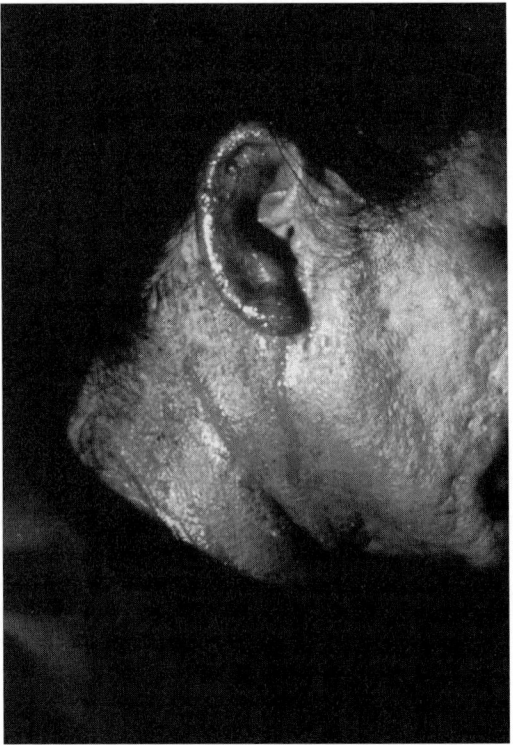

FIGURE 45–2. An acute weeping contact dermatitis on the ears and hair line caused by paraphenylenediamine in permanent hair dye.

TABLE 45–1. PERCENT POSITIVE PATCH TESTS PERFORMED ON 1200 PATIENTS WITH DERMATITIS

	% Concentration	% Positive
Nickel sulfate	2.5	11
Potassium dichromate	0.5	8
Paraphenylenediamine	1	8
Mercaptobenzothiazole	2	5
Thiuram	2	4

develop a secondary allergic contact dermatitis on a preexisting stasis, atopic, nummular, irritant, or neurodermatitis. Specific information should be sought regarding what a patient has used to treat the dermatitis. These questions should include:

1. Use of topical antibiotics?
2. Use of topical vitamin E and aloe vera? (Many over-the-counter aloe vera products contain vitamin E.)
3. Use of topical anesthetics?
4. Use of Mycolog cream? (Mycolog contains several common sensitizing chemicals such as neomycin, thiomerasol, ethylenediamine, and fragrances. Mycolog II does not contain ethylenediamine, neomycin, or thimerosal.)
5. Use of moisturizers? (These may contain preservatives, fragrances and lanolins.)

Topical antibiotics are potent sensitizers, particularly neomycin. In a large series of patients with dermatitis, 60 percent were patch test positive to neomycin (Rudner et al, 1973). In my opinion, topical neomycin never should be applied to any chronic dermatitis, especially not to stasis dermatitis. In fact, there is little reason to use this topical medication. Neomycin can be found in many otic, ophthalmic, and antiseptic ointments, creams, and solutions. In addition, many veterinary products including poultry feeds, pet foods and topical medications contain neomycin (Fisher, 1986). On rare occasions, neomycin has been added to antiperspirants. Some patients who are neomycin-sensitive may also be bacitracin-sensitive. This is because neomycin and bacitracin are often contained in the same preparations and are concurrently applied to acute and chronic dermatitis. Since bacitracin and neomycin are not structurally related, the contact sensitivity is coincidental and not due to cross-sensitization (Bjorkner and Moller, 1973).

When dealing with any patient with a chronic and recurrent dermatitis, it is a good idea to have the patient empty the medicine cabinet and bring to the office all topical medications, both prescription and over-the-counter, that may have been used in the past and in the present. On occasion, the patient will arrive at the next visit with several grocery sacks full.

A detailed occupational history should be taken. Approximately 30 percent of all occupational disorders involve skin disease. Specific allergens are often related to specific occupations (Table 45–2). Occupational skin disease may be irritant, allergic, or both. It can be difficult to distinguish between them on a purely clinical basis (Table 45–3).

Treatment for occupational allergic contact dermatitis consists of identification and complete avoidance of the offending antigen. Treatment of irritant dermatitis entails avoidance and the use of protective measures including safe work practices and protective gloves and clothing. The 4 H glove is imper-

TABLE 45–2. OCCUPATIONS AND SPECIFIC ANTIGEN EXPOSURES

Health care workers, pharmacists, veterinarians	Benzalkonium chloride, rubber (latex), formaldehyde, glutaraldehyde, antibiotics, phenothiazines, acrylics
Dentists	Balsam of Peru, caines, acrylics, epoxy resins, mercury, gutta percha, glutaraldehyde
Outdoor workers, florists, gardeners, wood workers	Poison ivy, exotic woods, chrysanthemum, tulips
Beauticians	Nickel, paraphenylenediamine, ammonium persulfate, glycerol thioglycolate, rubbers
Morticians, laboratory workers, insulation workers, paper mill workers, wood workers	Formaldehyde
Electric workers, electricians, painters, construction workers, aircraft assembly workers	Epoxy resins, chromates, synthetic rubber

TABLE 45–3. ALLERGIC VERSUS IRRITANT CONTACT DERMATITIS

Allergic	Irritant
Genetically predisposed	Every one
Low-molecular-weight antigen	Solvents, soaps, acids, alkalis
Low concentration of antigen	High concentration
Delayed hypersensitivity	A physical or chemical reaction
Onset 12–48 hours, after exposure and induction of sensitivity	Onset minutes, hours, days, weeks, or months—depending on irritant, exposure, and individual tolerance

meable to most solvents, hydrocarbons, ketones, and other chemicals. It has been tested for permeability against more than 250 chemicals and is impervious for more than 4 hours. It is available through Safety 4 Inc, 2920 Wolff Street, Racine, Wisconsin, 53404 (414) 632-8133.

The clinical pattern and distribution of a dermatitis presents clues to the offending antigen (Table 45–4). The acute phase of allergic contact dermatitis includes urticarial papules, edema, erythema with eventual vesiculation, bullae, serous oozing, and crusts. With chronic exposure the skin thickens (lichenifies), develops accentuation of skin markings, hyperkeratosis, fissures, cracks, scaling, secondary excoriations, and erosions. In severe cases new lesions may appear over 7 to 10 days, and the eruption may last for 3 to 4 weeks. Often the entire skin surface can become reactive with generalized itching and spread of the dermatitis to areas outside the original sites of contact (auto-eczematization) (Parish et al, 1965). This is a poorly understood immunologic phenomenon and is particularly common when patients with chronic stasis dermatitis become contact-sensitive. This raises the question whether certain contact antigens in some patients may function as superantigens, as happens with bacterial antigens (Leung et al, 1993).

TABLE 45–4. CLINICAL PATTERNS OF ALLERGIC CONTACT DERMATITIS AND PROBABLE OFFENDING ANTIGENS

Clinical Patterns	Offending Antigens
Blisters in lines and streaks	Poison ivy, oak, sumac, primrose, chrysanthemum, and other plants
Symmetric dorsal foot dermatitis	Shoe allergy, chromates, rubbers, paraphenylenediamine, nickel, glues
Exposed skin	Airborne contact dermatitis, plant oleoresins
Earlobe, neck, wrist dermatitis	Jewelry, nickel, cobalt
Axillary dermatitis; dome of axilla is usually spared	Deodorants, fragrances, zirconium (aluminum salts are primarily irritants)
Eyelid dermatitis	Formaldehyde in nail polish, nail hardeners, eye drops, particularly with neomycin, contact lens solutions (most reactions to cosmetics, particularly to eye shadows, are irritants)
Forehead, ears, scalp margins	Hair dyes, paraphenylenediamine
Acute dermatitis surrounding leg ulcers	Neomycin, Furacin, preservatives, other topical antibiotics
Neck, axilla, waist band, and groin dermatitis	Most commonly found in clothing due to permanent press formaldehyde resins
Genital dermatitis	Latex, synthetic rubbers, caines, hemorrhoidal medications, fragrances
Contact urticaria; can be due to type I hypersensitivity or to direct histamine release	Latex, animal saliva, plants, cobalt, foods, antibiotics, nitrogen mustard used to treat patients with mycosis fungoides, ammonium persulfate used for hair bleaching as a peroxide booster
Facial dermatitis, often irritant, may be allergic	Preservatives, fragrances, methacrylates in sculptured nails; some fragrances, especially musk ambrette, can be photo contact sensitizers
	Numerous antigens can be carried from the hands to the face
Dermatitis of palms and soles	Rarely allergic

Rarely, contact dermatitis may have an unusual clinical appearance (Fregert, 1974). Lichen planus–like eruptions can occur with exposure to color film developers, and purpuric eruptions have been reported from rubber exposure. Other unique presentations include vitiligo-like lesions from rubber accelerators and phenolic detergents; granulomatous reactions from zirconium and beryllium; contact uriticaria from numerous allergens including plants, metals, latex, and foods; and acneiform eruptions from dioxin, cooking oils, and pomades.

PATHOLOGY

From a practical point of view it is not possible to distinguish irritant from allergic contact dermatitis on histologic examination. Histologic patterns of contact dermatitis can be divided into acute, subacute, and chronic dermatitis. Acute dermatitis shows intra-epidermal multilocular vesicles, prominent intracellular edema, and inflammatory cells within both the epidermis and the superficial dermis. The cellular infiltrate is mixed, with the predominant cell being mononuclear. Basophils, eosinophils, neutrophils, and macrophages are also present in the inflammatory infiltrates. Chronic contact dermatitis shows varying patterns of hyperkeratosis, parakeratosis, acanthosis, and a predominately mononuclear cell infiltrate.

PATCH TESTING

Properly applied and interpreted patch tests are simple and are the only scientific proof of allergic contact dermatitis. There is no contraindication to patch testing, and significant side effects are rare. Occasionally, persistent dyspigmentation can be seen after markedly positive patch tests, but this rarely lasts more than a few months. Patch testing during pregnancy should only be done if clearly indicated. When patients are properly selected for patch testing, 50 percent will have one or more positive reactions, and half of these will be relevant to the patient's problem. Patch testing is simple, safe, rewarding, and underutilized. There are over two million known chemicals; over 100,000 are used in industry and over 2000 are synthesized each year (Fregert, 1986). The 20 most common allergens are available in the North American contact dermatitis tray (Table 45–5). The tray is continually updated, and the antigens that frequently cause severe reactions are dispersed so that it is rare to have two adjacent strongly positive reactions (Fig. 45–3). The screening tray will pick up 80 percent or more of all contact allergies.

TABLE 45–5. NORTH AMERICAN CONTACT DERMATITIS TRAY

Metals
  Nickel sulfate, 2.5%
  Potassium dichromate, 0.025%
Preservatives
  Quaternium 15, 2%
  Imidazolidinyl urea, 2%
  Formaldehyde, 1%
Medicaments
  Neomycin, 20%
  Benzocaine, 5%
  Wool alcohols (lanolin), 30%
Fragrances
  Balsam of Peru, 25%
  Cinnamic aldehyde, 1%
Rubbers
  Thiuram mix, 1%
  Mercaptobenzathiazole, 1%
  Carba mix, 3%
  Black rubber mix, 0.6%
  Mercapto mix, 1%
Resins
  P-Tert-Butyphenol, 1%
  Epoxy, 1%
Miscellaneous
  Paraphenylenediamine, 1%
  Colophony, 20%
  Ethylenediamine, 1%

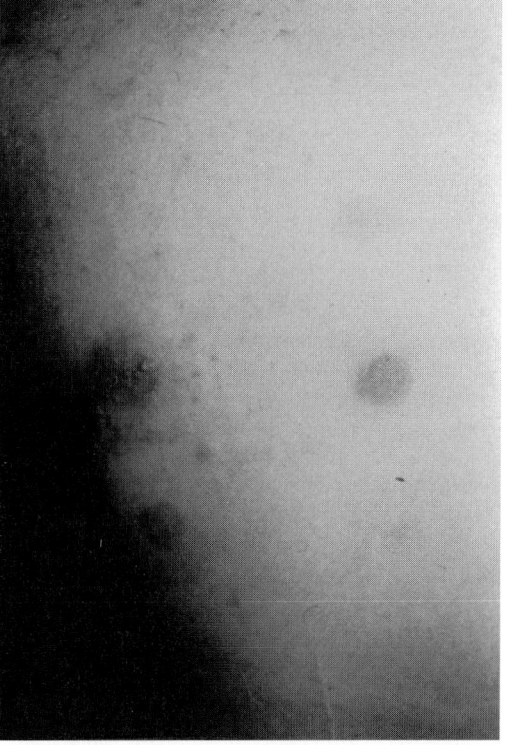

FIGURE 45–3. A 2+ and 3+ positive patch test.

TABLE 45–6. WHEN TO PATCH TEST

1. To confirm a suspected allergen
2. When a dermatitis is possibly work related
3. When the clinical pattern of dermatitis suggests a contact dermatitis
4. In cases of recurring facial dermatitis
5. When a dermatitis does not respond or is worse after topical therapy
6. When you think of it

Although other antigens are commercially available, for most practices it is not feasible to have all possible antigens available for testing. The antigens are expensive and should be replaced on a yearly basis. Most large cities have a center or physician who has a special interest in occupational dermatitis and contact allergy. If a product is suspect and is marketed to be used on the skin, or if it is frequently contacted, a use test can be recommended. This is particularly helpful with cosmetics, sun screens, and moisturizers. It is recommended that the suspect product be applied twice daily to the same quarter-size spot on the flexor forearm for 7 days. False-negative use tests can occur. If the use test is negative, a closed patch test can be done with little risk. Soaps, detergents, and shampoos are exceptions for open or closed patch tests. If these are clinical suspects, the individual ingredients should be tested separately. When one or more 3+ patch test reactions are encountered with several weak 1+ reactions, the patient may have an excited skin syndrome (angry back). Often the weak positive reactions are false-positives. These should be repeated as single tests after the original patch test reaction has subsided (Tables 45–6 and 45–7).

A simple patch test system (True Test) has been available in Europe for several years (Fig. 45–4) and should be available in the United States in the near future (Adams and Rietschel, 1989).

Table 45–8 lists rules for patch testing, and Table 45–9 lists sources of allergen patch test supplies.

Nickel is one of the most common sensitizers. Eleven percent of patients with dermatitis show a positive nickel patch test. Women have a higher frequency of positive tests due to sensitization at the time of ear piercing. Besides obvious metal exposures, nickel can be found in paints, dyes, duplicating fluids, plastics (Fig. 45–5), insecticides, wallpapers, and many other products. A dimethylglyox-

TABLE 45–7. HOW TO PATCH TEST

1. The patients should be in a relaxed but upright position.
2. Hairy skin should be shaved, preferably with an electric razor, prior to patch testing.
3. The patch test site should be free of dermatitis.
4. The upper back is the preferable site for patch testing, not over vertebrae. The upper arm can be used as an alternative.
5. Finn chambers with scanpor tape are the preferred application method.
6. Mark outline of test sites with a fluorescent marker.
7. Draw map of patch test location on patch test form.
8. Test sites should remain dry until removed. Frontal bathing only. No strenuous exercise or perspiration.
9. Remove tests at 48 hours. Remove immediately if severe itching, burning, or irritation occurs and call the office.
10. Read the patch tests no sooner than 72 hours and preferably at 96 hours after application. A delayed reading 7 days after application is recommended.
11. Patch test reading: 1+ (erythema), 2+ (erythema, papules, small vesicles), 3+ (confluent bullae, extends beyond application site), NT (not tested), IR (probable irritant reaction). Use a black light to identify the patch test site.

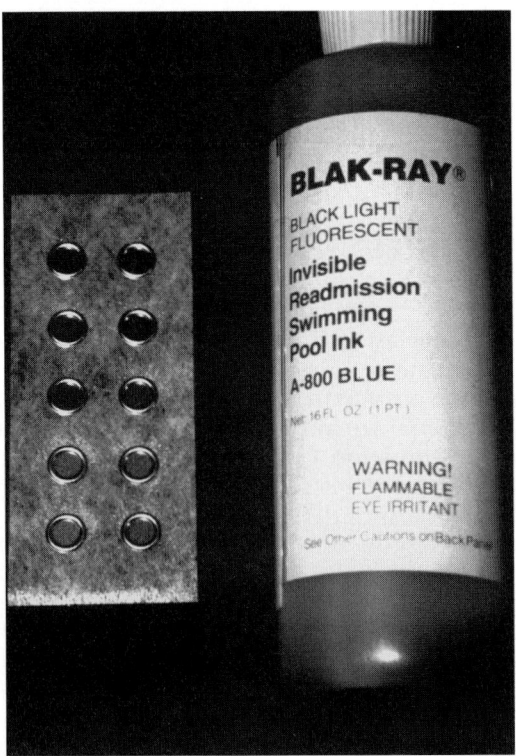

FIGURE 45–4. True Test system with Finn Chambers, scanpor tape, and ultraviolet ink.

TABLE 45–8. RULES OF PATCH TESTING

1. Use only known substances in standard concentrations.
2. Do not test if dermatitis is acute.
3. Discontinue topical steroids at the test site for at least one week prior to testing.
4. Prednisone at a dose of 30 mg daily or less does not significantly affect patch test results.
5. A positive patch test may be non-relevant.
6. A weak positive reaction may or may not be relevant.
7. Irritant reactions may be difficult to tell from allergic reactions. They may appear glazed, scalded, eroded, and limited to test site and often fade within 24 hours of patch test removal. Formaldehyde, potassium dichromate, and neomycin commonly cause irritant reactions.
8. Repeat any questionable positive or negative test results.
9. Petechial lesions (black rubber and cobalt) and pustular lesions (metals and atopics) are false-positive reactions.
10. If a substance is designed to be applied to the skin, open testing is usually safe. Soaps, detergents, and shampoos are exceptions.

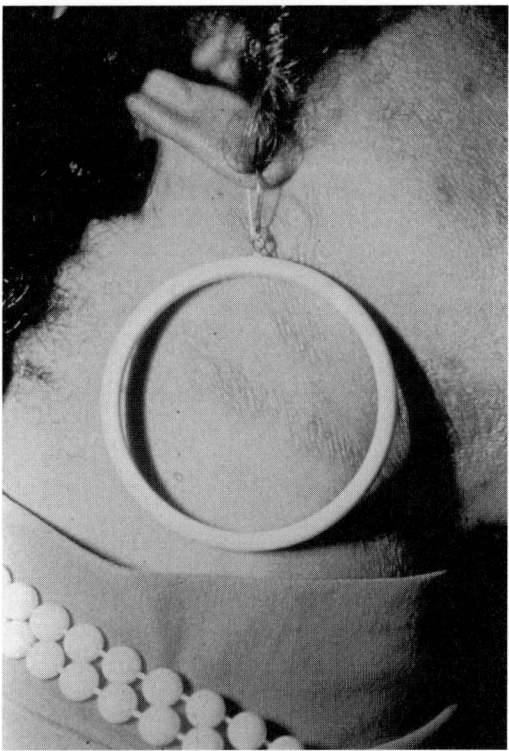

FIGURE 45–5. A patient with intermittent dermatitis of the lateral neck posed a diagnostic dilemma until her plastic earrings were discovered to be the antigenic culprit.

ene spot test for the detection of small amounts (1 part per 10,000) of nickel in jewelry can be obtained from Alerderm Laboratories, P.O. Box 931, Mill Valley, CA 94941.

Chromate dermatitis is the second most common metal sensitizer. Cement exposure is a common source of sensitization. Other exposures include leather, dyes, paints, wood stains, fireworks, wallpaper, sponges, safety matches, ceramic paints, plastics, glues, waxes, flypaper, green felt (blackjack dermatitis), photographic chemicals, catgut, radiator coolants, bleaches, and many others.

Quaternium 15 (Dowicil) is a formaldehyde-releasing preservative and the most common cause of preservative dermatitis, accounting for 2 to 3 percent of positive patch tests in patients with dermatitis. It is found in many cosmetics and over-the-counter skin products. Positive patch tests may represent an allergic reaction to Quaternium, the released formaldehyde, or both chemicals.

Formaldehyde is a ubiquitous chemical found in almost every environment. The degree of sensitivity varies greatly from person to person. Common exposures include glues, paper, insulation, fumigating chemicals, deodorizers, cleaners, polishers, explosives, permanent press fabrics, nail products, embalming fluids, and many others. Formaldehyde is still used as a preservative in shampoos. It is a rare cause of scalp or facial dermatitis because it is rapidly diluted and rinsed. However, it is a cause of hand dermatitis in beauticians.

TABLE 45–9. SOURCES OF ALLERGEN PATCH TEST SUPPLIES

Finn Chambers and scanpor tape:
  Hermal Pharmaceutical Inc.
  Route 134
  Oakhill, New York 12460

True Test System:
  Pharmacia, Inc.
  800 Centennial Avenue
  Piscataway, New Jersey 08854

Standard Tray of 20 Allergens:
  Hermal Pharmaceutical
  163 Delaware Ave
  Delmar, NY 12054 (800) 437-6251

Synthetic rubber-free undergarments for men and women:
  Natural Choice
  1365 Rufina Circle
  Santa Fe, New Mexico 87501
  (800) 621-2591

Imidazolidinyl urea (Germall) is a weak formaldehyde releaser. Most formaldehyde-sensitive patients can use over-the-counter products with this preservative. This is the third most commonly used preservative after methyl and propylparaben.

Neomycin is the most common over-the-counter topical antibiotic. It is found in many skin, eye, and ear products and in animal feeds and veterinary products.

Benzocaine is a common sensitizer and a para-aminobenzoic acid–related compound. Cross-reactions occur with sunscreens, sulfonamides, and paraphenylenediamine. It does not cross-react with lidocaine. It is found in poison ivy remedies, hemorrhoid preparations, burn remedies, sunburn topicals, and throat lozenges.

Wool alcohols contain the main antigens in lanolin, a wool grease. Other trade names for lanolin include Clearlin, Glossylan, Golden Dawn, Hychol, Nodorain, and Sparklein. Lanolin contains many sterols, fatty acids, and fatty alcohols. It can be found in both prescription and over-the-counter topical skin products. Other sources include furniture polishes, leather, paper, printing inks, shoe polishes, and textile finishes.

Balsam of Peru is a complex thick, transparent liquid obtained from trees in El Salvador. Fifty percent of patients with fragrance allergy will be patch test positive to balsam of Peru. These patients may also react to benzoin, rosin, benzoic acid, benzoic alcohols, cinnamic acids, orange peel, clove, cinnamon, and wood tars. They may also cross-react with resorcinol monobenzoate found in some plastics as an ultraviolet light stabilizer (Jordan, 1973).

Cinnamic aldehyde is the most common antigen found in fragrances. It is found naturally in cinnamon, hyacinth, and daffodils and is a common additive in chewing gums, mouthwashes, beverages, vermouths, toothpastes, and perfumes. There are many other antigenic chemicals in fragrances including musk ambrette, cinnamic alcohol, benzyl alcohol, oak moss, and hydroxycittronella.

Rubber antigens (Thiuram, Mercaptopenzathiazole, carba mix, and black rubber mix) are common antigens found in synthetic rubber and are contained in the standard tray. Natural rubber occurs in over 200 species of plants. Only two plants account for 99 percent of the world's natural rubber: the Hevea tree and the guayule bush. Allergic reactions to latex have become a serious health problem and have been increasingly reported since the mandatory implementation of universal precautions in 1988 (see Chapter 24). Recent reports estimate that 7.4 percent of surgeons and 5.6 percent of operating nurses are latex sensitive. The specific antigens that induce latex allergy have not been determined, but the reactions are known to be IgE-mediated and are reactions to latex proteins, which are found not only in surgical gloves but also in the powders on the gloves. Reactions to the antigens produce contact urticaria, asthma, and anaphylaxis (Beezhold and Beck, 1992). Synthetic rubbers are complex compounds that contain hundreds of chemicals. Mercaptobenzathiazole, a rubber accelerator, is the most common antigen responsible for delayed contact dermatitis. Thiurams, also accelerators, are the second most common antigen in synthetic rubbers. These compounds can also be found in lawn fungicides, germicides, pesticides, oils, paints, putty, soaps, and shampoos. Thiurams can be absorbed through the skin and cause an antabuse effect when alcohol is ingested.

P-Tert-Butyphenol is a formaldehyde resin found in many glues and adhesives. Sensitization occurs to the chemical and not to the formaldehyde. It is used in the shoe, leather, auto, textile, plywood, dental, and box-making industries. It has been reported to cause vitiligo-like syndromes.

Epoxy resin dermatitis is most commonly due to bisphenol A, which is the antigen in the standard tray. However, epoxy dermatitis can be caused by other epoxy-curing agents not found in the standard tray. These compounds are used widely in the home and in many industries.

Paraphenylenediamine is found in permanent hair dyes, leather, rubbers, ink, color film developers, lubricating oils, plastics, and gasoline antioxidants.

Colophony is a solid rosin obtained from distilled turpentine. The principal antigen is abietic acid. It can be found in adhesives, depilatories, nail polish, rosin, paper boxes, shoe wax, permanent press, solder flux, paper, floor polish, and many tacky substances used to improve grip and prevent slipping.

Ethylenediamine is a preservative and common sensitizer found in many creams, eye drops, nose drops, and antihistamines. The high incidence of contact sensitivity is believed to be due to the widespread use of

Mycolog cream. Mycolog II cream does not contain this compound. However, it is still present in generic Mycolog creams and in Fougera's Nystatin cream. Ethylenediamine is used to solubilize theophylline for intravenous administration. Travenol Laboratory's intravenous theophylline does not contain ethylenediamine. It is also found in epoxy resins and cutting oils.

PLANT DERMATITIS

Poison ivy is the most common cause of allergic contact dermatitis in the United States (Fig. 45–6). Fifty percent of the adult population in the United States is sensitive to this potent antigen, and 70 percent of the population in endemic areas will be patch test positive. The antigens found in poison ivy are pentadecylcatechols and heptadecylcatechols. These antigens are also present in related plants including poison oak, poison sumac, mango peel, cashew, ginkgo, Japanese lacquer, and dye from the India marking nut tree. The antigen is found in the leaves, berries, sap, fruits, and nuts of these plants and is extremely durable, persisting on animals and inanimate objects such as blankets, clothing, and utensils for several years. It also can be volatilized if it is burned. Some of the most severe cases of poison ivy result from chemical contact after the vines have been burned and an unfortunate, sensitive patient is downwind of the smoke.

The other common sensitizers found in plants are sesquiterpene lactones. These antigens are common to a large group of plants, which include chrysanthemum, ragweed, sage brush, artichoke, tansy weed, and many others. The best antigen for patch testing is alantolactone, 0.25 percent, in petrolatum (Mitchell and Rook, 1971).

Other plant antigens that frequently cause allergic contact dermatitis include rosin (colophony) obtained from pine stumps and pine trees. The principal sensitizer in rosin is abietic acid. Other sensitizers found in pine trees are turpenes found in turpentine and many related products.

PRESERVATIVE DERMATITIS

All topical preparations have some preservative system to prevent the overgrowth of bacteria and molds. The most common preservative systems are formaldehyde, formaldehyde-releasing chemicals, and parabens. In the mid-1960s, there were several reports implicating parabens as contact sensitizers. Because these compounds were so ubiquitous it became popular for manufacturers to promote their products as paraben-free—hence, the era of formaldehyde-releasing preservatives. Formaldehyde and formaldehyde-releasing preservatives account for the majority of contact dermatitis from preservative systems (Nethercott and Holness, 1991). Cross-reactions between formaldehyde and formaldehyde-releasing preservatives are common. The degree of allergy to these compounds is variable, with some patients being mildly sensitive and some exquisitely sensitive. Quaternium 15 (Dowicil) is the most common preservative to cause contact allergy. A partial list of moisturizers that are formaldehyde-free include Eucerin, Nivea oil, petroleum jelly, and plastibase. A simple test kit is available to detect free formaldehyde from Formalert (Organon Teknika [405] 682–4461).

TREATMENT

The mainstay of management for patients with allergic contact dermatitis is identification and avoidance of the offending antigen.

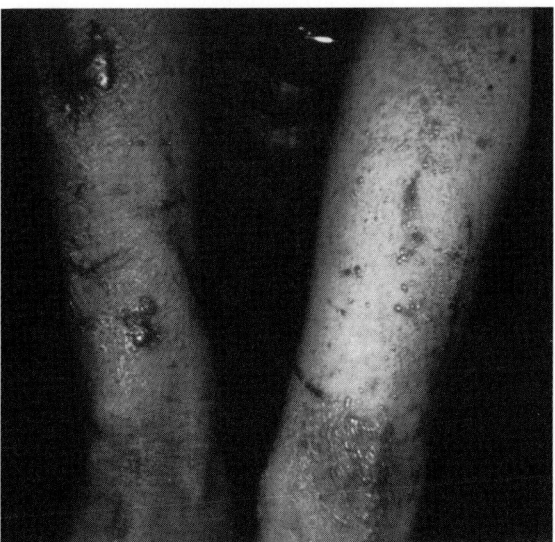

FIGURE 45–6. Blisters in lines and streaks typical of poison ivy dermatitis.

This is particularly true for contact urticaria, since repeated exposures can cause progressive symptoms and possible anaphylaxis.

For mild or limited delayed contact dermatitis, topical treatment with cool water compresses and moderate-strength topical corticosteroids is sufficient treatment. Recommending a moist compress applied over the topical steroid enhances the penetration of the steroid molecule and speeds recovery. A systemic antihistamine provides mild sedation and some relief of pruritus. Compress therapy helps dry blisters and oozing, removes crusts, and is soothing.

For extensive and/or severe allergic contact dermatitis, systemic prednisone is the treatment of choice. A tapering dose beginning with a 40- to 60-mg daily dose, tapered over 14 to 21 days, is recommended. A shorter taper period is not recommended and frequently results in a flare of the dermatitis. Attempts at desensitization programs have not been successful in most cases.

For chronic allergic contact dermatitis a more conservative approach should be taken. Often treatment will be required for several months. A mid-potency topical steroid ointment is usually recommended. A high-potency steroid can be used for 10 to 14 days and then downgraded to a mid- or low-potency topical once the itch-scratch cycle is broken. An exception would be allergic contact dermatitis of the face, axilla, or groin, where a low-potency topical steroid is the treatment of choice.

REFERENCES

Adams RM, Rietschel RL. Current concepts in clinical dermatologic allergy testing. J Am Acad Dermatol 21 (suppl):819, 1989.

Beezhold D, Beck WC. Surgical glove powders bind latex antigens. Arch Surg 127:1354–1357, 1992.

Bjorkner B, Moller H. Bacitracin: A cutaneous allergen and histamine liberator. Acta Derm Venereol (Stockh) 53:487, 1973.

Fisher AA. Contact Dermatitis. 3rd ed. Philadelphia, Lea & Febiger, 1986.

Fregert S. Contact allergens and prevention of contact dermatitis. J Allergy Clin Immunol 78:1071–1072, 1986.

Fregert S. Manual of Contact Dermatitis. Scandinavian University Books. Copenhagen, Munksgard, 1974.

Jordan WP. Resorcinol monobenzoate, Steering wheels, Peravian balsam. Arch Dermatol 108:178, 1973.

Leung DYM, Walsh P, Giorno R, et al. A potential role for superantigens in the pathogenesis of psoriasis. J Invest Dermatol 100:225–228, 1993.

Mitchell JC, Rook AJ. Diagnosis of contact dermatitis from plants. Int J Dermatol 16:257, 1971.

Nethercott JR, Holness DL. Patch testing with a routine screening tray in North America: 1985 through 1989. Am J Cont Derm 2:122–129, 1991.

Okamoto H, Horio T. The effect of 8-methoxypsoralen and long wave ultraviolet light on Langerhans' cell. J Invest Dermatol 77:345–346, 1981.

Parish WE, Rook AJ, Champion RH. A study of autoallergy in generalized eczema. Br J Dermatol 77:479–526, 1965.

Rudner EJ, Clendenning WE, Epstein E, et al. Epidemiology of contact dermatitis in North America. Arch Dermatol 108:537, 1973.

Chapter 46

Urticaria and Angioedema

Kathryn F. Hobbs, M.D., and Alan Schocket, M.D.

Urticaria and angioedema occur with an incidence of 15 to 20 percent. These fairly common and often frustrating problems can present alone (urticaria 40 percent, angioedema 11 percent) or in combination (49 percent). Although distressing for both patient and physician, they are rarely life-threatening. Urticarial lesions most commonly appear on the trunk, but may appear anywhere. The central area of superficial edema, or wheal, is surrounded by a variable amount of erythema. This flare may be flat or have a raised border. Hives are almost always pruritic and may last from 2 to 48 hours. Angioedema is a deeper, less circumscribed swelling, which more frequently affects areas of loose connective tissue such as the face, eyelids, lips, tongue, and extremities. It is rarely pruritic but may be painful, burning, or paresthetic. The time course of angioedema is similar to that of urticaria.

CLASSIFICATION

Urticaria can be divided into three main types: acute, chronic, and physical (Fig. 46–1).

ACUTE URTICARIA. Acute urticaria, the most frequent type, has been defined as episodes lasting for less than 6 weeks. Most patients have a single episode or a few recurring episodes. In general, a younger and atopic population usually is affected. There is often a specific cause, although one is not often readily identifiable. For a single episode, an extensive evaluation is hardly worthwhile.

CHRONIC URTICARIA. This form of urticaria has a peak incidence at ages 40 to 60 years, although children are also affected (Harris et al, 1983). Females are affected more often than males, and no atopic association is demonstrable. In most studies, a specific cause is identified in less than 20 percent of cases. Episodes may last from months to years. Other organ systems may be involved, such as gastrointestinal (nausea, vomiting, cramps, diarrhea), pulmonary (dyspnea), and musculoskeletal (myalgias, arthralgias). Malaise, fever, headache, and an elevated sedimentation rate may occur.

PHYSICAL URTICARIA. Physical urticaria includes a variety of syndromes induced by application of physical stimuli. Hives may be localized to the area of stimulus, or they may be diffuse. In most cases, urticaria develops within one half hour after the stimulus, although in rarer types—such as delayed pressure urticaria, vibratory angioedema, and familial cold urticaria—the lesions develop after several hours. In some cases, the involvement may be so diffuse that anaphylaxis may result (Kaplan et al, 1981).

C1 ESTERASE DEFICIENCY. Angioedema associated with this complement inhibitor may be either hereditary or acquired. Hereditary angioneurotic edema (HAE) is a rare, autosomal dominant disorder characterized clinically by recurrent attacks of acute circumscribed edema of deeper skin structures and subcutis and biochemically by reduced activity of the first component of the complement cascade, C1 esterase inhibitor. The edema is nonpitting and has a predilection for palms, soles, and periorbital-perioral areas. Local trauma may trigger an attack, which is unac-

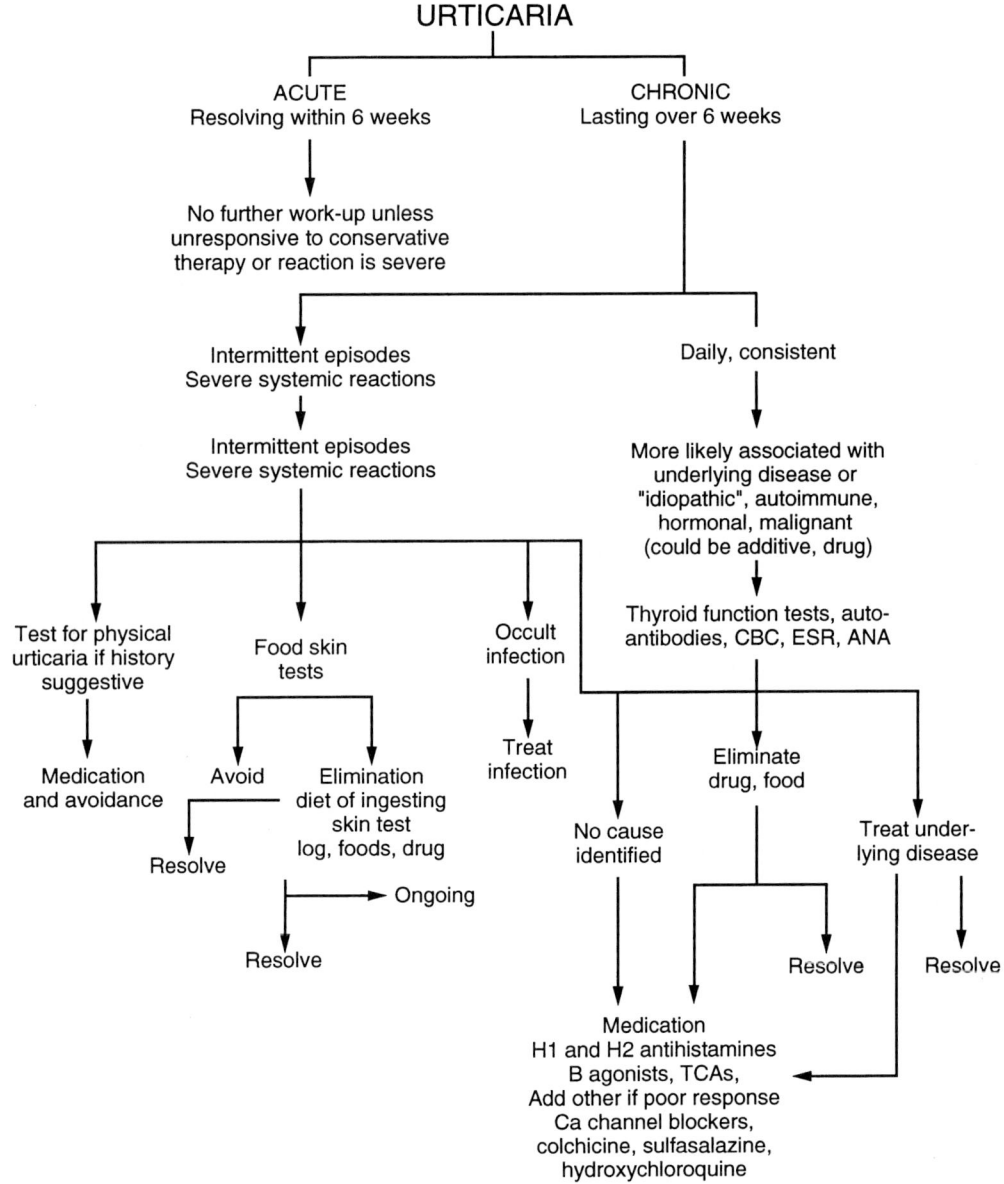

FIGURE 46–1

companied by urticaria. C1 INH inhibits activated Hageman factor, kallikrein, and plasmin in addition to its effects on C1. It is therefore possible that multiple biochemical pathways (e.g., bradykinin) are involved in the etiology of attacks.

Two variants have been described: type I, in which functional and antigenic C1 inhibitor deficiency is found, and type II, with normal or upper normal C1 INH antigenic levels but no functional activity. A minority of patients show genetic linkage with restriction fragment length polymorphisms (Agostoni, 1989). In comparison with the hereditary variant, the acquired deficiency of C1 INH is extremely rare. There are also two types. Type I is found in association with benign or malignant B cell lymphoproliferative disorders in which anti-idiotypic immune complexes consume massive amounts of C1 and, secondarily, C1 INH. Type II is not associated with underlying disease, but with anti-C1 INH autoantibodies, which render the inhibitor nonfunctional (Frigas, 1989; Alsenz and Loos, 1989).

DIFFERENTIAL DIAGNOSIS

There are several other cutaneous disorders that should be considered in the evaluation of the patient with urticaria and angioedema.

Papular urticaria is caused by insect bites (mosquitoes, gnats, ants). The lesions resemble hives, but are often associated with more local inflammation, persist longer, and are often on the lower legs. *Erythema multiforme* may resemble urticaria in its earlier stages. However, the lesions last longer than 48 hours, often involve the palms and soles, and progress to bullous or target lesions. *Scabies* is caused by infestation with mites, resulting in pruritic erythematous papules or secondary urticaria.

Pruritus alone should be included in the differential diagnosis of urticaria (Table 46–1). Generalized pruritus may be a manifestation of a systemic disease (Gilchrest, 1982).

Cellulitis may mimic angioedema as well as edema from cardiac, renal, or hepatic disease. Other uncommon possibilities include lymphedema, superior mediastinal syndrome, and periorbital edema associated with trichinosis. Rare diseases include Melkersson-Rosenthal syndrome (lip swelling, fissured tongue, recurrent facial palsies) and Muckle-Wells syndrome (urticaria, deafness, renal amyloidosis).

TABLE 46–1. TYPES AND CAUSES OF PRURITUS

Local
  Pruritus ani, pruritus vulvae
  Neurodermatitis
  Herpes zoster
Generalized
  Xerosis (dry skin)
  Endocrine dysfunction: hyper- and hypothyroidism, diabetes mellitus, hyperparathyroidism
  Biliary obstruction, cholestasis
  Uremia
  Neoplasm: lymphoreticular, polycythemia vera, carcinoma, carcinoid syndrome
  Pregnancy
  Parasitic infestations
  Allergic reactions
  (?) Psychogenic

PATHOPHYSIOLOGY

HISTOLOGY. Histologically, the lesions of acute urticaria demonstrate dermal edema with a sparse perivascular lymphocytic infiltrate. Eosinophils may be present. Collagen bundles in the superficial dermis are separated, with flattening of the rete pegs and widening of the dermal papillae. There may be small vessel dilatation. In chronic lesions, a more intense, non-necrotizing, mononuclear cell perivascular infiltrate may be seen (Phanuphak et al, 1980). Cutaneous mast cells can be increased tenfold (Natbony et al, 1983). Half of the biopsies will have major basic protein. Rarely, biopsies show changes consistent with vasculitis (Monroe, 1981), with a necrotizing venulitis with hypocomplementemia and a neutrophilic infiltrate, or normal complement with a lymphocytic infiltrate. The pathology of angioedema is characterized by these same alterations except that these changes occur in the deep dermis and subcutaneous tissue.

VASOACTIVE MEDIATORS AND MAST CELL ACTIVATION. The characteristic wheal and flare of the urticarial lesion was first reproduced in normal skin in 1927 by Sir Thomas Lewis with the intracutaneous injection of histamine. Histamine, and other vasoactive mediators, are stored in granules of mast cells. When these cells are activated, these granules are released, inducing increased capillary permeability (wheal), vasodilatation (flare), and irritation of nerve endings (pruritus). The neurogenic response then sends a stimulus back to the cutaneous nerve endings, which release substance P and other neuropeptides. The increased vascular permeability leads to activation of the plasma kinin-forming system and production of bradykinin, which is especially important in hereditary angioedema.

Mast cell activation can occur by IgE- or non-IgE-dependent mechanisms. In chronic idiopathic urticaria (CIU), there is increased histamine content and releasability in affected and unaffected skin. When CIU is in remission, mast cell histamine releasability following challenge with compound 48/80 is similar to that seen in normal controls (Jacques et al, 1992). The increased histamine content is not a result of an alteration in the metabolism of histamine (Smith et al, 1992). This suggests a transient functional imbalance rather than an intrinsic mast cell defect. The detection of circulating histamine-releasing autoantibodies with functional properties of anti-IgE has been reported in chronic urticaria (Grattan et al, 1991). These have been characterized recently in some patients as IgG autoantibodies against the alpha-subunit of the high-affinity IgE receptor (Hide et al, 1993).

Mast cells produce factors other than histamine, including tryptase, heparin, and chemotactic factors for neutrophils and eosinophils. Increased vascular permeability may also result from production of leukotrienes, prostaglandin D_2, platelet activating factor, and bradykinin. Mast cell cytokines such as GM-CSF, TNFa, IL-1, IL-3, IL-4, and IL-6 can activate inflammatory cells, stimulating T cell proliferation and self-degranulation of mast cells as well as causing autocrine mast cell growth. T cells are also believed to release the putative histamine releasing factor as well as cytokines (IL-3, GM-CSF), which can cause further mast cell and basophil degranulation through a positive feedback loop. Recently, histamine-releasing IgG autoantibodies against the alpha-subunit of the high-affinity IgE receptor have been found in the circulation of some patients with chronic urticaria (Hide et al, 1993). In these patients, intradermal injection of autologous serum induced a wheal and flare reaction, and *in vitro* the serum induced marked basophil histamine release.

Although eosinophils are not the most prominent cell type found in urticarial lesions, major basic protein deposition is often found. Other eosinophil products that may play a role in the wheal and flare response include eosinophil cationic protein and eosinophil-derived neurotoxin. Activated eosinophils also produce IL-3, GM-CSF, PAF, and LTC-4, which could all play a role in maintaining the inflammatory cascade.

Immune release via the action of complement activation components C3a, C4a, and C5a also occurs. These complement components are capable of directly activating mast cells. Complement and immunoglobulin are present in the immunofluorescent staining of venules in biopsies taken from cases of urticarial vasculitis. A necrotizing cutaneous vasculitis is seen with serum sickness as well as systemic lupus erythematosus, Sjögren's syndrome, or other systemic rheumatic diseases. In these cases, circulating immune complexes activate complement, which then activates mast cells in a nonspecific manner. This interplay of immune complexes and the complement system may be responsible for urticarial vasculitis seen in the prodrome of infectious hepatitis B (Alpert et al, 1971), infectious mononucleosis (Alfrick and Harprin, 1969), and Schnitzler's syndrome (chronic urticaria, vasculitis, monoclonal IgM spike, fever, and bone pain). Complement-mediated urticarial lesions have been reported after administration of blood, blood products, or immunoglobulins. Alternate complement pathway activation plays a role in the urticaria seen in reactions to radiocontrast media and cuprophane membrane dialysis.

There are several compounds that are capable of nonspecific activation of mast cells (Paton, 1957). Any individual, if exposed to sufficient levels, is susceptible. However, patients with increased numbers of mast cells (mastocytosis, urticaria pigmentosa) may be particularly vulnerable (Sutter et al, 1962). These compounds include drugs such as narcotics, curare, and polymixin B; detergents such as compound 48/80; certain foods such as strawberries and shellfish; and endogenous peptides such as endorphins, substance P, and vasoactive intestinal peptide (Foreman and Jordan, 1983).

ETIOLOGY. In all forms of urticaria, the underlying cause may be difficult to identify. For acute urticaria, unless the reaction is severe or recurs frequently, an extensive evaluation is neither useful nor cost-effective. This is not the case in chronic urticaria, for which medications with their side effects justify a more aggressive attempt to find an avoidable or treatable etiology. However, only a minority of patients (<20 percent in most reviews) have a determinable cause of their lesions. The following is a list of categories of etiologic factors to consider in the evaluation of patients with urticaria (Table 46–2).

Drugs are the most common identifiable cause of urticaria. Antibiotics such as penicillin may produce urticaria via IgE-mediated

TABLE 46–2. POSSIBLE CAUSES OF URTICARIA AND ANGIOEDEMA

Drugs	Infections
Foods and food additives	Collagen-vascular disease
Insect bites and stings	Malignancy
Contactants	Vasculitis
Immunotherapy	C1 esterase deficiency
Inhalants	syndromes
Systemic diseases	Physical urticaria
Endocrine disease	

allergic mechanisms or through a serum sickness syndrome. Other notable drugs that induce allergic reactions include hormones (insulin, ACTH, growth hormone) and larger heterologous proteins (horse serum, antitoxins). Almost any drug is capable of inducing urticaria. As noted previously, there exists a subset of medications that are capable of activating mast cells directly, such as morphine, codeine, curare, polymyxin B, vancomycin, thiamine, doxorubicin, and radiocontrast dye. Approximately 20 to 40 percent of patients with urticaria or angioedema will experience exacerbations with aspirin or other nonsteroidal anti-inflammatory agents (Doeglas, 1975). The mechanism is unknown. Angiotensin-converting enzyme inhibitors may cause angioedema by interfering with the degradation of bradykinin, autoantibody production, or complement-system components. The onset usually occurs within hours to one week after initiation of therapy (Israili and Hall, 1992). However, there are reports of ACEI-related angioedema occurring 3 months or longer into therapy (Jain et al, 1992).

Food and food additives are other commonly encountered causes of urticaria, especially acute urticaria. Children and atopic individuals are seen most frequently. Reactions usually are IgE-mediated. The most frequently implicated foods are peanuts, nuts, seafood, dairy products, wheat, soybeans, and fruits. As with drugs, some foods are capable of nonspecific mast cell activation. Consumed in sufficient quantities, foods such as tomatoes, strawberries, and shellfish can induce urticaria in the absence of "allergic" sensitivities. Several anecdotal reports and uncontrolled studies have implicated various preservatives (benzoates, sulfites, BHA, BHT), food dyes (tartrazine, coal-tar derivatives), yeasts (*Candida*, baker's), natural substances (salicylates), and flavorings (MSG, saccharin) as causes of acute and chronic urticaria (Michaelsson and Juhlin, 1973; Doeglas, 1975). There is no doubt that this occurs, but much less frequently than has been suggested.

The evaluation of food sensitivity must begin with a carefully taken, focused history. Problems arise when the reaction is delayed, occurs after several foods are ingested, or requires a concomitant factor such as exercise or pressure. If reactions occur less than two or three times weekly, keeping a food diary is cost-effective and may suggest an offending agent. For more frequent or daily symptoms, measures such as elimination diets, artificial nutrients (e.g., Vivonex, Nutramigen), or fasts of variable duration will provide useful information. Skin test results may be used to design an elimination diet, using those foods that do not induce a wheal and flare. If symptoms do not resolve over the period of elimination (3 to 7 days), an ingestant sensitivity can be virtually excluded. To establish cause, provocation tests are necessary (Genton et al, 1985). Double-blind challenge formats are the most definitive diagnostic method. It should be noted that it is difficult to make valid conclusions without a hive-free baseline. The choice of challenge foods may be guided by the results of food skin testing. A positive skin test is supportive, whereas a negative test eliminates causality. If a food or ingestant is identified, the most effective therapy is avoidance. Care should be taken to avoid nutritional deficiencies that may occur with severe elimination diets in patients with multiple sensitivities. Other treatments, such as rotating diets, sublingual drops, and injection therapy, have no scientific basis and should not be used until efficacy has been established.

Infectious causes are common in acute or self-limited urticaria. Some reports have related chronic urticaria to occult chronic bacterial infections, such as dental abscesses or vaginal infections, but these are uncommon. Other acute and chronic infections associated with urticaria include ECHO, coxsackie virus, and cytomegalovirus. Although an association between chronic urticaria and infestation with helminths (*Ascaris, Trichinella, Schistosoma*) and protozoa (ameba, *Giardia, Trichomonas* malaria) has been described, it is rare even in endemic areas (Pasricha et al, 1972).

Insect bites and stings may result in acute urticaria, which may appear as papular urticaria in children. These lesions can represent part of a systemic reaction to *Hymenoptera* or fire ants and may warrant evaluation and possible immunotherapy.

Contact urticaria is seen in highly sensitive individuals and has been described with latex, animals, food, plants, sea nettles, and caterpillars. Industrial chemicals, medications, and cosmetics can also cause contact urticaria. A positive response on patch testing with the appropriate antigen is diagnostic (Fisher, 1982). Inhalant allergens may, in rare instances, result in urticaria, and usually with the association of respiratory symptoms. Nevertheless, individuals extremely allergic to inhalants (such as grass pollen) may develop urticaria on contact with specific antigens.

Underlying *systemic diseases* can occasionally be associated with chronic urticaria. Major disease categories include infection, connective tissue disease, endocrine dysfunction, and malignancy. Seven percent of patients with systemic lupus erythematosus develop hives. Urticaria may be present in patients with rheumatoid arthritis. Endocrine disorders include hyper- and hypothyroidism, thyroiditis, diabetes, and hyperparathyroidism. Exacerbation of chronic urticaria with menses and pregnancy has been described, and allergic sensitivity to progesterone has been reported (Meggs et al, 1984) but is rare. An autoimmune process may underlie the urticaria seen in these patients, especially those with thyroid disorders (Leznoff and Sussman, 1989). Some patients with thyroid autoimmunity and normal thyroid function tests respond well to treatment with Synthroid (Katz et al, 1993). The association of occult malignancy and chronic urticaria is rare but has been reported with polycythemia vera, chronic myelogenous leukemia, mastocytosis, lymphoreticular malignancies, and carcinoma of the rectum, colon, and lung.

The syndrome of "urticarial vasculitis" is part of the differential diagnosis of chronic urticaria with systemic symptoms, especially when individual hives persist for over 48 hours. Lesions are often burning rather than pruritic and can resolve with residual pigmentation. Diagnostic skin biopsies will demonstrate vasculitis involving the postcapillary venules (Soter, 1977). Other manifestations include fever, arthralgias, arthritis, elevated sedimentation rate, nephritis (rarely), and hypocomplementemia (occasionally) (Monroe, 1981). Some patients have precipitins to Clq (Zeiss et al, 1980). Patients with severe disease often require corticosteroid therapy, although reports describe successful results with NSAIDs, hydroxychloroquine (Lopez et al, 1984), dapsone, and colchicine.

C1 esterase inhibitor deficiency syndromes have been described earlier. This inhibitor is important as a regulatory protein in the clotting, fibrinolytic, and inflammatory systems. Clinically, attacks are characterized by gradual onset of swelling in any part of the body. In contrast to allergic angioedema, which has a rapid onset, reaching its peak in less than one hour, hereditary angioedema peaks gradually over several hours. Urticaria is not a feature of this disease. The most common cause of mortality is from asphyxiation with laryngeal edema. Laryngeal involvement can be heralded by hoarseness, and tracheostomy may be lifesaving. Attacks are self-limited, lasting 2 to 3 days, and are unaffected by corticosteroids, antihistamines, or epinephrine. As C4 levels are consistently depressed in both types (HAE and AAE) even between attacks, measurement of C4 is a good screening test. Treatment of acute attacks is symptomatic and supportive. In HAE patients scheduled for surgical or dental procedures, prophylaxis with two units of fresh frozen plasma or the antifibrinolytic agents epsilon-aminocaproic acid (EACA) or tranexamic acid is advised. Postpubertal patients with HAE that require maintenance therapy should receive danazol or stanozolol, attenuated androgens. These agents enhance synthesis of C1 INH. Side effects include masculinization (minimal at doses used) and hepatitis. In children with HAE, treatment is not advised unless attacks are severe and frequent. Chronic therapy with EACA (Brickman and Hosea, 1983) or purified C1 INH is an effective alternative.

THERAPY

Treatment of urticaria depends on the severity of symptoms. Scattered or mild hives are self-limited and usually require no treatment or, at most, a mild antihistamine as needed. These may include any of the first- or, if sedation is to be avoided, second-generation antihistamines. In comparative trials between the various nonsedating agents (terfenadine, astemizole, loratadine, and cetirizine), no significant difference in efficacy has been noted. All these agents have good safety profiles, although astemizole has been correlated with increased appetite and weight gain in some, and cetirizine has a slight sedative effect when compared with placebo. Terfenadine and astemizole have caused a life-threatening cardiac arrhythmia (torsades de pointes), especially when taken with erythromycin or antifungal agents such as ketoconazole and fluconazole. The mechanism is believed to be due to extreme prolongation of the QT interval. Although H1/H2 antihistamine combinations are effective in some patients, some studies have produced mixed results (Monroe, 1981) (Table 46–3). If the urticaria is generalized and severe, as with angioedema, treatment should be similar to that for an anaphylactic reaction. In addition to antihistamines, the mainstay of therapy in this case is subcutaneous epinephrine or terbutaline until symptoms improve or side effects become unacceptable. Subcutaneous injection of epinephrine suspension (Sus-Phrine) can be used for prolonged therapy, as can oral ephedrine or terbutaline. Corticosteroid therapy is rarely necessary. If the episode was severe, the patient should be encouraged to carry and trained to use injectable epinephrine (Ana-Kit, Epi-Pen).

The ideal management for chronic urticaria would be avoidance of the offending agent. However, as the majority of cases remain idiopathic, chronic suppressive symptomatic therapy is often warranted. Regular use of antihistamines, first or second generation, is the mainstay of therapy. If longer-acting, more potent preparations are required, the tricyclic antidepressants, particularly Doxepin, 10 to 25 mg and increased as tolerated, should be administered at bedtime. If symptoms continue despite adequate H_1 blockade, then sympathomimetic preparations or H_2 blockers may deserve a trial (Harvey et al, 1981). Addition of an NSAID may be of benefit in some cases of delayed pressure urticaria (Sussman et al, 1982) and urticarial vasculitis (Milins et al, 1980). Corticosteroids should be used only as a last resort. Studies have shown effectiveness with ketotifen (antihistamine, calcium channel blocker, and mast cell stabilizer). Another medicine with calcium channel blockade properties, nifedipine, has also shown some benefit (Bressler et al, 1989).

The goal of symptomatic therapy is comfort until the disease remits. Approximately half of all urticaria patients have a single episode or a short, self-limited course. The majority of the remaining half will have active disease for 3 to 6 months. In 20 percent, the disease will last for 1 to 2 years. Urticaria will only rarely persist for up to 10 years (Champion et al, 1969).

PHYSICAL URTICARIA

By definition, physical urticaria is produced by a specific "physical" stimulus. Urticarial lesions usually develop within 30 minutes of exposure to the stimulus. Physical urticaria is relatively common, affecting up to 17 percent of all urticaria patients (Champion et al, 1969). Younger age groups are most often affected. The reaction is reproducible and often limited to the areas of stimuli. Mast cell mediators, especially histamine, have been

TABLE 46–3. DRUG THERAPY FOR CHRONIC URTICARIA

Drug	Brand Name	Dosage for Adults	Dosage for Children
Antihistamines			
H_1			
Hydroxyzine	Atarax Vistaril	25 mg. t.i.d. to q.i.d. or 25 to 50 mg h.s.	Under 6; up to 10 mg q.i.d. (elixir 1 tsp = 10 mg) Over 6: 25 mg t.i.d. to q.i.d. (if necessary)
Cyproheptadine	Periactin	4 mg q.i.d.	0.15 mg/kg/day; 2 mg b.i.d. to t.i.d. (syrup 1 tsp = 2 mg)
Doxepin	Sinequan Adapin	10 to 25 mg h.s. 25 mg b.i.d. to t.i.d. (liquid 10 mg/ml)	Not recommended under 12 by the manufacturer
Terfenadine	Seldane	60 mg b.i.d. or t.i.d.	Not recommended under 12 by the manufacturer
H_2			
Cimetidine	Tagamet	300 to 400 mg t.i.d.	Not recommended under 12 by the manufacturer
Ranitidine	Zantac	150 mg b.i.d.	Not recommended under 12 by the manufacturer
Sympathomimetics			
Ephedrine		25 mg t.i.d. to q.i.d.	10 to 25 mg t.i.d.
Terbutaline	Brethine Bricanyl	2.5 to 5 mg t.i.d.	Not recommended under 12 by the manufacturer

demonstrated in venous blood draining and in tissue taken from affected sites. The mechanism by which a physical stimulus results in mast cell activation is not well understood. It may be a direct effect by an unknown mechanism (such as imbalance in cytokines or neuropeptides resulting in an altered threshold) or by an immunologic mechanism. In some cases of physical urticaria, a passive transfer factor (usually IgE) has been shown (Jorizzo and Smith, 1982).

Dermatographism is the most common type of physical urticaria, occurring in up to 5 percent of the general population. It is defined as the production of a wheal larger than 2 mm on linear application of pressure (3600 gm/cm^2) to the skin by a dermographometer (or tongue blade). A small subset will develop associated pruritus and are classified as having symptomatic dermatographism. Females of any age are most often affected. Occasionally, dermatographism will develop following systemic allergic reactions such as penicillin reaction, multiple insect bites, or scabies. It then may persist for years afterward. Dermatographism may also be associated with endocrine disorders (diabetes, thyroid disease) and other forms of physical urticaria.

There are other distinct forms of pressure-induced lesions. Patients with chronic urticaria often develop lesions in areas of pressure (belt lines, bra straps) in the absence of demonstrable dermatographism. Delayed pressure urticaria (DPU) is another syndrome that was originally described as a rare familial disorder, but has also been seen in some patients with chronic urticaria (Sussman et al, 1982). Lesions are erythematous, swollen, and painful and develop 4 to 6 hours following a pressure stimulus (15 lb for 15 min over the shoulder). DPU is often mistaken for angioedema. Although IgE has not been implicated, the syndrome has been reported in association with specific food ingestion (Davis et al, 1984). This subgroup of patients will have delayed reactions to food skin tests, with or without immediate wheal and flare. Hereditary (autosomal dominant) vibratory angioedema is a variant of DPU. Inducing stimuli include motorcycling, toweling, and lawn mowing. IgE transfer has been negative in these patients, although histamine release after challenge has been demonstrated. These patients will have variable responses to H_1 blockade. DPU is usually unresponsive to antihistamine therapy. Some patients respond to NSAIDs. Over 50 percent of patients will require daily steroids, often in moderate doses. Alternate-day dosage should be tried but is often inadequate to control symptoms. Symptomatic dermatographism alone will respond to antihistamines or tricyclic antidepressants.

Cholinergic urticaria may comprise up to 7 percent of all forms of urticaria, occurring more frequently in teenagers and young adults. This syndrome is induced by exercise, "core heating," sweating, and emotional stress. The characteristic lesions are small, punctate, highly pruritic wheals surrounded by extensive erythema. These lesions may coalesce, however, forming a more classic hive. Patients sometimes have mild reversible obstructive changes on pulmonary function testing, and in rare cases, these changes will evolve into full-blown anaphylaxis (Kaplan et al, 1981). The cholinergic nervous system effector mechanisms involved in the compensatory responses in thermoregulation may lead to mast cell activation. Increases in histamine, neutrophil, and eosinophil chemotactic factors have been demonstrated in peripheral blood after provocative challenges (Soter et al, 1980). Intradermal injection of 0.1 mg of methacholine will produce satellite wheals in addition to that at the injection site (a positive response) in 33 to 50 percent of patients. Therefore, it is not a reliable diagnostic test. Therapy involves avoidance of exogenous heat provocation, cooling, and antihistamines, particularly hydroxyzine.

Exercise-induced anaphylaxis/urticaria differs from cholinergic urticaria in that raising the core temperature in the absence of exercise will not provoke an attack. Additionally, the lesions are usually larger. Mechanisms may involve an exaggerated response to factors such as endorphins, which are released during exercise and are capable of inducing mast cell degranulation. This syndrome has been reviewed in Chapter 26.

Temperature-related physical urticaria includes cold- and heat-induced urticaria. Heat-induced urticaria usually falls under the category of cholinergic urticaria, although there exists a rare subset in which the local application of heat will cause an isolated urticarial eruption (Delorme, 1969). Conflicting data on mediator abnormalities exist, but in all cases, this disorder could not be passively transferred. Cold urticaria is more common and may be life-threatening. Deaths have been described in patients who dived into cold water. Cold-induced urticaria may be either familial (autosomal dominant) or acquired ("essential"). The familial forms are not true urticarias, as biopsies have shown either polymorphonuclear or mononuclear infiltrates (immediate and late forms, respectively) (Tindall et al, 1969; Soter et al, 1977). Transfer does not occur. Acquired cold urticaria may develop following insect stings, viral infections, drug reactions, or even after childbirth. It has also been described in association with cryoglobulinemia, cryofibrinogenemia, cold agglutinin disease, or paroxysmal nocturnal hemoglobinuria.

Adrenergic urticaria has been described in which lesions develop at times of stress. These lesions are widespread, pruritic, and papular and are surrounded by a striking white halo. Plasma norepinephrine and epinephrine levels were increased. The halo hives are reproducible with an intradermal injection of norepinephrine, but not with acetylcholine. Treatment with a beta blocker prevented attacks (Shelley and Shelley, 1985).

Solar urticaria is rare (<1 percent of all urticarias) and occurs usually within 30 minutes of sun exposure (Ravits et al, 1982). It can be associated with drug ingestion (sulfonamides, tetracycline), sunburn, insect stings, infection, and underlying systemic diseases such as systemic lupus erythematosus or erythropoietic protoporphyria. Solar urticaria can occur at any age but predominates in the fourth and fifth decades. There are six types, depending on the wavelength of light to which the patient reacts. The most common is sensitivity to ultraviolet light (385 to 320 nm). The inciting wavelength spectrum may change over time. Some subjects with reactivity at 280 to 320 nm or 400 to 500 nm have a transferable factor (Sams et al, 1969). Within minutes of exposure, patients note erythema and pruritus, then urticaria in the exposed skin. The skin will normalize in a few hours, and then be tolerant to light for 12 to 24 hours. Chronically exposed areas such as the face and arms may become relatively resistant to light. Therapy includes topical sunscreen or blocking agents. Induction of tolerance with natural or artificial light may be of benefit (Ramsay, 1977).

Aquagenic urticaria, a very rare disorder, results from contact with water. Clinically, the lesions are indistinguishable from cholinergic urticaria. Some patients will have both forms. Topically applied scopolamine has been reported to suppress the lesions, suggesting a contribution from a cholinergic mechanism in some patients (Sibbald et al, 1981). A recent study suggests that a water-soluble epidermal antigen permeates the skin in the presence of water and activates cutaneous mast cells (Czarnetki et al, 1986). Therapy includes inert skin oils and antihistamines.

REFERENCES

Agostoni A. Inherited C1 inhibitor deficiency. Compl Inflamm 6:112, 1989.

Alfrick JA, Harprin KM. Infectious mononucleosis presenting as urticaria. JAMA 209:1524, 1969.

Alpert E, Isselbacher KJ, Schur PH. The pathogenesis of arthritis associated with viral hepatitis. N Engl J Med 285:185, 1971.

Alsenz J, Loos M. The acquired C1-INH deficiencies with autoantibodies. Behring Inst Mitt 84:165–172, 1989.

Bressler RB, Sowel K, Houston DP. Therapy of chronic idiopathic urticaria with nifedipine: Demonstration of beneficial effect in a double-blinded, placebo-controlled crossover trial. J Allergy Clin Immunol 83:756, 1989.

Brickman CNM, Hosea SW. Hereditary angioedema. Int J Dermatol 22:141, 1983.

Champion RN, Roberts SOB, Carpenter RG, Roger J. Urticaria and angioedema: A review of 554 cases. Br J Dermatol 81:588, 1969.

Czarnetzki BM, Breetholt KH, Traupe H. Evidence that water acts as a carrier for an epidermal antigen in aquagenic urticaria. J Am Acad Dermatol 15:623, 1986.

Davis KC, Mekori YA, Kohler PF, Schocket AL. Late cutaneous reactions in patients with delayed pressure urticaria. J Allergy Clin Immunol 73:183, 1984. (Abstract)

Delorme P. Localized heat urticaria. J Allergy 43:284, 1969.

Doeglas HM. Reactions to aspirin and food additives in patients with chronic urticaria, including the physical urticarias. Br J Dermatol 93:135, 1975.

Fisher AA. Contact urticaria due to medicaments, chemicals and foods. Cutis 30:171, 1982.

Foreman J, Jordan C. Histamine release and vascular changes induced by neuropeptides. Agents Actions 13:103, 1983.

Frigas E. Angioedema with acquired deficiency of the C1 inhibitor: A constellation of syndromes. Mayo Clin Proc 64:1269, 1989.

Genton C, Frei PC, Pecoud A. Value of oral provocation tests to aspirin and food additives in the routine investigation of asthma and chronic urticaria. J Allergy Clin Immunol 76:40, 1985.

Gilchrest BA. Pruritus: Pathogenesis, therapy and significance in systemic disease states. Arch Intern Med 142:101, 1982.

Grattan CE, Francis DM, Hide M, Greaves MW. Detection of circulating histamine-releasing autoantibodies with functional properties of anti-IgE in chronic urticaria. Clin Exp Allergy 21:695–704, 1991.

Harris A, Twarog FJ, Geha RS. Chronic urticaria in children: Course and etiology. Ann Allergy 51:161, 1983.

Harvey RP, Wegs J, Schocket AL. A controlled trial of therapy in chronic urticaria. J Allergy Clin Immunol 68:262, 1981.

Hide M, Francis DM, Grattan CEH, et al. Autoantibodies against the high-affinity IgE receptor as a cause of histamine release in chronic urticaria. N Engl J Med 328:1599, 1993.

Israili ZH, Hall WD. Cough and angioneurotic edema associated with angiotensin-converting enzyme inhibitor therapy. A review of the literature and pathophysiology. Ann Intern Med 117:234, 1992.

Jacques P, Lavoie A, Bédard PM, Brunet C, Hébert J. Chronic idiopathic urticaria: Profiles of skin mast cell histamine release during active disease and remission. J Allergy Clin Immunol 89:1139–1143, 1992.

Jain M, Armstrong L, Hall J. Predisposition to and late onset of upper airway obstruction following angiotensin-converting enzyme inhibitor therapy. Chest 102:871–874, 1992.

Jorizzo JL, Smith EB. The physical urticarias. Arch Dermatol 118:194, 1982.

Kaplan AP, Natbony SF, Tarvil AP, Frudster LF, Foster M. Exercise-induced anaphylaxis as a manifestation of cholinergic urticaria. J Allergy Clin Immunol 68:319, 1981.

Katz JL, Rumbyrt JS, Schocket AL. Resolution of chronic urticaria with thyroid hormone therapy in euthyroid patients. J Allergy Clin Immunol 93:281, 1993. (Abstract)

Leznoff A, Sussman GI. Syndrome of idiopathic chronic urticaria and angioedema with thyroid autoimmunity. A study of 90 patients. J Allergy Clin Immunol 84:66, 1989.

Lopez LR, Davis KC, Kohler PF, Schocket AL. The hypocomplementemic urticarial–vasculitis syndrome: Therapeutic response to hydroxychloroquine. J Allergy Clin Immunol 73:600, 1984.

Meggs WJ, Pescovitz OH, Metcalfe D, Loriaux DL, Cutler G, Kaliner M. Progesterone sensitivity as a cause of recurrent anaphylaxis. N Engl J Med 311:1236, 1984.

Michaelsson G, Juhlin L. Urticaria induced by preservatives and dye additives in food and drugs. Br J Dermatol 88:525, 1973.

Milins JL, Randle HW, Solley GO, Dicken CH. The therapeutic response of urticarial vasculitis to indomethacin. J Am Acad Dermatol 3:349, 1980.

Monroe EW. Urticarial vasculitis: An updated review. J Am Acad Dermatol 5:88, 1981.

Natbony SF, Phillips ME, Elias JM, Godfrey HP, Kaplan AP. Histologic studies of chronic idiopathic urticaria. J Allergy Clin Immunol 71:177, 1983.

Pasricha JS, Pasricha A, Prakash OM. Role of gastrointestinal parasites in urticaria. Ann Allergy 30:368, 1972.

Paton WDM. Histamine release by compounds of simple chemical structure. Pharmacol Rev 9:269, 1957.

Phanuphak P, Kohler PH, Stanford RE, Schocket AL, Carr RI, Claman HN. Vasculitis in chronic urticaria. J Allergy Clin Immunol 65:436, 1980.

Ramsay CA. Solar urticaria treatment by inducing tolerance to artificial radiation and natural light. Arch Dermatol 113:1222, 1977.

Ravits M, Armstrong RB, Harber LC. Solar urticaria: Clinical features and wavelength dependence. Arch Dermatol 118:288, 1982.

Sams WM Jr, et al. Solar urticaria: Investigation of pathogenetic mechanisms. Arch Dermatol 99:390, 1969.

Shelley WB, Shelley ED. Adrenergic urticaria: A new form of stress-induced hives. Lancet 2(8463):1031–1033, 1985.

Sibbald RG, Black AK, Eady RA, Jams M, Greaves MW. Aquagenic urticaria: Evidence of cholinerginic and histaminergic basis. Br J Dermatol 105:297–302, 1981.

Smith CH, Soh C, Lee TH. Cutaneous histamine metabolism in chronic urticaria. J Allergy Clin Immunol 89:944–950, 1992.

Soter NA. Chronic urticaria as a manifestation of necrotizing vasculitis. N Engl J Med 296:1440, 1977.

Soter NA, Joshi NP, Twarog FJ, Zeiger RS, Rothman PM, Colten HR. Delayed cold-induced urticaria: A dominantly inherited disorder. J Allergy Clin Immunol 59:294–297, 1977.

Soter NA, Wasserman SI, Austen KF, McFadden ER Jr. Release of mast-cell mediators and alterations in lung function in patients with cholinergic urticaria. N Engl J Med 302:604–608, 1980.

Sussman GL, Harvey RP, Schocket AL. Delayed pressure urticaria. J Allergy Clin Immunol 70:337, 1982.

Sutter MC, Beaulieu G, Birt AR. Histamine liberation by codeine and polymyxin B in urticaria pigmentosa. Arch Dermatol 86:217, 1962.

Tindall JP, et al. Familial cold urticaria: A generalized reaction involving leukocytosis. Arch Intern Med 124:129, 1969.

Zeiss CR, Burch FX, Marder RJ, Rurney NL, Schmid FR, Gewurz H. A hypocomplementemic vasculitic urticarial syndrome. Report of four cases and definition of the disease. Am J Med 68:867, 1980.

Chapter 47
Other Skin Disorders

Don Warren Printz, M.D.

In this chapter, common congenital and hereditary disorders of the skin, infectious dermatoses, and other skin disorders with features that sometimes raise the question of "allergy" are reviewed. Immune mechanisms have been implicated in the pathogenesis of some disorders. A more comprehensive review of these disorders can be found from the general references at the end of this chapter.

INFECTIOUS DERMATOSES

Fungal Infections

SUPERFICIAL FUNGAL INFECTIONS. Only three genera of fungi, *Tricophyton, Microsporum,* and *Epidermophyton,* account for virtually all superficial fungal disease from childhood to adulthood in North America. An interesting epidemiologic change has taken place in tinea capitis over the past 35 years. Whereas, formerly, almost all epidemic tinea capitis was caused by *M. audouinii,* in the past 35 years, this organism has been virtually replaced completely by *T. tonsurans.* This trend was first observed in the Southwestern United States and has now reached Canada. It is important to note that unlike *M. audouinii, T. tonsurans* exhibits no consistently reliable fluorescence under Wood's light examination, mandating the use of KOH preparations and culture for diagnostic confirmation. Furthermore, alopecia, which is sometimes cicatricial, can sometimes occur in *T. tonsurans* infections without the characteristic short broken-off hairs seen in *M. audouinii* infections. Thus, *T. tonsurans* infection should always be considered in a patient with otherwise unexplained hair loss.

Tinea capitis occurs chiefly before puberty, and it has been suggested that free fatty acids in sebum, which are first secreted at puberty, have an inhibitory effect on these fungi. Moreover, *T. tonsurans* is more likely to be involved in kerion formation in which a boggy, pustular faintly fluctuant lesion develops in the scalp. The lesion may be over 5 cm in diameter. It is important that the clinician realize that this lesion represents a delayed hypersensitivity reaction to the fungus. Because of its etiology, there is no response to antibiotics despite the purulence observed in this lesion. A brief course of systemic corticosteroid (e.g., prednisone, 0.9 mg/kg/day in three divided doses) may be necessary for prompt resolution of the lesion. Kerions often form shortly after the initiation of systemic antifungal therapy. Delayed hypersensitivity reactions also are seen in tinea corporis. Jones et al (1974) demonstrated a correlation between severity of disease and response to intradermal skin tests with purified *Tricophyton* antigen. In 1973, Jones showed a greater frequency of dermatophyte infections in individuals with atopic dermatitis.

Superficial fungal infections of the face are almost completely confined to patients in the pediatric age group. Often, the characteristic lesions on the malar areas are the result of holding infected household pets against the face.

Treatment of the superficial dermatophytic infections (except for tinea capitis) usually can be accomplished with use of topical therapy alone; the agents econazole nitrate and ciclopirox olamine applied twice daily are agents of choice. Tinea capitis requires systemic therapy. Griseofulvin (ultramicrosize) must be administered twice daily (10 mg/kg divided into two doses) for at least 3 weeks. Since it is fat-soluble, it should be administered with milk or peanut butter. Because of the high cost of the suspension, crushing the tablets in peanut butter is an economic and a practical method of giving the medication to younger children. From an epidemiologic standpoint, the concomitant use of selenium sulfide shampoos twice weekly (Selsun prescription, not Selsun Blue) renders the patient noninfectious much more rapidly than griseofulvin alone because of its sporicidal effect.

CANDIDOSIS. Candidosis may affect patients of all ages. Except in congenital candidosis, it appears as characteristic beef-red, faintly glistening and macerated, sharply demarcated lesions with satellite lesions separated from the main body of the eruption. Thrush is a uniform finding in neonatal candidosis, which appears in the second week after birth. In adolescent males, the scrotum is characteristically affected in candidosis and spared in tinea cruris. Diaper dermatitis complicated by *Candida* is a classic presentation. By contrast, congenital candidosis is present at birth or within 12 hours after delivery, presenting as a vesiculopustular eruption chiefly on the extremities; it rapidly desquamates, resulting in collarette scaling and diffuse erythroderma.

Using murine models, Ray (1985) has demonstrated the remarkable ability of *Candida* to adhere to the stratum corneum. In this system, the organism secretes an acid protease, which is keratolytic. The process is associated with the elaboration of a mucoid "cohesin," which is present within 10 minutes after experimental inoculation. Ray also demonstrated that cell wall extracts from *Candida* can activate complement by the alternative pathway. In addition, complement activation evokes neutrophil chemotaxis and promotes opsonization and subsequent phagocytosis of the organism.

Host defenses rest chiefly on cell-mediated immunity; when T-cell mechanisms are deranged, chronic *Candida* infections are frequent. Immunoglobulins, including IgG, IgA, IgM, and IgE, are produced in response to the organism but have no effect on the *in vitro* growth of homogenized organisms. Clinically, patients with immunoglobulin deficiencies do not appear to be unusually susceptible to *Candida* infections. Conversely, patients with chronic candidosis with T cell aberrations may have high immunoglobulin levels that are not protective.

Treatment involves topical agents; cycloprox olamine (Loprox), unlike the topical imidazoles such as clotrimazole, is candidicidal rather than candidistatic. It should be applied twice daily. Oral nystatin suspension, ½ teaspoonful administered every 2 hours while the patient is awake, is useful in treating thrush. Since 80 percent of nystatin is hydrolyzed by the low pH of the gastric contents, its systemic effect in the doses usually employed is questionable.

Local factors are critical in successful management. The affected areas must be kept as dry as possible. In infants, this is accomplished through avoidance of disposable diapers and use of cloth diapers without rubber pants. When the acute phase subsides, the use of methylcellulose-containing powder (ZeaSorb) can be an effective preventive measure because of its greater absorbency than pure talc.

Viral Infections

HERPES SIMPLEX. Grouped vesicles arising on an erythematous base should bring to mind the diagnosis of herpes simplex virus (HSV) in patients of any age. However, only 70 percent of neonates infected with HSV will exhibit the characteristic skin eruptions. Any history of maternal genital HSV infection should raise the clinician's index of suspicion in case of abnormal neonatal development. The virus is easily cultured from mucous membranes as well as skin. The Tzanck smear is reliable for a quick diagnosis if vesicles are present. The Sure-Cell test for HSV, an ELISA-type test available in kit form, enjoys a 99 percent specificity and sensitivity rate if performed in the vesicular stage of the eruption, making timely treatment possible on a diagnostic rather than an empiric basis for the clinician who is not proficient in performing Tzanck smears. Although viral cultures may be used for confirmation, they are of limited value in a therapeutic setting because of the necessity of prompt antiviral therapy.

In the majority of children and adults, primary HSV infections of the facial-oral type are asymptomatic. Primary inoculations in older adolescents or adults at either facial or genital locations are usually painful and accompanied by fever to 105°F and localized adenopathy.

Recurrent herpetic infections, triggered by a wide variety of factors, need no longer be the bane of existence for so many patients. Acyclovir, 18 mg/kg/day in five divided doses for 5 days, given early in the course of the recurrence (during the prodromal phase if possible) not only speeds the resolution of the current eruption, but after repeated courses seems to prolong the recurrence-free interval. Although not effecting a cure, the treatment helps to relieve pain and discomfort and may prevent recurrence.

VARICELLA AND ZOSTER. These two diseases are caused by members of the herpesvirus group. Herpes simplex types 1 and 2, cytomegalovirus, and Epstein-Barr virus of infectious mononucleosis are all members of the group.

Varicella, the most contagious of the "childhood" diseases, usually begins on the face and scalp and spreads rapidly to the extremities and trunk. The lesions quickly pass through several morphologic stages, beginning as erythematous macules that rapidly evolve into vesicles, pustules, and crusts. The entire process may take less than 24 hours. Lesions occur in varying stages of development in "crops," unlike variola, and resolve over 8 to 9 days. Varicella in children usually requires only supportive treatment, such as bland lotion.

Herpes zoster, caused by varicella virus, is a result of reactivation of latent virus, which resides in sensory ganglia. Unknown factors activate the virus, which then spreads antidromically down the sensory nerve, producing discomfort even before the characteristic grouped vesicles, arising on an erythematous base and arranged in dermatomal fashion, appear.

The immunology of varicella-zoster is complex. Although IgA, IgM, and IgG antibodies occur within a few days of visible varicellar lesions, with low levels of IgG persisting throughout life, children with agammaglobulinemia do not experience severe or recurrent varicella. On the other hand, children and immunosuppressed adults with deficient cell-mediated immunity develop severe or long-lasting varicella-zoster. Interestingly, varicella-zoster immunoglobulin greatly modifies the course of the disease in such patients and may be lifesaving. Since herpes zoster can occur relatively early in the course of HIV (human immunodeficiency virus) disease, even with CD4 cell counts well in excess of 300, it may be the first clinical manifestation of HIV disease. Accordingly, *it is imperative to determine the HIV status of any child or young adult presenting with herpes zoster,* and the presence of HIV infection should be considered in patients of any age with herpes zoster.

Although acyclovir is not as active against varicella-zoster virus as it is against herpes simplex virus, its use in immunocompromised patients, parenterally if necessary, can be lifesaving. Dosage is 80mg/kg/day divided into five doses orally.

In patients affected with zoster 70 years of age or older, the administration of prednisone, 20 mg three times a day for 6 days, followed by 20 mg every other day for 2 weeks, along with the application of potent topical steroids (clobetasol 0.05 percent twice a day) has been shown to limit the incidence of postherpetic neuralgia greatly. The application of firm pressure, such as an elastic bandage, to the trunk area overnight offers the patient considerable comfort without resorting to potentially addictive analgesics for this long-term complication.

WARTS. Warts come in all shapes and sizes, can occur anywhere there is stratified squamous epithelium, and are the bane of existence of countless patients, especially those suffering from painful plantar warts. The etiology is the papilloma virus, a DNA-containing virus that can be separated into numerous types, each demonstrating a striking site specificity. Types 6 and 11 have been associated with urogenital tumors, including verrucous carcinoma; types 16 and 18 may be the major causes of carcinoma of the cervix and urogenital Bowen's disease.

Immunity against this virus seems to depend on cell-mediated pathways. Patients with acquired immune deficiency syndrome (AIDS) frequently have large numbers of flat warts, particularly in the bearded area. Warts are common in immunosuppressed patients and are notoriously difficult to treat in these patients as well as in patients with advanced Hodgkin's disease.

A variety of treatment methods is available. Cryotherapy for multiple, relatively flat warts leaves no scarring and is almost painless under nitrous oxide analgesia. Electrodesiccation, excision, curettage, and final electrofulguration have a high rate of success, although they leave small scars and require the use of intralesional anesthesia. Laser treatment is similar in this regard. Podophyllin (25 percent) in a compound tincture of benzoin is useful for treatment of genital warts. The compound should not be left *in situ* more than 4 hours at the initial treatment; the time should be increased at weekly intervals. X-ray therapy is now infrequently employed. Occlusal-HP, a 17 percent salicylic acid solution in a polyacrylic vehicle, is especially useful for small new warts. Since the incubation period of warts can be at least 6 months, patients should be alerted to look for new lesions, especially lesions that had been removed previously. Occlusal HP offers a painless way to remove these new lesions.

MOLLUSCUM CONTAGIOSUM. This is an extremely common viral disease of children. The typical lesion is an umbilicated flesh-colored papule, 1 to 5 mm in diameter. Although "giant" molluscous bodies measuring up to 2 cm occur, these are more common in adults. The molluscum contagiosum virus is a member of the poxvirus group. The disease is transmissible both from person to person and by autoinoculation. It is not uncommon for patients to present with 50 or more lesions. Although multiple lesions of molluscum contagiosum are the norm on the body below the neck, the presence of multiple facial lesions may be an early sign of HIV disease.

The lesions are readily treated by simple curettage. Nitrous oxide analgesia greatly simplifies this procedure for both physician and patient when there are multiple lesions. The use of Keralyt, a 7 percent salicylic acid gel, twice daily for 2 weeks before the curettage of multiple lesions, makes the procedure much less painful. Several treatment sessions at monthly intervals are usually necessary to remove newly developing lesions.

HAND, FOOT, AND MOUTH SYNDROME. A number of rashes can be confused with allergy. One of the more dramatic is that of hand, foot, and mouth syndrome. It consists of an exanthem-exanthem syndrome, consisting of papulovesicles on the hands and feet associated with oral ulceration especially on the tongue. Usually the cutaneous papulovesicles arise on an erythematous base, and the vesicle is gray rather than clear. The etiologic agent is coxsackie virus A-16 and possibly other enteroviruses. The incubation period is 3 to 6 days, and the clinical manifestations are self-limited, running a course from 5 to 7 days.

Immunologically, serum-neutralizing antiviral antibody is present transiently, and complement-fixing antibodies are present during the convalescent stage. There is no specific treatment.

Bacterial Infections

BACTERIAL INFECTIONS OF THE SKIN (PYODERMA). A few years ago, virtually every adult patient presenting with impetigo or similar skin infections had direct contact with children. It was an occupational hazard in nursery school workers, baby sitters, and certainly pediatricians and their staffs. Now these superficial pyodermas seem to occur spontaneously in adults and children. Also, mosquitoes and other biting insects can serve as vectors for transmission of staphylococcal and streptococcal infections, especially during late summer.

The emergence of methicillin-resistant staphylococcal pyodermas in the past decade, along with the near-total resistance of the *Staphylococcus* to erythromycin, clindamycin, and the quinolones, has sharply limited the clinician's armamentarium. Topical therapy with mupirocin ointment has accordingly become prominent in the management of superficial bacterial skin infections. The medication is applied three times daily until total clearing results. Although mupirocin labeling indicates that it is not intended for use on mucous membranes, there is evidence that the application of mupirocin just inside the anterior nares twice daily for 2 weeks may lessen the tendency for recurrent pyodermas. The long-term use of Hibiclens (chlorhexidine gluconate) in any family that is prone to recurrent pyodermas may be of great help.

STAPHYLOCOCCAL SCALDED SKIN SYNDROME (SSSS). Formerly known as Ritter's disease, SSSS is principally a disease of infants; children under the age of 5 years are occasionally affected. Following a brief macular erythematous phase, the disease quickly progresses to an intensely erythematous eruption almost always with facial involvement. At this time the skin is extremely tender. Perinasal and perioral vesicles and bullae usually herald the development of the subsequent phase in which sheets of the epidermis are shed, leaving eroded, weeping lesions that are burn-like in appearance. There is little or no mucous membrane involvement, which serves to differentiate SSSS from the Stevens-Johnson syndrome. In case of doubt, histology reveals a characteristic separation at the granular-cell layer of the epidermis. The etiology is an infection with *Staphylococcus* group 2, phage type 71, which produces a potent epidermolytic toxin. Treatment is with dicloxacillin, 18 mg/kg/day in four divided doses.

LYME DISEASE. Lyme disease is a complex consisting of characteristic skin lesions (erythema chronicum migrans), mono- or oligoarticular arthritis of the large joints, and various constitutional symptoms. It is caused by a spirochete, *Borrelia burgdorferi*, and is transmitted by the bite of a tick of the genus *Ixodes*. Most cases have occurred in the Northeastern United States, although sporadic cases have been reported elsewhere in the United States and in Europe.

The characteristic erythema is extremely prolonged and may spread to involve wide areas. There is no scale; the erythema is deep, producing a blue tinge, and there is a tendency toward central clearing. Existing serology, because of the large number of both false-positives and false-negatives, is less valuable than the observations of the astute clinician. The lesions of Lyme disease are both larger (>5 cm) and more persistent (>5 days) than many other exanthemata. Penicillin, erythromycin, and the first-generation cephalosporins have all been used successfully in the treatment of Lyme disease; the newer cephalosporin and erythromycin derivatives offer no clear-cut advantage. Doxycycline has been used in older children and adults. Therapy is usually continued for a minimum of one month (Coyle, 1993). Untreated, the disease may persist for years.

Mites and Insects

SCABIES. The most frequently encountered mite infection in North America is that caused by *Sarcoptes scabiei*. Sites of predilection are the interdigital spaces and the genitalia. So-called Norwegian scabies, in institutionalized patients, often occurs with large erythematous papular lesions on the palms and soles. Mites involved in these cases number in the dozens rather than only a few.

Lindane currently is the treatment of choice. The medication is applied over the entire body surface from the neck down and left on for an absolute minimum of 12 hours. The lindane conundrum has been well discussed by Rasmussen (1981), who observed that (1) most cases of neurotoxicity have been associated with gross misuse of the drug and (2) the skin of children over 1 year of age absorbs much less of the medication. At the time of this writing, lindane remains fully effective in its scabicidal properties. However, the total resistance of *Pediculus humanus var. capitis* among Indian tribes in the San Blas Islands of Panama may bode ill for the future of lindane in other infestations. Permethrin 5 percent cream is an acceptable alternative to lindane; it is effective in lindane-resistant tropical pediculosis and carries no warnings for use on infants at least 2 months of age (Schultz et al, 1990). Crotamiton, unfortunately, has an unacceptably high failure rate as an alternative to lindane.

PAPULAR URTICARIA. Despite the name, this entity is in reality a delayed hypersensitivity reaction to arthropod bites, usually to that of the flea harbored by domestic animals. It manifests itself in an early age group, usually those under age 7. The changing immune response to insect bites, such as mosquitoes, with age can be seen in Table 47–1.

In intensely mosquito-infested areas, most adults are in the final stage of this scenario. Prevention of papular urticaria consists of the use of effective insect repellents. Treatment is application of a potent corticosteroid, such as clobetasol, on the papules twice a day for 5 days.

Kawasaki Disease

The formal name for this entity is mucocutaneous lymph node syndrome. However, the disease can occur without appreciable lymphadenopathy. The disease is diagnosed using the following clinical criteria: (1) fever of abrupt onset, persisting at least 5 days and unresponsive to treatment; (2) conjunctival injection without exudation; (3) oral changes, including fissuring cheilitis, "strawberry tongue," and diffuse erythema of the oropharynx; (4) erythema of the palms and soles, progressing to acral induration and distal desquamation of the digits; (5) a polymorphous exanthem of the trunk, which may resemble

TABLE 47–1. TEMPORAL DIFFERENCES IN IMMUNE RESPONSES TO INSECT BITES

STAGE	WHEAL	PAPULE
No exposure	0	0
Early exposure	+	0
Typical response in midlife	+	+
Delayed hypersensitivity	0	+
Full immunity	0	0

erythema multiforme; and (6) adenopathy, principally cervical (1.5 cm or more in diameter). Virtually all patients are under 10 years of age, and the majority are under the age of 5. The etiology remains unknown; a host of infectious agents have been suspect.

Laboratory findings are nonspecific. Elevation of IgE level has been reported during the first 2 weeks of illness, followed by a subsequent decline. Thrombocytosis during the second week of the disease is a consistent finding. Complications include aneurysms of the coronary arteries, thrombosis of which may prove fatal. Aspirin (acetylsalicylic acid [ASA]) is the keystone of therapy during the acute phase of the illness; its mechanisms are presumed to be both anti-inflammatory and antithrombotic. It should be initiated at doses of 80 to 100 mg/kg of body weight until a serum salicylate level of 20 to 25 mg/dl has been achieved. Intravenous gamma globulin (IVGG) has been shown to enhance the effectiveness of salicylate therapy in preventing coronary artery abnormalities and especially in preventing giant aneurysms, and has been recommended by the American Academy of Pediatrics in addition to salicylate therapy (AAP, 1988). For convenience, IVGG can be administered as a single dose of 2 gm/kg body weight (Newburger, 1990). The serum salicylate level should be maintained for 14 days, or until the sedimentation rate returns to normal, if longer.

BULLOUS DERMATOSES AND VASCULITIDES

ERYTHEMA MULTIFORME. Erythema multiforme is a cutaneous reaction pattern to a variety of etiologic factors rather than a separate disease entity. It varies in severity from a few transient skin lesions to fatal Stevens-Johnson syndrome. The most common infectious etiologic factors are herpes simplex, *Streptococcus,* and *Mycoplasma pneumoniae.* The most common drugs implicated in erythema multiforme are penicillin and the sulfonamides. Many episodes are idiopathic.

The characteristic lesion of erythema multiforme is the ''iris'' or ''target'' lesion, often observed on the palms, soles, and mucous membranes; unlike urticaria, the lesions persist for days or weeks. Such lesions exhibit a dusky red central maculopapule surrounded by erythematous concentric rings. In more severe forms of the disease, hemorrhagic mucosal erosions, affecting virtually every body orifice, may be present; these are accompanied by severe constitutional symptoms, high fever, and renal, cardiac, or pulmonary involvement. The cutaneous manifestations also may include bullae, with the entire clinical picture virtually indistinguishable from toxic epidermal necrolysis. Immunohistology reveals granular deposits of immunoglobulin M (IgM) and complement (C3) in superficial dermal blood vessels, provided a fresh lesion is obtained for biopsy. Treatment of mild cases of erythema multiforme is supportive. Patients with severe cases of Stevens-Johnson syndrome are managed essentially as patients with severe burns. The use of corticosteroids remains controversial. Although controlled studies are lacking, many clinicians employ pharmacologic doses of corticosteroids early in the disease. There is some retrospective evidence that corticosteroids may delay recovery, and some dermatologists believe they should not be used at all in this syndrome.

ERYTHEMA NODOSUM. Erythema nodosum is a vasculitis caused by various etiologic factors, as follows:

1. Streptococcal infection
2. Herpes simplex infection
3. Tuberculosis
4. Drugs (sulfonamides, penicillin, salicylates)
5. Coccidioidomycosis
6. Rare diseases (leprosy, lymphogranuloma venereum)

The disease manifests as tender nodules, particularly on the shins. Biopsy adds little to the clinical diagnosis. Treatment with prednisone, 1 mg/kg/day divided into three doses for 6 days, is dramatic in reducing signs and symptoms.

LINEAR IgA BULLOUS DISEASE OF CHILDHOOD. Until the development of immunofluorescent microscopy, this entity masqueraded under a variety of clinical names and classifications. Weston (1985) observes that this may be the most common nonhereditary bullous disease of childhood.

The vesicles and bullae in this disease are pleomorphic, ranging from pinhead-sized grouped lesions that mimic dermatitis herpetiformis, to large tense round or oval lesions, containing clear or hemorrhagic fluid. Distribution also is variable, although usually there is prominent involvement of the buttocks and inguinal region. Itching ranges from intense to total absence.

Direct immunofluorescence reveals linear IgA and C3 deposits in the basement membrane zone in both lesional and perilesional skin. Indirect immunofluorescence has revealed circulating antibasement membrane zone antibodies, also in the IgA class. Treatment is with sulfapyridine (3 mg/kg) or dapsone (1.5 mg/kg). Gluten-free diets are ineffective.

VASCULITIS. Vasculitis is an immune complex disease characterized by the presence of immunoreactive products (immunoglobulins, complement), circulating immune complexes, and neutrophils with varying degrees of leukocytoclasia. The immune complexes bind to blood vessel walls, and complement binding occurs, which is followed by erythrocytic diapedesis.

In Henoch-Schönlein (anaphylactoid) purpura, such changes occur in the capillaries and postcapillary venules. Immunofluorescent studies of skin biopsy specimens reveal the presence of IgA in the vessel walls. In addition, serum levels of IgA may be elevated. IgA deposition also may be observed in renal biopsy specimens. The clinical picture of an initially erythematous macular eruption that blanches on pressure evolving into a nonblanching purpuric lesion correlates with the extravasation of erythrocytes, as the lesion matures.

Some classifications of vasculitis would broaden the aforementioned criteria to include the lymphocytic infiltrative disorders, such as pityriasis lichenoides et varioliformis acuta, which similarly exhibits erythrocytic diapedesis and the presence of C3 and IgM in dermal blood vessel walls. Neutrophils characteristically are absent. Individual lesions heal within a few weeks, often with smallpox-like scarring, which reflects the severity of the vasculitic process.

EPIDERMOLYSIS BULLOSA. This constellation of diseases comprises nine major groups and some subgroups based on the site of skin cleavage involved. Recent advances in electron microscopy have provided the tools for organizing this group of diseases in this manner. The disorders will be considered briefly here, and the reader is referred to Cooper et al (1987) for more extensive discussion. As these investigators state, "Epidermolysis bullosa (EB) is the term applied to a group of disorders whose common primary feature is the formation of blisters following trivial trauma."

As mentioned, a convenient way of classifying these disorders is to group them according to the level of skin cleavage: (1) the nondystrophic diseases, in which the site of cleavage is in the epidermis (these are the only truly *epidermolytic* diseases in the epidermolysis bullosa group); (2) the atrophic diseases, in which the site of cleavage is at the dermoepidermal junction; and (3) the dystrophic diseases, which are dermolytic in nature.

The dystrophic diseases follow an autosomal dominant pattern of inheritance. Thus, families are generally affected by and familiar with many aspects of the disease; genetic counseling is mandatory. Epidermolysis bullosa simplex may be generalized or localized. The generalized disease tends to flare in warm weather and heals without scarring. The localized form, known as Weber-Cockayne disease, may become manifest only later in life, with blisters forming on the hands and feet following vigorous physical exercise, such as long hiking. Treatment of both conditions, which heal spontaneously, is based on removing the offending agents: heat, friction, and physical trauma. Saline soaks and topical antibiotics may be helpful in resolving the lesions.

The atrophic diseases, with cleavage occurring at the dermoepidermal junctions, are inherited in an autosomal recessive pattern. The blisters may be extensive at birth and generally heal without scarring, but with some residual atrophy. However, the prognosis is grave for patients affected by some variants, with mortality greater than 50 percent in the first 2 years of life, often accompanied by pyloric atresia and refractory anemia. Patients with these diseases generally require care by trained personnel at specialized medical centers.

Acquired epidermolysis bullosa is a nonhereditary adult-onset disease characterized by bullae forming over the joints after only minor trauma, accompanied by atrophic scarring and nail dystrophy. It has nothing in common with the inherited forms of the disease except for the clinical similarity. This is an autoimmune disorder, with direct immunofluorescence studies demonstrating a linear deposition of IgG along the basement membrane zone. IgG in the upper dermis is demonstrated through immunoelectron microscopy of perilesional skin. Light microscopic examination findings are identical to the findings in bullous pemphigoid and porphyria cutanea tarda.

ACNE

ACNE VULGARIS. Acne is virtually a universal occurrence at some time in every adolescent's life, varying in severity from a few evanescent lesions to severe cystic and pustular forms resulting in both cutaneous and psychologic scars.

Acne has a multifactorial etiology, as follows: (1) the effects of androgens on the maturation of the epidermal cells in the infundibulum of the pilosebaceous apparatus cause cellular adherence rather than orderly desquamation and thus begin comedo formation; (2) the effects of *Propionibacterium acnes,* an anaerobic diphtheroid, increase the content of free fatty acids in sebum and induce an inflammatory response either directly or indirectly through metabolic products; and (3) the effects of plugging of the pilosebaceous-follicular orifice result in the accumulation of neutrophils, complement, immunoglobulins (IgG, IgM, IgA), and other mediators of inflammation with development of pustular cysts, which often rupture. This frequently produces permanent scarring as the inflammatory process resolves. In addition, *P. acnes* probably activates the T cell system. Intradermally injected heat-killed organisms evoked a delayed hypersensitivity reaction in patients with acne.

The foundation for acne therapy is composed of antimicrobial agents and retinoids. Topical agents, such as benzoyl peroxide and clindamycin, and systemic antibiotics, such as tetracycline and erythromycin, are efficacious in eradicating *P. acnes*. These antibiotics, which also inhibit leukocyte migration, are more effective clinically than the penicillins, although *P. acnes* is sensitive to both groups of antibiotics.

The retinoids, either tretinoin (Retin-A) topically or 13-*cis* retinoic acid (Accutane) systemically, restore the epithelial maturation in the follicular infundibulum to its normal state, promoting orderly desquamation and preventing comedo formation. Accutane additionally reduces sebum production by 98 percent or more within 2 weeks after initiation of therapy. At least 25 percent of patients treated with Accutane for 4 months continue to exhibit decreased sebum production at least 1 year after cessation of the drug. Although this may be a desirable factor in the long-term effectiveness of the drug, the accompanying xerotic cheilitis and xerophthalmia causing difficulty in the wearing of hard contact lenses are long-term side effects that must be balanced against the benefits of the drug. In my experience, at least 70 percent of patients treated with full 4-month courses of Accutane must be maintained on topical tretinoin, or they must receive repeat courses of Accutane within 6 months after completing the initial course of the drug in order to maintain acceptable clinical clarity. The other side effects of Accutane, such as elevation of serum triglyceride levels with concomitant elevation of low-density lipoprotein levels and decrease of high-density lipoprotein levels, colitis, vertebral skeletal abnormalities, and teratogenicity, mandate that it be reserved for those patients who do not respond to other therapeutic modalities.

ACNE ROSACEA. Rosacea is distinctly unusual in the pediatric age group but common in adults. It is characterized by multiple closed comedos on the central portion of the face accompanied by rhinophyma.

The combination of systemic tetracycline, 250 mg three times a day, until the patient's skin is totally clear, along with topical metronidazole gel, 0.75 percent, twice a day for at least 4 months achieves long-lasting improvement (Bleicher et al, 1987). The exact mechanism of action is unknown, although metronidazole is toxic to both gram-positive and gram-negative organisms, yeasts, and *Demodex folliculorum,* an ectoparasite found in profusion in the dilated pilosebaceous apparatus of rosacea.

The most dramatic resolution of rhinophyma is with isotretinoin (Accutane) in a dosage of 1 mg/kg daily for 6 weeks. It is not unusual to see the size of the nose decrease 50 percent in this period of time. The therapy may be continued for 4 months if necessary.

ALOPECIA

ALOPECIA AREATA. The dense perifollicular accumulation of lymphocytes at the base of the hair shaft has been cited as the feature identifying this as an autoimmune disease. The treatment of alopecia areata by the deliberate development of delayed hypersensitivity, allegedly to bring in "normal" lymphocytes and reverse the "abnormal" process, is certainly in question, not only for its efficacy but its rationale. It must be remembered that purely irritant therapy (application of phenol, ultraviolet light) was employed decades ago with gratifying results.

The etiology of this disease remains controversial. Empiric treatment of the typical well circumscribed nummular areas of alopecia with intralesional corticosteroids (5 mg/ml triamcinolone with lidocaine, up to 20 mg/ml) and systemic corticosteroids (prednisone, 20 mg every second day for 2 to 3 months) is employed in extensive alopecia, particularly that which begins on the occipital or marginal (ophiasis) scalp areas. This therapy is accompanied by the use of potent topical corticosteroids (clobetasol, 0.05 percent twice a day) even to the point of atrophy to induce hair regrowth. The mutagenic effects of dinitrochlorobenzene (DNCB) have been a problem with long-term use (up to 5 years) (Muller, 1985).

If alopecia begins in the occiput or scalp margins, therapy should be instituted quickly, even if only with topical clobetasol. Bald patients may not appreciate therapeutic nihilism.

TRICHOTILLOMANIA. An irregular pattern of hair loss, with varying lengths of regrowing hair, should suggest the diagnosis of self-induced alopecia. Unlike factitial dermatitis, in which skin lesions are consciously produced with intent to deceive, the patient with trichotillomania may be almost unaware of hair plucking. Absent-minded twisting of the hair while reading or watching television is a common history. The clinician can play a valuable role in explaining to both patient and parent the nature of the disease and that it may be an expression of a deep-seated need for better family communication. Counseling, not drugs, is the treatment of choice. The physician's prime duty is to allay feelings of guilt by any party.

OTHER DISORDERS

MILIARIA. Miliaria crystallina, in which multiple tiny nonerythematous vesicles develop, is seen frequently in premature infants. It resolves in 1 to 3 days without treatment. Full-term and older infants develop sweat gland blockage at the midepidermis with rupture of the duct and resultant inflammation. Almost inevitably these children are in an overheated environment (miliaria rubra). Loosening or use of less clothing and blankets results in clearing. Bland shake lotions, such as milk of bismuth (NF), may dry the skin and afford faster clearing. The very brief use of corticosteroid *lotion* (Cordran Lotion three times a day, not to exceed 4 days) will resolve the erythema almost immediately and provide some drying simultaneously.

Infants and older children can be spared all manifestations of miliaria rubra if they are in an air-conditioned environment for only 8 hours of 24. This preventive practice is effective even in tropical areas; the United States Armed Forces installed air-conditioned barracks to avoid the serious morbidity associated with tropical miliaria.

KERATOSIS PILARIS. Keratosis pilaris is a familial hyperkeratosis of follicular orifices, with the plugging of the infundibulum of the hair follicle. It is thought to be inherited as an autosomal dominant disorder. It commonly appears in early childhood and persists through adolescence. The characteristic "goose-flesh" appearance is seen predominantly on the extensor surfaces of the arms and thighs, although it can appear on the face and eyebrows. Individual lesions are red papules with a dry, central scale. Treatment consists of avoiding tight clothes; using topical keratolytic agents, such as retinoic acids, alpha-hydroxy acids, or salicylic acid; and skin hydration by standard dermatologic hydration and lubrication techniques.

NUMMULAR ECZEMA. Sharply demarcated, excoriated, weeping, and occasionally crusted coin-shaped lesions (Latin *nummulus,* coin) are the hallmarks of this disorder. Many etiologic factors have been proposed, but the cause remains unknown. Basically, an itch-scratch cycle is developed. Many of the lesions persist for long periods because of unconscious rubbing and scratching of the lesions. Since serum IgE levels are normal (Krueger et al, 1973), it is not surprising that antihistamines have little or no effect. The brief short-term use, not to exceed 5 days, of a potent corticosteroid (clobetasol three times a day) is most effective in breaking the excoriation cycle. If the eruption is accompanied by xerosis, the use of superfatted soap and stratum corneum hydrating agents (Complex 15, UltraMide) applied to the moist skin after bathing may be invaluable in preventing recurrence.

PITYRIASIS ROSEA (PR). A member of the maculopapulosquamous group of diseases, this viral skin infection is frequently seen in the older pediatric and adolescent age groups. Clustering of cases, demonstration of picornavirus-like particles from the lesions by electron microscopy, recovery of a virus of the picornavirus series from tissue inoculation, and rapid improvement of the disease following injection of convalescent plasma are all indirect evidence of a viral etiology. Anticytoplasmic IgM antibodies to keratinocytes in 100 percent of patients with PR also have been demonstrated.

The initial "sentinel" lesion characteristically appears 5 to 21 days prior to the onset of the generalized eruption and is usually larger and more irregularly shaped than the subsequent lesions. Because of its peripheral scaling and accentuation of peripheral erythema, it often is misdiagnosed as tinea circinata.

The definitive eruption consists of an oval-shaped, erythematous, peripherally scaling primary lesion, with the long axis arranged parallel to the lines of skin cleavage, producing the typical "Christmas tree" pattern. The face and distal extremities characteristically are spared, although an "inverse" form of the disease occurs that affects these areas only. The eruption varies from asymptomatic to moderately pruritic; itching is often triggered by a hot bath or shower.

Untreated, the duration of the disease varies, as a rule, from 4 to 10 weeks although persistence for as long as 6 to 8 months occasionally may occur. A brief regimen of systemic steroids (prednisone, 0.5 to 1.0 mg/kg, three times a day for 5 days) and topical steroid lotions (Cordran Lotion, three times a day for 7 days) greatly shortens the course of the disease and alleviates itching.

PSORIASIS. While the majority of psoriasis patients develop the disease in adult life, psoriasis may appear at any age. As a general rule, psoriasis developing in children and adolescents tends to occur with a strong family history of the disease and often culminates in severe and refractory disease in adulthood.

Psoriasis, one disease of the maculopapulosquamous group, consists of the development of sharply demarcated plaques surmounted by a silvery, thick scale. The extensor surfaces generally show the greatest involvement, especially at sites of minor trauma, such as the elbows and knees. The scalp is another frequent site of involvement; there may be an overlap with seborrheic dermatitis in the adolescent age group that exacerbates the disease.

The Koebner phenomenon, the production of isomorphic lesions at sites of trauma, is triggered not only by physical trauma but also the trauma of other dermatologic disease. For example, the psoriatic patient who develops pityriasis rosea or poison ivy may be expected to develop lesions of psoriasis at these affected areas after several weeks. The patient should be forewarned to begin antipsoriatic therapy as soon as such new lesions develop (or to employ general measures, such as sunbathing, to act as preventives).

A variant of psoriasis seen frequently in childhood is guttate psoriasis. In this variant, multiple drop-like lesions smaller than 1 cm in diameter develop over the trunk and extremities with little accentuation on the extensor surfaces. Scales tend to be less thick and silvery than in the typical plaque type of psoriasis, with erythema predominating. This variant is often seen as a sequela to streptococcal infection, and a throat culture should always be performed on any patient with guttate psoriasis even in the absence of a history of pharyngitis. Guttate psoriasis is occasionally seen following viral illness, perhaps a koebnerization of a viral exanthem, as noted above.

Treatment of psoriasis generally begins with the use of topical corticosteroids. As a general principle, it is best to initiate therapy with a superpotent steroid, used for no more than 2 weeks to achieve control, and promptly shift to a low-potency steroid to maintain control. Attempts to achieve control with a mid-potency steroid are rarely successful, and worse, may make the patients tachyphylactic to further steroid therapy. When patients have achieved complete clearing, they should be instructed to stop all topical corticosteroid therapy and to use the superpotent steroids at the first sign of a recurrence. With this type of pulse dosing, the lesions of psoriasis can often be controlled within days, and the disease kept in remission with only occasional use of medication. The clinician must convey to the patient and family the concept that these powerful substances must be used exactly as directed, and the full gamut of side effects from misuse must be emphasized. This not only improves patient compliance, but dispels the notion that a medication administered topically need not be taken seriously. The therapist must keep close control of the quantity of medication at the patient's disposal in order to prevent overuse.

The use of the alpha-hydroxy acid ammonium lactate 12 percent in a lotion base (Lac-Hydrin) applied to the moist skin daily after bathing seems to prolong remission more than other emollients and is safe for long-term use. Adjunctive therapy that suppresses *Candida* in scalp involvement, such as ketoconazole shampoo (Nizoral), affords a measure of relief in some patients. Anthralin (Drithocreme), widely used in Europe, is often overlooked as an alternative to corticosteroids. The drug can conveniently be applied to all lesions for 30 minutes in the evening and washed off prior to retiring, thus avoiding the staining and potential accidental inoculation of the medication into the eye, which occasionally occurs when the drug is applied at bedtime. Calcipotriene ointment 0.005% (Dovonex), a synthetic vitamin D_3 derivative useful for treating plaque psoriasis in adults is not currently recommended in pediatric patients because of the potential for hypercalcemia. The use of ultraviolet radiation in any form in the pediatric and adolescent age group should be minimal, as this will be in addition to the effects of a lifetime of solar ultraviolet exposure. Recalcitrant thick plaques of the scalp, a variant of psoriasis called *Tinea amiantacea*, may respond to Baker's P&S Liquid left on overnight for several nights in succession and used as an adjunct to topical steroid scalp lotions. Systemic therapy in the form of methotrexate, etretinate, corticosteroids, or cyclosporine is associated with severe side effects and requires the expertise of a specialist familiar with these modalities.

From an immunologic standpoint, the fact that immunosuppressives such as those listed above have been demonstrated to have a beneficial effect on psoriasis has opened new etiologic and therapeutic vistas in the investigation of this perplexing disease.

URTICARIA PIGMENTOSA. This is the most common of the mastocytosis group of diseases. Inevitably, it occurs before the age of 2 years. Vesiculobullous lesions are common in the initial stages of the eruption. The lesions tend to occur in crops, later subsiding to papular or macular pigmented lesions. Darier sign, the production of a wheal by vigorous stroking of a lesion, is virtually diagnostic. Dermographism also may be present.

Prognosis is excellent, with spontaneous resolution occurring almost universally by late adolescence. If symptomatic (pruritus or overanxious parents), an H_1 blocker may be used to prevent whealing.

SUN SENSITIVITIES. The sun exposure clock begins running at birth. With the widespread consumption of vitamin D–fortified milk, the only rational indication for sun exposure is gone. All other effects, from skin cancer to aging, are deleterious and may be prevented with sunscreens with a sun protective factor (SPF) of 15.

Ultraviolet, midrange, UVB (280–320 nM), generally is responsible for sunburn and skin cancer. The longer wavelengths of UVA (320–344 nM) are responsible for most other sun sensitivity diseases, including erythropoietic protoporphyria, porphyria cutanea tarda, berloque dermatitis, polymorphous light eruption, discoid and systemic lupus erythematosus, and poikiloderma, to name but a few. Therefore affected patients require opaque blocking agents, such as Neutrogena chemical-free sunscreen, which uses titanium dioxide to block out all wavelengths of light, both UV and visible. Dura Screen is somewhat less effective, but is waterproof, unlike the Neutrogena product. The longer wavelengths of UVA also elicit the development of aggressive squamous cell carcinomas and, because of their deeper penetration in the skin, actually irradiate the blood circulating through the skin during the time of exposure. This effect, coupled by the death of the Langerhans' cells with any appreciable length of UVA or UVB exposure, is a potentially ominous situation, considering the presumptive role of the Langerhans' cells in detecting foreign antigens including malignancies. The rate of internal malignancy in patients who receive psoralen and UVA (PUVA) treatment for psoriasis for 6 years or more is increased, as is the rate of occurrence of aggressive squamous cell carcinoma. To paraphrase Thomas Jefferson, he does best who is irradiated least.

DISORDERS OF PIGMENTATION

VITILIGO. Vitiligo is an acquired idiopathic depigmentation, with borders sharply circumscribed by normal or hyperpigmented skin. The most frequently affected sites are the face, neck, sternal area, arms, and dorsal surface of the hands, but the condition may be generalized. It is thought to be due to an autoimmune mechanism. Antibodies to melanin-producing cells have been detected.

There is some association between vitiligo and hyperthyroidism, adrenocortical insufficiency, pernicious anemia, and diabetes. There also is a reportedly increased frequency of vitiligo associated with IgA deficiency syndromes, as well as an increased association with combined occurrence of antithyroid antibodies and the HLA-I3 haplotype. Histologically, there is a complete absence of dopa-positive melanocytes. Pruritus may occur after sunburn of vitiliginous areas but also can occur without sun exposure. Treatment is mainly supportive, but intralesional steroids, oral psoralens, artificial keratin staining, and tattooing all have been used with varying success.

LEUKODERMA. The acquired hypopigmentation of skin that is produced by specific substances or is secondary to dermatitis is known as leukoderma. This has been shown in association with occupational dermatitis (e.g., from rubber garments as well as phenolic detergent germicides). These forms are rarely seen in children. The postinflammatory form of leukoderma is seen with a variety of inflammatory skin diseases, including pityriasis rosea, herpes zoster, psoriasis, atopic dermatitis, secondary syphilis, and morphea. Resolution consists of removing the offending substance and treating the underlying dermatosis. Leukoderma usually is reversible.

PITYRIASIS ALBA. Pityriasis alba appears in children and adolescents as hypopigmented, scaly, oval patches, usually on the face, upper arms, neck, and shoulders. Histologically, a mild dermatitis is seen. Pruritus, when it occurs, usually is mild. Treatment consists of hydration and lubrication techniques or application of topical low-potency steroids.

INCONTINENTIA PIGMENTI. This uncommon dermatosis usually affects female infants. When it does affect males, it tends to be lethal. There are three characteristic stages of the disorder; vesiculobullous, verrucous or papillomatous, and hyperpigmented. The lesions tend to be arranged in a linear or grouped fashion, mainly on the flexor surfaces of the extremities and the lateral trunk. Eosinophil counts are elevated in most cases. Other ectodermal defects include those of skin, hair, and teeth; neurologic and ocular defects are found in 30 percent of patients with this disorder. Abnormalities in skin pigmentation tend to disappear by adulthood. There is no known treatment. Genetic counseling is important in families with this disorder.

REFERENCES

AAP (American Academy of Pediatrics: Intravenous gamma globulin use in children with Kawasaki disease. Pediatrics 82:122, 1988.

Bleicher PA, et al. Topical metronidazole therapy for rosacea. Arch Derm 123:609, 1987.

Cooper TW, Bauer EA, Briggaman RA. The mechano bullous diseases (epidermolysis bullosa). In Fitzpatrick TB, Eisen AZ, Wolff K, Freedberg IM, Austin KF (eds). Dermatology in General Medicine. New York, McGraw-Hill, 1987.

Coyle PK. Lyme Disease. St. Louis, Mosby–Year Book, 1993.

Krueger GG, Kahn G, Weston WL, Mandez MJ. IgE levels in nummular eczema and ichthyosis. Arch Derm 107:56–58, 1973.

Jones HE, Reinhardt JH, Rinaldi MG. A clinical, mycological and immunological survey for dermatophytosis. Arch Derm 108:61–65, 1973.

Jones HE, Reinhardt JH, Rinaldi MG. Model dermatophytosis in naturally infected subjects. Arch Derm 110:369–374, 1974.

Muller S. Dinitrochlorobenzene in treatment of alopecia areata. Paul O'Leary Seminar, Mayo Clinic, September, 1985.

Newburger JW. Intravenous gamma globulin use in children with Kawasaki disease with single infusion. Pediatr Res 17:22A, 1990.

Ray LL. Candidosis. In Stone E (ed). Dermatologic Immunity and Allergy. St. Louis, CV Mosby, 1985.

Rasmussen JE. The problem of lindane. J Am Acad Dermatol 5:507–516, 1981.

Schultz MW, et al. Comparative study of 5% Permethrin Cream and 1% Lindane Lotion for the treatment of scabies. Arch Derm 126:167, 1990.

Weston WL. Practical Pediatric Dermatology. Boston, Little, Brown & Company, 1985.

Section Nine
ADVERSE REACTIONS TO FOODS

Chapter 48
Evaluation and Management of Patients With Adverse Food Reactions

Kristina M. Hoffman, M.D., and Hugh A. Sampson, M.D.

When considering the diagnosis of food allergy, familiarity with the accepted nomenclature and hypersensitivity disorders ensures that the patient will be provided with the correct diagnosis, treatment plan, and prognostic information. The American Academy of Allergy and Immunology and the National Institute of Allergy and Infectious Diseases have attempted to standardize the terms used to describe reactions to food. An *adverse food reaction* is a general term that encompasses the various untoward reactions following the ingestion of a food or food additive. *Food allergy (hypersensitivity)* refers to an *abnormal immunologic* response attributed to exposure to a food but is unrelated to any physiologic effect of the food. *Food intolerances* refer to *abnormal physiologic* responses to food or food additives that are nonimmunologic in nature. They account for the majority of adverse food reactions and include responses due to toxic, pharmacologic, or metabolic etiologies. Examples of these various reactions are listed in Table 48–1.

PREVALENCE

The true prevalence of food allergy is unknown. Epidemiologic data differ by age cate-

TABLE 48–1. DIFFERENTIAL DIAGNOSIS OF ADVERSE FOOD REACTIONS

Gastrointestinal disorders (vomiting and/or diarrhea)
   Structural abnormalities
      Hiatal hernia
      Pyloric stenosis
      Hirschsprung's disease
      Tracheoesophageal fistula
   Enzyme deficiencies (primary versus secondary)
      Disaccharidase deficiency (lactase, sucrase-isomaltase, glucose-galactose)
      Galactosemia
      Phenylketonuria
   Malignancy
   Other
      Pancreatic insufficiency (cystic fibrosis, Shwachman-Diamond syndrome)
      Gallbladder disease
      Peptic ulcer disease
Contaminants and additives
   Flavorings and preservatives
      Sodium metabisulfite
      Nitrites/nitrates
      Monosodium glutamate
   Dyes
      Tartrazine, ? other azo dyes
   Toxins
      Bacterial *(Clostridium botulinum, S. aureus)*
      Fungal (aflatoxins, trichothecenes, ergot)
      Seafood associated
         Scombroid poisoning (tuna, mackerel)
         Ciguatera poisoning (grouper, snapper, barracuda)
         Saxitoxin (shellfish)
Infectious organisms
   Bacteria *(Salmonella, Shigella, Escherichia coli, Yersinia, Campylobacter)*
   Parasites *(Giardia, Trichinella)*
   Virus (hepatitis, rotavirus, enterovirus)
Mold antigens (?)
Accidental contaminants
   Heavy metals (mercury, copper)
   Pesticides
   Antibiotics (penicillin)
Pharmacologic agents
   Caffeine (coffee, soft drinks)
   Histamine (fish, sauerkraut)
   Serotonin (banana, tomato)
   Tyramine (cheeses, pickled herring)
   Glycosidal alkaloid solanine (potatoes)
   Alcohol
   Theobromine (chocolate, tea)
   Tryptamine (tomato, plum)
   Phenylethylamine (chocolate)
Psychologic reactions

From Sampson HA. Adverse reactions to foods. *In* Middleton E Jr, et al (eds). Allergy: Principles and Practice. 4th ed. St. Louis, Mosby Year-Book, 1993a, p 1676.

gories, country, public perception, and study methods. Results of community surveys have reported the perceived incidence of food allergy to be 14 to 33 percent. This wide disparity in statistics probably is due to a combination of improper terminology and public misconceptions and a lack of challenge-proven confirmation of symptoms (Sloan and Powers, 1986). In 1982, a Finnish study that evaluated 866 children from ages 1 to 6 years reported the prevalence of food allergy as 19 percent at 1 year of age, 27 percent at 3 years, and 8 percent at 6 years. Results were based on history, effect of an elimination diet, and nonblinded food challenges (Kajosaari, 1982). A more rigorous study looked prospectively at 1749 Danish infants for the development of cow's milk allergy during their first year. About 7 percent of the children had suggestive clinical symptoms, but only 2.2 percent actually were proved to have cow's milk allergy by food challenges in the hospital (Host and Halken, 1990). These results were similar to an earlier study from the Isle of Wight (2.5 percent) (Hide and Guyer, 1983) and a more recent study from the Netherlands (2.7 percent) (Schrander et al, 1993).

In a prospective study of children followed through 3 years of age in a general pediatric practice, Bock concluded that about 8 percent of children experience adverse food reactions, most of which are transient. It may be concluded that 4 to 6 percent of children experience food hypersensitivity in the first 3 years of life, but only 1 to 2 percent of the pediatric population is affected by their tenth birthday (Bock, 1987), figures similar to those for the adult population.

ANTIGEN HANDLING BY THE GASTROINTESTINAL TRACT

The main functions of the gastrointestinal tract are to block harmful foreign antigens (e.g., infectious organisms, toxins) from entering the body proper and to process ingested food into a form that can be absorbed and utilized for energy and cell growth. The "barrier" formed by the gastrointestinal tract is composed of several components, which may block or destroy foreign antigens, preventing their entry into the circulation. Nonimmunologic components include the secretion of gastric acid, intestinal enzymes and intestinal mucus; generation of intestinal epithelial cell lysozymes; and expulsion of harmful substances with increased intestinal peristaltic activity. The major immunologic component is composed of antigen-specific secretory IgA antibodies, which will block penetration of ingested antigens. However, immaturity of these mechanisms in infants may reduce the efficiency of the infant gastrointestinal barrier. Basal acid output is low in the first month of life; intestinal epithelial lysozyme activity does not reach adult levels until approximately 2 years of age; and immature mucin composition in infants may result in decreased binding of foreign proteins and organisms.

Despite the multiple components of the gastrointestinal barrier, intact antigens penetrate the gut and enter the circulation in normal individuals. Some studies have suggested that more food antigens can be found in the circulation of food-allergic infants following meals than in that of normal adults. However, when food antigens bound in antigen-antibody complexes are taken into account, food antigenemia is comparable to that seen in adults (Heyman et al, 1988). Therefore, it is not an increased absorption of food proteins that leads to increased food hypersensitivities in young children, but a failure to develop normal *tolerance* to these food antigens.

Although the gut-associated lymphoid tissue (GALT) must mount a rapid and potent response against potentially harmful foreign substances and pathogenic organisms, it also must remain unresponsive to enormous quantities of essential nutrient antigens. GALT is composed of the appendix and Peyer's patches (aggregates of lymphoid follicles located primarily in the distal small intestine), lymphocytes and plasma cells scattered throughout the lamina propria, intraepithelial lymphocytes (IELs) interdigitated between enterocytes, and mesenteric lymph nodes. Dendritic cells (dome cells) located above Peyer's patches transport macromolecules from the lumen to resident precursor B cells and T cells. Although antibodies of all immunoglobulin classes can be produced following oral administration of antigen, antigen presentation activates predominantly IgA-secreting B cell precursors while suppressing IgM-, IgG-, and IgE-secreting B cell precursors. Once stimulated, the majority of activated B and T cells exit Peyer's patches through intestinal lymphatics and "home" to the lymphoid compartments of the gut, respiratory tract, and skin, and to the mammary gland of the lactating female. IELs are composed mainly of T cells, of which 80 to 90 percent are the cytotoxic/suppressor phenotype (CD8+). Human IELs mostly lack the H366 antigen, which suggests that they function mainly as T suppressor cells (Brandtzaeg et al, 1989). However, the role of immunologic suppression in induction of tolerance remains controversial. IgA antibodies found in intestinal secretions are predominantly in the secretory form consisting of two IgA molecules covalently linked by a peptide "J chain," which is also synthesized by IgA plasma cells. During transport to the intestinal lumen, mucosal epithelial cells attach a secretory component to dimeric IgA, forming secretory IgA (s-IgA). The addition of the secretory component makes the IgA molecule more resistant to enzymatic degradation. In the gut lumen, antigen-specific s-IgA binds foreign antigens, forming complexes that become "hung-up" in the glycocalyx (mucus), blocking absorption and allowing additional time for proteolytic digestion of foreign antigens to take place.

Development of Oral Tolerance

Since intact food antigens penetrate the gastrointestinal tract in both normal children and adults, it is imperative that the GALT develop tolerance to these nutrient proteins. The development of oral tolerance is poorly understood, but recent studies in rodents provide some insight. Utilizing a mouse model, it has been shown that the effect of neonatal protein ingestion on later specific antibody responses depends on the antigen, the antigen dose, and the age of the mouse at the time of feeding (Hanson, 1981). A single feeding of a protein antigen results in suppression of systemic IgM, IgG, and IgE antibody responses as well as cell-mediated immune responses (Ngan and Kind, 1978). This appears to be the result of $CD8^+$ (suppressor) cell activation, since cyclophosphamide-induced depletion of suppressor cells prevents the development of tolerance. Antigen-presenting cells (APCs) in the reticuloendothelial system

(RES) also play a critical role in the development of oral tolerance. Agents that activate the RES, such as muramyl dipeptide or a graft-versus-host reaction, enhance APC activity, which interferes with generation of $CD8^+$ cells and the development of oral tolerance (Mowat, 1987). In addition, ingestion of one antigen by a naive mouse will transiently activate the RES and inhibit induction of tolerance to a second antigen. If similar immunologic responses occur in human infants, this might explain the observation that introducing several solid foods in the first 4 months of life increases the likelihood of developing food hypersensitivity.

It also has been shown in the mouse that processing of food antigens by the gut is essential for the development of oral tolerance. Shortly after feeding a mouse ovalbumin, a "tolerogenic ovalbumin" can be found in serum, and this substance induces suppression of cell-mediated responses to native ovalbumin in recipient mice. The tolerogenic ovalbumin is similar in molecular weight to native ovalbumin and can be adsorbed from the serum with anti-native ovalbumin antibodies, indicating that the tolerogenic ovalbumin has undergone only minor modification and that it continues to share common epitopes with native ovalbumin. The essential role of lymphoid cells in the processing of tolerogenic proteins was shown by the fact that irradiated mice lost their ability to form tolerogenic ovalbumin but that the infusion of normal spleen cells restored their ability to generate tolerogenic protein (Bruce et al, 1987).

Similar factors could also account for a failure to develop oral tolerance to ingested food proteins in human neonates and result in the development of food hypersensitivity. It appears that the increased susceptibility of young infants to food allergic reactions is mainly the result of immunologic immaturity and, to a lesser extent, immaturity of the gut. The newborn lacks IgA and IgM in exocrine secretions and salivary s-IgA concentrations at birth, and they remain low during the early months of life. The relatively low concentration of s-IgA (blocking antibody) in the intestine of young infants together with the relatively large quantities of ingested proteins contribute to the large amount of food antigens confronting the immature GALT. In genetically predisposed infants, these antigens may stimulate excessive production of IgE antibodies or other maladaptive immune responses.

Food Antigens

The major food allergens are water-soluble glycoproteins, which have molecular weights ranging from 10,000 to 60,000 daltons and are stable to treatment with heat, acid, and proteases. The antigens responsible for most of the morbidity and mortality owing to food allergy will be discussed individually. The importance of these food antigens varies in different countries, depending on dietary habits and amount of consumption.

Cow's Milk

Cow's milk is one of the most common food allergens in children, perhaps because it is usually the first foreign protein encountered by infants. About 2.5 percent of children <3 years of age experience a milk-allergic reaction. Cow's milk protein fractions are subdivided into casein and whey proteins. Although extensive heating may denature some of these proteins, it does not decrease significantly the allergenicity of most protein fractions. Casein fractions are used extensively in processed foods as well as cheeses. The whey fraction consists of β-lactoglobulin, α-lactalbumin, bovine immunoglobulins, bovine serum albumin, and small amounts of various other proteins. IgE antibodies to these whey proteins have been demonstrated in most milk-allergic patients. Cross-reactivity among milk proteins obtained from cows, goats, and sheep has been reported, and in one report, clinical reactivity to goat's milk was estimated to occur in 50 percent of children allergic to cow's milk (Clein, 1958).

Eggs

Probably the most common cause of food-allergic reactions in children is the egg of the chicken. The major protein allergens found in egg white are ovomucoid, ovalbumin, and ovotransferrin (Holen and Elsayed, 1990). Although the yolk is considered to be less allergenic than egg white, IgE antibodies to egg yolk protein can still be demonstrated (Anet et al, 1985). IgE antibodies from children allergic to chickens' eggs have been shown to cross-react with those of eggs from other species (Langeland, 1983). The presence of IgE antibodies to egg in young children is associated with a high risk of developing other atopic disorders, including asthma, multiple food allergies, atopic dermatitis, and allergic rhinitis (Buffum and Settipane, 1966).

Frequently, questions arise about the administration of the MMR vaccine in egg-allergic children. Most studies agree that the MMR vaccine, which is propagated on chicken embryo fibroblasts, may be given safely to egg-sensitive children (Fasano et al, 1992; Businco et al, 1991). The majority of children experiencing anaphylactic reactions to the MMR are *not* egg-allergic. The American Academy of Pediatrics Infectious Disease Committee (Redbook Committee) currently recommends that MMR skin tests be performed prior to administering the vaccine to children with histories of reacting to eggs. The vaccine can be administered if the patient has both negative prick and intradermal skin tests to appropriate dilutions of the MMR. Children with positive skin tests are supposed to receive the MMR utilizing a "desensitizing" regimen. However, the reliability of MMR skin tests in predicting MMR anaphylaxis in egg-allergic individuals is doubtful. The "bottom line" on this issue is that children should not be denied an MMR vaccine because of a history of egg allergy, but until the AAP Red Book Committee changes its recommendations, skin testing with MMR and use of the desensitization protocol in egg-allergic children with positive skin tests should be continued for medical-legal reasons. Safety measures, such as the presence of resuscitative equipment, oxygen, epinephrine, and trained personnel, should be observed in every vaccination setting, regardless of allergic history.

Soybeans

Soybeans are legumes that cause food-allergic reactions, mainly in children. Soybeans are used in many commercial foods, since they are an inexpensive source of high-quality protein. Of four major protein fractions identified, no fraction appeared to be more allergenic than the others in a study of eight children with IgE-mediated soy hypersensitivity (Burks et al, 1988a). Soy proteins have been identified in some soy oils, lecithin, and margarine, but the clinical significance of this finding has yet to be determined. Immunologic cross-reactivity among legumes has been demonstrated; however, symptomatic hypersensitivity to more than one legume is rare (Bernhisel-Broadbent and Sampson, 1989).

Peanuts

The peanut is responsible for food-allergic reactions in both children and adults. Peanut allergy is probably the most common cause of death by food anaphylaxis in the United States. In one study, 3.2 percent of 248 atopic patients had positive skin tests to peanuts, and of these, 62.5 percent had clinical reactivity to peanut (Kalliel et al, 1989). Peanut allergy is rarely outgrown and, once diagnosed, should be treated with a strict lifelong avoidance of peanuts (Bock and Atkins, 1989). Peanut proteins are classified as water-soluble albumins or non–water-soluble globulins. Sixteen allergenic protein fractions have been identified in unprocessed peanuts. Two major peanut allergens have been identified: *Ara h* I and *Ara h* II, with molecular weights of 63.5 kd and 17 kd, respectively (Burks et al, 1992b). Thermal denaturation does not alter the IgE-specific binding capacity of allergenic peanut proteins (Burks et al, 1992a). Peanuts may be included as a flavoring in a variety of foods, including chili, spaghetti sauce, gravies, candy, and egg rolls. An additional risk factor for the peanut-allergic individual is a commercial product consisting of deflavored, reflavored, and recolored peanuts, which have been processed to resemble walnuts, pecans, or almonds. Although commercial peanut oil elicited no clinical reaction in ten peanut-sensitive patients (Taylor et al, 1981), preparation methods vary, and some peanut oil products may contain allergenic peanut protein.

Tree Nuts

Tree nuts are frequently implicated in adult food allergy and also cause reactions in children. Walnuts, pecans, almonds, brazil nuts, cashews, filberts (hazel nuts), pine nuts (piñon nuts), pistachios, and hickory nuts have all been implicated as food allergens. Bock and Atkins studied 14 tree nut–allergic children and found none to be allergic to the peanut, a legume. Twelve children were allergic to only a single tree nut while two had multiple nut allergies (1989).

An association between certain tree pollen sensitivities and an increased risk of allergy to the tree nut has been reported. A plant "pan-allergen profilin" has been implicated in cross-reactivity studies in some patients, although its clinical importance has not been established (Hirschwehr et al, 1992).

Fish

Fish is another common cause of food hypersensitivity in adults and children, especially in countries where fish is consumed in large amounts. Cross-reactivity among fish species was reported as early as 1946 (Tuft and Blumstein, 1946). More recently, it has been demonstrated that *in vitro* evidence of IgE-specific cross-reactivity does not necessarily correlate with symptomatic fish allergy (Bernhisel-Broadbent et al, 1992a). Heat- and pressure-processing of canned tuna and salmon has been shown to reduce the allergenic properties of these fish compared with their raw or cooked counterparts (Bernhisel-Broadbent et al, 1992b).

Shellfish

Seafood allergy is a common food allergy in adults but is increasingly more frequent in children, especially in geographic regions where their consumption is high. Shellfish can be divided into mollusks and crustaceans. Included in the mollusk group are snails, mussels, limpets, oysters, scallops, clams, octopuses, and squid. Although mollusk hypersensitivity has been reported infrequently in the medical literature, there are studies that report cross-reactivity between mollusks and crustaceans.

Shrimp allergens have been the most extensively studied among crustaceans, which include lobsters, crabs, prawns, and shrimp. Two heat-stable shrimp allergens, SA-I and SA-II, have been characterized and found to have 54 percent homology (Nagpal et al, 1989). In a study of 30 shrimp-allergic patients, the predictive value of positive shrimp prick skin tests and elevated serum-specific IgE was found to be 87 percent in patients who eventually had positive open challenges to shrimp (Daul et al, 1988). In a follow-up study, the same group reported that seven of 11 patients who had positive double-blind, placebo-controlled shrimp challenges had persistent highly elevated shrimp-specific IgE in their sera 24 months later, despite shrimp avoidance (Daul et al, 1990). Although it should be assumed, no study has yet determined whether seafood allergy is a lifelong condition.

Wheat

Cereal grains include wheat, rice, corn, rye, barley, and oats. Wheat is the predominant grain in the American diet, but consumption of other grains may be higher in other parts of the world, such as rice in Asia. Forty different protein antigens have been identified in wheat, and half have been reported to cross-react with rye antigens (Yunginger, 1991b). One study suggested that specific protein fractions of wheat were involved in specific disease processes: globulin and glutenin in IgE-mediated reactions, gliadin in celiac disease, and albumin in baker's asthma (Sutton et al, 1982). Although cross-reactivity among cereal grains and grass pollens is frequently seen with RASTs and skin tests, clinical reactivity to each grain and grass generally does not correlate with these findings (Jones et al, 1993).

CLINICAL MANIFESTATIONS

Cutaneous Manifestations

Atopic Dermatitis

Atopic dermatitis is most prevalent during early childhood. Approximately 95 percent of all cases manifest by 5 years of age, with most (80 percent) being symptomatic before the age of 1 year (Queille-Roussel et al, 1985). The disorder is characterized by an intensely pruritic erythematous rash that progresses to a lichenified dermatitis. Food hypersensitivity has been implicated as an etiologic factor in a large subset of children with atopic dermatitis (Sampson, 1983). In one report, one third of children seen at a university dermatology and allergy clinic were found to have food allergies, which contributed to their eczema (Burks et al, 1988b).

Sampson has evaluated over 350 patients with atopic dermatitis for evidence of food hypersensitivity. Most children (95 percent) had significant family histories for atopy, and 45 percent of the patients had both asthma and allergic rhinitis at the time of evaluation. Food allergy was diagnosed by double-blind placebo-controlled food challenges (DBPCFC). In 75 percent of the positive challenges, cutaneous symptoms developed within minutes to 2 hours, but only 30 percent of the positive responses were isolated cutaneous symptoms alone. Most of the skin manifestations consisted of pruritus, erythema, and a morbilliform rash. Urticaria was rarely seen in the initial evaluation. However, it was seen more often in patients who had experienced clearing of their eczema after several months on an allergen-avoidance diet but had retained their food hypersensitivity. It is important to note that, although these patients were selected for their skin symptoms, systemic manifestations occurred in a high percentage after ingesting the offending food. One third of these patients developed laryngeal symptoms; 41 percent experienced gastrointestinal distress (pain, nausea, vomiting, diarrhea), and about 15 percent developed wheezing (James et al, 1994).

The pathogenesis of atopic dermatitis appears to involve both immediate and late-phase effects of food hypersensitivity reactions (Sampson, 1992). Biopsies obtained 8 to 14 hours after a positive food challenge reveal an eosinophilic infiltration and deposition of major basic protein. Repeated ingestion of food allergens in atopic dermatitis patients is associated with production of histamine releasing factor (HRF) from mononuclear cells *in vitro*. This production of HRF was also associated with increased spontaneous basophil histamine release *in vitro* (Sampson et al, 1989). HRF production and basophil releasibility decreased over several months when the patients adhered to a food-allergen elimination diet.

In a prospective study of 113 patients, marked improvement was noted in food-allergic patients with atopic dermatitis who strictly followed an allergen elimination diet when compared with those who did not (Sampson and McCaskill, 1985). After 1 to 2 years of such a restriction diet, about one third of symptomatic food allergies were lost ("outgrown") (Sampson and Scanlon, 1989). Even though clinical reactivity was lost, the results of prick skin tests (or RASTs) were not significantly different. The likelihood of food allergy "resolution" was influenced by the type of food allergen involved, strict adherence to the elimination diet, and to a lesser degree, the age of the child.

Urticaria and Angioedema

Acute urticaria may be one of the most common symptoms associated with food allergy. However, its true prevalence is uncertain since many patients will not seek medical attention if their hives are unaccompanied by other more life-threatening symptoms. Since the development of urticaria usually occurs within minutes following the ingestion of a food, the patient can readily pinpoint the causative food and then simply avoid it. Some foods may cause urticaria by contact and not by actual ingestion; this type of reaction may be seen more often with fish, raw meats, and fruits.

Food allergy is rarely the cause of chronic urticaria (symptoms lasting for more than 6 weeks). In studies of chronic urticaria, only 1.4 percent of 554 adults and 11 percent of 163 children were found to have food allergy (Champion et al, 1969; Kauppinen et al, 1984).

Oral Allergy Syndrome

The oral allergy syndrome (OAS) may be thought of as a contact urticaria/angioedema involving the oropharynx. Symptoms such as swelling and pruritus appear within a few minutes of contact and are usually localized to the mouth and lips. A small subset of these patients may also experience subsequent systemic symptoms, but this type of progression is rare. OAS is most often triggered by fresh fruits or raw vegetables (Ortolani et al, 1989). Many patients with allergic rhinitis triggered by certain pollens, such as birch or ragweed, develop symptoms after ingestion of celery, apples, hazelnuts, and potatoes (birch) or ingestion of melons and bananas (ragweed).

Dermatitis Herpetiformis

Dermatitis herpetiformis (DH) appears as an intensely pruritic erythematous, papulovesicular rash that is localized over extensor surfaces, buttocks, and posterior hairline. Except for its distribution pattern, it can be easily mistaken for atopic dermatitis. Gluten-sensitive enteropathy (celiac disease) is found in 85 percent of DH patients (Hall, 1992). Over 80 percent of patients with DH have the HLA-B8 haplotype, and more than 90 percent have the HLA-Dw3 antigen. Skin biopsy findings in DH reveal IgA deposits at the dermo-epidermal junction. Histologic changes in the small bowel are similar to those in the skin. Treatment with sulfones will rapidly alleviate the skin symptoms but will not affect the gastrointestinal disease (Hall, 1992). Avoidance of dietary wheat will lead to resolution of the skin and GI abnormalities over time.

Gastrointestinal Manifestations

Gastrointestinal Anaphylaxis

Gastrointestinal anaphylaxis is a type of IgE-mediated reaction that often accompanies other systemic manifestations of a food-allergic reaction (Sampson, 1993b). Symptoms of abdominal cramping, nausea, vomiting and/or diarrhea usually develop within minutes to 2 hours of ingesting the offending food allergen. As in other types of immediate hypersensitivity reactions, mast cells play a major role in this clinical manifestation of food allergy. Degranulated mast cells and decreased tissue histamine levels have been demonstrated in gastric biopsy specimens obtained after food antigen challenges, findings consistent with mast cell degranulation (Reimann and Lewin, 1988). Increased amounts of IgE found in feces of food-allergic children are not necessarily correlated with increased serum IgE but may be due to the presence of local IgE-secreting plasma cells in the intestinal mucosa (Kolmannskog and Haneberg, 1985).

Diagnosis of gastrointestinal anaphylaxis is usually based on clinical symptoms observed following a food challenge in a controlled setting. Using gastroscopy to directly observe mucosal changes in food-allergic patients before and after food challenges, investigators have described hyperemia, a lumpy or nodular appearance, edema and thickening of the rugal folds with diminished peristalsis, and copious mucus clinging to the mucosa (Pollard and Stuart, 1942; Reimann and Lewin, 1988). They also observed that only food-allergic patients with clinical gastrointestinal symptoms (e.g., pain, cramps) had these mucosal changes. Food-allergic patients with only respiratory symptoms had mild mucosal hyperemia, and the non-food-allergic asthmatic control patients had no mucosal changes (Pollard and Stuart, 1942).

Food-Induced Enterocolitis Syndrome

Food-induced enterocolitis syndrome is a disorder characterized by protracted vomiting and/or diarrhea in infants, usually <3 months old, and is commonly associated with ingestion of cow's milk and/or soy protein. The clinical spectrum of this disorder may vary widely; patients may present with malabsorption and poor weight gain or acutely ill with severe dehydration. The term "cow's milk allergy" often appears in the literature indicating this entity, which leads to confusion when distinguishing this entity from IgE-mediated cow's milk allergy. Although cow's milk and soy are most often responsible for this syndrome, other food antigens have occasionally been implicated (Sampson, 1993a). It is occasionally seen in breast-fed infants and, rarely, in infants taking casein hydrolysate formulas.

Laboratory findings in this syndrome usually include increased stool leukocytes and occult blood, as well as an increase in the peripheral blood polymorphonuclear leukocyte (PML) count. The diagnosis is established by feeding affected infants up to 0.6 gm of the offending protein per kilogram of body weight (Powell, 1978). Clinical symptoms usually develop within 2 to 4 hours following ingestion but, in rare instances, may take as long as 24 hours. PMLs will increase >3000 cells/mm^3 in a blood sample obtained 6 to 8 hours after a positive oral challenge compared with a sample drawn just prior to challenge. PMLs, eosinophils, Charcot-Leyden crystals, and RBCs can generally be found in the stool. Challenges need to be conducted in a clinic setting with prolonged observation, since about 15 percent of these infants may become hypotensive and require aggressive medical therapy (Goldman et al, 1963).

Prick skin tests and RASTs to the offending food protein are negative. Jejunal biopsies reveal villus atrophy and increased numbers of lymphocytes, eosinophils, and mast cells, similar to biopsy findings in allergic eosinophilic gastroenteritis (Katz et al, 1984). The immunopathophysiology of this syndrome is not well understood. *In vitro* evidence for peripheral lymphocyte sensitization to specific food proteins in this syndrome has been demonstrated in infants with positive challenges (Van Sickle et al, 1985), but the significance of these findings in determining the etiology of the food-induced enterocolitis syndrome has not yet been established.

Dietary removal of the causative food antigen results in clinical resolution within 24 to 72 hours. Children can be orally rechallenged in a clinic setting in 6 to 12 months, depending on the interim history of any accidental ingestions with reactions. Between 20 and 50 percent of infants with cow's milk–induced enterocolitis will develop similar reactions to soy if placed on a soy formula. Reactivity to soy tends to persist longer than reactivity to cow's milk, and so it is recommended that cow's milk–sensitive patients be placed on a casein hydrolysate formula. Most children will have clinical resolution by the age of 3 years (Katz et al, 1984; Host and Halken, 1990).

Food-Induced Colitis

Food-induced colitis usually presents in the first few months of life in healthy appearing infants with occult or gross blood in their stools. Typically these infants have normal weight gain. Cow's milk protein is most often the offending antigen, although soy, beef, and food antigens present in maternal breast milk have been reported (Jenkins et al, 1984). Colonic biopsies reveal mucosal edema with an eosinophilic infiltrate in the epithelium and lamina propria. Polymorphonuclear leukocytes may be found in severe lesions with crypt destruction (Goldman and Proujansky, 1986). Symptoms generally resolve within 3 days after dietary elimination of cow's milk or other causative protein. Reintroduction of dietary cow's milk is usually possible within 6 to 24 months, although no definitive investigation has evaluated this aspect of the disorder. It is possible that food-induced colitis may not be a distinct clinical entity, but may be part of a spectrum that includes the food-induced enterocolitis syndrome and allergic eosinophilic gastroenteropathy.

Allergic Eosinophilic Gastroenteritis

Allergic eosinophilic gastroenteritis (or gastroenteropathy) (AEG) is characterized by eosinophilic infiltration of the gastrointestinal wall, peripheral eosinophilia, and gastrointestinal symptoms such as abdominal cramping, nausea, vomiting, and/or diarrhea. Peripheral eosinophilia is present in about half the patients, and the clinical manifestations may sometimes be limited to weight loss, or failure to thrive. Approximately half of the patients diagnosed with eosinophilic gastroenteritis are atopic, and a subset of these have been found to have specific food allergies.

Previous reports have classified this disease based on the level of eosinophilic infiltration in the gastrointestinal tract (mucosa, muscle layer, serosa) (Klein et al, 1970). However, since tissue eosinophilia may involve multiple layers of the bowel wall, and endoscopic biopsies are usually limited to the superficial layers, this classification may be artifactual and of limited usefulness in the clinical setting (Wershil and Walker, 1992). Pathologic findings in AEG may be similar to those found in children with milk-induced enterocolitis but generally have more prominent tissue eosinophils. Gastrointestinal biopsies reveal marked eosinophilic infiltration with patchy, flat villus lesions in the small intestine (Katz et al, 1984). AEG patients may have positive skin tests or RASTs to foods that can be implicated in the pathogenesis, but in young children these tests are not reliable. Patients improve when the causative food(s) are identified and eliminated from the diet. Sometimes multiple foods are implicated, and the patient must adhere to a strict diet consisting only of an elemental formula and one or two foods. Adults often do not have a good response to an elimination diet and must be treated with systemic corticosteroids.

Additional laboratory studies that may be helpful in this diagnosis include Charcot-Leyden crystals in the stools, anemia, hypoalbuminemia, and abnormal D-xylose tests (Sampson, 1993a). The erythrocyte sedimentation rate is normal in AEG, an important consideration when excluding other diagnoses such as polyarteritis nodosa and malignancies. Obviously, further studies would be indicated to rule out diseases other than AEG, as tissue eosinophilia may occur in other pathologic states including intestinal parasitic infection and the hypereosinophilic syndrome.

Colic

Infantile colic is a poorly defined syndrome of paroxysmal irritability characterized by inconsolable crying, abdominal distention, and leg flexion. Symptoms typically begin at 3 to 4 weeks of age and may persist until the age of 4 months. The etiology of this disorder is unknown, although much attention has been directed toward implicating cow's milk protein as a possible factor.

A number of studies have attempted to address this difficult issue. One group in Sweden has reported improvement in colicky symptoms in 35 to 88 percent of selected colicky infants with removal of dietary cow's milk

(Jakobsson and Lindberg, 1983; Lothe and Lindberg, 1989). In the United States, 17 colicky infants were studied in a double-blind, multiple crossover study with cow's milk formula and Nutramigen (Mead-Johnson), a hypoallergenic formula. There was a great day-to-day variability in colicky symptoms, as reported by the infants' mothers; however, there was a subset of infants who seemed improved with removal of dietary cow's milk (Forsyth, 1989). A study that included all-night polygraphic recordings of sleep patterns in infants found that only 13 of 31 cow's milk–allergic infants with overt symptoms (eczema or GI symptoms) actually had normal sleep patterns. The remaining 18 patients became "good sleepers" within 4 weeks of initiation of a milk-free diet (Kahn et al, 1987).

The difficulty in any study relating to colic is apparent when one considers the subjective and self-limited nature of the disorder. The subjective "complaint" of colic represents a wide variety of parent and physician perceptions; therefore, strict attention to diagnostic criteria and study design needs to be addressed. On the basis of the recent studies mentioned, the following conclusions may be reached: (1) infantile colic is a short-lived disorder of heterogeneous origins, one of which is food allergy or intolerance; (2) food allergy or intolerance may cause increased crying in some colicky infants; (3) a 2- to 3-month trial of hypoallergenic formula may be warranted in some colicky infants, but parents should not be left with the idea that their infant will have "lifelong" food allergy problems; (4) in a disorder as subjective as colic, more than one food antigen trial will be necessary to establish a cause-and-effect relationship between a food ingestion and the development of symptoms (Sampson, 1989).

Celiac Disease

Celiac disease is defined as a permanent intolerance of the small bowel mucosa to gluten. Traditionally, the diagnosis is based on the presence of marked villus atrophy seen on jejunal biopsy while the patient is on a gluten-containing diet, resolution of abnormal bowel histology seen on repeat biopsy after treatment with a gluten-free diet, and recurrence of the pathologic lesion with reintroduction of gluten (Kagnoff, 1992).

Children typically present in the first 3 years of life with steatorrhea, crampy abdominal pain with or without vomiting, and failure to thrive. They may be irritable and hypotonic with some degree of muscle wasting. Adolescents and adults may present with episodic diarrhea and weight loss. Vague abdominal discomfort and bloating may lead to an erroneous diagnosis of irritable bowel syndrome. Recurrent, severe aphthous stomatitis may be the sole clinical complaint. Patients with unexplained recurrent iron deficiency anemia, especially in combination with folate deficiency, should undergo a small bowel biopsy (Kelly et al, 1990).

Celiac disease is more common in those of Western European descent, especially in individuals of Irish ancestry. There is a predominance of HLA-DR4, HLA-B8, HLA-DRw17 (formerly termed DR3) haplotype in patients with celiac disease. Approximately 5 percent of celiac patients have concurrent dermatitis herpetiformis (DH), a skin manifestation discussed previously (Kagnoff, 1992).

The immunopathogenesis of celiac disease is poorly understood. Plasma cell and lymphocytic infiltration of the intestinal lamina propria have been described, as well as infiltration of the epithelium with intraepithelial lymphocytes. Increased numbers of mast cells may also be present (Kagnoff, 1992). Many different pathologic mechanisms have been implicated in celiac disease including both cellular and complement-mediated cytotoxicity and lymphokine-induced damage (Kelly et al, 1990). The HLA associations in conjunction with the specific protein trigger (i.e., gliadin) might suggest an abnormal antigen-processing mechanism. It is probably a combination of events that leads to the disease manifestations.

After diagnosis, patients usually respond well to the removal of gluten from their diets. Gluten is a major protein found in wheat, barley, rye, and oats and is composed of two types of proteins: alcohol-soluble gliadins and alcohol-insoluble glutenins. It is the gliadins that are believed to cause damage to the intestinal mucosa (Kelly et al, 1990).

Although not necessarily a primary phenomenon, patients with active celiac disease usually have high levels of serum antibodies, especially IgA, to gluten. Anti-gliadin antibodies are elevated in about 90 percent of untreated celiac patients but may be present in other intestinal disorders and rarely in normal patients (Scott and Brandtzaeg, 1985).

IgA anti-gliadin antibody levels are used as a screening test but should not be considered diagnostic. In many patients, anti-gliadin antibodies may be used to follow the course of the disease and patient compliance with the gluten-free diet. As celiac disease is a lifelong disorder, patients must continue their gluten-free diet, not only to avoid clinical manifestations of the disease, but to decrease their risk of malignancy, which is significantly higher than that of the general population if the diet is not maintained (Kelly et al, 1990).

Respiratory Manifestations

Lower Respiratory Reactions

Isolated respiratory symptoms in the absence of other clinical manifestations of food hypersensitivity are rare (Bock and Atkins, 1990; Sampson, 1993a). Measurements of pulmonary function—including FVC, FEV_1, and MMEF—may decrease significantly during a positive oral food challenge in some children. In one study of 140 children with asthma followed in a pulmonary clinic, asthmatic symptoms occurred in 5.7 percent of patients during positive oral food challenges (Novembre et al, 1988). Another study found 24 of 284 (8.5 percent) asthmatic children to have food allergy as the etiology for their asthma symptoms (Oehling and Cagnani, 1980). Changes in airway hyperreactivity were evaluated in 11 adult asthmatic patients with methacholine challenges before and 24 hours after DBPCFCs. No significant difference in bronchial hyperresponsiveness was noted between food and placebo challenges (Zwetchkenbaum et al, 1991). In a recent study, 17 food-allergic asthmatic children underwent methacholine inhalation challenges before and after DBPCFCs. Fourteen patients had positive DBPCFCs. In five of the eight patients who developed chest symptoms (wheezing in one, deep cough in four), there were significant increases in airway reactivity as determined by the methacholine challenge. One of six patients with positive DBPCFCs but without chest symptoms also had a significant change in airway reactivity. These findings indicated that food-induced allergic reactions could increase airway reactivity in some asthmatic patients (James et al, 1994).

Upper Airway Reactions

Nasal congestion, sneezing, and rhinorrhea may occur during a food allergic reaction. Again, as in lower respiratory reactions, these symptoms are unlikely to occur as an isolated clinical manifestation of food allergy (Bock and Atkins, 1990; Sampson, 1993a).

The phenomenon of "gustatory rhinitis" (clear, watery rhinorrhea) is sometimes seen following ingestion of hot spicy foods, such as chili peppers and horseradish. Gustatory rhinitis does not involve nasal mast cells or histamine; the clinical manifestations are not due to allergic etiologies but are secondary to chemicals in the food that have irritant and/or neuronal effects in the nose. Treatment involves avoidance or prophylactic application of topical nasal atropine (Raphael et al, 1989).

Heiner's Syndrome

Cow's milk–induced pulmonary hemosiderosis (Heiner's syndrome) is a rare condition, usually occurring in young children and characterized by chronic cough, wheezing, recurrent lung infiltrates, and a microcytic hypochromic anemia. In affected patients' sera, precipitins to cow's milk proteins are detectable by diffusion of reactants in agar using the Ouchterlony technique (Heiner and Sears, 1960). Removal of dietary cow's milk protein results in symptomatic improvement, and reintroduction of cow's milk protein results in symptom recurrence, a worsening clinical course, and often death. Although primary pulmonary hemosiderosis may be idiopathic or associated with glomerulonephritis (Goodpasture's syndrome), the presence of severe anemia should raise the suspicion of a cow's milk–induced etiology.

The immunopathophysiology of this disease is not understood. Elevated specific IgD antibodies have been reported in one patient, but the significance of this finding remains unknown. No consistent *in vitro* immunologic laboratory studies have been demonstrated in this disorder, including lymphocyte proliferation tests, RASTs, or complement-fixation assays. Further studies must be done to elucidate the immunologic mechanisms responsible for this disease.

Generalized Manifestations

Systemic Anaphylaxis

Systemic anaphylaxis, in the "classic" sense, is an acute allergic reaction due to the rapid release of pharmacologically active mediators from peripheral blood basophils and tissue mast cells, leading to a life-threatening reaction with cardiopulmonary involvement. The clinical manifestations may or may not involve urticaria, angioedema (oral and/or laryngeal), nausea, abdominal cramps, vomiting, nasal congestion, rhinorrhea, dyspnea, wheezing, arrhythmias, and/or hypotension. "Anaphylactoid" reactions may be clinically indistinguishable from anaphylaxis but are not mediated by IgE antibodies (Yunginger, 1992). Food proteins are not uncommonly implicated as triggers for anaphylaxis in susceptible individuals.

In a review of fatal and near-fatal anaphylactic reactions to food in 13 children, all but one of the survivors had received epinephrine within the first 30 minutes of allergen ingestion. Six of the 13 children experienced biphasic and/or protracted reactions. Five of the six fatalities occurred in public settings (most in school), whereas all the near-fatal reactions took place in private homes. One of six patients with fatal anaphylaxis developed cutaneous symptoms compared with seven of seven with near-fatal reactions (Sampson et al, 1992). In another series of fatalities (seven patients, aged 11 to 43 years) owing to food-induced anaphylaxis, Yunginger and colleagues (1988) found that none of the victims received epinephrine immediately after the onset of symptoms. They emphasize that these cases illustrate the need for patient education and prescription with instruction for self-injectable epinephrine.

Laboratory findings in food-induced anaphylaxis are not consistent. Although elevated mast cell–derived serum tryptase levels are usually found in anaphylaxis owing to Hymenoptera or drugs (Yunginger et al, 1991), this is not the case for food-induced anaphylaxis (Sampson et al, 1992). Specific IgE antibodies to food antigens have been found to be elevated in postmortem serum from victims of food-induced anaphylaxis; however, this finding proves prior sensitization, which may or may not be related to an anaphylactic death (Yunginger et al, 1991).

Food-Dependent Exercise-Induced Anaphylaxis

A variant of exercise-induced anaphylaxis is a clinical entity known as food-dependent exercise-induced anaphylaxis. This unusual phenomenon is characterized by anaphylactic symptoms that occur in certain individuals when exercise and ingestion of food occur within 2 hours of each other. These patients do not have anaphylaxis with exercise alone or with food consumption alone. Exercise may precede or follow food consumption for the reaction to occur. There are two subsets of patients who are affected by this syndrome. The one group has reactions with exercise and food consumption, regardless of the foods eaten. The second and probably larger group has symptoms only with exercise and ingestion of a specific food. These patients will often identify the offending food and have positive prick skin tests to the responsible food. The pathogenic mechanisms involved in this syndrome are unknown. Treatment involves avoidance of food ingestion for at least 2 hours before and after exercise, carrying a self-injectable epinephrine device during exercise, and exercising with a companion (Kidd et al, 1983).

Food Additive Reactions

A complete discussion of preservatives, thickeners, colorings, flavorings, and antioxidants that are added to food is beyond the scope of this chapter. Although reactivity to dyes and additives are rare, this issue often comes up in practice, and so it is useful to be aware of the more common additives reported to be associated with adverse clinical reactions. The pathophysiologic mechanisms of these reactions are unclear and are often not proved to have an allergic etiology. Treatment, as with most adverse reactions to food, involves avoidance of the implicated substance.

Sulfites are used in many foods as an antioxidant and antimicrobial agent. In susceptible individuals, they have been reported to induce bronchospasm or even anaphylaxis. Patients with this reaction are usually nonatopic and have severe asthma. Sulfites may be contained in some medications as well as in processed food and beverages (Simon and Stevenson, 1993).

Tartrazine (FD&C Yellow #5) and other dyes, parabens, and benzoates may exacerbate chronic urticaria but have not been implicated as its underlying cause. Past reports linking aspirin sensitivity and tartrazine reactions are suspect. In a recent study of more than 150 single-blind challenges with tartrazine in aspirin-sensitive asthmatic patients, six patients had a 20 percent or greater decline in FEV_1. On follow-up double-blind placebo-controlled challenge, no patients experienced any change in their FEV_1 values. Given these results, it is doubtful that any cross-reactivity between aspirin and tartrazine exists (Simon and Stevenson, 1993).

BHA and BHT have been reported to be the cause of isolated cases of urticaria but have not been shown to produce asthma exacerbations. Nitrates and nitrites (often added to processed meats) are not causative factors in angioedema, urticaria, or anaphylaxis (Simon and Stevenson, 1993).

Monosodium glutamate (MSG) is a flavor enhancer which, in large quantities, is reported to cause a burning sensation, facial pressure, chest pain, and sometimes headache in certain people. Originally dubbed the "Chinese restaurant syndrome" because these symptoms often occurred after eating a meal of Chinese food (Kwok, 1968), MSG reactions have been reported following ingestion of other Asian foods containing MSG. Processed meat, soups, and diet foods also contain MSG and should be avoided by susceptible individuals (Simon and Stevenson, 1993).

Other Food-Induced Reactions

There are several disorders in which foods have been implicated as an associative or causative factor, yet no convincing proof of immunologic mechanisms has been forthcoming. Perhaps the one that has received the most media attention is hyperactivity and its relationship to food additives. In the early 1970s, Feingold proposed that hyperkinetic activity and learning disabilities in children were associated with dietary food additives and salicylates (Feingold, 1975). He claimed a large majority of these children would improve on an avoidance diet, but his claims were largely anecdotal. Later studies showed that Feingold's findings were probably exaggerated, but that there may be an occasional child who may benefit from an additive-free diet (Stevenson et al, 1991).

Migraine is another disorder in which the role of adverse food reactions has been suspected. Foods that contain tyramine (cheese, chocolate, and red wine) have been reported to provoke migraines in some migrainous patients (Moffett et al, 1972). In a large study of adults with at least three migraines per week, food-induced symptoms were documented in 15 percent of patients (Weber and Vaughan, 1991). Another study showed that an oligoantigenic diet could benefit children with migraine and epilepsy, but not children with epilepsy alone (Egger et al, 1989). However, no evidence for immune mechanisms in the pathogenesis of this disorder has been demonstrated.

In some patients with irritable bowel syndrome (IBS), food intolerance has been shown to provoke clinical symptoms. Of 21 patients with IBS, six underwent double-blind food challenges which confirmed the presence of a food intolerance. Serum IgE and peripheral eosinophil counts were normal, and there was no evidence of specific histamine release by peripheral blood basophils to the implicated foods. The patients had normal breath hydrogen excretion after challenge and control foods. Rectal prostaglandin E_2 was found to increase following challenge. Some of these patients could prevent symptoms by prior administration of prostaglandin-synthetase inhibitors (Alun-Jones et al, 1982). However, the best treatment was complete elimination of the causative food.

The notion that food allergy, especially cow's milk allergy, is linked to some autoimmune disorders has been discussed in the medical literature. Rheumatoid arthritis, for example, has been allegedly associated with food allergy, although most published studies on this subject "do not meet acceptable standards of modern medical research" (van de Laar and van der Korst, 1991), and only one case documenting symptom provocation by DBPCFC has been published (Panush et al, 1986). Circumstantial evidence surrounding milk allergy and certain types of steroid-responsive nephrotic syndrome, especially IgA nephropathy, has been reported (Sandberg et al, 1977). However, despite a reportedly high incidence of atopy in nephrotic syndrome patients, there is no definitive proof of a cause-and-effect relationship in this disorder relating to milk allergy. Insulin-dependent diabetes mellitus (IDDM) is another autoimmune disorder in which circumstantial evidence suggests an association between milk allergy and IDDM pathogenesis. In countries where cow's milk consumption is high, there is a proportional increase in the incidence of IDDM (Scott, 1990). A serum antibody to bovine serum albumin that cross-reacts with a surface antigen in pancreatic beta cells was reported to be elevated in newly diagnosed IDDM patients compared with controls (Karjalainen et al, 1992). However, the significance of this finding remains in doubt. Probably the most compelling evidence for a cause-and-effect relationship between a food substance and IDDM comes from an Icelandic study, which suggests that consumption of high quantities of smoked mutton by a mother around the time of conception puts the male progeny at much higher risk of developing IDDM later in childhood (Helgason and Jonasson, 1981). This effect probably is due to a toxic effect of the N-nitroso compounds contained in smoked foods and is not an immunologically mediated phenomenon.

DIAGNOSIS

A thorough medical history is the initial step in diagnosing an adverse food reaction. Questions should be directed toward pinpointing the food involved and toward elucidation of the character, duration, reproducibility, frequency, and timing of the symptoms. Both the history and physical examination should be performed to help focus the differential diagnosis (see Table 48–1). Any laboratory studies or subspecialty referrals will depend on the physician's ability to distinguish between food-induced hypersensitivity and other disorders. Once other etiologies have been ruled out, various laboratory studies (Table 48–2) may be performed, depending on the individual patient and his or her medical history (Bock et al, 1988).

TABLE 48–2. METHODS USED IN THE EVALUATION OF FOOD ALLERGIC REACTIONS

Medical history
Diet diary
Elimination Diet
Prick Skin Testing [PST]
Radioallergosorbent Tests [RAST]
Basophil Histamine Release [BHR] Assays
Intestinal Mast Cell Histamine Release [IMCHR]
Intragastral Provocation Under Endoscopy
Double-Blind Placebo-Controlled Food Challenge [DBPCFC]
Intestinal Biopsy Following Allergen Elimination and Feeding

From Sampson HA. Adverse reactions to foods. *In* Middleton E Jr, et al (eds). Allergy: Principles and Practice. 4th ed. St. Louis, Mosby Year-Book, 1993a, p. 1675.

Although the medical history is extremely useful, especially in acute reactions, it can be unreliable in chronic disorders such as atopic dermatitis, asthma, eosinophilic gastroenteritis, and chronic urticaria. In several studies, less than 50 percent of reported food-allergic reactions could be confirmed by double-blind placebo-controlled food challenges (Sampson, 1983; Bock et al, 1978).

The following information should be gleaned from the history in order to design the appropriate blind challenge: (1) the suspected food that may have caused the reaction, (2) the quantity of the suspected food that was ingested, (3) the length of time between ingestion and development of the reaction, (4) symptom description, (5) whether symptoms occurred every time the food was ingested, (6) whether other factors, such as exercise, are necessary for the symptoms to occur, and (7) when the most recent reaction to the food occurred (Sampson, 1993a). Although many foods have been reported to cause allergic reactions, about 85 percent of reactions may be attributed to eggs, milk, peanuts, soy, and wheat in American children and to peanuts, nuts, fish, and shellfish in adults.

A sometimes useful adjunct to detect food allergens involves the patient's keeping a record of all ingested foods and of subsequent symptoms if they occur. These diaries should also include items such as chewing gum, mouthwash, toothpaste, and medications. The timing and description of any symptoms are also recorded. This approach is more dependable than the patient's memory, but lacks objectivity.

Elimination diets alone are usually insufficient to make a definitive diagnosis of food allergy. However, they are often used in the management of adverse food reactions and are usually recommended for specific periods of time prior to oral food challenges. The success of the diet depends on the choice of the correct causative food proteins, the patient's ability to avoid all forms of the food antigen(s), and the assumption that other factors will not trigger allergic reactions during the period of the diet. These conditions are often difficult to achieve.

Prick skin tests are frequently used to screen patients with suspected IgE-mediated food hypersensitivity. They are not useful in the diagnosis of non–IgE-mediated diseases such as food-induced enterocolitis syndrome, food-induced colitis, or celiac disease. Negative prick skin tests virtually rule out IgE-mediated reaction with a negative predictive accuracy of greater than 95 percent, provided good-quality food extracts are utilized and the prick technique is performed properly with negative (saline) and positive (histamine) controls. The positive predictive accuracy of prick skin tests is generally less than 50 percent. A positive prick skin test simply indicates the presence of food antigen–specific IgE antibodies and indicates foods that should be investigated as the cause of food-allergic reactions (Bock and Atkins, 1990; Sampson and Albergo, 1984).

Some important caveats must be considered in interpreting prick skin test results: (1) skin tests with commercially prepared extracts may be negative in some patients with IgE-mediated sensitivity to fruits or vegetables (Ortolani et al, 1989); (2) skin tests may be negative in some infants less than one year of age who have IgE-mediated food reactions; (3) skin test wheals may be smaller in children less than 2 years old (Menardo et al, 1985); and (4) a positive prick skin test to a single food that provoked a life-threatening anaphylactic reaction may be considered diagnostic.

A prick/puncture skin test wheal 3 mm in diameter or greater than the negative control using food extracts of 1:20 w/v concentration has been shown to indicate the degree of hypersensitivity likely to be associated with clinically significant hypersensitivity reactions to food. Intradermal skin tests are too sensitive and have not been shown to identify additional patients with positive DBPCFC who did not already have positive prick skin tests. Intradermal skin testing for food allergens is unwarranted and only increases the risk of causing a systemic reaction when compared with prick skin testing.

Radioallergosorbent tests (RASTs) detect the presence of food-specific IgE antibodies in patient sera and are often used by practitioners as a screen for IgE-mediated food hypersensitivity. Standard RASTs are slightly less sensitive than prick skin tests, depending on the quality of the laboratory and the methods used. A study which compared outcomes of DBPCFCs and Phadebas RAST found that RASTs and PSTs had similar specificity and sensitivity if a Phadebas score of 3 or greater (on a scale of 4) was considered positive (Sampson and Albergo, 1984). Using scores of 2 or greater to indicate positivity greatly reduced the specificity of the test. Other studies, which are utilized primarily in research settings, are basophil histamine release assays, intestinal mast cell histamine release, and intragastral provocation under endoscopy. Lymphocyte proliferation assays are not useful as a diagnostic test (Hoffman et al, 1994).

The "gold standard" for the diagnosis of food allergies is the DBPCFC (Sampson, 1988; Bock et al, 1978). The selection of foods to be investigated will depend on the history and PST or RAST results. In the clinical setting, an open or single-blind food challenge may be utilized with foods that have a low probability of inducing a reaction or to screen large numbers of foods. However, if several positive reactions occur, they need to be confirmed by a DBPCFC, except in cases in which the reaction was life-threatening or in children less than one year of age. Considerations regarding the conduct of DBPCFC are delineated in Table 48–3. DBPCFCs should not be undertaken if the patient has a concurrent illness, such as a viral illness, or if a chronic illness, such as asthma, is not under good control. Recommendations for an office evaluation of food allergy with a single-blind challenge are outlined in Table 48–4.

Food challenges should be performed after the patient has fasted. Small doses are given at first (125 to 500 mg of lyophilized food); then the dose is doubled approximately every

TABLE 48–3. CONSIDERATIONS WHEN CONDUCTING A DBPCFC

Eliminate suspected foods for 7–14 days prior to challenge.
Discontinue antihistamines; minimize other medications.
Administer challenge to patient on an empty stomach.
An equal number of food and placebo challenges need to be administered; randomized by non-interested party (dietitian).
Lyophilized foods are blinded in liquid or capsules.
Administer 10 gm over 1 hr; 1st dose ≤500 mg.
Utilize a standardized scoring system.
The length of the observation period is dependent on type of reaction being studied.
Appropriate equipment should be available to treat systemic anaphylaxis.

ALL NEGATIVE CHALLENGES *MUST* BE CONFIRMED BY AN OPEN FEEDING UNDER OBSERVATION

From Sampson HA. Adverse reactions to foods. *In* Middleton E Jr, et al (eds). Allergy: Principles and Practice. 4th ed. St. Louis, Mosby Year-Book, 1993a, p 1677.

TABLE 48-4. OFFICE EVALUATION OF FOOD HYPERSENSITIVITY

1. History and physical examination
2. Prick skin tests with appropriate antigens
   − Further work-up generally unnecessary if IgE-mediated sensitivity suspected
   + Go to next step
3. Strict allergen avoidance diet for 2 weeks
   Unequivocal improvement and only 1 "major" or 1 or 2 "minor" foods involved
   CONTINUE RESTRICTED DIET
   Improvement equivocal and/or more than 2 foods involved, go to next step
4. Single-blind challenge in office
   If −, discontinue restricted diet
   If + to only 1 "major" food or <4 "minor" foods in total, institute appropriate restricted diet
   If + to only 1 "major" food or >4 foods in total, to next step
5. Double-blind placebo-controlled challenge in hospital setting

From Sampson HA. Immunologically mediated food allergy: The importance of food challenge procedures. Ann Allergy 60:267, 1988.

15 minutes. If the patient begins to develop symptoms, the challenge is terminated and the patient treated. If the patient tolerates a total of 10 gm (in dehydrated form) of the suspected food, the challenge is deemed negative. However, an open challenge with a generous portion of food in its natural state must be consumed in its usual form under observation to identify the rare patient with a false-negative DBPCFC.

A number of variables need to be monitored during the performance of a DBPCFC utilizing a standard scoring system: time of observation (2 to 4 hours for IgE-mediated reactions; at least 8 hours for food-induced enterocolitis), equal numbers of placebo and test food challenges, adequate wash-out periods between challenges, and the participation of an individual not involved in scoring the challenge to randomize the order of test substance administration (such as a dietician). DBPCFCs for chronic disorders (e.g., atopic dermatitis, chronic asthma) are best performed in an inpatient setting where environmental factors and dietary components are strictly regulated. However, as mentioned, blind challenges may be performed as an office procedure if the proper personnel and resuscitative equipment are present. If anaphylactic symptoms are suspected from the patient's history, the challenge, if necessary for identifying the suspected food or to document the development of tolerance for the suspected food, should be performed in an ICU setting.

The diagnostic accuracy of DBPCFCs is excellent. Excluding challenges with lyophilized fish protein, the false-negative rate on over 500 DBPCFCs from three centers was between 0.5 and 4.6 percent, and the false-positive rate between 0.5 and 1.5 percent. Use of dehydrated fish resulted in a false-negative rate of 21 to 27 percent and therefore is not appropriate for food challenges.

An algorithm for an approach to evaluation of food allergy has been provided in Figure 48-1. Except in cases of severe anaphylaxis to a single food, presumptive diagnoses of food hypersensitivity based on skin tests and/or RASTs are no longer adequate.

TREATMENT

The only proven therapy for food hypersensitivity is complete avoidance of the causative food protein. Therapeutic elimination diets should be prescribed only if the offending food allergens have been identified with appropriate diagnostic methods. It is often helpful to consult a dietician knowledgeable about food allergy to ensure the nutritional content of the diet. Elimination diets, if not utilized and supervised properly, may lead to untoward side effects such as malnutrition or eating disorders (Bierman et al, 1978). Patients rarely react to more than one food in a botanical family or animal species, and therefore it is usually not necessary to restrict large groups of foods unless each specific food has been proved to cause a reaction. Institution of an elimination diet will result in symptomatic improvement and may lead to resolution of the food allergy within a few years. DBPCFCs may be performed at 12- to 24-month intervals, depending on the food, type of reaction provoked, and the patient's dietary compliance. Although most food allergies resolve over time, sensitivity to peanuts, nuts, and seafood is rarely lost, and therefore repeated DBPCFCs for these foods are generally not indicated.

Patients and parents must be educated on how to read food labels and to identify vague or alternative terms on ingredient labels, which may indicate the presence of the offending foods. Examples would include using the words "caseinate," "whey," or "natural

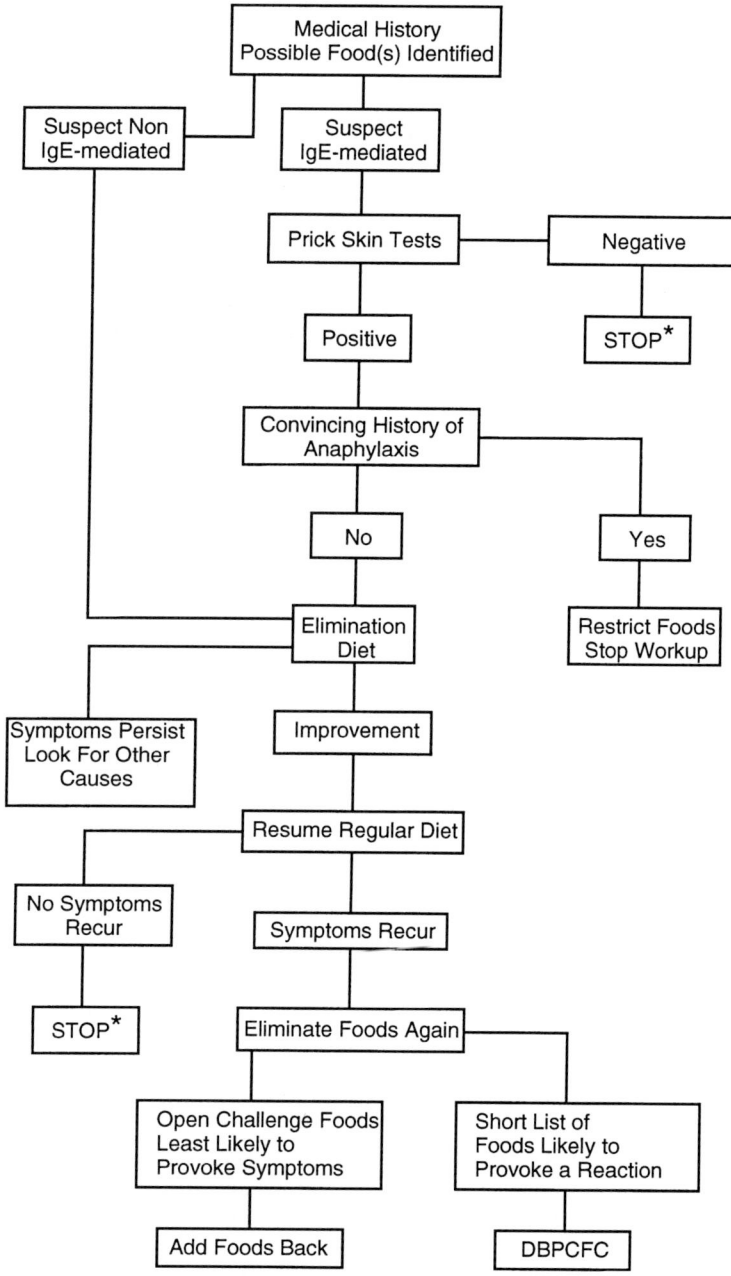

FIGURE 48–1. Diagnosing food hypersensitivity. (From James JM, Sampson HA. Overview of food hypersensitivity. Pediatr Allergy Immunol 3:67–78, 1992.)

flavoring" instead of "milk." Organizations such as the Food Allergy Network (4744 Holly Ave, Fairfax VA 22030; phone (703) 691-3179) are extremely helpful in offering educational material and counseling for patients and their families.

When food allergen avoidance fails, anaphylaxis may result. Accidental ingestion of an offending food allergen is most likely to occur away from home in a restaurant or at school. Patients, their family members, and adult caregivers (e.g., teachers, school nurses, baby-sitters) should all be familiar with the use of self-injectable epinephrine.

Early symptoms of anaphylaxis should be discussed at length with patients diagnosed with IgE-mediated food allergy and their family members, so that an immediate subcutaneous dose of epinephrine may be administered by the patient or an adult caretaker in the event of an accidental ingestion. The dose of aqueous epinephrine (1:1000/mg/ml) is 0.01 mg/kg body weight, up to 0.3 ml. Physicians should prescribe a self-injectable device with instructions for use by the food-allergic patient. Also, patients with asthma on chronic glucocorticoid therapy may be at higher risk because of adrenal suppression; these patients should receive "stress" doses of intravenous hydrocortisone during a resuscitation (Yunginger et al, 1988).

The concept of uniphasic, biphasic, and protracted anaphylactic reactions is an important consideration for physicians, especially in an emergency department setting. Anaphylaxis is usually thought to be uniphasic, with rapid progression of symptoms from the initiating event. However, some patients may have mild initial symptoms, which are subsequently followed by life-threatening symptoms. Other patients may have a biphasic picture in which the initial symptoms respond readily to epinephrine, but a second wave of symptoms may follow. Protracted anaphylaxis may also occur and may require vasopressors and ventilator support for more than 24 hours, as three patients did in the review by Sampson and colleagues (1992). Given the varied reaction kinetics in these cases, food-allergic patients need to be observed for a minimum of 4 hours in the emergency department or hospital despite an apparent good response to initial therapy.

In young children who have no history of asthma or no respiratory or anaphylactic symptoms, and whose reactions are strictly confined to skin symptoms, liquid diphenhydramine in doses of 1 to 2 mg/kg body weight up to 75 mg may be administered for an accidental food-allergen ingestion. For any anaphylactic symptoms, respiratory compromise, or angioedema, the patient should receive subcutaneous epinephrine and be taken to a hospital emergency department immediately.

Prophylactic pharmacotherapy with a variety of drugs has been attempted in food-allergic patients. Some of these medications may modify the milder symptoms, but overall they have minimal efficacy, have unacceptable side effects, or mask early cutaneous symptoms. Reliance on a drug to prevent food allergic symptoms may also give the patient the false impression that an elimination diet is of lesser importance in the management of the disorder. Some of the medications proposed as preventive in food allergy include antihistamines, ketotifen, corticosteroids, and prostaglandin synthetase inhibitors (Sogn, 1986). Most of the studies reporting the efficacy of these drugs failed to use appropriate study design or to prove the diagnosis of food allergy in their patients. In one study, which did use a double-blind placebo-controlled cross-over trial of cromolyn in 10 children with DBPCFC-proven food allergy, the investigators found no difference in the effect of oral cromolyn compared to placebo (Burks and Sampson, 1988). Another study showed that oral disodium cromoglycate may reduce local intestinal responses (i.e., carbohydrate marker absorption) in children with cow's milk allergy but *does not* prevent the extraintestinal reactions (Van Elburg et al, 1993).

Although avoidance of food allergens is the treatment of choice for oral allergy syndrome (OAS), one study showed promising results using pharmacotherapy for OAS when avoidance was not possible. In 1991, Bindslev-Jensen and co-workers prospectively evaluated 30 birch-allergic patients with OAS due to hazelnuts; these patients had localized oral symptoms only. In a randomized, double-blind protocol, the patients received placebo or astemizole, a long-acting antihistamine, for 2 weeks and then underwent two oral challenges. Patients on the antihistamine had a significant reduction in their symptoms when compared with the placebo group. However, the investigators did stress that this type of therapy for oral allergy syndrome is not appropriate for patients with any history of systemic reactions to hazelnuts such as laryngeal edema, asthma, or anaphylaxis (Bindslev-Jensen et al, 1991).

Immunotherapy has not proved to be of benefit in the treatment of food allergy. Preliminary results in one discontinued study of rush immunotherapy for peanut allergy are promising (Oppenheimer et al, 1992). However, the dangers inherent in such a clinical trial preclude this type of study from being conducted anywhere but in an allergy research unit with ICU capability. Immunotherapy with food extracts should not be used in a practice setting because of its unproven efficacy and potential for serious reactions.

UNCONVENTIONAL AND/OR NONVALIDATED METHODS IN DIAGNOSIS AND TREATMENT OF FOOD ALLERGY

In a survey of unproven methods utilized in the diagnosis and treatment of food allergy, the following methods were reviewed and determined to be of no therapeutic value: radionics, intradermal testing, pulse test, leukocyte cytotoxicity, hair trace metal analysis, sublingual food extracts, subcutaneous injection of food extracts, "yeast-free" diets with nystatin enemas, and the rotating elimination diet (David, 1985). One well-controlled study of subcutaneous provocation and neutralization demonstrated no therapeutic efficacy for these procedures (Jewett et al, 1990). Claims for the success of these techniques need to be substantiated with convincing scientific evidence. The responsibility to produce this evidence lies with the proponents of the methods. The existence of these nonvalidated practices provides "fuel for the many doctors who are skeptical about the existence or relevance of food allergy" (David, 1985). Perhaps patients will be less likely to seek out these unconventional methods when physicians seriously consider food allergy in the differential diagnosis of patients with symptoms such as atopic dermatitis, urticaria, asthma, vomiting, diarrhea, failure to thrive, or weight loss. An appropriate early allergy referral can make a significant difference in reducing the morbidity of this clinical entity.

NATURAL HISTORY

Food hypersensitivity is commonly "outgrown" in the first few years of life. In a prospective study of milk-allergic children, the milk allergy had resolved in 87 percent of children by 3 years of age (Host and Halken, 1990). Children who have their food allergy diagnosed at older ages may be less likely to outgrow their allergies (Bock, 1982), although this may reflect the greater number of peanut, nut, and seafood allergies in older patients. Both children and adults have a better chance of developing tolerance if the offending foods are completely eliminated from their diets (Bock, 1982; Pastorello et al, 1989; Sampson et al, 1989). Prick skin tests and RASTs generally remain positive even in the face of clinical resolution and are therefore not useful in predicting outcome unless they are negative (Pastorello et al, 1989; Sampson et al, 1989). As mentioned previously, peanut, tree nuts, fish, and shellfish allergy tend to persist indefinitely.

Non–IgE-mediated food-induced reactions also are likely to resolve over time, although this aspect has not been formally studied. Celiac disease is a lifelong diagnosis, but less is known about the other diagnoses in this category.

PREVENTION

Avoidance of allergenic foods in infants at high risk for atopic disease has been shown to reduce food sensitization and atopic dermatitis during the first years of life (Zeiger et al, 1992). Avoidance diets include elimination of cow's milk, eggs, and peanuts in infants and in mothers who are breast-feeding. Halken and co-workers (1992) showed a reduction in the prevalence of atopy in "high-risk" infants who were fed breast milk or hypoallergenic formula and avoided solid foods until the age of 6 months, when compared with infants not in the prevention group. Another study reported parental atopy and increased numbers of solid foods introduced in the first 4 months of life as being risk factors for developing childhood eczema (Fergusson et al, 1990).

Based on these studies, it seems reasonable to recommend the following guidelines for the "high-risk" infant: (1) no maternal dietary restrictions during pregnancy; (2) exclusive breast-feeding for the first 4 to 6 months of life or use of a hypoallergenic formula if breast-feeding is not possible or supplementation is required (mothers should eliminate all peanuts and tree nuts from their diet and, if highly motivated, consider eliminating eggs and milk); (3) delay introduction of solid foods until after 4 to 6 months of age; and (4) delay introduction of cow's milk until 1 year of age, eggs until 2 years, and peanuts, nuts, and fish until 3 years of age.

SUMMARY

In most individuals, tolerance will develop to the myriad foreign food proteins ingested over their lifetime. However, in approximately 8 percent of children less than 3 years of age and in 1 to 2 percent of the general population, food hypersensitivity will occur.

Symptoms may include a variety of cutaneous, gastrointestinal, respiratory, and/or systemic manifestations.

Research studies have characterized these disorders, yet the underlying immunologic mechanisms are often still obscure. Application of strict scientific method in exploring these mechanisms will lead to useful information in this field and, it is hoped, to new diagnostic techniques and therapies. Until then, the clinician must be aware of the manifestations of food allergy, the appropriate diagnostic steps as well as diagnostic pitfalls, and the correct management of the food-allergic patient.

REFERENCES

Alun-Jones V, McLaughlan P, Shorthouse M, Workman E, Hunter JO. Food intolerance: A major factor in the pathogenesis of irritable bowel syndrome. Lancet 2:1115–1117, 1982.

Anet J, Back JF, Baker RS, et al. Allergens in the white and yolk of hen's egg. Inter Arch Allergy Appl Immunol 77:364–371, 1985.

Bernhisel-Broadbent J, Sampson HA. Cross-allergenicity in the legume botanical family in children with food hypersensitivity. J Allergy Clin Immunol 83:435–440, 1989.

Bernhisel-Broadbent J, Scanlon SM, Sampson HA. Fish hypersensitivity. I. In vitro and oral challenge results in fish-allergic patients. J Allergy Clin Immunol 89:730–737, 1992a.

Bernhisel-Broadbent J, Strause D, Sampson HA. Fish hypersensitivity. II. Clinical relevance of altered fish allergenicity caused by various preparation methods. J Allergy Clin Immunol 90:622–629, 1992b.

Bierman CW, Shapiro GG, Christie DL, VanArsdel PO, Furukawa CF, Ward BH. Eczema, rickets and food allergy. J Allergy Clin Immunol 61:119–127, 1978.

Bindslev-Jensen C, Vibits A, Skov PS, Weeke B. Oral allergy syndrome: The effect of astemizole. Allergy 46:610–613, 1991.

Bock SA, Lee W-Y, Remigio LK, May CD. Studies of hypersensitivity reactions to foods in infants and children. J Allergy Clin Immunol 62:327–334, 1978.

Bock SA. The natural history of food sensitivity. J Allergy Clin Immunol 69:173–177, 1982.

Bock SA. Prospective appraisal of complaints of adverse reactions to foods in children during the first 3 years of life. Pediatrics 79:683–688, 1987.

Bock SA, Sampson HA, Atkins FM, Zeiger RS, Lehrer S, Sachs M, Bush RK, Metcalfe DD. Double-blind placebo-controlled food challenge (DBPCFC) as an office procedure: A manual. J Allergy Clin Immunol 82:986–997, 1988.

Bock SA, Atkins FM. The natural history of peanut allergy. J Allergy Clin Immunol 83:900–904, 1989.

Bock SA, Atkins FM. Patterns of food hypersensitivity during sixteen years of double-blind, placebo-controlled food challenges. J Pediatr 117:561–676, 1990.

Brandtzaeg P, Halstensen TS, Kett K, Krajci P, Kvale D, Rognum TO, Scott H, Sollid LM. Immunobiology and immunopathology of human gut mucosa: Humoral immunity and intraepithelial lymphocytes. Gastroenterology 97:1562–1584, 1989.

Bruce MG, Strobel S, Hanson DG, et al. Irradiated mice lose the capacity to "process" fed antigen for systemic tolerance of delayed-type hypersensitivity. Clin Exp Immunol 70:611–618, 1987.

Buffum WP, Settipane GA. Prognosis of asthma in childhood. Am J Dis Child 112:214–217, 1966.

Burks AW, Brooks JR, Sampson HA. Allergenicity of major component proteins of soybean determined by enzyme-linked immunosorbent assay (ELISA) and immunoblotting in children with atopic dermatitis and positive soy challenges. J Allergy Clin Immunol 81:1135–1142, 1988a.

Burks AW, Mallory SB, Williams LW, Shirrell MA. Atopic dermatitis: Clinical relevance of food hypersensitivity reactions. J Pediatr 113:447–451, 1988b.

Burks AW, Sampson HA. Double-blind placebo-controlled trial of oral cromolyn in children with atopic dermatitis and documented food hypersensitivity. J Allergy Clin Immunol 81:417–423, 1988.

Burks AW, Williams LW, Thresher W, Connaughton C, Cockrell G, Helm RM. Allergenicity of peanut and soybean extracts altered by chemical or thermal denaturation in patients with atopic dermatitis and positive food challenge. J Allergy Clin Immunol 90:889–897, 1992a.

Burks AW, Williams LW, Connaughton C, Cockrell G, O'Brien T, Helm RM. Identification and characterization of a second major peanut allergen, *Ara h* II, with use of the sera of patients with atopic dermatitis and positive peanut challenges. J Allergy Clin Immunol 90:962–969, 1992b.

Businco L, Grandolfo M, Bruno G. Safety of measles immunization in egg-allergic children. Pediatr Allergy Immunol 4:195–198, 1991.

Champion RH, Roberts SOB, Carpenter RG, Roger JH. Urticaria and angio-oedema. A review of 554 patients. Br J Dermatol 81:588–597, 1969.

Clein NW. Cow's milk allergy in infants and children. Int Arch Allergy 13:245–256, 1958.

Daul CB, Morgan JE, Hughes J, Lehrer SB. Provocation-challenge studies in shrimp-sensitive individuals. J Allergy Clin Immunol 81:1180–1186, 1988.

Daul CB, Morgan JE, Lehrer SB. The natural history of shrimp hypersensitivity. J Allergy Clin Immunol 86:88–93, 1990.

David TJ. The overworked or fraudulent diagnosis of food allergy and food intolerance in children. J R Soc Med 78(suppl):21–31, 1985.

Egger J, Carter CM, Soothill JF, Wilson J. Oligoantigenic diet treatment of children with epilepsy and migraine. J Pediatr 114:51–58, 1989.

Fasano MB, Wood RA, Cooke SK, Sampson HA. Egg hypersensitivity and adverse reactions to measles, mumps, and rubella vaccine. J Pediatr 120:878–881, 1992.

Feingold BF. Hyperkinesis and learning disabilities linked to artificial food flavors and colors. Am J Nursing 75:797–803, 1975.

Fergusson DM, Horwood LJ, Shannon FT. Early solid feeding and recurrent childhood eczema: a 10-year longitudinal study. Pediatrics 86:541–546, 1990.

Forsyth BWC. Colic and the effect of changing formulas: A double-blind multiple-crossover study. J Pediatr 115:521–526, 1989.

Goldman AS, Anderson DW, Sellers WA, Saperstesin S, Kniker WT, Halpern SR. Milk allergy. I. Oral challenge with milk and isolated milk proteins in allergic children. Pediatrics 32:425–433, 1963.

Goldman H, Proujansky R. Allergic proctitis and gastroenteritis in children. Am J Surg Pathol 10:75–86, 1986.

Halken S, Host A, Hansen LG, Osterballe O. Effect of an allergy prevention programme on incidence of atopic symptoms in infancy. A prospective study of 159 "high-risk" infants. Allergy 47:545–553, 1992.

Hall RP. Dermatitis herpetiformis. J Invest Dermatol 99:873–881, 1992.

Hanson DG. Ontogeny of orally induced tolerance of soluble proteins in mice. I. Priming and tolerance in newborns. J Immunol 127:1518–1524, 1981.

Heiner DC, Sears JW. Chronic respiratory disease associated with multiple circulating precipitins to cow's milk. Am J Dis Child 100:500–502, 1960.

Helgason T, Jonasson MR. Evidence for a food additive as a cause of ketosis-prone diabetes. Lancet 1:716–720, 1981.

Heyman M, Grasset E, Ducroc R, Desjeux J-F. Antigen absorption by the jejunal epithelium of children with cow's milk allergy. Pediatr Res 24(2):197–202, 1988.

Hide DW, Guyer BM. Cow's milk intolerance in Isle of Wight infants. Br J Clin Prac 37:285–287, 1983.

Hirschwehr R, Valenta R, Ebner C, Ferreira F, Sperr WR, Valent P, Rohac M, Rumpold H, Scheiner O, Kraft D. Identification of common allergenic structures in hazel pollen and hazelnuts: A possible explanation for sensitivity to hazelnuts in patients allergic to tree pollen. J Allergy Clin Immunol 90:927–936, 1992.

Hoffman KM, Lederman HM, Sampson HA. Cellular responses to soy and cow milk antigens in children with soy and cow milk allergy. J Allergy Clin Immunol 93:192, 1994.

Holen E, Elsayed S. Characterization of four major allergens of hen egg-white by IEF/SDS-PAGE combined with electrophoretic transfer and IgE-immunoautoradiography. Int Arch Allergy Appl Immunol 91:136–141, 1990.

Host A, Halken S. A prospective study of cow milk allergy in Danish infants during the first 3 years of life. Allergy 45:587–596, 1990.

Jakobsson I, Lindberg T. Cow's milk proteins cause infantile colic in breast-fed infants: A double-blind crossover study. Pediatrics 71:268–271, 1983.

James JM, Eggleston PA, Sampson HA. Food allergy increases airway reactivity. Am J Crit Care Resp Med 149:59–64, 1994.

Jenkins HR, Pincott JR, Soothill JF, Milla PJ, Harries JT. Food allergy: The major cause of infantile colitis. Arch Dis Childh 59:326–329, 1984.

Jewett DL, Fein G, Greenberg MH. A double-blind study of symptom provocation to determine food sensitivity. N Engl J Med 323:429–433, 1990.

Jones SM, Cooke SK, Sampson HA. Immunologic cross-reactivity among cereal grains and grasses in children with food hypersensitivity. J Allergy Clin Immunol 91:343, 1993.

Kagnoff MF. Celiac disease. A gastrointestinal disease with environmental, genetic, and immunologic components. Gastroenterol Clin North Am 21:405–425, 1992.

Kahn A, Rebuffat E, Blum D, Casimir G, Duchateau J, Mozin MJ, Jost R. Difficulty in initiating and maintaining sleep associated with cow's milk allergy in infants. Sleep 10:116–121, 1987.

Kajosaari M. Food allergy in Finnish children aged 1 to 6 years. Acta Paediatr Scand 71:815–819, 1982.

Kalliel JN, Klein DE, Settipane GA. Anaphylaxis to peanuts: Clinical correlation to skin tests. Allergy Proc 10:259–260, 1989.

Karjalainen J, Martin JM, Knip M, Ilonen J, Robinson BH, Savilahti E, Akerblom HK, Dosch HM. A bovine albumin peptide as a possible trigger of insulin-dependent diabetes mellitus. N Engl J Med 327:302–307, 1992.

Katz AJ, Twarog FJ, Zeiger RS, Falchuk ZM. Milk-sensitive and eosinophilic gastroenteropathy: Similar clinical features with contrasting mechanisms and clinical course. J Allergy Clin Immunol 74:72–78, 1984.

Kauppinen K, Juntunen K, Lanki H. Urticaria in children. Retrospective evaluation and follow-up. Allergy 39:469–472, 1984.

Kelly CP, Feighery CF, Gallagher RB, Weir DG. Diagnosis and treatment of gluten-sensitive enteropathy. Adv Intern Med 35:341–364, 1990.

Kidd JM, Cohen SH, Sosman AJ, Fink JN. Food-dependent exercise-induced anaphylaxis. J Allergy Clin Immunol 71:407–411, 1983.

Klein NC, Hargrove RL, Sleisenger MH, Jeffries GH. Eosinophilic gastroenteritis. Medicine 49:299–319, 1970.

Kolmannskog S, Haneberg B. Immunoglobulin E in feces from children with allergy. Evidence of local production of IgE in the gut. Int Arch Allergy Appl Immunol 76:133–137, 1985.

Kwok RHM. Chinese-restaurant syndrome. N Engl J Med 278:796, 1968.

Langeland T. A clinical and immunological study of allergy to hen's egg white. VI. Occurrence of proteins cross-reacting with allergens in hen's egg white as studied in egg white from turkey, duck, goose, seagull, and in hen egg yolk, and hen and chicken sera and flesh. Allergy 38:399–412, 1983.

Lothe L, Lindberg T. Cow's milk whey protein elicits symptoms of infantile colic in colicky formula-fed infants: A double-blind crossover study. Pediatrics 83:262–266, 1989.

Menardo JL, Bousquet J, Rodiere M, Astruc J, Michel F-B. Skin test reactivity in infancy. J Allergy Clin Immunol 75:646–651, 1985.

Moffett A, Swash M, Scott DF. Effect of tyramine in migraine: A double-blind study. J Neurol Neurosurg Psychiat 35:496–499, 1972.

Mowat AM. The regulation of immune responses to dietary protein antigens. Immunol Today 8:93–98, 1987.

Nagpal S, Rajappa L, Metcalfe DD, Rao PVS. Isolation and characterization of heat-stable allergens from shrimp (Penaeus indicus). J Allergy Clin Immunol 83:26–36, 1989.

Ngan J, Kind LS. Suppressor T cells for IgE and IgG in Peyer's patches of mice made tolerant by the oral administration of ovalbumin. J Immunol 120:861–865, 1978.

Novembre E, de Martino M, Vierucci A. Foods and respiratory allergy. J Allergy Clin Immunol 81:1059–1065, 1988.

Oehling A, Cagnani CEB. Food allergy and child asthma. Allergol Immunopathol 8:7–14, 1980.

Oppenheimer JJ, Nelson HS, Bock SA, Christensen F, Leung DYM. Treatment of peanut allergy with rush immunotherapy. J Allergy Clin Immunol 90:256–262, 1992.

Ortolani C, Ispano M, Pastorello EA, Ansaloni R, Magri GC. Comparison of results of skin prick tests (with fresh foods and commercial food extracts) and RAST in 100 patients with oral allergy syndrome. J Allergy Clin Immunol 83:683–690, 1989.

Panush RS, Stroud RM, Webster EM. Food-induced (allergic) arthritis. Inflammatory arthritis exacerbated by milk. Arthritis Rheum 29:220–226, 1986.

Pastorello EA, Stocchi L, Pravettoni V, Bigi A, Schilke ML, Incorvaia C, Zanussi C. Role of the elimination diet in adults with food allergy. J Allergy Clin Immunol 84:475–483, 1989.

Pollard HM, Stuart GJ. Experimental reproduction of gastric allergy in human beings with controlled observations on the mucosa. J Allergy 13:467–473, 1942.

Powell GK. Milk- and soy-induced enterocolitis of infancy. Clinical features and standardization of challenge. J Pediatr 93:553–560, 1978.

Queille-Roussel C, Raynaud F, Saurat J-H. A prospective computerized study of 500 cases of atopic dermatitis in childhood. I. Initial analysis of 250 parameters. Acta Derm Venereol 114(S):87–92, 1985.

Raphael G, Raphael MH, Kaliner M. Gustatory rhinitis: A syndrome of food-induced rhinorrhea. J Allergy Clin Immunol 83:110–115, 1989.

Reimann H-J, Lewin J. Gastric mucosal reactions in patients with food allergy. Am J Gastroenterol 83:1212–1219, 1988.

Sampson HA. Role of immediate food hypersensitivity in the pathogenesis of atopic dermatitis. J Allergy Clin Immunol 71:473–480, 1983.

Sampson HA, Albergo R. Comparison of results of skin tests, RAST, and double-blind, placebo-controlled food challenges in children with atopic dermatitis. J Allergy Clin Immunol 74:26–33, 1984.

Sampson HA, McCaskill CC. Food hypersensitivity and atopic dermatitis: Evaluation of 113 patients. J Pediatr 107:669–675, 1985.

Sampson HA. Immunologically mediated food allergy: The importance of food challenge procedures. Ann Allergy 60:262–269, 1988.

Sampson HA, Broadbent KR, Bernhisel-Broadbent J. Spontaneous release of histamine from basophils and histamine-releasing factor in patients with atopic dermatitis and food hypersensitivity. N Engl J Med 321:228–232, 1989.

Sampson HA, Scanlon SM. Natural history of food hypersensitivity in children with atopic dermatitis. J Pediatr 115:23–27, 1989.

Sampson HA. Infantile colic and food allergy: Fact or fiction? J Pediatr 115:583–584, 1989.

Sampson HA, Mendelson L, Rosen JP. Fatal and near-fatal anaphylactic reactions to food in children and adolescents. N Engl J Med 327:380–384, 1992.

Sampson HA. The immunopathogenic role of food hypersensitivity in atopic dermatitis. Acta Derm Venereol 176(suppl):34–37, 1992.

Sampson HA. Adverse reactions to foods. In Middleton E Jr, et al (eds). Allergy: Principles and Practice. 4th ed. St. Louis, Mosby-Year Book, 1993a, pp 1661–1686.

Sampson HA. Food allergies. In Sleisenger MH, Fordtran JS (eds). Gastrointestinal Disease: Pathophysiology/Diagnosis/Management. 5th ed. Philadelphia, WB Saunders, 1993b, pp 1233–1240.

Sandberg DH, McIntosh RM, Bernstein CW, Carr R, Strauss J. Severe steroid-responsive nephrosis associated with hypersensitivity. Lancet 1:388–391, 1977.

Schrander JJP, van den Bogart JPH, Forget PP, Schrander-Stumpel CTRM, Kuijten RH, Kester ADM. Cow's milk protein intolerance in infants under 1 year of age: A prospective epidemiological study. Eur J Pediatr 152:640–644, 1993.

Scott H, Ek J, Brandtzaeg P. Changes of serum antibody activities to various dietary antigens related to gluten withdrawal or challenge in children with coeliac disease. Int Arch Allergy Appl Immunol 76:138–144, 1985.

Scott FW. Cow milk and insulin-dependent diabetes mellitus: Is there a relationship? Am J Clin Nutr 51:489–491, 1990.

Simon RA, Stevenson DD. Adverse reactions to food and drug additives. In Middleton E, et al (eds). Allergy: Principles and Practice. 4th ed. St. Louis, MO, Mosby-Year Book, 1993, pp 1687–1704.

Sloan AE, Powers ME. A perspective on popular perceptions of adverse reactions to foods. J Allergy Clin Immunol 78:127–133, 1986.

Sogn D. Medications and their use in the treatment of adverse reactions to foods. J Allergy Clin Immunol 83:435–440, 1986.

Stevenson DD. Tartrazine, AZO, and non-AZO dyes. In Metcalfe DD, Sampson HA, Simon RA (eds). Food Allergy: Adverse Reactions to Foods and Food Additives. Oxford, Blackwell Scientific, 1991, pp 267–287.

Sutton R, Hill DJ, Baldo BA, Wrigley CW. Immunoglobulin E antibodies to ingested cereal flour components: Studies with sera from subjects with asthma and eczema. Clin Allergy 12:63–74, 1982.

Taylor SL, Busse WW, Sachs MI, Parker JL, Yunginger JW. Peanut oil is not allergenic to peanut-sensitive individuals. J Allergy Clin Immunol 68:372–375, 1981.

Tuft L, Blumstein GI. Studies in food allergy. J Allergy 17:329–339, 1946.

Van de Laar MAF, van der Korst JK. Rheumatoid arthritis, food, and allergy. Semin Arthritis Rheum 21:12–23, 1991.

Van Elburg RM, Heymans HSA, DeMonchy JGR. Effect of disodiumcromoglycate on intestinal permeability changes and clinical response during cow's milk challenge. Pediatr Allergy Immunol 4:79–85, 1993.

Van Sickle GJ, Powell GK, McDonald PJ, Goldblum RM. Milk- and soy protein-induced enterocolitis: Evidence for lymphocyte sensitization to specific food proteins. Gastroenterology 88:1915–1921, 1985.

Weber RW, Vaughan TR. Food and migraine headache. Immunol Allergy Clin North Am 11:831–841, 1991.

Wershil BK, Walker WA. The mucosal barrier, IgE-mediated gastrointestinal events, and eosinophilic gastroenteritis. Gastroenterol Clin North Am 21:387–404, 1992.

Yunginger JW, Sweeney KG, Sturner WQ, Giannandrea LA, Teigland JD, Bray M, Benson PA, York JA, Biedrzycki, Squillace DL, Helm RM. Fatal food-induced anaphylaxis. JAMA 260:1450–1452, 1988.

Yunginger JW, Nelson DR, Squillace DL, Jones RT, Holley KE, Hyma BA, Biedrzycki L, Sweeney KG, Sturner WQ, Schwartz LB. Laboratory investigation of deaths due to anaphylaxis. J Forensic Sci 36:857–865, 1991.

Yunginger JW. Food antigens. In Metcalfe DD, Sampson HA, Simon RA (eds). Food Allergy: Adverse Reactions to Food and Food Additives. Oxford, Blackwell Scientific, 1991b, pp 36–51.

Yunginger JW. Anaphylaxis. Ann Allergy 69:87–96, 1992.

Zeiger RS, Heller S, Mellon MH, Halsey JF, Hamburger RN, Sampson HA. Genetic and environmental factors affecting the development of atopy through age 4 in children of atopic parents: A prospective randomized study of food allergen avoidance. Pediatr Allergy Immunol 3:110–127, 1992.

Zwetchkenbaum JF, Skufca R, Nelson HS. An examination of food hypersensitivity as a cause of increased bronchial responsiveness to inhaled methacholine. J Allergy Clin Immunol 88:360–364, 1991.

Chapter 49

Inflammatory Bowel Diseases

Douglas S. Levine, M.D.

Among all inflammatory bowel diseases, Crohn's disease and ulcerative colitis are the most common of the idiopathic varieties and together are estimated to affect approximately two million individuals in the United States. Crohn's disease may affect any portion of the alimentary tract from mouth to anus, whereas ulcerative colitis is confined to the large intestine. These diseases affect adolescents and young adults predominantly, but individuals of any age may be stricken. The idiopathic inflammatory bowel diseases are chronic, and because of their predilection for relatively young patients in their second and third decades, these diseases impact significantly upon their life styles and productivity. The specific etiologies of these disorders are unknown, but ongoing research that includes clinical observations focused on patients who have received a wide variety of treatment interventions (Levine, 1994) is leading to a holistic concept of disease pathogenesis. At the present time, immune stimulation by intestinal lumenal antigens, altered permeability of the intestinal mucosal barrier, disordered regulation of host gut mucosal and systemic immune systems, generation of various soluble pro-inflammatory mediators within intestinal mucosa, and other local gut physiologic and anatomic factors are all suspected, individually or in combination, in the etiology and pathogenesis of the idiopathic inflammatory bowel diseases in genetically susceptible individuals (Fig. 49–1).

The type and severity of the symptomatic manifestations of Crohn's disease and ulcerative colitis are related to the intensity of inflammation and repair in those portions of the alimentary tract that are affected, and include gastrointestinal bleeding, abdominal pain, nausea, anorexia, vomiting, diarrhea, weight loss, malabsorption, growth failure, anemia, fevers, other constitutional symptoms, site-specific inflammatory complications such as fistulas and abscesses, secondary infections, the development of intestinal epithelial malignancies, and extraintestinal manifestations such as arthritis, spondylitis, sacroiliitis, hepatitis, cholelithiasis, pancreatitis, nephrolithiasis, skin disorders, inflammatory disorders of the eyes, hematologic disorders, amyloidosis, reactive depression, anxiety, neuroses, and other psychosocial problems.

Medical therapies for Crohn's disease and ulcerative colitis can acutely suppress intestinal inflammation, thereby improving the associated symptoms, and induce temporary remissions of disease. Although medications do not provide an absolute cure for these diseases, some can be used chronically to prevent symptomatic relapses. The commonly used drug therapies for the idiopathic inflammatory bowel diseases include aminosalicylates, steroids, immunosuppressive agents, and antibiotics, which may be administered as oral, rectal, or parenteral formulations. Unfortunately, such therapies can be ineffective in a substantial proportion of patients or can be associated with deleterious side effects. In some cases, side effects of these drugs may preclude their use. Patients with ulcerative colitis can be essentially cured by surgical resection of the entire large intestine (proctocolectomy with ileostomy). However, such operations are often thought to be disfiguring by patients and/or their families, and these

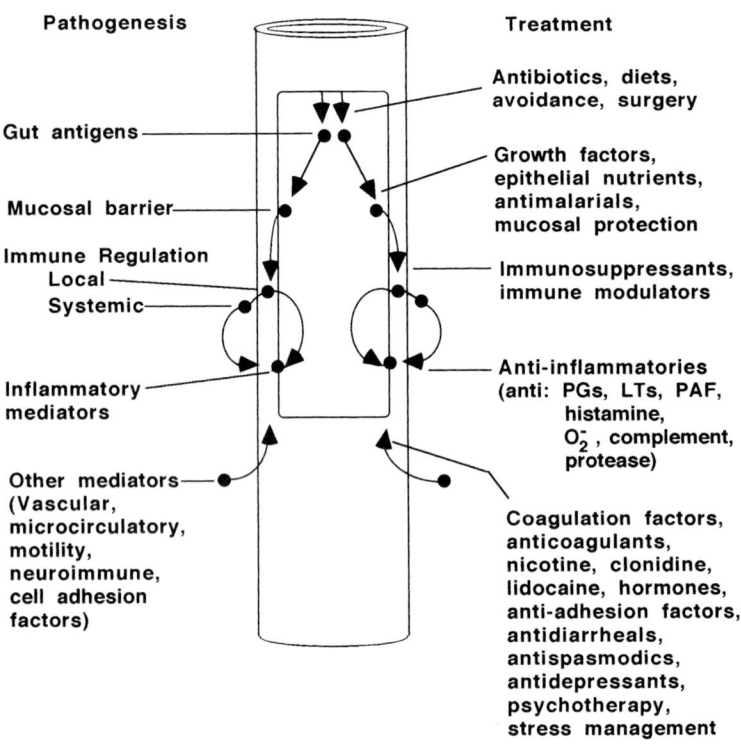

FIGURE 49–1. Immunopathogenetic mechanisms of idiopathic inflammatory bowel diseases paired with treatment strategies. (From: Levine DS. Medical and surgical options for ulcerative colitis. Curr Opin Gastroenterol 11:29–35, 1995. Reprinted with permission from Current Science, Philadelphia, PA.)

may not be accepted by patients who are relatively young. In addition, among those patients with ulcerative colitis who do agree to undergo either total or subtotal colectomy, with subcutaneous ileal pouch or ileoanal pouch anastomosis, respectively, in order to avoid a permanent ileostomy with an accessory fecal collection appliance, a subset of individuals will continue to have intermittent inflammation in the surgically constructed subcutaneous or pelvic pouch. Surgical intervention in patients with Crohn's disease is appropriate as care for specific complications, but it is not curative and is frequently followed by disease recurrences.

A combination of factors is leading to a heightened interest in drug development for patients with idiopathic inflammatory bowel diseases. The lack of effectiveness of available drugs in some patients, the adverse effect profiles of some of the available agents, and the poor response to, or the lack of acceptance for, surgical intervention for these diseases by some patients is stimulating more basic investigations of the etiology and pathogenesis of Crohn's disease and ulcerative colitis.

The effects of this research activity are an improved understanding of the molecular and cell biologic mechanisms of immune-mediated inflammatory damage to the alimentary tract that characterizes these diseases, and the development of new therapeutic strategies and better drug products that can prevent, inhibit, or otherwise interfere with immune reactions, and thereby suppress inflammatory damage to the gastrointestinal tract with fewer adverse effects in patients.

In this chapter, the common clinical disease manifestations of Crohn's disease and ulcerative colitis are first summarized for readers who do not routinely provide clinical care to such patients. Second, the hypothesized interactive immunopathogenetic mechanisms of these idiopathic inflammatory bowel diseases are discussed (Fig. 49–1). This classification of immunopathogenetic mechanisms was proposed originally in order to provide a foundation for a description of available or potential immune modulating therapies for patients with idiopathic inflammatory bowel diseases (Levine, 1994), but it also may serve as a framework for new clinical approaches to, and investigational studies of, the immunology and immunogenetics of Crohn's disease and ulcerative colitis, as well as other less common types of inflammatory bowel diseases and malabsorption syndromes.

CLINICAL MANIFESTATIONS OF IDIOPATHIC INFLAMMATORY BOWEL DISEASES

The two most common forms of idiopathic inflammatory diseases affecting the human alimentary tract are usually classified into two major categories: Crohn's disease and ulcerative colitis. These two diseases share many clinical, pathologic, and epidemiologic features, but there are usually sufficient differences to allow their separation as distinct clinical entities. The cause(s) of Crohn's disease and ulcerative colitis are unknown (Targan and Shanahan, 1994). When differentiation between these two categories is not possible in some patients, a diagnosis of "indeterminate" is applied. Other varieties of idiopathic inflammatory bowel diseases, which are variably well defined by mucosal pathology and clinical characteristics and are less common than Crohn's disease and ulcerative colitis, include collagenous colitis, microscopic or lymphocytic colitis, diversion colitis, Behcet's syndrome, eosinophilic gastroenterocolitis, solitary rectal ulcer syndrome, colitis cystica profunda, nonspecific intestinal ulcer syndromes, AIDS enteropathy, nonspecific jejunoileal inflammatory disease, and postcolectomy pouchitis. The idiopathic inflammatory bowel diseases are differentiated from inflammatory bowel diseases resulting from known causes, such as host deficiency states, foods, infections, toxins, ischemia, diverticulitis, neoplasia, drugs, radiation, other physical agents, or intestinal graft-versus-host disease following allogeneic bone marrow transplantation.

What we classify as "Crohn's disease" or "ulcerative colitis" may in fact be several different diseases that may become defined molecularly in the future (Yang et al, 1993). Ongoing immunogenetic investigations of idiopathic inflammatory bowel diseases may confirm observations suggesting that patients with these disorders seem to conform to a wide variety of subsets with different clinical presentations, pathologic manifestations, medical or surgical treatment responses, and tendencies toward disease recurrence. Classically, Crohn's disease may affect any portion of the alimentary tract from mouth to anus, disease involvement of which may be transmural. Ulcerative colitis is generally limited to the relatively superficial mucosa of the large intestine. These diseases may vary in both the inflammatory intensity and the total surface area of involvement of the alimentary tract. Only a small portion of the ileum or rectum may be involved in their most limited forms. However, in their more severe forms a large portion of the small intestine or the entirety of the colon is affected. Therefore, the spectrum of clinical symptoms and diagnostic abnormalities that reflect these varying pathologic manifestations is diverse (Targan and Shanahan, 1994). In some patients, inflammation may be so minimal it may only be detectable by endoscopic visualization and biopsy. In other patients, severe ulceration and hemorrhage are obvious, and in still others, inflammation may involve the entire bowel wall thickness and lead to formation of strictures or progression to perforation, fistulous tracts or sinuses, and abscesses with the potential for septicemia.

The clinical courses of patients with Crohn's disease or ulcerative colitis are highly variable and usually relate in part to the anatomic sites of involvement within the alimentary tract and the intensity of inflammation. Most patients give a history of periodic exacerbations of disease interspersed with normal or near-normal health during time intervals that vary from months to a few years. In other patients, their disease is chronic and unremitting with continuous bloody diarrhea, anemia, abdominal discomfort, and generalized or constitutional symptoms. Still others have an initial acute attack followed by apparent good health for periods ranging up to several years before they experience recurrent symptoms. Some patients develop small or large intestinal epithelial dysplasia and adenocarcinoma independent of the inflammatory intensity and the course of their disease.

The cardinal symptoms of Crohn's disease are abdominal pain and nonbloody diarrhea, which reflect the tendencies for the disease to produce transmural inflammation, narrowing of the intestinal lumen, and partial bowel obstruction. The most common symptoms of ulcerative colitis include tenesmus, hematochezia, and crampy abdominal pain because of the typical intestinal mucosal erosions involving the rectum and a variable extent of the large intestine proximal to the rectum. Symptoms of idiopathic inflammatory bowel diseases are mild or moderate in the majority of patients, with some increase in the number of bowel movements per day, clinically insignificant intestinal blood loss, and tolerable levels of abdominal pain. For others, symptoms are severe with disabling diarrhea, anemia due to intestinal blood loss, abdominal pain, fevers, and/or significant extraintestinal manifestations. Fulminant disease occurs in the minority of patients who must be hospitalized for a variety of complications, including severe intestinal hemorrhage, vomiting, abdominal pain, fevers, malnutrition, dehydration, electrolyte imbalances, and infection. A subset of this group may develop toxic colitis with gross dilatation (megacolon) or intestinal perforation and require emergent surgical intervention to prevent peritonitis and sepsis.

Ulcerative colitis generally is most easily and safely diagnosed by use of rigid or flexible sigmoidoscopy with superficial mucosal biopsies to differentiate this disease from other forms of colitis. Other diagnostic tests that provide imaging of the entire large intestine, such as air contrast barium enema or colonoscopy, are potentially hazardous and more uncomfortable for patients with active disease. However, such examinations may become necessary in some patients to allow differentiation between ulcerative colitis and Crohn's disease, or to assess the proximal extent of large intestinal involvement and the intensity of mucosal inflammation as part of therapeutic planning and monitoring. These examinations also identify complications of colitis such as strictures, pseudopolyposis, or adenocarcinoma. Diffuse, contiguous colonic mucosal involvement is characteristic of ulcerative colitis. Patients with active disease have loss of normal mucosal vascular detail, mucosal friability, erosions, and/or ulcers, and the presence of an inflammatory exudate composed of pus, mucus, and blood. The diagnosis of Crohn's disease may be challenging insofar as symptoms and diagnostic results may mimic those of ulcerative colitis. Differentiating features of Crohn's disease may be suggested by findings on barium enema, and sigmoidoscopy or colonoscopy with mucosal biopsies, of focal or segmental colitis rather than contiguous colorectal disease. Evidence of active inflammatory disease involving other portions of the alimentary tract, which may be provided by upper endoscopy or by roentgenologic studies of the upper gastrointestinal tract and small intestine, with or without disease affecting the large intestine, and the presence of fissures, fistulous tracts, mesenteric sinuses, or intra- or extra-abdominal abscesses also suggest a diagnosis of Crohn's disease.

The loss of mucosal integrity, as demonstrated endoscopically and histologically, is perhaps the most obvious feature of the inflamed intestinal mucosa in patients with idiopathic inflammatory bowel diseases. The differention between Crohn's disease and ulcerative colitis is difficult if Crohn's disease involvement is limited to the large intestine. However, radiologic and endoscopic observations and certain histologic features of mucosal biopsies may help to differentiate these two disorders. Barium enema and total colonoscopy establish the presence of a diffuse, contiguous mucosal inflammatory process consistent with ulcerative colitis. Histologic evaluation of colonic mucosal biopsies of patients with ulcerative colitis reveals diffuse inflammatory involvement with increased mucosal neutrophils, plasma cells, lymphocytes, and eosinophils. Crypt architecture is distorted, the epithelial surface loses its integrity and develops erosions, and crypt abscesses appear. In Crohn's disease of the colon, radiologic and colonoscopic examination may reveal segmental disease, focal rather than diffuse inflammatory changes, and small aphthous or larger, irregularly shaped stellate, elliptical, and serpiginous ulcerations. Colonoscopic biopsies of patients with Crohn's colitis may share the same histologic features of ulcerative colitis, but the presence of focal rather than diffuse inflammation or of noncaseating, epithelioid granulomas is more consistent with a diagnosis of Crohn's disease. Other radiologic, endoscopic, and histologic features help to differentiate Crohn's disease and ulcerative colitis from the less common categories of idiopathic inflammatory bowel diseases and inflammatory bowel diseases of known causes.

INTERACTIVE IMMUNOPATHOGENETIC MECHANISMS OF IDIOPATHIC INFLAMMATORY BOWEL DISEASES

Until recently, research investigations of the pathogenesis of Crohn's disease and ulcerative colitis, as well as observations of beneficial clinical responses in patients who received a variety of empiric therapies, have led to traditional hypotheses concerning the etiologies of these disorders. Two main theories have been proposed for the causes of idiopathic inflammatory bowel diseases: (1) the immunologic hypothesis; and (2) the infectious hypothesis. Immunoregulatory, autoimmune, and infectious mechanisms have been proposed (Targan and Shanahan, 1994), leading to the use of immunosuppressive or immune modulating agents, anti-inflammatory drugs, and antibiotics in patients with these disorders (Levine, 1994).

For the immunologic hypothesis, it is proposed that the immune systems of patients afflicted with Crohn's disease or ulcerative colitis are reacting abnormally or inappropriately against one or more antigens to which everyone is commonly exposed such as, for example, intestinal bacterial, viral, dietary, or other environmental agents. The manifestations of these idiopathic inflammatory bowel diseases were believed to be based on immunologic mechanisms because of the pathology of involved portions of the alimentary tract, beneficial clinical responses to immunosuppressive drugs, systemic extraintestinal complications that occur in patients with Crohn's disease and ulcerative colitis, and various laboratory observations of cell-mediated and humoral immune abnormalities, including circulating immune complexes (Targan and Shanahan, 1994).

For the infectious hypothesis, it is proposed that an undiscovered pathogen is causing the idiopathic inflammatory bowel diseases and the immune systems of affected patients are responding appropriately to the infectious agent. Although extensive investigation has not led to the identification of a consistent transmissible agent in patients with Crohn's disease or ulcerative colitis, new candidate organisms are periodically considered such as, most recently, atypical mycobacterial species and the measles virus.

Many types of host immune system abnormalities have been demonstrated in patients with Crohn's disease or ulcerative colitis. Whether or not these represent primary immunoregulatory abnormalities or secondary epiphenomena is vigorously debated. Nevertheless, altered immunoreactivity may be clinically significant and thus be responsible for disease manifestations in patients with idiopathic inflammatory bowel diseases, either as a primary etiologic factor or as a secondary manifestation that leads to intestinal tissue damage. The various immunopathogenetic mechanisms of these diseases are probably interactive in genetically susceptible patients and may be broadly classified (see Fig. 49–1) as follows: (1) stimulation by intestinal lumenal antigens; (2) dysfunction of intestinal barrier epithelium; (3) defects in intestinal mucosal and/or systemic immunoregulation; (4) generation of mediators of intestinal inflammatory damage; (5) other factors affecting immune-mediated intestinal inflammatory damage; and (6) factors leading to complications of Crohn's disease and ulcerative colitis, such as neoplastic progression in intestinal epithelium and various extraintestinal manifestations. This classification system is presented as a succinct summary of the immunopathogenetic mechanisms of idiopathic inflammatory bowel diseases and may be of practical use to both clinicians and researchers. It is hoped that the following review of these mechanisms will serve as a stimulus for continued basic investigations of the etiologies of the idiopathic inflammatory bowel diseases and the development of safer, more effective therapeutic interventions.

Stimulation by Intestinal Lumenal Antigens

Any of a variety of lumenal antigens within the alimentary tract may trigger an immune-mediated inflammatory response in the intestinal mucosa of susceptible individuals who develop idiopathic inflammatory bowel diseases. Such antigens may include dietary antigens; viral particles; cellular structural proteins or toxins from bacteria, environmental agents, or proteins; carbohydrate residues; or lipid moieties from sloughed intestinal epithelial cells. Evidence in support of this hypothesis includes several different investigations of the association of idiopathic inflammatory bowel diseases with exogenous agents that may trigger disease development, including: disease exacerbations following respiratory tract or enteric infections with bacterial or viral pathogens (Kangro et al, 1990); geographic and seasonal patterns of disease incidence and prevalence that further suggest the influence of infections or other unknown environmental agents (Sonnenberg et al, 1991); and disease incidence related to smoking, diet, and drug ingestion habits (Boyko et al, 1987; Sutherland et al, 1990).

The significance of gut mucosal stimulation by intestinal lumenal content as a proposed mechanism for the pathogenesis of the idiopathic inflammatory bowel diseases is further suggested by observations of clinical improvement in patients following treatments that modify the intralumenal antigenic load or content. Such therapeutic interventions include antimicrobial agents, mechanical modulation, modification of diet and ingestion of other substances, and surgical procedures.

Antibiotics that are administered to patients with idiopathic inflammatory bowel diseases may reduce and/or alter intestinal bacterial populations. Bacteria elaborate chemotactic peptides that may be pathogenic in patients because of dysfunction of their intestinal barrier epithelium. Several antibiotics have been evaluated as therapeutic agents. Randomized controlled trials of oral metronidazole administered to patients with Crohn's disease demonstrate therapeutic effectiveness (Sutherland et al, 1991). The use of antituberculous therapies in Crohn's disease stems from reports of the isolation of atypical mycobacterial organisms from intestinal tissues of some patients (Van Kruiningen et al, 1986). Various antimycobacterial treatment protocols have been investigated with varying conclusions regarding their benefits in Crohn's disease. Continued clinical investigation of antimycobacterial agents has been advocated using drug combinations that are effective against the proposed Crohn's organism, *Mycobacterium paratuberculosis*, because single-drug therapy can lead to antibiotic resistance and treatment failure. It is debatable whether the observed beneficial effects of antimycobacterial agents in some studies are related to neutralization and eradication of disease-causing atypical mycobacterial organisms or to suppression of other lumenal microorganisms or immune-mediating effects. A variety of other broad-spectrum antibiotics also have been investigated as therapies for idiopathic inflammatory bowel diseases, predominantly Crohn's disease, with differing conclusions regarding their effectiveness. As an alternative to antibiotic therapy, mechanical methods have been used to alter the intestinal lumenal content and, at least theoretically, might provide therapeutic benefit to patients with these diseases.

Exclusion of substrate from the bacterial flora of the intestinal lumen may lessen the potential antigenic burden to intestinal mucosal sites affected by idiopathic inflammatory bowel diseases. This may be achieved by dietary alterations, including bowel rest (with parenteral nutrition), consumption of elemental diets, or use of highly assimilable, low-residue diets. The effects of nutritional support, bowel rest, and elemental or low-residue diets may not only reduce antigens and bacterial populations, but may improve immune function (Culpepper-Morgan and Floch, 1991). Complete bowel rest and provision of total parenteral nutrition can be therapeutically effective in patients with Crohn's disease. Elemental diets also are effective for patients with Crohn's disease, possibly by decreasing intestinal permeability and intestinal inflammation (Teahon et al, 1991).

Although surgical resection or bypass of diseased portions of the alimentary tract is most likely to produce clinical improvement on a mechanical basis, the potential immunologic effects of these procedures should not be overlooked. Surgical resection of diseased bowel segments may eliminate a potent immunologic stimulus. Such phenomena may explain the observed tendency for more frequent disease recurrences in patients with Crohn's disease of the colon who undergo subtotal colectomy and ileoproctostomy (i.e., leaving an intact rectal remnant) rather than complete proctocolectomy and ileostomy. Surgical bypass of portions of the bowel that are involved in Crohn's disease may lead to diminished exposure of the mucosa to antigens and thus reduce the number of relapses.

Dysfunction of Intestinal Barrier Epithelium

An intact intestinal epithelium forms the most basic host defense mechanism against the large number of microbial populations and other antigens that are present within the intestinal lumen. Abnormalities in intestinal mucin species have been demonstrated in patients with ulcerative colitis (Podolsky and Isselbacher, 1984), and these may be correlated with intestinal macrophage production of a mucin secretagogue (Sperber et al, 1993). Whether or not primary abnormalities of intestinal epithelial permeability are responsible for the pathogenesis of idiopathic inflammatory bowel diseases is controversial because of varying results of different investigations (Munkholm et al, 1994). However, other abnormalities of intestinal epithelial function could contribute to the development of these diseases (Mayer, 1990; McKay and Perdue, 1993). In addition, intestinal epithelial destruction that is mediated by specific immune mechanisms or nonspecific inflammatory mediators leads to the secondary loss of integrity of the barrier epithelium (for example, epithelial erosions and mucosal ulcerations are commonly present in intestinal sites involved by active Crohn's disease and ulcerative colitis). Such breaches of intestinal mucosal defense presumably allow increased entry of microorganisms and lumenal antigens into the mucosa, thereby permitting propagation of immune stimulating and inflammatory processes.

Factors that enhance intestinal epithelial regrowth and healing of the epithelium damaged by idiopathic inflammatory bowel diseases might be expected to produce ameliorative effects simply by achieving restitution of the barrier epithelium. One possible interventional strategy may involve administration of intestinal epithelial energy substrates to inflamed intestinal tissues. Short-chain fatty acids (acetate, propionate, butyrate) are known to be essential sources of energy for colonocytes, which presumably permit intestinal epithelial proliferation. Impaired metabolism of butyrate by reducing sulfur compounds has been demonstrated in ulcerative colitis (Roediger et al, 1993). Retention enemas of butyrate are effective in treating diversion colitis (Harig et al, 1989), and preliminary open-label trials report that short-chain fatty acid enemas reduce colorectal mucosal inflammation and improve symptoms in patients with distal ulcerative colitis.

The development of the idiopathic inflammatory bowel diseases also may be related to defective presentation of antigens in the intestine. In the intestinal mucosa of normal individuals, lumenal antigens stimulate suppressor T lymphocyte activity, but in patients with idiopathic inflammatory bowel diseases, this does not occur appropriately (Mayer and Eisenhardt, 1990). Hypothetically, the combination of heightened antigen presentation in patients with altered gut mucosal immunoreactivity would lead to the development of Crohn's disease and ulcerative colitis. Therefore, another treatment strategy might involve the administration of antimalarial compounds, such as chloroquine and hydroxychloroquine, which change the pH of intracellular lysosomes and thus disrupt intracellular digestion and processing of antigens (Mayer, 1990). Antimalarials might benefit patients with Crohn's disease or ulcerative colitis by limiting intestinal mucosal antigenic immune stimulation.

Other gut mucosal protective agents have been reported to vary in their therapeutic effectiveness in Crohn's disease and ulcerative colitis. For example, acid antisecretory agents, such as anticholinergic agents, H_2-receptor blockers, and proton pump inhibitors, as well as acid-neutralizing buffers, are effective agents for the treatment of peptic ulcers of the stomach and duodenum. These agents are often prescribed for patients with Crohn's disease involvement of the upper gastrointestinal tract; they may help to heal mucosal erosions of the stomach and duodenum and can produce improvement in clinical symptoms. Sucralfate, a mucopolysaccharide that has mucosal protective properties in the upper gastrointestinal tract, also is an effective agent for the treatment of peptic ulcers of the stomach and duodenum. However, controlled trials of sucralfate enemas in patients with ulcerative colitis reveal them to be inferior to standard treatment (Riley et al, 1989). Lastly, exogenously administered prostaglandins have mucosal protective properties in the upper gastrointestinal tract and are effective agents for the treatment of peptic ulcers of the stomach and duodenum. However, therapeutic trials of prostaglandins as potential mucosal protective agents for idiopathic inflammatory bowel diseases produce disease worsening or diarrheal side effects (Goldin and Rachmilewitz, 1983; Johnson et al, 1992).

Defects in Intestinal Mucosal and/or Systemic Immunoregulation

The previous hypotheses regarding genetic susceptibility to idiopathic inflammatory bowel diseases are now supported by the reports of HLA class II gene associations with Crohn's disease and ulcerative colitis (Toyoda et al, 1993; Sugimura et al, 1993; Yang et al, 1993), as well as associations between alleles of the interleukin-1 receptor antagonist and ulcerative colitis (Mansfield et al, 1994). Abnormalities of cell-mediated and humoral immunity in patients with idiopathic inflammatory bowel diseases have been demonstrated, examples of which include: abnormal T lymphocyte function (Kramer et al, 1988); disease-specific autoantibodies (Fiocchi et al, 1989; Saxon et al, 1990; Das et al, 1992); aberrations in B lymphocyte function and immunoglobulin secretion (MacDermott et al, 1989a); and elaboration of cytokines and cytokine receptors (Sartor, 1991). The relationship between disordered immune regulation and the development of inflammatory bowel diseases is being further investigated through the use of recently developed rodent models characterized by HLA-B27 expression, deficiencies of interleukin-2 or interleukin-10, and mutant T cell receptors.

The distribution of inflammatory changes and microscopic pathology in the intestinal tract of patients with idiopathic inflammatory bowel diseases is similar to that in patients with other immunologically mediated diseases affecting the alimentary tract, an example of which is intestinal graft-versus-host disease following allogeneic bone marrow transplantation. Intestinal graft-versus-host disease may serve as a human model of idiopathic inflammatory bowel diseases. The pathogenesis of the mucosal necrosis, edema, and protein loss that is characteristic of this complication of allogeneic marrow grafting is believed to result from the activity of donor T lymphocytes, leading to immune destruction of intestinal epithelial cells, local release of cytokines (particularly tumor necrosis factor, interleukin-1, and interferon-gamma), breakdown of the intestinal barrier epithelium, massive intestinal wall edema, and secondary microbial invasion of the intestinal mucosa (McDonald et al, 1986). Although the primary inciting events in Crohn's disease and ulcerative colitis are unknown, dysfunction of T lymphocytes, among other primary host immune abnormalities, is hypothesized (Matsuura et al, 1993; Targan and Shanahan, 1994), and the resulting cascade of inflammatory events leading to intestinal mucosal destruction is similar to that in intestinal graft-versus-host disease. Therefore, it is not surprising that the therapeutic approaches to intestinal graft-versus-host disease, Crohn's disease, and ulcerative colitis are similar, often involving the use of systemic immunosuppressive and anti-inflammatory medications.

The appreciation of immune regulatory disturbances as key pathogenetic factors in idiopathic inflammatory bowel diseases is reinforced by clinical observations of remission induction or significant objective improvement in disease-related symptoms in patients treated with immune modulating drugs. Azathioprine and 6-mercaptopurine are purine biosynthesis inhibitors, and immune effector cells (lymphocytes and plasma cells) seem to be particularly susceptible to the antiproliferative effects of these agents. These agents are known to be clinically beneficial therapeutic agents for patients with Crohn's disease or ulcerative colitis (Present, 1989). Azathioprine and 6-mercaptopurine can reduce the number of plasma cells in the rectal mucosa and suppress the enhanced cytotoxic T lymphocyte activity associated with idiopathic inflammatory bowel diseases. Cyclosporine may be effective as treatment for idiopathic inflammatory bowel diseases because of several drug actions, including binding of cyclophilin, thereby producing an antiproliferative effect on lymphocytes and specifically suppressing helper T lymphocytes because of an inhibition of interleukin-2 release, leading to the suppression of induction and amplification of the immune response (Sawyerr et al, 1991). Methotrexate, a folic acid analog that inhibits the activity of dihydrofolate reductase, has different mechanisms of action, which may contribute to its effectiveness as an immunosuppressive therapy in idiopathic inflammatory bowel diseases. Dihydrofolate reductase has structural homology to interleukin-1, and thus methotrexate interferes with the functions of this cytokine, which promote activation of an immune response and inflammation (Miller et al, 1988).

Elaboration of cytokines is essential to the stimulation of an immune response and the generation of an inflammatory reaction. Cytokines are molecules that include lymphokines or interleukins, interferons, tumor necrosis factor, and peptide growth factors such as epidermal growth factor. Cytokines are soluble proteins that, at low concentrations, regulate host cellular function through ligand binding to specific receptors. Several specific alterations in cytokines have been identified in patients with idiopathic inflammatory bowel diseases. Loss of interleukin-2-producing T helper lymphocytes in the intestinal mucosa may contribute to the immunopathogenesis of Crohn's disease and ulcerative colitis (Kusugami et al, 1991). In patients with Crohn's disease, there is evidence of inhibitors of interleukin-1 that induce T lymphocyte activation (Brynskov et al, 1991). Enhanced interleukin-6 synthesis was measured in involved intestinal tissue in patients with Crohn's disease or ulcerative colitis (Stevens et al, 1992), and increased serum interleukin-6 was measured in patients with Crohn's disease (Gross et al, 1992). Increased interleukin-8 was measured in ulcerative colitis (Mahida et al, 1992) and Crohn's disease (Izzo et al, 1993). Enhanced production of granulocyte colony-stimulating factor and interleukin-1 by intestinal mucosal mononuclear cells was detected in patients with idiopathic inflammatory bowel disease, and *in vitro* suppression of cytokine production was achieved with supplemented hydrocortisone and 5-aminosalicylic acid, but not with cyclosporine (Pullman et al, 1992). An imbalance of interleukin-1 and interleukin-1 receptor antagonist exists in the intestinal mucosa of patients with Crohn's disease or ulcerative colitis, and provision of an antagonist to the interleukin-1 receptor improves experimental rabbit colitis (Cominelli et al, 1992). Exogenously administered interleukin-1 receptor antagonist is predicted to be beneficial in patients with these diseases, and clinical trials of this agent are in progress.

Mediators of Intestinal Inflammatory Damage

Epithelial cell destruction in idiopathic inflammatory bowel diseases may occur via an innocent bystander reaction as well as by primary intestinal epithelial damage caused by specific cell- or antibody-mediated immune mechanisms. Nonspecific inflammatory processes in Crohn's disease and ulcerative colitis have been shown to be mediated by local generation of soluble mediators of inflammation in intestinal mucosa. Increased secretion of immunoglobulins activates complement components that attract macrophages and neutrophils to the intestinal mucosa, thereby initiating release of injurious tissue proteases and free oxygen radicals. Activation of macrophages and neutrophils produces phospholipase-mediated release of arachidonic acid, the substrate for cyclooxygenase and lipoxygenase enzymatic action that generates the production of prostaglandins, leukotrienes, and thromboxanes (Lauritsen et al, 1986; Rampton and Collins, 1993). Prostaglandins and leukotrienes are known to be mediators of the inflammatory response of the body, causing vasodilation, hyperemia, and edema, which are features of the mucosal inflammation of idiopathic inflammatory bowel diseases and are believed to be important contributors to the inflammatory processes of these disorders.

Corticosteroids, sulfasalazine, and its aminosalicylate derivative, 5-aminosalicylic acid, are the most commonly used and extensively investigated therapeutic agents for idiopathic inflammatory bowel diseases, and their multifarious modes of therapeutic action provide insights into the immunopathogenesis of these disorders.

Systemically active adrenocorticosteroids have multiple anti-inflammatory and immunosuppressive effects (Routes and Claman, 1987; Schleimer et al, 1989; Sawyerr et al, 1991), which include (1) inhibition of chemotaxis, (2) inhibition of antibody-dependent cytotoxicity, (3) inhibition of phagocytosis, (4) promotion of a natural phospholipase A2 inhibitor, lipocortin, to stabilize cell membranes and prevent phospholipid release, and (5) stimulation of the production of an endogenous cyclooxygenase inhibitor; all of the foregoing lead to reduced synthesis of prostaglandins and leukotrienes. The therapeutic effects of corticosteroids in autoimmune disorders and asthma may have relevance for Crohn's disease and ulcerative colitis. These effects include a beta-adrenergic response to relieve smooth muscle spasm, decreased mucosal edema, decreased vascular permeability via vasoconstrictive effects, an eosinopenic effect, inhibition of chemotaxis, reduced mucus secretion by interference with cytokine release by macrophages, and inhibition of leukotriene release. Corticosteroids inhibit adhesion of leukocytes to endothelium by inhibiting production of interleukin-1, tumor necrosis factor, interferon-gamma, leukotrienes, and platelet activating factor; induce lymphopenia by a shift to the bone marrow compartment; lower peripheral eosinophil and monocyte counts due to changes in cellular adherence and chemotaxis; increase the numbers of circulating neutrophils due to altered margination and reduced release into the tissues from the vascular compartment; reduce mast cell numbers in intestinal mucosa; suppress IgG and C3 receptor function; reduce interleukin-1 production; reduce lymphocyte reactions both *in vivo* and *in vitro*; reduce suppressor T lymphocyte function; reduce serum immunoglobulins (IgG, IgA, and IgM); induce lymphocyte death; diminish lymphocyte proliferation; diminish lymphocyte production of interleukin-2; interfere with lymphocyte function; inhibit production of platelet activating factor; and inhibit secretion of free oxygen radicals by neutrophils.

Lipid peroxidation is an initiating process in the formation of soluble mediators of inflammation, which produce intestinal mucosal damage in idiopathic inflammatory bowel diseases. Sulfasalazine and 5-aminosalicylic acid inhibit hemoglobin-catalyzed, hydrogen peroxide–dependent peroxidation of phospholipid. Arachidonic acid, which is released from cell membranes during intestinal inflammation, is further metabolized, via cyclooxygenase and lipoxygenase enymatic pathways, to the inflammatory mediators, prostaglandins and leukotrienes (Lewis et al, 1990). Sulfasalazine administration produces inhibition of cyclooxygenase and lipoxygenase and thus reduces the generation of prostaglandins, leukotrienes, thromboxane, and other hydroxy fatty acids (Hawkey et al, 1985). Aminosalicylates possess an antioxidant effect as scavengers of the free oxygen radicals that are generated in intestinal inflammation (Emerit et al, 1989; Ahnfelt-Ronne et al, 1990). They also inhibit the respiratory burst of neutrophils by attentuating the generation of active oxygen species from these cells and being scavengers of active oxidants (Suematsu et al, 1987). Aminosalicylates possess several other properties that may reduce intestinal inflammation in patients with idiopathic inflammatory bowel diseases, including enhancement of colonocyte utilization of short-chain fatty acids (Roediger et al, 1989) and inhibition of interleukin-1 production, neutrophil chemotaxis, leukotriene production, adhesion of leukocytes to endothelium (Sawyerr et al, 1991), myeloperoxidase activity (Kettle and Winterbourn, 1991), platelet activating factor (Eliakim et al, 1988), and histamine release by mast cells (Fox et al, 1991). The therapeutic action of sulfasalazine in other immune-mediated disorders may be of relevance in the idiopathic inflammatory bowel diseases. For example, in psoriatic arthritis, treatment with this drug resulted in clinical improvement and lowering of previously increased B lymphocyte counts and immunoglobulin levels (Newman et al, 1991). Sulfasalazine and 5-aminosalicylic acid inhibit antibody secretion (MacDermott et al, 1989b), natural killer cell function (Gibson and Jewell, 1985), and spontaneous cell-mediated cytotoxicity (MacDermott et al, 1986).

Oxidants, such as free oxygen radicals, are generated by inflammatory reactions and mediate further intestinal damage in patients with idiopathic inflammatory bowel diseases (Grisham and Granger, 1988). Babbs (1992) theorizes that activated leukocytes produce superoxide and hydrogen peroxide, which combine with lumenal iron and denatured hemoglobin to amplify inflammation. "Oxidative stress" leads to continued propagation of intestinal mucosal inflammation, cell membrane disruption, lipid peroxidation, and further amplification of inflammatory processes. Therefore, continued therapeutic trials with superoxide dismutase mimetics, iron chelators, and antioxidants are advocated. Scavengers of free oxygen radicals have been shown to ablate intestinal inflammation in experimental animal models of inflammatory bowel disease, further suggesting a role for such agents in patients with Crohn's disease or ulcerative colitis (Emerit et al, 1989). Otamiri and Sjodahl (1991) theorize that in idiopathic inflammatory bowel diseases the rate of formation of superoxide and hydroxyl radicals exceeds the capacity of antioxidant defenses that are naturally present in intestinal tissues, such as cellular antioxidant enzymes and scavengers. Several deficits have been demonstrated in intestinal resection specimens from patients with Crohn's disease or ulcerative colitis: decreased superoxide dismutase was measured in inflamed intestinal mucosa compared to uninvolved or normal control mucosa; decreased copper and zinc metallothionein proteins were measured in inflamed intestinal mucosa compared to uninvolved mucosa; and metallothionein levels in uninvolved mucosa were less than in those of control tissues (Mulder et al, 1991).

Increased numbers of mast cells are present in the colorectal mucosa of patients with ulcerative colitis (Balazs et al, 1989), leading to investigations of antihistamines such as cromoglycate as a potential therapeutic agent for patients with idiopathic inflammatory bowel diseases. Increased platelet activating factor is measured in the feces and intestinal tissues of patients with Crohn's disease or ulcerative colitis (Denizot et al, 1992). Platelet activating factor activity is increased in the colonic mucosa of patients with ulcerative colitis, and *in vitro* inhibition of this activity is achieved with corticosteroids and aminosalicylates (Eliakim et al, 1988). Complement proteins are established mediators of intestinal inflammatory damage, and local intestinal production of complement components appears to be increased in patients with Crohn's disease (Ahrenstedt et al, 1990). Prostaglandins are generated as inflammatory mediators in the intestinal mucosa of patients with active idiopathic inflammatory bowel diseases. Therapeutic trials of prostaglandin synthesis–inhibitor nonsteroidal anti-inflammatory drugs were initiated on the premise that these would be therapeutically effective in patients with these diseases. However, such drugs lead to worsening of colitis in patients with ulcerative colitis (Rampton and Sladen, 1981). Consumption of nonsteroidal anti-inflammatory drugs may exacerbate ulcerative colitis (Kaufmann and Taubin, 1987) or produce alimentary tract damage that may be confused with manifestations of Crohn's disease.

Other Factors Affecting Immune-Mediated Intestinal Inflammatory Damage

Several other factors may influence immune-mediated inflammatory damage to intestinal mucosa in idiopathic inflammatory bowel diseases. The local access of immune effector cells to the intestinal mucosa is controlled by intestinal vascular conditions, adhesion to vascular endothelium, and egress from the vascular compartment into the mucosal tissue. Intestinal mucosal immunoreactivity may be affected by a variety of neuropeptides and other molecules, the release of which may be initiated by psychologic phenomena and the central nervous system. The contact of immunostimulating lumenal microorganisms and other antigens with the intestinal mucosa may be influenced by disordered intestinal smooth muscle function and motility.

Immune-mediated inflammatory damage to the intestinal mucosa in idiopathic inflammatory bowel diseases may be ameliorated or worsened by local circulatory functions that affect access of immune effector cells and vascular clearance. Disturbances of fibrinolysis and hemostasis that could affect local circulation have been reported in patients with Crohn's disease and ulcerative colitis, and were demonstrated in both the plasma and colonic mucosa of patients (De Jong et al, 1989). Thrombotic manifestations and hemostatic abnormalities observed in patients with idiopathic inflammatory bowel diseases include hypofibrinolysis or impaired fibrinolytic capacity, decreased tissue-type plasminogen activator antigen release, absence of significant Von Willebrand antigen release, residual plasminogen activator inhibitor activity after venous occlusion (Gris et al, 1990), activation of the fibrinolytic system with high plasminogen activator inhibitor-1 levels and natural anticoagulants with low antithrombin III activity, increased plasma fibrinogen levels, and increased anticardiolipin antibodies (Vecchi et al, 1991). In patients with Crohn's disease, signs of platelet and blood coagulation activation were identified, including increased serum beta thromboglobulin, platelet factor 4, and fibrinopeptide (Chamouard et al, 1990). Increased platelet activation and aggregation are present in patients with Crohn's disease or ulcerative colitis (Collins et al, 1994). Deficient factor XIII and factor XIII subunit A were measured in patients with active Crohn's disease (Galloway et al, 1983) or ulcerative colitis (Stadnicki et al, 1991).

An inverse correlation between cigarette smoking and disease activity in patients with ulcerative colitis has been reported (Boyko et al, 1987), whereas smoking is directly correlated with recurrence of Crohn's disease (Sutherland et al, 1990). It was hypothesized that the observations in ulcerative colitis relate to the ingestion of nicotine that accompanies cigarette smoking, and it has been shown that administration of transdermal nicotine ameliorates ulcerative colitis (Pullan et al, 1994). Nicotine has a variety of effects that could be potentially beneficial to patients with ulcerative colitis and are possibly mediated by its known physiologic effects, including stimulated release of neurotransmitters such as catecholamines and serotonin. In addition, nicotine induces a decrease in rectal blood flow, which may be pathophysiologically relevant in patients with ulcerative colitis (Srivastava et al, 1990). Available evidence on the effect of cigarette smoking on intestinal permeability is debated.

Intestinal inflammation in idiopathic inflammatory bowel diseases may be influenced by neuroimmune modulation of intestinal epithelial cell function (Perdue et al, 1992). A local anesthetic, lidocaine, has been investigated as a therapy for patients with ulcerative colitis based on the hypothesis that hyperreactive autonomic nerves may be the basis for intestinal inflammatory disease in these patients. Lidocaine also may act as a scavenger of free oxygen radicals (Siminiak and Wysocki, 1992). Nitric oxide may mediate inflammatory responses in the gut via vascular, neurologic, and immune mechanisms (Lowenstein et al, 1994).

A variety of neuropeptides may mediate the intestinal inflammatory response in patients with idiopathic inflammatory bowel diseases, suggesting that a relationship may exist between stress and disease exacerbations (Shanahan and Anton, 1988). In Crohn's disease and ulcerative colitis, alterations in receptor levels for substance P and vasoactive intestinal peptide were measured in inflamed tissues, suggesting that these may be important in regulating inflammatory and immune responses in idiopathic inflammatory bowel diseases. Other sensory neurotransmitter receptors that were assayed, but were not altered, included those for bombesin, calcitonin gene-related peptide-alpha, cholecystokinin, galanin, glutamate, somatostatin, and neurokinin A (substance K) (Mantyh et al, 1991). Furthermore, the potential role of neuroimmune mechanisms in the pathogenesis of these diseases is suggested by reports of autonomic vagal nerve dysfunction in ulcerative colitis (Lindgren et al, 1993) and increased expression of receptors for somatostatin neuropeptide in intestinal intramural veins of patients with active ulcerative colitis or Crohn's disease (Reubi et al, 1994). Future therapeutic interventional strategies may involve the design of agents that inhibit or modulate neurotransmitter production or block neurotransmitter receptors.

Endothelial leukocyte adhesion molecule-1 (ELAM-1) is expressed in the vascular endothelium of intestinal tissues from patients with Crohn's disease or ulcerative colitis, but not in that from normal controls. ELAM-1 also is expressed in neutrophils migrating into crypt abscesses in inflamed intestinal mucosa, suggesting some pathogenetic significance (Koizumi et al, 1992). Intercellular adhesion molecule-1 (ICAM-1) expression by mononuclear phagocytes is greater in patients with Crohn's disease or ulcerative colitis than in normal controls, suggesting some importance in the propagation of inflammation by facilitating T lymphocyte interactions and T lymphocyte antigen recognition (Malizia et al, 1991). A treatment strategy for patients with idiopathic inflammatory bowel diseases may involve the development of monoclonal antibodies to adhesion molecules in order to interrupt leukocyte-mediated inflammatory damage in intestinal tissues (Podolsky et al, 1993). Other evidence suggests that disruption of vascular and connective tissue sulfated glycosaminoglycans may contribute to disease pathogenesis by extravasation of protein and fluid (Murch et al, 1993). Intestinal vascular injury by anti–endothelial cell antibodies is hypothesized to be involved in the pathogenesis of idiopathic inflammatory bowel diseases (Stevens et al, 1993), and it has been proposed that persistent measles virus infection may produce a granulomatous vasculitis that is key to the pathogenesis of Crohn's disease (Inflammatory Bowel Disease Study Group, 1993).

A variety of symptomatic agents are prescribed for patients with idiopathic inflammatory bowel diseases. Categorized as antimotility agents, antispasmodics, or antidiarrheal agents, these drugs may produce therapeutic improvement via immune-mediated mechanisms by modulating antigenic contact between lumenal contents and the intestinal mucosal immune system, or by affecting other neuroimmune processes (Mayer et al, 1988). Symptoms of incontinence and diarrhea that accompany exacerbations of ulcerative colitis have been hypothetically attributed to a motility disturbance of the colon, possibly mediated by free oxygen radicals that affect smooth muscle function (Snape and Kao, 1988).

A variety of measures that do not overtly reduce intestinal inflammation are nevertheless helpful to patients with idiopathic inflammatory bowel diseases. Additional research may clarify the physiology of psychologic and neuroendocrine modulation of immune systems and the effects on intestinal inflammation in patients whose disease activity occasionally improves with such measures. Advances in psychoimmunology may effect altogether new therapeutic strategies in the future.

Factors Leading to Complications (Intestinal Cancer, Extraintestinal Manifestations)

Intestinal adenocarcinomas may develop in patients with Crohn's disease and ulcerative colitis. Extraintestinal complications may develop in up to 40 percent of patients with idiopathic inflammatory bowel diseases (Targan and Shanahan, 1994). It is not known whether the same immunoregulatory disturbances that predispose patients to the development of idiopathic inflammatory bowel diseases are responsible for intestinal epithelial neoplastic progression and nonintestinal complications, or whether other immune-mediated disturbances are operative. A complete discussion of the theoretic basis for these complications is beyond the scope of this chapter.

LESS COMMON TYPES OF INFLAMMATORY BOWEL DISEASE AND MALABSORPTION SYNDROMES

A variety of other, less common inflammatory bowel diseases and malabsorptive states should be considered by clinicians when they are confronted by patients with cardinal signs and symptoms of intestinal illness (Yamada, 1991; Sleisenger and Fordtran, 1993). These conditions may be approached diagnostically and therapeutically in a manner analogous to that for Crohn's disease and ulcerative colitis. Moreover, the disease manifestations of, as well as the treatments for, these less common disorders offer opportunities for furthering our understanding of the more common idiopathic inflammatory bowel diseases.

Short bowel syndrome, with loss of considerable lengths of the small intestine, may result from congenital conditions, surgical resection of necrotic intestines resulting from vascular catastrophes, surgical resection of diseased bowel (as, for example, from severe Crohn's jejunoileitis), or widespread inflammatory disease that affects small bowel absorptive function. Clearly, short bowel syndrome is the crudest example of a host deficiency state in which disease manifestations of malabsorptive diarrhea and malnutrition result from deficient function, if not complete absence, of the small intestine. *Iatrogenic disease* from treatment modalities for other diseases, such as radiation therapy and drugs, may lead to similarly gross damage to the intestinal mucosa and accompanying absorptive dysfunction. Potentially more subtle disease manifestations result from a variety of *mucosal protein deficiency states*, which are characterized by the absence of specific digestive enzymes or mucosal transport proteins responsible for the absorption of specific nutrients. Carbohydrate malabsorption may result from deficiencies in the intestinal brush border hydrolytic enzymes lactase, sucrase-isomaltase, or trehalase, congenital deficiencies of intestinal glucose and galactose transporters, infectious or other inflammatory illness that temporarily reduces or eradicates these mucosal proteins, or other less well-characterized intolerances to carbohydrates. Protein malabsorption may result from deficiency of enterokinase or specific amino acid transporters. Fat malabsorption results from abetalipoproteinemia. Other miscellaneous host deficiency states include deficiencies of cellular proteins that lead to electrolyte, bile salt, and vitamin malabsorption. Another unusual condition is microvillous inclusion disease, which is characterized by a congenital defect in the microvillous structure of enterocytes. For all of these host deficiency states, therapy usually involves provision of individually defined diets or nutritional support via the parenteral route.

Other immune-mediated inflammatory bowel diseases have more similarities to the idiopathic inflammatory bowel diseases than host deficiency states. *Intestinal graft-versus-host disease* resulting from allogeneic bone marrow transplantation, as discussed above, probably results from T cell mediated attack and inflammatory damage of the gut, which is managed by institution of immunosuppressive and anti-inflammatory drug therapies. Congenital or acquired *immune deficiency states* have primary and secondary intestinal disease manifestations. More commonly, secondary infection results, leading to malabsorptive or overtly inflammatory dysfunction with diarrhea and malabsorption. Primary enteropathy, as well as secondary infection, is managed by efforts to augment the immune system (e.g., provision of parenteral immunoglobulins) and treatment with appropriate antibiotics for treatable infections. *Celiac disease* manifests as small intestinal mucosal inflammatory disease in genetically susceptible individuals who are exposed to dietary gluten. Although mucosal inflammation can be suppressed and clinical improvement in symptoms of malabsorptive diarrhea results from anti-inflammatory treatments, withdrawal of exposure to gluten is in most circumstances curative. *Eosinophilic gastroenterocolitis* is truly an idiopathic inflammatory bowel disease and is characterized by eosinophilic inflammatory infiltrates in the intestine and peripheral eosinophilia. Although an immune or allergic basis for this condition has been sought, elimination diets are rarely helpful, and treatment approaches must usually include the use of steroid anti-inflammatory drugs. *Food allergy* is a distinctive, immune-mediated clinical syndrome that must be differentiated from food intolerances. Identification of food allergens, documentation of systemic manifestations, and appropriate diagnosis using a double-blind placebo-controlled food challenge and elimination diets make this a challenging clinical problem. However, removal of offending substances from the diet of affected individuals is usually more effective than the use of anti-inflammatory, antihistamine, or immunosuppressive therapies.

CONCLUSION

Improvements in our fundamental understanding of the pathobiology and etiologies of the idiopathic inflammatory bowel diseases—including Crohn's disease, ulcerative colitis, and less common disorders—ultimately will form the basis for new therapeutic strategies that may be more successful than those currently available. The availability of powerful molecular genetic and cell biologic laboratory investigational techniques has created opportunities to uncover basic causes of these diseases, which may lead to singular curative therapies. Drugs that more specifically interrupt immune-mediated intestinal tissue destruction will become available as knowledge of the regulation of local mucosal and systemic immune response is further dissected. Alternatively, a better appreciation of the environmental factors, microbial ecology of the intestinal lumen, and altered mucosal barrier function—all of which may trigger these diseases in genetically susceptible individuals—may lead to other treatment approaches. These approaches should include more specific preventive measures involving isolation of patients from exogenous disease triggers and a coupling of the first-line immune-modulating and anti-inflammatory therapies with, perhaps, antibiotics and other agents that help to restore the mucosal barrier epithelium.

REFERENCES

Ahnfelt-Ronne I, Nielsen OH, Christensen A, et al. Clinical evidence supporting the radical scavenger mechanism of 5-aminosalicylic acid. Gastroenterology 98:1162–1169, 1990.

Ahrenstedt O, Knutson L, Nilsson B, et al. Enhanced local production of complement components in the small intestines of patients with Crohn's disease. N Engl J Med 322:1345–1349, 1990.

Babbs CF. Oxygen radicals in ulcerative colitis. Free Radic Biol Med 13:169–181, 1992.

Balazs M, Illyes G, Vadasz G. Mast cells in ulcerative colitis: Quantitative and ultrastructural studies. Virch Arch Cell Pathol 57:353–360, 1989.

Boyko EJ, Koepsell TD, Perera DR, et al. Risk of ulcerative colitis among former and current cigarette smokers. N Engl J Med 316:707–710, 1987.

Brynskov J, Hansen MB, Reimert C, et al. Inhibitor of interleukin-1 alpha and interleukin-1 beta-induced T-cell activation in serum of patients with active Crohn's disease. Dig Dis Sci 36:737–742, 1991.

Chamouard P, Grunebaum L, Duclos B, et al. Biological manifestations of a prethrombotic state in developmental Crohn's disease. Gastroenterol Clin Biol 14:203–208, 1990.

Collins CE, Cahill MR, Newland AC, et al. Platelets circulate in an activated state in inflammatory bowel disease. Gastroenterology 106:840–845, 1994.

Cominelli F, Nast CC, Duchini A, et al. Recombinant interleukin-1 receptor antagonist blocks the proinflammatory activity of endogenous interleukin-1 in rabbit immune colitis. Gastroenterology 103:65–71, 1992.

Culpepper-Morgan JA, Floch MH. Bowel rest or bowel starvation: Defining the role of nutritional support in the treatment of inflammatory bowel disease. Am J Gastroenterol 86:269–271, 1991.

Das KM, Squillante L, Chitayet D, et al. Simultaneous appearance of a unique common epitope in fetal colon, skin, and biliary epithelial cells: a possible link for extracolonic manifestations in ulcerative colitis. J Clin Gastroenterol 15:311–316, 1992.

De Jong E, Porte RJ, Knot EA, et al. Disturbed fibrinolysis in patients with inflammatory bowel disease: A study in blood plasma, colon mucosa, and faeces. Gut 30:188–194, 1989.

Denizot Y, Chaussade S, Nathan N, et al. PAF-acether and acetylhydrolase in stool of patients with Crohn's disease. Dig Dis Sci 37:432–437, 1992.

Eliakim R, Karmeli F, Razin E, et al. Role of platelet-activating factor in ulcerative colitis: Enhanced production during active disease and inhibition by sulfasalazine and prednisolone. Gastroenterology 95:1167–1172, 1988.

Emerit J, Droy-Lefaix MT, Likforman J, et al. Oxygen free radicals and inflammatory diseases of intestines. J Chir (Paris) 126:287–293, 1989.

Fiocchi C, Roche JK, Michener WM. High prevalence of antibodies to intestinal epithelial antigens in patients with inflammatory bowel disease and their relatives. Ann Intern Med 110:786–794, 1989.

Fox CC, Moore WC, Lichtenstein LM. Modulation of mediator release from human intestinal mast cells by sulfasalazine and 5-aminosalicylic acid. Dig Dis Sci 36:179–184, 1991.

Galloway MJ, Mackie MJ, McVerry BA. Reduced levels of factor XIII in patients with chronic inflammatory bowel disease. Clin Lab Haematol 5:427–428, 1983.

Gibson PR, Jewell DP. Sulphasalazine and derivatives, natural killer activity and ulcerative colitis. Clin Sci 69:177–184, 1985.

Goldin E, Rachmilewitz D. Prostanoids cytoprotection for maintaining remission in ulcerative colitis: Failure of 15(R),15-methylprostaglandin E2. Dig Dis Sci 28:807–811, 1983.

Gris JC, Schved JF, Raffanel C, et al. Impaired fibrinolytic capacity in patients with inflammatory bowel disease. Thromb Haemost 63:472–475, 1990.

Grisham MB, Granger DN. Neutrophil-mediated mucosal injury: role of reactive oxygen metabolites. Dig Dis Sci 33(suppl):6S–15S, 1988.

Gross V, Andus T, Caesar I, et al. Evidence for continuous stimulation of interleukin-6 production in Crohn's disease. Gastroenterology 102:514–519, 1992.

Harig JM, Soergel KH, Komorowski RA, et al. Treatment of diversion colitis with short-chain fatty acid irrigation. N Engl J Med 320:23–28, 1989.

Hawkey CJ, Boughton-Smith NK, Whittle BJR. Modulation of human colonic arachidonic acid metabolism by sulphasalazine. Dig Dis Sci 130:1161–1165, 1985.

Inflammatory Bowel Disease Study Group. Evidence of persistent measles virus infection in Crohn's disease. J Med Virol 39:345–353, 1993.

Izzo RS, Witkon K, Chen AI, et al. Neutrophil-activating peptide (interleukin-8) in colonic mucosa from patients with Crohn's disease. Scand J Gastroenterol 28:296–300, 1993.

Johnson JS, Karboski JA, Williams GO. Profuse diarrhea after misoprostol use in a patient with a history of Crohn's disease. Ann Pharmacother 26:1092–1093, 1992.

Kangro HO, Chong SKF, Hardiman A, et al. A prospective study of viral and mycoplasma infections in chronic inflammatory bowel disease. Gastroenterology 98:549–553, 1990.

Kaufmann HJ, Taubin HL. Nonsteroidal anti-inflammatory drugs activate quiescent inflammatory bowel disease. Ann Intern Med 107:513–516, 1987.

Kettle AJ, Winterbourn CC. Mechanism of inhibition of myeloperoxidase by anti-inflammatory drugs. Biochem Biopharmacol 41:1485–1492, 1991.

Koizumi M, King N, Lobb R, et al. Expression of vascular adhesion molecules in inflammatory bowel disease. Gastroenterology 103:840–847, 1992.

Kramer JK, Depew WT, Szewczuk MR. T-cell immunoregulation in patients with inflammatory bowel disease. I. Differential helper T-cell function in ulcerative colitis and Crohn's disease. J Clin Lab Immunol 25:9–17, 19–27, 1988.

Kusugami K, Matsuura T, West GA, et al. Loss of interleukin-2-producing intestinal CD4+ T cells in inflammatory bowel disease. Gastroenterology 101:1594–1605, 1991.

Lauritsen K, Laursen LS, Bukhave K, et al. Effects of topical 5-aminosalicylic acid and prednisolone on prostaglandin E_2 and leukotriene B_4 levels determined by equilibrium in vivo dialysis of rectum in relapsing ulcerative colitis. Gastroenterology 91:837–844, 1986.

Levine DS. Immune modulating therapies for idiopathic inflammatory bowel diseases. Adv Pharmacol 25:171–234, 1994.

Lewis RA, Austen KF, Soberman RJ. Leukotrienes and other products of the 5-lipoxygenase pathway: Biochemistry and relation to pathobiology in human disease. N Engl J Med 323:645–655, 1990.

Lindgren S, Stewenius J, Sjolund K, et al. Autonomic vagal nerve dysfunction in patients with ulcerative colitis. Scand J Gastroenterol 28:638–642, 1993.

Lowenstein CJ, Dinerman JL, Snyder SH. Nitric oxide: A physiologic messenger. Ann Intern Med 120:227–237, 1994.

MacDermott RP, Kane MG, Steele LL, et al. Sulfasalazine inhibits spontaneous cell-mediated cytotoxicity by peripheral blood and intestinal mononuclear cells from control and inflammatory bowel disease patients. Immunopharmacology 11:101–109, 1986.

MacDermott RP, Nash GS, Auer IO, et al. Alterations in serum immunoglobulin G subclasses in patients with ulcerative colitis and Crohn's disease. Gastroenterology 96:764–768, 1989a.

MacDermott RP, Schloemann SR, Bertovich MJ, et al. Inhibition of antibody secretion by 5-aminosalicylic acid. Gastroenterology 96:442–448, 1989b.

Mahida Y, Ceska M, Eggenberger F, et al. Enhanced synthesis of neutrophil-activating peptide-1/interleukin-8 in active ulcerative colitis. Clin Sci 82:273–275, 1992.

Malizia G, Calabrese A, Cottone M, et al. Expression of leukocyte adhesion molecules by mucosal mononuclear phagocytes in inflammatory bowel disease. Gastroenterology 100:150–159, 1991.

Mansfield JC, Holden H, Tarlow JK, et al. Novel genetic association between ulcerative colitis and the anti-inflammatory cytokine interleukin-1 receptor antagonist. Gastroenterology 106:637–642, 1994.

Mantyh PW, Catton M, Maggio JE, et al. Alterations in receptors for sensory neuropeptides in human inflammatory bowel disease. Adv Exp Med Biol 298:253–283, 1991.

Matsuura T, West GA, Youngman KR, et al. Immune activation genes in inflammatory bowel disease. Gastroenterology 104:448–458, 1993.

Mayer EA, Raybould H, Koelbel C. Neuropeptides, inflammation, and motility. Dig Dis Sci 33:71s–77s, 1988.

Mayer L. The role of the epithelial cell in immunoregulation: Pathogenetic and therapeutic implications. Mt Sinai J Med 57:279–282, 1990.

Mayer L, Eisenhardt D. Lack of induction of suppressor T cells by intestinal epithelial cells from patients with inflammatory bowel disease. J Clin Invest 86:1255–1260, 1990.

McDonald GB, Shulman HM, Sullivan KM, et al. Intestinal and hepatic complications of human bone marrow transplantation. Gastroenterology 90:460–477, 770–784, 1986.

McKay DM, Perdue MH. Intestinal epithelial function. Dig Dis Sci 38:1377–1387, 1735–1745, 1993.

Miller LC, Cohen SE, Orencole SF, et al. Interleukin-1 is structurally related to dihydrofolate reductase: Effect of methotrexate on Il-1. Lymphokine Res 7:272, 1988.

Mulder TP, Verspaget HW, Janssens AR, et al. Decrease in two intestinal copper/zinc containing proteins with antioxidant function in inflammatory bowel disease. Gut 32:1146–1150, 1991.

Munkholm P, Langholz E, Hollander D, et al. Intestinal permeability in patients with Crohn's disease and ulcerative colitis and their first-degree relatives. Gut 35:68–72, 1994.

Murch SH, MacDonald TT, Walker-Smith JA, et al. Disruption of sulphated glycosaminoglycans in intestinal inflammation. Lancet 341:711–714, 1993.

Newman ED, Perruquet JL, Harrington TM. Sulfasalazine therapy in psoriatic arthritis: Clinical and immunologic response. J Rheumatol 18:1379–1382, 1991.

Otamiri T, Sjodahl R. Oxygen radicals: Their role in selected gastrointestinal disorders. Dig Dis 9:133–141, 1991.

Perdue MH, Kosecka U, Crowe S. Antigen-mediated effects on epithelial function. Ann NY Acad Sci 664:325–334, 1992.

Podolsky DK, Isselbacher KJ. Glycoprotein composition of colonic mucosa. Specific alterations in ulcerative colitis. Gastroenterology 87:991–998, 1984.

Podolsky DK, Lobb R, King N, et al. Attenuation of colitis in the cotton-top tamarin by anti-alpha 4 integrin monoclonal antibody. J Clin Invest 92:372–380, 1993.

Present DH. 6-Mercaptopurine and other immunosuppressive agents in the treatment of Crohn's disease and ulcerative colitis. Gastroenterol Clin North Am 18:57–71, 1989.

Pullan RD, Rhodes J, Ganesh S, et al. Transdermal nicotine for active ulcerative colitis. N Engl J Med 330:811–815, 1994.

Pullman WE, Elsbury S, Kobayashi M, et al. Enhanced mucosal cytokine production in inflammatory bowel disease. Gastroenterology 102:529–537, 1992.

Rampton DS, Collins CE. Review article. Thromboxanes in inflammatory bowel disease—pathogenic and therapeutic implications. Aliment Pharmacol Ther 7:357–367, 1993.

Rampton DS, Sladen GE. Prostaglandin synthesis inhibitors in ulcerative colitis: Flurbiprofen compared with conventional treatment. Prostaglandins 21:417–425, 1981.

Reubi JC, Mazzucchelli L, Laissue JA. Intestinal vessels express a high density of somatostatin receptors in human inflammatory bowel disease. Gastroenterology 106:951–959, 1994.

Riley SA, Gupta I, Mani V. A comparison of sucralfate and prednisolone enemas in the treatment of active distal ulcerative colitis. Scand J Gastroenterol 24:1014–1018, 1989.

Roediger WEW, Deakin EJ, Walker G, et al. Assessment of salicylate derivatives for potential use in ulcerative colitis: Proposal for a new action of 5-aminosalicylic acid? Pharmacology 39:39–45, 1989.

Roediger WE, Duncan A, Kapaniris O, et al. Reducing sulfur compounds of the colon impair colonocyte nutrition: Implications for ulcerative colitis. Gastroenterology 104:802–809, 1993.

Routes J, Claman HN. Corticosteroids in inflammatory bowel disease: A review. J Clin Gastroenterol 9:529–535, 1987.

Sartor RB. Pathogenetic and clinical relevance of cytokines in inflammatory bowel disease. Immunol Res 10:465–471, 1991.

Sawyerr AM, Wakefield AJ, Hudson M, et al. Review article. The pharmacological implications of leucocyte-endothelial cell interactions in Crohn's disease. Aliment Pharmacol Ther 5:1–14, 1991.

Saxon A, Shanahan F, Landers C, et al. A distinct subset of antineutrophil anticytoplasmic antibodies is associated with inflammatory bowel disease. J Allergy Clin Immunol 86:202–210, 1990.

Schleimer RP, Claman HN, Oronsky AL (eds). Anti-Inflammatory Steroid Action: Basic and Clinical Aspects. New York, Academic Press, 1989.

Shanahan F, Anton P. Neuroendocrine modulation of the immune system: Possible implications for inflammatory bowel disease. Dig Dis Sci 33:41s–49s, 1988.

Siminiak T, Wysocki H. The effect of lidocaine on oxygen free radical production by polymorphonuclear neutrophils. Agents Actions 1992 (Special Conference Issue):C104–C105.

Sleisenger MH, Fordtran JS (eds). Gastrointestinal Disease: Pathophysiology/Diagnosis/Management. 5th ed. Philadelphia, WB Saunders Co, 1993.

Snape Jr WJ, Kao HW. Role of inflammatory mediators in colonic smooth muscle function in ulcerative colitis. Dig Dis Sci 33:65s–70s, 1988.

Sonnenberg A, McCarty DJ, Jacobsen SJ. Geographic variation of inflammatory bowel disease within the United States. Gastroenterology 100:143–149, 1991.

Sperber K, Ogata S, Sylvester C, et al. A novel human macrophage-derived intestinal mucin secretagogue: Implications for the pathogenesis of inflammatory bowel disease. Gastroenterology 104:1302–1309, 1993.

Srivastava ED, Russell MA, Feyerabend C, et al. Effect of ulcerative colitis and smoking on rectal blood flow. Gut 31:1021–1024, 1990.

Stadnicki A, Kloczko J, Nowak A, et al. Factor XIII subunits in relation to some other hemostatic parameters in ulcerative colitis. Am J Gastroenterol 86:690–693, 1991.

Stevens C, Walz G, Singaram C, et al. Tumor necrosis factor-alpha, interleukin-1-beta, and interleukin-6 expression in inflammatory bowel disease. Dig Dis Sci 37:818–826, 1992.

Stevens TR, Harley SL, Groom JS, et al. Anti-endothelial cell antibodies in inflammatory bowel disease. Dig Dis Sci 38:426–432, 1993.

Suematsu M, Suzuki M, Miura S, et al. Sulfasalazine and its metabolites attenuate respiratory burst of leukocytes: A possible mechanism of anti-inflammatory effects. J Clin Lab Immunol 23:31–33, 1987.

Sugimura K, Asakura H, Mizuki N, et al. Analysis of genes within the HLA region affecting susceptibility to ulcerative colitis. Human Immunol 36:112–118, 1993.

Sutherland LR, Ramcharan S, Bryant H, et al. Effects of cigarette smoking on recurrence of Crohn's disease. Gastroenterology 98:1123–1128, 1990.

Sutherland LR, Singleton J, Sessions J, et al. Double-blind, placebo-controlled trial of metronidazole in Crohn's disease. Gut 32:1071–1075, 1991.

Targan SR, Shanahan F (eds). Inflammatory Bowel Disease From Bench to Bedside. Baltimore, Williams & Wilkins, 1994.

Teahon K, Smethurst P, Pearson M, et al. The effect of elemental diet on intestinal permeability and inflammation in Crohn's disease. Gastroenterology 101:84–89, 1991.

Toyoda H, Wang S-J, Yang H-Y, et al. Distinct associations of HLA class II genes with inflammatory bowel disease. Gastroenterology 104:741–748, 1993.

Van Kruiningen HJ, Chiodini RJ, Thayer WJ, et al. Experimental disease in infant goats induced by a *Mycobacterium* isolated from a patient with Crohn's disease: A preliminary report. Dig Dis Sci 31:1351–1360, 1986.

Vecchi M, Cattaneo M, de Franchis R, et al. Risk of thromboembolic complications in patients with inflammatory bowel disease: Study of hemostasis measurements. Int J Clin Lab Res 21:165–170, 1991.

Yamada T (ed). Textbook of Gastroenterology. Philadelphia, JB Lippincott Co, 1991.

Yang H, Rotter JI, Toyoda H, et al. Ulcerative colitis: A genetically heterogeneous disorder defined by genetic (HLA class II) and subclinical (anti-neutrophilic cytoplasmic antibodies) markers. J Clin Invest 92:1080–1084, 1993.

ACKNOWLEDGMENTS: This work was supported in part by Food and Drug Administration Office of Orphan Products Development grant FD-R-000827.

Section Ten
SPECIAL ISSUES

Chapter 50
Allergic Disorders of the Eye

Mitchell H. Friedlaender, M.D.

THE OCULAR IMMUNE RESPONSE

The eye resists foreign invaders through a variety of specific and nonspecific defense mechanisms. Like other parts of the body, the eye is constantly exposed to a flood of microorganisms but is capable of warding off most of these with little or no alteration of its structure or function. Much of the eye's natural resistance depends on anatomic and physiologic properties of its external structures—the lids, tears, conjunctiva, and cornea (Friedlaender, 1979; Friedlaender and Allansmith, 1975). Once a foreign substance (such as a bacterium) has entered the eye, the defense mechanisms are far less effective than at the eye's outer surface, and destructive effects are more likely to occur. In this chapter, we consider the specific and nonspecific defense mechanisms that characterize the different ocular tissues. We are concerned not only with the way the eye responds under normal circumstances, but also with the immunologic responses of the eye when it is exposed to various infectious agents and antigenic stimuli.

EYELIDS

The eyelids have the obvious function of protecting the eye from trauma by the blink mechanism and by screening out small particles through the action of the cilia. In addition, the lids keep the eye lubricated with tears and help to sweep foreign substances from the eye and into the tear drainage. The skin of the eyelids possesses the same antimicrobial properties that skin has elsewhere in the body. In addition, the lids possess a number of glands whose secretions contribute to the tear film and also contain numerous antimicrobial substances.

TEARS

The tear film consists of three layers:

1. An outer, oily layer, composed of phospholipids, is produced by the meibomian glands. This layer retards evaporation of the tear film and aids the spreading of the tears over the surface of the cornea.
2. The middle layer of the tear film comprises aqueous secretions from the lacrimal and accessory lacrimal glands of Krause and Wolfring. This layer, which contains lysozyme and immunoglobulins, is deficient in Sjögren's syndrome.
3. The innermost layer of the tear film is a thin, mucoid layer that is derived mainly from the goblet cells of the conjunctiva. The mucoid layer facilitates spreading of the aqueous layer over the surface of the eye. We have become more aware of mucoid deficiencies in recent years, particularly in cases of cicatricial pemphigoid and in the Stevens-Johnson syndrome.

Lysozyme

The tears contain both antibody and lysozyme (Drutz and Mills, 1978). Lysozyme is a cationic, low-molecular-weight enzyme that reduces the local concentration of susceptible bacteria by attacking the mucopeptides of their cell walls. Although most gram-positive bacteria are affected by lysozyme, *Staphylococcus aureus* is not, since the lysozyme-susceptible site on this organism's cell wall is blocked structurally from lysozyme attack.

Tear lysozyme is believed to be produced by the lacrimal gland and is present in a much higher concentration in tears than in serum (Horwitz et al, 1978). Tear lysozyme concentration is elevated during the morning and reduced during sleep (Greiner et al, 1977). Lactoferrin, another major tear protein, has bacteriostatic properties, presumably due to its ability to make certain metals unavailable for microorganisms (Broekhuyse, 1974).

Immunoglobulins

All of the major immunoglobulin classes except IgD have been detected in human tears. IgA is the major immunoglobulin in tears, and as in other external secretions, it is the 11S, dimeric variety containing secretory piece that predominates (Bluestone et al, 1975; Chandler et al, 1974; Josephson and Weiner, 1968; McClellan et al, 1973; Sen et al, 1976). IgG is usually detectable in only small amounts, and IgM is only rarely detectable (Chandler et al, 1974). IgD has not been detected in any study of tears. IgE is detectable by radioimmunoassay (McClellan et al, 1973; Brauninger and Centifanto, 1971), and this immunoglobulin may be increased in patients suffering from allergic disorders of the external eye (Brauninger and Centifanto, 1971).

Tear immunoglobulin seems to be produced by plasma cells within the lacrimal gland, whereas secretory component is produced within the acinar epithelial cells of the gland (Franklin et al, 1973). Various studies have shown that the level of IgA in tears varies from 7 to 85 mg/100 ml and that IgG concentrations range from trace amounts to 14 mg/100 ml. Ninety-three percent of tear IgA is in the polymeric form (Allansmith et al, 1985). In the inflamed eye, tear immunoglobulins are generally increased and resemble more closely the distribution of the immunoglobulins in serum. This is probably due to a transudation of serum proteins into the tears (McClellan et al, 1973). In rats, IL-5 and IL-6 augment tear IgA antibody responses (Pockley and Montgomery, 1991). The exact mechanism by which secretory IgA works is not known. Its clearest role is in bacterial disease, where in some way it prevents the attachment of bacteria to mucosal cells (Drutz and Mills, 1978). A T helper cell in the lacrimal gland can influence B lymphocytes to differentiate into IgA-producing plasma cells (Franklin, 1989). No specific immunoglobulin changes can currently be correlated with specific disease entities other than an increase in IgE in some allergic conditions (Chandler et al, 1974; McClellan et al, 1973).

Complement is detectable in human tears, and both C3 (Bluestone et al, 1975) and C4 (Chandler et al, 1974) have been quantitated. In humans with conjunctivitis, the concentration of C3 in tears is proportional to the severity of inflammation (Imanishi et al, 1982). The relationship of complement to specific ocular diseases requires further study.

CONJUNCTIVA

Normal Structure and Function

The normal conjunctiva forms a natural barrier to invasion by exogenous substances.

Inflammatory cells present from birth have been studied in several animal species (McMaser et al, 1967), and the quantity of leukocytes seems to increase with age and antigenic exposure. The normal human conjunctiva contains an extraordinary number of infiltrative inflammatory cells, among which lymphocytes, plasma cells, and neutrophils are found. Fixed-tissue mast cells are also found in great numbers in the conjunctiva, as in other vascularized tissue (Allansmith et al, 1977). No doubt many of the inflammatory cells normally present in the conjunctiva are engaged in phagocytosis and in processing antigen for its elimination and for the individual's immunologic memory. The epithelial cells of the conjunctiva may also participate in phagocytosis (Zimianshi et al, 1974). Epithelial phagocytosis is active in conjunctival infection with *Listeria* and *Chlamydia*. Both epithelial cells and leukocytes possess lysosomes containing acid hydrolases that have a strong antimicrobial effect.

The normal palpebral conjunctiva varies a great deal in its surface morphology from a satin-smooth appearance to a uniform or nonuniform papillary appearance (Greiner et al, 1977). Papillae represent collections of nonspecific inflammatory cells and tissue elements that are bound closely to the tarsal plate or the limbus. Follicles may also be seen in the normal conjunctiva, especially in the lower fornix. These are not related to disease and are especially common in childhood. Conjunctival follicles represent tightly packed collections of lymphocytes in various stages of development. Lymphoid aggregates containing mature and immature lymphocytes are found just below the epithelium in the conjunctiva of adult rabbits after 10 weeks of age (Axelrod and Chandler, 1978).

The conjunctiva is endowed with several other nonspecific protective mechanisms. Constant epithelial turnover and a cool temperature due to tear evaporation may serve a protective function. In addition, certain unknown factors make the conjunctiva usually resistant to certain viruses (such as those that cause the common cold), yet highly susceptible to the gonococcus and the agent of inclusion conjunctivitis. (In contrast, the nasal mucosa is highly susceptible to cold viruses yet resistant to the gonococcus.) The prominent vascularity of the conjunctiva and the frequently observed dilatation of its vessels suggest that the exchange of substances across the vessel walls is a fundamental response of the conjunctiva to noxious substances. The resident normal flora, intrinsic anatomic barriers, secretion of mucous and antibacterial substances, local humoral and cellular immune responses, and a highly efficient amplification system provide the conjunctiva with a complex system of defense (Chandler and Gillette, 1983).

Pathologic Responses

The conjunctiva can undergo a variety of morphologic changes in response to microorganisms, toxins, and various antigens. The type of response depends largely on the nature of the stimulus. Hyperemia occurs in response to physical stimuli such as wind, sun, or smoke or in response to allergens, toxins, and infectious agents. A brilliant red appearance suggests a bacterial conjunctivitis, whereas a milky appearance suggests an allergic conjunctivitis. Tearing often accompanies hyperemia and may be increased by transudation across the vessel walls. Exudation is seen in all types of acute conjunctivitis. A purulent exudate is characteristic of bacterial conjunctivitis, whereas a stringy exudate is more often seen in allergic conjunctivitis. Drooping of the upper eyelid (pseudoptosis) may be due to increased weight of the lid from cellular infiltration and edema. Chemosis, or edema of the conjunctiva, is often associated with an acute allergic response and several other types of conjunctivitis.

Papillary hypertrophy occurs when inflammatory cells accumulate within the conjunctiva, causing it to heap up in mounds that are bound to the tarsal plate by strong connective tissue fibrils. A tuft of vessels forms in the substance of the papilla and branches over it like the spokes of an umbrella. When the papillae are small, the conjunctiva frequently has a smooth, velvety appearance, as in bacterial conjunctivitis. In allergic conditions, such as vernal and atopic keratoconjunctivitis, the papillae of the upper tarsus may be large, flat-topped, polygonal, and milky in appearance. These giant papillae may also form at the limbus, where they appear as gelatinous excrescences. Follicles are characteristics of viral chlamydial infections and also of toxic conjunctivitis due to the application of certain topical medications. When they are located on the upper palpebral conjunctiva or at the limbus, they are strongly suggestive of chlamydial disease. Those located in the lower fornix or at the lateral margins of the upper tarsus have limited diagnostic value. The follicle is rounded, whitish gray, and avascular, although small vessels may encircle it (Vaughan and Asbury, 1978).

Pseudomembranes and membranes result from a coagulation process on the surface of the conjunctiva. A true membrane involves the entire epithelium, and when it is removed a raw bleeding surface remains. A pseudomembrane is a coagulum on the surface of the epithelium, and when it is removed the epithelium remains intact and bleeding does not occur. Both membranes and pseudomembranes accompany various types of bacterial conjunctivitis, erythema multiforme major (Stevens-Johnson syndrome), and chemical burns. Neutrophils are abundantly present in smears taken from such cases.

Granulomas appear on the conjunctiva in response to various infectious agents or in the form of a chalazion (lipogranuloma). A grossly visible preauricular node may accompany such a granulomatous response.

Conjunctival scrapings are often helpful in determining the etiology of an inflammatory response (Kimura and Thygeson, 1955; Thygeson, 1946). A predominantly neutrophilic reaction is characteristic of fungal infections and all but two bacterial infections *(Branhamella catarrhalis* and *Moraxella)*. Several diseases of unknown etiology also produce a neutrophil response, including erythema multiforme and Reiter's syndrome. An eosinophil response is characteristic of allergic inflammation, such as vernal conjunctivitis, hay fever, and drug-related allergies. Mast cells are also characteristically seen in conjunctival smears from patients with vernal conjunctivitis. Mononuclear cells predominate in conjunctival scrapings from viral conjunctivitis, whereas neutrophils are usually seen in response to chlamydial infections.

Humoral Immune Responses

All five immunoglobulins are routinely found in the human conjunctiva (Allansmith and Hutchison, 1967). Most are present in the subepithelial tissue, and almost none is found in the epithelium. Immunoglobulin-producing plasma cells are not routinely identified in the perilimbic conjunctiva with the use of immunofluorescent techniques (Allansmith et al, 1973). Immediate hypersensitivity reactions have been studied in the guinea pig conjunctiva following systemic sensitization with normal rabbit serum (Dwyer et al, 1974). Topical conjunctival challenge produces edema, hyperemia, and infiltration by a large number of eosinophils and neutrophils. Both IgE and IgG homocytotropic antibody can be demonstrated in serum, and when these are passively transferred to normal guinea pigs, conjunctival hypersensitivity can be demonstrated by topical challenge (Dwyer et al, 1974). Leukotrienes (Bisgaard et al, 1985) and trypase (Abelson et al, 1990) can be demonstrated in tears after allergen challenge and other stimuli. Other mediators, such as kinins, histamine, tame-esterase, and prostaglandins, have also been demonstrated after allergen challenge (Friedlaender, 1990). Antihistamines, cromolyn (disodium cromoglycate), and steroids do not modify the clinical signs, but they do inhibit the neutrophil and eosinophil response (Dwyer et al, 1976).

Cellular Immune Responses

Cellular immune responses have not been well studied in the conjunctiva, and it is often stated that these responses can be elicited on mucous membranes only with great difficulty. We recently studied a model of contact sensitivity in the guinea pig conjunctiva in which a nontoxic hapten, oxazolone, elicits a delayed-onset reaction 5 to 7 days after topical cutaneous sensitization (Friedlaender and Cyr, 1979). The conjunctival response contains predominantly mononuclear cells, but a large number of eosinophils is also seen. A reaction that is widely believed to represent delayed hypersensitivity in the conjunctiva is the phlyctenule, a transient, nodular lesion seen in response to a variety of microbial agents. Both B and T lymphocytes have been identified in human conjunctiva and lacrimal gland taken from patients with phlyctenular conjunctivitis and Sjögren's syndrome (Belfort and Mendez, 1978). B cells are generally found in higher numbers but are more concentrated in the central follicles, whereas T cells are found mainly in peripheral follicles and scattered throughout the tissue.

ALLERGIC DISORDERS
Allergic Rhinoconjunctivitis

Conjunctivitis is the chief ocular manifestation of many allergies to common airborne substances. Pollens of trees, grasses, and weeds; house dust; animal dander; and molds have been implicated in these recurrent and often seasonal allergies. Such reactions are a manifestation of type I hypersensitivity and are mediated by immunoglobulin E. Mucous membranes, including the nasal mucosa and conjunctiva, are generally affected.

Conjunctivitis is the chief ocular manifestation of many allergies to common airborne substances (Fig. 50–1). The conjunctival mucosa may act in a manner similar to the nasal mucosa in sensitized individuals. Itching of the eyes is a common symptom. It is often said that itching is pathognomonic of ocular allergy. Attacks are usually seasonal; however, with perennial allergens such as house dust, the symptoms may occur year-round. Chronic allergic conjunctivitis has been associated with the house dust mite. The conjunctiva is edematous and appears pale and boggy. The lids may also be edematous and hyperemic. Installation of the offending pollen into the conjunctival sac produces typical signs of hay fever conjunctivitis. A scraping of the conjunctiva for eosinophils may be helpful. Under normal circumstances, eosinophils are not found in conjunctival scrapings, and the presence of even one eosinophil or of eosinophil granules is considered diagnostic (Friedlaender et al, 1984).

Antihistamines may be given systemically to relieve allergic symptoms involving the eye. Topical antihistamines, sometimes combined with vasoconstrictors, may also be useful. Corticosteroid drops may be extremely effective in relieving symptoms of allergic conjunctivitis, but since the disease is chronic, recurrent, and a benign condition, these drugs should be used with extreme caution. The installation of a mast cell stabilizer eyedrop may be effective in reducing ocular signs and symptoms. Because these drops drain into the nose, a secondary benefit may be relief of nasal symptoms.

Atopic Dermatitis

The skin of the eyelids is susceptible to the same types of hypersensitivity disorders and infections that involve the skin of other parts of the body. Because of anatomic factors, the lids are especially prone to show evidence of inflammation. The eyelid skin is thinner than any other skin of the body and is frequently subjected to trauma, allergens, and toxic substances. The loose subcutaneous tissues allow accumulation of fluid, which becomes walled off from the surrounding structures by the orbital septum, creating prominent periorbital edema.

Atopic dermatitis is one of the eczematous skin eruptions. It often occurs in childhood but may be seen in adolescents and adults as well. The incidence in children under 5 yr of age is estimated to be 3 percent. Frequently, patients with atopic dermatitis have a history of respiratory allergy or allergic reactions to certain foods. Although immunologic abnormalities have been noted in atopic dermatitis, this condition also seems to represent an abnormal reactivity of the skin to various stimuli. This abnormal skin reactivity may be genetically determined, and it is considered by some to represent a metabolic or biochemical defect. Although patients with atopic dermatitis undergo extensive allergic testing, frequently it is difficult to find a relationship between this condition and a known allergen. Allergy to house dust mites and hypersensitivity to staphylococcal antigens have been associated with atopic dermatitis.

Ocular Findings

The skin of the eyelids may be involved with erythematous and exudative lesions. In later stages, scaling and crusting may occur. Secondary staphylococcal blepharitis requiring treatment may also occur. Atopic keratoconjunctivitis may be observed in patients with atopic eczema (Fig. 50–2). Clinically, there may be hyperemia, chemosis, and filamentous discharge. Less commonly, giant papillary hypertrophy ("cobblestones") may

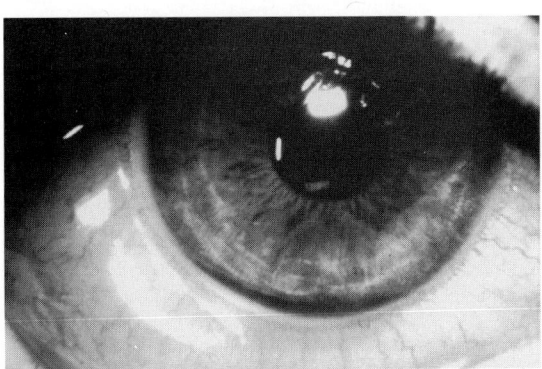

FIGURE 50–1. Allergic rhinoconjunctivitis. Note mild redness and prominent edema giving the conjunctiva a boggy appearance.

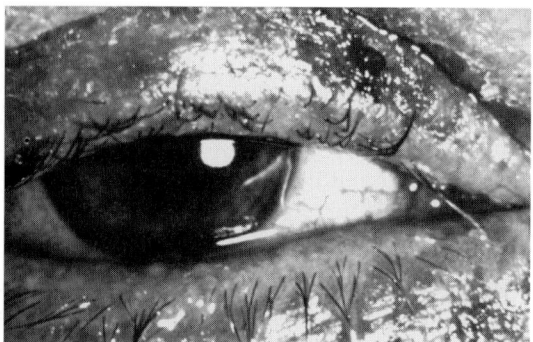

FIGURE 50–2. Atopic keratoconjunctivitis in a patient with atopic dermatitis.

be observed on the palpebral conjunctiva; in contrast to vernal conjunctivitis, the lower tarsus is more frequently involved in atopic dermatitis (Spencer and Fisher, 1959). Trantas' dots (Fig. 50–3), which consist of localized deposits of eosinophils, can occur at the limbus. Linear or stellate scarring may be present on the palpebral conjunctiva. In vernal conjunctivitis, no scarring is seen. According to Thygeson (personal communication), papillary hypertrophy of the lower palpebral conjunctiva is so unusual in vernal conjunctivitis that it helps to differentiate this condition from atopic conjunctivitis. Vernal conjunctivitis will frequently become arrested by age 18. It is not uncommon to see atopic conjunctivitis in older patients. Occasionally, shrinkage of the fornices is noted in atopic keratoconjunctivitis.

Punctate staining of the cornea may be present, and if the disease is severe, scarring and vascularization of the cornea may occur. Keratoconus is sometimes associated with atopic dermatitis. Copeman (1965) reviewed 100 patients with keratoconus and found that 32 had some form of eczema. The incidence of atopic eczema in the general population is about 3 percent compared with an incidence of 16 percent in this group of keratoconus patients. Karseras and Ruben (1976) also found a strong association between keratoconus and atopic conditions. It has been suggested that local irritation of the eyelids due to eczema or hay fever may lead to excessive eye rubbing. This, coupled with a congenitally thinned and weakened cornea, may be associated with the development of keratoconus.

Atopic cataracts (Fig. 50–4) have been described as a complication of atopic dermatitis (Beethan, 1940). Their incidence has been estimated to be 8 to 10 percent. They are seen mainly in severe chronic forms of the disease, especially in children and young adults. Atopic cataracts usually appear at least 10 years after the onset of skin involvement. Once the cataract is detected, however, it may evolve rapidly into complete opacification within 6 months. These cataracts are frequently bilateral, and involvement may be symmetric. Occasionally, however, a unilateral cataract is seen. Classically, atopic cataracts have a shield-like opacification affecting the anterior cortex. Frequently, the cataract begins as a posterior subcapsular opacity. Histologically, a localized degeneration and proliferation of the subcapsular epithelium is seen. Degeneration of the adjacent cortex may occur and may lead to widespread opacification of the lens.

Spontaneous retinal detachment is said to be more common in patients with atopic dermatitis than in the general population (Ingram, 1965). Whether this is associated with

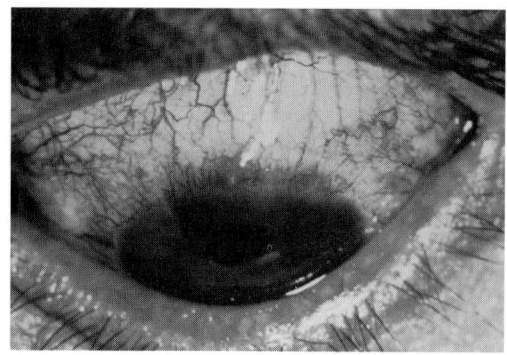

FIGURE 50–3. Trantas' dots at the superior limbus. These contain deposits of eosinophils.

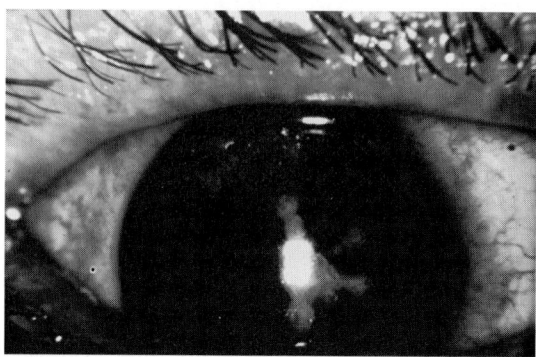

FIGURE 50–4. Atopic cataract in severe atopic keratoconjunctivitis.

continued rubbing of the eyes or with degenerative vitreous change is uncertain.

In atopic keratoconjunctivitis, if an inciting antigen can be identified it should be eliminated. Topical corticosteroids may be used for shorter periods; however, their long-term usage should be avoided. Some recent success has been obtained with the use of a mast cell stabilizer eyedrop. This medication prevents the release of mast cell mediators.

Surgery of atopic cataracts should not be undertaken lightly. Several investigators have reported complications such as severe hemorrhage, retinal detachment, iridocyclitis, and corneal edema. A relatively high incidence of pre- and postoperative retinal detachment has also been reported (Ingram, 1965; Coles and Laval, 1952). In patients with keratoconus associated with atopic eczema, penetrating keratoplasty may be carried out with a high degree of success.

Contact Dermatitis

Contact dermatitis is probably the most common immunologic disease encountered by dermatologists. It results from exposure of the skin to a wide variety of substances commonly found in the environment, including drugs, dyes, plant resins, preservatives, cosmetics, and metals. There are two varieties of contact dermatitis: irritant (the more common form) and allergic. *Irritant contact dermatitis* is caused by excessive moisture or by acids, alkalis, resins, or chemicals capable of injuring any person's skin if persistent contact is allowed. Allergy or hypersensitivity plays no role in irritant contact dermatitis. *Allergic contact dermatitis*, unlike the irritant variety, occurs only in sensitized individuals and involves the mechanism of cell-mediated immunity. In allergic contact dermatitis, an individual becomes sensitized to a given chemical or other sensitizing substance, and upon reexposure to the same chemical, an erythematous delayed skin reaction is elicited.

The eye is a frequent site of involvement in contact dermatitis (Duke-Elder, 1974). Drugs including neomycin sulfate (Fig. 50–5), atropine and its derivatives, chloramphenicol, penicillin, and related compounds may all act as sensitizers. Antazoline, an ophthalmic antihistamine solution, is also a potential sensitizer. Besides the skin lesions of contact dermatitis, contact sensitizers may produce a conjunctivitis characterized usually by papillary response, pronounced vasodilatation, chemosis, and watery discharge. An erythematous blepharitis may also occur, and in very severe cases, a keratitis typified by small yellow necrotic opacities just inside the limbus may develop. Primary irritant conjunctivitis can produce similar findings. The fine epithelial punctate keratitis produced by chronic use of gentamicin, topical anesthetics, echothiophate (phospholine iodide), phenylephrine, and epinephrine is well known to the ophthalmologist. In 1979, Mathias et al reported a convincing case of contact dermatitis and conjunctivitis associated with the use of tetracaine and two unusual allergens, echothiophate iodide and phylephrine hydrochloride.

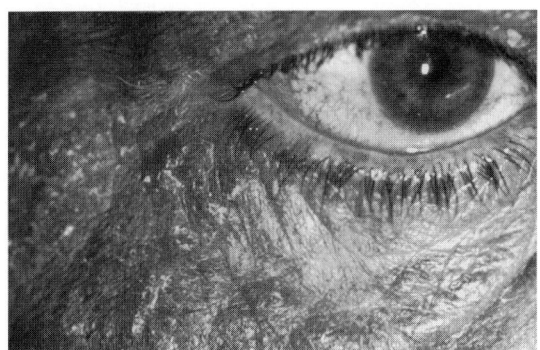

FIGURE 50–5. Contact dermatitis and conjunctivitis caused by eyedrops containing neomycin.

Rubbing the eyes after handling soaps, detergents, or chemicals may provoke a contact dermatitis reaction. Allergic reactions to cosmetics affect primarily the eyebrows and upper lids because of the method of application. Mascara, eyebrow pencil, and face creams all may act as allergens. Nail polish can cause sensitization around the eye by accidental touching of the area. Lip gloss and eye gloss cosmetics contain lanolin fractions that may also act as sensitizers.

Parabens are used in a great many lotions, creams, and cosmetics because they are excellent antimicrobial agents that prevent spoilage from bacterial and fungal growth. Paraben allergy was first reported in 1966 (Schorr and Mohajerin, 1966) and is now thought to be one of the leading causes of contact dermatitis. Nickel sulfate is a common sensitizer found in jewelry and undergarments. Chromates, which are used in costume jewelry, leather products, bleaches, industrial chemicals, fabrics, and automobile products, are common offenders. *p*-Phenylenediamine is widely used in hair dyes, clothing, and shoes. It contains a benzamide nucleus and may cross-react with a variety of therapeutic agents including sulfonamides, benzocaine, and hydrochlorothiazide.

The basis of treatment in contact dermatitis is the removal of the allergen or irritant.

For the conjunctivitis or keratoconjunctivitis that is associated with drugs that are primary irritant substances or contact allergens, the best treatment is withdrawal of the drug and substitution of an appropriate, non-irritating medication.

Vernal Keratoconjunctivitis

Vernal keratoconjunctivitis ("vernal") is a bilateral and often severe disease, occurring mainly in children and associated with climatic factors. It is characterized by a stringy, mucinous discharge and giant papillae of the upper palpebral conjunctiva. Many features of vernal keratoconjunctivitis suggest an allergic etiology. A recently described entity with similar but milder manifestations has been described in individuals who wear hard or soft contact lenses.

Immunopathology

Patients with vernal keratoconjunctivitis frequently have a history of atopic disease such as hay fever, atopic eczema, or asthma (Frankland and Easty, 1971). Sometimes, a history of atopy can be elicited only in a member of the patient's family. Increased levels of IgG can be detected in the tears of patients with vernal (Brauninger and Centifanto, 1971; Allansmith et al, 1976); even when the mean level of IgE in tears is not significantly greater than in control subjects, the serum IgE levels are significantly increased (Allansmith et al, 1976). In patients with vernal keratoconjunctivitis, IgA, IgD, and IgE are synthesized locally by conjunctival plasma cells in a ratio of approximately 4:1:2, respectively.

Histologically, the conjunctiva of patients with vernal keratoconjunctivitis contains many eosinophils, plasma cells, and fixed-tissue mast cells. Eosinophils and mast cells can also be demonstrated in scrapings of the conjunctiva. Additional histologic features have recently been described in this disease, including the presence of basophils, microvascular alterations of endothelial cells, and the deposition of fibrin. These features have suggested the possibility of a delayed hypersensitivity component in vernal because they are similar to the typical histologic features of cutaneous basophil hypersensitivity reactions (Collin and Allansmith, 1977). Other histologic features of vernal include infiltration by lymphocytes and neutrophils and epithelial invasion by mast cells and eosinophils.

Similar although milder histopathologic changes are present in the giant papillary conjunctivitis associated with the wearing of hard or soft contact lenses (Henley et al, 1973). In contrast to vernal conjunctivitis, this syndrome may not be more common in atopic patients and itching is mild, whereas in vernal it is severe. The inciting antigen in this condition is the material that accumulates over a period of time on the surface of the contact lens. This material may incite a hypersensitivity reaction with both humoral and cellular immune components.

Clinical Features

Vernal keratoconjunctivitis begins in the prepubertal years and is more common in boys than in girls. After the age of 20, the incidence in the two sexes is about the same. The peak incidence is between the ages of 11 and 13, and the disease is rare after age 30. Vernal is more common in warm climates than in temperate zones and is rarely seen in cold climates. Because of this geographic pattern, heat and other physical factors have been thought to contribute to the pathogenesis of the disease.

Patients complain of extreme itching and a ropy mucous discharge. The hallmark of vernal keratoconjunctivitis is the presence of giant papillae on the palpebral conjunctiva (Fig. 50–6). These papillae are polygonal and flat-topped and contain tufts of capillaries. The conjunctiva has a milky appearance, and many fine papillae may be present on the lower palpebral conjunctiva. A pseudomembrane may be present in severe cases (Maxwell-Lyons sign).

Corneal findings include superficial corneal ulcers and plaque-like deposits in the anterior cornea (Fig. 50–7). These contain mucus or many compacted layers of epithelial cells. The white dot-like deposits located at the limbus are known as Trantas' dots. They contain large numbers of eosinophils, and their presence parallels the activity of the disease.

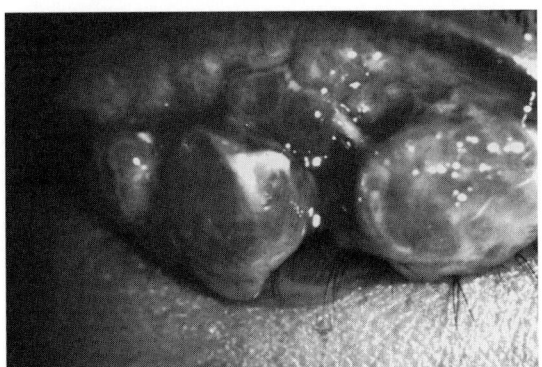

FIGURE 50–6. Giant papillae on the tarsal conjunctiva in a child with vernal keratoconjunctivitis.

Other corneal complications include a diffuse epithelial keratitis, a micropannus, and a pseudogerontoxon that is often adjacent to a limbic papilla. Conjunctival scarring does not occur in vernal unless the papillae have been treated with cryotherapy, irradiation, surgical removal, or other damaging procedures.

A limbic form of vernal keratoconjunctivitis with less involvement of the palpebral conjunctiva may also be seen. It is characterized by gelatinous swellings at the limbus. This form of vernal is said to be more common in blacks.

Treatment

Vernal keratoconjunctivitis is a self-limited disease that runs a 5- to 10-year course. Treatment, therefore, should be conservative and aimed at relieving symptoms without producing serious iatrogenic side effects. Topical and systemic corticosteroids are frequently used in treating this condition. Although they decrease the symptoms, they do not significantly affect the corneal complications or shorten the duration of the disease, and they may be associated with serious side effects. A short course of topical steroids is useful in breaking the inflammatory cycle. Their use should be supplemented with vasoconstrictors, cold compresses, ice packs, and climatotherapy. Having the patient move to a cool, moist climate or sleep in a cool or air-conditioned room has been associated with marked relief of symptoms in many cases. Hyposensitization therapy with grass pollens and other antigens may be helpful in some instances but in general has not been rewarding.

Mast cell stabilizer eyedrops have been used topically with good results (Henley et al, 1973; Tabbard and Arafat, 1977). This drug reduces itching, hyperemia, and mucous discharge. The giant papillae do not decrease in number with this therapy, but corneal complications seem to be lessened. The mast cell stabilizer, lodoxamide tromethamine, has recently become available as an eyedrop. Antihistamines, such as the potent H_1-receptor antagonist (Davis et al, 1990) levocabastine, may be helpful. Topical cyclosporine has also been used for short periods with encouraging results. However, long-term administration of this potent immunosuppressive drug has yet to be evaluated.

REFERENCES

Abelson MB, Chambers WA, Smith LM. Conjunctival allergen challenge. A clinical approach to studying allergic conjunctivitis. Arch Ophthalmol 108:84, 1990.

Allansmith MR, Hahn GS, Simon MA. Tissue, tear and serum IgE concentrations in vernal conjunctivitis. Am J Ophthalmol 81:506, 1976.

Allansmith MR, Hutchison D. Immunoglobulins in the conjunctiva. Immunology 12:225, 1967.

Allansmith MR, Korb DR, Greiner JV, et al. Giant papillary conjunctivitis in contact lens wearers. Am J Ophthalmol 83:697, 1977.

Allansmith MR, Radl J, Haaijman JJ, et al. Molecular forms of tear IgA and distribution of IgA subclasses in human lacrimal glands. J Allergy Clin Immunol 76:569, 1985.

Allansmith MR, Whitney CR, McClellan BH, et al. Immunoglobulins in the human eye: Location, type, and amount. Arch Ophthalmol 89:36, 1973.

Axelrod AJ, Chandler JW. Morphologic characteristics of conjunctival-associated lymphoid tissue in the rabbit. Invest Ophthalmol Vis Sci 17(suppl):182, 1978.

Beethan WP. Atopic cataract. Arch Ophthalmol 24:21, 1940.

Belfort R Jr, Mendez NF. T and B lymphocytes in the human conjunctiva and lacrimal gland. Invest Ophthalmol Vis Sci 17(suppl):182, 1978.

Bisgaard H, Ford-Hutchinson AW, Charleston S, et al.

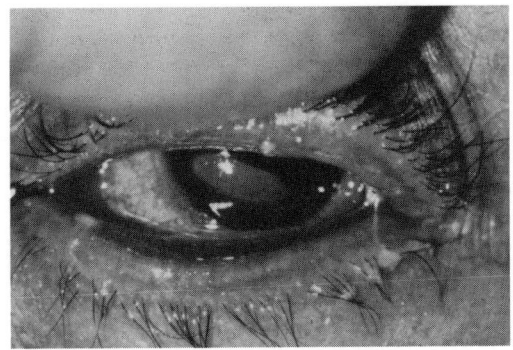

FIGURE 50–7. Corneal plaque (consisting of mucin and epithelial cells) in vernal keratoconjunctivitis.

Production of leukotrienes in human skin and conjunctival mucosa after specific allergen challenge. Allergy 40:417–423, 1985.

Bluestone R, Easty DL, Goldberg LS, et al. Lacrimal immunoglobulins and complement quantified by counter-immunoelectrophoresis. Br J Ophthalmol 59:279, 1975.

Brauninger GE, Centifanto YM. Immunoglobulin E in human tears. Am J Ophthalmol 72:558, 1971.

Broekhuyse RM. Tear lactoferrin: A bacteriostatic and complexing protein. Invest Ophthalmol 13:550, 1974.

Chandler JW, Gillette TE. Immunologic defense mechanisms of the ocular surface. Ophthalmology 90:585, 1983.

Chandler JW, Leder R, Kaufman HE, et al. Quantitative determinations of complement components in tears and aqueous humor. Invest Ophthalmol 13:151, 1974.

Coles RS, Laval J. Retinal detachments occurring in cataract associated with neurodermatitis. Arch Ophthalmol 48:30, 1952.

Collin HB, Allansmith MR. Basophils in vernal conjunctivitis in humans: An electron microscopic study. Invest Ophthalmol 16:858, 1977.

Copeman PWM. Eczema and keratoconus. Br Med J 2:977, 1965.

Davis JL, Mittal KK, Freidlin V, et al. HLA associations and ancestry in Vogt-Koyangi-Harada disease and sympathetic ophthalmia. Ophthalmology 97:1137, 1990.

Drutz DJ, Mills J. Immunity and infection. In Fudenberg HH, Stites DP, Caldwell JL, Wells JV (eds): Basic and Clinical Immunology. Los Altos, Lange, 1978.

Duke-Elder S. The ocular adnexa. In System of Ophthalmology. London, Henry Kimpton, 1974, Vol 13, Part I, p 58.

Dwyer RStC, Darougar S, Jones BR. Immediate hypersensitivity in the guinea pig conjunctiva. II. Effect of treatment with antihistamines, steroids and disodium cromoglycate. Mod Probl Ophthalmol 16:186, 1976.

Dwyer RStC, Turk JL, Darougar S. Immediate hypersensitivity in the guinea pig conjunctiva. I. Characterisation of the IgE and IgG antibodies involved. Int Arch Allergy Appl Immunol 46:910, 1974.

Frankland AW, Easty D. Vernal keratoconjunctivitis: An atopic disease. Trans Ophthalmol Soc UK 91:479, 1971.

Franklin RM. The ocular secretory immune system: A review. Curr Eye Res 8:599, 1989.

Franklin RM, Kenyon KR, Tomasi TB Jr. Immunohistologic studies of human lacrimal gland: Localization of immunoglobulins, secretory component and lactoferrin. J Immunol 110:984, 1973.

Friedlaender MH. Ocular allergy and immunology. J Allergy Clin Immunol 63:51, 1979.

Friedlaender MH. Conjunctival provocation tests: A model of human ocular allergy. Trans Am Ophthalmol Soc 87:577, 1990.

Friedlaender MH, Allansmith MR. Ocular allergy. Ann Ophthalmol 7:1171, 1975.

Friedlaender MH, Cyr R. Contact sensitivity in the guinea pig eye. Invest Ophthalmol Vis Sci 18(suppl):95, 1979.

Friedlaender MH, Ohashi Y, Kelley J. Diagnosis of allergic conjunctivitis. Arch Ophthalmol 102:1198–1199, 1984.

Greiner JV, Covington HI, Allansmith MR. Surface morphology of the human upper tarsal conjunctiva. Am J Ophthalmol 83:892, 1977.

Henley WL, Okas S, Leopold IH. Cellular immunity in chronic ophthalmic disorders. 4. Leukocyte migration inhibition in diseases associated with glaucoma. Am J Ophthalmol 76:60, 1973.

Horwitz BL, Christensen GR, Ritzman SR. Diurnal profiles of tear lysozyme and gamma A globulin. Ann Ophthalmol 10:75, 1978.

Imanishi J, Takahashi F, Inatomi A, et al. Complement levels in human tears. Jpn J Ophthalmol 26:299, 1982.

Ingram RM. Retinal detachment associated with atopic dermatitis and cataract. Br J Ophthalmol 49:96, 1965.

Josephson AS, Weiner RS. Studies of the proteins of lacrimal secretions. J Immunol 100:1080, 1968.

Karseras AG, Ruben M. Aetiology of keratoconus. Br J Ophthalmol 60:522, 1976.

Kimura SJ, Thygeson P. The cytology of external ocular disease. Am J Ophthalmol 39:137, 1955.

Mathias CGT, Maibach HI, Irvine A, et al. Allergic contact dermatitis to echothiophate iodide and phenylephrine. Arch Ophthalmol 97:286, 1979.

McClellan BH, Whitney CR, Newman LP, et al. Immunoglobulins in tears. Am J Ophthalmol 76:89, 1973.

McMaser PRB, Aronson SB, Bedford MJ. Mechanisms of the host response in the eye. IV. The anterior eye in germ-free animals. Arch Ophthalmol 77:392, 1967.

Pockley AG, Montgomery PC. In vivo adjuvant effect of interleukin 5 and 6 on rat tear IgA antibody responses. Immunology 73:19, 1991.

Schorr WF, Mohajerin AH. Paraben sensitivity. Arch Dermatol 93:721, 1966.

Sen DK, Sarin GS, Mani K, et al. Immunoglobulin in tears of normal Indian people. Br J Ophthalmol 60:302, 1976.

Spencer WH, Fisher JJ. The association of keratoconus with atopic dermatitis. Am J Ophthalmol 47:332, 1959.

Tabbara KF, Arafat NT. Cromolyn effects on vernal keratoconjunctivitis in children. Arch Ophthalmol 95:2184, 1977.

Thygeson P. The cytology of conjunctival exudates. Am J Ophthalmol 29:1499, 1946.

Vaughan D, Asbury T. General Ophthalmology. Los Altos, Lange, 1978.

Zimianski MC, Dawson CR, Togni B. Epithelial cell phagocytosis of *Listeria monocytogenes* in the conjunctiva. Invest Ophthalmol 13:623, 1974.

Chapter 51
Chronic Cough

Richard S. Irwin, M.D.

According to data obtained from a recent national medical care survey, cough is the most common complaint for which patients seek medical attention and the second most common reason for a general medical examination (Schappert, 1993). In addition, referrals of patients with chronic cough of unknown etiology have been shown to account for 10 to 36 percent of a pulmonologist's outpatient practice (Irwin et al, 1981; Irwin et al, 1990).

From a symptom standpoint, cough can be divided into two categories that are not mutually exclusive. It can be acute, lasting less than 3 weeks, or chronic, lasting 3 weeks or more. Acute cough is most commonly transient and of relatively minor consequence, as in the common cold. However, it can reflect a potentially life-threatening disorder such as pneumonia, congestive heart failure, pulmonary embolism, and aspiration syndromes, or it can persist and become a chronic problem. The duration of 3 weeks or more as the definition of chronic cough was initially chosen as a way of distinguishing the cough of the common cold from that of other more serious conditions. It is the management of the persistently troublesome, chronic cough on which this chapter will primarily focus.

DIAGNOSTIC EVALUATION

ANATOMIC DIAGNOSTIC APPROACH. In 1977, a systematic method for evaluating patients with chronic cough was proposed, based on the location of the afferent limb of the cough reflex (Irwin et al, 1977) (Fig. 51–1). This approach evolved as a result of a review of animal histologic data, case reports of clinical observations in man, and a few prospective, epidemiologic studies. From this review, it was reasoned by the author that cough could be caused by a multiplicity of conditions located in a variety of anatomic locations and that an anatomic diagnostic protocol would provide a framework for systematically evaluating patients with chronic cough. The validity of this approach has been verified on multiple occasions. Most importantly the anatomic diagnostic protocol has allowed us to discover and appreciate that extrapulmonary as well as pulmonary conditions commonly cause cough and that they need to be routinely considered as potential causes.

ANATOMIC DIAGNOSTIC PROTOCOL. The diagnostic protocol that I use and recommend is as follows.

1. Perform a history and physical exami-

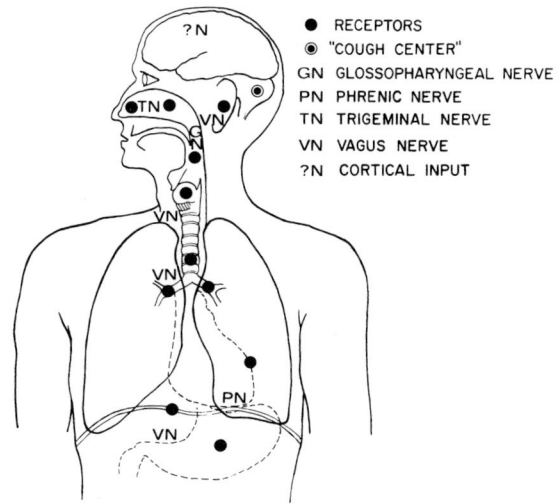

FIGURE 51–1. Schematic representation of the anatomy of the cough reflex. (From Irwin RS, et al. Cough: A Comprehensive review. Arch Intern Med 137:1186, 1977.)

nation, concentrating on the anatomy of the afferent limb of the cough reflex, specifically the most common causes of chronic cough. These are postnasal drip syndrome (PNDS), asthma, and gastroesophageal reflux disease (GERD).

2. Order a chest roentgenogram in all cases. It is extremely useful for initially ranking differential diagnostic possibilities and directing laboratory testing. A normal roentgenogram points to PNDS, asthma, and/or GERD as a likely diagnosis, and to bronchogenic carcinoma, sarcoidosis, and bronchiectasis as unlikely diagnoses.

3. Do not order additional laboratory tests in smokers or in patients taking an angiotensin converting enzyme inhibitor (ACEI) until the response to cessation of smoking or discontinuation of the drug for 4 weeks can be assessed.

4. Depending on the results of the initial evaluation, smoking cessation, or discontinuation of the ACEI, the following studies may be ordered.

  Sinus roentgenograms and allergy evaluation
  Spirometry pre- and post-bronchodilator (BD) or methacholine inhalational challenge (MIC)
  Barium esophagography (BaE) and/or 24-hour esophageal pH monitoring (EPM)
  Sputum for microbiology and/or cytology
  Fiberoptic bronchoscopy
  Noninvasive cardiac studies

Sinus roentgenograms and allergy evaluation are utilized to determine the possible causes of a PNDS, spirometry pre- and post-BD or MIC to diagnose asthma, and BaE or EPM to diagnose GERD. If the chest roentgenogram is normal or shows nothing more than inconsequential, stable scarring, evaluation should proceed according to the above order. If the chest roentgenogram is abnormal (e.g., shows a mass or localized/diffuse infiltrate), sputum studies and bronchoscopy should be performed sooner.

5. Determine the cause(s) of cough by observing which specific therapy eliminates cough as a complaint. Specific therapy is defined as therapy directed at the etiology or presumed operant pathophysiologic mechanism (e.g., the drip in PNDS). If the evaluation suggests more than one possible cause of cough, therapies should be initiated in the same sequence that the abnormalities were discovered. Since cough can be simultaneously caused by more than one condition, do not stop therapy that appears to be partially successful, but rather, sequentially add to it.

RESULTS OF THE ANATOMIC DIAGNOSTIC APPROACH. The anatomic diagnostic approach has been utilized in managing immunocompetent children as well as adults with chronic cough (Irwin et al, 1981; Poe et al, 1982; Poe et al, 1989; Irwin et al, 1990; Holinger and Sanders, 1991). The results can be summarized as follows.

1. The cause could be determined from 88 to 100 percent of the time, leading to specific therapy with success rates between 84 and 98 percent.

2. Although cough was most commonly due to a single cause in 73 to 82 percent of cases, it was due to multiple conditions up to 26 percent of the time (Fig. 51–2). Cough from multiple causes was reported to have three explanations 3 percent of the time.

3. Although most smokers have a cough, they were not the group of patients who commonly sought medical attention for cough.

4. In children above the age of 1 year, adults of all ages, and the elderly, PNDS, asthma, and GERD were the three most common causes of chronic cough.

5. Cough in adults was due most commonly to PNDS, asthma, GERD, and chronic bronchitis from cigarette smoking in 91 to 94 percent of cases.

6. Cough in adults who were nonsmokers, were not taking ACEI, and had normal or nearly normal chest roentgenograms was due to PNDS, asthma, and/or GERD 100 percent of the time.

7. Chronic cough can be the sole clinical manifestation of asthma and GERD up to 57 percent and 43 percent of the time respectively. MIC and 24-hour EPM were singularly helpful in diagnosing these patients.

8. Unless the chest roentgenogram is abnormal, an uncommon finding (4 to 7 percent), fiberoptic bronchoscopy will have a low diagnostic yield (4 percent).

9. The principal strength of the anatomic diagnostic protocol is in ruling out suspected conditions (Table 51–1). The limitation is that a positive test does not necessarily establish the diagnosis and cannot consistently predict a favorable response to specific therapy. For example, the negative and positive predictive values of an MIC for predicting that asthma

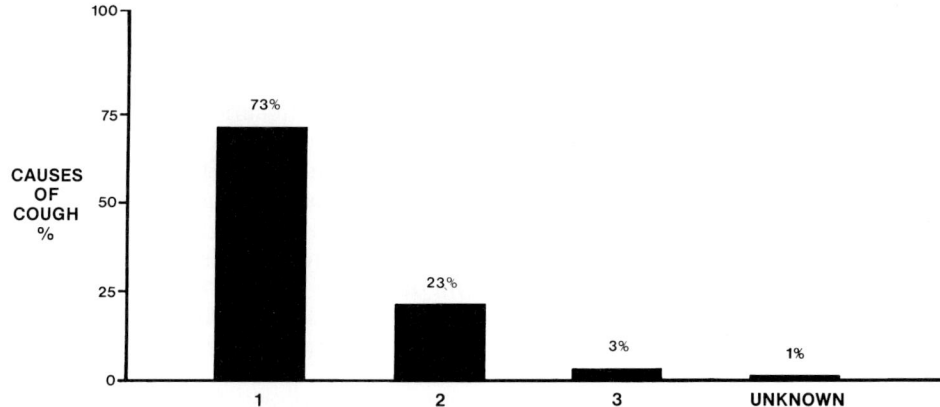
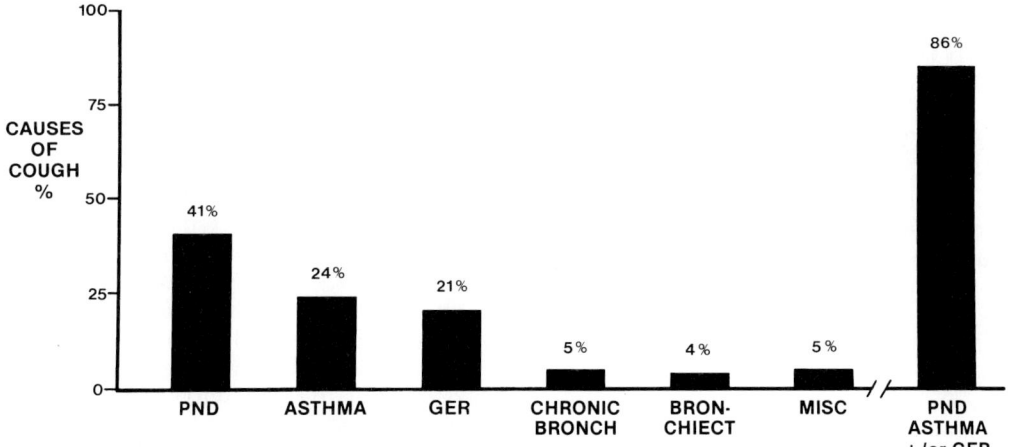

FIGURE 51-2. Representative causes of chronic cough from a prospective study. *Top panel*, The cause was determined in 99 percent of patients; it was due to a single condition in 73 percent and to multiple disorders in 26 percent. *Bottom panel*, The spectrum and frequency of the 131 causes (PND = postnasal drip syndrome; GER = gastroesophageal reflux; bronch = bronchitis; bronchiect = bronchiectasis; misc = miscellaneous). The miscellaneous conditions included bronchogenic carcinoma in two, left ventricular failure in one, stage 3 pulmonary sarcoidosis in one, angiotensin converting enzyme inhibitor drug in one, and aspiration from a Zenker's diverticulum in one. (From Irwin et al. Chronic cough: The spectrum and frequency of causes, key components of the diagnostic evaluation, and outcome of specific therapy. Am Rev Respir Dis 141:640–647, 1990.)

TABLE 51-1. TESTING CHARACTERISTICS OF COUGH PROTOCOL

Tests	N	Sens	Spec	PPV	NPV
Chest x-ray	100	100	76	36	100
Sinus x-ray	98	100	79	57	100
MIC	86	100	67	60	100
Barium esophagography	54	48	76	63	63
Esophageal pH	25	100	100	100	100
Bronchoscopy	23	100	92	89	100

Abbreviations: Sens = sensitivity; spec = specificity; PPV = positive predictive value; NPV = negative predictive value; MIC = methacholine inhalational challenge. (Modified from Irwin RS, et al. Chronic cough: The spectrum and frequency of causes, key components of the diagnostic evaluation, and outcome of specific therapy. Am Rev Respir Dis 141:640–647, 1990.)

is the cause of cough have been reported to be 100 percent and 60 percent respectively. In other words, when an MIC is negative, asthma is essentially ruled out as the cause of cough, except for the patient who may have occupational asthma in its earliest stage. In this circumstance, the test usually becomes positive as the exposure continues. However, since MICs can be falsely positive for predicting that asthma is causing the patient's cough, it must be stressed that a positive test by itself, without observing a favorable response to treatment, is only consistent with and not diagnostic of asthma as the cause of cough.

DIFFERENTIAL DIAGNOSIS AND SPECIFIC TREATMENT

POSTNASAL DRIP SYNDROME (PNDS). The diagnosis of PNDS is made when respiratory complaints such as cough, dyspnea, or wheeze are due to a postnasal drip. PNDS has been found to be the most common cause of chronic cough in adults of all ages and the second most common cause in children of all ages in most studies to date. Data from prospective studies suggest that the cough results from the stimulation of the afferent limb of the cough reflex in the upper respiratory tract (Curley et al, 1988). Causes include allergic, perennial nonallergic, postinfectious, environmental irritant, drug-induced (e.g., ACEI), and vasomotor rhinitis as well as sinusitis. PNDS should be considered when patients describe a sensation of having something drip down into the throat, a frequent need to clear the throat, and/or frequent nasal discharge. It should also be considered when physical examination of the oropharynx reveals mucoid or mucopurulent secretions or a cobblestone appearance of the mucosa. Cough due to the postnasal drip is also associated with an extrathoracic upper airway obstruction that can be demonstrated by flow-volume loops (Irwin et al, 1984; Curley et al, 1988). This obstruction disappears when postnasal drip and cough abate.

Allergic, perennial nonallergic, postinfectious, environmental irritant, and vasomotor rhinitis can be treated with intranasal corticosteroids and/or antihistamine-decongestant or antihistamine alone, and sometimes avoidance of environmental precipitating factor(s). Vasomotor rhinitis that fails to respond to the aforementioned measures can be treated with intranasal ipratropium bromide. Sinusitis should be treated with a combination of an antibiotic and an oral antihistamine-decongestant for at least 3 weeks, and decongestant nasal spray for 5 days. The newer, relatively nonsedating H_1 antagonists appear to be helpful only in the treatment of chronic cough due to those conditions known to be mediated by histamine, such as allergic rhinitis. It is likely that these newer agents have failed in non–histamine-mediated conditions, such as the common cold, when the older, potentially more sedating H_1 antagonists have succeeded because the newer drugs possess relatively little if any anticholinergic activity (Irwin et al, 1993a). The PNDS caused by ACEIs should respond to discontinuation of the drug.

ASTHMA. Asthma is the most common cause of chronic cough in children of all ages, the second in adults of all ages, and the third in the elderly. It should be considered as the cause of cough when patients complain of episodic wheezing and shortness of breath in addition to their cough, and when wheezing is heard on auscultation. Alternatively, it should be considered when reversible airflow obstruction is demonstrated by pulmonary function testing and when MIC is positive in the setting of normal spirometry and absence of wheeze.

Uncomplicated cough-variant asthma is easily treated. If bronchodilators and inhaled corticosteroids do not easily control the cough, either the cough is not due to asthma or it is due to asthma plus a condition making asthma difficult to control. A systematic protocol for managing difficult to control asthma can be found elsewhere (Irwin et al, 1993b) (see also Chapter 35). Occasionally, inhaled medications (e.g., bronchodilators and corticosteroids) provoke coughing. If the use of spacer devices and the switching of brands are to no avail, treatment with oral bronchodilators should be initiated.

GASTROINTESTINAL REFLUX DISEASE (GERD). The third most common cause of chronic cough in children of all ages and the third and second in adults of all ages and in the elderly is gastrointestinal reflux disease. Stimulation of the afferent limb of the cough reflex in the distal esophagus is believed to be the most likely reason for the development of cough in these patients, although reflux to the hypopharynx and larynx or frank aspiration can also contribute in some cases (Irwin et al, 1993c). GERD should be considered the cause of cough when patients complain of heartburn, a sour taste, or regurgitation, when upper gastrointestinal contrast roentgenograms demonstrate reflux of barium to the mid-esophagus or higher, when esophagoscopy shows esophagitis, or when esophageal pH monitoring shows cough to be associated with reflux episodes even in the absence of gastrointestinal symptoms.

Although some investigators have occasionally found it necessary to resort to antireflux surgery, our group has found an intensive antireflux medical regimen to be highly efficacious. The regimen has multiple components: (1) a high protein, low fat (45 gm) antireflux diet consisting of three daily meals, abstinence from foods and beverages that have the potential for decreasing the lower esophageal sphincter pressure and are of low acidity, and abstinence from food or beverage (except for medications) between meals or for 2 hours prior to reclining; (2) a 4-inch elevation of the head of the bed; and (3) medications that include metoclopramide, cisapride, H_2 antagonists, and/or sucralfate. Since it has been our bias that the diet is the most important component of the regimen, most patients see a nutritionist in consultation and receive detailed verbal and written instructions on the diet each time they are seen in clinic. Patients with cough due to GERD have been successfully treated with this regimen after they had failed to improve with H_2 antagonist therapy alone. Successful therapy for chronic cough due to GERD is usually relatively prolonged, averaging 5 to 6 months (Irwin et al, 1989; Irwin et al, 1990), and it may take up to 2 to 3 months of treatment before the cough even begins to improve.

BRONCHIECTASIS. Bronchiectasis should be suspected when cough is associated with expectoration of more than 30 ml of purulent sputum in 24 hours, fever, hemoptysis, weight loss, and malaise. The plain chest roentgenogram is suggestive of bronchiectasis in 90 percent of cases. Occasionally, high-resolution CT scanning of the chest is necessary to confirm the diagnosis. Bronchiectasis is treated with antibiotics, chest physiotherapy and postural drainage, and drugs that stimulate mucociliary clearance (e.g., theophylline, beta-adrenergic agonists).

CHRONIC BRONCHITIS. Chronic bronchitis is diagnosed as the cause of cough when the following four criteria are met: (1) the patient expectorates phlegm on most days during periods spanning at least 3 consecutive months, and such periods have occurred for more than 2 consecutive years; (2) alternative cough-phlegm syndromes such as PNDS, asthma, and bronchiectasis have been ruled out; (3) the patient is known to be exposed to irritating dust, fumes, or smoke; and (4) the cough goes away when the respiratory irritant is eliminated. In cases of cigarette smoking, cough goes away or markedly decreases in 94 percent of cases after abstinence for at least 4 weeks.

ANGIOTENSIN CONVERTING ENZYME INHIBITORS (ACEIs). Cough attributable to ACEI should be suspected when cough begins within 1 year after the initiation of the drug. It is well documented that a substantial number of patients using ACEIs will develop cough (Irwin et al, 1993a). Recent studies suggest that the pathogenesis in some way involves prostaglandins, mainly through the accumulation of bradykinin in the tracheobronchial tree. Evidence supporting this comes from studies showing that sulindac, nifedipine, and indomethacin attenuate the cough associated with ACEIs. Since cough should disappear within 4 weeks of discontinuance of the drug, the most definitive treatment is to discontinue its use altogether. Nifedipine is a dihydropyridine calcium channel antagonist that may inhibit prostaglandin synthesis. While reducing the severity of the cough, it also acts to further lower blood pressure. Therefore, in patients with troublesome cough who have cardiovascular disorders that have responded to an ACEI, combining nifedipine and an ACEI may be an alternative to withdrawing the ACEI.

MISCELLANEOUS CONDITIONS. There is an almost endless number of miscellaneous causes of chronic cough. From a purely statistical standpoint, these causes are much less commonly encountered than those conditions discussed above. By following the anatomic diagnostic protocol, it is possible to diagnose them with a high degree of success and then institute specific therapy. For instance, the cough due to pulmonary embolism responds to intravenous anticoagulation, resectable bronchogenic carcinoma to surgery, sarcoidosis to corticosteroids, and left ventricular failure associated with atrial fibrillation to digitalis and diuretics. The psychogenic or tic-related cough is a diagnosis of exclusion; its delineation and treatment may be more difficult.

SUMMARY

Chronic cough is one of the most common symptoms that physicians have to manage. If one utilizes a systematic, anatomic diagnostic protocol, the cause can be determined in most cases. Once the specific etiology has been identified, specific therapy should be prescribed because it has a high likelihood of being successful. Since specific therapy should be successful in the greatest majority of cases, there should be little need to prescribe nonspecific antitussive therapy. A recent review of nonspecific antitussive therapy can be found elsewhere (Irwin et al, 1993a).

REFERENCES

Curley FJ, Irwin RS, Pratter MR, et al. Cough and common cold. Am Rev Respir Dis 138:305–311, 1988.

Holinger LD, Sanders AD. Chronic cough in infants and children: An update. Laryngoscope 101:596–605, 1991.

Irwin RS, Corrao WM, Pratter MR. Chronic persistent cough in the adult: The spectrum and frequency of causes and successful outcome of specific therapy. Am Rev Respir Dis 123:413–417, 1981.

Irwin RS, Curley FC, Bennett FM. Appropriate use of antitussives and protussives: A practical review. Drugs 46:80–91, 1993a.

Irwin RS, Curley FC, French CL. Difficult to control asthma: Contributing factors and outcome of a systematic management protocol. Chest 103:1662–1669, 1993b.

Irwin RS, Curley FJ, French CL. Chronic cough: The spectrum and frequency of causes, key components of the diagnostic evaluation, and outcome of specific therapy. Am Rev Respir Dis 141:640–647, 1990.

Irwin RS, French CL, Curley FC, et al. Chronic cough due to gastroesophageal reflux: Clinical, diagnostic, and pathogenetic aspects. Chest 104:1511–1517, 1993c.

Irwin RS, Pratter MR, Holland PS, et al. Postnasal drip causes cough and is associated with reversible upper airway obstruction. Chest 85:346–352, 1984.

Irwin RS, Rosen JM, Braman SS. Cough: A comprehensive review. Arch Intern Med 137:1186–1191, 1977.

Irwin RS, Zawacki JK, Curley FC, et al. Chronic cough as the sole presenting manifestation of gastroesophageal reflux. Am Rev Respir Dis 140:1294–1300, 1989.

Poe RH, Harder RV, Israel RJ, et al. Chronic persistent cough: Experience in diagnosis and outcome using an anatomic diagnostic protocol. Chest 95:723–728, 1989.

Poe RH, Israel RH, Utell MJ, et al. Chronic cough: Bronchoscopy or pulmonary function testing? Am Rev Respir Dis 126:160–162, 1982.

Schappert SM. National Ambulatory Medical Care Survey: 1991. Summary. Vital and Health Statistics No. 230. U.S. Department of Health and Human Services, March 29, 1993, pp 1–20.

Chapter 52

Headaches

Roger M. Katz, M.D., and Sheldon C. Siegel, M.D.

Headache is a common medical complaint and a frequent reason for seeking medical advice. The most common headaches in childhood are migraine, tension, and probably sinus related. It has been estimated that 4 percent of school children suffer from migraine and/or vascular headaches (Bille, 1962). In the adult, migraine is more common than in children, as are sinus-related headaches, skeletal muscular spasm, temporomandibular joint syndrome, anxiety, and other psychogenic causes. It is not the purpose of this chapter to discuss headaches stemming from serious central nervous system conditions such as brain tumors and meningitis. The cost of treatment and quality of life from headache can be over $2 billion dollars per 6 million sufferers in the United Kingdom (Editorial, 1992). The cost of treatment in the United States will obviously be much higher.

MIGRAINE HEADACHE

Migraine-type headaches can be subclassified as classic, common, cluster, or complicated (Shinnar and D'Souza, 1982). These headaches differ from each other. *Classic migraine* is characterized by contralateral neurologic manifestations (visual) with both unilateral and contralateral pulsatile pain. *"Common"* migraines are associated with hours or days of disturbances such as edema, irritability, pallor, dizziness, and sweating, along with bilateral pain. *Cluster migraines* are characterized by unilateral facial pain of high intensity lasting less than 2 hours (Duvoisin, 1972). Concomitant ipsilateral tearing, nasal congestion, and conjunctival injection may occur. The bouts may be frequent with total freedom of pain in between. *Complicated* migraines often include all of the above plus disturbances in speech as well as ocular and hemiplegic occurrences. Migraines have been triggered by hypoglycemia causing reflex vasodilatation.

MUSCLE TENSION HEADACHE

Muscle tension or muscle contraction headache involves the insertions of those muscles at the occiput (e.g., sternocleidomastoid) and scalp, including the muscles of the temporomandibular joint (TMJ). These headaches are generalized, achy, and nonpulsatile and are described as tightness (band-like or vise-like). The muscle contraction is accompanied by vascular spasm and local ischemia resulting in tenderness and local "pain" as well (Pikoff, 1984). Pressure applied to these tender localities may aggravate the headache "pain" or soreness and cause it to spread to adjacent portions of the head. This may be triggered by the simple act of combing one's hair.

COUGH SYNCOPE

Headaches frequently occur after cough syncope attacks related to bronchospasm owing to transient hypoxemia and decreased blood flow to the CNS during the syncopal episode. This may also occur during seizure disorders.

MEDIATORS

Vasoactive mediators can also cause painful dilated arteries. These mediators, such as tyramine and phenylethylamine (monoamines), and serotonin may be byproducts of ingested foods such as milk products, chocolate, and bananas. Monosodium glutamate, caffeine, nitrates, metabisulfites, steroid, ethanol, and sulfonylureas are chemicals that can be associated with headaches induced through both vasoconstriction and vasodilation (Egger et al, 1983). Rebound headaches occur with coffee (caffeine) withdrawal, typified by the "executive weekend" headache. Headaches are often associated with drugs taken for other systemic problems. These include decongestants, antibiotics, beta blockers, calcium channel blockers, diuretics, and bronchodilators.

SINUS HEADACHE

Headache of sinus origin generally is due to inflammation and fluid retention in the sinus, which in turn cause a stretching of the mucosal membranes. These headaches are described as either painful or tender to external sinus pressure, or as a pressure or binding-type headache most commonly over the frontal and/or temporal and/or maxillary areas bilaterally. The symptoms are directly proportional to the degree of obstruction of the ostiomeatal complex (Graham, 1990). An apparent vacuum-type headache occurs when the ostiomeatal complex acts like a valve and the air within the sinus is absorbed, resulting in local hypoxia (Stammberger, 1986). It is not known whether this deep ache is related to the stretch receptors or other mucosal receptors.

ANXIETY

Psychogenic headaches are frequently observed in depressed children and adults. This mood disorder is characterized by withdrawal, irritability, aggression, lack of energy, somatic complaints, poor school or work performance, feeling of worthlessness, and poor eating and sleeping habits. Anxiety disorders may also be associated with headaches. At times anxiety and tension can cause headaches via muscle spasm. Neurologic examination of these individuals usually results in normal findings.

EVALUATION OF THE PATIENT WITH HEADACHE

The approach to the subject with headache is similar to that for other conditions beginning with a history and physical examination, appropriate laboratory tests, and therapy. Important historical clues to the origin of headaches include the intensity and quality (pounding, aching, pressure, or pain), location, frequency, duration, aggravating factors, and distinguishing features such as blurred vision, sixth nerve palsy, and ataxia. Headaches in which factors are suspected to be related to allergy require an additional history pertinent to allergen exposures.

Headaches occur with a variety of historical characteristics, which may overlap in their presentation (Table 52–1). The physical examination often is helpful in making a more definitive diagnosis. Point tenderness elicited over the maxillary, external, and frontal sinuses may confirm acute sinus disease although it is not a consistent or necessary indication of disease. Examination of the mucosal membrane can show inflammatory lesions such as granulomata, cysts, or polyps. Fundoscopic examination for papilledema as well as sixth nerve evaluation for nerve palsies may suggest brain tumors or pseudotumor cerebri. Meningeal irritation or inflammation is often associated with nuchal rigidity. Headaches owing to trauma are often associated with hemiparesis, somnolence, irritability, loss of vision or visual fields and brain stem signs, personality changes, dizziness, and depression. A localized bruit may suggest a vascular abnormality. Headaches associated with the finding of hypertension may lead to a suspicion of renal, endocrine, or cardiovascular disease as an underlying cause. An endoscopic nasal examination can be helpful in identifying sinus ostiomeatal blockage as well as drainage from specific sinus ostia.

Laboratory and imaging evaluation are strongly dependent on history and physical examination. Nasal cytology may show eosinophils if an allergic mechanism is present. A predominance of polymorphonuclear cells may suggest an underlying sinusitis. Sinus roentgenogram or CT scans can be helpful in diagnosing sinusitis. CT and/or MRI brain scans should be considered if there is elevated intracranial pressure or meningismus, or if significant neurologic changes occur with a

TABLE 52–1. HEADACHE EVALUATION

	Frequency	Intensity	Location	Course	Duration	Associated Signs/Symptoms	Common Key Physical Findings	Lab Considerations
Migraine	1–3 times/year to 2–4 times/week	Moderate to severe throbbing	Unilateral to diffuse	Fluctuates	Hours to ≥24 hours	GI, Aura Fm Hx	Bruit Light sensitivity, blindness, hemiplegia, ataxia, vertigo	Differential diagnosis
Seizure	Variable	Mild to severe	Frontal to diffuse	Sudden onset	Minutes to hours	Fm Hx febrile Neonatal distress Other seizure events	Ictal event	EEG CT scan
Increased CNS pressure	Wax/wane with increases daily	Day to day change	Generalized	Progressive	Hours	Blurred or double vision	Fundoscopic neurologic exam	CT scan or MRI LP
Meningeal irritation	Acute	Mild to moderate	Occiput to paracervical	Acute	Hours	Memory loss Poor balance Blurred vision Fever	Nuchal rigidity	LP CT scan
Trauma	Acute to 2 weeks after accident	Moderate to severe	Occiput Paracervical Bifrontal Generalized	Progressive	Hours to constant	Dizziness Irritability Depression Anxiety Loss of taste/smell Increased by exertion, noise, heat, light	Hemiparesis Somnolence Blindness Brain stem	CT scan or MRI
Sinus	Occasional to frequent	Mild to severe	Directly over sinus to temporal to diffuse	Sudden onset to insidious onset	Hours to constant	Respiratory allergy, PND, cough (originally at night) Recurrent URI and O.M.	Point tenderness in acute disease Endoscopic exam of nasal passages	Sinus Water's x-ray vs. CT scan vs. MRI
TMJ	Infrequent to daily	Mild to moderate	TMJ to temporal to frontal	Fluctuates	Hours to constant	Tension, abnormal TMJ, teeth grinding	Auscultatory click over TMJ	X-ray of TMJ
Tension (muscle contraction)	Daily	Mild to moderate	Local to general	Variable	Hours to days	None	Loose muscle tenderness	None

DRUG THERAPY

Over the past three decades there have been advances in our understanding of the pathophysiology of head pain. Recent pharmacology has made many medicines available for the management of headaches. Several newer classes of drugs are specific in alleviating various types of headaches. Hence, the physician must try to identify the cause of headache in order to select the most appropriate agent and optimize the response to pharmacotherapy.

Migraine

The drug treatment of migraine headaches has been reviewed by Welch, Gallagher, and Matthew (Welch, 1993; Gallagher et al, 1990; Matthew, 1990). The goals of migraine treatment are twofold: (1) to relieve the symptoms of an acute attack, and (2) to suppress the frequency and severity of further attacks by behavioral or pharmacologic means. The behavioral approach commonly involves regular sleep and meals and avoidance of triggering factors.

Treatment of Acute Migraine

The acute episode of migraine usually can be aborted if medication is taken either during the aura or at the first inkling of onset of migraine without aura. The most effective drugs for this purpose are ergot preparations, nonsteroidal anti-inflammatory agents, sumatriptan, dopamine antagonists, and analgesic drugs (Table 52–2). The latter include aspirin, acetaminophen, propoxyphene, and codeine—all of which have been shown to be more effective than placebo in relieving the pain of migraine (Hakkarainen et al, 1989). Combinations of isometheptene with acetaminophen and dichloral phenazone (Midrin) and aspirin in combination with caffeine and butalbital (Fiorinal) may be helpful in some patients who are unresponsive to other analgesic drugs. Major narcotic analgesics are also useful for emergency treatment of severe migraine attacks. Because of their addictive properties, they should be limited to patients who have infrequent attacks, patients with peripheral vascular or coronary artery disease, and pregnant women in whom antimigraine drugs may be contraindicated.

Recently, sumatriptan (Imitrex), a serotonin receptor agonist, has been shown to be highly effective for treating acute attacks of migraine. In three collaborative studies, a subcutaneous dose of 6 mg resulted in 70 to 80 percent improvement within 1 to 2 hours of treatment (Cady et al, 1991; Stammberger, 1986). When it was given orally in 100-mg doses, 75 percent of patients reported relief of headache and other symptoms within 4 hours (Oral Sumatriptan International Multiple-Dose Study Group, 1991). Because of its vasoconstrictor properties, sumatriptan should not be administered to patients with a history of coronary artery disease and should not be used with ergotamine preparations or other vasoconstrictor drugs. Sumatriptan is not indicated for prophylaxis of migraine.

Protracted Migraine

For protracted migraine attacks the dopamine antagonists—metoclopramide (Reglan), chlorpromazine (Thorazine), or prochlorperazine (Compazine)—are useful agents. In one double-blind, randomized trial, chlorpromazine was superior to dihydroergotamine in relieving acute migraine (Jones et al, 1989). Infrequent side effects of the three drugs include dystonia and tardive dyskinesia, drowsiness, nausea, vomiting, dizziness, and hypotension. The mechanism by which these drugs relieve headache remains unknown. It has been postulated that they are effective via (1) adrenergic blockade, (2) antiserotonin activity, (3) antiemetic action, and (4) modulation of pain systems (Bell et al, 1990).

PROPHYLACTIC MEASURES

Efforts to prevent migraine are warranted if attacks occur two or more times a month, if the headaches are incapacitating, if the attacks are complicated by prolonged neurologic signs, or if nonpharmacologic measures have failed. Because patients respond in a variable manner to prophylactic agents, prophylactic therapy may require more than one

TABLE 52-2. DRUG TREATMENT OF ACUTE MIGRAINE ATTACKS

Type of Drug	Adult Dosage (mg)	Pediatric Dosage	Important Side Effects
Analgesics			
Aspirin	500–650 bid	10–15 mg/kg q4–6h	Dyspepsia, GI hemorrhage
Acetaminophen	500 3–4×/24 hr	5–10 mg/kg q4–6h	Dyspepsia
Propoxyphene	65 q4h	Not recommended	Addiction
Codeine	60 q4h	Not recommended	Addiction, constipation
Nonsteroidal anti-inflammatory drugs (NSAID)			
Naproxen Na	275 bid-tid	2.5–5 mg/kg q12h	Dyspepsia, GI hemorrhage
Tolmetin Na	200–400 tid-qid	Not recommended	Dyspepsia, GI hemorrhage
Fenoprofen Ca	300–600 tid-qid	Not recommended	Dyspepsia, GI hemorrhage
Meclofenamate Na	50 q4–6h	Not recommended	Dyspepsia, GI hemorrhage
Flubiprofen	100 bid-tid	Not recommended	Dyspepsia, GI hemorrhage
Diclofenac Na	50–75 bid-tid	Not recommended	Dyspepsia, GI hemorrhage
Ibuprofen	400–800 tid-qid	Not recommended	Dyspepsia, GI hemorrhage
Ketorolac tromethamine (IM)	30–60 qd	Not recommended	Dyspepsia, GI hemorrhage
			All NSAID are contraindicated in aspirin-intolerant asthmatic patients
5-Hydroxytryptamine (5-HT)			
Ergotamine			
Oral	2 tabs stat, 1 tab q 1/2 hr.	Not recommended	Nausea, vomiting, abd pain, diarrhea
Suppository	1 suppos hourly (max dosage 2 suppos)	Not recommended	Muscle cramps, limb paresthesia, vasoconstriction
Sublingual	1 sublingually, may repeat in 1/2 hr (max dosage 3 in 24 hr)	Not recommended	
Dihydroergotamine (IM)	1 ml q hr (max 3 inj/24hr)	Not recommended	
Sumatriptan Subcutaneous	6 mg max dose 2 inj/24 hr 1 hr apart	Not recommended	Flushing, heat, tingling, neck pain, chest heaviness, pressure pain
Dopamine antagonist			
Metoclopramide IV	10 qd	Not recommended	Dystonia
Chlorpromazine IM	12.5–25 mg q4h until vomiting stops		Tardive dyskinesia
Prochlorperazine IV	2.5–10 mg qd slow IV injection for nausea and vomiting	0.03 mg/kg IM	

GI = gastrointestinal.
Modified from Welch KMA. Drug therapy of migraine. N Engl J Med 329:1476–1483, 1993.

agent. Administration of each agent is initiated at a relatively low dose and the dose gradually increased over several weeks, depending on the patient's tolerance and response. Drugs used in prophylactic treatment of migraine are shown in Table 52-3.

The medications most commonly used and considered the treatment of choice for prophylaxis are the beta-adrenergic blocking drugs. Propranolol is the agent most widely studied for the prevention of migraine; however, other beta-adrenergic antagonists are also effective. Their mechanism of action in the treatment of headaches is poorly understood. These drugs are contraindicated in patients with bronchospasm, cardiac arrhythmias, or a history of depression.

Tricyclic antidepressants have central analgesic actions unrelated to their antidepressant effects and can be useful in preventing migraine (Couch and Hassanein, 1979). The combination of a beta blocker and tricyclic antidepressant has been shown to be more beneficial than either drug alone.

TABLE 52-3. PROPHYLACTIC DRUG TREATMENT OF MIGRAINE

Type of Drug	Dosage (mg)	Important Side Effects
5-HT-influencing*		
Methysergide	2–8 qd	Muscle cramps, insomnia, tissue fibrosis
Amitriptyline	10–150 qd	Weight gain, drowsiness, dry mouth, blurred vision, cardiac arrhythmias, urinary retention, muscle cramps
Beta-adrenergic antagonists		
Propranolol	80 1–4×/24 hr	Fatigue, nausea, depression, bradycardia, hypotension, bronchospasm
Metroprolol	100 bid	
Atenolol	50–100 qd	
Nadolol	40–80 qd	
Calcium channel blockers		
Nifedipine	10–30 tid	Headache, tachycardia, depression
Nimodipine	60 tid	Headache, tachycardia, depression, weight gain, constipation
Verapamil	80–120 tid	Headache, bradycardia, depression, weight gain, constipation
NSAID†		
Naproxen Na	275 bid-tid	Dyspepsia, gastritis, GI bleeding, diarrhea
Tolmetin	200–400 tid-qid	
Fenoprofen	300–600 tid-qid	
Meclofenamate Na	50 q4-6h	
Flurbiprofen	100 bid-tid	
Diclofenac	50–75 bid-tid	
Ibuprofen	400–800 tid-qid	
Aspirin	500–650 bid	
Miscellaneous		
Valproic acid	15 mg/kg/24 hr initial dose max 60 mg/kg/24 hr	Hair loss, weight gain, hepatic dysfunction, neural-tube defect

*5-hydroxytryptamine (serotonin).
†NSAID = nonsteroidal anti-inflammatory drugs.
Modified from Welch KMA. Drug therapy of migraine. N Engl J Med 329:1476–1483, 1993.

The effectiveness of calcium channel blockers in the prevention of migraine has been more controversial (McArthur et al, 1989). In general, they tend to decrease the frequency of attacks but have little effect on their severity.

Methysergide (Sansert), a serotonin antagonist, is a potent prophylactic agent but has limited usefulness because of its tendency to cause retroperitoneal, cardiac valvular, and pleural fibrosis with prolonged usage. It is also contraindicated in patients with vascular disease because of its vasoconstrictor action.

In a small clinical trial, valproate sodium (800 mg daily) was shown to be moderately effective in reducing the severity, frequency, and duration of migraine headache (Hering and Kuritzky, 1992). Agents used to treat acute attacks of migraine may also be helpful in preventing recurrent attacks. Repeated doses of nonsteroidal anti-inflammatory drugs (NSAID) or ergotamine preparations administered in divided doses or as long-acting preparations have proved useful.

OTHER HEADACHES

A cluster headache is considered to be a variant of migraine but may be responsive to corticosteroids and lithium (Couch, 1982; Ekbom, 1981). The use of histamine desensitization, H_1 and H_2 antagonists, to treat cluster headaches has been controversial with few well-designed studies to support their use. Treatment of other types of headaches is based on the etiology of the headache. Muscle contraction headache usually responds to analgesics. However, persistent use of these agents has also been reported to perpetuate this type of headache, and such agents should be withdrawn before other medications are tried (Speed, 1990). Tricyclic antidepressants, tranquilizers, and muscle relaxants in addition to other drugs used in the management of migraine may be of benefit. When associated with depression, a psychiatric evaluation should be considered.

Ingestant Related Headaches

Although it has been recognized since Hippocrates that ingestion of food may provoke headaches, the role of food allergy in causing headaches has been controversial. This is largely due to the subjective nature of evaluating headaches and because few double-blind trials with suspected foods have been carried out.

Many anecdotal reports have appeared in the literature claiming that a migraine headache may be produced by food hypersensitivity reactions. Monro, in a chapter entitled Food-Induced Migraine, has referred to many of these early reports (Monro, 1987; Mansfield et al, 1985; Egger et al, 1983). Double-blind, placebo-controlled studies suggest that in some patients migraine might be related to an underlying specific IgE food allergy. More commonly and more likely, migraine headaches are exacerbated by pharmacologic properties of foods, either an endogenous component of the food itself or an exogenous chemical that has been added to the food.

The vasoactive amines (histamine and monoamines, tyramine, phenylethylamine, and serotonin) are contained in many foods and are in many instances known to precipitate migraine headaches. Because histamine released by IgE-mediated mechanisms plays a major role as a mediator in virtually all atopic diseases, it is not unusual for a histamine-mediated pharmacologic reaction that includes headaches to be mistaken for an allergic reaction induced by a food. Recently, Wanthe et al (1993) have suggested that some patients have diminished histamine degradation based on a deficiency of diamine oxidase and that the ingestion of histamine-rich foods causes headache in these patients; symptoms of headache reportedly decreased when these subjects were placed on a histamine-free diet. Their histamine-free diet eliminated some fishes, cheeses, hard cured sausages, pickled cabbage, spinach, tomato ketchup, and some wines and beer.

The vasoactive amine tyramine is also found in large quantities in several foods and beverages that have been recognized to trigger acute migraine (Hanington, 1967) and produce severe headache in patients receiving monoamine oxidase (MAO) inhibitors. The headache has been postulated to be due to the sharp rise in blood pressure that follows the ingestion of tyramine in such patients, presumably owing to high levels of tyramine, which is vasoconstrictive. Another monoamine, phenylethylamine, is found in various cheeses, especially Gouda and Stilton, in red wine, and in chocolate. Other substances that have been reported to precipitate migraine include nitrates, sodium nitrite, monosodium glutamate (Chinese restaurant syndrome), and aspartame (Perkin, 1990).

REFERENCES

Bell R, Montaya D, Shudib A, Lee MA. A comparative trial of three agents in the treatment of acute migraine headache. Ann Emerg Med 19:1079–1082, 1990.

Bille B. Migraine in school children. Acta Paediatr Scand 5:136, 1962.

Cady RK, Wendt JD, Kirchner JR, Sargent SD, Rothrock JF, Skaggs H Jr. Treatment of acute migraine with subcutaneous sumatriptan. JAMA 265:2831–2835, 1991.

Couch JR, Hassanein RS. Amitriptyline in migraine prophylaxis. Arch Neurol 36:695–699, 1979.

Couch JR. Cluster headache: Characteristics and treatment. Semin Neurol 2:30–49, 1982.

Duvoisin RC. The cluster headache. JAMA 222:1403–1404, 1972.

Editorial. Sumatriptan, serotonin, migraine and money. Lancet 339:151–152, 1992.

Egger J, Wilson J, Carter CM, Turner MW, Soothill JF. Is migraine food allergy? A double-blind controlled diet of oligoantigenic diet treatment. Lancet 2:865–869, 1983.

Ekbom K. Lithium for cluster headache: Review of the literature and preliminary results of long-term treatments. Headache 21:132–139, 1981.

Gallagher RM, Meyer JS, Ichijo M, Kobari M, Lofti J, Rose FC, Davies PTG, Solomon GD. Prophylactic treatment of migraine. In Gallagher RM (ed). Drug Therapy for Headache. New York, Marcel Dekker, 1990, pp 65–94.

Graham JK. Headache of nasal origin. J Louisiana Med Soc 122:(2)375–379, 1990.

Hakkarainen H, Quiding H, Stockman O. Mild analgesics as an alternative to ergotamine in migraine: A comparative trial with acetylsalicylic acid, ergotamine tartrate, and dextropropoxyphene compound. J Clin Pharmacol 20:590–595, 1989.

Hanington E. Preliminary report on tyramine headache. Br Med J 2:550–551, 1967.

Hering R, Kuritzky A. Sodium valproate in the prophylactic treatment of migraine: A double-blind study versus placebo. Cephalgia 12:81–84, 1992.

Jones S, Sklar D, Dougherty J, White W. Randomized double-blind trial of intravenous prochlorperazine for the treatment of acute headache. JAMA 261:1174–1176, 1989.

Mansfield LE, Vaughn TR, Waller SF, Haverly RW, Ting

S. Food allergy and adult migraine double-blind and mediator confirmation of an allergic etiology. Ann Allergy 55:126–129, 1985.

Matthew NT. The abortive treatment of migraine. *In* Gallagher RM (ed). Drug Therapy for Headache. New York, Marcel Dekker, 1990, pp 95–113.

McArthur JC, Marek K, Pestronk A, McArthur J, Perouka SJ. Nifedipine in the prophylaxis of classic migraine: A crossover, double-masked, placebo-controlled study of headache frequency and side effects. Neurology 23:266–277, 1989.

Monro J. Food-induced migraine. *In* Brostoff J, Challacombe SJ (eds). Food Allergy and Intolerance. London, Baillière Tindall, 1987, pp 633–665.

Oral Sumatriptan International Multiple-Dose Study Group. Evaluation of a multiple-dose regimen of oral sumatriptan for the acute treatment of migraine. Eur Neurol 31:306–313, 1991.

Perkin JE. Adverse food reactions: Relationship to arthritis and migraine. *In* Perkin JE (ed). Food Allergies and Adverse Reactions. Gaithersburg, Maryland, Aspen Publishers, 1990, pp 171–187.

Pikoff H. Is the muscular model of headache still viable? Headache 24:186, 1984.

Shinnar S, D'Souza B. Migraine in children and adolescents. Pediatrics in Review. 3:8, 1982.

Speed WG. Treatment of muscle contraction (tension) headache. *In* Gallagher RM. Drug Therapy for Headache. New York, Marcel Dekker, 1990, pp 151–161.

Stammberger H. Nasal and paranasal sinus endoscopy—a diagnostic and surgical approach to recurrent sinusitis. Endoscopy 6:213–218, 1986.

Wanthe F, Gotz M, Jarisch R. Histamine-free diet: Treatment of choice for histamine-induced food intolerance and supporting treatment for chronical headaches. Clin Exp Allergy 23:982–985, 1993.

Welch KMA. Drug therapy of migraine. N Engl J Med 329:1476–1483, 1993.

Chapter 53

Asthma and Allergy During Pregnancy

Michael Schatz, M.D., and Robert S. Zeiger, M.D., Ph.D.

Asthma complicates approximately 4 percent of pregnancies (National Asthma Education Program Report of the Working Group on Asthma and Pregnancy, 1992), and allergic disease occurs in approximately 20 percent of women of childbearing age. These disorders probably represent the most common group of medical conditions that complicate pregnancy. The coexistence of these illnesses with pregnancy raises a number of important questions: (1) What is the effect of the specific disorder on the course and outcome of pregnancy? (2) What is the effect of pregnancy on the course of the specific illness? (3) What is the optimal management of these disorders during pregnancy and lactation with respect to the welfare of both the mother and the baby? This chapter will attempt to provide practical answers to these questions.

RELEVANT PHYSIOLOGY OF NORMAL PREGNANCY

Maternal Pulmonary Physiology

Increased placental progesterone production is believed to be responsible for the increase in tidal volume and resulting relative hyperventilation of pregnancy (Schatz et al, 1993). This hyperventilation leads to an increased Po_2 (100 to 106 mm Hg) and decreased Pco_2 (28 to 30 mm Hg) in normal pregnant women. Although other lung volume changes occur during pregnancy (most prominently decreased functional residual capacity), these are of doubtful significance to patients with asthma, and measures of airway obstruction (FEV_1, FEV_1/FVC ratio or maximum mid-expiratory flow rates) do not change during normal pregnancy (National Asthma Education Program Report of the Working Group on Asthma and Pregnancy, 1992; Schatz et al, 1993).

Fetal Oxygenation

The human placenta acts as a simple concurrent exchanger. Fetal umbilical vein blood leaving the placenta exists in oxygen equilibrium with maternal uterine vein blood (Schatz et al, 1993; Cousins and Catanzarite, 1993). As a consequence, fetal umbilical vein blood has the highest fetal Po_2 and can never exceed maternal venous Po_2. The fetus, however, normally tolerates this relatively low Po_2 (30 to 37 mm Hg) because of increased oxygen-carrying capacity of fetal hemoglobin, differences between adult and fetal oxygen-hemoglobin dissociation curves, high fetal cardiac output, and a unique distribution of fetal cardiac output. Nonetheless, maternal hypoxia (especially <60 mm Hg), reduced uteroplacental blood flow (e.g., from hypotension), and even hypocapnia and alkalosis (such as may occur with early acute asthma) may compromise fetal oxygenation. It is important to point out that, because maternal compensatory mechanisms tend to maintain systemic arterial pressure and oxygenation of vital maternal organs at the expense of uteroplacental blood flow, fetal distress can occur even in the absence of maternal hypotension or hypoxia (National Asthma Education Program Report of the Working Group on

Asthma and Pregnancy, 1992). This dictates the necessity for aggressive monitoring of fetal well-being during critical maternal illness. Finally, it is reassuring to know that when fetal hypoxia is a consequence of maternal hypoxia, maternal oxygen therapy has the potential to significantly increase fetal oxygen content (Cousins and Catanzarite, 1993).

Immunologic Changes

Some maternal immunologic changes have been reported during pregnancy (Table 53-1). It is not clear, however, whether any of these is clinically relevant to maternal health or illness during pregnancy (Schatz et al, 1993; Galbraith and Galbraith, 1993).

GENERAL THERAPEUTIC PRINCIPLES

Psychologic Support

Asthma and allergies may add to the stress of normal pregnancy, and conversely, this stress may aggravate asthma and allergies. It is important that anxiety in pregnant women regarding their illness and its interrelationships with pregnancy be reduced by (1) giving them the opportunity to express their concerns, and (2) educating them regarding their illness and its interactions with pregnancy (Stone and Brown, 1993). Such education should also improve patient compliance.

Although the vast majority of pregnant women with asthma or allergic disease require no additional psychologic intervention, an occasional patient with unusual stress or impaired coping mechanisms may require psychiatric consultation. This may be necessary either for the psychologic symptoms themselves or because of a substantial adverse effect of the psychologic state on the medical illness, or both.

Immunologic Management

The first tenet of immunologic therapy is avoidance, and this is particularly important during pregnancy, since avoidance procedures increase the likelihood of physical well-being without pharmacologic intervention (Kershaw-McLennan and Spector, 1993). Full information on antigen avoidance (see Chapter 15) and irritant avoidance should be given

TABLE 53-1. SUMMARY OF MATERNAL IMMUNOLOGIC CHANGES DURING PREGNANCY

Parameter	Change During Pregnancy
Cell counts	
Total white count	Increased
Neutrophils	Increased
Lymphocytes	No change (absolute count)
Monocytes	Increased
T/B cell ratio	No change
CD4/CD8 ratio	No change
Immunoglobulins	
IgG	Decreased
IgA	Some decrease (hemodilution)
IgM	Some decrease (hemodilution)
IgE	No consistent change
Antigen-specific antibody response	No change
Autoantibodies	
Rheumatoid factor	No change in titer
Immune complexes	No increase in titer
In vivo lymphocyte responsiveness	
Allograft rejection	No change
Delayed skin tests	No change
In vitro lymphocyte responsiveness	
PHA	Unchanged in majority of studies
Antigen	Conflicting data
Mixed lymphocyte	No change
In vitro functional changes	
Suppresser cell activity	Increased
Interleukin-2 producton	Decreased in some studies
Natural killer function	Decreased
Pregnancy serum	
Effect on lymphocyte responsiveness	Decreased (to PHA, viral antigens, alloantigens)
Effect on monocyte responsiveness	Decreased

From Galbraith GMP, Galbraith RM. Maternal immunologic changes in pregnancy. *In* Schatz M, Zeiger RS (eds). Asthma and Allergy in Pregnancy and Early Infancy. New York, Marcel Dekker, 1993.

to the patient. The patient should be convinced that a decision to trade symptoms and possibly medication for an avoidable adverse exposure is extremely unwise during pregnancy when both she and the baby stand to suffer. This is particularly important regarding cigarette smoking, which may directly adversely affect the pregnancy as well as exacerbate the rhinitis or asthma (Schatz et al, 1993).

Abortions associated with systemic reactions following allergen immunotherapy have been reported (Francis, 1941). In experienced hands, however, allergy immunotherapy during pregnancy appears to be safe. A study of 121 pregnancies in 90 women receiving inhalant allergen immunotherapy reported no increase in abortions, fetal deaths, neonatal deaths, prematurity, toxemia, or congenital malformations in the treated patients in comparison with a nontreated pregnant allergic control group and with the general population (Metzger et al, 1978). In addition, preliminary information suggests that continuation of venom immunotherapy during pregnancy does not increase the risk of perinatal complications (Schwartz et al, 1990).

Based on this information, it is recommended that allergen immunotherapy be carefully continued during pregnancy in patients already receiving it if they (1) appear to be deriving benefit, (2) are not prone to systemic reactions, and (3) are at maintenance or at least receiving a therapeutic dosage. Dose reduction is usually appropriate to further decrease the risk of a systemic reaction, and for the same reasons, patients early in their course of immunotherapy may be best served by discontinuing their treatment during pregnancy. Benefit/risk considerations do not favor beginning immunotherapy during gestation for most patients owing to (1) the undefined propensity for systemic reactions in such patients, (2) the increased likelihood that systemic reactions will occur during initiation of immunotherapy, (3) the latency of immunotherapy effect, and (4) the frequent difficulty in predicting which allergic patients will benefit from immunotherapy, especially for asthma (Schatz et al, 1993; Kershaw-McLennan and Spector, 1993).

Because skin testing with potent antigens may also be associated with systemic reactions, some physicians defer routine allergy skin testing until the postpartum period. Even in patients not previously skin tested, historical information will often suggest dust, mold, dander, or pollen sensitivities for which avoidance instructions may be empirically given. Determination of specific IgE antibodies could be safely performed by sensitive *in vitro* assay (i.e., RAST, ELISA) if confirmation of historically relevant allergens seems necessary during pregnancy (Kershaw-McLennan and Spector, 1993).

Pharmacologic Management

Drug-induced congenital malformations remain the major concern for the physician prescribing a medication to the pregnant patient. In this regard, it is important to realize that congenital malformations are recognized in 3 to 8 percent of all newborns, and of these, only 1 percent or fewer can be attributed to drug exposure (National Asthma Education Program Report of the Working Group on Asthma and Pregnancy, 1992). Other potential adverse effects of medication administered during pregnancy include (1) abortion, (2) fetal death, (3) reduced intrauterine growth, (4) adverse effect on function of developing organs, such as the central nervous system, (5) effect on maternal or uteroplacental vasculature or uterine smooth muscle, and (6) effect of transplacentally administered drugs in the newborn (Abrams, 1993).

Because of the aforementioned possible effects, the ideal pharmacologic therapy during pregnancy is *no* pharmacologic therapy, especially during the first trimester. However, pregnant patients with medical complications must be evaluated for pharmacologic therapy with a thorough appreciation of the adverse effects on reproductive outcome of untreated or poorly treated disease. Thus, a number of women with asthma or allergic diseases require pharmacologic therapy during pregnancy to prevent disease severe enough to be life-threatening to the mother or to be threatening to the fetus through hypoxemia. In addition, many women with asthma or allergic diseases require gestational pharmacologic therapy to provide an adequate level of comfort so that the illness does not adversely affect the pregnancy indirectly through interference with sleeping, eating, or emotional well-being.

The choice of a specific medication for use during pregnancy is based on a number of considerations:

1. *Human data*. Although statistical and ethical considerations make it unlikely that any drug will be "proven safe" based on experimental human studies, negative observational human data are reassuring (Scialli and Lione, 1993).

2. *Animal data*. If an agent is appropriately tested in animals and found not to be a developmental toxicant, its potential for developmental toxicity in humans is low (Scialli and Lione, 1993). Positive data in animal studies are not as useful because it is often not possible to know whether the effects on the offspring were caused by the high doses used,

maternal toxicity, or species differences (National Asthma Education Program Report of the Working Group on Asthma and Pregnancy, 1992).

3. *FDA categories.* In 1979, the United States Food and Drug Administration (FDA) established five categories to indicate a drug's potential for causing adverse effects during pregnancy (Table 53–2) and mandated that newly approved drugs introduced after November 1, 1980, be classified into one of these categories in the package insert. These categories are based on the available animal studies, the available human data, and a consideration as to whether the benefit of the drug's use during pregnancy outweighs its risk. No asthma or allergy medication labeled to date meets the requirements for pregnancy category A. One may wish to choose class B versus C drugs among equally effective alternatives owing to the reassuring animal studies. Some authorities believe that because a large amount of information of varying quality may not be adequately represented by a single-letter designation, the FDA category system is not useful for making therapeutic decisions (Scialli and Lione, 1993).

4. *Other considerations.* A topical medication would appear to be preferable to a systemic one owing to a reduced likelihood of fetal penetration. An older medication for which there is more experience in gestational use may be preferable to a newer medication. Finally, efficacy must also be considered in the choice of a medication for use during pregnancy.

Based on the foregoing considerations, the National Asthma Education Program Report of the Working Group on Asthma and Pregnancy (1992) has recommended the asthma and allergy medications in Table 53–3 as "preferred for use during pregnancy." The Working Group recommends that alpha-adrenergic compounds (other than pseudoephedrine), epinephrine (other than for anaphylaxis), iodides, sulfamonamides (in late pregnancy), tetracyclines, and quinolones be avoided during pregnancy. The data on which these recommendations are based are presented elsewhere in the literature (Schatz et al, 1993; Scialli and Lione, 1993). Because less drug reaches the infant through breast milk than reaches the fetus through the placenta, and based on the recommendations of the American Academy of Pediatrics Committee on Drugs (1989), the Working Group's recommendations apply to the lactating mother as well.

In our litigious society, the medicolegal implications of prescribing asthma and allergy medications during pregnancy must be considered. A number of steps have been recommended to reduce medicolegal jeopardy in managing gestational asthma and allergies (Schatz et al, 1993):

1. Discuss with the patient that, while relatively few medications of any kind have been *proved* harmful during pregnancy, no asthma/allergy medication can be considered to be *proved* absolutely safe.

2. Discuss with the patient the potential direct and indirect consequences for the mother and for the baby of inadequately controlled disease.

TABLE 53–2. FOOD AND DRUG ADMINISTRATION PREGNANCY CATEGORIES INDICATING DRUG RISK

Category	Animal Studies	Human Data	Benefit May Outweigh Risk
A	Negative*	Studies† negative	Yes
B	Negative	Studies not done	Yes
B	Positive‡	Studies negative	Yes
C	Positive	Studies not done	Yes
C	Not done	Studies not done	Yes
D	Positive or negative	Studies or reports positive	Yes
X§	Positive	Studies or reports positive	No

*No teratogenicity demonstrated
†Adequate and well-controlled studies in pregnant women
‡Teratogenicity demonstrated
§Drug is contraindicated during pregnancy

From Schatz M, Hoffman CP, Zieger RS, et al. The course and management of asthma and allergic diseases during pregnancy. *In* Middleton E Jr, Reed CE, Ellis EF, et al (eds). Allergy: Principles and Practice. St Louis, Mosby-Year Book, 1993.

TABLE 53-3. PREFERRED DRUGS FOR ASTHMA AND ASSOCIATED CONDITIONS DURING PREGNANCY

Drug Class	Specific Drug	Rationale
Anti-inflammatory	Cromolyn sodium	Topical; reassuring animal and human data
	Beclomethasone dipropionate	Topical; reassuring human data; longer duration of experience than alternatives; efficacy
	Prednisone	Reassuring human data; benefits outweigh risks
Bronchodilator	Inhaled β_2-agonist	Topical; reassuring human data
	Theophylline	Reassuring human data; long duration of experience
Antihistamine	Chlorpheniramine	Reassuring animal and human data; long duration of experience
	Tripelennamine	Reassuring animal and human data; long duration of experience
Decongestant	Pseudoephedrine	Reassuring animal and human data
	Oxymetazoline	Topical; reassuring human data

Recommendations of the Working Group on Asthma and Pregnancy (1992) of the National Asthma Education Program.

3. Discuss with the patient the concept that there are medications that appear safe enough to permit their use in preference to the uncontrolled illness that would result if they are not used.

4. Discuss the alternative medication choices available for the patient's particular situation and the rationale for choosing among those alternatives.

5. Clearly document in the chart that the above discussion has taken place—that the benefits, risks, and alternatives of the specific pharmacologic approach have been discussed with the patient and her informed consent to that approach has been obtained.

COURSE AND MANAGEMENT OF SPECIFIC ILLNESSES DURING PREGNANCY

Asthma

DIFFERENTIAL DIAGNOSIS. The differential diagnosis of asthma during pregnancy includes those entities that must be excluded in nonpregnant patients (see Chapter 35). In addition, there are several conditions unique to pregnancy that must be considered. Pulmonary edema, typically associated with nocturnal dyspnea but occasionally associated with wheezing, may be caused during pregnancy by *tocolytic therapy* or *peripartum cardiomyopathy*. The latter entity usually presents during the last 2 months of gestation or in the immediate postpartum period but is otherwise indistinguishable from other forms of dilated congestive cardiomyopathy (Elkayam et al, 1992). *Dyspnea of early or late pregnancy* is not associated with wheezing, cough, or airway obstruction. *Amniotic fluid embolism* usually presents with acute respiratory distress during labor or delivery with cyanosis, shock and bleeding, but wheezing may occasionally occur (Schatz and Zeiger, 1992).

EFFECT OF ASTHMA ON PREGNANCY. Eight controlled studies have been published over the past two decades comparing the outcomes of pregnancy in women with asthma with outcomes in nonasthmatic women. All of the studies except one have reported an increase in one or more of the following adverse outcomes in the pregnancies of asthmatic compared with control women: perinatal mortality (Gordon et al, 1970; Bahna and Bjerkedal, 1972), low-birth-weight infants (Bahna and Bjerkedal, 1972; Lao and Huengsberg, 1990; Perlow et al, 1992), preterm births (Bahna and Bjerkedal, 1972; Perlow et al, 1992), preeclampsia (Bahna and Bjerkedal 1972; Stenius-Aarniala et al, 1988), and chronic gestational hypertension (Dombrowski et al, 1986; Schatz et al, in press). In addition, more severe asthma has been associated with a greater risk in most (Gordon et al, 1970; Mabie et al, 1992; Perlow et al, 1992) but not all (Lao and Huengsberg, 1990) studies.

The mechanism(s) of these adverse effects of maternal asthma are not totally clear. An important role for the degree of control of the asthma is suggested by the observations that (1) asthma managed by specialists did not increase the risk of perinatal mortality compared with nonasthmatic controls (Stenius-Aarniala et al, 1988; Schatz et al, in press), and (2) uncontrolled asthma as defined by hospitalization for asthma (Greenberger and

Patterson, 1988) or lower gestational pulmonary function (Schatz et al, 1990) was associated with poorer intrauterine growth. However, other factors associated with more severe asthma cannot be easily excluded.

For example, pregnancies in asthmatic women receiving oral corticosteroids compared with those not receiving such therapy have been reported to be more frequently complicated by preeclampsia (Stenius-Aarniala et al, 1988), delivery of low-birthweight and preterm infants (Perlow et al, 1992), and intrauterine growth retardation (Mabie et al, 1992). Although these data were poorly controlled for potential confounding factors such as smoking, race, other medication use, and degree of asthma control, a more recent study designed to control for these factors did not prove to be definitive. In the Kaiser Permanente study of 486 asthmatic women compared with 486 matched controls (Schatz et al, in press), an increased risk of preeclampsia and low-birthweight infants in the pregnancies of asthmatic women requiring corticosteroids could neither be confirmed nor reliably excluded. Moreover, even if women requiring corticosteroids are at increased risk for these complications, the available data cannot differentiate the relative roles of the corticosteroid medication, less well-controlled asthma, or potentially other factors, such as autonomic nervous system–related vascular hyperreactivity in asthmatic women (Kaliner et al, 1982), in causing these adverse outcomes.

Effect of Pregnancy on Asthma. Studies addressing the effect of pregnancy on asthma have been recently reviewed (Juniper and Newhouse, 1993). In the reported studies with sample sizes ranging from 16 to 366, asthma improved in 0 to 69 percent of patients, worsened in 0 to 44 percent, and remained unchanged in 6 to 100 percent. The discrepancies between study results were attributed to differences in outcome measures and different definitions of clinically important changes in the course of the disease. In addition, differences in asthma severity between study populations may also play a role since it has been reported that patients with more severe asthma prior to pregnancy may be more likely to experience a worsening of their disease during pregnancy than patients with milder asthma (Williams, 1967; Gluck and Gluck, 1976). The variable effect of pregnancy on the course of asthma appears to be more than just random fluctuation in the natural history of the disease, since the changes women attribute to pregnancy generally revert to the prepregnancy course within 3 months postpartum (Schatz et al, 1988). It is also of interest that the course of asthma is often consistent in an individual woman during successive pregnancies (Williams, 1967; Schatz et al, 1988).

Additional observations have been made concerning the course of asthma during pregnancy. Upper respiratory tract infections appear to be the most common precipitants of severe asthma during pregnancy (Williams, 1967). Patient noncompliance may also be associated with poor asthma control during pregnancy, especially in adolescents (Apter et al, 1989). The peak incidence of flares during pregnancy appears to be between the twenty-fourth and thirty-sixth weeks of gestation (Gluck and Gluck, 1976), particularly in women whose asthma worsens with pregnancy (Schatz et al, 1988). In contrast, asthma usually improves during the last 4 weeks of pregnancy and is generally quiescent during labor and delivery (Schatz et al, 1988).

The exact mechanisms responsible for the altered asthma course during pregnancy are unknown. There are multiple biochemical, physiologic, and psychologic factors that could potentially ameliorate or exacerbate gestational asthma (Table 53–4). It seems probable that the importance of individual factors varies from patient to patient, and it is presumably the combination of these factors that determines what effect, if any, pregnancy will have on the course of asthma.

Management of Chronic Asthma During Pregnancy. It should be emphasized at the outset that frequent, regular historical, auscultatory, and spirometric follow-up by physicians skilled in managing asthma is essential to ensure optimal success and safety of asthma management during pregnancy. Home monitoring of peak expiratory flow rates should be considered in women with particularly severe or labile disease; in women with high or low panic-fear asthma coping styles; or in women experiencing substantial dyspnea of pregnancy, which is confounding their assessment of their asthma. All pregnant patients with asthma should have facilitated access to their asthma physician for increased symptoms (Patterson et al, 1990).

The goals of outpatient asthma therapy in pregnant women are not different from such

TABLE 53-4. PHYSIOLOGIC CHANGES DURING PREGNANCY THAT MAY AFFECT THE COURSE OF ASTHMA

Factors that may improve asthma	Factors that may worsen asthma
Progesterone-mediated bronchodilation	Pulmonary refractoriness to cortisol effects because of competitive binding to glucocorticosteroid receptors by progesterone, aldosterone, or deoxycorticosterone
Estrogen or progesterone-mediated potentiation of β-adrenergic bronchodilation	
Decreased plasma histamine-mediated bronchoconstriction (due to increased circulating histaminase)	Prostaglandin F_{2a}–mediated bronchoconstriction
	Decreased functional residual capacity with resultant airway closure during tidal breathing and altered ventilation-perfusion ratios
Pulmonary effects of increased serum free cortisol	
Glucocorticosteroid-mediated increased β-adrenergic responsiveness	Increased placental major basic protein reaching the lung
Prostaglandin E–mediated bronchodilation	Increased viral or bacterial respiratory infection-triggered asthma
Prostaglandin I_2–mediated bronchial stabilization	
Atrial natriuretic factor–induced bronchodilation	Increased gastroesophageal reflux–induced asthma
Increased half-life or decreased protein binding of endogenous or exogenous bronchodilators	Increased stress

From Schatz M. Asthma during pregnancy: Interrelationships and management. Ann Allergy 68:123, 1992.

goals in nonpregnant patients: (1) prevention of severe asthmatic episodes, (2) prevention of asthma that interferes with sleep or normal activity, and (3) maintenance of optimal pulmonary function. The immunologic and psychologic therapy previously discussed is particularly applicable to the management of asthma during pregnancy. It is particularly important that pregnant patients with asthma be educated regarding their illness and its interaction with pregnancy in order to reduce anxiety and to improve compliance. Several examples of educational material for pregnant asthmatic patients have been published (Ziment, 1989; Patterson et al, 1990; National Asthma Education Program, 1993). It is also important that effective three-way communication exists among the physician managing the asthma, the patient, and the obstetrician.

The recommendations of the National Asthma Education Program Report of the Working Group on Asthma and Pregnancy (1993) regarding pharmacologic step therapy of chronic asthma are summarized in Table 53–5. The emphasis on the use of inhalational therapy seems appropriate during pregnancy, but respiratory tract penetration of the drugs must be optimized by appropriate inhaler technique and the use of spacer devices (Newhouse and Dolovich, 1986).

Two medications, salmeterol and nedocromil, have become available in this country since the Working Group completed its report. Animal studies with nedocromil have been reassuring (FDA class B), whereas those with salmeterol have not (FDA Class C), but there are no published human data with either drug. Although these drugs would not generally be recommended for use during pregnancy instead of older $beta_2$ agonists,

TABLE 53-5. PHARMACOLOGIC STEP THERAPY OF CHRONIC ASTHMA DURING PREGNANCY

Category	Frequency/Severity of Symptoms	Pulmonary Function† (Untreated)	Step Therapy
Mild	<3 times per week Nocturnal symptoms <2/month	>80%	Inhaled $β_2$-antagonists as needed
Moderate	≥3 times per week Exacerbations affect sleep or activity	60–80%	Inhaled cromolyn Substitute inhaled beclomethasone Add oral theophylline
Severe	Daily Limited activity Frequent nocturnal symptoms Frequent acute exacerbations	<60%	Above + oral corticosteroids (burst for active symptoms, alternate day or daily if necessary)

*Based on the recommendations of the National Asthma Education Program Report of the Working Group on Asthma During Pregnancy (1993).
†FEV_1 or PEFR based on the norm for the patient, which may be standardized norms or personal best.

cromolyn or beclomethasone, benefit-risk considerations may favor their continuation during pregnancy in patients who have demonstrated a good therapeutic response to either of these medications prior to becoming pregnant.

MANAGEMENT OF ACUTE ASTHMA DURING PREGNANCY. Objective as well as subjective parameters must be evaluated in pregnant women presenting with acute asthma. Although the resting pulse in pregnant women may be somewhat elevated, pulse rates greater than 120 in afebrile pregnant women with acute asthma generally reflect severe disease and less often are due to sympathomimetic excess, anxiety, anemia, or combinations of factors. The amount of pulsus paradoxus correlates with asthma severity in nonpregnant patients (see Chapter 35). Although this sign has not been systematically evaluated in acute gestational asthma, a pulsus paradoxus greater than 18 mm Hg in a pregnant woman with acute asthma must be considered to represent more severe asthma until proved otherwise.

Expiratory flow measurements (peak expiratory flow rate or FEV_1) and pulse oximetry should be obtained in pregnant women presenting with acute asthma. Since a pulse oximetry measurement of less than 95 percent may be associated with a PO_2 of less than 60 mm Hg (Ries, 1987), arterial blood gases should be obtained in women whose oxygen saturation determined by pulse oximetry is less than 95 percent. Arterial blood gases should also be obtained in patients with persisting severe disease (PEFR <200 L/minute or FEV_1 <1.0 L) after the first hour of treatment. Appropriate fetal monitoring is also an essential aspect of the management of acute gestational asthma (Cousins and Catanzarite, 1993; National Asthma Education Program Report of the Working Group on Asthma and Pregnancy, 1993).

Supplemental oxygen (initially 3 to 4 L/min by nasal cannula) should be immediately administered to pregnant women presenting with acute asthma and the FIO_2 adjusted to maintain a PaO_2 ≥70 and/or O_2 saturation by pulse oximetry ≥95 percent. The recommendations of the National Asthma Education Program Report of the Working Group on Asthma and Pregnancy (1993) regarding the pharmacologic management of acute asthma during pregnancy are summarized in Table 53–6.

Parenteral corticosteroids should be administered along with initial therapy to patients on regular corticosteroids. In addition, parenteral corticosteroids should be administered to subjects with severe initial impairment in whom no improvement is observed after the initial dose of β_2-agonist and in those patients with persisting severe airflow obstruction (PEFR <200 L/min, FEV_1 <40 percent predicted) after 1 hour of intensive beta-agonist therapy (National Asthma Education Program Report of the Working Group on Asthma and Pregnancy, 1993). There are no data on the pharmacokinetics of exogenous corticosteroids administered during pregnancy, and dosages of corticosteroids recommended for pregnant patients are not generally different from those recommended for nonpregnant patients.

Since it has been demonstrated that intravenous aminophylline provides no additional benefit to optimal inhaled β_2-agonist therapy in the first 4 hours of treatment, and that it may increase the side effects, intravenous aminophylline is not generally recommended in the emergency room management of acute

TABLE 53–6. PHARMACOLOGIC MANAGEMENT OF ACUTE ASTHMA DURING PREGNANCY

1. Nebulized β_2-agonist bronchodilator
    Up to 3 doses in first 60–90 minutes
    Every 1–2 hours thereafter until adequate response
2. Intravenous methylprednisone, with initial therapy in patients on regular corticosteroids and for those with poor response during the first hour of treatment (see text)
    1 mg/kg every 6–8 hours
    Taper as patient improves
	3. Consider intravenous aminophylline (generally only if patient requires hospitalization). If it is to be used:
	    6 mg/kg loading dose
	    0.5 mg/kg/hour maintenance dose
	    Adjust rate to keep theophylline level between 8 and 12 µg/ml
	4. Consider subcutaneous terbutaline 0.25 mg if patient is not responding to the above therapy

Based on the recommendations of the National Asthma Education Program Report of the Working Group on Asthma During Pregnancy (1993).

gestational asthma (National Asthma Education Program Report of the Working Group on Asthma and Pregnancy, 1993). It may be considered for patients who require hospitalization, particularly those in impending or frank respiratory failure. If it is to be used, pharmacokinetic studies during pregnancy support the dosage recommendations in Table 53–6.

For patients who are not helped by the initial therapy, blood gases must be carefully observed. Pregnant patients with a Po_2 less than 70 or Pco_2 greater than 35 must be monitored particularly closely (Hollingsworth et al, 1989). Criteria for hospital admission of the pregnant woman with status asthmaticus probably should be more lenient than for a patient in the nongravid state. When the pregnant asthmatic is hospitalized, both medical and obstetrical supervision are required. The use of intubation and assisted ventilation for life-threatening asthma during pregnancy is occasionally necessary; the management of respiratory failure during pregnancy is described elsewhere in the literature (Hollingsworth and Irwin, 1992).

MANAGEMENT OF ASTHMA DURING LABOR AND DELIVERY. Although asthma exacerbations during labor are uncommon, it is recommended that patients taking inhaled cromolyn, inhaled corticosteroids, or oral theophylline continue this therapy during labor (National Asthma Education Program Report of the Working Group on Asthma and Pregnancy, 1993). Patients experiencing some asthma symptoms during labor usually either require no medication or are adequately controlled by inhaled beta-agonists. If the patient's asthma responds poorly to inhaled beta-agonists, intravenous methylprednisone should be administered (Table 53–6). Patients on regular corticosteroids or who have received frequent courses during pregnancy should receive supplemental steroids for the stress of labor, delivery, and the puerperium: 100 mg hydrocortisone intravenously at admission, followed by 100 mg intravenously every 8 hours for 24 hours or until the absence of complications is established (National Asthma Education Program Report of the Working Group on Asthma and Pregnancy, 1993). Methylprednisolone is used in the acute situation to minimize salt and water retention, whereas hydrocortisone is used during labor for its mineralocorticoid effects, which are desirable for adrenal stress prophylaxis.

Rhinitis and Sinusitis

Approximately 30 percent of randomly selected pregnant women develop troublesome nasal symptoms (Mabry, 1986). The high frequency of pregnancy rhinitis relates in part to the high incidence of allergic rhinitis in the general population and the nearly sixfold increased incidence in sinusitis during pregnancy (Sorri et al, 1980). Any of the recognized causes of rhinitis may preexist and therefore also occur during pregnancy. In some women, nasal symptoms may begin for the first time during pregnancy. Such symptoms may be attributed to the initial onset allergic rhinitis, sinusitis, rhinitis medicamentosa, or "vasomotor rhinitis of pregnancy." This latter syndrome, which results in varying degrees of nasal congestion and vasomotor instability, tends to be most prominent during the second half of pregnancy and remits by 5 days postpartum (Mohun, 1943). Superimposed rhinitis medicamentosa or acute sinusitis may complicate preexisting nasal conditions during pregnancy. Patulous eustachian tubes may occur during the second trimester owing to hormonal influences leading to ear fullness and hearing of one's own breathing sounds (autophony) in the upright position (Plate et al, 1979).

INTERRELATIONSHIPS BETWEEN RHINITIS AND PREGNANCY. Pregnancy-associated hormones, including estrogen and progesterone, may increase nasal swelling by increasing (1) nasal glandular activity, (2) nasal blood volume resulting from greater circulatory volume, and (3) nasal vascular smooth muscle relaxation (Schatz and Zeiger, 1988). Preexisting nasal symptoms have been reported to worsen in 34 percent, improve in 15 percent, remain unchanged in 45 percent, and be unevaluable in 6 percent of pregnant women (Schatz and Zeiger, 1988).

DIAGNOSIS. As in the nongravid state, the etiology of rhinitis during pregnancy can usually be determined by directed history, physical examination, nasal cytologic analysis, and, when necessary, specific IgE determination (as discussed above) (Table 53–7). Since classic symptoms and signs of sinusitis may be absent in 50 percent of pregnant women with documented sinusitis (Sorri et al, 1980), clinical findings must be supplemented with a high index of suspicion. The usefulness of A-mode ultrasonography is limited by unacceptable false-positive and false-negative rates. Si-

TABLE 53-7. CLINICAL AND NASAL CYTOLOGIC FEATURES OF THE COMMON TYPES OF RHINITIS OCCURRING DURING PREGNANCY

Type	Major Symptoms	Exacerbating Factors*	Nasal Cytology
Allergic rhinitis	Sneezing, runny nose, nasal itching, eye itching	Seasonal Grass, house dust, animals Pregnancy in ⅓ of women	Eosinophils ± basophilic cells
Bacterial rhinosinusitis	Postnasal drainage, sinus distribution pain, purulent discharge	Following an upper respiratory infection Pregnancy (increased incidence)	Neutrophils ± bacteria (may be normal)
Rhinitis medicamentosa	Congestion	Vasoconstricting nose spray abuse	Normal
Nonspecific postnasal drainage	Postnasal drainage, clear or white mucus	Pregnancy	Normal
Vasomotor rhinitis	Congestion (particularly alternating nostril)	Pregnancy	Normal
Eosinophilic nonallergic rhinitis	Congestion, nose blowing, sneezing	None (nonseasonal)	Eosinophils ± basophilic cells
Nasal polyps	Obstruction, anosmia	None (nonseasonal)	Eosinophils ± basophilic cells

*Other than nonspecific precipitants such as aerosols, alcohol, temperature changes, smoke.
From Schatz M, Zeiger RS. Diagnosis and management of rhinitis during pregnancy. Allergy Proc 9:545, 1988.

nus radiographs during pregnancy, though ideally avoided, may be necessary in recalcitrant sinusitis. Sinus irrigations may serve both diagnostic and therapeutic purposes in selected patients unresponsive to medical treatment.

TREATMENT. A summary of the treatment of specific rhinitis entities during pregnancy can be found in Table 53-8. Nonpharmacologic therapy should be maximally utilized to minimize the need for medication, especially during the first trimester. Symptoms interfering with sleep or quality of life or adversely affecting asthma should be aggressively treated. With regard to antihistamines, based on the available data, tripelennamine or chlorpheniramine is recommended. Sneezing, itching, and rhinorrhea respond to antihistamines, whereas congestion responds best to alpha-agonist decongestants (e.g., pseudoephedrine). The combination of the two may be more efficacious in some patients. Intermittent symptoms are best treated by oxymetazoline as necessary or intermittent oral antihistamines and/or decongestants. More chronic or frequently recurring nasal symptoms may require intranasal cromolyn (allergic rhinitis) or intranasal beclomethasone diprorionate (other eosinophilic nasal conditions, or allergic rhinitis unresponsive to cromolyn). Patients with particularly severe eosinophilic rhinitis, nasal polyps, or rhinitis medicamentosa often require combinations of intranasal beclomethasone and regular oral therapy with antihistamines and/or decongestants. Oral glucocorticosteroids should be reserved for the rare patient with recalcitrant debilitating nasal symptoms.

With respect to sinusitis, one must recognize that expansion of maternal extravascular volume, increases in maternal glomerular filtration rate, and rapid passage of some antibiotics across the placenta contribute to reduced serum antibiotic levels, and these changes must be compensated for by more generous dosages of antibiotics during pregnancy. Dosages of 500 mg of amoxicillin (first choice in those not allergic to penicillin), cephalosporins, or erythromycin three to four times daily may be necessary to eradicate the most common organisms found in sinus aspirates during pregnancy (*H. influenzae* and *S. pneumoniae*) (Sorri et al, 1980). In the penicillin-allergic patient, erythromycin may be started and sulfasoxazole added in early or mid-pregnancy if improvement does not occur within 5 to 7 days. A 3-week course of antibiotic therapy appears to be superior to shorter courses during pregnancy. Oxymetazoline topically for 3 to 5 days twice a day and/or pseudoephedrine 120 mg orally twice a day may be useful adjuvants for symptom relief during gestational sinusitis. Amoxicillin/clavulanate or cefaclor may be helpful for resistant sinusitis. Should symptoms not respond to these second-line antibiotics, sinus irrigation should be considered.

TABLE 53-8. TREATMENT OF SPECIFIC RHINOLOGIC ENTITIES DURING PREGNANCY

Type of Rhinitis	Nonpharmacologic Therapy	Pharmacologic Therapy
Allergic rhinitis	Avoidance of antigens Immunotherapy (continuation, not initiation)	Intranasal cromolyn (1–2 sprays b.i.d.–t.i.d.) Antihistamine* ± pseudoephedrine† Intranasal beclomethasone‡
Bacterial rhinosinusitis	Sinus irrigation for recalcitrant disease	Topical oxymetazoline (2 b.i.d.) ≤5 days Pseudoephedrine† Antibiotics for 3 weeks (see text)
Rhinitis medicamentosa	Discontinue vasoconstrictive nose spray	Intranasal beclomethasone‡ Pseudoephedrine† ± antihistamine*
Nonspecific postnasal drip	Saline lavage	Antihistamine*
Vasomotor rhinitis	Exercise (commensurate with prepregnancy) Nasal saline spray	Pseudoephedrine†
Eosinophilic nonallergic rhinitis	—	Intranasal beclomethasone‡ Antihistamine* ± pseudoephedrine† Treatment of complicating infection
Nasal polyps	Polypectomy under local anesthesia	Intranasal beclomethasone‡ Antihistamine* ± pseudoephedrine† Treatment of complicating infection Prednisone for recalcitrant disease

*Tripelennamine 25–50 mg q6h or 100 mg sustained-release b.i.d.; chlorpheniramine 4 mg q6h or 8–12 mg sustained-release b.i.d.
†60 mg b.i.d.–q.i.d. or 120 mg sustained-release b.i.d.
‡Two sprays b.i.d. and taper to lowest effective dosage.
Modified from Schatz M, Zeiger RS. Diagnosis and management of rhinitis during pregnancy. Allergy Proc 9:545, 1988.

Anaphylaxis

Anaphylaxis during pregnancy is uncommon and is caused by etiologic agents similar to those in the nongravid state (see Chapter 21) (Huff and Hayashi, 1980). In early studies, penicillin and procaine were the most frequent causes during pregnancy, but recently many agents, including intravenous iron, bee venom, snake antivenom, shellfish, oxytocins, human serum albumin, modified polygelatin solution, intravenous conjugated estrogens, endogenous progesterone, and strenuous activity encountered during labor and delivery have been reported (Schatz et al, 1993).

EFFECT OF ANAPHYLAXIS ON PREGNANCY. The fetus may be partially protected from anaphylaxis since (1) increased levels of circulating histaminase can catalyze released histamine more effectively, and (2) the placenta tends to exclude maternal IgE antibody. However, hypoxia and/or hypotension in the mother may exert catastrophic effects on both mother and fetus. Maternal anaphylaxis has been associated with fetal distress documented by repetitive late decelerations in fetal heart rate and multicystic fetal or infantile encephalomalacia (Entman and Moise, 1984). Prompt and aggressive therapy may reverse anaphylaxis completely with no maternal or fetal compromise, whereas inadequate treatment may lead to fetal or neonatal death despite maternal survival, the latter due to diminished uteroplacental perfusion.

DIFFERENTIAL DIAGNOSIS. The clinical features and differential diagnosis of anaphylaxis during pregnancy resemble those observed in the nonpregnant patient with anaphylaxis (see Chapter 21). Such conditions as vasovagal collapse, hyperventilation, and acute cardiac/pulmonary/cranial catastrophes should be differentiated from anaphylaxis (see Chapter 21).

Laryngeal stridor, often seen during anaphylaxis, must be distinguished from the laryngeal edema reported during *preeclampsia* (Seager and MacDonald, 1980) and that associated with *laryngopathia gravidarum* (Bhatia et al, 1981) or *hereditary angioedema* (HANE) (discussed below) (Frank et al, 1976). In preeclampsia, hypertension, peripheral edema, and urinary abnormalities predominate. In laryngopathia gravidarum, laryngeal symptoms appear less abruptly, with the acute form occurring immediately prior to parturition. In HANE, stridor is slower in onset, associated with abdominal pain, generally diagnosed previously, and free of hypotension and urticaria.

PREVENTION AND TREATMENT. Active prevention is both mandatory and rewarding.

Measures that should reduce anaphylaxis include (1) identification of a previous history of adverse reactions to the myriad anaphylaxis-causing agents, (2) education of at-risk gravid women regarding their condition and the necessity for avoidance of exposure, (3) prescription of an auto-injection form of epinephrine (Epipen, Ana-Kit) to those with noniatrogenic anaphylaxis potential, (4) avoidance of parenteral medications, if possible, (5) observation of patients for at least 30 minutes after parenteral injections, (6) determination of sensitivity to heterologous sera prior to use, and (7) referral of presumptively allergic gravid patients requiring the suspected agent to an allergist for evaluation.

With regard to the hymenoptera-sensitive pregnant patient in whom anaphylaxis risk is high, the following suggestions may be useful: (1) renew insect avoidance precautions (avoidance, ice, tourniquets), (2) ensure proper technique with the auto-injectable epinephrine devices (which should be carried at all times), and (3) consider providing tripelennamine or chlorpheniramine. Those patients already receiving maintenance venom immunotherapy should not stop such therapy (Schwartz et al, 1990). In the diagnosis of venom sensitivity during pregnancy, an *in vitro* assay may be preferable to skin testing since the potential for anaphylaxis will be avoided. Benefit-risk considerations may not favor initiating venom immunotherapy in most venom-allergic pregnant women, although exceptions may be necessary for the especially sensitive patient at increased risk of exposure.

Reversal of anaphylaxis during pregnancy must be particularly speedy, employing the same medication used in nonpregnant patients. Intravascular volume repletion and oxygenation are especially important during pregnancy because of altered maternal circulatory and respiratory physiology and the needs of the fetus. Although both epinephrine and diphenhydramine have been implicated as possible causes of fetal malformations (Schatz et al, 1993), the tentative nature of the data and the absence of suitable alternatives compel one to use these drugs during pregnancy for anaphylaxis. A protocol for the treatment of anaphylaxis during pregnancy is presented in Table 53–9.

A minimum maternal systolic blood pressure of 90 mm Hg must be maintained during pregnancy to avoid hypotension and provide adequate placental perfusion (Witter and Niebyl, 1983). The pregnant hypotensive patient should be placed on her left side to prevent additional positional hypotension, which may occur from compression of the inferior vena cava by the gravid uterus. Some obstetricians and obstetric anesthesiologists prefer ephedrine to treat hypotension during pregnancy, owing to its greater beta-adrenergic activity and reduced likelihood of decreasing uterine blood flow compared with epinephrine (Eng et al, 1971), but subsequent reports demonstrate the greater efficacy of epinephrine compared with ephedrine in reversing anaphylaxis-induced hypotension during pregnancy, and thus epinephrine must be the agent of first choice to treat gestational anaphylaxis (Barach et al, 1984).

As noted elsewhere, corticosteroids may be helpful for prolonged, refractory, or recurrent anaphylaxis, but they do not reverse acute anaphylaxis symptoms. Early institution of corticosteroids is recommended in the treatment of more severe anaphylaxis to obtain earlier benefit from their anti-allergic effects. Intubation and, rarely, tracheostomy may be necessary. Although prompt and aggressive treatment should successfully reverse anaphylaxis and its potential insult on both mother and fetus, prevention remains the best way to avoid the potential dire consequences of anaphylaxis.

Urticaria and Angioedema

Urticaria and angioedema represent common dermatologic responses to diverse physical, allergic, chemical, infectious, and emotional triggers. During pregnancy, urticaria/angioedema can occur from any of the various causes, agents, and mechanisms responsible during the nonpregnant state (see Chapter 46). Urticaria/angioedema limited to pregnancy and recurring with subsequent pregnancies was noted in 0.5 percent of 554 consecutive patients with urticaria and was thought to be possibly due to allergic sensitization to endogenous hormones, particularly progesterone (Champion et al, 1969). Another form of sensitivity to progesterone during pregnancy, "autoimmune progesterone dermatitis of pregnancy," is characterized by a papulopustular eruption associated with transient arthritis, peripheral and tissue eosinophilia, miscarriage, and delayed intradermal sensitivity to aqueous progesterone (Bier-

TABLE 53-9. KAISER-PERMANENTE SEVERE ANAPHYLAXIS PROTOCOL

Modify as desired, cross off nonapplicable orders.
1. Call a doctor STAT.
2. P, R, B/P q5min or q2min if B/P <90 mm Hg.
3. Patient wt _____ kg.
4. O₂ at 6 L/min by nasal cannula.
5. If systolic B/P <90 mm Hg, use Trendelenburg position, place patient on left side, and monitor EKG.
6. Continue ice and tourniquets if reaction secondary to injection, skin test, or sting.
7. Continue epinephrine (1:1000) 0.3 ml IM in deltoid, repeat q10min if reaction persists. In addition, give either half or equivalent dose into site of skin test injection or sting.
8. Start IV with 18- or 19-gauge needle or intracath; infuse Ringer's lactate; start wide open, then check with doctor for rate or volume (may require 3–10 L).

Consider:

9. Benadryl (50 mg/ml): 1 ml IV piggyback in 50 ml over 5 min.
10. Methylprednisolone (125 mg/2 ml) 2 ml in 50 ml IV piggyback over 5 min. Do not mix with Benadryl.
11. If wheezing, use albuterol (5 mg/ml) 0.5 ml added to 2 ml saline and nebulize.
12. If symptoms persist, ranitidine (50 mg/2 ml) 2ml in 50 ml IV piggyback infused in 5 min.
13. If systolic BP less than 90 mm Hg and pulse less than 60 beats per min, give atropine (1 mg/10 ml saline) 5 ml IV push; may repeat 10 ml if necessary in 5–10 min.
14. If still hypotensive, or hypotension recurs, use intravenous epinephrine: 1 ml epinephrine (1:1000) to 10 ml saline and infuse over 10 min. Consider repeating if still hypotensive, perfusing immediately after previous dose.
15. If still hypotensive, or hypotensive recurs, use maintenance epinephrine: 1 ml epinephrine (1:1000) in 250 ml D₅W (4 µg/ml) and infuse at 15 ml/h (1 µg/min). Titrate q5min to maintain systolic B/P ≥90 mm Hg. Maximum dose 60 ml/h = 4 µg/min.
16. If still hypotensive, DC maintenance epinephrine and infuse dopamine (400 mg/5 ml): mix 5 ml with 250 ml IV solution (1.6 mg/ml) and start infusion at 0.15 × _____ kg (4 µg/kg/min) = _____ ml/h to maintain systolic B/P ≥90 mm Hg (usual maximum dose 5 × infusion rate = 20 µg/kg/min).
17. If ventricular dysrhythmia occurs, use lidocaine (100 gm/50 ml) acutely: 0.05 × _____ kg = _____ ml IV bolus, which may be repeated in 5 min. Consider twice the dose in 15 min if necessary.
18. If dysrhythmia persists, lidocaine (2 gm/50 ml) maintenance dosage: add 50 ml to 500 ml D₅W, and start infusion at 30 ml/h (2 mg/min).
19. Consider glucagon if patient on beta blocker and anaphylaxis persists. Add 1 ml glucagon diluting solution to glucagon vial and infuse 0.5 ml IV push. May repeat if necessary.
20. If wheezing persists and no previous theophylline given for past 24 hours, give bolus of aminophylline (500 mg/20 ml) 0.2 × _____ kg = _____ ml IV in 50 ml IV solution over 20 min.

P = pulse; R = respiration; B/P = blood pressure; DC = discontinue.
From Schatz M, Zeiger RS. Allergic diseases. *In* Gleicher N (ed). Principles and Practice of Medical Therapy in Pregnancy. 2nd ed. Norwalk, Appleton and Lange, 1992, p 446.

man, 1973). Progesterone sensitivity has also been implicated in anaphylaxis during pregnancy (Meggs et al, 1984).

HEREDITARY ANGIOEDEMA (HANE). Differentiation of HANE-induced abdominal crises from an obstetric abdominal emergency is crucial to prevent needless exploratory surgery. HANE during pregnancy was associated with markedly fewer attacks, or an absence of attacks, from the fourth to ninth months in 23 of 25 pregnant women with HANE (Frank et al, 1976). Most fortunately, HANE symptoms did not appear during vaginal delivery in these 25 pregnancies. This rather profound amelioration of HANE during pregnancy is most characteristic, although recurrent worsening during multiple pregnancies and postpartum exacerbations have been described (Schatz et al, 1993). Tragically, HANE has triggered localized perineal swelling after delivery, resulting in secondary irreversible shock and death (Postnikoff and Pritzker, 1979).

DIAGNOSIS. A thorough history and careful physical examination may reveal the cause of urticara/angioedema, if one is to be found. Should a cause not be readily identified, laboratory evaluation of chronic urticaria/angioedema during pregnancy should be limited to screening with a CBC, urinary analysis, and ESR, with more extensive diagnostic tests reserved for unusual or particularly severe symptoms.

Gestational urticaria/angioedema should be differentiated from such dermatologic entities as (1) autoimmune progesterone dermatitis of pregnancy, (2) polymorphic eruption of pregnancy, (3) other pruritic dermatoses of pregnancy, and (4) laryngopathia gravidarum (Schatz et al, 1993). Laryngopathia gravidarum is an acute or chronic noninfectious, somewhat inflammatory disorder of the larynx seen in multigravidas (Bhatia et al, 1981). The acute form presents prior to parturition, whereas the chronic entity occurs throughout pregnancy, recurring with subsequent pregnancies and spontaneously resolving postpartum. Symptoms include (1) progressive dyspnea, sporadically requiring artificial ventilation, (2) hoarseness, (3) nonfebrile sore throat and odynophagia, (4) malaise, (5) lymphadenopathy, (6) cough, and (7) elevated erythrocyte sedimentation rate (40 to 60 mm/hour) with normal white blood count. Patchy edema and congestion occur in the larynx and frequently in the epiglottis, but not in the aryepiglottic folds, arytenoids, vestibular region, or true vocal cords. Microscopic abnormalities are limited to the submucosa, which appears edematous owing to infiltration with lymphocytes and plasma cells. Owing to its resolution postpartum, pregnancy hormones have been implicated in its causation.

PREVENTION AND TREATMENT. Triggering agents or causes should be identified and avoided. Such prevention is the hallmark of treatment in order to obviate pharmacologic intervention. During pregnancy, tripelennamine (25 to 50 mg every 6 hours or 100 mg sustained-release form twice a day) or chlorpheniramine (4 mg every 6 hours or 8 to 12 mg sustained-release form twice a day) is the recommended initial H_1-antihistamine for symptomatic control of urticaria/angioedema. Substitution with hydroxyzine (10 to 25 mg every 6 hours), which, though teratogenic in animals, has not increased the risk of congenital malformations in human studies (Schatz et al, 1993), may be considered for refractory cases. Occasionally, systemic corticosteroids are required for severe, recalcitrant urticaria or angioedema. Acute, severe urticaria/angioedema requires aggressive therapy modeled after that used for anaphylaxis (Table 53–9).

Attenuated androgen prophylaxis generally is not required or warranted for the treatment of HANE during pregnancy (Frank et al, 1976) since the potential for drug-related fetal damage includes female masculinization, pseudohermaphroditism, and spontaneous abortion (Stiller et al, 1984). Vaginal deliveries are safe for HANE patients (Frank et al, 1976). In contrast, cesarean section requires preoperative transfusion of two units of fresh frozen plasma or purified C1-esterase enzyme preparations to prevent episodes (Stiller et al, 1984). Regional is preferred to general anesthesia to avoid endotracheal intubation, which could trigger laryngeal edema. Life-threatening laryngeal edema from HANE during pregnancy requires timely and aggressive treatment including (1) androgenic therapy (stanozolol, 4 mg four times a day), (2) standard emergency measures for airway obstruction (endotracheal intubation and, if necessary, tracheostomy), and (3) intravenous fluid replacement if hypovolemia develops (Stiller et al, 1984). The usual therapeutic modalities for angioedema (epinephrine, antihistamines, and corticosteroids) typically are ineffective in most patients during acute HANE attacks, but may be helpful in a minority of cases (Frank et al, 1976). Postpartum episodes of HANE must be recognized rapidly and aggressive therapy instituted, including large-volume fluid replacement of third-space losses and reinstitution of androgenic therapy (Postnikoff and Pritzker, 1979; Stiller et al, 1984).

Atopic Dermatitis

The characteristic features of atopic dermatitis, an eczematous disorder that occurs in about 1 to 2 percent of adults, include (1) pruritus, (2) chronicity, (3) typical morphology and distribution, and (4) a genetic predilection to develop allergic rhinitis, asthma, and food allergy. To aid in the diagnosis of atopic dermatitis, specific diagnostic criteria have been formulated and should be used during pregnancy (see Chapter 44).

INTERRELATIONSHIPS BETWEEN PREGNANCY AND ATOPIC DERMATITIS. Older data suggested that pregnancy exerts no demonstrable effect on atopic dermatitis since definite improvement (3 percent) or definite exacerbation (1 percent) occurred in only a minority of women with mild-to-severe atopic dermatitis (Roth and Kierland, 1964). In contrast, a recent study reported that atopic dermatitis worsened in 52 percent, improved in 24 percent, and remained unchanged in 24 percent of pregnancies (Kemmett and Tidman, 1991).

PREVENTION AND TREATMENT. The treatment of atopic dermatitis during pregnancy must focus on avoidance of triggering factors, including known (1) food and inhalant allergens, (2) irritating agents such as wools and chemicals, (3) excessive perspiration and heat, (4) unwarranted stress, (5) occlusive clothing, and (6) other known exacerbating agents. The topical therapy proved efficacious for atopic dermatitis includes (1) moisturizers and lubricants to alleviate dryness, (2) cleansers such as Cetophil lotion instead of soaps, and (3) aluminum acetate (Burow's solution) or baking soda soaks to reduce inflammation, weeping, and pruritus. Oral antihistamines should be administered at the lowest effective dose, if necessary, initiating therapy with tripelennamine or chlorpheniramine in doses similar to those given for urticaria/angioedema. Hydroxyzine may be necessary for recalcitrant pruritus. A similar conservative approach should be followed for topical corticosteroid usage. Corticosteroid treatment should be initiated, when clinically indicated, with the preparation with the least potential for suppressing the adrenals, such as hydrocortisone (0.5 to 2.5 percent). Use of the more potent topical corticosteroid preparations should be reserved for the more recalcitrant areas or cases. Administration of corticosteroids by intralesional or systemic injections should be avoided. Infectious exacerbations, generally secondary to *Staphylococcus aureus* colonization, should be treated with penicillinase-resistant synthetic penicillins, cephalosporins, or erythromycin in those allergic to penicillin (see Chapter 44) (Schatz et al, 1993).

Drug Allergy

The incidence of drug reactions during pregnancy is lower than in the nonpregnant state, owing to the reduced frequency of drug use during pregnancy. Their diagnosis, prevention, and treatment in pregnant women are similar in most respects to those in nonpregnant patients (see Chapter 22). Although avoidance of drugs to which sensitization has been documented can be achieved most of the time, occasionally such a drug must be used. During pregnancy, both penicillin and insulin desensitization protocols have been developed and used successfully (Wendel et al, 1985; Gossain et al, 1985). Avoidance is the mainstay of drug allergy prevention in pregnancy, and history is the key to avoidance. When needed in the rare instance, desensitization may be safely achieved in pregnant women when overseen by experienced clinicians.

REFERENCES

Abrams RS. Use of medication during pregnancy and lactation: General considerations. *In* Schatz M, Zeiger RS (eds). Asthma and Allergy in Pregnancy and Early Infancy. New York, Marcel Dekker, 1993, p 109.

American Academy of Pediatrics Committee on Drugs. Transfer of drugs and other chemicals into breast milk. Pediatrics. 84:924, 1989.

Apter AJ, Greenberger PA, Patterson R. Outcome of pregnancy in adolescents with severe asthma. Arch Intern Med 149:2571, 1989.

Bahna SL, Bjerkedal T. The course and outcome of pregnancy in women with bronchial asthma. Acta Allergol 27:397, 1972.

Barach E, Nowak R, Tennyson G, et al. Epinephrine for treatment of anaphylactic shock. JAMA 251:2118, 1984.

Bhatia PL, Singh MS, Jha BK. Laryngopathia gravidarum. Ear Nose Throat J 60:408, 1981.

Bierman SM. Autoimmune progesterone dermatitis of pregnancy. Arch Dermatol 107:896, 1973.

Champion, RH, Roberts, SOB, Carpenter, RG, et al. Urticaria and angioedema. Br J Dermatol 81:588, 1969.

Cousins L, Catanzarite VA. Fetal oxygenation and acid-base balance as it relates to the pregnancy complicated by asthma or anaphylaxis. *In* Schatz M, Zeiger RS (eds). Asthma and Allergy in Pregnancy and Early Infancy. New York, Marcel Dekker, 1993, p 25.

Dombrowski MR, Bottoms SF, Boike GM, et al. Incidence of preeclampsia among asthmatic patients lower with theophylline. Am J Obstet Gynecol 155:265, 1986.

Elkayam U, Ostizega EL, Shoten A. Peripartum cardiomyopathy. *In* Gleicher N (ed). Principles and Practice of Medical Therapy in Pregnancy. 2nd ed. Norwalk, Appleton and Lange, 1992, p 812.

Eng M, Berges PV, Voland K, et al. The effect of methoxamine and ephedrine in normotensive pregnant primates. Anesthesiology 35:354, 1971.

Entman SS, Moise KJ. Anaphylaxis in pregnancy. South Med J 77:402, 1984.

Francis N. Abortion after grass pollen injection. J Allergy 12:559, 1941.

Frank MM, Gelfand JA, Atkinson, JP. Hereditary angioedema: The clinical syndrome and its management. Ann Intern Med 4:580, 1976.

Galbraith GMP, Galbraith RM. Maternal immunologic changes in pregnancy. *In* Schatz M, Zeiger RS (eds). Asthma and Allergy in Pregnancy and Early Infancy. New York, Marcel Dekker, 1993, p 63.

Gluck JC, Gluck, PA. The effects of pregnancy on asthma: A prospective study. Ann Allergy 37:164, 1976.

Gossain VV, Rovner DR, Mohan K. Systemic allergy to human (recombinant DNA) insulin. Ann Allergy 55:116, 1985.

Gordon M, Niswander KR, Berendes H, et al. Fetal morbidity following potentially anoxigenic obstetric conditions. VII. Bronchial asthma. Am J Obstet Gynecol 106:421, 1970.

Greenberger PA, Patterson R. The outcome of pregnancy complicated by severe asthma. Allergy Proc 9:539, 1988.

Hollingsworth HM, Irwin RS. Acute respiratory failure in pregnancy. Clin Chest Med 13:723, 1992.

Huff RW, Hayashi RH. Emergency care in pregnancy. *In* Queenan JT (ed). Management of High Risk Pregnancy. Oradell, NJ, Medical Economics Co., 1980, p 411.

Juniper EF, Newhouse MT. Effect of pregnancy on asthma: A critical appraisal of the literature. *In* Schatz M, Zeiger RS (eds). Asthma and Allergy in Pregnancy and Early Infancy. New York, Marcel Dekker, 1993, p 223.

Kaliner M, Shelhammer JH, David PB, et al. Autonomic nervous system abnormalities and allergy. Ann Intern Med 96:349, 1982.

Kemmett O, Tidman MJ. The influence of the menstrual cycle and pregnancy on atopic dermatitis. Br J Dermatol 125:59, 1991.

Kershaw-McLennen J, Spector SI. Immunological diagnosis and therapy during pregnancy. In Schatz M, Zeiger RS (eds). Asthma and Allergy in Pregnancy and Early Infancy. New York, Marcel Dekker, 1993, p 77.

Lao TT, Huengsburg M. Labor and delivery in mothers with asthma. Eur J Obstet Gynecol Reprod Biol 35:183, 1990.

Mabie WC, Barton JR, Wasserstrum N, et al. Clinical observations on asthma in pregnancy. J Maternal-Fetal Med 1:45, 1992.

Mabry RI. Rhinitis of pregnancy. South Med J 79:965, 1986.

Meggs WJ, Pescouitz OH, Metcalfe D, et al. Progesterone sensitivity as a cause of recurrent anaphylaxis. N Engl J Med 311:1236, 1984.

Metzger WJ, Turner E, Patterson R. The safety of immunotherapy during pregnancy. J Allergy Clin Immunol 61:268, 1978.

Mohun M. Incidence of vasomotor rhinitis during pregnancy. Arch Otol 37:699, 1943.

National Asthma Education Program Report of the Working Group on Asthma and Pregnancy. Management of Asthma During Pregnancy (Executive Summary). NIH Publication Number 93-3279A, Oct. 1992.

National Asthma Education Program Report of the Working Group on Asthma and Pregnancy. Management of Asthma During Pregnancy. NIH Publication Number 93-3279, Sept. 1993.

Newhouse MT, Dolovich MC. Control of asthma by aerosols. N Engl J Med 315:870, 1986.

Patterson R, Greenberger PA, Frederiksen MC. Asthma and pregnancy: Responsibility of physicians and patients. Ann Allergy 65:469, 1990.

Perlow JH, Montgomery D, Morgan MA, et al. Severity of asthma and perinatal outcome. Am J Obstet Gynecol 167:963, 1992.

Plate S, Johnsen NJ, Pedersen SN, et al. The frequency of patulous eustachian tubes in pregnancy. Clin Otolaryngol 4:393, 1979.

Postnikoff IM, Pritzker KP. Hereditary angioneurotic edema: An unusual case of maternal mortality. J Forensic Sci 24:473, 1979.

Ries AL. Oximetry—know thy limits. Chest 91:316, 1987.

Roth HL, Kierland RR. The natural history of atopic dermatitis. Arch Dermatol 89:209, 1964.

Schatz M. Asthma during pregnancy: Interrelationships and management. Ann Allergy 68:123, 1992.

Schatz M, Harden K, Forsythe A, et al. The course of asthma during pregnancy, postpartum, and with successive pregnancies. A prospective analysis. J Allergy Clin Immunol 81:509, 1988.

Schatz M, Hoffman CP, Zeiger RS, et al. The course and management of asthma and allergic diseases during pregnancy. In Middleton E Jr, Reed CE, Ellis EF, et al (eds). Allergy: Principles and Practice. St. Louis, Mosby-Year Book, 1993, p 1301.

Schatz M, Zeiger RS. Diagnosis and management of rhinitis during pregnancy. Allergy Proc 9:545, 1988.

Schatz M, Zeiger RS. Allergic diseases. In Gleicher N (ed). Principles and Practice of Medical Therapy in Pregnancy. 2nd ed. Norwalk, Appleton and Lange, 1992, p 446.

Schatz M, Zeiger RS, Hoffman CP, et al. Intrauterine growth is related to gestational pulmonary function in pregnant asthmatic women. Chest 98:389, 1990.

Schatz M, Zeiger RS, Hoffman CP, et al. Perinatal outcome in the pregnancies of asthmatic women: A prospective controlled analysis. Am J Respir Crit Care Med (in press).

Schwartz HJ, Golden DBK, Lockey RF. Venom immunotherapy in the Hymenoptera-allergic pregnant patient. J Allergy Clin Immunol 85:709, 1990.

Scialli AR, Lione A. The reproductive effects of specific medications for asthma and allergy. In Schatz M, Zeiger RS (eds). Asthma and Allergy in Pregnancy and Early Infancy. New York, Marcel Dekker, 1993, p 127.

Seager SJ, MacDonald R. Laryngeal oedema and pre-eclampsia. Anesthesia 35:360, 1980.

Sorri M, Bortikanen-Sorri AL, Karja J. Rhinitis during pregnancy. Rhinology 18:83, 1980.

Stenius-Aarniala R, Piirila P, Teramo K. Asthma and pregnancy: A prospective study of 198 pregnancies. Thorax 43:12, 1988.

Stiller RJ, Kaplan BM, Andreoli JW. Hereditary angioedema and pregnancy. Obstet Gynecol 64:133, 1984.

Stone AB, Brown WA. Psychologic changes during pregnancy: Implications for medical care. In Schatz M, Zeiger RS (eds). Asthma and Allergy in Pregnancy and Early Infancy. New York, Marcel Dekker, 1993, p 89.

Wendel GD, Stark BJ, Jamison RB, et al. Penicillin allergy and desensitization in serious infections during pregnancy. N Engl J Med 312:1229, 1985.

Williams DA. Asthma and pregnancy. Acta Allergol (Kbh.) 22:311, 1967.

Witter FR, Niebyl JR. Drug intoxication and anaphylactic shock in the obstetric patient. In Berkowitz, RL (ed). Critical Care of the Obstetric Patient. New York, Churchill Livingstone, 1983, p 527.

Ziment I. Taking care of asthma when you're pregnant. J Resp Dis 10:91, 1989.

ACKNOWLEDGMENTS: We would like to thank Pat Stanwood for typing the manuscript and the Kaiser Foundation Hospital Medical Library staff for assistance with the references.

Chapter 54

Surgery in Allergic and Asthmatic Patients

John Latall, M.D., and Leslie C. Grammer, M.D.

This chapter's primary purpose is to provide guidelines for the perioperative management of the asthmatic patient. Special cases will also be considered, including the pregnant asthmatic patient, emergency surgery, the perioperative management of idiopathic anaphylaxis, and hereditary angioedema. These are important areas of interest because perioperative morbidity and mortality due to complications of these diseases can approach that of the general population if proper management is instituted. The approach outlined in this chapter is the one used at Northwestern University and has been associated with safety and success. However, other variations on this approach also exist which may also be efficacious; since we do not have experience with such approaches, it is difficult for us to comment on them.

One of the first reports of this optimistic outcome was an asthma and surgery study from the Mayo Clinic in the late 1950s, in which the pulmonary complication rate was comparable to that of the general population. These favorable outcomes were attributed to aggressive perioperative treatment with corticosteroids, bronchodilators, and antibiotics, if needed. Studies performed at Northwestern in the 1970s and 1980s reported minimal pulmonary or other complications and no perioperative mortality in severe asthmatics who underwent major surgery. These studies reported that asthma, if optimally controlled before surgery, does not constitute an excessive risk.

This chapter will not attempt to detail every aspect of perioperative concern in allergic patients. Such areas include the well-established risks of surgery in patients with chronic obstructive pulmonary disease (COPD) and the growing concern regarding latex allergy. Nor will we discuss drug allergies such as those to certain neuromuscular blocking agents or antibiotics. The definition of asthma that we will use in this chapter is that proposed by a recent expert panel: Asthma is a disease with the following characteristics: (1) airway obstruction that is reversible either with treatment or spontaneously; (2) airway hyperresponsiveness; and (3) airway inflammation.

Postoperative complications comprise the majority of pulmonary complications in asthmatic patients. However, intraoperative bronchospasm has been reported as a potentially life-threatening complication. It occurs most frequently in patients undergoing minor endoscopic or major surgical procedures via the oral route.

Although all of the principles reported here are important to optimum perioperative care of these patients, none is more important than the coordinated team of the physicians managing the asthma, the anesthesiologist, and the surgeon with regard to preparation for surgery, timing and choice of surgical procedures, anesthesia type, and postoperative care. Only with such a well informed, skilled, and committed effort, in concert with a compliant patient, can the care of such patients be optimized.

PERIOPERATIVE ASSESSMENT AND PREPARATION FOR SURGERY

The physician caring for the preoperative asthmatic patient should see the patient approximately one week prior to surgery for assessment and institution of a proper preoperative regimen (Jackson, 1988; Kingston and Hirshman, 1984). The history should focus on current symptoms as well as recent emergency room visits, hospitalizations, and intubations. It is important to inquire about recent upper respiratory infection, which is well known to increase morbidity due to bronchospasm, mucous plugging, and atelectasis.

The patient's pharmacologic regimen should be detailed, focusing on the need for inhaled and systemic corticosteroids to maintain good control of asthma. By using Table 54–1, specific recommendations can be given based on current asthma control and what medications are ordinarily required to control a patient's asthma.

National Heart, Lung and Blood Institute (NHLBI) guidelines recommend the use of pulmonary function testing in asthmatic patients scheduled for surgery. Pulmonary function testing may have particular utility in selected cases, as in patients with significant irreversible lung disease or in patients in whom clinical assessment is inconclusive.

Recommendations for the use of perioperative corticosteroids are based on their reported efficacy and safety in prospective trials. There are many reasons that corticosteroids aid in the perioperative management of asthmatic patients. First, they have been shown to decrease airway mucus production. They also alleviate airway inflammation and reduce bronchial hyperreactivity. Asthmatic patients receiving corticosteroids demonstrate lessened ventilation-perfusion mismatch and reduced alveolar-arterial oxygen gradient. Corticosteroids have also been shown to potentiate the bronchodilator response to adrenergic agonists. Finally, concerns about life-threatening adrenal insufficiency are eliminated by the administration of sufficient corticosteroid. Despite the widespread fear about the risks of delayed wound healing and wound infection with corticosteroid therapy, these effects have yet to be definitely demonstrated in asthmatic patient populations.

The discontinuation of theophylline preparations before surgery may be preferable with supervision and appropriate substitution of other drugs. Therapeutic levels of theophylline may have serious interactions with other common intraoperative drugs. Halothane and ketamine, each having some desirable properties in asthmatic patients, can interact with therapeutic theophylline to produce ventricular tachyarrhythmias and grand mal seizures, respectively. Also, theophylline preparations reduce the lower esophageal sphincter tone, predisposing to intraoperative aspiration. Finally, with hepatic perfusion reduced by up to 30 percent during inhalational anesthesia, the metabolism of theophylline is reduced and predisposes to its toxicity. Patients receiving a beta-adrenergic blocker for cardiovascular disease may benefit from a change to a calcium channel blocker, which should not have adverse effects on airway function.

CHOICE OF ANESTHESIA

There are many deleterious alterations in pulmonary physiology in the asthmatic patient receiving general anesthesia. Premedication with sedatives predisposes to pre-induction hypoventilation. Intubation is a potent stimulus for parasympathetic bronchospasm. Inhalational anesthetics depress ciliary func-

TABLE 54–1. RECOMMENDED PREPARATIVE MEDICATIONS FOR ELECTIVE SURGERY IN NONGRAVID ASTHMATIC PATIENTS, STRATIFIED BY SEVERITY OF ASTHMA*†

OUTPATIENT REGIMEN	RECOMMENDATION
No episode past year, no asthma medications, normal physical examination	No specific intervention
On bronchodilators, no history of corticosteroid use	Beclomethasone dipropionate,‡ 400 µg/day or equivalent × 5–7 days preoperatively
On inhaled or systemic corticosteroids now or in past	Prednisone,‡ 1 mg/kg/day × 5 days preoperatively
Already on prednisone 1 mg/kg/day	Substantially increase‡ dose × 5 days preoperatively

*Assumes good control of asthma on regimen
†*Note:* If poor control or recent upper respiratory infection then delay surgery if possible. If not possible, see discussion under "Emergency Surgery" in this chapter.
‡All patients treated preoperatively with inhaled or systemic corticosteroids should receive hydrocortisone, 100 mg IV, starting preoperatively and continuing every 8 hours until respiratory status is stable.

tion and cough reflex. General anesthesia causes decreased functional residual capacity (FRC) and propensity for atelectasis, reduced compliance, and ventilation-perfusion mismatch. Ventilation may also be impaired by accumulated secretions. The gastroesophageal reflux associated with general anesthesia predisposes to aspiration as well as increased acidity in the mid-esophagus, with resultant reflex bronchoconstriction.

Given the aforementioned drawbacks to general anesthesia, regional anesthesia is preferable for the asthmatic individual, when feasible. The exception to this is in children, because poor cooperation and either inadequate or excessive sedation have been problematic. All patients for whom regional anesthesia is planned should be prepared in the same way as those for general anesthesia, since inadequate regional anesthesia may necessitate the implementation of general anesthesia.

ANESTHETIC AGENTS

Although there are general guidelines for the management of anesthetic agents and techniques for the asthmatic patient, the approach to any given case depends primarily on the judgment and experience of the anesthesiologist. The relationship between psychologic stress and asthma is ill-defined, but decreased anxiety improves patient cooperation and reduces the tendency for hyperventilation. Therefore, control of anxiety is an important preoperative consideration for the asthmatic patient. Cautious premedication with hydroxyzine, a benzodiazepine, or low-dose narcotics may be useful.

Opiates can be potent nonspecific histamine-releasing agents. Morphine is of particular concern in this regard. Both intravenous and inhaled histamine have been reported to precipitate rapid bronchoconstriction in asthmatic patients. This effect is only partially blocked by H_1 antagonists and is possibly enhanced by H_2 antagonists. However, narcotics are used regularly in asthmatic surgical patients without apparent bronchospasm. Interestingly, fentanyl, a frequently used intravenous anesthetic, has opiate properties up to 200 times that of morphine, yet no known histamine-releasing effect.

Intravenous lidocaine is a useful pre-intubation drug because of documented reflex-induced bronchospasm prophylaxis. There are also reports of efficacy in treating intraoperative bronchospasm. Note that the aerosol route offers no advantage and indeed has been associated with mild bronchospasm.

Atropine's anticholinergic effect may counteract both the reflex bronchoconstriction caused by upper airway manipulation and that caused by stimulation of lower airway irritant receptors. Intravenous ketamine is the preferred agent for induction in asthmatic patients because it possesses a sympathomimetic bronchodilating effect. Some authorities believe that barbiturates predispose to reflex bronchoconstriction and thus are undesirable induction agents for asthmatic patients.

After induction, but before intubation, neuromuscular blocking agents are commonly administered. Vecuronium and pancuronium are the safest nondepolarizing muscle relaxants in the asthmatic patient. Others, such as D-tubocurarine, may precipitate bronchospasm via histamine release. A cholinergic mechanism is invoked to explain depolarizing agent–induced bronchoconstriction. The fact that atropine prevents this effect supports this assertion.

Succinylcholine is useful to differentiate true bronchospasm from inadequate muscle relaxation (i.e., "tight chest syndrome"). It is interesting to note that only rare reports of bronchospasm related to succinylcholine exist.

Fortunately, the inhalational anesthetic agents halothane, isoflurane, and enflurane are all prophylactic against bronchoconstriction. Widely accepted mechanisms explaining these phenomena include direct bronchial smooth muscle relaxation, enhancement of $beta_2$-adrenergic receptor response, and blockade of parasympathetic reflexes. For most asthmatic patients, halothane is the agent of choice in this category. Through many years of successful experience, it has been reported to induce minimal secretions and is not irritating.

Enflurane and isoflurane may be at times preferable as they do not cause myocardial sensitization to theophylline or catecholamines. Additionally, isoflurane has the least negative inotropic effect. However, both agents are airway irritants, and enflurane has been reported on rare occasion to induce bronchospasm. Interestingly, all three agents have been successfully employed in the treatment of refractory status asthmaticus.

VENTILATOR MANAGEMENT

The only absolutely contraindicated aspect of ventilator management in asthmatic patients is high-frequency ventilation, as it can result in lung hyperexpansion and hyperventilation. Rather, volume-limited ventilation, with slow inspiratory flow rates and expiratory times long enough to prevent air trapping, is indicated. The inhaled oxygen concentration (FIO_2) should be at least 35 percent to ensure adequate oxygenation, given the variable ventilation-perfusion mismatch in these patients. Nitrous oxide concentrations above 65 percent in inspired gases may allow nitrous oxide to diffuse preferentially into poorly ventilated air spaces, with resultant dilution of oxygen concentration and increased ventilation-perfusion mismatch. Inspired gases should also be humidified and warmed, as cold, dry air can induce bronchospasm. Finally, the use of positive end-expiratory pressure should be avoided to prevent limitation of adequate exhalation.

INTRAOPERATIVE BRONCHOSPASM

The diagnosis of intraoperative bronchospasm is associated with each of the following clinical findings: prolonged expiratory time; slow filling of the reservoir bag; increased peak pressures with volume-limited ventilation; and audible wheezing. It is imperative to establish the correct diagnosis in an expedient fashion, as other life-threatening problems such as pneumothorax or pulmonary edema may also cause wheezing and/or increased peak pressures. Other conditions that are included in this differential are upper airway secretions, inadequate muscle relaxation, and light levels of anesthesia.

Treatment for intraoperative bronchospasm includes inhaled $beta_2$-adrenergic agonists and increased FIO_2. Transient V/Q mismatch and compromise of oxygenation due to reversal of hypoxic pulmonary vasoconstriction out of proportion to bronchodilatation may occur with administration of $beta_2$-agonist. Additional interventions of potential benefit include repositioning of the endotracheal tube, administration of intravenous lidocaine, or increased inhaled anesthetic concentration. Hydrocortisone, 200 mg IV, should follow the initial bronchodilator therapy regardless of whether preoperative corticosteroids were administered. The benefit of aminophylline for intraoperative bronchospasm is questionable and may result in the drug interactions discussed previously.

POSTOPERATIVE MANAGEMENT

Early extubation, after thorough suctioning, while reflexes are still suppressed is ideal. It must be appreciated, however, that the lingering effects of anesthetics, narcotics, or muscle relaxants (Gold and Helrich, 1963) may cause hypoventilation. Pulse oximetry, with supplemental oxygen as needed, is important because postoperative hypoxemia is common during the recovery period in the asthmatic patient. All patients treated preoperatively with corticosteroids should receive hydrocortisone, 100 mg IV, every 8 hours until respiratory status is stable.

Postoperative bronchospasm may be treated with aerosolized $beta_2$-agonists or subcutaneous epinephrine or terbutaline. Hydrocortisone should be increased to 200 mg IV every 6 hours until the patient is stable. Some clinicians may recommend intravenous aminophylline in this setting. Adequate analgesia, especially after upper abdominal surgery, to allow adequate cough, hydration to allow thinner secretions, and early patient mobilization will all act to minimize the risk of postoperative atelectasis. Early antibiotic therapy for pyrexia in the setting of atelectasis may be of benefit. Patients with COPD may benefit from chest physical therapy. Finally, regional rather than general anesthesia may be preferable in patients with low ventilatory reserve because of the increased risk of anesthesia-induced ventilatory suppression in these patients.

EMERGENCY SURGERY

Asthmatic patients who undergo emergency surgery are at increased risk for perioperative pulmonary complications. Control of bronchospasm and aspiration are key goals in this setting. Factors such as poorly controlled asthma, dehydration, fever, or sepsis may contribute to perioperative complications and should be treated as early as possible. Any patient receiving chronic asthma medications requiring emergency surgery should receive the equivalent of 200 mg hydrocortisone stat. and every 6 hours until stable. As in elective cases, the agent of choice for induction of general anesthesia is ketamine, both to control bronchospasm and to minimize the risk of aspiration. Transient hypertension is a potential adverse effect of ketamine rapidly infused for emergency induction.

THE PREGNANT ASTHMATIC PATIENT

The physiologic changes that occur in the pregnant asthmatic patient may lead to poor maternal or neonatal outcome. Total lung capacity, functional residual capacity, and residual volume all decrease, while vital capacity is essentially unchanged and minute ventilation increases. There is an increase in the alveolar-arterial oxygen gradient as term approaches. Maternal $P{CO_2}$ in the third trimester is approximately 30 mm Hg. This baseline respiratory hypocarbia may be exaggerated by hyperventilation leading to inadequate fetal oxygenation. The presence of a $P{CO_2}$ above 35 mm Hg and a pH less than 7.35 in the setting of an asthma exacerbation are indicative of impending ventilatory failure. It is essential to keep in mind that the pregnant asthmatic patient has decreased pulmonary reserve, and that control of asthma is of paramount importance in this setting.

The details of specific drug therapy in the pre-labor asthmatic patient have been delineated elsewhere. In women who have used inhaled or systemic corticosteroids during the previous year, systemic corticosteroids (see Table 54–1) should be administered on admission for labor and delivery. This is important because of the potential necessity for cesarean section.

Regional anesthesia and supplemental oxygen are indicated during labor and delivery to minimize pain-induced hyperventilation and to ensure adequate fetal oxygenation. Epidural or spinal anesthesia is preferable to general anesthesia for operative delivery because of the greater risk of fetal cardiac and respiratory depression and increased risk of uterine bleeding (via decreased uterine tone) with general anesthesia. If regional anesthesia is not possible, rapid induction and intubation are indicated because of the risk of aspiration of stomach contents.

First-line therapy for bronchospasm during labor is inhaled beta-adrenergic agonists. Subsequently, the equivalent of 200 mg hydrocortisone should be administered and continued every 4 hours until labor is completed and the patient is stable. If the response to inhaled beta-agonist is inadequate, aminophylline may be administered. However, this has occasionally resulted in neonatal theophylline toxicity. Inhaled anticholinergic agents have little apparent adverse effect but little apparent benefit in the therapy of asthma.

In situations in which bronchospasm is unresponsive to inhaled beta-agonist and is likely to compromise the fetus or inhibit labor, subcutaneous administration of epinephrine or terbutaline is indicated. Maternal arterial blood gases must be assessed frequently to ensure prompt recognition of impending ventilatory failure, which would require immediate intubation, ventilation, and subsequent operative delivery.

PERIOPERATIVE IDIOPATHIC ANAPHYLAXIS MANAGEMENT

Idiopathic anaphylaxis may be defined as life-threatening reactions consisting of urticaria or angioedema accompanied by upper airway obstruction, bronchospasm, or hypotension without an identifiable antigen or other stimulus (Stoloff et al, 1992). Some patients experience these episodes frequently, others infrequently, with unpredictable onset of episodes.

This is a well-described and well-characterized patient population. Both acute and maintenance therapy have proved safe and effective. Northwestern's treatment protocol of prednisone, 60 mg daily, almost always controls disease activity within 2 weeks, as reported by Orfan et al (1991).

The goal of perioperative management of idiopathic anaphylaxis is to reduce the risk of anaphylaxis. An episode of anaphylaxis during general anesthesia or recovery greatly increases the risk of complications. For instance, hypotension related to blood loss may be exacerbated or bronchospasm could contribute to hypoxemia. At Northwestern, we routinely administer prophylactic preoperative corticosteroids in patients with idiopathic anaphylaxis and have had no perioperative anaphylaxis.

Elective surgery should be delayed if a patient is having frequent episodes (more than one every 2 months) of idiopathic anaphylaxis. A 5-day preoperative course of 40 to 60 mg of prednisone per day should be given to a patient who has had an episode of idiopathic anaphylaxis or who has been treated for same in the past year. Additionally, hydrocortisone, 100 mg IV, should be given preoperatively and every 8 hours throughout the recovery period. Emergency surgery for these patients dictates the use of 200 mg of intravenous hydrocortisone stat. followed by 100 mg every 8 hours throughout the recovery period. Intraoperative anaphylaxis is treated with subcutaneous epinephrine, intravenous corticosteroids, and parenteral H_1 antagonists along with requisite airway and fluid management.

PERIOPERATIVE MANAGEMENT OF HEREDITARY ANGIOEDEMA

Hereditary angioedema is characterized by recurrent episodes of angioedema due to a quantitative or qualitative defect of C1 esterase inhibitor. Trauma, including surgery, is a well-known trigger for episodes of hereditary angioedema. Patients scheduled for elective surgery should receive stanozolol, 4 mg PO, every 6 hours beginning 5 days prior to surgery. Epsilon-aminocaproic acid 5 mg every 6 hours beginning 5 days prior to surgery may be used as an alternative to stanozolol. Some clinicians advocate the use of 2 units of fresh frozen plasma the day prior to the procedure. In the event of acute angioedema intra- or postoperatively, subcutaneous epinephrine, diphenhydramine, and intravenous hydrocortisone may be added in addition to appropriate airway management maneuvers.

REFERENCES

Gold MI, Helrich M. A study of the complications related to anesthesia in asthmatic patients. Anesth Analg 42:283–293, 1963.

Jackson CV. Preoperative pulmonary evaluation. Arch Intern Med 148:2120–2127, 1988.

Kingston HGG, Hirshman CA. Perioperative management of the patient with asthma. Anesth Analg 63:844–855, 1984.

Orfan N, Greenberger PA, Patterson R. Perioperative management of asthma and idiopathic anaphylaxis. Ann Allergy 67:377–385, 1991.

Stoloff R, Adams SL, Orfan N, Harris KE, Greenberger PA, Patterson R. Emergency medical recognition and management of idiopathic anaphylaxis. J Emerg Med 10:693–698, 1992.

ACKNOWLEDGMENTS: We would like to acknowledge the secretarial and editorial assistance of Ms. Senta Berggruen, Ms. Wanda Gray, Ms. Martha A. Shaughnessy, Ms. Michelle Tosi, and Ms. Donna Watkins.

DEDICATION: This chapter is dedicated to the memory of Robert Charles Latall.

Chapter 55

Controversial Concepts in Allergy and Clinical Immunology

Abba I. Terr, M.D., and John E. Salvaggio, M.D.

Allergic diseases are among the most common chronic disorders, particularly in childhood and adolescence where they are an important cause of morbidity. Diagnostic procedures and treatment methods that are of proven efficacy in allergy are readily available today. These are based on well-established scientific principles, basic research, and controlled clinical trials. Present and future research will undoubtedly add new procedures to the existing ones for allergy management. In spite of this, some practitioners adhere to certain nonscientific theories that give rise to diagnostic tests and therapeutic strategies of unproven efficacy. This chapter will describe and assess these controversial procedures and their theories. A distinction will be made between those procedures that have not been shown to be effective under any circumstances and those that are inappropriate for allergy but may nevertheless be useful in other diseases.

From time to time various theories have been offered to explain the etiology and pathogenesis of various conditions or constellations of symptoms of unknown etiology. Usually these theories propose some alternative form of hypersensitivity, but to date the proponents of these theories have come forth with no experimental proof that the presumed sensitivity to environmental substances is mediated through the immune system in these patients. Evidence is based entirely on anecdotal case reports and "clinical experience."

CONTROVERSIAL THEORIES

Allergic Toxemia

Allergic toxemia, also called the allergic tension-fatigue syndrome, has been proposed as a disease caused by multiple food sensitivities (Speer, 1954). Although it has not been precisely defined, symptoms include recurrent headaches, abdominal pains, fatigue, musculoskeletal pains, respiratory complaints, and general malaise. It is usually diagnosed in children. Symptoms are chronic and variable. Fatigue and listlessness may alternate with hyperactivity, and insomnia with hypersomnia. The condition is believed to be more symptomatic in winter than in summer, but there has been no explanation for this or documentation that this occurs. Pain may involve muscles, joints, bones, abdomen, chest, and head at different times. Less common complaints are lymph node enlargement, low-grade fever, urinary frequency, bladder discomfort, excessive colds, tachycardia, hives, difficulty concentrating, and "allergic shiners," the term used to describe bluish discoloration of the suborbital areas.

Allergic toxemia or allergic tension-fatigue syndrome is believed to result from sensitivities to multiple foods; milk, chocolate, corn, and wheat are listed as the most common causes.

Physical examination in this condition is unrevealing, and even the symptoms that can be verified rarely are confirmed by examination. Routine laboratory testing shows no abnormalities.

The diagnosis is made on the basis of symptoms (Rowe, 1950). Proponents of the concept of food-induced allergic toxemia believe that the onset of symptoms after ingestion of foods is often delayed by hours, days, or even weeks, and the connection is often made retrospectively. The diagnosis is confirmed by trial elimination diets, but generally the dietary eliminations are done without the use of placebo controls, so that it is impossible to state that subsidence of symptoms relates to the elimination of a particular food or to a spontaneous event. If the child fails to improve after certain foods are avoided, additional foods are eliminated from the diet. If symptoms recur or if the response to the elimination diet is not satisfactory, the lack of response may be attributed to poor cooperation by the patient, trace quantities of food allergens in the diet, or to intercurrent infections.

The symptoms described for this condition occur commonly in certain children. They are nonspecific and not consistent with those of allergic inflammation, particularly in the absence of objective physical findings. A definitive double-blind placebo-controlled clinical trial would be necessary to support the existence of food-induced allergic toxemia. Controlled food challenges have successfully reproduced food-induced immediate reactions that are clinically consistent with IgE-mediated allergic mechanisms, but reactions that are reportedly delayed by 2 hours or more after eating the food and that consist of nonspecific symptoms have not been confirmed (Bock et al, 1978).

Although some patients suffering from organ-specific allergic or other chronic diseases may secondarily experience fatigue, difficulty in concentration, and lethargy, the concept that these represent primary allergic manifestations is unproven. Furthermore, there have been no definitive clinical trials showing that therapeutic elimination diets have successfully controlled the multitude of symptoms in so-called allergic toxemia. Support for the concept comes from anecdotal reports only.

Food Additive Sensitivity

Attention deficit disorder is not an uncommon childhood condition. It consists of excessive motor activity, inattention, impulsivity, discipline problems, and poor school performance. The natural history is unpredictable. Some children become asymptomatic during puberty, and others continue to manifest the disease throughout life. The etiology is unknown, although it probably involves constitutional, genetic, environmental, and psychosocial factors.

In 1973 it was proposed that attention deficit disorder was an allergic disease caused by sensitivity to food coloring agents (Feingold, 1975). Naturally occurring salicylates in foods were also proposed as allergens causing this disease. Based on this hypothesis, many children with attention deficit disorder were subjected to a diet in which all food dyes and preservatives, other food additives, and salicylates in foods and medications were restricted. Initially, there were reports that up to 50% of children with attention deficit disorder experienced improved behavior and school performance, but these results were based on uncontrolled trials and anecdotal reports.

Nevertheless, the Feingold diet, named after its original proponent, was enthusiastically supported by parents of affected children, and it was endorsed by a few mental health workers, educators, and some physicians. Eventually controlled clinical trials were undertaken. Because of differing protocols, results are not uniform. Different criteria have been used for patient selection and for measurement of behavioral changes. Some of these trials employed dietary exclusion, which is subject to the uncertainties of compliance and difficulties in blinding, whereas others used challenges with dyes or dye mixtures. A consensus conference by the Office for Medical Applications for Research of the National Institutes of Health concluded that only a few children—at most 2 percent—might benefit by improvement in behavior from a defined diet and that furthermore there is no direct evidence that toxicity, idiosyncrasy, or allergic hypersensitivity from food additives cause direct effects on the central nervous system (Consensus, 1982).

The hypothesis that naturally occurring food salicylates and artificial food or drug additives such as dyes and preservatives cause attention deficit disorder is unproven. There is no evidence that any food additive affects behavior in children through an immunologic or allergic mechanism. The behavioral and cognitive features of attention deficit disorder are not consistent with allergy. An additive-free diet cannot be recommended for children with this condition.

Multiple Chemical Sensitivities

The concept of multiple chemical sensitivities, also called environmental illness, is that of an illness in which ordinary, every-day exposure to numerous, environmental substances results in numerous multisystemic symptoms in the absence of positive physical findings, pathology, or abnormal laboratory tests (Randolph and Moss, 1980). Patients with this diagnosis are almost always adults, usually women, and they experience varying degrees of disability in their work and everyday activities. The concept of this illness is fostered by a small group of physicians who use many of the unproven diagnostic procedures discussed in this chapter, particularly provocation-neutralization. The patient typically is intolerant to numerous foods and drugs as well.

A number of theories have been proposed to explain the illness. Most of these theories are based on the concept that the immune system has been damaged by environmental chemicals, and the symptoms are explained as those of allergy, autoimmunity, or immunodeficiency (Terr, 1987). However, the wide ranging symptoms, absence of physical findings, and absence of objective evidence of immunologic disease in multiple chemical sensitivities differs significantly from these diseases. There has never been any proof that these patients have antibody or cellular immunity to the various environmental chemicals to which they apparently react. A recent theory proposes that these common environmental chemicals are toxic to the central nervous system, causing unspecified and unconfirmed damage to higher centers in the brain, which result in somatic symptoms.

The list of environmental chemicals to which the patients react adversely is extensive and includes ethanol, phenol, formaldehyde, and ammonia, as well as such agents as pesticides, perfumes, solvents, paints, synthetic building materials and clothing, carpets, fuels, and exhaust fumes. In some cases, electromagnetic fields, such as those found around power lines, are believed to provoke symptoms. The pattern of symptomatology is similar to that experienced by a patient with the psychiatric disorder known as somatoform illness, and it is not unlike the clinical presentation of other poorly defined syndromes such as the chronic fatigue syndrome and fibromyalgia. In fact, the only factor that separates multiple chemical sensitivities from other syndromes is the fact that the patient attributes symptoms to the environment. However, blinded challenges suggest that the response to chemicals is based on suggestion. Treatment is largely based on avoidance. Patients go to extreme measures to avoid chemicals, and they often follow special elimination diets. In some cases neutralization therapy with sublingual drops or injections of chemical extracts is recommended.

A number of investigators have examined the multiple chemical sensitivity phenomenon. Clinical evaluation of the patients indicates a high prevalence of current and prior psychiatric illness and/or psychosocial stress (Black et al, 1990; Sparks et al, 1994). Immunologic evaluation has failed to show any consistent abnormalities that would explain the symptoms (Terr, 1987).

Candida Hypersensitivity

A popular theory has surfaced in recent years that certain people develop hypersensitivity to a toxin produced by the yeast *Candida albicans*, which normally exists in the gastrointestinal tract and vagina (Truss, 1981; Crook, 1989). The illness is described as one of numerous wide-ranging symptoms without positive physical findings or laboratory abnormalities. It has even been proposed that behavioral problems in teenagers are caused by sensitivity to *Candida albicans* (Crook, 1989). Therefore, the clinical presentation cannot be distinguished from that of multiple food and chemical sensitivities. In fact, many patients are diagnosed with the combination of food, chemical, and *Candida* sensitivity. The popular acceptance of *Candida* hypersensitivity as an "illness" can be traced to a series of books written for the lay public and geared to self-diagnosis and self-treatment.

Candida albicans is frequently a part of the normal flora of the skin and the mucosa of the respiratory, gastrointestinal, and female genitourinary tracts. Because of its commensal status with humans, there is virtually universal exposure to *Candida* antigens, and immune responses with low levels of antibody and cell-mediated immunity are detectable in a high percentage of normal individuals.

The so-called *Candida* hypersensitivity syndrome contrasts sharply with local or systemic opportunistic candidiasis in patients with impaired natural or acquired immunity (Edwards et al, 1978). Thrush or localized infection of the buccal mucosa is not an unusual illness in infants, and it may complicate antibiotic or topical inhaled corticosteroid therapy. Thrush and/or *Candida* vulvovaginitis can be a complication of diabetes mellitus, pregnancy, progesterone therapy, or a temporary residual effect of antibiotic therapy. Systemic candidiasis is seen most commonly in children with therapeutic immunosuppression for cancer, chronic granulomatous disease, chronic mucocutaneous candidiasis, and immunodeficiency disorders with impaired cell-mediated immunity.

The *Candida* hypersensitivity syndrome has been applied most often to persons with numerous subjective symptoms but without objective evidence of pathology. It is also claimed—without any clinical or scientific justification—to be a potentiating factor for a number of other diseases such as multiple sclerosis, arthritis, psoriasis, schizophrenia, depression, and various behavioral and emotional conditions. The syndrome therefore lacks a specific definition. Proponents of *Candida* hypersensitivity blame current or past use of antibiotics, corticosteroid therapy, birth control pills, and dietary sugar as potentiating factors.

UNPROVEN DIAGNOSTIC METHODS

Skin End-point Titration

The value of prick/intradermal skin testing to identify specific IgE antibody sensitivities is thoroughly established as the most reliable and sensitive method for this purpose as part of the overall diagnostic procedure, including a history and physical examination. It is a simple two-tiered procedure that is safe and rapid. It is suitable for the vast majority of cases of suspected atopic or anaphylactic diseases. For certain special circumstances, such as *Hymenoptera* insect venom anaphylaxis, tenfold serial intradermal tests (following preliminary prick testing) are recommended to minimize a possible systemic reaction to the test. Most allergists would use a similar form of serial intradermal testing when dealing with a new allergen of uncertain potency. In any event, the end point or titer (the lowest concentration of allergen that produces a positive skin test) is not necessarily a reliable indicator of clinical sensitivity.

Some clinicians perform routine serial end-point intradermal testing for all patients with suspected atopy. The end-point or titer is then used to determine both the starting dose for allergen immunotherapy and an "optimal dose" for treatment, i.e., an anticipated maintenance dose claimed to provide maximal benefit. The method described by Rinkel (1949) is generally used. It is complicated and based on uncontrolled empiric observations. Increasing fivefold serial concentrations of allergen are injected intradermally, usually in a dose of 0.01 ml. The test site is read by measuring the size of the wheal at 10 minutes without regard for the presence or absence of erythema. Results of testing are called "end points," the injected dose that initiates a series 2-mm incremental increase in wheal diameter with increasing fivefold concentrations. However, test results that do not fit into this defined pattern are considered "bizarre." "Hourglass" patterns of decreasing and then increasing wheal diameter, "flash response," which refers to a nonreproducible wheal, and "plateau" responses of unchanging wheal diameters with increasing dose are attributed to a variety of extraneous factors such as infection, exposure to airborne pollen, exposure to food allergens, immunotherapy treatment, and peculiarities of specific allergens. Since each allergen must be tested with as many as nine serial intradermal injections, the total number of such injections and the time involved are considerable. If the patient fails to improve as expected, re-testing is recommended to establish a new "end point" during the course of immunotherapy.

Serial titration has been shown to be a safe method in determining the starting dose of immunotherapy in order to avoid a possible systemic reaction to the first subcutaneous dose (Hirsch et al, 1981). However, the method frequently underestimates the initial tolerated dose, especially for patients highly sensitive to the allergen (Van Metre et al, 1980). This results in many unnecessary injections and lost time before achieving the maintenance level for high-dose immunotherapy that has been shown by double-blind controlled studies to be effective for ameliorating pollen rhinitis.

The "optimal" dose is calculated at various multiples of the end point, usually between 25 and 50 times the quantity of allergen producing the end point, but this may vary with the particular allergen. However, several controlled clinical trials have shown that a calculated "optimal" immunotherapy dose based on the end point is almost always too low, and the therapeutic effect is no more effective than placebo (Van Metre, 1980).

Failure to include the presence of erythema at the skin test site is a critical fault in the methodology. Wheal diameter in the presence of accompanying erythema is an efficient indication of the degree of skin test reactivity to an allergen, but its presence in the absence of erythema is of unknown significance and is likely to lead to clinically false-positive test results, since some allergens might cause a nonspecific irritant wheal in the absence of specific immunologic sensitivity.

While serial end-point titration using common atopic allergens produces increasing wheal diameter with increasing doses of intradermal test allergen, the method of Rinkel and his followers cannot be recommended as a reliable diagnostic test for IgE-mediated skin sensitivity, and there is evidence that the method is not capable of establishing *a priori* an optimal immunotherapy dose to control atopic disease.

Provocation-Neutralization Testing

The procedure consists of the administration to the patient of a test dose of a food, chemical, hormone, or allergen extract by the intracutaneous, subcutaneous, or sublingual route. This is called "provocation." The patient records any and all subjective sensations for a period of 10 minutes after the challenge. *Any* reported sensation is considered a positive test. Once a positive result is "provoked," further challenges with the same substance at different doses (higher or lower) are given until the patient reports no sensations. This is called "neutralization." The "neutralizing" dose of the substance is then recommended for therapy (to be discussed).

The rationale for this type of testing cannot be defended scientifically. The items used for testing are usually selected from a predetermined group of materials without reference to the patient's history. They include such chemicals as formaldehyde, phenol, ethanol, foods, inhalant allergens, and hormones such as progesterone. Some proponents of this procedure test patients with "extracts" of air, water, saline, automobile exhaust fumes, chlorine, gasoline, and other substances. In some cases, a positive "result" from a single chemical is believed to reveal sensitivities to a range of other chemicals, e.g., a positive response to ethanol (or phenol) indicates that the patient is allergic to all "petrochemicals." The subjective and uncontrolled nature of provocation-neutralization is inconsistent with any mechanism known to operate in the pathogenesis of allergic disease. Jewett et al (1990) evaluated the method, using a well-designed double-blind placebo-controlled protocol. They showed that responses to sublingual food extract were no different from placebo responses in 18 patients who had previously responded positively to the same food extracts and negatively to controls in an unblinded setting. The study clearly exposes the role of suggestion in provocation-neutralization and similar tests.

The Pulse Test

A theory that allergy causes a change in the pulse has led to the so-called pulse test for food allergy (Coca, 1982). An increase in the pulse rate of 10 beats per minute or more after a test dose of a food is eaten is considered a positive test. Some proponents of this bizarre theory consider either a rise or a fall in pulse rate to be equally diagnostic. There is no prescribed time interval in performance of the test.

There is no reasonable theory and no scientific evidence to support this theory. Changes in pulse rate can occur from many physiologic and pathologic conditions, but there is no basis for its role in the pathogenesis of any allergic disease. There has never been a controlled clinical trial of pulse testing in allergy.

The Cytotoxic Food Test

The cytotoxic test for food allergy consists of applying one drop of diluted whole blood or buffy coat to a microscope slide that was previously coated with a dried film of a food extract. A cover slip is placed on the sample, and the slide is observed microscopically for swelling, vacuolation, crenation, or other distortion of leukocytes. Any such change in cell morphology is said to indicate "food allergy."

The test is performed without standardization of time, temperature, pH, or osmolarity (Black, 1956; Bryan and Bryan, 1960).

Based on current knowledge of the immune pathogenesis of allergic disease, there is no theoretic basis for this test. Allergic reactions to foods are not caused by cytotoxicity of leukocytes. Exposure of a food substance to white cells *in vitro* is an unlikely diagnostic replica of an *in vivo* allergic response to a food. Typically, reports from those few laboratories offering this test indicate that up to 150 foods have been tested on a single blood sample, a feat that is logistically unlikely. Attempts to substantiate the validity of the cytotoxic tests have revealed that results are random and not reproducible (Franklin and Lowell, 1949).

Applied Kinesiology

Applied kinesiology is the application of an unfounded and scientifically illogical theory that an allergic reaction, especially to a food, causes weakening of skeletal musculature. The method consists of a subjective estimate by a technician of the muscle strength in an extremity before and after exposure of the patient to an allergen (Garrow, 1988). The exposure consists of placing a vessel such as a glass vial containing allergen extract on the patient's skin. Even though there is no pathophysiologic rationale for this "test" and no basis whatsoever for its diagnostic efficacy, it is widely used because of its simplicity. Many patients accept the results when they are presented and endorsed with enthusiasm and confidence by the practitioner. For testing infants and small children, the procedure is done by proxy by having a parent hold the hand of the child during the testing.

Electrodiagnosis

Various diagnostic procedures have been propounded based on the theory that allergy produces a change in electrical resistance of the skin. In general, food extracts are placed in containers that are connected to an electric circuit, which makes contact with the patient's skin with a galvanometer for measuring the electrical resistance of the skin. Skin contact is made with a metal probe that can contact different parts of the body (Voll, 1980).

This and other unproven diagnostic procedures, no matter how bizarre and incredible, may impress suggestible and gullible patients when presented by enthusiastic proponents along with assurance of success in alleviating illness. In addition, equipment used for electrodiagnosis provides for the presentation of "results" in the form of a computer printout. It is a painless procedure advertised as being superior to the old-fashioned "outmoded" painful skin testing.

Serum IgG Antibodies

Although some have postulated that IgG antibodies to specific foods may be responsible for delayed symptoms or vague intolerance to foods, there is yet no proof for this. The radioallergosorbent test (RAST) and similar technology are capable of detecting minute quantities of such antibodies, and it is likely that low levels of IgG antibodies to foods circulate normally, but they are of no known pathogenic significance.

IgG antibodies are not involved in the pathogenesis of atopic disease. However, allergen immunotherapy with extracts of aeroallergens does induce specific IgG blocking antibodies, which reflect the treatment, not the disease. Many years of research have so far failed to show that quantifying immunotherapy-induced IgG blocking antibodies is a useful marker of successful treatment.

High-level specific IgG antibodies are involved in the pathogenesis of serum sickness and possibly certain stages of hypersensitivity pneumonitis and allergic bronchopulmonary aspergillosis. Thus, measurement of specific IgG antibodies to the relevant allergen may be diagnostically helpful in these particular diseases, but they are not useful in the diagnosis or management of patients with atopic disease.

Some clinical laboratories provide quantitative measurement of circulating IgG antibodies to food and mold allergens. Antibodies are usually measured by radioallergosorbent test (RAST) or enzyme-linked immunosorbent assay (ELISA), or by a modification of these techniques.

Although some have postulated that IgG antibodies may be responsible for delayed symptoms or vague intolerance to foods, there is currently no proof of this. RAST and similar technology are capable of detecting minute quantities of such antibodies, and it is likely that low-level IgG antibodies to foods circulate normally (Djurup et al, 1984), but they are of no known pathogenic significance.

Food Immune Complexes

Circulating immune complexes containing food antigen molecules combined with, or coupled to, specific antibodies can be detected by a two-site immune assay. As in the case of IgG antibodies to foods, low levels of such immune complexes can be detected in normal individuals (Dannaeus et al, 1979; Husby et al, 1985), particularly after a meal, but there are no studies to indicate that any form of allergic disease is related to food immune complexes.

"Biomarker" Tests

There is an increasing trend among certain practitioners who espouse controversial and unproven allergy theories and practices to utilize the clinical immunology laboratory for an extensive battery of immunologic blood tests. Certain abnormal results are said to be "biomarkers" of environmental or chemical-induced disease. This approach is especially popular among those who tout the concept that low levels or minute amounts of numerous environmental chemicals produce a host of subjective complaints or sensations. Although the individual tests may be legitimately applicable to certain defined immunologic diseases, misuse of the biomarker concept comes from interpreting either an abnormal test result in itself or slight and clinically insignificant variations in a test result as evidence of overt disease or illness.

These practitioners claim, without objective evidence or physical examination or functional tests and on the basis of belief only, that a slightly abnormal laboratory test by itself indicates that chemicals or related agents existing in trace amounts have damaged the immune system and caused disease in man. Suppression of the immune system would theoretically result in an increased incidence of infections or a decrease in immune tumor surveillance mechanisms. Activation of the immune system by a putative environmental agent could theoretically result in autoantibody formation and the possibility of autoimmune disease or some other form of hypersensitivity such as IgE-mediated extrinsic asthma, rhinitis, or urticaria. At present, there is no basis in fact to substantiate these claims in man other than anecdotal reports. In spite of this lack of evidence, many individuals who have been allegedly exposed to such chemicals are being referred to laboratories or laboratory-based physicians for assessment of possible "immunotoxic" effects on cellular or humoral components of the immune system.

Assaying of immune cell populations and subpopulations requires the use of expensive automated methodology and monoclonal antibodies against a variety of CD differentiation antigens on the surface of T cells, B cells, NK cells, and various T cell phenotypic subsets. Cells are counted by flow cytometry using a fluorescent-activated cell sorter (FACS) (Jones, 1989). In this process a fluent stream of cells passes in single file through sensors capable of measuring their physical characteristics, particularly the cell size. Flow cytometry is widely used in the identification and characterization of immune cell subpopulations and can also measure lymphocyte activation for clinical purposes, including assessment for the activity of autoimmune disease processes and susceptibility of transplanted tissue to host rejection. The surface expression of several antigens appearing on the cell surface after mitogenic stimulation can also be assessed.

B Cell and T Cell Phenotypic Subset Analysis by Flow Cytometry

Quantitation of peripheral blood lymphocytes has been performed in a wide variety of human disease states, but only rarely do the results provide diagnostic information. When used in a clinical context, these assays are difficult to interpret because of many confounding variables, among which are a wide range of normal values, varying normal ranges among different laboratories, and age- and time-related differences (Biologic Markers, 1992). Other variables such as concurrent viral infections, cigarette smoking, the influence of drugs, stress, and associated disease states can all affect the quantity and function of lymphocyte cell populations. The extent of these variations can easily obscure alterations that might otherwise be of diagnostic help. For example, the number of CD4 helper T cells can vary by 50 percent or more, depending on the time of day that a blood sample is drawn. It should also be remembered that the lymphocyte composition of the blood differs from that of most body organs and tissues, where they function in normal and pathologic immune response. Thus, peripheral lymphocyte numbers do not necessarily reflect the pathologic changes occurring in specific organs. In addition, the peripheral blood contains only approximately 2 percent of the total lymphocyte pool in the adult human body, and small alterations in lymphocyte numbers within lymphoid organs can cause major alterations in peripheral blood numbers. Thus, it is obvious that one cannot make clinical evaluations based on results of isolated *in vitro* assessment of quantity and function of immune system cellular components without considering all of these variables and without knowledge of the complete case history and physical examination. This is especially true when a test subject with alleged environmental injury, "environmental illness," or "multiple chemical sensitivity," has no symptoms characteristic of immune deficiency or no abnormal signs on physical examination, as often is the case. If attention is not paid to the aforementioned variables, patients can be misdiagnosed as having various forms of "immune dysregulation," "immune dysfunction," "low NK cell syndrome," or even "chemical AIDS" in the absence of evidence of overt clinical disease by history and physical examination, on the sole basis of minor deviations in quantitative cellular and functional assays of lymphoid cell populations.

Proven indications for such biomarker lymphoid analysis are limited to diagnosis and classification of immunodeficiency diseases; follow-up of patients who have undergone immune reconstitution; clinical suspicion of AIDS; determination of type and source of malignant lymphocytes in lymphocytic leukemia and lymphoma; monitoring of cellular changes following bone marrow and other organ transplantation; and monitoring of patients on immunosuppressive drug regimens.

In cases involving alleged exposure to trace amounts of environmental chemicals, there is no sound experimental evidence that has revealed abnormal quantities or function of any specific cellular component of the immune system, including cell phenotypic subsets, following these types of environmental exposure. In the few cases in which exposure to environmental chemicals in trace amounts has been associated with slight abnormalities of lymphoid cell numbers or function, such effects have no meaningful value in terms of diagnosing such a disease state or of predicting a certain clinical course.

Cytokine quantitation has also been used by some as a diagnostic aid in alleged environmentally induced immunoregulatory disorders. However, to date there have been no properly controlled studies definitively showing altered production of cytokines in individuals exposed to trace amounts of environmental chemicals. As in the case of cell quantitation by flow cytometry, levels of these cytokines vary widely, and random measurements in any given individual neither support nor refute the presence of illness in themselves (Campden et al, 1988). The interleukin-2 receptor (IL-2R) and its beta chain component referred to as the high-affinity receptor or soluble IL-2R (sIL-2R) have been used by some as a diagnostic aid for certain forms of alleged environmental injury, even though there is no evidence for increased sIL-2R levels in individuals with any type of alleged environmental illness.

Tests for Autoantibodies

A panel of autoantibodies is often part of the diagnostic laboratory armamentarium of those who endorse the concept of "multiple chemical sensitivities." Circulating autoantibodies are markers of many autoimmune diseases, including the so-called connective tissue disorders (Tan, 1982). In some cases, such as autoimmune thyroiditis, autoimmune hemolytic anemias, and myasthenia gravis, the autoantibody is directly involved in disease pathogenesis, whereas in other cases, the autoantibody may be an epiphenomenon but a potential diagnostic marker of a disease. In the clinical evaluation of circulating autoantibodies, it is critical to remember that they exist normally in low titer, which increases with age.

Certain metallic salts such as mercuric chloride (Pelletier et al, 1988), cadmium (Ohsawa et al, 1988), and gold thiomalate (Robinson et al, 1983) can induce non–organ-specific autoantibody formation, autoimmune disease, hypergammaglobulinemia, and other immune abnormalities in experimental animals. In some other cases, drugs and chemicals may cause immunoregulatory aberrations. For example, alpha methyl-dopa has been shown to have effects on T suppressor cells, silicon dioxide can induce autoimmune phenomena and autoantibody formation in man, and asbestos fibers are known to act simultaneously as polyclonal B cell stimulants and as suppressors of certain T cell functions. At present, however, there is no sound evidence that autoantibodies are operative in the pathogenesis of diseases of man associated with exposure to environmental chemicals or pollutants or that autoantibodies are in fact induced by such exposure in man.

Blood and Tissue Chemical Analyses

The controversial concept of multiple chemical sensitivities has resulted in a recent trend of some laboratories to offer analyses of blood, fat, or other body tissue samples for the presence of pesticides, hydrocarbons, and various organic and inorganic chemicals. Analytic techniques for detecting these chemicals are available with extreme sensitivity so that detection at the level of parts per billion or parts per trillion can be accomplished easily. As a result, such minute amounts of xenobiotic chemicals can be detected in virtually all human beings living in civilized countries where synthetic chemical products are a way of life. This type of chemical analysis can be used to confirm disease caused by toxic overexposure to a specific chemical. However, analyses of a broad range of chemicals are being done indiscriminately in patients with so-called multiple chemical sensitivities under the assumption that any detectable level of any chemical can support that diagnosis. There has been no documentation that extremely low levels of these chemicals in blood, fat, or other body tissue are diagnostic of multiple chemical sensitivities or any recognized disease.

UNPROVEN TREATMENTS

Neutralization Therapy

Following the provocation-neutralization testing described earlier, a "neutralizing" dose of the test substance is recommended for therapeutic use. Treatment consists of sublingual (Morris, 1969) or injected (Rea et al, 1984) neutralizing doses of one substance or a combination of substances to theoretically "neutralize" or to produce tolerance as a way of promptly relieving symptoms. "Neutralizing" or "relieving" therapy is administered with little regard for the specificity of the administered substance to the patient's clinical symptoms. Furthermore, there is no rational explanation for the relief of symptoms using such a procedure. Proponents of neutralization therapy justify the treatment by comparing it with allergen immunotherapy. However, the doses used in neutralization are far too low to have a significant immunologic impact, and there is no scientific explanation for immediate symptom relief, other than suggestion. The treatment has been recommended for use both before and after exposure, and it has been recommended both on an ad lib basis or as maintenance therapy. No reliable study has confirmed efficacy and safety of neutralization.

Acupuncture

Acupuncture is an ancient form of "healing" that has no scientific or logical basis. Nevertheless, it is a commonly used form of alternative practice employed by nonphysicians and by a few physicians as well. It is often combined with other forms of treatment such as homeopathy, naturopathy, psychotherapy, and even medications. Acupuncture is often recommended for the treatment of allergic diseases, based on a completely unfounded and unproven theory that it activates or inhibits a variety of cell mediators and enzymes. No controlled clinical trial has shown efficacy and safety in the treatment of any form of allergic disease. Any reported beneficial effect is most likely to be explained on the basis of suggestion (Skrabanek, 1984).

Homeopathy

Homeopathy is an alternative medical practice in which exceedingly minute quantities of substances believed to cause disease are administered to the patient to cure the disease. These substances are referred to as "remedies," and they are usually given orally. Patients will sometimes take as many as 50 different extracts daily. The extracts are made from plants and animal organs. The basic theory of homeopathy is that "like cures like," although current-day homeopathists often claim that they cure diseases by inducing immunity.

There is a superficial similarity between homeopathic treatment and allergen immunotherapy. However, the latter procedure requires that specific environmental allergens be identified objectively for each allergic patient, and successful immunization against atopic or anaphylactic allergic disease requires injection of allergens over a period of time and at a sufficient dosage to alter favorably the specific immunologic hypersensitivities. Clinical effectiveness of allergen immunotherapy in atopy and in *Hymenoptera* venom anaphylaxis has been repeatedly demonstrated in double-blind trials. No such evidence exists for homeopathic remedies.

Elimination Diets

Dietary and nutritional advice is a frequent concomitant of most forms of unconventional or alternative therapy. The advice may range from a sensible approach to maintaining a balanced diet of necessary nutrients to bizarre, faddish, and dangerous diets. In medical practice, scientifically based diets are required for demonstrated nutritional deficiencies and some metabolic disorders, as well as for short-term use before and after surgery. Specific food elimination is the only currently effective treatment for allergy to a food, but in most cases of a proven food allergy, individual patients are allergic to one food or a small number of foods, so that the required diet usually has no nutritional consequence.

Unfortunately, highly restrictive diets are a frequent accompaniment of a treatment program based on some of the unconventional theories of allergy. Because unproven tests such as provocation-neutralization, the cytotoxic test, and tests utilizing IgG antibodies or immune complexes to foods incorrectly diagnose multiple food allergies, the resulting recommendation for multiple food eliminations places the patient in jeopardy of eventual nutritional deficiency. Supplemental vitamins and minerals will not necessarily correct these deficiencies. Some practitioners recommend a "rotary diversified diet," in which foods in the diet are rotated in such a way that the same food is not eaten more often than once every 4 to 5 days (Dickey, 1976). In theory this might alleviate some of the problems of a highly restrictive diet, but the rotary plan is complicated and time-consuming. Some proponents of this diet recommend that rotating foods prevents the induction of food allergy, based on an erroneous concept that allergy to a food is caused by eating that food too frequently. Others claim that a variety of foods have an immunosuppressive effect, a completely unsubstantiated theory.

The concept of food additive sensitivity has attained a certain amount of popular appeal. Avoiding chemical food additives or pesticides usually entails purchasing "natural" foods from health food stores. There have been no research studies showing that a rotary diversified diet, a diet based on health foods, or multiple food eliminations not based on reliable allergy testing are efficacious or safe.

Chemical Avoidance Therapy

The concept of multiple chemical sensitivities or environmental illness includes a recommendation that patients avoid a wide range of environmental chemicals (Dickey, 1976). The list almost always includes all pesticides, perfumes, new carpets, gasoline, synthetic clothing, plastic materials used in furniture, common household cleaners and detergents, and many other substances. The practical effect of avoiding such substances can be an extreme departure from the patient's usual life style. This may entail extensive renovation of the home, work modification, and often loss of job and friends. In contrast to reasonable measures to avoid exposure to house dust, indoor fungi, and animals in patients with demonstrated allergy to these substances, the widespread avoidance of chemicals in multiple chemical sensitivities is based on unreliable diagnostic tests or presumption of sensitivity. The psychological impact of extensive environmental avoidance has never been addressed by proponents of this procedure, and there have been no control studies to show improvement. In fact, there is evidence that patients who pursue extensive environmental avoidance measures become more symptomatic rather than less (Terr, 1986).

Enzyme-Potentiated Immunotherapy

Enzyme-potentiated desensitization is a recently introduced procedure that is claimed to offer therapeutic results superior to conventional allergen immunotherapy (Fell and Brostoff, 1990). It consists of mixing allergen with the enzyme beta-glucuronidase. The combination is injected in a very small quantity, and proponents claim that seasonal allergy can be controlled with a few preseasonal injections (or even a single injection). Perennial allergy symptoms are usually treated with injections given every 2 to 6 months. Some practitioners treat food allergies by this method.

There are claims that enzyme-potentiated desensitization can be used to treat successfully all forms of allergy, as well as autoimmune disease and even epilepsy.

The theoretic basis is a claimed immunosuppressant action of beta-glucuronidase, presumably through activation of lymphocytes. However, no such effect has yet been demonstrated to occur in humans, and it is unlikely that the minute amount of enzyme used in this procedure would have a pharmacologic effect, since the dose given is a small fraction of the amount of the same enzyme normally present in the body.

There is a single report in which 44 grass pollen–allergic patients showed significant improvement over a placebo effect when measured by overall patient preference and lessened requirement for drug therapy, although daily symptom records showed no effect (Fell and Brostoff, 1990). All other reports are anecdotal. Enzyme-potentiated desensitization at this time must be considered highly experimental.

REFERENCES

Biologic markers in immunotoxicology. Subcommittee on Immunotoxicology, Committee on Biologic Markers, Washington, DC, National Academy Press, 1992.

Black AP. A new diagnostic method in allergic disease. Pediatrics 17:716, 1956.

Black DW, Rathe A, Goldstein RB. Environmental illness: A controlled study of 26 subjects with "20th century disease." JAMA 264:3166, 1990.

Bock SA, Lei Y, Remigo LK, et al. Studies of hypersensitivity reactions to foods in infants and children. J Allergy Clin Immunol 62:327, 1978.

Bryan WTK, Bryan M. The application of in vitro cytotoxic reactions to clinical diagnosis of food allergy. Laryngoscope 70:810, 1960.

Campden DH, Horwitz DA, Quismorio FP, et al. Serum levels of interleukin-2 receptor and activity of rheumatic disease characterized by immune system activation. Arthritis Rheum 31:1358, 1988.

Coca AF. The Pulse Test. New York, Carol Publishing Group, 1982.

Consensus Conference. Defined diets and childhood hyperactivity. JAMA 248:290, 1982.

Crook WG. The Yeast Connection. 3rd ed. Jackson, Tenn., Professional Books, 1989.

Dannaeus A. Iganas M, Johansson SGO, Foucard T. Intestinal intake of ovalbumin in malabsorption and food allergy in relation to serum IgE antibody and orally administered sodium cromoglycate. Clin Allergy 9:263, 1979.

Dickey LD (ed). Clinical Ecology. Springfield, Ill, Charles C Thomas, Publisher, 1976.

Djurup R, Kappelgaard E, Skov PS, et al. Determination of IgE-containing immune complexes in human sera. Evaluation of polyethylene glycol precipitation of monomeric and complex IgE and of the detectability of IgE in the complexes. Allergy 39:395, 1984.

Edwards JE Jr, Lehrer RI, Stiehm ER, et al. Severe candidal infections: Clinical perspective, immune defense mechanisms and current concepts of therapy. Ann Intern Med 89:91, 1978.

Feingold B. Why Your Child Is Hyperactive. New York, Random House, 1975.

Fell P, Brostoff J. A single-dose desensitization for summer hayfever. Results of a double-blind study—1988. Eur J Clin Pharmacol 38:77, 1990.

Franklin W, Lowell FC. Failure of ragweed pollen extract to destroy white cells from ragweed-sensitive patients. J Allergy 20:375, 1949.

Garrow JS. Kinesiology and food allergy. Br Med J 296:1573, 1988.

Hirsch SR, Kalbfleisch JH, Golbert TM, et al. Rinkel injection therapy: A multicenter controlled study. J Allergy Clin Immunol 68:133, 1981.

Husby S, Oxelius VA, Teisner B, et al. Humoral immunity to dietary antigens in healthy adults. Occurrence, isotype and IgG subclass distribution of serum antibodies to protein antigens. Int Arch Allergy Appl Immunol 77:416, 1985.

Jewett DL, Fein G, Greenberg MH. Double-blind study of symptoms provocation to determine food sensitivity. N Engl J Med 323:429, 1990.

Jones S. Flow cytometry: Applications in research and medicine. Immunochemica 3:1–4, 1989.

Morris DL. Use of sublingual antigen in diagnosis and treatment of food allergy. Ann Allergy 27:289, 1969.

Ohsawa M, Takahashi K, Otsuka F: Induction of antinuclear antibodies in mice orally exposed to cadmium at low concentrations. Clin Exp Immunol 73:98, 1988.

Pelletier L, Pasquier R, Rossert J, Vial MC, Chantal M, Druet P. Autoreactive T cells in mercury-induced autoimmunity: Ability to induce the autoimmune disease. J Immunol 140:750, 1988.

Randolph TG, Moss RW. An Alternative Approach to Allergies: The New Field of Clinical Ecology Unravels the Environmental Cause of Mental and Physical Ills. New York, Harper and Row, 1980.

Rea WJ, Podell RN, Williams M, et al. Elimination of oral food challenge reaction by injection of food extract. Arch Otolaryngol 110:248, 1984.

Rinkel HJ. Inhalant allergy. I. The whealing response of the skin to serial dilution testing. Ann Allergy 7:625, 1949.

Robinson C, Egorov I, Balazo T. Strain differences in the induction of antinuclear antibodies by mercuric chloride, gold sodium thiomalate, and D-penicillamine in inbred mice. Fed Proc 42:1213, 1983.

Rowe AH. Allergic toxemia and fatigue. Ann Allergy 8:72, 1950.

Skrabanek P. Acupuncture and the age of unreason. Lancet 1:1169, 1984.

Sparks PJ, Daniell W, Black DW, Kipen HM, Altman LC, Simon GE, Terr AI. Multiple chemical sensitivity syndrome: A clinical perspective. I. Case definition, theories of pathogenesis, and research needs. J Occup Med 36:718, 1994.

Speer F. The allergic tension fatigue syndrome. Pediatr Clin North Am 1:1029, 1954.

Tan ED. Autoantibodies to nuclear antigens (ANA): Their immunobiology and medicine. Adv Immunol 33:167, 1982.

Terr AI. Environmental illness: A clinical review of 50 cases. Arch Intern Med 146:145, 1986.

Terr AI. "Multiple chemical sensitivities": Immunologic critique of clinical ecology theories and practice. State Art Rev Occup Med 2:683, 1987.

Truss CO. The role of *Candida albicans* in human illness. J Orthomol Psychiatr 10:228, 1981.

Van Metre TE, Adkinson NF, Lichtenstein LM, et al. A controlled study of the effectiveness of the Rinkel method of immunotherapy for ragweed pollen hay fever. J Allergy Clin Immunol 65:288, 1980.

Voll R. The phenomenon of medicine testing in electro-acupuncture according to Voll. Am J Acupuncture 8:87, 1980.

Chapter 56

Allergies in the School

Clifton T. Furukawa, M.D.

Approximately one of every five school children has allergy and/or asthma problems. During the school year it can be expected that one of every ten children will have an episode of wheezing. It is estimated that about one in 250 children may be sensitive to bee stings. Approximately 1 to 3 percent of school children suffer from food allergy. Thus, allergic diseases are important, not only because of their prevalence, but because allergic reactions may occur during the school session which may require emergency action.

These special problems for the child and the school can be anticipated, and concrete solutions do exist. The special issues in the school revolve around allergic emergencies including anaphylaxis and acute asthma, health conditions that limit full participation in scholastic or sport activities, factors that may affect learning, and health risks that are the consequence of the school environment.

ALLERGIC EMERGENCIES

A program dealing with anaphylaxis occurring at school is critically important. Anaphylaxis can be caused by foods, insect stings, medications, or exercise. For patients who are allergic to insect stings or who have anaphylactic reactions to food, situations requiring epinephrine actually occur once every 1 to 3 years (Grabenstein and Smith, 1989). Concerns about unavailability of epinephrine are well founded, since omission of epinephrine correlates with death from accidental food ingestion in highly allergic individuals. One study reported that four of six fatal anaphylactic reactions to foods occurred within the school setting, where epinephrine was not available (Sampson et al, 1992). Since neither the physician nor the parent has direct authority within the school system, cooperation and communication with the school system are essential to ensure the existence of an emergency action plan.

There are issues in terms of who in the school setting is the responsible person for administering epinephrine. Key individuals must be identified, and written permission and explicit information from the student's parent and physician must be provided.

The Committee on School Health of the American Academy of Pediatrics (1990) has suggested that two or more members of the school staff should be designated and trained to handle anaphylaxis recognition and treatment. Furthermore, the Section on Allergy and Immunology of the American Academy of Pediatrics (1993) has pointed out five important recommendations.

1. Prevention of exposure to relevant etiologic agents is the cornerstone of the management of anaphylaxis and requires close communication among school personnel, family members, and medical authorities.

2. The treatment of choice of anaphylaxis is the subcutaneous injection of epinephrine, which has been shown to be well-tolerated in children and adolescents.

3. Children and adolescents with a history of anaphylaxis should have ready access to epinephrine while at school. Preferably, the student should carry epinephrine with him or her at all times and self-administer it if a reaction occurs. If this is not feasible, epinephrine should be available in the classroom, physical education facility, and cafeteria, where it is most likely to be needed. Following such treatment, the child should receive prompt medical evaluation to deter-

mine whether there is any need for further treatment.

4. If a school does not have a full-time nurse, other school personnel should be trained in the recognition of anaphylaxis and the administration of epinephrine in the event of an anaphylactic emergency. Cafeteria personnel and the classroom teacher of any student with a history of anaphylaxis should be trained to recognize the symptoms of anaphylaxis and in the administration of epinephrine.

5. Legislation is needed in many states to provide a mechanism for certifying nonmedical persons to administer epinephrine.

Acute severe asthma may also represent an emergency within the classroom setting. Certainly, those students with sufficient maturity to control their own medications should be allowed to carry their inhalers to school, keep them nearby, and self-administer medication. With acute asthma, the student would be allowed to use his or her inhaler and to notify the teacher or nurse if medication fails to provide sufficient relief. In cases in which the student might be unable to make his or her own decision, the parent and doctor should provide the school with an action plan that could use objective parameters, such as peak flow readings, to determine when to use medication, when to contact the parent, and when to consider this an emergency that requires immediate transport to an emergency facility.

CONDITIONS LIMITING FULL PARTICIPATION IN SCHOOL ACTIVITIES

Full and unrestricted participation in all school activities is the general goal for all children with allergies and asthma. There are instances, however, when it may be best to limit a student from full participation, for example, from strenuous activity in severe, difficult-to-control asthma, especially when school personnel cannot be adequately educated about the disorder or cannot be relied upon to use good judgment. All efforts should be made to effectively prevent exercise-induced asthma and to openly communicate recommendations to the physical education teacher or coach, as recommended by the statement on Exercise and the Asthmatic Child from the American Academy of Pediatrics Section on Allergy and Immunology and the Section on Diseases of the Chest (1989). Perhaps the issue most in need of resolution has to do with the student's self-administration of inhaled bronchodilators during school time. A position statement by the American Academy of Allergy and Immunology Committee on Drugs recommends that ". . . students with asthma be permitted to have in their possession inhaled medications for the treatment and prevention of asthma symptoms when they are provided by that student's physician."

Since most states consider inhaled medications to fall in the same category as oral drugs, it is necessary for the physician to provide the school with clear indications and directions for the use of such medications. The National Asthma Allergy Network/Mothers of Asthmatics have written recommendations as to what schools should and should not do, a statement that was supported by both the Section on Allergy and Immunology and the Section on Diseases of the Chest of the American Academy of Pediatrics (Furukawa and Murphy, 1990) (Table 56–1).

These measures should help in the control of allergic and asthmatic symptoms, optimize school performance, maximally normalize participation in regular physical education, and minimize allergen and irritant exposure of the child at school.

CONDITIONS AFFECTING LEARNING BY THE CHILD IN SCHOOL

Poorly controlled asthma or allergic disease can have substantial impact on the ability of the child to learn within the classroom. Additionally, side effects of medications may be detrimental to the learning of some children. Antihistamines can cause tiredness and inattention. Decongestants may result in hyperactivity or poor sleeping patterns. Asthma medications may cause tremor, jitteriness, or agitation. These and other drug side effects can affect the child's attention, performance and learning, yet the physician must optimize the control of asthma, allergic rhinitis, sinus disease, otitis and subsequent hearing loss, and eczema in order to have the child as physically well as possible. Poor control of the health conditions noted can result in discom-

TABLE 56–1. STATEMENT OF NATIONAL ASTHMA ALLERGY NETWORK AND THE MOTHERS OF ASTHMATICS

Schools should:
1. Provide necessary medical support for students' health-related needs (such as managing medications) that enable them to control their condition and benefit from regular education
2. Have a system of administering medications which is medically timely and nondisruptive of classroom or athletic activities
3. Provide necessary staff education and medical support for health-related emergencies
4. Consider a student's condition, medications, or their side effects when assessing performance
5. Provide a modified regular or adapted physical education program when it is medically necessary
6. Allow temporary adjustments for students who sometimes require restrictions on vigorous gym, sports, or outdoor play, especially in cold weather
7. Provide advance notice of field trips and special class events so that parents can make accommodations for their children's allergies, diet restrictions, medications, or limited stamina

Schools should not:
1. Send children home to exclude them from field trips and other activities instead of providing prescribed medications
2. Impose waiting periods that disqualify students with frequent and/or intermittent absences from receiving home or hospital tutoring, back-up tutoring, or make-up assistance
3. Penalize students with chronic illnesses for missing class or gym

fort and fatigue, which in turn result in poor attention span and loss of concentration. Hearing loss has an obvious impact on auditory learning. Itching or skin lesions from eczema or urticaria can be preoccupying and behavior altering, and may even discourage school attendance altogether. Medications may affect behavior or attention by inducing drowsiness, irritability, or nervousness. Every attempt should be made to minimize or modify dosage or to change to medications that minimize side effects. Specific inquiry by the physician into the performance of the child in school is necessary to detect difficulties that need attention. In addition, objective assessment of hearing should be performed periodically. Tympanometry, which identifies negative middle ear pressure and fluid, may help to identify those with intermittent hearing difficulties, even in the face of normal screening audiometry. Those with intermittent hearing loss should be placed closer to the front of the classroom, and the teacher should be aware that inattention may occur at times due to hearing loss. Of course, the child's family must be informed so that medical assessment and intervention can occur.

SCHOOL HEALTH RISKS

Since it is not feasible for the physician to evaluate each school's program and environment, it is necessary that the parent communicate to the physician specifics about the child's school environment and activities. Especially relevant are the presence of animals within the classroom or renovations at the school that may involve the use of paints or the installation of new carpets. The types and maintenance of the heating and humidification systems may need to be explored, particularly if dust mite or mold allergy appears to be a significant problem for the patient. Special activities such as parties, which may expose a food-allergic child to dangerous foods, need to be dealt with. Special school activities (such as visits to a zoo) may expose a student to risks that need to be specifically addressed. The physician may need to communicate with the school concerns about specific allergens (such as animals in the classroom) and irritant exposures (such as wood dust or fumes from science projects), which need to be reduced for the sake of a specific student.

PHYSICIAN COMMUNICATION WITH THE SCHOOL

Since the physician has no direct authority within the school system, the parent(s) must take an active role in communicating health concerns. This is especially important for children who are at risk of anaphylaxis while at school. The physician can help with clearly marked prescriptions, a written emergency plan, and even with lectures and training of school personnel, particularly in the administration of epinephrine.

For asthma therapy, many special forms for the school are available. The Student Asthma Action Card (Fig. 56–1), developed by the Asthma and Allergy Foundation of America (AAFA) and endorsed by the National Asthma Education Program, is available at no charge from AAFA, or may be reproduced for office use. The National Heart, Lung and Blood Institute's publication, Managing Asthma: A Guide for Schools (NHLBI, 1991),

Text continued on page 768

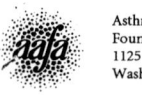

STUDENT ASTHMA ACTION CARD

Asthma and Allergy Foundation of America
1125 15th St., N.W., Suite 502
Washington, DC 20005

Endorsed by
National Asthma Education Program

Name: _____ Grade: _____ Age: _____

Teacher: _____ Room: _____

Parent/Guardian Name: _____ Ph: (H) _____

                 Address: _____ Ph: (W) _____

Parent/Guardian Name: _____ Ph: (H) _____

                 Address: _____ Ph: (W) _____

Emergency Phone Contact #1 _____
                           Name   Relationship   Phone

Emergency Phone Contact #2 _____
                           Name   Relationship   Phone

Physician Student Sees for Asthma: _____ Ph: _____

Other Physician: _____ Ph: _____

ID Photo

DAILY ASTHMA MANAGEMENT PLAN

- **Identify the things which start an asthma episode** (Check each that applies to the student.)

  ☐ Exercise   ☐ Strong odors or fumes   ☐ Other _____
  ☐ Respiratory infections ☐ Chalk dust   _____
  ☐ Change in temperature ☐ Carpets in the room
  ☐ Animals   ☐ Pollens
  ☐ Food _____   ☐ Molds
  Comments _____

- **Control of School Environment**

  (List any environmental control measures, pre-medications, and/or dietary restrictions that the student needs to prevent an asthma episode.)
  _____
  _____
  _____

- **Peak Flow Monitoring**

  Personal Best Peak Flow number: _____
  Monitoring Times: _____ _____ _____

- **Daily Medication Plan**

	Name	Amount	When to Use
1.	_____	_____	_____
2.	_____	_____	_____
3.	_____	_____	_____
4.	_____	_____	_____

FIGURE 56–1. Student Asthma Action Card. (From Asthma and Allergy Foundation of America.)

Emergency Plan

Emergency action is necessary when the student has symptoms such as _____, _____, _____, _____ or has a peak flow reading of _____.

- **Steps to take during an asthma episode:**
  1. Give medications as listed below.
  2. Have student return to classroom if _____
     _____
  3. Contact parent if _____
  4. Seek emergency medical care if the student has any of the following:
     - ✔ No improvement 15-20 minutes after initial treatment with medication and a relative cannot be reached.
     - ✔ Peak flow of _____
     - ✔ Hard time breathing with:
       - Chest and neck pulled in with breathing
       - Child is hunched over
       - Child is struggling to breathe
     - ✔ Trouble walking or talking
     - ✔ Stops playing and can't start activity again
     - ✔ Lips or fingernails are gray or blue

  } *If This Happens, Get Emergency Help Now!*

- **Emergency Asthma Medications**

	Name	Amount	When to Use
1.	_____	_____	_____
2.	_____	_____	_____
3.	_____	_____	_____
4.	_____	_____	_____

Comments / Special Instructions

_____
_____
_____

For Inhaled Medications

- ☐ I have instructed _____ in the proper way to use his/her medications. It is my professional opinion that _____ should be allowed to carry and use that medication by him/herself.
- ☐ It is my professional opinion that _____ should not carry his/her inhaled medication by him/herself.

_____   _____
Physician Signature   Date

_____   _____
Parent Signature   Date

FIGURE 56–1 *Continued*

TABLE 56–2. MANAGING ASTHMA IN THE SCHOOL

ACTIONS FOR THE PRINCIPAL

- Involve your staff in the asthma management program. A school asthma management program is a cooperative effort that involves the student, parents, teachers, school staff, and physicians. Many members of the school staff can play a role in maintaining your school's asthma management program, although the principal or the school nurse may be most instrumental in getting a program started. Take the steps listed below to help set up an asthma management program in your school.

- Develop a clear policy on taking medication during school hours. Work with parents, teachers, the school nurse (if available), and others to provide the most supportive policy that your school system allows so that the student can get the medication he/she needs.

- Designate one person on the school staff to be responsible for maintaining each student's asthma action plan.

- Provide opportunities for staff to learn about asthma and allergies by setting up inservice courses. You may get assistance from your school nurse, or a local hospital or medical society. Other sources of information are the American Lung Association, Asthma and Allergy Foundation of America, National Jewish Center for Immunology and Respiratory Medicine, and the Mothers of Asthmatics.

- Establish an asthma resource file of pamphlets, brochures, and other publications for school personnel to provide an opportunity for the staff to get additional information about asthma. Many of the organizations cited above offer materials for this purpose. Make general information available to students as well.

- Schedule any extensive building repairs or cleaning to avoid exposing students to fumes, dust, and other irritants. When possible, try to schedule painting and major repairs during long vacations or the summer months.

- Support and encourage communication with parents to improve school health services.

ACTIONS FOR THE SCHOOL NURSE OR OTHER HEALTH PERSONNEL

- Maintain the asthma action plan for every student with asthma. Include information on medications, dosages, triggers, and emergency procedures.

- Alert staff members about students with a history of asthma.

- Use the warning signs presented in the publication, *Managing Asthma: A Guide for Schools*, to help identify students with uncontrolled asthma. Provide this information to parents with the encouragement to see a physician.

- Assist with the administration of medication in accordance with school policy.

- Monitor response to treatment using a peak flow meter.

- Communicate with parents about acute episodes, if any, and about the student's general progress in controlling asthma at school.

- Conduct inservices on asthma, and consult with staff to help develop appropriate school activities for students with asthma.

- Collaborate with the PTA to consider offering a family asthma education program in school. Consult organizations on the resource list in the publication, *Managing Asthma: A Guide for Schools*, for assistance.

- If there is no nurse at the school, these tasks should be assigned to an appropriate staff member.

TABLE 56–2. MANAGING ASTHMA IN THE SCHOOL *Continued*

ACTIONS FOR THE CLASSROOM TEACHER

- Know the early warning signs of an asthma episode.
- Have a copy of the asthma action plan in the classroom. Review it with the student and parents. Know what steps to take in case of an asthma episode.
- Develop a clear procedure with the student and parent for handling schoolwork missed due to asthma.
- Understand that a student with asthma may feel:
  Drowsy or tired,
  Different from the other kids,
  Anxious about access to medication,
  Embarrassed about the disruption to school activities that an asthma episode causes, and/or
  Withdrawn.
- Help the student feel more comfortable by recognizing these feelings. Try to maintain confidentiality. Educate classmates about asthma so they will be more understanding.
- Know the possible side effects of asthma medications and how they may impact the student's performance in the classroom. Refer any problem to the school nurse and parent(s). Common side effects of medicine that warrant referral are nervousness, nausea, jitteriness, hyperactivity, and drowsiness.
- Reduce known allergens in the classroom to help students who have allergies. Common allergens found in classrooms include chalk dust, animals, and strong odors (perfumes, paints).
- Encourage the student with asthma to participate fully in physical activities.
- Allow a student to engage in quiet activity if recovery from an acute episode precludes full participation.

ACTIONS FOR THE PHYSICAL EDUCATION INSTRUCTOR AND COACH

- Encourage exercise and participation in sports for students with asthma. When asthma is under good control, students with the disease are able to play most sports. A number of Olympic medalists have asthma.
- Appreciate that exercise can cause acute episodes for many students with asthma. Exercise in cold dry air and activities that require extended running appear to trigger asthma more readily than other forms of exercise. However, medicines can be taken before exertion to help avoid an episode. This preventive medicine enables most students with exercise-induced asthma to participate in any sport they choose. Warm-up and cool-down activities appropriate for any exercise will also help the student with asthma.
- Support the student's treatment plan if it requires premedication before exercise.
- Understand what to do if an asthma episode occurs during exercise. Have the child's asthma action plan available.
- Encourage students with asthma to participate actively in sports but also recognize and respect their limits. Permit less strenuous activities if a recent illness precludes full participation.
- Refer your questions about a student's ability to fully participate in physical education to the parents and school nurse.

ACTIONS FOR THE GUIDANCE COUNSELOR

- Help all school personnel understand that asthma is not an emotional or psychological disease—it is not "all in the child's head." Strong emotions such as laughing or crying can trigger an acute episode because this irritates and constricts the sensitive airways of a person with asthma.
- Recognize that learning to cope with asthma, as with any chronic illness, can be difficult. Teachers may notice low self-esteem, withdrawal from activities, discouragement over the steps needed to control asthma, or difficulty making up school work. Special counseling with the student and/or parents may help the student handle problems more effectively.

Data from National Heart, Lung, and Blood Institute and U.S. Department of Education: Managing Asthma: A Guide for Schools, 1991.

TABLE 56-3. RESOURCE MATERIALS FOR SCHOOL PERSONNEL AND PARENTS

- **American Academy of Allergy and Immunology,** 611 E. Wells St., Milwaukee, WI 53202. 414/276-6071.
  The AAAI has many public education resources on asthma and allergies. Among the many offerings are "Tips to Remember" booklets (Tip #19: Asthma and the School Child), a quarterly newsletter for patients and "Helpful Hints" and other written resources. Videotapes on asthma and allergies are also available.

- **American Lung Association,** 1740 Broadway, New York, NY 10019-4374. 212/315-8700.
  These Are Solutions for the Student with Asthma—4 page leaflet; *What School Personnel Should Know About Asthma*—11 minute video and booklet.

- **Asthma and Allergy Foundation of America,** 1125 Fifteenth Street NW, Suite 502, Washington, DC 20005. 202/466-7643.
  Asthma and Allergies in the Schools: The Importance of Cooperative Care—14 minute video designed to show parent and school groups the importance of communication and cooperation in the management of asthma and allergies in the school setting.
  School Poster—full color action poster with asthma information for school on the reverse side.
  School Support Group Resource Kit—how to start and maintain a support group, tips for starting school-based support groups.
  Asthma in the Schools: Improving Control with Peak Flow Monitoring—peak flow monitoring and asthma management in the school.
  Student Asthma Action Card—form for use at school (Fig. 56-1).

- **Eczema Association for Science and Education**—prints newsletter, *EA Advocate*—1221 SW Yambill, Suite 303, Portland, OR 97205.

- **Food Allergy Network,** 4744 Holly Avenue, Fairfax, VA 22030. 703/691-3179.
  Food Allergy News, bimonthly newsletter, and other materials for food-allergic families.
  Off to School with Food Allergies—A guide for parents and teachers.

- **National Allergy and Asthma Network/Mothers of Asthmatics,** 3554 Chain Bridge Road, Suite 200, Fairfax, VA 22030-2709. 703/385-4403.
  MA Report—monthly newsletter, *School Information Packet.*
  A Parent's Guide to Asthma by Nancy Sander—practical advice for school, home, play.
  Asthma in the School: Improving Control with Peak Flow Monitoring—a guide to help the school nurse.

- **National Institutes of Health-National Asthma Education Program,** PO Box 30105, Bethesda, MD 20824-0105. 301/496-5717.
  Managing Asthma: A Guide for Schools—booklet designed to provide school personnel with basic guidelines.

---

recommends actions that are useful for the principal, school health personnel, teacher, coach, and guidance counselor (see Tables 56-1 and 56-2).

Many organizations have already developed materials that are useful for assisting in educating school personnel about allergies and asthma (Table 56-3). Use of these materials should improve considerably the knowledge base and readiness of the school to appropriately handle students with allergies or asthma.

REFERENCES

American Academy of Pediatrics, Committee on School Health. Guidelines for Urgent Care at School. Pediatrics 86:999-1000, 1990.

American Academy of Pediatrics, Section on Allergy and Immunology, Ad Hoc Committee on Anaphylaxis in School. Anaphylaxis at School: Etiologic Factors, Prevalence, and Treatment. Pediatrics 91:516, 1993.

American Academy of Pediatrics, Section on Allergy and Immunology, Section on Diseases of the Chest. Exercise and the Asthmatic Child. Pediatrics 84:392-393, 1989.

Furukawa CT, Murphy S (Chairpersons), Section on Allergy and Immunology, Section on Diseases of the Chest. Asthma and exercise—What schools should and should not do. Pediatrics 85:386, 1990. (Letter)

Grabenstein JD, Smith LJ. Incidence of anaphylactic self-treatment in an outpatient population. Ann Allergy 63:184-188, 1989.

National Heart, Lung and Blood Institute (NHLBI), National Institute of Health, U.S. Dept. of Health and Human Services, and the Fund for the Improvement and Reform of Schools and Teaching, Office of Educational Research and Improvement (OERI), U.S. Dept. of Education. Managing Asthma: A Guide for Schools. Bethesda MD, NIH Publication No. 91-2650, September, 1991.

Sampson HA, Mendelson L, Rosan JP. Fatal and near-fatal anaphylactic reactions to food in children and adolescents. N Engl J Med 327:380-384, 1992.

Chapter 57

Industrial Hygiene Aspects of Preventing Occupational Asthma

Michael S. Morgan, Sc.D., and Leonard C. Altman, M.D.

Minimizing or eliminating occupational asthma requires the full use of all levels of preventive strategies: primary, secondary, and tertiary. Industrial hygiene methods focus on primary prevention—the control of worker exposure to the causative agent. They are directed in a coordinated manner toward: (1) reducing or eliminating release of the causative agent from the source, (2) controlling its transmission through the environment to the worker, and (3) preventing contact of the agent with the worker through use of protective barriers. Figure 57–1 shows a schematic example of the transmission of an industrial contaminant from the source, through the environment, to the worker, illustrating the points in the process of exposure where control techniques can be applied. Industrial hygiene control methods assume that inhalation is the most important route of worker exposure to the etiologic agent, and therefore the control of air movement, together with the allergen contaminant it bears, is the major goal. The exposure may be to particulate matter, to gaseous low–molecular-weight compounds, or, in some cases, to agents that occur in both gaseous and particulate phases simultaneously. Di-isocyanates exemplify this two-phase occurrence, and consequently they pose special problems for control and monitoring (Lesage et al, 1992) because gases and particles behave so differently in air. Despite the assumption that inhalation exposure is of primary importance, most control methods can address other routes of exposure such as ingestion or skin contact, as these methods extend to work practices and worker hygiene, which also affect non-inhalation routes of exposure.

The prospect for successful reduction of occupational asthma through industrial hygiene is good, provided the causative agent is known and its source or sources in the workplace can be identified. These requirements may present difficulties in the case of expo-

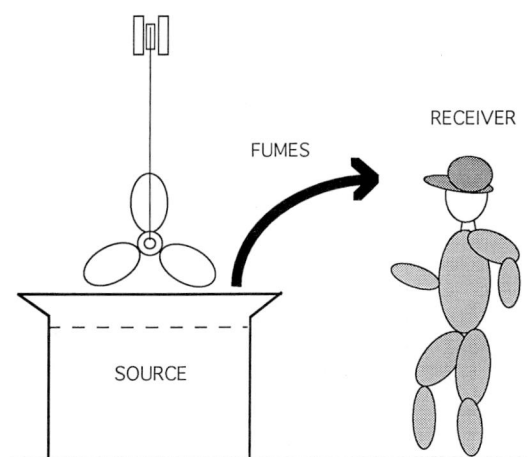

FIGURE 57–1. Schematic diagram of the typical mechanism of exposure to airborne agents in the workplace. Agents are released at the *source* as the result of heating and mechanical processes. They are conducted as fumes to the worker via motion of the ambient air in the workplace, the *transmission pathway*. The agents contact the worker, the *receiver*, by inhalation and deposition in the respiratory system, by direct contact with the skin, and less often by ingestion.

sure to biologic agents, many of which are released by multiple sources and at infrequent or irregular intervals (Agarwal et al, 1983; Corn, 1983; Cullen, 1990; Lacey and Crook, 1988). In such cases complete elimination of exposure may not be possible, but minimization of exposure and risk to workers may still be accomplished. In any case, effective control requires cooperative action by employers, workers, and health professionals.

Industrial hygiene methods of prevention should be regarded as complementary to medical screening and medical surveillance. The latter procedures are valuable in confirming the effectiveness of any primary prevention strategy (Juniper et al, 1977) and may also reveal evidence of previously unknown exposures requiring primary control. In particular, because of the variable periods between the time of first exposure and sensitization in occupational asthma (Burge, 1991; Cox et al, 1988), continuing medical surveillance of workers plays a critical role both in identifying sources of sensitizing agents and in assessing workplace environmental control measures.

Table 57–1 presents a summary of the industrial hygiene control methods, organized into categories based on their involvement of engineering and work practices, method of exposure measurement, or supplemental techniques. In general these apply to the source, the transmission pathway, and the worker, respectively.

CONTROL AT THE SOURCE

Preventing or minimizing release of etiologic agents at the source is based on engineering principles and on carefully chosen work practices. The design and operation of machinery and hardware involved with the process, as well as the industrial process itself, are the domain of the engineer. Engineers must be prepared to cooperate and consult with the industrial hygienist and other occupational health professionals when worker exposure has been uncovered, and the decision has been made to control it. The term "work practices" refers to the procedures used by the workers in carrying out their assigned tasks. Standard operating procedures are commonly written out and form a part of the training materials used in developing a skilled work force. Having written procedures available is of great value to the industrial hygienist in evaluating and revising hazardous work practices.

Engineering Control Methods

Industrial ventilation systems deliver fresh, uncontaminated air to the workplace (dilution ventilation) and/or withdraw air from the region at or near the source, before a contaminant can reach the worker's breathing zone (local exhaust ventilation). For example, dilution ventilation has been used to reduce mold spore concentrations in mushroom-growing operations (Lenhart and Cole, 1993); however, it has been well established that local exhaust ventilation provides better contaminant control where it can be installed (Hinds, 1991). The use of local exhaust hoods at or close to the source, together with associated duct work, blower, and air cleaning devices, is preferable because this method can virtually eliminate exposures, whereas dilution ventilation can only reduce the airborne agent to a concentration determined by the volume of clean air available and the contaminant emission rate. Figure 57–2 illustrates the application of local exhaust ventilation to a particular source of airborne fumes, showing the aim of the system to capture fumes before they enter the general workplace environment and the air the worker is breathing.

TABLE 57–1. SUMMARY OF PREVENTIVE MEASURES

I. Control at the source
  A. Engineering control methods
    1. Industrial ventilation
    2. Substitution
    3. Isolation
    4. Elimination
    5. Enclosure
    6. Air cleaning devices
    7. Process modification
  B. Work practices
II. Monitoring airborne concentrations
III. Biologic monitoring
IV. Additional preventive measures
  A. Workplace management
    1. Housekeeping
    2. Workplace maintenance
    3. Dust suppression
    4. Worker-education
    5. Administrative control
  B. Personal protective equipment
    1. Respiratory protective devices
    2. Skin protection

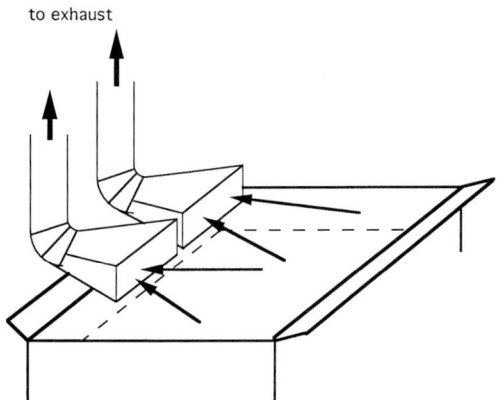

FIGURE 57–2. Control of agent release by the source is best accomplished by engineering methods, of which local exhaust ventilation is an example. The ventilation system inlets are placed as close to the source as possible, to ensure complete capture of the fumes rising from the tank, before they can enter the ambient air of the workplace. Note that the ventilation system must also be located in a way that does not interfere with the industrial operation.

One should note that local exhaust ventilation systems can often be added after a plant or process has been in operation and a hazard has been discovered ("retrofitting"). However, it is also not uncommon to find that there are serious physical impediments to placing the inlet of the exhaust system close enough to the source to achieve effective control. Clearly, the employer will not look favorably on an engineering control system which interferes with production by getting in the way.

Substitution of one material or process for another can effectively eliminate the exposure. Examples from the occupational asthma literature range from simply replacing colophony (rosin) with paraffin-based flux in the solder used to assemble electronic devices (Burge et al, 1980) to replacing a batch, or open, process with one in which the operation is continuous and automated so that open containers and manual transfers of materials are not required (Corn, 1983). The latter method was used with great success in controlling worker exposure to vinyl chloride in the plastics industry, once that chemical was confirmed as causing cancer.

Isolation uses distance or shielding of the source to reduce or eliminate worker exposure. This may include use of robotic manipulation of hazardous materials and sources, as is now done routinely in the handling of nuclear materials, or other forms of remote-controlled processing.

Elimination of the process or material responsible for release of the causative agent has been described in a case of slime allergen exposure arising from the air conditioning system in a nylon manufacturing plant. In this case it was shown that carefully controlled chlorination of the water recycled through the system eradicated the slime (Reed, 1990).

Enclosure, for example by encapsulating the material or using process barriers, has been used to reduce worker exposure to allergens in a variety of operations. Filter top cages and filtration of exiting air in animal housing facilities have accomplished important reductions of exposures to laboratory animal allergens (Gordon et al., 1992; Ziemann et al, 1992).

Air cleaning devices may be added to workplace ventilation systems to remove contaminants as the air is circulated. Electrostatic precipitators have been used to reduce mold spore levels (Kozak et al, 1979), and high-efficiency particulate air (HEPA) filters incorporated in the dilution ventilation system have been reported to provide partial control of laboratory animal allergens (Reed, 1990).

Process modifications include adopting wet methods of manipulating powdered materials to avoid airborne releases or making the product in coarse instead of fine particles, where this does not impair the commercial use of the product (Corn, 1983). Another example is the processing of enzyme detergents using large aggregate pellets instead of finely divided powders, thus reducing both the amount of airborne material (since large particles do not remain airborne for long) and, through a change in particle size, reducing access of the sensitizing agent to the workers' respiratory system (Liss et al, 1984).

As a cautionary note, in all applications of engineering methods, certain information about the workplace environment is necessary before modification can be developed. This information includes knowledge of the current levels of exposure in the workplace and the level of exposure reduction necessary to protect the workers (Reed, 1990). If this information is absent or incomplete, an arbitrary decision must be made as to the amount of exposure reduction needed. The engineer must be given a "target" concentration of the contaminant in air, in order to design a device or measure to keep exposures low enough. In many instances of exposure to agents causing asthma, although the causal association has been established, the level of exposure below which a clinical response would be avoided in sensitized individuals is not known (Dutkiewicz et al, 1988), and thus full protection by engineering methods cannot be completely assured.

Work Practices

These consist of standard operating procedures planned to minimize release of allergens from the source. For example, in the manufacture of enzyme-containing detergent powders, reaction vessels are not opened unless the contents are moist, and until the internal pressure is relieved. Methods of animal handling have been described which have reduced worker exposure, including use of absorbent pads instead of loose wood chips under rodent cages (Gordon et al, 1992) and the addition of fat to swine feed to act as an agglomerating agent to reduce dust (Chiba et al, 1985).

Assessment and Outlook

Apart from complete isolation and elimination or substitution of materials, engineering controls cannot reduce worker exposure to zero. The extent of exposure reduction to a given substance is limited by economic and technical considerations, but it can be sufficient to prevent sensitizing new workers and, in many instances, to prevent eliciting reactions in already sensitized workers. The economic benefits of installing engineering controls are only realized in the long term, in the form of reduced workers' compensation insurance expenditures, improved productivity, reduced work time lost to occupational asthma, and improved worker satisfaction. The costs of engineering controls, however, are borne principally in the short term and thus are more visible to financial officers. Employers who resist this form of prevention must be persuaded of the less tangible benefits of using engineering and source controls. These include the aforementioned economic factors and the knowledge that such preventive methods offer protection to all workers, including those who are not, or cannot be, adequately protected by personal equipment such as face masks. A further advantage of engineering controls above all other methods is that their effectiveness is much less dependent on human behavior (Corn, 1983; Hinds, 1991). This is because engineered systems are generally automated to at least some degree, using fixed hardware whose purpose is not easily defeated, either intentionally or accidentally, by workers.

The choice of which combination of source controls is best for a particular problem of allergen exposure should be made by qualified industrial hygienists and engineers. Useful information on how to locate such persons is available from several professional organizations, including the American Industrial Hygiene Association (AIHA), the American Board of Industrial Hygiene (ABIH), and the American Society of Heating, Refrigeration and Air Conditioning Engineers (ASHRAE). Each group maintains up-to-date geographic listings of specialists they regard as competent in hazard control; ABIH also conducts the national certification program in industrial hygiene, which includes a rigorous examination covering hazard control procedures.

MONITORING AIRBORNE CONCENTRATIONS

Goals

Regardless of the preventive methods chosen, air monitoring for the concentration of contaminant is an essential component of the preventive strategy. The goals of air sampling and analysis are to assess the performance of the source control measures, to confirm their function, and to evaluate worker exposure levels so that the remaining health risks can be determined.

Methods

Air sampling techniques for determining inhalation hazards must provide a representative sample of the air being inhaled by the worker, and they must account for the differential effect of particle size distribution on deposition in the respiratory system. The most representative samples are taken in the "breathing zone" of the individual worker, using a device worn by the worker with the sampler inlet placed within 30 cm of the nose and mouth and usually operated by a battery-powered pump (Corn, 1983). Figure 57-3 shows an example of a sampling "train" designed to be worn by the worker, in which the sampler inlet is clipped to the worker's collar or lapel. Because such sampling devices are limited to relatively low air flow rates and therefore relatively small air samples, they cannot measure concentrations at very low levels unless they are coupled with a very sensitive analytic technique (Newman-Taylor and Tee, 1990). The anticipated development of more sensitive immunochemical assays should permit the expanded use of breathing zone sampling methods in the future. As an alternative, "area" sampling with a much larger device may be used, but this must be conducted at a stationary location. Area samples are not representative of any individual's exposure, but may still be used to evaluate the performance of control methods and to estimate the average exposure to the workers.

The distribution of an allergenic agent according to airborne particle size is of major importance in evaluating worker exposure and risk. Particle size has a strong influence on the fraction of airborne material that is inhaled and on the site and magnitude of surface deposition within the respiratory system (Farant and Moore, 1978; Licorish et al, 1985; Liss et al, 1984; Phalen et al, 1986; Smid et al, 1992). It is now established, for example, that almost 50 percent of particles up to 100 μm in diameter may be inspired at least as deeply as the nasopharynx, and thus particles of relatively large size may present some risk, despite earlier suggestions to the contrary (Hinds, 1991). In addition, detailed information is now available on the site and extent of deposition of particles with diameters from 10 μm to less than 0.1 μm, permitting assessment of potential exposure and reactions in the large and small airways and alveolar region of the lungs (Phalen et al, 1986). Methods for sampling airborne particles and determining their size distribution have been described, and convenient portable devices are available (Corn, 1983; Smid et al, 1992).

Results of air sampling measurements may be compared to reference values, when they exist, to support decisions on worker health risk. Occupational exposure recommendations exist for more than 15 agents recognized as allergens, and federal Occupational Safety and Health Administration (OSHA) regulations have been established for several of these (ACGIH, 1990; ACGIH, 1991; OSHA, 1988). Threshold limit values (TLV, recommended guidelines) and OSHA permissible exposure limits (PEL, enforceable standards) for such agents as grain dust, phthalic anhydride, and subtilisins (alcalase) specifically address the risk of occupational asthma. Exposure control strategies should maintain airborne concentrations well below these guidelines or standards. A rule of thumb commonly used by the industrial hygienist is to keep measured exposures below one half the guideline or standard, to provide a margin of safety and to account for sampling and analytical errors.

The absence of reliable dose-response relationships for sensitization and for eliciting re-

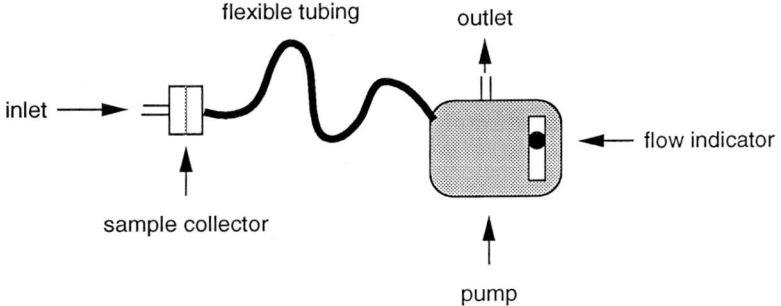

FIGURE 57-3. The important components of a personal air sampling system. The inlet and sample collector are clipped to the worker's pocket or lapel, so that air is sampled from the breathing zone, a space within 12 inches of the mouth and nose. Flexible tubing leads from the sampler to the battery-powered pump mounted on the worker's belt or on a shoulder harness. Modern pumps weigh less than two pounds and are well tolerated by workers for periods of 8 hours or more.

actions in sensitized workers is a major obstacle to the development of useful exposure guidelines for occupational allergens (Eggleston et al, 1990). This difficulty notwithstanding, it is possible to use the limited amount of dose-response information available to estimate the proportion of risk that can be reduced by any achievable reduction in exposure. To illustrate, when the slope of the dose-response relationship is known to be steep, modest reductions in exposure would be expected to produce large reductions in health risk for workers; examples have been described for such agents as flour dust (baker's asthma) and machining fluids (Kennedy et al, 1989; Tee et al, 1992).

An additional complication in assessing the risk of occupational allergens is the observation that high-level exposures of short duration ("peaks") may be of critical importance; at the same time, they are difficult to monitor owing to technical impediments associated with the sampling equipment (Cullen, 1990): most instruments cannot respond instantly to changing concentrations and many require sampling durations of 15 to 30 minutes or more. Finally, for many allergens the spatial and temporal variation in concentration is large (Eggleston et al, 1990; Lacey and Crook, 1988; Licorish et al, 1985). Consequently, in workplaces where the mean observed concentration may be within existing guidelines, extreme variability in time and space means that there is likely to be a significant fraction of concentrations well in excess of the mean. In one example of grain dust exposure measurements, the average worker's breathing zone concentration was below 5 mg/m^3, but 10 percent of workers had breathing zone concentrations above 50 mg/m^3 (Farant and Moore, 1978). Depending on the shape of the dose-response curve, the 10 percent of workers with the higher exposures could have very much higher risks than average.

In summary, air monitoring is a critical element in an integrated strategy for prevention of occupational asthma. Present limitations to its application are being addressed by developing immunochemical methods with improved sensitivity, permitting measurement of air samples collected over short time periods to characterize brief, peak exposures. At the same time, new data are being developed which should prompt the establishment of additional exposure guidelines and standards aimed specifically at preventing or minimizing the incidence of occupational asthma.

BIOLOGIC MONITORING

A second component of exposure monitoring of growing importance is biologic monitoring of individual workers. Biologic monitoring is the sampling and analysis of body fluids or tissues for quantitative evidence of occupational exposure. Common examples used currently are blood analyses for lead or porphyrins, as evidence of workplace exposure to this element, and measurement of aromatic solvents in exhaled breath, as evidence of exposure to those compounds. These methods are complementary to air monitoring, adding information regarding individual absorption and disposition of workplace agents, but they do not reveal the source of the exposure. Additional benefits of biologic monitoring include the ability to detect events such as non-inhalation exposure, failure of personal protective equipment, or non-occupational exposures.

Biologic monitoring procedures and guidelines currently exist for two agents known to cause occupational asthma—cobalt and chromium. The American Conference of Governmental Industrial Hygienists (ACGIH) has developed sampling and analytic methods and biologic exposure indices for appropriate sampling and analysis of these metals in the blood of workers at increased risk of sensitization (ACGIH, 1991; ACGIH, 1993).

The development of additional biologic monitoring techniques and guidelines is dependent on the progress of current research and will be limited in most cases to agents that produce sensitization over relatively long exposure periods. This is because the pharmacokinetics of rapid-acting sensitizing agents are not compatible with biologic monitoring, since the appearance of such an agent or its metabolite in blood or urine would occur too late to be useful in prevention. Exposure to isocyanates is an example whereby the detection of the compounds in body fluids occurs, but well after sensitization has already taken place. Further, the exposure level of many allergens associated with the induction of sensitivity corresponds to an extremely low level of the material or its metabolite in body fluids, compounding the analytic problem. However, newer methods of immune system surveillance, including measurements of anti-chemical antibodies and detection of changes in lymphocyte populations (Simon et al, 1993), may enhance the value of biologic monitoring as a technique of secondary prevention.

ADDITIONAL PREVENTIVE MEASURES

Because of the limitations inherent in the source control methods described earlier, it will often be necessary to use supplementary control techniques when peak exposures occur or in any other instance in which source controls are demonstrably inadequate to prevent occupational asthma. Supplementary controls include management practices and the use of personal protective equipment.

Workplace Management

Housekeeping and workplace maintenance procedures may be adjusted to prevent or minimize exposure to allergens. Replacement of dry sweeping of settled dust with wet sweeping or vacuum collection (with an appropriate HEPA air filter in the vacuum system) has been shown to be effective in reducing exposure to alcalase (Juniper et al, 1977). The importance of careful planning and monitoring of maintenance work has been underlined by several studies showing that maintenance workers have higher exposures than most other job categories (Farant and Moore, 1978). This stems in part from the fact that maintenance work requires that processes which are closed while operating be opened during repairs, thus creating conditions leading to much higher exposures for the worker carrying out the repairs.

Dust suppression by wetting down settled material has also been shown to be effective in reducing exposure of grain-handling facility workers (Farant and Moore, 1978).

Worker education in the nature of the dangers posed by workplace materials, and in proper work practices for minimizing hazardous exposures, is an important element of industrial hygiene. A well-executed educational program offers the potential benefit of showing workers that they have some control over their own fates by acting in a manner that prevents exposure. Physicians, nurses, and other health care professionals should take an active role in the education of workers.

Administrative control refers to limiting individual worker exposure by rotating workers among tasks and by scheduling tasks to take advantage of known fluctuations in exposure. For tasks having known high exposure levels, assigning several workers in turn will reduce the exposure duration and hence the absorbed dose to any individual. Careful assignment of job tasks has contributed to reduction in occurrence of asthma in the animal feed and laboratory animal research industries (Eggleston et al, 1990; Smid et al, 1992).

Personal Protective Equipment

Although regarded by many as the least desirable method of preventing occupational exposures, use of protective equipment is nonetheless widespread. Employers commonly view protective gear as the fastest and cheapest route to solving an exposure problem, without due regard for the important limitations inherent in this strategy. Industrial hygiene professionals, on the other hand, firmly rate the effectiveness of protective gear below that of source controls and workplace management techniques, owing largely to the critical dependence on worker behavior for efficacy of protective devices and the serious potential for interference of these devices with work processes (Hinds, 1991). Thus protective equipment is appropriate only where source controls and management methods: (1) are shown to provide inadequate protection, (2) are not technically feasible, or (3) require time to install, and protection is needed in the interim.

Respiratory protective devices offer a wide range of exposure reduction, depending on the proper selection of the device and the ability of the wearer to achieve an adequate seal to the face or head. Figure 57–4 shows the sensitive points on a typical respiratory protective device, indicating the routes by which air contaminants may breach the expected barrier. The important routes for "leakage" are the face seal, the exhalation valve, and the purifying cartridge itself. The most problematic of these routes is the face seal, since its performance is highly dependent on facial shape, movement of facial muscles, and the willingness of the wearer to keep it in place. The degree of protection is described using the workplace protection factor (WPF), which is the ratio of the concentration of airborne agent outside the device to that inhaled by the worker. WPF values have been determined by the U.S. National

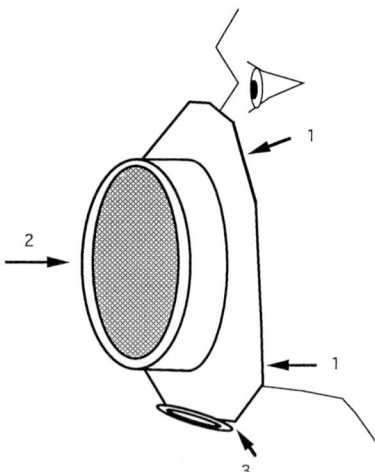

FIGURE 57-4. A typical Air-Purifying Device for respiratory protection has three points at which airborne agent may enter the worker's respiratory tract, thus reducing the degree of protection provided. Point 1 represent leakage across the face seal, which can occur intermittently as the worker moves his or her head, talks, or even smiles. Point 2 represents breaching of the air purifying element of the device. Ordinarily this does not occur in well-maintained devices, but all such elements have a fixed lifetime, after which they are unable, owing to saturation, to remove additional contaminant from the incoming air. Point 3 represents failure of the exhalation valve that is incorporated into most respiratory protective devices, so that inhaled air enters by this route and thus bypasses the primary air purifying elements.

Institute for Occupational Safety and Health (NIOSH) for a variety of respiratory protective devices, and examples are listed in Table 57–2. The tabulated values represent the anticipated degree of protection offered by each device when worn by most workers for up to 8 hours, after proper training. The highest protective values are assigned to devices that provide a separate air supply independent of the immediate surroundings (Air Supply Respirators) or have a built-in pump to draw workplace air through a filter and deliver it to the worker's helmet or facepiece (Powered Air-Purifying Respirators). A key point is that no protective device is able to eliminate exposure completely and that the worker's exposure while using the device depends on the concentration of agent in the workroom air. Thus, the use of source controls to minimize air concentration, combined with a respiratory protective device to provide additional protection, may reduce exposure to levels at which the risk is negligible (Anderson et al, 1989; Bollinger and Schutz, 1987; Muller-Wening and Repp, 1989; Newill et al, 1989).

TABLE 57–2. WORKPLACE PROTECTION FACTORS FOR RESPIRATORY PROTECTIVE DEVICES

Respirator Type	Workplace Protection Factor*
I. Air purifying	
A. Particulate removing	
Single use, dust	5
Half-mask (covering nose and mouth), dust	10
Half-mask or quarter-mask (mouth only), high-efficiency filter	10
Full facepiece, high-efficiency filter	50
Powered, high-efficiency-filter, all enclosures	1000
B. Gas and vapor removing	
Half-mask	10
Full facepiece	50
II. Atmosphere supplying	
A. Supplied air	
Demand regulator, half-mask	10
Demand regulator, full facepiece	50
Pressure demand regulator, half-mask	1000
Pressure demand regulator, full facepiece	2000
Continuous flow, hood, helmet or suit	2000
B. Self-contained breathing apparatus (SCBA)	
Open circuit, demand regulator, full facepiece	50
Open circuit, pressure demand regulator, full face	10,000

*Workplace Protection Factor = $\dfrac{\text{Concentration of airborne agent outside the device}}{\text{Concentration inhaled by the worker}}$

From Bollinger N, Schutz R. NIOSH Guide to Industrial Respiratory Protection. Cincinnati, OH, National Institute for Occupational Safety and Health, 1987.

Care must be exercised in selecting a vendor, once the general category of respiratory protective device has been determined, since not all manufacturers produce devices of equal effectiveness, even within a category. It is strongly recommended that only devices tested and approved by NIOSH or the Mine Safety and Health Administration (MSHA) be used. Manufacturers who have obtained such approval place a clear indication of this on their product packaging, and purchasers should request evidence of approval.

Clearly, the higher the value of the WPF, the better. However, as the WPF of the devices increases, so do problems associated with their use. The more effective devices are heavier, less comfortable to wear, and generally have shorter service periods, after which their protective value is drastically reduced (Muller-Wening and Repp, 1989; Slovak et al, 1985). These factors serve to emphasize the importance of worker cooperation in achieving the level of protection suggested by the WPF values.

Skin protection consists of gloves and protective clothing. Proper selection of materials will afford significant protection from airborne and direct contact exposure, as long as the clothing is worn. This qualification is important because, as with respiratory protective devices, protective clothing is often uncomfortable and it may interfere with the work operations themselves. Special problems arise with the use of skin protection, related to heat stress associated with work for extended periods when significant portions of the skin are covered. In addition, once clothing and gloves are contaminated, removing them at the end of the task can present serious exposure risk, as material deposited on outer surfaces is dislodged during removal (Lenhart and Cole, 1993). Decontamination of protective clothing before removal is now recognized as an important component of worker protection and one that poses formidable difficulties.

CONCLUSIONS

Engineering and other source controls are the first and most effective strategy for preventing exposure to workplace allergens. However, their effectiveness may be limited in certain circumstances. Important factors contributing to these limits are: (1) problems in identifying the causative agent and its source; (2) inadequate information regarding the dose-response relationship and the level of exposure at which risk is eliminated or is negligible; (3) inadequate methods for air sampling and analysis, which are critical to the verification of exposure control methods. Recent research relating exposure levels to worker sensitization, and to elicitation of reactions in sensitized workers, and new immunochemical analyses suggest that some of these limitations will be overcome in the near future.

In cases in which source controls are not adequate to the task, additional strategies for prevention include workplace management and, where appropriate, use of personal protective equipment. In the case of exposure to allergens where sensitized workers may react at very low levels, or where sensitization may be induced by low levels of exposure or by very brief exposure, use of multiple preventive strategies is necessary. The industrial hygienist and all other occupational health professionals, as well as other members of the broader professional health care community, must be fully aware of the limitations of each of the strategies discussed, and must take advantage of all available techniques for worker health surveillance in order to provide the maximum prevention possible.

REFERENCES

ACGIH (American Conference of Governmental Industrial Hygienists). Documentation of the Threshold Limit Values. Cincinnati, OH, ACGIH, 1990.

ACGIH (American Conference of Governmental Industrial Hygienists). Documentation of the Threshold Limit Values. Cincinnati, OH, ACGIH, 1991.

ACGIH (American Conference of Governmental Industrial Hygienists). 1993–1994 Threshold Limit Values for Chemical Substances and Physical Agents and Biological Exposure Indices. Cincinnati, OH, ACGIH, 1993.

Agarwal M, Swanson M, Reed C, Yunginger J. Immunochemical quantitation of airborne short ragweed, Alternaria, antigen E and alt-1 allergens: Two-year prospective study. J Allergy Clin Immunol 72:40–45, 1983.

Anderson K, Walker A, Boyd G. The long-term effect of a positive pressure respirator on the specific antibody response in pigeon breeders. Clin Exper Allergy 19:45–49, 1989.

Bollinger N, Schutz R. NIOSH Guide to Industrial Respiratory Protection. Cincinnati, OH, National Institute for Occupational Safety and Health, 1987.

Burge P. New developments in occupational asthma. Br Med Bull 48:221–230, 1991.

Burge P, Harries M, O'Brien I, Pepys J. Bronchial provocation exposure in workers exposed to the fumes of electronic soldering fluxes. Clin Allergy 10:137–149, 1980.

Chiba L, Peo E, Lewis A, Brumm M, Fritschen R, Crenshaw J. Effect of dietary fat on pig performance and dust levels in modified open front and environmentally regulated confinement buildings. J Animal Sci 61:763–781, 1985.

Corn M. Assessment and control of environmental exposure. J Allergy Clin Immunol 72:231–241, 1983.

Cox A, Folgering H, van Griensven L. Extrinsic allergic alveolitis caused by spores of the oyster mushroom Pleurotus ostreatus. Eur Respir J 1:466–468, 1988.

Cullen M. Clinical surveillance and management of occupational asthma. Tertiary prevention by the primary practitioner. Chest 98(suppl):196S–201S, 1990.

Dutkiewicz J, Jablonski L, Olenchock S. Occupational biohazards: A review. Am J Ind Med 14:605–623, 1988.

Eggleston P, Ansari A, Ziemann B, Adkinson N, Corn M. Occupational studies with laboratory workers allergic to rats. J Allergy Clin Immunol 86:63–72, 1990.

Farant J, Moore C. Dust exposures in the Canadian grain industry. Am Ind Hyg Assoc J 39:177–194, 1978.

Gordon S, Tee R, Lowson D, Wallace J, Newman-Taylor A. Reduction of airborne allergenic urinary proteins from laboratory rats. Br J Ind Med 49:416–422, 1992.

Hinds W. The role of industrial hygiene in preventing occupational lung disease. Occupational Medicine: State of the Art Reviews 6:29–42, 1991.

Juniper C, How M, Goodwin B, Kinshott A. *Bacillus subtilis* enzymes: A 7-year clinical, epidemiological and immunological study of an industrial allergen. J Soc Occup Med 27:3–12, 1977.

Kennedy S, Greaves I, Kriebel D, Eisen E, Smith T, Woskie S. Acute pulmonary responses among automobile workers exposed to aerosols of machining fluids. Am J Ind Med 15:627–641, 1989.

Kozak P, Gallup J, Cummins L, et al. Factors of importance in determining the prevalence of indoor molds. Ann Allergy 43:88–94, 1979.

Lacey J, Crook B. Fungal and actinomycete spores as pollutants of the workplace and occupational allergens. Ann Occ Hyg 32:515–533, 1988.

Lenhart S, Cole E. Respiratory illness in workers of an indoor shiitake mushroom farm. Appl Occup Environ Hyg 8:112–119, 1993.

Lesage J, Goyer N, Desjardins F, Vincent J-Y, Perrault G. Workers' exposure to isocyanates. Am Ind Hyg Assoc J 53:146–153, 1992.

Licorish K, Novey H, Kozak P, et al. Role of *Alternaria* and *Penicillium* spores in the pathogenesis of asthma. J Allergy Clin Immunol 76:819–825, 1985.

Liss G, Kominsky J, Gallagher J, Melius J, Brooks S, Bernstein I. Failure of enzyme encapsulation to prevent sensitization of workers in the dry bleach industry. J Allergy Clin Immunol 73:348–355, 1984.

Muller-Wening D, Repp H. Investigation on the protective value of breathing masks in farmer's lung using an inhalation provocation test. Chest 95:100–105, 1989.

Newill C, Koegel A, Prenger V, Evans R, Corn M. Utilization of personal protective equipment by laboratory personnel at a large medical research institution. Appl Ind Hyg 4:205–209, 1989.

Newman-Taylor A, Tee R. Environmental and occupational asthma. Chest 98:209S–211S, 1990.

OSHA (Occupational Safety and Health Administration), US Dept. of Labor. Code of Federal Regulations, Title 29: Labor. Section 1910.1000: Air Contaminants pp. 705–711. Washington, DC, Office of the Federal Register, 1988.

Phalen R, Hinds W, John W, et al. Rationale and recommendations for particle size-selective sampling in the work place. Appl Ind Hyg 1:3–14, 1986.

Reed C. Clinical management when the environment can be changed. Chest 98:216S–219S, 1990.

Simon GE, Daniell W, Stockbridge H, Claypoole K, Rosenstock L. Immunologic, psychological, and neuropsychological factors in multiple chemical sensitivity. A controlled study. Ann Intern Med 19:97–103, 1993.

Slovak A, Orr R, Teasdale E. Efficacy of the helmet respirator in occupational asthma due to laboratory animal allergy (LAA). Am Ind Hyg Assoc J 46:411–415, 1985.

Smid J, Heederik D, Mensink G, Houba R, Boleij J. Exposure to dust, endotoxins, and fungi in the animal feed industry. Am Ind Hyg Assoc J 53:362–368, 1992.

Tee R, Gordon D, Gordon S, Crook B, Nunn A, Musk A, Venables K, Newman-Taylor A. Immune response to flour and dust mites in a United Kingdom bakery. Br J Ind Med 49:581–587, 1992.

Ziemann B, Corn M, Ansari A, Eggleston P. The effectiveness of the Duo-Flo BioClean unit for controlling airborne antigen levels. Am Ind Hyg Assoc J 53:138–145, 1992.

INDEX

Note: Page numbers in *italics* refer to illustrations; page numbers followed by t refer to tables.

Acaricide(s), for dust mite control, 199
  for indoor environmental control, 118
Acid anhydride(s), in occupational asthma, 541–542
Acne rosacea, 660
Acne vulgaris, 660
Acquired immunodeficiency syndrome. See *HIV infection*.
Acrodermatitis enteropathica, immunodeficiency in, 39
Acupuncture, 757
ADA (adenosine deaminase) deficiency, 28
  treatment of, 52
Additive(s), drug, 339, 556
  food. See *Food additive(s)*.
Adenosine deaminase (ADA) deficiency, 28
Adhesion molecule(s), in asthma, 464–465
Adrenergic urticaria, 651
Aeroallergen(s), in atopic dermatitis, 620, 625
  sampling of, 93–96
    fungal cultures for, 94–96, *96*
    gravity slides and plates for, 94
    methods for, 94–96
    uses and limitations of, 93–94
    volumetric samplers for, 94, *95*
Agammaglobulinemia, infections in, 22
  X-linked, 22–23
    immunologic findings in, 23
    infections in, 22–23
    late onset, 23
AIDS. See *HIV infection*.
Air pollution, as risk factor, in infantile atopy, 285
  indoor, 130–131
  outdoor, 124–130
    airway hyperresponsiveness and, 174
    asthma and, 86
    asthma statistics and, 124, *125*
    economic burden of, 131
    Federal Air Quality Standards on, 124, 126t
    nitrogen dioxide as, 126–127
    ozone as, 127–129
    particulate matter (PM_{10}) as, 129–130
    statistics on, 124, *125*, 126t
    sulfur dioxide as, 124–126, 127t
    wood smoke as, 129–130
Air-filtration system(s), for indoor environmental control, 118–119
Airway hyperresponsiveness, air pollution and, 174

Airway hyperresponsiveness *(Continued)*
  allergic sensitization and, 173
  bronchial challenge test in. See *Bronchoprovocation challenge(s)*.
  definition of, 173
  effect of age on, 173, *174*
  exercise challenge test in, 165, 184
  in COPD, 602
  viral infections and, 173–174
Airway obstruction. See also *Laryngeal and tracheal obstruction*.
  in asthma, 484t, 484–486
  in COPD, 603–604
  reversible, pulmonary function testing in, 164, *165*
Airway responsiveness. See also *Airway hyperresponsiveness*.
  in asthma, 474–475, *475*
  in general population, 473–474, 474t
Airway smooth muscle spasm, in asthma, 485
Albuterol, chemical structure of, *219*
Alcohol flush, anaphylaxis vs., 308–309
Alimentum, characteristics of, 291t
Allergen extract(s), for immunotherapy, 239–240
  for skin testing, 148–149
Allergen(s), cloning of, 91
  exposure to, monitoring of, 91–92
  individual, quantitation of, 91
  indoor, asthma and, 118
    sources of, 196, 196t
  isolation and characterization of, 90
  major, 96
  minor, 96
  nomenclature for, 89–90, 96–97
  of cockroaches, 116
  of house dust mites, 116, 116t
Allergenicity, factors influencing, 89, *90*
Allergic toxemia, 749–750
Allergy. See also specific allergy, e.g., "Food allergy"
  definition of, 321
  prevention of, in infants. See *Prevention of allergy (in infants)*.
Alopecia areata, 660–661
Alpha-1-antitrypsin, in COPD, 601–602
Alpha-1-antitrypsin deficiency, treatment of, 606
Alternaria, characteristics of, 109t
Amniotic fluid embolism, 731

779

Anaphylactoid reaction(s), anaphylaxis vs., 301–302, 307t, 308
  causes of, 301–302
  definition of, 321
  due to drug therapy, 323, 327, 327t
  due to food. See also *Food allergy, anaphylactic and anaphylactoid.*
  due to food allergy, 366–375, 675–676
  management of, drug therapy for, 312t
  pathophysiology of, 301t
  to radiocontrast media, 355, 357–358
Anaphylatoxin(s), 17
Anaphylaxis, 297–319
  abnormal physiologic events in, 305–306
  acute, management of, 311–315
    antihistamines in, 314
    β-adrenergic blockade and, 315
    corticosteroids in, 314
    drug therapy for, 312t
    epinephrine in, 313–314
    equipment and medication for medical office in, 313, 313t
    in schools, 761–762
    initial step in, 313
    intravascular volume restoration in, 314–315
    MAST suit in, 315
    steps in, 313t
    vasopressors in, 315
  anaphylactoid reactions vs., 301–302, 307t, 308
  biphasic, 307–308, 315
  challenge testing for, 193
    controls for, 193
    criteria for positive reaction in, 193
    medications in, 193
  differential diagnosis of, 307t, 308–311
    autonomic epilepsy in, 309
    chronic urticaria vs., 310
    flush in, 308–309
    hereditary angioedema in, 310
    laboratory diagnosis in, 310–311
    MSG ingestion in, 309
    Munchausen's stridor in, 309
    postprandial syndromes in, 309
    progesterone in, 310
    scombroidosis vs., 309
    thyroid carcinoma in, 309
    vasopressor reactions in, 308
    vocal cord dysfunction in, 309
  due to drug therapy, 326–327, 327t
  due to food, 366–375. See also *Food allergy, anaphylactic and anaphylactoid.*
  exercise-induced, 367, 376–383. See also *Exercise-induced anaphylaxis.*
  gastrointestinal, 672
  historical, 297
  in pregnancy, 737–738
  incidence of, 297–299
    factor(s) affecting, 298–299, 300t
      age as, 298, 300t
      atopy as, 298–299, 300t
      route of administration as, 298, 300t
      sex as, 298, 300t
      time since last reaction as, 298, 300t
    overall, 297–298
  pathologic finding(s) in, 299–301, 301t
    allergen-specific IgE in, 300–301
    cardiovascular collapse as, 299
    respiratory obstruction as, 299
    serum tryptase in, 300–301

Anaphylaxis *(Continued)*
  pathophysiology of, 301t, 301–306
    basophil degranulation in, 302–305
    complement system in, 304, 305t
    histamine in, 302–304, 304t
    kallikrein-kinin system, 304–305, 305t
    mast cell degranulation in, 302–305, 303t
    recruitment of various inflammatory pathways in, 304–305, 305t
  perioperative, 747–748
  prevention of, 311, 311t
  sign(s) and symptom(s) of, 306t, 306–308
    angioedema as, 306–307
    cardiovascular, 308
    timing of, 307
    urticaria as, 306–307
  to insect stings, 349
Anemia, Fanconi's, immunodeficiency diseases in, 39
  hemolytic, 333–334
Anemophilous plant(s), 97, *97*
Anesthesia, in allergy and asthma patients, 744–745
  agents for, 745
  routes of, 744–745
  local, 358–361
    adverse reaction to, 359–361
      allergic, 359–360
      chemotoxic, 360
      classification of, 359t, 359–360
      diagnostic tests for, 360, 360t
      idiosyncratic, 360
      management of, 343, 360–361
      non-drug-related, 360
      pseudoallergic, 359–360
    classification of, 359, 359t
    solutions of, 359
Angiitis, allergic (hypersensitivity), due to drug therapy, 338
Angioedema, 643–652. See also *Urticaria.*
  classification of, 643–645
  complement activation in, 646
  differential diagnosis of, 645
  eosinophil products in, 646
  etiology of, 646t, 646–648
    drugs in, 646–647
    food additives in, 647
    foods in, 647
    infectious agents in, 647
    insect bites and stings in, 647
  hereditary, anaphylaxis vs., 310
    complement deficiency in, 38
    in pregnancy, 739
    surgery and, 748
    vibratory, 650
  histologic pathology in, 645
  in anaphylactic and anaphylactoid reactions to food additives, 370–371
  in anaphylaxis, 306–307
  in C1 esterase deficiency, 643–645, 648
  in pregnancy, 738–740
  pathophysiology in, 645–648
  treatment of, 648–649
  vasoactive mediators and mast cell activation in, 645–646
Angiotensin-converting enzyme (ACE) inhibitor(s), asthma due to, 555
  chronic cough in, 717
  side effects of, 324
Animal(s), farm, 117
Animal dander(s), 117–118

Animal dander(s) *(Continued)*
    as risk factor, in infantile atopy, 285
    in occupational asthma, 540
Ankylosing spondylitis, 63
Ant(s), fire, 349
    venom of, 350
Anther sac(s), *96*, *97*
Anthesis, 97
    of northern and southern grasses, 101, *102*
    of trees, *103*, 103
    of weeds, 105, *105*
Anti-allergic agent(s), 208–211. See also *Cromolyn; Nedocromil sodium.*
Antibiotic sensitivity, topical, in contact dermatitis, 635
Antibody deficiency, 22–24
    evaluation of, 49
    infections in, 22
    polysaccharide, 25–27
    therapy in, 51
    with normal immunoglobulin concentrations, 24
Antibody level(s), in children, determination of, 50
    in evaluation of immunodeficiency disease, 49
Antibody system, qualitative function of, 142–143
Antigen-presenting cell(s) (APC), 5, 55–56, *56*, 89, *90*
Antigen(s), for bronchoprovocation challenge, 183
    gastrointestinal tract and, 666–670
    presentation of, for T cells, 5, *6*, 55–56, *56*
Antihistamine(s), 227–231
    adverse effects of, 230–231
    clinical uses of, 230
    for allergic rhinitis, 406
    mechanisms of action of, 228
    pharmacokinetics/pharmacodynamics of, *229*, 229–230
    structure and activity of, 227–228, *228*
Antihypertensive agent(s), side effects of, 324
Antinuclear antibody(ies), in SLE, 57
Antiphospholipid antibody(ies), in SLE, 57–58
Antisynthetase antibody, in myositis, 62
Anxiety disorder(s), in asthma, 260
Anxiety headache, 720
Aquagenic urticaria, 651
Arthritis, inflammatory bowel disease and, 64
    psoriatic, 64
    reactive, 63–64
    rheumatoid, complement deficiency in, 38
ASA/NSAID-induced asthma, 491, 549–553
    cross-sensitivities in, 550–551
    diagnosis of, 550
    mechanisms of, 551, *552*
    presentation and clinical features of, 549
    prevalence of, 549–550
    therapy in, 552–553
Aspergillosis, allergic bronchopulmonary, 566–571
    clinical features of, 566
    cystic fibrosis and, 569, 580
    definition of, 566
    diagnostic criteria in, 567t, 567–569
    hypersensitivity pneumonitis vs., 564
    IgE antibodies in, 567–568
    pathophysiology of, 569
    precipitins in, 567
    roentgenographic findings in, *568*, 568–569
    skin testing in, 567
    staging of, 569–570, 570t
    treatment of, 570–571
Aspergillus, characteristics of, 109t
Aspirin, anaphylactoid reactions due to, 301–302
    asthma and. See *ASA/NSAID-induced asthma.*

Aspirin *(Continued)*
    desensitization to, 345
Astemizole, chemical structure of, *228*
Aster(s), pollens of, 106–107
Asthma, acute, treatment of, 506–508, 507t
    in adult, with hospitalization, 509–510
    in children, with hospitalization, 508–509
  air pollution and, statistics on, 124, *125*
  airway obstruction in, 484t, 484–486
    airway smooth muscle spasm in, 485
    alterations in respiratory secretions in, 485
    edema of airway mucosa in, 485
    factors contributing to, 484, 485t
    inflammation in, 485–486
    mucous plugging in, 485
  airway responsiveness in, 473–475, 474t, *475*
  allergy and, 86, 475–478
    allergen exposure in, 476–477
    environmental antigens and, 476
    laboratory evaluation of, 502
  approaches for patient identification in, 473, 473t
  atopy and, 86, 476, 477–478
  bakers', 121
  basophils in, 452–454
    mediators of, 453–454
    recruitment and activation of, 453
  bronchial epithelium in, 457–460
    damage to, 457–459, *458–459*
    mediator(s) and cytokine(s) of, 459–460, *460*
      endothelins as, 459
      15-HETE as, 459
      ICAM-1 as, 460
      neutral endopeptidase as, 460
      nitric oxide as, 459–460
  bronchial hyperresponsiveness in, 487–488
    allergen exposure in, 489, *489*
  bronchoprovocation challenges in, 173–186. See also *Bronchoprovocation challenge(s).*
  challenge testing in, 191–193
    controls in, 191
    criteria for positive reaction in, 191–193, *192*
    medications in, 191
    safety in, 191
  chronic, treatment of, 506t, 513–517
    allergen immunotherapy in, 516
    cromolyn-like NSAIDs in, 514
    inhaled corticosteroids in, 515–516
    intermittent, 513
    metered-dose inhalers in, 513–514
    oral corticosteroids in, 515–516
    regular regimen for, 514
    severe disease and, 514–515
    theophylline in, 515
  complication(s) of, 510–513
    atelectasis as, 510–511
    cardiorespiratory arrest with brain damage as, 512–513
    death as, 513, 513t
    extrapulmonary, 512–513
    neuromyopathy as, 512
    pneumomediastinum as, 511–512, *511–512*
    pneumothorax as, 511–512, *512*
    pulmonary, 510–512
    respiratory failure as, 510
    vasopressin excess (inappropriate ADH secretion) as, 512
  COPD and, 517–518
  COPD vs., 605
  cystic fibrosis and, 579–580

Asthma *(Continued)*
  definition of, 84, 472–473
  determinant(s) of inflammatory response in, 461–468
    adhesion molecules as, 464–465
    autonomic nerves and receptors in, 465–466
    chemokines as, 463
    cytokines as, 461–463
    excitatory NANC neurotransmitters in, 467–468
    IL-3, IL-5, GM-CSF as, 462
    IL-4 and IFN-gamma as, 462–463
    inhibitory NANC neurotransmitters in, *466*, 466–467
    neurogenic, 465–468
  diagnosis of, histamine challenge testing in, 179–180, 501
    methacholine challenge testing in, 179–180, 501
  differential diagnosis of, 492, 492t
  drug therapy for, 505t, 505–506
    antihistamines in, 230
    cromolyn in, 210, 514
    histamine challenge testing for evaluation of, 180, *180*
    inhaled glucocorticoids in, 214–215
    ipratropium bromide in, 226
    methacholine challenge testing for evaluation of, 180, *180*
    nedocromil sodium in, 210, 514
    theophylline in, 223–225
  drug-induced, 549–558. See also *Drug-induced asthma*; individual drugs.
  due to drug therapy, 336
  emotional triggers of, 256–257
  environmental history in, 499
  eosinophils in, 447, 447–450
    mediators of, 447–448
    recruitment and activation of, 448–450, *449*
    studies on, 447
  epidemiology of, 84–87, 472–483, 486–487
  etiology of, 443–471, 488–489, *489*. See also specific mediators.
  evaluation in, 498–502
  exercise-induced. See *Exercise-induced asthma*.
  family clustering of, 86
  history in, 498–499
  IgE-mediated LPR in, 75
  immunotherapy for, clinical trials of, 241
  in anaphylactic and anaphylactoid reactions to food additives, 371–372
  in pregnancy, 516
  incidence of, 84
  indoor allergens and, 118
  inflammatory mediators in, 447–461
  investigation of pathology and mediators in, 443–446
    bronchial mucosal biopsy for, 443–444
      autopsy studies in, 444
      fiberoptic bronchoscopic studies in, 444
      immunohistochemical studies in, 444, *445*
      nonatopic patients and, 444–445
      rigid bronchoscopic studies in, 444
    early asthmatic response and, 445–446
    late asthmatic response and, 446
  laboratory evaluation in, 499–502, 500t
    allergy testing in, 502
    bronchodilator response in, 501
    chemical challenge tests in, 501. See also *Bronchoprovocation challenge(s)*.
    chest X-ray examination in, 502
    exercise tolerance tests in, 501
    nasal and sputum cytology in, 501–502

Asthma *(Continued)*
  pulmonary function testing in, 167t, 499–501
  spirometry in, 500–501
  total serum IgE in, 502
  lymphocytes in, 454–456
  macrophages in, 457
  mast cells in, *450*, 450–451
  morbidity and mortality in, 86, 495–496
    death and, 86
    hospitalization and, 86
    poverty and, 86
  natural course of, 487
  neutrophils in, 456–457
  occupational, 529–548. See also *Occupational asthma*.
  pathology in, 484t, 484–486
  patient education in, 268–281. See also *Patient education, in asthma*.
  patterns of, 491–492, 494t
  physical examination in, 499
    in children, 499
  physiology of, 487–488, *488*
  platelet activating factor in, 460–461
  pregnancy and, 731t, 731–735, 733t–734t. See also *Pregnancy, asthma in*.
  presentation of, 492–494, *493*
  prevalence of, 84–86, 473, *474*
    age-related factors in, 84
    by demographic characteristics, 84, 85t
    disease definition and, 84, 84t
    increases in, 85–86
    race/ethnic factors in, 84
    socioeconomic status in, 84–85
  principles of diagnosis and treatment of, 484–497
  prognosis in, 480–481, 494–496
  psychosocial factors in, 256–267, 518. See also *Psychosocial factor(s), in asthma*.
  risk factor(s) for, 478–480, 489
    age as, 478
    cigarette smoke as, 86, 130, 479–480, 504
    gender as, 478
    mechanical, 478
    prematurity as, 479
    race as, 479
    respiratory illness as, 478–479
    socioeconomic status as, 479
    viral infections as, 86–87
  severity of, 493–494, 494t
  sinusitis and, 434
  sleep or nocturnal, 491
  sulfur dioxide inhalation and, 125
  surgery in, 516–517
  T_{H1} and T_{H2} lymphocytes in, 455–456
  therapy consideration(s) in, 502–506
    compliance and, 503
    dust mite avoidance as, 504
    environmental control and, 503–505
    goals of, 503
    home peak-flow monitoring in, 504–505
    management philosophy in, 502–503
    pet removal as, 504
  trigger(s) (aggravating factors) for, 86–87, 489–491
    allergens as, 86, 489–490
    allergic rhinitis as, 490
    emotional factors as, 490
    endocrine factors as, 491
    exercise as, 490
    gastroesophageal reflux as, 490
    interaction of, 491
    irritants as, 490

Asthma *(Continued)*
    nonallergic hypersensitivity to drugs and chemicals as, 490–491
    pollution as, 86
    pulmonary function testing for evaluation of, 166–168, *167*
    sinusitis as, 490
    sleep or nocturnal asthma and, 491
    upper respiratory infection as, 490
    viral infections as, 86–87, 490
    weather changes as, 490
  unstable, as contraindication in immunotherapy, 245
  wheezing in, 492–493
Ataxia-telangiectasia, 32–33
  clinical findings in, 32–33
  immune abnormalities in, 33
Atelectasis, in asthma, 510–511
Athlete(s), exercise-induced asthma in, 526–527, 527t
Atopic cataract(s), 708, *708*, 709
Atopic dermatitis, 613–632. See also *Eczema.*
  aeroallergens in, 620
  antihistamines for, 230
  chronic inflammation in, *623*, 623–624
  clinical features of, 613–617, 614t
  complication(s) of, 616–617
    atopic diathesis and, 616
    cutaneous infection as, 616–617
      Pityrosporum ovale in, 617
      Staphylococcus aureus, 617
      Trichophyton rubrum in, 617
      bacterial, 616–617
      fungal, 617
      herpes simplex, 616
      viral, 616
    ichthyosis as, 616
    xerosis as, 616
  diagnostic features of, 614, 641t
    in infants, 614, 641t
  differential diagnosis of, 617, 618t
  distribution of, 615–616
  emotional and family dysfunction in, 617
  foods in, 619–620
  histopathology in, 617–619
  IgE-mediated LPR in, 75
  immunologic features of, 622–623
  in pregnancy, 740–741
  management of, 624–630
    allergen immunotherapy in, 629–630
    antimicrobials for, 628–629
    controlling itch in, 626
    corticosteroids for, 627–628
      systemic, 628
      topical, 627t, 627–628
    cyclosporine in, 630
    education/emotional support in, 629
    exacerbating factor(s) in, 624–626
      aeroallergens as, 625
      allergens as, 624–625
      foods as, 624–625, 670–671
      irritants as, 625–626
    hydration in, 626–627
    IFN-γ in, 630
    immunomodulators in, 629–630
    phototherapy in, 630
    tars for, 628
    thymopentin in, 630
  morphology of, 614–615, *614–615*
    acute eczema in, 614, *614*
    chronic eczema in, 614–615, *615*

Atopic dermatitis *(Continued)*
    pigmentary disorders in, 615, *615*
    subacute eczema in, 614, *615*
  ocular finding(s) in, 707–709, *708*
    atopic cataracts in, 708, *708*
    eyelids in, 707–708
    punctate staining of cornea in, 708
    retinal detachment in, 708–709
    Trantas' dots in, 708
  patch testing in, 620–622
  pathophysiology in, 617–624
  prevalence of, 613
  RAST testing in, 620
  skin prick testing in, 620
  symptoms in, 616
Atopic keratoconjunctivitis, 707–708, *708*, 709
Atopy, as factor affecting incidence of anaphylaxis, 298–299, 300t
  asthma and, 86, 476, 477–478
  family history of, food allergy and, 82
  in infants, breast milk and, 284–285
    cord blood IgE and, 283
    inhalants as risk factor for, 285–286
    prediction of, 282–286
  penicillin allergy and, 83
Atropine, for anesthesia in asthma and allergy, 745
  structure and activity of, 225, *225*
Attention deficit disorder, food additives and, 677, 750–751
Audiometry, in otitis media, 417
Aureobasidium, characteristics of, 109t
Autoantibody(ies), tests for, controversial, 756–757
Autoimmune disease, 55–67. See also individual diseases.
  as contraindication, in immunotherapy, 245
  in complement deficiency, 38
  mechanism of, 56
  organ-specific, 64–65
  systemic, 56–64
Autoimmune reaction(s), in drug hypersensitivity, 325
Avoidance diet, during lactation, effect of, on infantile atopy, 288–290, 289t–290t
  during pregnancy, effect of, on infantile atopy, 288, 289t–290t
Avoidance principle(s), 195–207
  allergens and, 196–203
  environment and, 203–205
  for animals, 202
  for cats, 200–201, *201*, 201t
  for cockroaches, 202
  for combustion byproducts, 205
  for dogs, 201–202
  for dust mites, 196–200. See also *Dust mite(s), avoidance of.*
  for infections, 204
  for molds, 203
  for pests, 202
  for pollens, 202–203
  for tobacco smoke, 204–205
  home and office construction and, 203–204
  problems with, 205–206
  strategies for, 195
  targets of, 195, *195*

B cell(s), 3
  activation of, 7
  differentiation of, 3

B cell(s) *(Continued)*
   phenotypic subset analysis of, flow cytometry for, 755–756
B-cell deficiency, in X-linked agammaglobulinemia, 23
B lymphocyte(s). See *B cell(s)*.
Bacterial infection(s), in immunodeficiency disease, 22
   of skin, 656–657
Bacterial vaccine(s), clinical trials of, 242
Bakers' asthma, 121
Balsam of Peru sensitivity, 640
Bare lymphocyte syndrome, 29
Basophil degranulation. See also *Histamine*.
   in anaphylaxis, 302–305
   inflammatory pathways activated by, 302
   pathophysiologic events due to, 302
Basophil(s), allergen-induced cross-linking of IgE and, 70
   chemoattractants of, 453
   functions of, 4–5
   histamine-releasing factors in, 453
   IL-4 and, 453
   in asthma, 452–454
   mediators of, 453–454
   modulation of, with immunotherapy, 237–238
   priming and activating factors of, 453
   recruitment and activation of, 453
Beclomethasone dipropionate, chemical structure of, *212*
   pharmacokinetics of, 213–214
Bee sting(s). See *Insect sting(s)*.
Beech(es), pollens of, 104
Benzalkonium chloride, asthma due to, 556
Benzoate(s), asthma due to, 556
Benzocaine sensitivity, 640
Benzyl benzoate, for dust mite control, 199
   for indoor environmental control, 118
Beta blocker(s). See *Beta-adrenergic antagonist(s)*.
Beta-adrenergic agonist(s), 218–223
   adverse effects of, 223
   clinical effects of, 220–223
   for COPD, 607
   mechanism of action of, 218–220
   structure and activity of, 218, *219*
Beta-adrenergic antagonist(s), as contraindication, in immunotherapy, 244–245
   asthma due to, 553
Biology of allergens, 89–92
Bird(s), 117
   pet, allergen avoidance techniques for, 202
Blood chemical analysis, controversial, 757
Bloom syndrome, immunodeficiency diseases in, 39
Body plethysmography, for lung volume and capacity measurement, 160
Bone marrow transplantation, for cellular immune defects, 52
Botrytis, characteristics of, 109t
Bread mold(s), 110
Breast milk, allergic disease in infants and, 283–284
   studies on, 286–288, 287t
   atopy in infants and, 284–285
   infantile eczema and, 81
Bronchial hyperresponsiveness. See also under *Airway*.
   in asthma, 487–488
   nonspecific, tests for, 141
Bronchial mucosal biopsy, for investigation of asthma, 443–444
Bronchiectasis, chronic cough in, 717
   in allergic bronchopulmonary aspergillosis, 568
   in cystic fibrosis, 583–584

Bronchiolitis (small airways disease), in COPD, 601
Bronchitis, chronic, chronic cough in, 717
   in COPD, 600
Bronchodilator response, in asthma evaluation, 501
Bronchodilator(s), future types of, 234
   in bronchopulmonary dysplasia, 596
Bronchoprovocation challenge(s), 164–166, *165*
   in airway hyperreactivity, 166
   in asthma, 501
   in COPD, 166
   in occupational asthma, 538–539
   inhalation, 173–186. See also *Histamine challenge testing; Methacholine challenge testing*.
      antigen for, 183
      cold air hyperventilation for, 181, 184
      comparisons of, 183–185, 184t
      nebulized water, 181–182, 182t, 184
      nonpharmacologic, 181–183
      pharmacologic, 175–181
      purposes for, 174t, 174–175
      research avenues for, 183
      ultrasonic saline for, 182–183, 184
Bronchopulmonary dysplasia, 592–599
   clinical findings in, 594
   complications of, 596–597, 597t
   definition of, 592
   gastroesophageal reflux in, 597
   long-term prognosis in, 597–598
   medical management of, 594–596
      acute and chronic, 596
      anti-inflammatory agents in, 596
      bronchodilators in, 596
      conventional ventilation in, 594–595, 595t
      cromolyn sodium in, 595–596
      disease prevention and, 594–596
      diuretics in, 596
      steroids in, 595
      surfactant therapy in, 594
   pathogenesis of, 592–593
      hyaline membrane disease in, 592–593
   pathology in, 593–594
   pulmonary hypertension in, 597
   tracheobronchomalacia in, 597
Bronchospasm, due to radiocontrast reaction, 357
Budesonide, chemical structure of, *212*
   pharmacokinetics of, 214
Bullous reaction(s), due to drug therapy, 330

C1 esterase deficiency, angioedema in, 643–645, 648
C1 inhibitor deficiency, 38
C1q deficiency, 38
C2 deficiency, autoimmune diseases in, 38
   recurrent infections in, 38
C3 deficiency, autoimmune diseases in, 38
   recurrent infections in, 38–39
Caddis fly, 119
Candida, characteristics of, 109t
Candida hypersensitivity syndrome, 751–752
Candidiasis, chronic mucocutaneous, 31–32
   immune defect in, 31–32
   infections in, 31
   superficial, 654
Captopril, side effects of, 324
Carboxylase deficiency, biotin-dependent, immunodeficiency in, 39–40
Carcinoid syndrome, anaphylaxis vs., 308
Cardiac reaction(s), to drug therapy, 337

Cardiorespiratory arrest, in asthma, 512–513
Cardiovascular collapse, due to radiocontrast reaction, 358
  in anaphylaxis, 299
Cardiovascular system, physical examination of, 139
Carrier, definition of, 321
Cartilage-hair hypoplasia, 33
Castor bean, 121
Cat(s), 117
  allergen avoidance techniques for, 200–201, *201*, 201t
  exposure to, control methods for, 118
Cataract(s), atopic, 708, *708*, 709
Catecholamine, chemical structure of, *219*
CD11a/CD18 (leukocyte function antigen–1, LFA-1) deficiency, 37, 39
CD11b/CD18, functions of, 37
CD11c/CD18 (CR4), functions of, 38
CD3, in T-cell activation, 6
CD4. See under *T cell(s)*.
CD8. See under *T cell(s)*.
Celiac disease, 674–675, 699
Cellulitis, angioedema vs., 645
Cerumen, impaction of, 411
Cetirizine, chemical structure of, *228*
Challenge (provocation) testing. See *Bronchoprovocation challenge(s)*.
  exercise. See *Exercise challenge testing*.
  for drug allergy, 343
  histamine. See *Histamine challenge testing*.
  methacholine. See *Methacholine challenge testing*.
Chédiak-Higashi syndrome, 35
Chemical avoidance therapy, 758
Chemical sensitivity(ies), multiple (environmental illness), 751
Chemokine(s), in asthma, 463
Chemotactic factor(s), 17
Chemotoxic reaction(s), to local anesthetics, 360, 360t
  to radiocontrast media, 355–356, 356t, 358
Chest, physical examination of, 138–139
Chest radiography. See *Radiography, chest*.
Childhood depression, in asthma, 261
Children. See also *Infant(s)*.
  AIDS in, *Pneumocystis carinii* pneumonia in, 43
    diagnosis of, 43–44
    lymphoid interstitial pneumonia in, 43
    progression of HIV infection to, 43
  asthma in. See *Asthma*.
  chronic pulmonary disease in, 572–591. See also *Cystic fibrosis*.
    types of, 573t
  immunodeficiency diseases in, evaluation of, 50
  laryngeal and tracheal obstruction in, 439–440
  methacholine challenge testing for, 177–178, *179*
  pulmonary function values in, 171t
Chinese restaurant syndrome, 677
Chloride channel blocker(s), 233
Chlorpheniramine, chemical structure of, *228*
Choanal atresia, 394
Cholestatic reaction(s), to drug therapy, 335–336
Cholesteatoma, in otitis media, 422
Cholinergic antagonist(s), 225–227
  adverse effects of, 226–227
  clinical use of, 226
  mechanisms of action of, 226
  pharmacokinetics of, 226
  structure and activity of, *225*, 225–226
Chromate dermatitis, 639
Chromium salt(s), in occupational asthma, 543
Chromosomal abnormality(ies), immunodeficiency diseases in, 39

Chronic allergic disease, cytokines in, 76
  pathogenesis of, 75–76
  T cells in, 76
Chronic obstructive pulmonary disease (COPD), 600–612
  asthma vs., 605
  bronchial challenge test in, 166
  clinical characteristics of, 603–605
    airway obstruction in, 603–604
    diffusing capacity in, 604–605
    electrocardiography in, 603
    lung volumes in, 604
    maximal exercise performance in, 605
    pulmonary function testing in, 603–604
    radiologic findings in, 603
    signs and symptoms in, 603
    spirometry in, 604
  definitions and pathology in, 600–601
    chronic bronchitis in, 600
    emphysema in, 600–601
    small airways disease (bronchiolitis) in, 601
  differential diagnosis of, 605
  etiology and pathogenesis of, 601–603, *602*
    airway hyperresponsiveness in, 602
    alpha-1-antitrypsin in, 601–602
    childhood respiratory illnesses in, 602
    cor pulmonale, 602–603
    occupational exposures in, 602
    tobacco smoking in, 601
  in asthma, 517–518
  preventive therapy in, 606
  prognosis in, 611
  treatment of, 605–611, *606*
    alpha-1-antitrypsin deficiency and, 606
    anticholinergics in, 607
    β_2-agonists in, 607
    corticosteroids in, 608
    in acute exacerbations, 610–611
    low-flow oxygen in, 608–609
    lung transplantation in, 609–610
    metered dose inhalers in, 607
    pharmacologic, 607–609
    pulmonary rehabilitation in, 609
    theophylline in, 607–608
    vaccination in, 606–607
    various options for, 610
Chronomid midge(s), 119
Chymopapain, allergy to, 83
Cigarette smoke (smoking), asthma and, 86, 130, 479–480, *480*, 504
  avoidance techniques for, 204–205
  Crohn's disease and, 697
  environmental, 130
  in COPD, 601
  in infantile atopy, 285
  in medical history, 137
  ulcerative colitis and, 697
Ciliary dyskinesia syndrome, 587–589
  clinical manifestations of, 587
  diagnosis of, 588
  management of, 588–589
  pathogenesis of, 587–588
  respiratory manifestations of, 588
  sinusitis in, 439
Cinnamic aldehyde sensitivity, 640
Cladosporium, characteristics of, 109t
Clubbing of fingers and toes, in cystic fibrosis, 581–582, 582t
Cluster headache, 724–725

Cobalt salt(s), in occupational asthma, 543
Cockroach(es), 116
   allergen avoidance techniques for, 202
   allergens of, 116
   asthma therapy and, 504
Cold air hyperventilation, for bronchoprovocation challenge, 181, 184
Colic, 673–674
Colitis, food-induced, 673
   ulcerative. See *Ulcerative colitis*.
Colony stimulating factor–granulocyte (G-CSF), immunologic properties of, 15t, 16
Colony stimulating factor–granulocyte macrophage (GM-CSF), immunologic properties of, 15t, 16
Colony stimulating factor–macrophage (M-CSF), immunologic properties of, 15t, 16
Colophony dermatitis, 640
Colophony fume(s), in occupational asthma, 543
Common variable immune deficiency (CVID), 23–24
   clinical manifestations of, 24
   immune defect in, 24
Complement, activation of, 17–18, *18*
   alternative pathway of, 17, *18*
   classical pathway of, 17, *18*
   in angioedema, 646
   in occupational asthma, 536
   in pseudoallergic drug reactions, 323–324
   in urticaria, 646
   in immunity, 16–17
   in tears, 704
Complement component(s), cell surface, defects in, 39
Complement deficiency, 38–39
   autoimmune diseases due to, 38
   infections in, 22, 38–39
   laboratory evaluation in, 48t, 49–50
Complement receptor(s), deficiencies in, 39
Complement system, in anaphylaxis, 304, 305t
Complementarity determining region (CDR), 8
Computed tomography, in laryngeal and tracheal obstruction, 438
   in sinusitis, 432
Conifer(s), pollens of, 102
Conjunctiva, 704–706
   cellular immune response of, 706
   granulomas of, 706
   humoral immune response of, 706
   hyperemia of, 705
   inflammatory response of, 706
   normal structure and function of, 704–705
   papillary hypertrophy of, 705–706
   pathologic responses of, 705–706
   pseudomembranes and membranes of, 706
Contact dermatitis, 633–642
   allergic, eyes in, 709
   allergic eczematous, in drug hypersensitivity, 328–329, 329t
   clinical pattern and distribution of, 636t, 636–637
   clinical presentation in, *634*, 634–637
   history in, 634
   immunology in, 633
   immunopathogenesis in, 633–634
   irritant, allergic dermatitis vs., 635, 636t
   eyes in, 709–710
   occupational history in, 635, 635t
   ocular findings in, *709*, 709–710
   patch testing in, 634, 635t, 637–641
      balsam of Peru for, 640
      benzocaine, 640
      chromate for, 639

Contact dermatitis *(Continued)*
      cinnamic aldehyde for, 640
      colophony for, 640
      epoxy resin for, 640
      ethylenediamine for, 640–641
      formaldehyde for, 639–640
      imidazolidinyl urea for, 640
      method for, 638, 638t
      neomycin for, 640
      nickel for, 638–639, *639*
      North American tray for, 637, *637*t
      paraphenylenediamine for, 640
      p-tert-butyphenol for, 640
      quarternium 15 for, 639
      rubber antigens for, 640
      rules of, 638, 639t
      sources of supplies for, 638, 639t
      timing of, 638, 638t
      True test system for, 638, *638*
      wood alcohols for, 640
   pathology in, 637
   plant, 641
   preservative, 641
   self-treatment in, 634–635
   topical antibiotic sensitivity in, 635
   treatment of, 641–642
Controversial concepts in allergy and immunology, 749–760
   diagnostic method(s) in, 752–757
      applied kinesiology as, 754
      autoantibody test as, 756–757
      B-cell and T-cell phenotype subset analysis as, 755–756
      biomarker tests as, 755
      blood and tissue chemical analyses as, 757
      cytotoxic food test as, 753–754
      electrodiagnosis as, 754
      food immune complexes as, 755
      provocation-neutralization testing as, 753
      pulse test as, 753
      serum IgG antibodies as, 754–755
      skin end-point titration as, 752–753
   etiologic theory(ies) in, 749–752
      allergic toxemia as, 749–750
      candida hypersensitivity as, 751–752
      food additive sensitivity as, 750–751
      multiple chemical sensitivities as, 751
   treatment(s) in, 757–759
      acupuncture as, 757
      chemical avoidance as, 758
      elimination diets as, 758
      enzyme-potentiated immunotherapy as, 758–759
      homeopathy as, 757–758
      neutralization therapy as, 757
Cor pulmonale, in COPD, 602–603
   therapy in, 609
Cord blood, total serum IgE in, 154–155
   as predictor of atopy, 283
Corticosteroid(s), for allergic rhinitis, 406–407
   for atopic dermatitis, 627–628
      systemic, 628
      topical, 627t, 627–628
   for bronchopulmonary dysplasia, 595, 596
   for chronic asthma, 515–516
   for COPD, 608
Cotton, 120
Cottonseed, 121
Cough, chronic, 713–718
   anatomic diagnostic evaluation in, *713*, 713–716

Cough (Continued)
  protocol for, 713–714
  results of, 714–716, 715
  testing characteristics of, 714, 715t
 differential diagnosis of, 716–718
  ACE inhibitors in, 717
  asthma in, 716
  bronchiectasis in, 717
  chronic bronchitis in, 717
  gastrointestinal reflux disease in, 716–717
  miscellaneous conditions in, 717–718
  postnasal drip syndrome in, 716
 in medical history, 136
Cough syncope headache, 719
Cow's milk. See Milk.
Cow's milk formula, in prevention of allergy in infants, 286–288, 287t
CR4 (CD11c/CD18), functions of, 38
CREST syndrome, 62
Crohn's disease, 687–702
 arthritis and, 64
 clinical manifestations of, 689–690
 diagnosis of, 690
 immunopathogenesis of, 690–699
  adhesion molecules in, 698
  cigarette smoking and, 697
  complications and, 698–699
  hemostatic abnormalities in, 697
  intestinal barrier epithelium dysfunction in, 692–693
  intestinal luminal antigens in, 691–692
  intestinal mucosal defects in, 693–695
  mediators of intestinal inflammatory damage in, 695–697
  neuroimmune modulation in, 697–698
  systemic immunoregulation in, 693–695
 proposed cause(s) of, 691
  immunologic hypothesis as, 691
  infectious hypothesis as, 691
 therapy in, medical, 687
 ulcerative colitis vs., 690
Cromolyn, 208–211
 adverse effects of, 211
 chemical structure of, 208, 208
 in allergic rhinitis, 210–211, 406
 in asthma, 210, 514
 in bronchopulmonary dysplasia, 595–596
 mechanism of action of, 208–210, 209
 pharmacokinetics of, 210
Cross-reaction, definition of, 321
Croup (acute laryngotracheobronchitis), 440
 spasmodic, 440
Curvularia, characteristics of, 109t
Cyclosporine, in atopic dermatitis, 630
Cystic fibrosis, 572–587
 allergic bronchopulmonary aspergillosis and, 569, 580
 allergic complications of, 579–581
 allergy skin testing and, 579–580
 altered immune processes in, 581
 asthma and, 579–580
 chronic sinusitis in, 580
 clinical presentation in, 577–579
  external manifestations of, 577–578
  gastrointestinal manifestations of, 578–589
  internal manifestations of, 578
 complication(s) of, 573, 574t
  Pseudomonas infection as, 581
  resembling immune disease, 580–581
 diagnosis of, 573–575

Cystic fibrosis (Continued)
 genetics of, 575–576, 576t
 incidence of, 573
 management of, 585–587
  approaches to therapy in, 586, 586t
  cystic fibrosis centers in, 585, 585t
  lung transplantation for, 586–587
 nasal polyps in, 580
 pathogenesis of, cystic fibrosis transmembrane regulator in, 576–577
 pulmonary complications of, 581–585
  bronchiectasis in, 583–584
  clubbing of fingers and toes in, 581–582, 582t
  hemoptysis in, 582–583, 583t
  pneumothorax in, 584–585
 pulmonary function testing in, 167t
 sweat testing in, 141, 574, 574t
 treatment of, new strategies for, 577, 577t
Cystic fibrosis transmembrane regulator (CFTR), 576–577
Cytokine(s), 14–16. See also individual types.
 as hematopoietic growth factors, 16
 as lymphocyte activators, 16
 as nonspecific inflammatory mediators, 14, 16
 eosinophils and, 461–462
 in asthma, 461–463
 in chronic allergic disease, 76
 in modulation of IgE synthesis, 72t, 72–73
 LPR, 75
 mast cells and, 451–452
 T_{H1}- and T_{H2}-cell secretion of, 73
Cytomegalovirus infection, in AIDS, treatment of, 45
Cytotoxic anaphylactoid reaction(s), 302
Cytotoxic food test, controversial, 753–754

Dander(s), animal, 117–118
 in infantile atopy, 285
 human, 117–118
Deafness, sudden, 424
Decongestant(s), 231–233
 adverse effects of, 232–233
 clinical usage of, 232
 for allergic rhinitis, 406
 mechanism of action of, 231
 pharmacokinetics/pharmacodynamics of, 231–232
 structure and activity of, 231, 231
Depression, childhood, in asthma, 261
Dermatitis, atopic. See Atopic dermatitis.
 contact. See Contact dermatitis.
 diaper, 654
 exfoliative, due to drug therapy, 330, 337–338, 338t
Dermatitis herpetiformis, 671–672
Dermatitis medicamentosa, 330
Dermatographism, 650
Dermatomyositis, 62–63
 in X-linked agammaglobulinemia, 23
Dermatophytic infection(s), superficial, 653–654
Dermatosis, bacterial, 656–657
 bullous, 658–660
 fungal, 653–654
 infectious, 653–658
 insect, 657
 viral, 654–656
Desensitization, for drug hypersensitivity, 344t, 344–345
 to aspirin, 345
 to insulin, 344–345
 to penicillin, 344, 344t

Desensitization *(Continued)*
  to sulfasalazine, 344
  to xenogenic serum, 344
Diabetes mellitus, type I, 64
Diagnostic challenge(s), 187–194. *See also Bronchoprovocation challenge(s).*
  dietary avoidance in, 187
  dosage for, 187t, 187–188
  general principles of, 187–188
  in asthmatic patients, 191–193. *See also Asthma; Bronchoprovocative challenge(s).*
  in patients with anaphylaxis, 193
  in patients with other symptoms, 193
  in urticaria/angioedema patients, 188–191. *See also Urticaria/angioedema.*
  site of challenge in, 187
  substance vehicles for, 188
  timing of, 188
Diagnostic testing, 139t, 139–143
  for immunologic function, 142–143
  for lower airway disease, 140–141
  for suggestive and specific allergy, 141
  for upper airway disease, 139–140
  performance indices for, 152t
Diaper dermatitis, 654
Diet, elimination, 680, 758
  in eczema, 81
Diisocyanates, in occupational asthma, 541
Diphenhydramine, chemical structure of, *228*
Diphtheria vaccine, adverse reactions to, 388–389
Dipyridamole, asthma due to, 554–555
Diuretic(s), in bronchopulmonary dysplasia, 596
Dog(s), 117
  allergen avoidance techniques for, 201–202
  exposure to, control methods for, 118
Double-stranded DNA antibody(ies), in SLE, 57
Down syndrome, immunodeficiency diseases in, 39
Downy mildew(s), 110
Drug(s). *See also Drug therapy;* individual drugs.
  never or rarely causing skin eruptions, 330t
Drug abuse, in medical history, 137
Drug additive(s), asthma due to, 556
  pseudoallergic reactions to, 339
Drug allergy. *See Drug hypersensitivity, allergic.*
Drug hypersensitivity/hypersensitivity reaction(s), 320–347
  accelerated, 83
  allergic, 321t, 321–323
    background in, 321
    characteristics of, 321t, 321–322
    classification of, 326, 326t
    in AIDS, 323
    in pregnancy, 741
    incidence of, 322
    provocative challenge test in, 322
    risk factors for, 322–323
    sensitivity testing in, 321–322
  angioedema in, 646–647
  autoimmune reaction(s) in, 332–333
    other types of, 333
    systemic lupus erythematosus as, 332–333
  classification of adverse reactions in, 320t, 320–321
  cutaneous, 329–331
    allergic eczematous contact dermatitis as, 328–329, 329t
    fixed drug eruptions as, 329–330
    generalized skin rashes as, 330
    photodermatitis as, 329, 329t
    toxic epidermal necrolysis as, 330–331

Drug hypersensitivity/hypersensitivity reaction(s) *(Continued)*
  definitions in, 321
  epidemiology of, 83–84
  erythema multiforme in, 337
  exfoliative dermatitis in, 337–338, 338t
  fever in, 331–332
    nonallergic causes of, 331, 331t
    without other signs of allergy, 332, 332t
  general aspects of, 321–324
  immediate, 83
  immune pathogenesis of, 324–326
    autoimmune reaction in, 325
    cell-mediated conditions in, 326
    cytotoxic antibody reactions in, 325
    hapten-cell reaction in, 325
    IgE antibodies in, 325
    immune complex reactions in, 325–326
    immunochemical principles in, 324–325
    mechanisms of, 325–326
  late, 83
  management of, 340–345
    in patient with positive history, 341–345
      alternative drugs for, 341–342
      assessment in, 341, *341*
      desensitization in, 344t, 344–345
      immunologic testing in, 342–343
      premedication in, 343–344
      provocative testing in, 343
  mast cell–mediated, 326–328
    cutaneous reactions as, 327
    serum sickness as, 327–328
    systemic anaphylaxis as, 326–327, 327t
    urticaria as, 327, 328t
  nonallergic, asthma in, 490–491
    fever in, 331, 331t
  organ system reaction(s) in, 333–337
    asthma as, 336
    cardiac, 337
    eosinophilia as, 333, 333t
    granulocytopenia as, 335
    hematologic, 333–335
    hemolytic anemia as, 333–334
      autoimmune, 334
      hapten-cell type, 333–334
      immune complex type, 334
    hepatic, 335t, 335–336
    pulmonary, 336t, 336–337
      fibrotic, 336–337
      infiltrative, 336, 336t
    renal, 337
      glomerular injury as, 337
      interstitial nephritis as, 337
    thrombocytopenia as, 334t, 334–335
  prevention of, 340–341
    patient history in, 340
    product refinements in, 340
    reducing drug exposure in, 340
    routine testing or premedication in, 341
  pseudoallergic reactions in, 323t, 323–324, 338–339
    to food and drug additives, 339
    to NSAIDs, 338–339
    to radiocontrast media, 339
    to sulfites, 339
  T-cell mediated, 328–329
  treatment of, 345
  types of, 83, 326–339
  urticaria in, 646–647
  vasculitis in, 338

Drug reaction(s), adverse, classification of, 320t, 320–321
  psychophysiologic, 321
Drug therapy, 208–236. See also under individual disorders.
  anti-allergic, 208–211
  β-adrenergic agonists, 218–223
  bronchodilators as, 234
  chloride channel blockers as, 233
  cholinergic antagonists as, 225–227
  decongestant(s) as, 231–233
  enzyme inhibitor(s) as, 233
  glucocorticoid, 211–218
  H$_1$-receptor antagonist(s) as, 227–231. See also Antihistamine(s).
  immunomodulator(s) as, 233–234
  mediator antagonist(s) as, 233
  methylxanthine(s) as, 223–225
Drug-induced asthma, 549–558
  angiotensin-converting enzyme inhibitors in, 555
  aspirin and NSAID in, 491, 549–553. See also ASA/NSAID-induced asthma.
  benzalkonium chloride in, 556
  benzoate in, 556
  beta-adrenergic antagonist in, 553
  dipyridamole in, 554–555
  drug additive in, 556
  intraoperative agent in, 553–554
  miscellaneous agents in, 556–557
  parabens in, 556
  pentamidine in, 555–556
  radiocontrast media in, 555
  sulfite in, 556
  tartrazine in, 556
Drug-induced lupus syndrome, 58, 58t
Dust mite(s), as risk factor, in infantile atopy, 285
  avoidance of, 196–200
    dust collectors and, 199
    from birth, 199–200
    in asthma, 504
    in bedroom, 198
    in carpeting, 198–199
    in upholstery, 198–199
    studies on, 197
    techniques for, 198t, 198–199
    temperature and humidity and, 199
  biology of, 197
  control methods for, 118
  levels of infestation of, in different localities, 197, 197t
  temperature and humidity for growth of, 199, 200

Ear(s), physical examination of, 138
Ear disease(s), 411–427
  external, 411–412
    cerumen impaction in, 411
    foreign bodies in, 411
    furuncles in, 412
    tumors in, 412, 412t
  inner, 423–425
    benign paroxysmal positional vertigo as, 424–425
    labyrinthitis as, 424
    Meniere's disease as, 423
    perilymphatic fistula as, 423–424
    sudden deafness as, 424
  middle, 412–423. See also Otitis media.
    tumors as, 423

EBV, in IL-4 dependent IgE synthesis, 71–72
Eczema. See also Atopic dermatitis.
  diet in, 81
  epidemiology of, 80–81
  family history in, 81
  influences on development of, 81
  nummular, 661
  prevalence of, 80
Egg(s), allergy to, 668–669
Electrocardiography, in COPD, 603
Electrodiagnosis, controversial, 754
Elemental amino acid–derived formula, characteristics of, 291t
Embolism, amniotic fluid, 731
Emotional factor(s), in asthma, 490
Emphysema, centriacinar, 600
  centrilobular, 600
  distal acinar, 600–601
  in COPD, 600–601
  panacinar, 601
  pulmonary function testing in, 167t
Endoscopy, for laryngeal and tracheal obstruction, 438
Enflurane, asthma due to, 554
  for anesthesia in asthma and allergy, 745
Entemophilous plant(s), 97
Enterocolitis syndrome, food-induced, 672–673
Environment, indoor. See Indoor environment.
Environmental control, for asthma, 503–505
Environmental factor(s), allergen avoidance techniques for, 203–205
  nonallergenic, 124–133
    indoor air pollution as, 130–131
    outdoor air pollution as, 124–130
Environmental history, in medical history, 137
Environmental illness (multiple chemical sensitivities), 751
Enzyme inhibitor(s), 233
Enzyme-potentiated immunotherapy, 758–759
Eosinophil count, total, 142
Eosinophil peroxidase, 447
Eosinophil-derived neurotoxin, 447
Eosinophil(s), cytokines and, 461–462
  functions of, 4
  in allergic drug reactions, 333, 333t
  in angioedema, 646
  in asthma, 447, 447–450
  in LPR, 75–76
  in urticaria, 646
  mediators of, in asthma, 447–448
  recruitment and activation of, chemoattractants for, 448
    cytokines for, 448
    in asthma, 448–450, 449
    initial step in, 448, 449
    on site regulation in, 449
    priming in, 450
    rolling adhesion in, 449, 449
Eosinophilic cationic protein, 447
Eosinophilic gastroenteritis, allergic, 673
Eosinophilic gastroenterocolitis, 699–700
Eosinophilic myocarditis, drug-induced, 337
Eosinophilic pneumonitis, due to drug therapy, 336
L-Ephedrine, chemical structure of, 231
Epicoccum, characteristics of, 109t
Epidemiology, 79–88
Epidermolysis bullosa, 659–660
  acquired, 659–660
  atrophic, 659
  dystrophic, 659

Epiglottitis, 439–440, 440
Epilepsy, autonomic, anaphylaxis vs., 309
Epinephrine, chemical structure of, 219
  in acute anaphylaxis, 313–314
Epoxy resin dermatitis, 640
Epstein-Barr virus infection, in X-linked lymphoproliferative syndrome, 26
Erythema multiforme, 658
  due to drug therapy, 337
  urticaria vs., 645
Erythema nodosum, 658
E-selectin, 464
Ethmoid sinus(es), 428
Ethylenediamine dermatitis, 640–641
Exercise challenge testing. See also *Bronchoprovocation challenge(s)*.
  in airway hyperreactivity, 165, 184
  in asthma evaluation, 501
  in exercise-induced anaphylaxis, 378–379
  in exercise-induced asthma, 525, 525t
Exercise-induced anaphylaxis, 376–383
  additional factors in, 377
  cholinergic urticaria vs., 379t, 379–380, 650
  classification of, 379, 379t
  clinical features of, 376–378
  differential diagnosis of, 379–380
  exercise challenge in, 378–379
  exercise-induced asthma vs., 524
  family history in, 378
  food-dependent, 367, 378, 676
  historical, 376
  inconsistent development of, 376–377
  management of, 381–382
  pathophysiology of, 380–381
  premonitory symptoms of, 377
  prevention of, 382
Exercise-induced asthma, 490, 520–528
  asthmatic response in, 520–521
  clinical management of, 524–527
  diagnosis of, 524–526
  differential diagnosis of, 524, 524t
  drug effects in, 523t, 523–524
  epidemiology and diagnosis in, 522–523
  exercise challenge in, 525, 525t
  exercise-induced anaphylaxis vs., 524
  in athletes, 526–527, 527t
  pathophysiology of, 521–522
    initiating stimulus in, 521–522
    modulating factors in, 522
    obstructive response in, 522
    transitional events in, 522
  refractory period in, 521, 521
  severity of attack in, 521
  therapy for, 525–526
Exercise-induced laryngospasm, exercise-induced asthma vs., 525
Exfoliative dermatitis, due to drug therapy, 330, 337–338, 338t
Expiratory reserve volume, 158
Extract(s), choice of, based on pollen and spore prevalence, 93
Eye(s), allergic disorders of, 703–712
  immune response of, 703
  in atopic dermatitis, 707–709, 708
  in contact dermatitis, 709, 709–710
  physical examination of, 138
Eyelid(s), functions of, 703
  in atopic dermatitis, 707–708

Facial nerve paralysis, in otitis media, 422

Fanconi's anemia, immunodeficiency diseases in, 39
Farm animal(s), 117
Feather(s), 117
Feingold diet, 750
Felty's syndrome, 59
Ferret(s), allergen avoidance techniques for, 202
Fever, in drug hypersensitivity, 331–332
Ficus tree(s), 120
Finger(s), clubbing of, in cystic fibrosis, 581–582, 582t
Fire ant immunotherapy, 247–248, 352–353
  dosage schedule for, 247–248, 249t
  optimum duration of therapy for, 248
Fire ant(s), 349
Fire ant venom, 350
Fireplace(s), 205
Fish, allergy to, 670
Fixed drug eruptions, in drug hypersensitivity, 329–330
Flax, 120
Flaxseed, 121
Flour dust, in occupational asthma, 540
Flow-volume curve(s), for pulmonary function, 159, 160–161
  spirograms vs., 161–163, 163
Flower, wind-pollinated, 96, 97
Flunisolide, chemical structure of, 212
  pharmacokinetics of, 213
Flush, anaphylaxis vs., 308–309
Fluticasone propionate, chemical structure of, 212
  pharmacokinetics of, 214
Food additive(s), anaphylactic and anaphylactoid reactions to, 676–677
  asthma in, 371–372
  laboratory studies in, 372–373
  prevalence of, 367–368
  prevention of, 373–374
  treatment of, 372
  types of allergens in, 369t, 370–372
  urticaria and angioedema in, 370–371, 647
  hyperactivity and, 677, 750–751
  pseudoallergic reactions to, 339
Food allergy, 665–686
  anaphylactic and anaphylactoid, 366–375, 675–676
    biphasic, 367
    clinical manifestations of, 366–367
    definition of, 366
    differential diagnosis of, 367
    laboratory studies in, 372–373
    prevalence of, 367–368
    prevention of, 373–374
    protracted, 367
    treatment of, 372, 682
    types of allergens in, 368–370, 369t
    uniphasic, 367
  antigen handling by gastrointestinal tract and, 666–670
  clinical manifestation(s) of, 670–678
    angioedema as, 647, 671
    atopic dermatitis as, 619–620, 670–671
    cutaneous, 670–672
    dermatitis herpetiformis as, 671–672
    gastrointestinal, 672–675
    generalized, 675–677
    respiratory, 675
    urticaria as, 647, 671
  diagnosis of, 678t, 678–680
    algorithm for, 680, 681
    diary for, 678
    double-blind placebo-controlled food challenge in, 679t, 679–680

Food allergy (Continued)
  elimination diets for, 678
  prick skin tests in, 678–679
  RASTs in, 679
  single-blind placebo-controlled food challenge in, 680t
  epidemiology of, 81–82
  family history of atopy and, 82
  food antigens in, 668
  food intolerance vs., 81
  immunotherapy for, clinical trials of, 241–242
  inhalant, 121
  laboratory studies in, 678, 678t
  medical history in, 678
  natural history of, 82, 683
  oral tolerance and, 667–668
  prevalence of, 81–82, 665–666
  prevention of, 683
  skin testing for, 82
  to cow's milk, 668
  to eggs, 668–669
  to fish, 670
  to peanuts, 669
  to shellfish, 670
  to soybeans, 669
  to tree nuts, 669–670
  to wheat, 670
  treatment of, 680–682
    avoidance and, 680–681
    elimination diets for, 680
    for accidental ingestion, 681–682
    for anaphylactic reactions, 682
    immunotherapy, 682
    prophylactic, 682
  unconventional or nonvalidated diagnosis and treatment of, 683
  various disorders associated with, 677–678
Food challenge, double-blind placebo-controlled, 679t, 679–680
  single-blind placebo-controlled, 680t
Food immune complex(es), controversial, 755
Food intolerance, 665
  food allergy vs., 81
Food reaction, adverse, 665
  differential diagnosis of, 666t
Food-induced colitis, 673
Food-induced enterocolitis syndrome, 672–673
Food(s), avoidance of, in atopic dermatitis, 624–625
  fungi in, 112
  in exercise-induced anaphylaxis, 367, 378
  infant atopy and, prophylaxis for, 624
  irritable bowel syndrome and, 677
  migraine and, 677
  solid, allergic disease in infants and, 284
    delayed introduction of, in prevention of allergy in infants, 292
    infantile eczema and, 81, 624
Forced vital capacity, 160, 161–162
Foreign body(ies), in ear, 411
Formaldehyde dermatitis, 639
Formoterol, activity of, 218
  chemical structure of, 219
  clinical effects of, 220
Formula, cow's milk, in prevention of allergy in infants, 286–288, 287t
  elemental amino acid–derived, characteristics of, 291t
  protein hydrolysate, characteristics of, 291t
    for prevention of allergy in infants, 291t, 291–292
  soy, for prevention of allergy in infants, 290–291

Frontal sinus(es), 429
Functional residual capacity, 158
Fungal culture(s), for aeroallergen sampling, 94–96, 96
Fungal infection, in atopic dermatitis, 617
  of skin, 653–654
Fungus(i), 108–113
  allergen avoidance techniques for, 203
  basic characteristics of, 108, 108–109, 109t, 110
  classes of, 110–113
  distribution and clinical relevance of, 111–113
  downy mildew(s), 110
  imperfect, 108, 109t, 110
  in foods, 112
  indoor(s), 111–112
  mushroom(s), 111
  outdoor(s), 111
  puffball(s), 111
  rust(s), 111
  sac, 111
  sensitivity to, clinical significance of, 112–113
  smut(s), 111
  sugar and bread mold(s), 110
Furuncle(s), of ear canal, 412
Fusarium, characteristics of, 109t

Gamma globulin therapy, for antibody deficiency, 51
  for HIV infection in children, 45
  risks of, 51
Gas dilution technique, for lung volume and capacity measurement, 159–160
Gastroenteritis, allergic eosinophilic, 673
Gastroenterocolitis, eosinophilic, 699–700
Gastroesophageal reflux, chronic cough in, 716–717
  in asthma, 490
  in bronchopulmonary dysplasia, 597
Gastrointestinal anaphylaxis, 672
Gastrointestinal tract, antigen handling by, 666–670
  physical examination of, 139
Geotrichum, characteristics of, 109t
Gliocladium, characteristics of, 109t
Glomerular injury, due to drug therapy, 337
Glucocorticoid(s), 211–218
  inhaled, adverse effects of, 217–218
    in asthma, 214–215
  intranasal, adverse effects of, 218
    in rhinitis, 215–217
  mechanism of action of, 212–213, 214
  pharmacokinetics of, 213–214
  relative binding affinity for human lung receptor of, 212, 213t
  topical blanching potency of, in human skin, 212, 213t
Glucose-6-phosphate dehydrogenase deficiency, 37
Glutathione peroxidase deficiency, 37
Glutathione reductase deficiency, 37
Good Start Formula, characteristics of, 291t
Goosefoot order, pollens of, 105–106
Grain dust, in occupational asthma, 540
Granulocyte-macrophage colony–stimulating factor (GM-CSF), eosinophils and, 461
  in asthma, 462
Granulocytopenia, in allergic drug reactions, 335
Granulomatous disease, chronic, 35–36
  clinical findings in, 35
  diagnosis of, 36
  gamma-interferon for, 36
  treatment of, 36

Grass allergen(s), diversity in, 100
  molecular characterization of, 100, 101t
Grass(es), northern and southern, anthesis of, 101, *102*
  pollens of, 99–102
    structure of, 97, *97*, 101–102
    timing of action of, 100–101, *102*
Grass ally(ies), pollens of, 102
Graves' disease, 64–65
Gravity slides and plates, for aeroallergen sampling, 94
Green coffee bean allergy, inhalant, 121
Guinea pig(s), allergen avoidance techniques for, 202
Gustatory rhinitis, 675

Halothane, for anesthesia in asthma and allergy, 745
Hand, foot, mouth syndrome, 656
Hapten(s), 89
  definition of, 321
Hapten-cell reaction(s), in drug hypersensitivity, 325
Hashimoto's thyroiditis, 64–65
Hay fever. See *Rhinitis, allergic, seasonal*.
Headache(s), 719–726
  anxiety, 720
  cluster, 724–725
  cough syncope, 719
  drug therapy in, 722, 723t
  ingestant-related, 725
  mediators of, 719–720
  migraine, 719
  muscle tension, 719
  patient evaluation in, 720–722, 721t
  prophylactic measures in, 722–724, 724t
  sinus, 720
Health care worker(s), transmission of HIV infection to, 41t, 41–42
Hearing loss, in otitis media, 422
Helminthosporium, characteristics of, 109t
Hemangioma(s), subglottic, 439
Hematopoietic growth factor(s), 16
Hemoglobinuria, paroxysmal nocturnal, 39
Hemolytic anemia, in allergic drug reactions, 333–334
    autoimmune, 334
      hapten-cell type, 333–334
      immune-complex type, 334
Hemoptysis, in cystic fibrosis, 582–583, 583t
Hemosiderosis, pulmonary, cow's milk–induced (Heiner's syndrome), 675
Hemp, 120
Henoch-Schönlein purpura, 659
Hepatic reaction(s), to drug therapy, 335t, 335–336
Hepatitis, cholestatic, due to drug therapy, 336
  chronic active, due to drug therapy, 336
  granulomatous, due to drug therapy, 336
  in X-linked agammaglobulinemia, 23
Hepatitis B virus vaccine, adverse reactions to, 389
Herbal product(s), drug sensitivity and, 340
Herpes simplex infection, cutaneous, 654–655
  in atopic dermatitis, 616
Herpes zoster, 655
Histamine, actions of, 302–304, 304t
    on extravascular smooth muscle, 303
    on glandular secretion, 303
    on heart, 303
    on vascular bed, 302–303
  in anaphylaxis, 302–304, 304t
Histamine challenge testing, 175–181
  abbreviated protocol for, 177, 179t
  clinical uses of, 178–180, *180*

Histamine challenge testing *(Continued)*
  current measures of, *175*, 175–176
  dosing schedules for, 177, 178t
  in diagnosis of asthma, 179–180, 501
  in evaluation of asthma therapy, 180, *180*
  methacholine challenge vs., 183–184
  technique(s) for, 176–177
    continuous generation method as, 176
    dosimeter method as, 176–177
History, 135–137
  chief complaint in, 136
  cigarette smoke exposure in, 137
  drug abuse in, 137
  environmental, 137
  family, 137
  of past illness, 136–137
  of present illness, 136
HIV infection, 40–47.
  determination of risk for, 45t
  diagnosis of, 43–45
    counseling for, 44–45
    in adults and children, 43–44
    in infants, 44
  drug hypersensitivity in, 323
  epidemiology of, 40
  in infants vs. adults, 42–43, 42t
  management of, 45, 47
  primary, treatment of, 45, 47
  progression of, and development of AIDS, 42–43
  seroprevalence of, 40
  transmission of, 41
    casual contact and, 42
    in clinical setting, 41t, 41–42
    sexual practices and, 41
    to infants, 42
  viral mutations and, 41
HIV-1, biology of, 40–41
HIV-2, biology of, 40–41
HLA. See also *Human leukocyte antigen(s) (HLAs)*.
HLA-B27, in spondyloarthropathies, 63
HLA-B8, in SLE, 56
HLA-DR1, in rheumatoid arthritis, 59
HLA-DR2, in SLE, 57
HLA-DR4, in rheumatoid arthritis, 59
  in SLE, 57
HLA-DR5, in SLE, 57
Home construction, allergen avoidance techniques and, 203–204
Homeopathy, 757–758
Honeybee venom, 350
House dust mite(s), 115–116, 116t
  allergens of, 116, 116t
  life cycle of, 116
  species of, 115
H_1-receptor antagonist(s), 227–231. See also *Antihistamine(s)*.
Human dander(s), 117–118
Human immunodeficiency virus infection. See *HIV infection*.
Human leukocyte antigen(s) (HLAs). See also *HLA* entries for specific antigens.
  class I, 10, *12*, 55, 56t
  class II, 10–11, *12*, 55, 56t
  class III, 10, 56, 56t
  deficiency in, 29
  diseases associated with, 10t
Hyaline membrane disease, in bronchopulmonary dysplasia, 592–593
Hydration, for atopic dermatitis, 626–627

Hydrocortisone, in IL-4 dependent IgE synthesis, 72
Hydroxyzine, chemical structure of, *228*
Hymenoptera, 349. See also *Insect sting(s)*.
Hymenoptera venom, 350
   testing for, 350
Hyper-IgE recurrent infection syndrome, 155
Hyper-IgE syndrome, 32
   chemotactic defects in, 35
Hyper-IgM, X-linked, 23
Hyperactivity, food additives and, 677, 750–751
Hypertension, pulmonary, in bronchopulmonary dysplasia, 597
Hyperventilation syndrome, exercise-induced asthma vs., 524
Hypogammaglobulinemia, incidence of, 20
Hypogammaglobulinemia of infancy, transient (THI), 26
Hypotension, due to radiocontrast reaction, 357

ICAM-1, 463–464
   in asthma, 464–465
ICAM-2, 463–464
ICAM-3, 463–464
Ichthyosis, in atopic dermatitis, 616
Idiosyncrasy, definition of, 321
IFN-α, immunologic properties of, 14, 15t
IFN-β, immunologic properties of, 14, 15t
IFN-gamma, dysregulation of, in human allergic disease, 74
   for chronic granulomatous disease, 36
   immunologic properties of, 14, 15t
   in asthma, 462–463
   in atopic dermatitis, 622
   in IgE synthesis inhibition, 72–73
IgA, structure and function of, 8, 8t
IgA deficiency, selective, 25–26
   clinical manifestations of, 25
   etiology of, 25–26
   incidence of, 20, 25
IgD, structure and function of, 8t, 9
IgE, allergen-specific. See *IgE antibody*.
   cross-linking of, allergen-induced, 70
   decreased, with immunotherapy, 237, *239*
   interaction with cellular FcERI receptors, 69–70
   interaction with cellular FcERII receptors, 70–71
   structure and function of, 8t, 9
   T cells in regulation of, 9
IgE antibody, in anaphylaxis, 300–301
   in vitro assays for, 150–153
      advantages and disadvantages of, 152–153
      diagnostic value of, 151–152, *152*
      other uses for, 153
      principles of, *150*, 150–151
      quality of results of, 151
      scoring results of, 151
      skin testing vs., 152, 153t
   in vitro determination of, 142
   in vivo determination of, 142
   skin tests for, 144–150. See also *Skin testing*.
   tests for, 144–156
      historical, 144
IgE level determination, total, 142, 153–155
   in allergic bronchopulmonary aspergillosis, 567–568
   in allergic disease, 154
   in asthma, 502
   in cord blood, 154–155
      as predictor of atopy, 283
   in nonallergic disease, 155

IgE level determination *(Continued)*
   in skin test–negative persons, 154, 154t
   methods for measurement of, 153–154, 154t
   two-site immunometric assay for, 153–154
IgE melanoma, 155
IgE receptor(s), high-affinity (FcERI), 70–71
   low-affinity (FcERII or CD23), 70–71
IgE synthesis, cytokine inhibition of, 72t, 72–73
   cytokine modulation of, 72t, 72–73
   regulation of, 71–74
   requirements for induction of, 71
   T-cell cytokine secretion patterns and, 73–74
   T-cell independent induction of, 71–72
   T-cell induction of, 71
   T_{H1}/T_{H2} cells in, 73–74
IgG, allergen-specific, for immunotherapy, 237, *238*
   biology and structure of, 69–71
   in allergic disease, controversial, 754–755
   properties of, 69, 69t
   structure and function of, 8, 8t
IgG deficiency, subclass, 24–25
IgG2 deficiency, polysaccharide antigen response and, 25
IgM, structure and function of, 8t, 8–9
IL-1, immunologic properties of, 14, 15t
IL-2, immunologic properties of, 15t, 16
   recombinant, for cellular immune defects, 52
IL-2 deficiency, in severe combined immunodeficiency, 16
IL-3, eosinophils and, 461
   immunologic properties of, 15t, 16
   in asthma, 462
IL-4, basophils and, 453
   dysregulation of, in human allergic disease, 74
   immunologic properties of, 15t, 16
   in asthma, 462–463
   in atopic dermatitis, 622
   in IgE synthesis, 71
   mast cells and, 451–452, *452*
IL-5, eosinophils and, 461
   immunologic properties of, 15t, 16
   in asthma, 462
   in IgE synthesis, 72
IL-6, immunologic properties of, 15t, 16
   in IgE synthesis, 72
IL-7, immunologic properties of, 15t, 16
IL-8, immunologic properties of, 15t
   in IgE synthesis inhibition, 73
IL-9, immunologic properties of, 15t
IL-10, immunologic properties of, 15t
IL-11, immunologic properties of, 15t
IL-12, immunologic properties of, 15t
   in IgE synthesis inhibition, 73
IL-13, immunologic properties of, 15, 16
IL-14, immunologic properties of, 15t
IL-15, immunologic properties of, 15t
Imidazolidinyl urea dermatitis, 640
Immediate allergic reaction(s), pathophysiology of, 74–76
Immune aggregate(s), anaphylactoid reactions due to, 302
Immune complex(es), as contraindication, in immunotherapy, 245
   food, controversial, 755
   in drug hypersensitivity, 325
   in SLE, 57
Immune response(s), allergic, 68–78. See also *IgE*.
   historical, 68
   diversity of, 14

Immune response(s) *(Continued)*
  normal, 1–19
Immune system evaluation, in otitis media, 417, 418t
Immunization. See *Vaccination.*
Immunoblotting, 90–91
Immunodeficiency disease(s), 20–54
  as contraindication, in immunotherapy, 245
  combined, 30–33
    severe. See *Severe combined immunodeficiency (SCID).*
  common variable. See *Common variable immune deficiency (CVID).*
  congenital, 20–40
    incidence of, 20
  history and physical examination in, 47–48
  in atopic dermatitis, 622
  in otitis media, 418–419, 419t
  infections in, 22
  laboratory evaluation in, 48t, 48–50
  patient evaluation in, 47–50
  primary, classification of, 20, 21t
  therapy in, 50–52
  with cellular immunity defect, 27–30
    evaluation of, 49
    therapy in, 51–52
  with chromosomal abnormalities, 39
  with complement disorders, 38–39
    evaluation of, 49–50
  with humoral immunity defect, 22–24. See also *Antibody* entries.
    evaluation of, 49
    therapy in, 51
  with intracellular adhesion molecule defects, 37–38
  with intracellular killing defects, 35–37
  with metabolic diseases, 39–40
  with nutritional disorders, 39
  with phagocytic disorders, 33–34
    evaluation of, 49–50
  with thymoma, 26–27
Immunoelectrophoresis, 91
Immunogenetic(s), 9–14
Immunoglobulin(s). See also individual types, e.g., *IgA.*
  classes of, 8t, 8–9
  diversity of, 14
  in B-cell differentiation, 3
  in tears, 704
  quantitative, 142
  structure and function of, 7, 7–9
Immunoglobulin gene(s), rearrangements of, 11–13, *13*
  heavy chains and, 12–13
  isotope exclusion in, 12
  kappa light chains and, 12, *13*
  lambda light chains and, 12
Immunologic function, diagnostic testing for, 142–143
Immunomodulator(s), 233–234
  in atopic dermatitis, 629–630
Immunosuppression, drug hypersensitivity in, 323
Immunotherapy, 237–255
  administration of, 245–250
  adverse effects of, 250–251
  allergen extracts for, 239–240
  allergen selection for, 244
  alum-precipitated allergen extract, 249–250
  bacterial vaccines for, clinical trials of, 242
  blocking antibody (allergen-specific IgG) production in, 237, *238*
  clinical applications of, 243–245
  contraindication(s) to, 244–245
    beta blocker treatment as, 244–245
    immune complex and autoimmune disease as, 245

Immunotherapy *(Continued)*
    immunodeficiency as, 245
    non-IgE hypersensitivity conditions as, 245
    pregnancy as, 245
    unstable asthma as, 245
  decrease in IgE with, 237, *239*
  effects of, 237–239
  efficacy of, 240–243
    dose dependency and, 242
    in asthma, 241
    in food allergy, 241–242
    in insect sting anaphylaxis, 241
    in rhinoconjunctivitis, 240–241
    ineffective methods and, 242
  historical, 237
  in asthma, 516
  in atopic dermatitis, 629–630
  in food allergy, 682
  indications for, 243–244, 244t
  inhalant extracts for, 245–247, *247*
    dosage schedule for, 246–247, 247t
    optimum duration of therapy for, 247
    subcutaneous injections for, 245–246
  local nasal, 248
  low-dose, clinical trials of, 242
  mast cell and basophil modulation with, 237–238
  modified aeroallergen extract, 250
  oral aeroallergen, 248
  patient consent form for, 251
  suppressor lymphocyte activity with, 238–239
  venom. See *Venom immunotherapy.*
Impetigo, 656
Inappropriate ADH secretion, in asthma, 512
Inclusion body myositis, 62
Incontinentia pigmenti, 664
Indoor air pollution, 130–131
Indoor allergen(s), asthma and, 118
  sources of, 196, 196t
Indoor environment, 115–119
  control method(s) for, 118–119
    air filtration systems as, 118–119
    benzyl benzoate as, 118
    dust mites and, 118
    pets and, 118
    tannic acid as, 118
Industrial hygiene, 769–778. See also *Occupational asthma, prevention of.*
Infant(s). See also *Children.*
  AIDS in, diagnosis of, 44
    progression of HIV infection to, 42–43
  allergic disease in, cord blood IgE and, 283
    effect of breastfeeding on, 283–284, 286–288, 287t
    effect of ingestants on, 283–284
    effect of solid foods on, 283–284
    family history and, 282–283
    risk factors for, 282, 283t
  at risk for HIV infection, evaluation of, 46t
  atopic dermatitis in, diagnosis of, 614, 641t
    foods and, 624
  atopy in, breast milk and, 284–285
    cord blood IgE and, 283
    inhalants as risk factor for, 285–286
    prediction of, 282–286
  characteristics of, 291t
  HIV infection in, transmission of, 42
  laryngeal and tracheal obstruction, 438–439
  prevention of allergy in, 282–296. See also *Prevention of allergy (in infants).*
Infection(s), in complement deficiency, 22, 38–39

Infection(s) *(Continued)*
  in immunodeficiency disease, 22
Infectious mononucleosis, in X-linked lymphoproliferative syndrome, 26
Inflammatory bowel disease, 687–702. See also *Crohn's disease; Ulcerative colitis.*
  arthritis and, 64
  immunopathogenesis of, 687, *688*, 690–699
  less common types of, 699–700
Inflammatory mediator(s), nonspecific, 14, 16
Inhalation challenge(s). See *Bronchoprovocation challenge(s).*
Inhibition radioimmunoassay(s), 90
Insect allergy. See also *Insect sting(s).*
  epidemiology of, 82–83
  inhalant, 119
  in occupational asthma, 540
Insect sting(s), 348–354. See also *Insect allergy.*
  anaphylaxis due to, 349
    immunotherapy for, clinical trials of, 241
    in pregnancy, 738
  diagnosis of, 350–351
  epidemiology of, 348–349
  etiology of, 349–350
  history in, 350
  immune responses to, 657, 657t
  natural history of, 348–349
  repeated, effect of, on allergy, 82–83
  signs and symptoms of, 349, 349t
  treatment of, 351
  urticaria due to, 647
  venom immunotherapy in, 351–354
Inspiratory reserve volume, 158
Insulin, allergy to, 83
  desensitization to, 344–345
Interferon (IFN). See *IFN* entries.
Interleukin(s). See *IL* entries.
Intestinal graft-vs.-host disease, 699
Intolerance, definition of, 321
Intracellular adhesion molecule(s) (ICAMs), in asthma, 464–465
Intracellular killing, disorders of, 35–37
Intradermal skin test, 147, *147*
  grading system for results of, 148, 148t
Intraoperative agent(s), asthma due to, 553–554
Ipratropium bromide, clinical uses of, 226, *227*
  for allergic rhinitis, 226
  for asthma, 226
  for COPD, 607
  inhaled, adverse effects of, 227
  intranasal, adverse effects of, 227
  pharmacokinetics of, 226
  structure and activity of, 225, *225*
Irritable bowel syndrome, foods and, 677
Isoflurane, for anesthesia in asthma and allergy, 745
Itching. See *Pruritus.*

Jute, 120
Juvenile rheumatoid arthritis, 60, 60t

Kallikrein-kinin system, in anaphylaxis, 304–305, 305t
Kapok, 120
Kartagener syndrome, 34–35, 587–589
  clinical manifestations of, 587
  diagnosis of, 588

Kartagener syndrome *(Continued)*
  management of, 588–589
  pathogenesis of, 587–588
  respiratory manifestations of, 588
Kawasaki disease, 657–658
Keratoconjunctivitis, atopic, 707–708, *708*, 709
  vernal, 710–711
    clinical features of, 710–711, *711*
    immunopathology in, 710
    treatment of, 711
Keratosis pilaris, 661
Kidney, reaction(s) of, to drug therapy, 337
Kinesiology, applied, controversial, 754
Koebner phenomenon, in psoriasis, 662
Kostmann's syndrome, 33–34
Kupffer's cell(s), 4

Labor and delivery, asthma in, 735
Labyrinthitis, 424
Lactation, avoidance diet during, effect of, on infantile atopy, 288–290, 289t–290t
Lambs quarters, pollens of, structure of, 97, *98*
Langerhans' cell(s), epidermal, IgE-bearing, 70
  in atopic dermatitis, 622–623
Laryngeal and tracheal obstruction, 436–441
  clinical assessment of, 436–438
  endoscopy for, 438
  management of, 438–441
    in adults, 440–441
    in neonates, 438–439
    in older children, 439–440
  radiologic examination in, 437–438
  symptoms and signs of, 436–437, 437t
  traumatic, 440
    external, 440
    internal, 440
Laryngeal stridor, in pregnancy, 737
Laryngeal tumor(s), 441
Laryngomalacia, in neonates, 438
Laryngopathia gravidarum, 737
Laryngospasm, exercise-induced, exercise-induced asthma vs., 525
Laryngotracheobronchitis, acute (croup), 440
  spasmodic, 440
Larynx, congenital abnormalities of, 439
  vascular anomalies of, 439
Late phase response (LPR), 68
  cytokines in, 75
  in chronic allergic disease, 75
  local accumulation of inflammatory cells in, 75
  pathophysiology of, 74–76
Latex, 119–120, 361–364
  adverse reactions to, 362–364
    clinical presentation of, 362
    diagnostic tests in, 362–363
    historical, 361
    management of, 363–364
    risk factors in, 362, 362t
  antigens of, 361–362
  asthma due to, 553–554
  common sources of, 363t, 364
  contact dermatitis due to, 640
Leukocyte adhesion molecule defect(s), 37–38
Leukocyte function antigen-1 (LFA-1, CD11a/CD18) deficiency, 37, 39
Leukoderma, 664
Levocabastine, chemical structure of, *228*

LFA-1 (leukocyte function antigen–1, CD11a/CD18) deficiency, 37, 39
Lidocaine, for anesthesia in asthma and allergy, 745
Liliopsida, 99, *100*, 102
Linear IgA bullous disease of childhood, 658–659
Linseed, 121
Liver. See *Hepatic, Hepatitis* entries.
Loratadine, chemical structure of, *228*
Lower respiratory disease, chest radiography for, 140–141
 determination of nonspecific bronchial hyperresponsiveness for, 141
 diagnostic testing for, 140–141
 pulmonary function evaluation for, 141
 sputum cytology for, 140
 sweat test for, 141
Lower respiratory reaction(s), in food allergy, 675
LPR. See *Late phase response (LPR)*.
Lung capacity, definition of, 157–158, *158*
 measurement of, *158*, 158–160
Lung transplantation, in COPD, 609–610
 in cystic fibrosis, 586–587
Lung volume(s), definition of, 157–158, *158*
 in COPD, 604
 measurement of, *158*, 158–160
Lupus. See *Systemic lupus erythematosus (SLE)*.
Lupus syndrome, drug-induced, 58, 58t
Lyme disease, 657
Lymphocyte count, in evaluation of immunodeficiency disease, 49
Lymphocyte(s), 2–4
 B. See *B cell(s)*.
 cytokine activators of, 16
 function of, 5–7
 in asthma, 454–456
 large granular (LGL), functions of, 4
 T. See *T cell(s)*.
Lymphoid interstitial pneumonia, in AIDS in children, 43
Lymphoid stem cell(s), lineage of, 2
Lymphoproliferative syndrome, X-linked, 26
Lymphotoxin. See *TNF-β (lymphotoxin)*.
Lysozyme, in tears, 704

Macrophage(s), 4
 in asthma, 457
Magnetic resonance imaging, in laryngeal and tracheal obstruction, 438
 in sinusitis, 432
Magnoliopsida, 99, *101*
Major basic protein, eosinophilic, 447
Major histocompatibility complex (MHC), 55–56. See also *Human leukocyte antigen(s) (HLAs)*.
 disease associations and, 9, 10t
 in antigen presentation, 2, 3, 5, 55–56, *56*
 molecular map of, *11*
Malabsorption syndromes, 699–700
Maple(s), pollens of, 104
Mast cell degranulation. See also *Histamine*.
 in anaphylaxis, 302–305, 303t
 inflammatory pathways activated by, 302
 pathophysiologic events due to, 302
Mast cell(s), allergen-induced cross-linking of IgE and, 70
 cytokines and, 451–452
 functions of, 4–5
 in asthma, *450*, 450–451

Mast cell(s) *(Continued)*
 inflammatory mediators of, 451
 modulation of, with immunotherapy, 237–238
Mastoid, tumors of, 423
Mastoiditis, in otitis media, 422
Maxillary sinus(es), 428
Mayfly, 119
Measles B virus vaccine, live, adverse reactions to, 389
Mechanical ventilation, in bronchopulmonary dysplasia, 594–595, 595t
Meconium ileus, in cystic fibrosis, 578
Mediator antagonist(s), 233
Melanoma, IgE, 155
Membrane attack complex (MAC), 17, *18*
Meniere's disease, 423
Meningitis, in otitis media, 422–423
Meningoencephalitis, chronic, in X-linked agammaglobulinemia, 23
Mental health care provider(s), in asthma, 262
Metabolic disease, immunodeficiency diseases in, 39–40
Metal fume fever, in occupational asthma, 543
Metallic salt(s), in occupational asthma, 542–543
Metaproterenol, chemical structure of, *219*
Metazoan parasitic infection(s), total serum IgE in, 155
Methacholine challenge testing, 175–181
 baseline airway caliber and, 177, *177*
 clinical uses of, 178–180, *180*
 current measures of, *175*, 175–176
 dosing schedules for, 177, 178t
 histamine challenge vs., 183–184
 in diagnosis of asthma, 179–180, 501
 in evaluation of asthma therapy, 180, *180*
 in young children, 177–178, *179*
 technique(s) for, 176–177
  continuous generation method as, 176
  dosimeter method as, 176–177
 truncated protocol for, 177, 178t
Methylxanthine(s), 223–225
 adverse effects of, 225
 clinical effects of, 224
 mechanism of action of, 224
 pharmacokinetics of, 225
 structure and activity of, *223*, 223–224
Mice, pet, allergen avoidance techniques for, 202
 wild, allergen avoidance techniques for, 202
Microbial detergent enzyme(s), in occupational asthma, 541
Microglia, 4
Midge(s), chronomid, 119
Migraine headache, 719
 foods and, 677
 prophylaxis for, 722–724, 724t
 treatment of, 722
Mildew(s), downy, 110
Miliaria, 661
Milk, allergy to, 668
 breast. See *Breast milk*.
 in infantile eczema, 81
 pulmonary hemosiderosis (Heiner's syndrome) due to, 675
Mixed connective tissue disease, 61
Mold(s), allergen avoidance techniques for, 203
 as risk factor, in infantile atopy, 285
 bread, 110
 sugar, 110
Molluscum contagiosum, 656
Monocyte(s), 4
Mononuclear phagocyte(s), development of, 4
Mononucleosis, infectious, in X-linked lymphoproliferative syndrome, 26

Monosodium glutamate, ingestion of, anaphylaxis vs., 309
  sensitivity to, 677
Moth(s), 119
Mouth, physical examination of, 138
Mucous plugging, in asthma, 485
Mucus, nasal, 398–399
Munchausen's stridor, anaphylaxis vs., 309
Muscle relaxant(s), asthma due to, 553–554
Muscle tension headache, 719
Musculoskeletal system, physical examination of, 139
Mushroom(s), 111
Myasthenia gravis, 65
Myeloid stem cell(s), lineage of, 4–5
Myeloperoxidase deficiency, 36–37
Myocarditis, eosinophilic, drug-induced, 337
Myopathy, inflammatory, 62–63
  clinical manifestations of, 62
  etiology and pathogenesis of, 62
  treatment of, 62–63
Myositis, 62–63

Nasal anatomy, 393–399
  developmental, disorders of, 394, 394t
    embryonic, 393–394
  external, 394
  innervation, 397
    nonadrenergic, noncholinergic, 397
    parasympathetic, 397
    sensory, 397
    sympathetic, 397
  mucosal, 397–398
    basal cells of, 398
    ciliated epithelium of, 398
    columnar cells of, 398
    goblet cells of, 398
    lamina propria of, 398
    mucociliary action of, 399
  vascular, 395–397, *396*
Nasal cavity, anatomy of, 394–395, *395–396*
  meatus in, 395
  nasal valves in, 394
  septum in, 395
  turbinates in, 395
Nasal cytology, 139–140, 403
  in asthma, 501–502
Nasal disease, 401–404. See also *Rhinitis*.
  classification of, 402–403
  diagnosis of, 403–404
    allergy testing for, 403
    fiberoptic rhinoscopy for, 403–404
    nasal cytology for, 403
  differential diagnosis of, 402, 402t
  history of, 401–402
  physical examination in, 402
Nasal function, 399–401
  air conditioning as, 400
  airflow as, 399–400
  olfaction as, 399
Nasal gland(s), 398
  anterior, 398
  seromucous, 398
Nasal mucosal immunity, 401
Nasal mucus, 398–399
Nasal polyp(s), 409–410
  in cystic fibrosis, 580
  in pregnancy, 736t, 737t

Nasal polyp(s) *(Continued)*
  management of, 410
  pathogenesis of, 409–410
Nasal protective reflex(es), 400–401
Nasal provocation study(ies), in otitis media, 414
Nasal valve(s), 394
Nausea, due to radiocontrast reaction, 357
Nedocromil sodium, 208–211
  adverse effects of, 211
  chemical structure of, 208, *208*
  in allergic rhinitis, 210–211
  in asthma, 210, 514
  mechanism of action of, 208–210
  pharmacokinetics of, 210
Neomycin sensitivity dermatitis, 635, 640
Neonate(s). See *Infant(s)*.
Nephritis, interstitial, due to drug therapy, 337
Nettle(s), pollens of, 102–103, 105
Neurologic system, physical examination of, 139
Neutralization therapy, controversial, 757
Neutropenia, congenital, 33–34
  cyclic, 34
Neutrophil(s), chemotaxis of, abnormalities of, 34
  in asthma, 456–457
  migration of, abnormalities of, 34
  polymorphonuclear, functions of, 4
Nezelof's syndrome (T-cell dysfunction with immunoglobulins), 29
Nickel dermatitis, 638–639, *639*
Nitrogen dioxide, 126–127
  controlled laboratory studies on, 126–127
  epidemiologic studies on, 127
Non-IgE hypersensitivity, as contraindication, in immunotherapy, 245
Nonallergic disease, total serum IgE in, 155
Nonorthodox medicine(s), drug sensitivity and, 340
Nose. See also *Nasal* entries.
  physical examination of, 138
NSAID(s), 550t
  anaphylactoid reactions due to, 301–302
  asthma and. See *ASA/NSAID-induced asthma*.
  pseudoallergic reactions to, 338–339
Nummular eczema, 661
Nutramigen, characteristics of, 291t
Nutritional disorder(s), immunodeficiency diseases in, 39

Occupational asthma, 529–548
  cause(s) of, complement activation in, 536
    high-molecular weight, 531–532, 533t
    low-molecular weight, 532, 534t–535t, 535
    nonimmunologic toxins or irritants as, 535–536
    pharmacologic, 536
  classification of, 531, 532t
  clinical approach to diagnosis of, 537–540
    algorithm for, 538, *539*
    environmental/employment history in, 538
    history in, 537–538
    immunologic studies in, 539–540
    inhalation challenge test in, 538–539
    preexisting pulmonary conditions in, 538
    serum-specific IgE assays in, 540
  definition of, 530
  epidemiology in, 536–537
  historical, 529
  latency period and, 530
  mechanisms of, 531–536

Occupational asthma *(Continued)*
    airborne agents in, 769, *769*
    pathologic findings in, 530–531
    pathophysiology of, 530–531, *531*
    prevalence of, 529–530
    prevention of, 544
        administrative control for, 775
        air cleaning devices for, 771
        assessment and outlook for, 772
        biologic monitoring for, 774–775
        control at source for, 770–772
        dust suppression in, 775
        elimination of process or materials for, 771
        enclosure for, 771
        engineering methods for, 770–772
        housekeeping and, 775
        industrial hygiene for, 769–778
        industrial ventilation for, 770–771, *771*
        isolation for exposure reduction for, 771
        monitoring airborne concentrations for, 772–774
            goals of, 772
            methods for, 772–774, *773*
        personal protective equipment for, 775–777
        process modification for, 771
        respiratory protective equipment for, 775–776, *776*, 776t
        skin protection for, 777
        substitution of materials for, 771
        summary of measures for, 770, 770t
        work practices for, 772
        worker education for, 775
        workplace management for, 775
    risk factors in, 536–537
    specific cause(s) of, 540–543
        acid anhydrides as, 541–542
        animal sources as, 540
        colophony fumes as, 543
        diisocyanates as, 541
        flour dust as, 540
        food processing as, 540–541
        grain dust as, 540
        high-molecular weight agents as, 540–541
        insect sources as, 540
        latex products as, 540
        low-molecular weight agents as, 541–543
        metallic salts as, 542–543
        microbial contaminates of wood dust as, 542
        microbial detergent enzymes as, 541
        plant sources as, 540
        vegetable gums as, 541
        western red cedar wood dust as, 542
        wood dusts as, 542
    treatment of, 543–544
Occupational exposure(s), in contact dermatitis, 635, 635t
    in COPD, 602
Office construction, allergen avoidance techniques and, 203–204
Olfaction, 397, 399. See also *Nasal* entries.
Olive(s), pollens of, 104–105
Omenn's syndrome, 30
Opiate(s), for anesthesia in asthma and allergy, 745
Opsonization, 17
Oral allergy syndrome (OAS), 367, 671, 682
Oral tolerance, development of, 667–668
Organic toxic dust syndrome, 564
Orotic aciduria, type I hereditary, immunodeficiency in, 40
Orris root, 120

Otitis externa, 411–412
    causes of, 411
    circumscribed, 412
    malignant, 412
    treatment of, 411–412
Otitis media, 412–423
    acute, 412
        treatment of, 420
    chronic suppurative, 412
    classification of, 412
    complication(s) of, 422–423
        cholesteatoma as, 422
        facial nerve paralysis as, 422
        hearing loss as, 422
        mastoiditis as, 422
        meningitis as, 422–423
        tympanic membrane perforation as, 422
        tympanosclerosis as, 422
    diagnosis of, 416–419
    history in, 416
    immune system evaluation in, 417, 418t
    immunodeficiency testing in, 418–419, 419t
    in vivo and in vitro allergy tests in, 417, 418t
    laboratory studies in, 417–419, 418t–419t
    pathogenesis of, 412
    pathophysiology of, 413–416, *415*
        H. influenzae in, 414
        M. catarrhalis in, 414
        S. pneumoniae in, 415
        allergy in, 414
        bacteria in, 414–415, *415*
        eustachian tube dysfunction in, 413–414
        immune system dysfunction in, 415–416
        nasal provocation studies in, 414
        viral infection in, 414
    physical examination in, 416–417
        audiometry in, 417
        pneumatic otoscopy in, *416*, 416–417, 417t
        tympanometry in, 417
    prevalence of, 412–413
    recurrent acute, treatment of, 421
    social impact of, 413
    with effusion, 412
        treatment of, 421–422
Otosclerosis, 423
Otoscopy, pneumatic, in otitis media, *416*, 416–417, 417t
Oxygen therapy, for COPD, 608–609
Ozone, 127–129
    controlled laboratory studies on, 128–129
    epidemiologic studies on, 129

Pancuronium, for anesthesia in asthma and allergy, 745
Papain, allergy to, 83
Papillomatosis, respiratory, recurrent, 439
Papular urticaria, 657
Parabens, asthma due to, 556
Paranasal sinus(es), development, structure, function of, *428*, 428–429
    ethmoid, 428
    frontal, 429
    maxillary, 428
Paraphenylenediamine dermatitis, 640
Parasitic infection(s), metazoan, total serum IgE in, 155
Paroxysmal nocturnal hemoglobinuria, 39
Particulate matter (PM_{10}), in air pollution, 129–130
    controlled laboratory studies on, 129

Particulate matter (PM$_{10}$) *(Continued)*
   epidemiologic studies on, 129
Patch test, in atopic dermatitis, 620–622
   in contact dermatitis, 634, 635t, 637–641. See also *Contact dermatitis, patch testing in.*
   in drug allergy, 343
Patient education, in asthma, 268–281
   clarifying expectations in, 270
   creating partnership for, 268–269
   developing treatment plan together for, 270
   five Rs of teaching in, 269–278
   integrating education into medical practice, 278–279
   negotiating details in, 270–271
   patient record for, 279, *280*
   providing written plan for, 271, *272–273*
   reaching agreement on goals in, 269–271
   rehearsing asthma management skills in, 273–274
   reinforcing appropriate behavior in, 274–276, *276–277*
   repeating messages in, 274
   resources for, 279
   reviewing in, 276, 278
Patient evaluation, 135–143
   diagnostic testing in, 139t, 139–143
      for immunologic function, 142–143
      for lower airway disease, 140–141
      for suggestive and specific allergy, 141
      for upper airway disease, 139–140
   history in, 135–137. See also *History.*
   physical examination in, 137–139. See also *Physical examination.*
   prior to skin testing, 145
Peak expiratory flow, 160
   testing for, 141
Peak-flow monitoring, home, in asthma, 504–505
Peanut(s), allergy to, 669
Penicillin allergy, atopy and, 83
   desensitization in, 344, 344t
   epidemiology of, 83
   management of, 342–343
   prevalence of, 83
Penicillium, characteristics of, 109t
Pentamidine, asthma due to, 555–556
Pertussis vaccine, adverse reactions to, 389
Pet(s), allergen avoidance techniques for, 200–202
   exposure to, control methods for, 118
   in asthma, 504
Phagocyte(s), deficiency of, infections in, 22
   mononuclear, development of, 4
Phagocytic disorder(s), 33–34, 34t
   evaluation of, 49–50
   of chemotaxis, 34
   of migration, 34
   of production, 33–34
Pharmacology and therapeutics, 208–236. See also individual drugs; *Drug therapy.*
Phenylephrine, chemical structure of, *231*
Phenylpropanolamine, chemical structure of, *231*
Phoma, characteristics of, 109t
Photodermatitis, in drug hypersensitivity, 329, 329t
Phototherapy, in atopic dermatitis, 630
Physical examination, 137–139
   cardiovascular system in, 139
   chest in, 138–139
   cutaneous, 138
   ears in, 138
   eyes in, 138
   gastrointestinal system in, 139

Physical examination *(Continued)*
   mouth in, 138
   musculoskeletal system in, 139
   neurologic system in, 139
   nose in, 138
Pigmentary disorder(s), 663–664
   in atopic dermatitis, 615, *615*
Pinophyta, *99*, 99
Pityriasis alba, 664
Pityriasis rosea, 662
Plant dermatitis, 641, *641*
Plantain(s), pollens of, 107
Plasma cell, development of, 3
Platelet-activating factor, in asthma, 460–461
Platinum salt(s), in occupational asthma, 542–543
Plethysmography, body, for lung volume and capacity measurement, 160
Pneumomediastinum, in asthma, 511–512, *511–512*
Pneumonia, *Pneumocystis carinii*, in AIDS in children, 43
   treatment of, 45
   lymphoid interstitial, in AIDS in children, 43
Pneumonitis, eosinophilic, due to drug therapy, 336
   hypersensitivity, 559–565
      acute, 562
      causative agents in, 560, 560t
      chest radiography in, 563, *563*
      chronic, 562–563
      clinical features of, 561–563, *562–563*
      diagnosis in, 563–564
      differential diagnosis of, 564
      etiology of, 560t, 560–561
      historical, 559–560
      laboratory tests in, 562
      pathogenesis of, 561
      prognosis in, 565
      pulmonary function testing in, 562
      therapy in, 565
Pneumothorax, in asthma, 511–512, *512*
   in cystic fibrosis, 584–585
Poaceae, 99, *100*
Poison ivy dermatitis, 641, *641*
Poliovirus infection, in X-linked agammaglobulinemia, 23
Poliovirus vaccine, adverse reactions to, 389
   in X-linked agammaglobulinemia, 23
Pollen(s), 97–108
   allergen avoidance techniques for, 202–203
   basic characteristics of, 97–98
   classification of, botanical taxonomy in, 99, *99–101*
      traditional, 98
   distribution of, 107
   in reproductive biology, *96–97*, 97
   of asters, 106–107
   of beeches, 104
   of conifers, 102
   of goosefoot order, 105–106
   of grass allies, 102
   of grasses, 99–102
      structure of, *97*, 97, 101–102
      timing of pollination of, 100–101, *102*
   of lambs quarters, structure of, 97, *98*
   of maples, 104
   of nettles, 102–103, 105
   of olives, 104–105
   of plantains, 107
   of ragweed, 106–107
   of short ragweed, structure of, 97, *98*
   of trees, 102–105
   of walnuts, 104

Pollen(s) *(Continued)*
   of weeds, *105*, 105–107
   of willows, 103–104
   prevalence of, aeroallergen sampling for, 93–96
     extracts and, 93
   reducing exposure to, 107–108
     indoors, 107
     outdoors, 107
     refuge option for, 107–108
   sources and similarities of, 98–107
   structure of, 97–98, *97–98*
Pollen count(s), 94
Pollution, air. See *Air pollution*.
Polymorphonuclear neutrophil(s), functions of, 4
Polymyositis, 62–63
Polyp, nasal. See *Nasal polyp(s)*.
Pooideae, 99
Postmenopausal flush, anaphylaxis vs., 308
Postnasal drip, in pregnancy, 736t, 737t
Postnasal drip syndrome, 716
Postprandial syndrome(s), anaphylaxis vs., 309
Preeclampsia, anaphylaxis vs., 737
Pregnancy, 727–742
   allergic conditions in, 728–741
     immunologic management of, 728–729
     pharmacologic management of, 729–731, 730t–731t
     psychologic support for, 728
   anaphylaxis in, 737–738
     differential diagnosis of, 737
     effect of, on pregnancy outcome, 737
     prevention and treatment of, 737–738
     protocol for, 739t
   as contraindication, in immunotherapy, 245
   asthma in, 516, 731t, 731–735, 733t–734t
     acute, management of, 734t, 734–735
     chronic, management of, 732–734, 733t
     differential diagnosis of, 731
     effects of, on pregnancy outcome, 731–732
     labor and delivery and, 735
     pregnancy effects on, 732, 733t
     surgery in, 747
   atopic dermatitis in, 740–741
   avoidance diet during, effect of, on infantile atopy, 288, 289t–290t
   drug allergy in, 741
   fetal oxygenation in, 727–728
   immunologic changes in, 728, 728t
   maternal pulmonary physiology in, 727
   rhinitis in, 735–736, 736t
   sinusitis in, 735–736
   urticaria and angioedema in, 738–740
     diagnosis of, 738–739
     prevention and treatment of, 740
Preservative dermatitis, 641
Prevention of allergy (in infants), 282–296
   avoidance of both ingested and inhaled allergens in, 293
   breastfeeding vs. cow's milk formula feeding in, 286–288, 287t
   combined maternal and infant avoidance of allergenic foods and, 292–293
   delayed introduction of solid foods for, 292
   maternal avoidance diets during lactation and, 288–290, 289t–290t
   maternal avoidance diets during pregnancy and, 288, 289t–290t
   prediction of atopy in, 282–286
   protein hydrolysate formula for, 291t, 291–292
   recommendations for, 293, 294t

Prevention of allergy (in infants) *(Continued)*
   soy formula for, 290–291
Prick skin test, 146, *146*
Progesterone-related anaphylaxis, 310
Propofol, asthma due to, 554
Protamine, side effects of, 324
Protein hydrolysate formula, characteristics of, 291t
   for prevention of allergy in infants, 291t, 291–292
Protozoal infection(s), in immunodeficiency disease, 22
Provocation-neutralization testing, controversial, 753
Prurigo nodularis, in atopic dermatitis, 615, *615*
Pruritus, in atopic dermatitis, control of, 626
   urticaria vs., 645, 645t
Pseudoanaphylaxis, 310
D-Pseudoephedrine, chemical structure of, *231*
Psoriasis, 662–663
   guttate, 662
   Koebner phenomenon in, 662
   treatment of, 662–663
Psoriatic arthritis, 64
Psychological referral, for asthma, 262–265
   assessment in, 263
   cognitive/behavioral therapy in, 264
   family therapy in, 264–265
   pharmacotherapy in, 263–264
   treatment in, 263–265
Psychosocial factor(s), in asthma, 256–267
   anxiety and, 257–258
   anxiety disorders and, 260
   childhood depression and, 261
   co-morbidity of, 260–261
   daily functioning in, 257
   depression and, 260–261
   emotional triggers in, 256–267
   interfering with disease management, 259–260
   mental health care providers and, 262
   predicting death, 259, 259t
   problems for physician in, 261–265
   psychological development and, 257–258
   psychological referral for, 262–265
   questions suggesting potential problems in, 261, 261t
   social support in, 258–259
   suicidal ideation and, 261, 262t
Psychosocial issue(s), in asthma, 518
Psyllium, 120–121
   p-tert-butyphenol, contact dermatitis due to, 640
Puffball(s), 111
Pulmonary disease, interstitial, pulmonary function testing in, 167t
   obstructive, pulmonary function testing in, 164, *165*
   restrictive, pulmonary function testing in, 164, *165*
Pulmonary function testing, 157–172
   as aid in diagnosis, 164–166, *165*
   caveats in, 169–170
   clinical applications of, 157, 157t
   definitions of lung volumes and capacities in, 157–158, *158*
   dynamic changes with age in, 169
   equipment for, 170, 171t, *172*
   flow rates in, *158–159*, 160–161, *161–162*
   for following disease course, 168–169
   in antigen challenge, 166–167, *167*
   in asthma, 167t, 400–501
   in children, 171t
   in COPD, 603–604
   in cystic fibrosis, 167t
   in emphysema, 167t
   in evaluation of asthma precipitants, 166–168, *167*

Pulmonary function testing *(Continued)*
  in evaluation of therapy, 168, *168*
  in hypersensitivity pneumonitis, 562
  in infants and small children, 170
  in interstitial lung disease, 167t
  in lower airway disease, 141
  in obstructive lung disease, 164
  in restrictive lung disease, 164
  in reversible airway obstruction, 164–166, *165*
  in vocal cord dysfunction, 167t
  indications for, 164–169
  limitations of, 157, 157t
  measurements of lung volumes and capacities in, *158–159*, 158–160
  other tests for, 163–164
  patient cooperation in, 169–170
  personnel and environment for, 170–171
  spirograms vs. flow-volume curves in, *159*, 161–163, *163*
  terminology and technique for, 157–164
  wide range of normal values in, 169
Pulmonary hemosiderosis, cow's milk–induced (Heiner's syndrome), 675
Pulmonary hypertension, in bronchopulmonary dysplasia, 597
Pulmonary reaction(s), to drug therapy, 336t, 336–337
  fibrotic, 336–337
  infiltrative, 336, 336t
Pulse test, controversial, 753
Puncture skin test, 146, *146*
Purine nucleoside phosphorylase deficiency, 29–30
Purpura, allergic, due to drug therapy, 338
Pyoderma, 656
Pyrethrum, 120

Quarternium 15 dermatitis, 639

Rabbit(s), pet, allergen avoidance techniques for, 202
Radiocontrast media, 355–358
  adverse reactions to, 355–356
    anaphylactoid, 355, 357–358
      prevention of, 358
      treatment of, 357–358
    chemotoxic, 355–356, 356t
      treatment of, 358
    classification of, 355–356, 356t
    prevalence of, 356
    prevention of, 358
    risk factors in, 356, 356t
    treatment of, 356–358, 357t
      in anaphylactoid reactions, 357–358
      in bronchospasm, 357
      in cardiovascular collapse, 358
      in hypotension, 357
      in nausea and vomiting, 357
      in seizures, 358
      in urticaria, 357
      in vasovagal reactions, 358
  asthma due to, 555
  frequency of, 355
  hyperosmolar, allergy to, 83
  pseudoallergic reactions to, 339
Radiography, chest, in allergic bronchopulmonary aspergillosis, *568*, 568–569
  in asthma, 502

Radiography *(Continued)*
  in COPD, 603
  in hypersensitivity pneumonitis, 563, *563*
  in laryngeal and tracheal obstruction, 437–438
  in lower airway disease, 140–141
  sinus, in upper respiratory disease, 140
Radioimmunoassay(s), inhibition, 90
Ragweed, false, 106
  giant, 106
    as wind-pollinated species, 97, *97*
    pollens of, 106–107
  short, 106
    pollens of, 97, *98*
  western, 106
Rat(s), pet, allergen avoidance techniques for, 202
  wild, allergen avoidance techniques for, 202
Reactive airways dysfunction syndrome, 530
Reiter's syndrome, 64
Renal reaction(s), to drug therapy, 337
Reserpine, side effects of, 324
Residual volume, 158
Respiratory failure, in asthma, 510
Respiratory infection, asthma and, 478–479
Respiratory obstruction, in anaphylaxis, 299
Respiratory papillomatosis, recurrent, 439
Reticular dysgenesis, 30
Retinal detachment, in atopic dermatitis, 708–709
Retrovirus(es), biology of, 40–41
Rheumatic disease, MHC class I and II alleles in, 56t
Rheumatoid arthritis, 59–60
  ARA criteria for diagnosis of, 59, 59t
  clinical manifestations of, 59
  complement deficiency in, 38
  etiology and pathogenesis of, 59
  juvenile, 60, 60t
  treatment of, 59–60, 60t
Rheumatoid factor, 59
Rhinitis, acute vs. chronic, 402
  allergic, 404–407
    antihistamines for, 406
    approach to management of, 405, *406*
    avoidance for, 405–406
    complications of, 80
    corticosteroids for, 406–407
    cromolyn for, 210–211, 406
    decongestants for, 406
    epidemiology of, 79–80, 405
    IgE-mediated LPR in, 75
    immunotherapy for, 407
    in asthma, 490
    in pregnancy, 736t, 737t
    intranasal glucocorticoids for, 215–217
    ipratropium bromide for, 226, *227*
    natural history of, 80
    nedocromil sodium for, 210–211
    nonallergic vs., 403
    pathophysiology of, 404–405
    perennial, epidemiology of, 80
    prevalence of, 80
    seasonal, epidemiology of, 80
      prevalence of, 80
      vs. perennial, 405
    surgery for, 407
    treatment of, 405–407
    vasomotor, in pregnancy, 736t, 737t
  chronic, 402–403
  differential diagnosis of, 402, 402t
  eosinophilic nonallergic, in pregnancy, 736t, 737t
  gustatory, 675

Rhinitis *(Continued)*
  in pregnancy, 735–736, 736t
  nonallergic, 407–409
    differential diagnosis of, 407–408, 408t
    management of, 409
    pathophysiology of, 408–409
    signs and symptoms of, 408
Rhinitis medicamentosa, in pregnancy, 736t, 737t
Rhinoconjunctivitis, allergic, 706–707, *707*
  antihistamines for, 230, 707
  immunotherapy for, clinical trials of, 240–241
Rhinoscopy, fiberoptic, 140, 403–404
  in sinusitis, 431
Rhinosinusitis, bacterial, in pregnancy, 736t, 737t
Rhodotorula, characteristics of, 109t
Rodent(s), 117
  pet, allergen avoidance techniques for, 202
Rubber antigen sensitivity, 640
Rubella virus vaccine, live, adverse reactions to, 389
Rust(s), 111

Saline, ultrasonic, for bronchoprovocation challenge, 182–183
Salmeterol, activity of, 218
  chemical structure of, *219*
  clinical effects of, 220–223, *221–222*
Scabies, 657
  urticaria vs., 645
Scalded skin syndrome, staphylococcal, 331
Schools and allergies, 761–768
  allergic emergencies and, 761–762
  conditions affecting learning and, 762–763
  limitation on activity participation and, 762, 763t
  management guidelines for, 766t–767t
  physician communication and, 763, 768
  resource materials for, 768t
  school health risks and, 763
  student asthma action card for, 763, *764–765*
SCID. See *Severe combined immunodeficiency (SCID)*.
Scleroderma, 61
Scombroidosis, anaphylaxis vs., 309
Seasonal rhinitis. See *Rhinitis, allergic, seasonal.*
Seizure(s), due to radiocontrast reaction, 358
Serum sickness, 325–326
  due to drug therapy, 327–328
Severe combined immunodeficiency (SCID), 27
  adenosine deaminase deficiency in, 28
  autosomal recessive, 27–28
  cellular immunodeficiency with immunoglobulins in, 29
  defective expression of MHC antigens in, 29
  IL-2 deficiency in, 16
  incidence of, 20
  Omenn's syndrome in, 30
  purine nucleoside phosphorylase deficiency in, 29–30
  reticular dysgenesis in, 30
  T-cell receptor deficiency in, 29
  therapy for, 52
  X-linked, 27–28
Shellfish, allergy to, 670
Short bowel syndrome, 699
Sick building syndrome, 130–131, 564
Silk, 120
Silo filler's disease, 564
Sinus headache, 720
Sinus radiography, 140
Sinus(es), paranasal, development, structure, function of, *428*, 428–429

Sinusitis, 428–435
  asthma and, 434
  chronic, in cystic fibrosis, 580
  CT in, 432
  diagnosis of, 431–432
  epidemiology of, 428
  fiberoptic rhinoscopy in, 431
  history in, 431
  imaging studies in, 431–432
  in asthma, 490
  in pregnancy, 735–736
  laboratory tests in, 431
  microbiology in, 430
  MRI in, 432
  pathogenesis of, 429t, 429–430
    immune defects in, 430
    mucociliary function in, 429–430
    ostial patency in, 429
    predisposing factors in, 429, 429t
    secretory mucus blanket in, 430
  physical examination in, 431
  sinus aspiration in, 432
  transillumination in, 431
  treatment of, 432–434
    ancillary, 433
    immunologic disease and, 433
    medical, 432–433
    surgical, 434
  ultrasonography in, 432
Sisal, 120
Sjögren's syndrome, 60–61
  clinical manifestations of, 61
  etiology and pathogenesis of, 61
  treatment of, 61
Skin, physical examination of, 138
Skin end-point titration, controversial, 752–753
Skin infection, in atopic dermatitis, 616–617
  bacterial, 616–617
  fungal, 617
  viral, 616
Skin rash(es), in drug hypersensitivity, 330
Skin testing, 144–150
  advantages and disadvantages of, 152–153
  allergen extracts for, 148–149
  contraindications to, 145
  diagnostic value of, 149
  epicutaneous, *146*, 146–147
  epidemiology of, 81
  ideal, 145
  in allergic bronchopulmonary aspergillosis, 567
  in atopic dermatitis, 620
  in cystic fibrosis, 579–580
  in food allergy, 82, 678–679
  in insect sting allergy, 350–351
  in local anesthetic reactions, 360, 360t
  in vaccination sensitivity, in egg-sensitive patients, 387–388
  in vitro assays for IgE antibody vs., 152, 153t
  intradermal, 147, *147*
  number needed for patient evaluation in, 149–150
  patient evaluation prior to, 145
  percutaneous, *146*, 146–147
  physiology of, 144–145
  positive and negative controls for, 147
  prick test for, 146, *146*
  puncture test for, 146, *146*
  quality control of, 149
  recording and scoring results of, 147–148, 148t
  techniques for, 146–150
SLE. See *Systemic lupus erythematosus (SLE)*.

Small airways disease (bronchiolitis), in COPD, 601
Smoke, cigarette. See Cigarette smoke (smoking).
    wood, 129–130
        asthma and, 504
        avoidance techniques for, 205
Smut(s), 111
Solar urticaria, 651
Solid food, allergic disease in infants and, 284
    delayed introduction of, in prevention of allergy in infants, 292
    infantile eczema and, 81
Soy formula, for prevention of allergy in infants, 290–291
Soybean(s), allergy to, 669
Spirometry, for asthma, 500–501
    for COPD, 604
    for lung volume and capacity, 158, *158*
    for pulmonary function, 160, *161–162*
        flow-volume curves vs., 161–163, *163*
Spondylitis, ankylosing, 63
Spondyloarthropathy(ies), seronegative, 63t, 63–64
Spore(s), prevalence of, 93–96
    aeroallergen sampling for, 93–96
    extracts and, 93
Spore count(s), 94
Sporobolomyces, characteristics of, 109t
Sputum cytology, 140
    in asthma, 501–502
SS-A antibody(ies), in SLE, 57
SS-B antibody(ies), in SLE, 57
Stamen, *96*, *97*
Staphylococcal scalded skin syndrome, 331, 656–657
Stem cell factor, mast cells and, 451
Stemphylium, characteristics of, 109t
Still's disease, 60
Sting(s). See Insect allergy; Insect sting(s).
Streptokinase, allergy to, 83
Stridor, laryngeal causes of, 436, 437t
    nonlaryngeal causes of, 436, 436t
Subglottic hemangioma(s), 439
Subglottic stenosis, 439
Sugar mold(s), 110
Suicidal ideation, in asthma, 261, 262t
Sulfasalazine, desensitization to, 344
Sulfite(s), asthma due to, 556
    pseudoallergic reactions to, 339
    sensitivity to, 676
Sulfur dioxide, 124–126, 127t
    controlled laboratory studies on, 124–125, 127t
    epidemiologic studies on, 126
Sun sensitivity(ies), 663
Surfactant therapy, in bronchopulmonary dysplasia, 594
Surgery, in allergy and asthma patients, 516–517, 743–748
    anesthesia in, 744–745
        agents for, 745
        routes of, 744–745
    emergency surgery and, 746–747
    in pregnancy, 747
    intraoperative bronchospasm in, 746
    perioperative anaphylaxis and, 747–748
    perioperative assessment in, 743–744, 744t
    perioperative hereditary angioedema and, 748
    postoperative management in, 746
    ventilator management in, 746
Sweat testing, in cystic fibrosis, 141, 574, 574t
Systemic lupus erythematosus (SLE), 56–58
    classification of, 58t
    clinical manifestations of, 58
    complement deficiency in, 38

Systemic lupus erythematosus (SLE) *(Continued)*
    drug-induced, 58, 58t
    etiology and pathogenesis of, 56–58
    immunologic abnormalities in, 57–58
    in drug hypersensitivity, 332–333
    serologic testing in, 57, 57t
    treatment of, 58
Systemic sclerosis, 61–62
    clinical manifestations of, 61–62
    etiology and pathogenesis of, 61
    treatment of, 62

T cell(s), activation of, 5–7
    adhesion of, 7
    antigen presentation for, 5, *6*
    $CD4^+$ (helper), 2
        antigen presentation to, 5, 55–56, *56*
        in APC-binding, 89, *90*
        in asthma, 454–455
        in IgE regulation, 9
    $CD4^+CD8^+$ (double positive), 3
    $CD4^-CD8^-$ (double negative), 2
    $CD8^+$ (cytotoxic), 2
        antigen presentation to, 5
    development of, 2, 2–3
    in IgE synthesis, 71
    negative selection of, 3
    phenotypic subset analysis of, flow cytometry for, 755–756
    positive selection of, 3
    suppressor, in immunotherapy, 238–239
    T_{H0}, in human allergic disease, 74
    T_{H1}, cytokine secretion patterns of, 73–74
        in asthma, 455–456
        in human allergic disease, 74
    T_{H2}, cytokine secretion patterns of, 73–74
        in asthma, 455–456
        in chronic allergic disease, 76
        in human allergic disease, 74
T lymphocyte(s). See T cell(s).
T-cell deficiency, infections in, 22
T-cell dysfunction, with immunoglobulins (Nezelof's syndrome), 29
T-cell–mediated drug reaction(s), 328–329
T-cell receptor(s), diversity of, 14
    function of, 3
    genetic rearrangements of, 13–14
    structure of, 2
T-cell receptor/CD3 complex deficiency, 29
Tannic acid, for dust mite control, 199
    for indoor environmental control, 118
Tar(s), for atopic dermatitis, 628
Tartrazine, asthma due to, 556
    sensitivity to, 676–677
Tear(s), 704
    complement in, 704
    immunoglobulins in, 704
    lysozyme in, 704
Tear film, 704
Temperature-related urticaria, 650–651
Terbutaline, chemical structure of, *219*
Terfenadine, chemical structure of, *228*
Tetanus vaccine, adverse reactions to, 388–389
TGF-β, immunologic properties of, 15t
    in IgE synthesis inhibition, 73
Theophylline, adverse effects of, 225
    clinical effects of, 224
    for COPD, 607–608

Theophylline *(Continued)*
   in chronic asthma, 515
     mechanism of action of, 224
     pharmacokinetics of, 224
     structure and activity of, *223*, 223–224
Thiobarbiturate(s), asthma due to, 553–554
Throat, physical examination of, 138
Thrombocytopenia, immune, in allergic drug reactions, 334t, 334–335
Thrush, 654
Thymic hypoplasia (DiGeorge anomaly), 27
Thymoma, immunodeficiency in, 26–27
Thymopentin, in atopic dermatitis, 630
Thyroid carcinoma, medullary, anaphylaxis vs., 309
Thyroid disease, autoimmune, 64–65
Thyroiditis, Hashimoto's, 64–65
Tidal volume, 158
Tinea capitis, 653
Tissue chemical analysis, controversial, 757
TNF-α, immunologic properties of, 14, 15t, 16
   mast cells and, 451, 452, *452*
TNF-β (lymphotoxin), immunologic properties of, 15t, 16
Tobacco, 120. See also *Cigarette smoke.*
Toe(s), clubbing of, in cystic fibrosis, 581–582, 582t
Total lung capacity, 158
Toxemia, allergic, 749–750
Toxic epidermal necrolysis, in drug hypersensitivity, 330–331
Trachea, congenital abnormalities of, 439
   vascular anomalies of, 439
Tracheal obstruction. See *Laryngeal and tracheal obstruction.*
Tracheitis, 440
Tracheobronchomalacia, in bronchopulmonary dysplasia, 597
Tracheomalacia, in neonates, 438
Transforming growth factor–β (TGF-β), immunologic properties of, 15t
Transillumination, in sinusitis, 431
Trantas' dot(s), in atopic dermatitis, 708, *708*
Tree nut(s), allergy to, 669–670
Tree(s), anthesis of, *103*, 103
   beech order, 104
   conifers, 102
   maples, 104
   nettle order, 102–103
   olive family, 104–105
   pollens of, 102–105
   walnut family, 104
   willow family, 103–104
Triamcinolone acetonide, chemical structure of, *212*
   pharmacokinetics of, 213–214
Trichoderma, characteristics of, 109t
Trichotillomania, 661
Tryptase, as mast cell inflammatory mediator, 451
   serum, in anaphylaxis, 300–301
Tumor necrosis factor. See *TNF-α; TNF-β.*
Tumor(s), of ear canal, 412, 412t
   of larynx, 441
   of mastoid, 423
   of middle ear, 423
Tympanic membrane perforation, in otitis media, 422
Tympanometry, in otitis media, 417
Tympanosclerosis, in otitis media, 422

Ulcerative colitis, 687–702
   arthritis and, 64
   clinical manifestations of, 689–690

Ulcerative colitis *(Continued)*
   Crohn's disease vs., 690
   diagnosis of, 690
   immunopathogenesis of, 690–699
     adhesion molecules in, 698
     cigarette smoking and, 697
     complications and, 698–699
     hemostatic abnormalities in, 697
     intestinal barrier epithelium dysfunction in, 692–693
     intestinal luminal antigens in, 691–692
     intestinal mucosal defects in, 693–695
     mediators of intestinal inflammatory damage in, 695–697
     neuroimmune modulation in, 697–698
     systemic immunoregulation in, 693–695
   proposed cause(s) of, 691
     immunologic hypothesis as, 691
     infectious hypothesis as, 691
   therapy in, medical, 687
     surgical, 687–688
Upper respiratory disease, diagnostic testing for, 139–140
   fiberoptic rhinoscopy for, 140
   in asthma, 490
   nasal cytology for, 139–140
   sinus radiography for, 140
Upper respiratory reaction(s), in food allergy, 675
Urticaria, 643–652. See also *Angioedema.*
   acute, 643
   adrenergic, 651
   aquagenic, 651
   cholinergic, 650
     exercise-induced anaphylaxis vs., 379t, 379–380, 650
     exercise-induced asthma vs., 524–525
   chronic, 643
     antihistamines for, 230
     drug therapy for, 649, 649t
   chronic idiopathic, anaphylaxis vs., 310
   classification of, 643–645, *644*
   complement activation in, 646
   contact, 647–648
   delayed pressure, 650
   differential diagnosis of, 645
   due to drug therapy, 327, 328t
     treatment of, 345
   due to radiocontrast reaction, 357
   eosinophil products in, 646
   etiology of, 646t, 646–648
     drugs in, 646–647
     food additives in, 647
     foods in, 647, 671
     infectious agents in, 647
     insect bites and stings in, 647
     systemic disease in, 648
   histologic pathology in, 645
   in anaphylactic and anaphylactoid reactions to food additives, 370–371
   in anaphylaxis, 306–307
   in pregnancy, 738–740
   papular, 645, 657
   pathophysiology in, 645–648
   physical, 643, 649–651
   pruritus vs., 645, 645t
   solar, 651
   temperature-related, 650–651
   treatment of, 648–649, 649t
   vasoactive mediators and mast cell activation in, 645–646

Urticaria pigmentosa, 663
Urticaria/angioedema. See also *Angioedema; Urticaria.*
   challenge testing in, 188–191
      activity of urticaria during, 188–189
      baseline observation in, 189–190
      controls in, 190–191, 191t
      medications in, 189
      patient selection for, 188
      placebo in, 190
      reaction criteria in, 189, *190*
Urticarial vasculitis, 648

Vaccination, adverse reaction(s) to, 384–391
   adequacy of sample size and, 385
   appropriateness of time interval and, 385
   biologic plausibility of observed reaction in, 385
   confirming vaccine effect in, 385
   diphtheria toxoid and, 388–389
   Haemophilus influenzae type B vaccine and, 389
   hepatitis B virus vaccine and, 389
   identifying putative factor in, 386
   infection as, 388
   inherent susceptibility of host and, 385–386
   live measles virus vaccine and, 389
   live mumps virus vaccine and, 389
   live rubella virus vaccine and, 389
   mechanism(s) producing, 386–388
      immunologic events as, 386–388
      mechanical or toxic events as, 386
      type I reactions as, 386–387
      type II reactions as, 387
      type III reactions as, 387
      type IV reactions as, 387
   pertussis vaccine and, 389
   polio vaccine and, 389
   questions pertaining to, 384–386
   skin testing in egg-sensitive patients and, 387–388
   specific vaccines and, 388–390
   tetanus toxoid and, 388–389
  bacterial, clinical trials of, 242
  in COPD, 606–607
  in X-linked agammaglobulinemia, 23
  poliovirus, in X-linked agammaglobulinemia, 23
Varicella, 655
Vasculitis, 659
  due to drug therapy, 338
     leukocytoclastic, 338
  urticarial, 648
Vasopressin excess, in asthma, 512
Vasopressor reaction(s), anaphylaxis vs., 308
Vasovagal reaction(s), due to radiocontrast reaction, 358
VCAM-1, 464
  in asthma, 465
Vecuronium, for anesthesia in asthma and allergy, 745
Vegetable gum(s), 121
  in occupational asthma, 541
Venom, fire ant, 350
  honeybee, 350
  Hymenoptera, 350
    testing for, 350
  vespid, 350
Venom immunotherapy, 247–248, 351–354
  adverse reactions to, 353
  dosage schedule for, 247–248, 249t
  duration of, 353–354
  extract selection for, 352
  in children and adults, 352, *352*
  indications for, 351

Venom immunotherapy *(Continued)*
  initial, 352
  maintenance therapy in, 353
  modified rush, 352
  optimum duration of therapy for, 248
  risks of, 351–352
Ventilation, mechanical, in bronchopulmonary dysplasia, 594–595, 595t
Vernal keratoconjunctivitis, 710–711
  clinical features of, 710–711, *711*
  immunopathology in, 710
  treatment of, 711
Vertigo, benign paroxysmal positional, 424–425
Vespid venom, 350
Vibratory angioedema, hereditary, 650
Viral dermatosis, 654–656
Viral infection(s), avoidance techniques for, 204
  in airway hyperresponsiveness, 173–174
  in asthma, 86–87, 490
  in atopic dermatitis, 616
  in immunodeficiency disease, 22
  in otitis media, 414
Vital capacity, 158
Vitiligo, 663–664
VLA-4, 464
Vocal cord dysfunction, anaphylaxis vs., 309
  pulmonary function testing in, 167t
Vocal cord paralysis, in adults, 440t, 440–441
  in neonates, 438
Volumetric sampler(s), for aeroallergens, 94, *95*
Vomiting, due to radiocontrast reaction, 357

Walnut(s), pollens of, 104
Wart(s), 655–656
Water, nebulized, for bronchoprovocation challenge, 181–182, 182t
Weed(s), anthesis of, 105, *105*
  pollens of, *105*, 105–107
Western red cedar, in occupational asthma, 542
Wheat, allergy to, 670
Wheezing, in asthma, 492–493
Willow(s), pollens of, 103–104
Wiskott-Aldrich syndrome, 30–31
  cutaneous anergy in, 31
  immunologic abnormalities in, 30–31
  infections in, 30
Wood dust(s), in occupational asthma, 542
Wood smoke, 129–130
  asthma and, 504
  avoidance techniques for, 205
Wood stove(s), 205
  asthma and, 504
Wool, 120
Wool alcohol sensitivity, 640

Xenogenic serum, desensitization to, 344
Xeroderma pigmentosa, immunodeficiency diseases in, 39
Xerosis, in atopic dermatitis, 616

Young syndrome, 589

Zidovudine, for primary HIV infection, 47

ISBN 0-7216-5587-4

RC
584
.A424
1996

SOUTH UNIVERSITY
709 MALL BLVD.
SAVANNAH, GA 31406